ENTEROIMMUNO

A Guide to the Prevention and Treatment of Chronic Inflammatory Disease

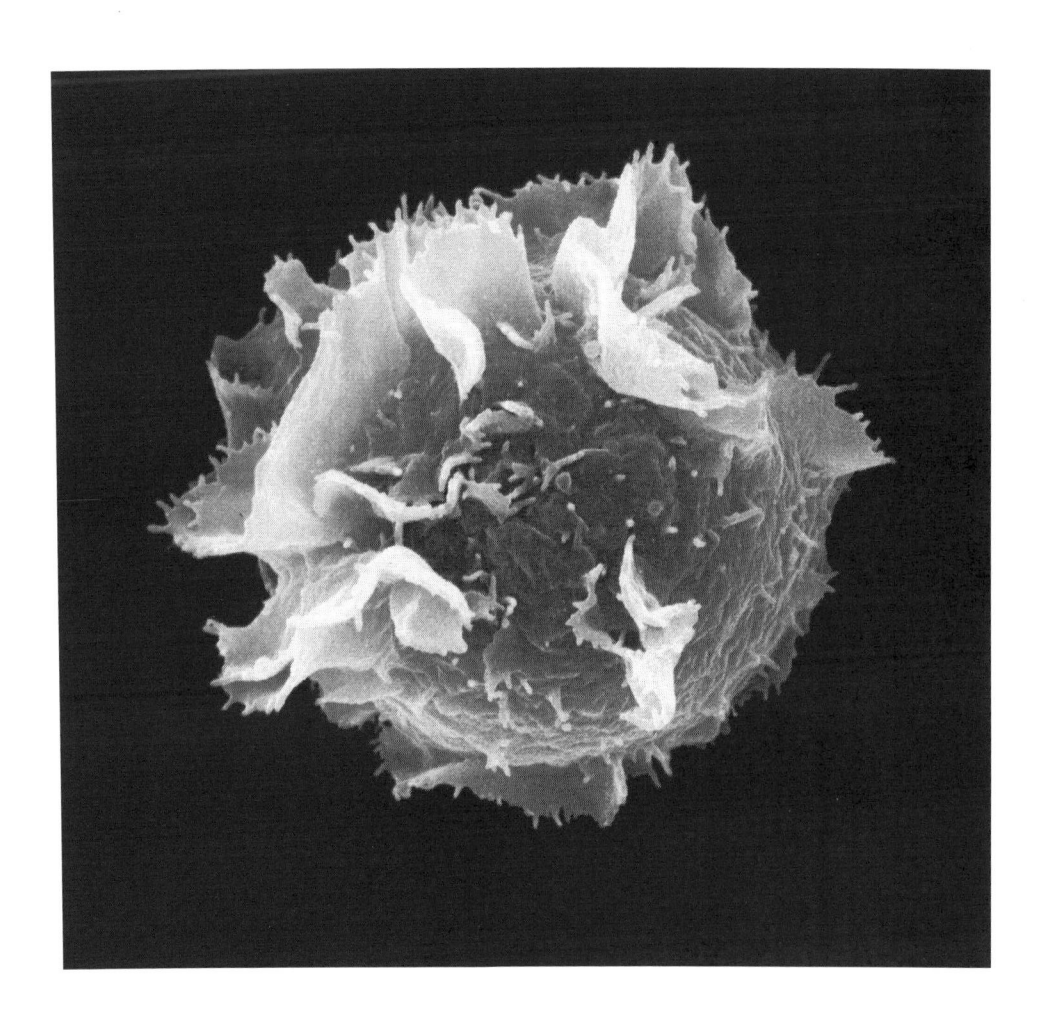

Charles Lewis, MD, MPH

Third Edition

Psy Press
Est. 1978

Copyright © 2015, by Charles A. Lewis

ALL RIGHTS RESERVED. This book contains material protected under U.S. Federal and International Copyright Laws and Treaties. Any unauthorized use or reprinting of this material is prohibited. No part of this book may be transmitted or reproduced in any form or by any means, electronic or mechanical, including photocopying, recording, or by any information storage or retrieval system without prior written permission of the publisher, except for the case of brief quotations embodied in critical reviews and certain other noncommercial uses permitted by copyright law

LIMIT OF LIABILITY AND DISCLAIMER OF WARRANTY: The author has presented information and opinions in this book he believes reflect information available to him accurately, according to his personal judgment. The information given herein is provided "as is." The author and publisher make no representation or warranties with respect to the accuracy or completeness of the contents of this book and specifically disclaims any implied warranties.

Nothing contained within this book should be construed as medical advice or is intended to replace the need for services and judgment provided by a medical professional. Information contained herein is intended only as educational material to supplement the professional acumen of medical professionals.

The readers should consult appropriate health professionals on any matter relating to their health and wellbeing. Readers who fail to consult appropriate health authorities assume the risk of any injuries.

Title page and back cover electron micrograph:
Activated Mast Cell, by Janet M Oliver

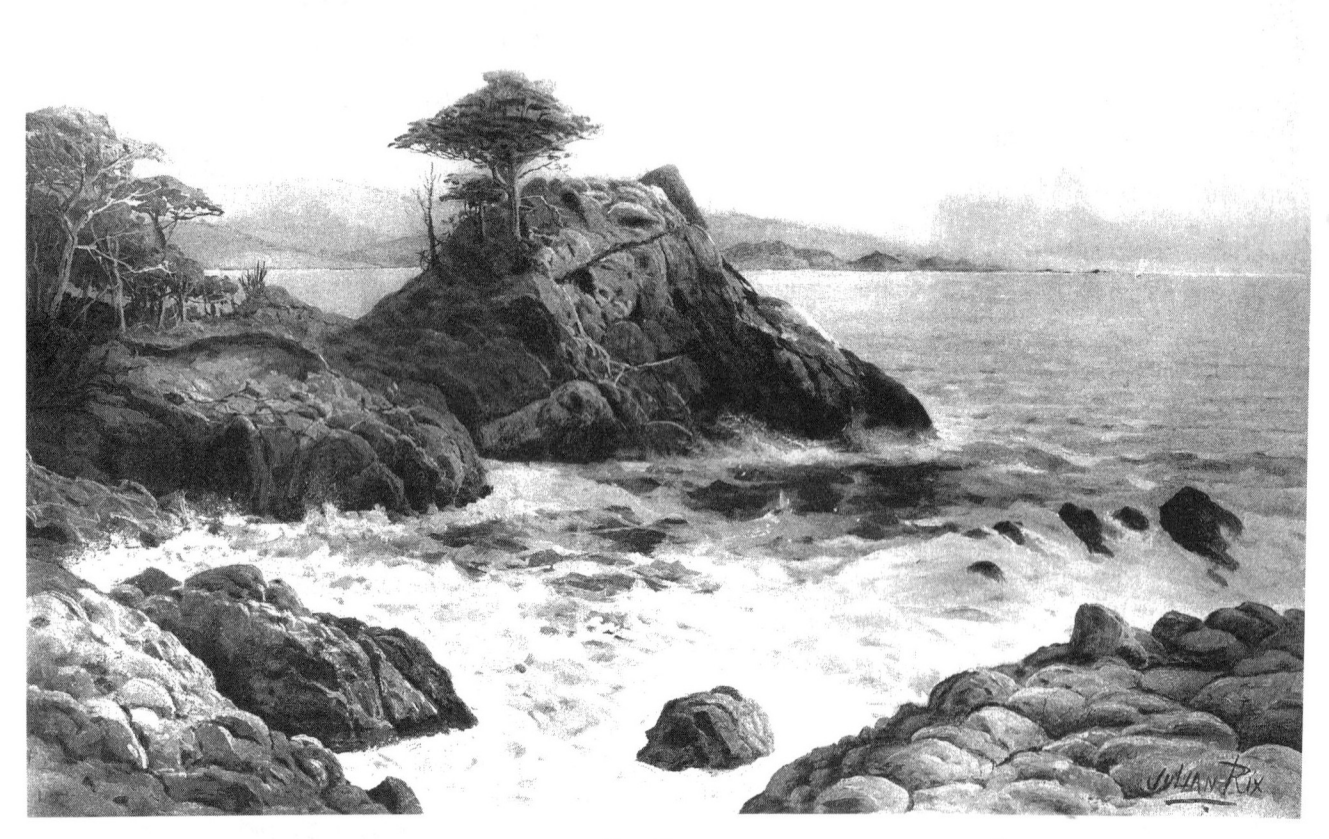

Psy Press
Carrabelle Florida
PsyPress email.com
Edition: 3.03 July 2015

On Demand Publishing
IBSN 978-1502706942

Table of Contents

1: Introduction to Enteroimmunology....1

2: The GI Primer...4

3: Carbohydrates...15

4: The Colon and its Inhabitants...18

5: Meteorism, Trots and Foul Winds...32

6: Fats: Essential to Health...43

7: Proteins...57

8: Appetite, Satiation, Satiety, and Pancreatic Exocrine Function...68

9: Obesity, Syndrome X, and the Company it Keeps...80

10: Immune Cells...93

11: Type I Hypersensitivity and IgE Food Allergies...107

12: Mast Cell Activation Disorders...116

13: Bioactive Amine Induced Pseudoallergy...125

14: Mast Cell Degranulation Induced Pseudo Allergy...142

15: Leukotriene Associated Hypersensitivity...148

16: Reactions to Enzymes in Food and Effects of Cooking...159

17: Chocolate and Wine: The Dark Side...161

18: Immune Hypersensitivity...168

19: Immune Hypersensitivity to Food...172

20: Vitamin D3...183

21: Mitochondria, Oxidation, Aging and Disease...192

22: Gluten Disease...208

23: Biofilms and Dysbiosis...218

24: Small Intestinal Bacterial Overgrowth...231

25: Leaky Gut Syndrome...243

26: Irritable Bowel Syndrome...254

27: Interstitial Cystitis/ Bladder Pain Syndrome and Chronic Prostatitis...263

28: Headaches...267

29: Stress and the Hypothalamic Pituitary Axes...278

30: Immunoexcitotoxic CNS Injury...292

31: Mood and Thought Disorders...322

32: Fibromyalgia, Pain Sensitization, Chronic Fatigue and Anxiety...351

33: Autoimmune Disease...370

34: Inflammatory Bowel Disease...376

35: Autism...387

36: Rage...397

37: Acne...406

38: Sexual Dysfunction and Male Infertility....419

39: Food Additives...423

40: Nutritional Supplements...427

41: Cancer Prevention...448

42: Osteoimmunology...476

43: Sleep...487

44. Hearing and Balance...506

45: Enteroimmune Disease and Public Health...515

Appendixes A to M: ...520 to 538

Index...539

Dedication: To Susana, for indulging me the opportunity to pursue this endeavor

"Let your food be medicine and your medicine be food."

Hippocrates

1. Introduction to Enteroimmunology

The intestines are the largest exposed surface of our bodies, and they are in constant exposure to trillions of bacteria, to toxins and immunogenic proteins. These exposures and the body's immune reaction to them underlie the pathology of a much of the chronic disease experienced in our society. Enteroimmunology is the emerging field of medicine that focuses on understanding, treating and preventing diseases initiated through inappropriate immune response in the gut.

Over half of the immune cells in the body are contained in the mucosa of the intestine, and these cells have the enormous task of protecting us from the 100 trillion bacteria, yeast, viruses and parasites that inhabit or try to infiltrate the intestine. Although these immune cells generally protect us, there are many disease conditions caused by the immune response of these cells. The mucosal barrier which separates the lumen of the intestine from the immune cells is a single cell thick, and if compromised, the immune cells must defend the body from infection. Parasites that burrow into the wall of the intestine need to be stopped. Bacteria that enter the body and can colonize the blood need to be eliminated. The immune system is a potent weapon against these invaders; however, collateral damage can occur. Intestinal immune cells may react to food as foreign antigens, setting up a self-destructive defense.

Enteroimmunology provides a framework for understanding a wide range of diseases, such as fibromyalgia, rage, and irritable bowel syndrome and allows for an approach to prevention and treatment of chronic inflammatory diseases. Enteroimmunology gives insight to the causation of obesity, cancer, migraine, and other disorders, whose inflammatory basis is initiated by the enteric immune system.

Many chronic diseases seem unrelated to the gastrointestinal (GI) tract; such as neurological diseases, including multiple sclerosis, depression, autism, and epilepsy. These commonly have enteroimmunopathic etiologies. It becomes less surprising that neurologic diseases share immune activation with the gut when it is understood that the central nervous system (CNS) evolved from the enteric nervous system. They thus share many hormones, cytokines, neurotransmitters, and receptors.

Many systemic immune mediated diseases result from the immune response in the gut through activation of specialized immune cells: the T17 helper (T_H17) cells that are adapted to respond to infections by the anaerobic bacteria that thrive in the colon. These immune cells are involved in most autoimmune disorders. By understanding the enteric immune system and the pathophysiology of these diseases, treatment for secondary and tertiary prevention, with the possible reversal of established disease processes, can be designed.

This text has three main sections. The early chapters (Chapter 2 through Chapter 10) provide a review of the organization of the digestive system and its hormones, basic nutritional components, the microbiota of the intestine, and immune cells. It is not intended for readers to dedicate effort to memorize details given in these chapters. Information in these chapters has placed into tables for easy referencing between chapters.

Chapters 11 through 19 discuss various immune and immune-like reactions to foods. The effect of food on the immune system, as well as the effect of food on the microbes that inhabit the intestines, is central to understanding the field of enteroimmunology. Many diseases can be controlled by altering the diet.

Chapters 20 through 25 further explain the pathophysiology of enteroimmune diseases. The final chapters (Chapters 26 through 43) discuss prominent examples of enteroimmunopathic diseases, their pathophysiology and treatment modalities. This is not an exhaustive list of enteroimmune diseases, but rather a sampling, with each chapter designed to build understanding of inflammatory and enteroimmune disease.

Each of these chapters also acts as a guide for the treatment of the diseases discussed. Chapters 29 and 43 discuss stress and sleep. Management of stress and sleep is integral to treating enteroimmunopathic diseases as stress disorders, and sleep disturbances can exacerbate these diseases, and enteroimmune response in the intestine can cause sleep disturbances and stress responses.

Inflammatory Diseases

With half of the body's immune cells housed in the intestine, it should be no surprise that the intestine is a major source of inflammatory cytokines. Inflammatory diseases, such as asthma, can be exacerbated by what happens in the GI immune system. Cytokines that promote T_H17 immune cell lineage proliferation in the GI tract also promote it other areas of the body and impede the development of other T helper cell lineages. This makes it more difficult for the body to fight other challenges, such as the control and elimination of respiratory viruses or cancer cells. Chronic inappropriate immune activation promotes cancer by inhibiting the apoptosis of unneeded cells (Chapter 41). Thus, chronic inflammation of the GI immune complex diverts the immune system, and indirectly allows the development of some infectious diseases and cancers.

Neurologic Diseases

Perhaps most unexpected is that autism is one of several enteroimmunopathic diseases affecting the nervous system. Recently, autism has been linked to intestinal inflammation and elevation of cytokines. Treatment and prevention of autism are discussed in Chapter 35.

Table 1-1: Examples of Neuro-inflammatory Diseases Associated with Enteroimmunopathies

- Autism
- Alzheimer's Disease
- Parkinson's Disease
- Multiple Sclerosis
- Depression
- Bipolar Disorder
- Schizophrenia
- Migraine Headaches
- Cerebellar Ataxia
- Certain Seizure Disorders

Autoimmune Disease

Enteroimmunopathies underlie the pathology of many, if not most, autoimmune diseases. In recent years, it has become clear that T17 helper (T_H17) cells are involved in multiple sclerosis, Crohn's disease, rheumatoid arthritis, psoriasis, and many other autoimmune conditions. Most of the body's T_H17 cells reside in the intestinal mucosa; this is the etiological ground zero for autoimmune disease. The enteroimmunopathic disease model provides a framework for moving autoimmune diseases into remission. (Chapter 32)

"Functional Diseases"

It is only in recent years that the pathophysiology of functional diseases has been understood. This group of diseases includes fibromyalgia, irritable bowel syndrome and interstitial cystitis. These diseases often have a prominent affective comorbidity, which share the underlying pathology; an aberrant enteroimmune reactivity.

Table 1-2: Common Nonspecific Symptoms in Enteroimmune Disease

Area Affected	Symptoms
Cognitive	Mental fog, poor concentration, learning disabilities, poor memory, lethargy, apathy, rage, restlessness, hyperactivity
Sensory	Vertigo, lightheadedness, tinnitus
Emotional	Anxiety, moodiness, depression, aggressiveness, irritability
Somatic	Headaches, insomnia, fatigue, joint pain, muscle pain, stiffness, weakness, weight gain, fluid retention, non-ischemic chest pain
Gastrointestinal	Dyspepsia, bloating, belching constipation, abdominal cramping nausea, excessive flatulence
Systemic	Palpitations, urinary urgency, sweating, flushing, hair loss, itching
Respiratory	Congestion, excessive phlegm and mucous, dyspnea, chronic cough, gagging

The prominence of nonspecific or non-localizing symptoms and the lack of accessible diagnostic tests have made in enteroimmunopathies difficult to treat and at times, difficult to diagnosis. Mast cell activation disorders are an example of conditions which are notoriously difficult to diagnose and which cause multiple nonspecific symptoms. Mast cell activation syndromes are caused by clones of mast cells in the intestinal lamina propria, or other areas of the body, and may cause multiple disease syndromes. (Chapter 12)

Nutrition and Health

While metabolic syndrome and obesity have long been understood as having a nutritional basis, they are predominantly inflammatory diseases, and successful treatment depends on understanding them as such.

Enteroimmunology and Metabolic Syndrome

Obesity, diabetes, coronary artery disease and stroke are some of the diseases that develop as part of the Metabolic Syndrome, discussed in Chapter 9. Metabolic syndrome and the diseases it causes are commonly considered to be lifestyles disease, caused by overeating and lack of exercise. Although these diseases are attributed to sloth and gluttony, these diseases have an inflammatory cause.

In a study, 120 individuals interested in weight loss, subjects were tested for IgG reacting foods, (Chapter 19) and the reacting food items were eliminated from each subject's diet.

> The subjects were not asked to go hungry; they were free to eat as much as they liked, just avoiding the foods they had IgG reactions to. Individuals in this study, on average, had IgG sensitivities to 15 foods. There was excellent (94.7%) compliance to the diet; in large part perhaps because the diet did not restrict caloric intake.
>
> Avoidance of the IgG reactive foods over a 90-day period was associated with an average 5-kg (11- pound) weight loss and a 7.4-cm (2.9-inch) reduction in waist circumference; the participants' blood pressures came down, cholesterol levels fell, and mental health improved[1]. This magnitude of weight loss is often sufficient to control type 2 diabetes.
>
> Understanding the mechanisms that control appetite (Chapter 8) and the effect of inflammation on them, allows treatment and interventions that can successfully prevent metabolic syndrome, by undoing its root causes.

The function of mitochondria in health and aging, and how they are affected by diet, immune function and exercise are discussed in Chapter 21. The role and interactions of stress and diet are discussed in Chapter 29. The benefits and harms of nutritional supplements are discussed in Chapter 40. The role of diet in cancer is discussed in Chapter 41.

Traumatic Injury

Perhaps seemingly most out of place for a text focusing on nutritional and immune disease, Traumatic Brian Injury (Chapter 31) and noise-induced hearing loss, (Chapter 21) are explained as inflammatory conditions. Similarly, osteoporosis and the success of orthodontic treatment are covered in Chapter 42.

Enteroimmunology is a guide to primary, secondary, and tertiary prevention and treatment for many of the most common chronic diseases afflicting our population. It gives a basis for secondary prevention, and for low cost, non-toxic treatments for diseases, including many that can be debilitating or deadly. Perhaps most importantly, this model provides treatment for the underlying causes of the disease, rather than attempting to control symptoms. This allows for systemic improvement in health, beyond the organ system targeted and thus provides relief for causally associated secondary diseases and symptoms.

> **Note:** Citations are given at the end of each chapter. A PMID number, given for most journal articles, allows easy access to the reference at the U.S. National Library of Medicine, at http://www.ncbi.nlm.nih.gov/pubmed/.
>
> PUBMED references that are shown with the title underlined have free access to the complete journal article linked through the National Library of Medicine website.

---

[1] Eliminating Immunologically-Reactive Foods from the Diet and its Effect on Body Composition and Quality of Life in Overweight Persons. Lewis JE, Woolger JM, Melillo A, Alonso Y, Rafatjah S, et al. J Obes Weig los Ther. (2012) 2:112. http://omicsgroup.org/journals/2165-7904/2165-7904-2-112.pdf

2. A GI Primer

The Gastrointestinal (GI) system has a large ecological footprint on the body. Diabetes and heart disease are understood to be nutritionally based disorders. It is less appreciated that disease conditions as diverse as autism, migraine, acne, and rheumatoid arthritis have pathologies arising from inflammatory derangements within the GI tract. The GI tract has a surprisingly large surface area, an independent nervous system, musculature, a specialized immune system, and a complex endocrine system producing dozens of hormones.

This chapter is an overview of the anatomy, enzymes, and hormones which are important features of the GI system. It provides a basis for the subsequent chapters that explain how the GI system and food affect health.

Saliva and Digestion in the Mouth

Digestion begins in the mouth, with mastication mechanically breaking food into smaller parts and mixing it with saliva. Saliva wets the food and adds mucin, which acts as a lubricant for swallowing. Saliva also contains the enzyme α-amylase, which begins the breakdown of carbohydrates; and lingual lipase, which begins the digestion of fats. Table 2-1 lists some important components of saliva and their functions.

Cells of Stomach

Delta cells (also known as D cells,) present in the antrum of the stomach, as well as in the small intestine and in the islets of Langerhans in the pancreas, produce the inhibitory hormone *somatostatin*. Somatostatin output is increased by the hormones VIP and gastrin, and inhibited by acetylcholine. Somatostatin acts in a feedback loop preventing excess acid production. It also has other inhibitory effects, as shown in Table 2-7. Efferent stimulation by the vagus nerve increases hydrochloric acid production by parietal cells.

ECL cells in the stomach produce histamine under the influence of vagal nerve stimulation. Somatostatin inhibits the release of histamine from these cells. ECL cells look similar to enterochromaffin cells of the intestine but contain and release histamine rather than the neurotransmitter serotonin.

G cells in the antrum of the stomach, the area just proximal to the pyloric sphincter, produce the hormone *gastrin*. This hormone stimulates the production of gastric juices and the proenzyme pepsinogen. Together with histamine, gastrin stimulates the production of stomach acid by parietal cells.

Table 2-1: Saliva

Saliva	Activity
Water	Promotes mixing of foods and lubrication.
Mucin	Lubricates the teeth so that the incisors slide by each other more easily and allows easier passage of food through the esophagus.
Potassium bicarbonate	Neutralizes acidity in the mouth. Prevents damage to the enamel of the teeth. It may also neutralize some bacterial toxins.
Lingual Lipase	This enzyme hydrolyses a portion of the triglycerides, resulting in free fatty acid and diglyceride. Lingual lipases are important for the perception of the flavor of fat[1]. Some of these fatty acids are directly absorbed through the buccal mucosa. Lingual lipase is resistant to an acid environment and does not require bile salts for its activity; thus, its activity continues in the stomach.
Salivary α-amylase	Cleaves starch and some other carbohydrates. It randomly cleaves α(1-4) glycosidic linkages of amylose to yield dextrin and maltose. With mastication, α-amylase breaks starch down enough to yield a mildly sweet flavor from these sugars. Salivary amylase is inactivated by stomach acid within a few minutes.
Haptocorrin	Produced by salivary glands. Binds to vitamin B_{12} and protects it from destruction by stomach acid.
Lysozyme	Protects the oral cavity through its antimicrobial activity and offers some protection from food-borne pathogens including *E. coli* and *Salmonella*.
IgA	Binds to bacteria, making them less adherent to cells lining the GI track and marks them for phagocytosis by immune cells.

Parietal cells in the stomach produce hydrochloric acid under the influence of histamine, the hormone gastrin and under post-ganglionic vagal acetylcholine stimulation. The parietal cells also produce *intrinsic factor* that binds to vitamin B_{12} in the duodenum and is required for vitamin B_{12} absorption.

Gastric acid is not essential for survival; however, it helps with the digestion of protein and the absorption of calcium, and iron. Stomach acid also helps prevent bacterial overgrowth and enteric infection.

Goblet cells in the stomach produce *mucin*. Mucin protects the stomach from acids, enzymes, and irritants in the chime, the mix of food and digestive juices.

Chief cells of the stomach produce the inactive proenzyme *pepsinogen*. Pepsinogen is released under the influence of gastrin under vagal stimulation. The acid environment triggers a conformational change in pepsinogen that allows it to be cleaved into *pepsin*, the active form of the enzyme. Pepsin is the first proteolytic enzyme to act in the digestion of food.

Pepsin cleaves peptide bonds between hydrophobic and, preferably, aromatic amino acids such as phenylalanine, tryptophan, and tyrosine. The acid environment of the stomach denatures many proteins, exposing sites for cleavage. Pepsin is most active at a pH of about 2.0. Once the chyme has entered the duodenum and the pH rises above 5.0, pepsin itself is denatured and inactivated.

The chief cells also produce gastric lipase, which like lingual lipase, is active in an acid environment. Combined, lingual and gastric lipases are responsible for hydrolysis of about one-third of dietary fat, converting them into fatty acids and monoglyceride, which can then be absorbed[2]. These fats are thus absorbed without needing bile acids.

Table 2-2: Gastric Digestive Enzymes

Pepsin	Hydrolysis of aromatic amino acids in acidic pH
Lipase	Hydrolysis of triglycerides in acidic environment

The Pancreas

The pancreas is both an endocrine gland and exocrine gland. As an endocrine gland, the pancreas produces the hormones insulin and glucagon that are released into the circulatory system and regulate blood glucose metabolism. The pancreatic hormone amylin slows gastric emptying, and pancreatic polypeptide helps regulate energy balance. Pancreatic hormones are outlined in Table 2-7, below.

Pancreatic exocrine activity is essential to digestion. The ductal cells of the pancreas produce bicarbonate that neutralizes stomach acid; raising the pH of the chyme to a level above a pH of 5 as it enters the jejunum. Bicarbonate is formed in response to gastrin in the blood stream that acts as a signal that hydrochloric acid is being created in the stomach. The **acinar cells** of the pancreas produce zymogens that are inactive proenzymes. These proenzymes could easily digest the pancreas itself if they were in their active form. Cholecystokinin (CCK), which acts as a hormone and neurotransmitter, promotes the release of the pancreatic zymogens into the duodenum. There are over a dozen pancreatic enzymes (Table 8-4). The most dominant of these enzymes are the proteases trypsin and chymotrypsin; lipase for the digestion of triglycerides; and α-amylase for the digestion of starches. Pancreatic exocrine function is discussed in detail in Chapter 8.

Bile and the Gallbladder

The liver produces close to a liter of bile a day. It drains into the duodenum through the common bile duct. In most individuals, the common bile duct joins the pancreatic duct at the ampulla of Vater, and here the bile and pancreatic fluids flow into the duodenum. There is a sphincter here (the sphincter of Oddi) that restricts the flow of bile and pancreatic fluids into the duodenum between meals. The sphincter relaxes; allowing flow, under the stimulus of the hormone VIP triggered by cholecystokinin in response to the presence certain nutrients in the duodenum.

The gallbladder is a small pouch, about three inches long, located below the liver, which collects up to about 50 ml (1.7 oz) of bile. Between meals when the sphincter of Oddi is closed, bile backs up into the gallbladder from the common hepatic duct.

Bile formed in the liver is concentrated to about five times its original strength in the gallbladder. Therefore, 250 ml of bile can be concentrated to about 50 ml over several hours between meals. Upon stimulation by CCK, the muscular layers in the wall of the gallbladder contract, the sphincter relaxes, and bile empties into the duodenum where along with the pancreatic fluids, it digests nutrients. Prior to concentration in the gallbladder, bile is made up of about 85% water and ten percent bile acids. Bile also contains pigments (bilirubin), mucous, organic salts, vitamins, cholesterol, and steroid hormones.

Bile Acids

Bile acids (BA) are essential for the emulsification of dietary fat. BA have a lipophilic (hydrophobic) side and a polar (hydrophilic) side. This allows a lipid molecule and a water molecule to adhere to opposite sides of the bile acid, thus allowing bile acids to act as surfactants. Bile helps to disperse fats in the diet and form micelles; tiny disk-shaped particles with a lipid bilayer center surrounded by a hydrophobic ring of bile salts, allowing lipids to be suspended in the aqueous chyme. Since the micelles are tiny, it provides a much greater surface area for the fats to interact with the enzyme pancreatic lipase. Pancreatic lipase can reach the fats in the center of the bile/lipid micelle disk and digest the triglycerides into two free fatty acids (FFA) and a monoglyceride. The FFA are released from the micelle and transported through the enterocyte membrane by carriers specific to the class of fatty acid.

Without bile, pancreatic lipase and colipase, very little fat and no fat-soluble vitamins are absorbed. Instead, fats pass into the colon and then into the feces causing fat malabsorption, steatorrhea, and vitamin deficiencies.

Most BA is reabsorbed, mainly in the distal ileum, and circulated back to the liver via the portal vein for reuse. A small amount of bile escapes into the colon; here, it is fermented by bacteria and converted into secondary BA. These too are mostly reabsorbed and reused. About 20 percent of the BA pool is composed of secondary bile acids. Normally, less than five percent of the BA pool is lost into the stool each day. The BA pool is maintained by new synthesis of BA from cholesterol in the liver. When BA are absorbed by mucosal cells in the distal ileum, the cells make fibroblast growth factor-19 (FGF-19). The liver increases BA synthesis when FGF-19 levels fall, signaling a shrinking pool of BA.

Two primary bile acids are synthesized in the liver: cholic and chenodeoxycholic acids. Bile is then conjugated in the liver to either glycine or taurine before its secretion. In conjugation, a covalent bond is formed with a small polar molecule, such as glycine, taurine, glucuronide or sulfate, resulting in a water-soluble compound. BA are released from the gallbladder under stimulation from CCK in response to feeding.

Table 2-3: Bile Acids

Primary Bile Acids	Secondary Bile Acids
Cholic Acid	Lithocholic acid
Chenodeoxycholic acid	Deoxycholic acid (DCA)
	Ursodeoxycholic acid

Secondary BA have additional properties. Lithocholic acid is cytotoxic and carcinogenic. This cytotoxic effect can damage enterocytes and promote intestinal inflammation. Deoxycholic acid is theorized to modulate immunity but also inhibits primary bile acid-induced apoptosis; thus it can prevent cells with DNA damage from being eliminated. Ursodeoxycholic acid lowers the production of bile acids by the liver, and thus participates in the feedback mechanisms that regulate BA production.

Digestive enzymes, especially proteolytic enzymes and lipases, kill bacteria in the small intestine. Bile and stomach acid also kill bacteria and maintain a very low bacteria count in the small intestine. The antibacterial enzyme lysozyme is not only found in the saliva but is also produced by the small intestine. It is produced in even higher concentrations by the mucosa lining the trachea[3].

The Intestine

The small intestine is divided into three functional regions. The first region is the duodenum, the area where the stomach empties into the small intestine. The name duodenum means 12 finger-lengths, as it is about 12 inches long. The duodenum is the location where the bile and pancreatic ducts open into the intestine.

The stomach contents enter the duodenum having been mixed with hydrochloric acid, and have a pH of about 2. The addition of sodium bicarbonate from the pancreas neutralizes the chyme to a pH of 5 to 6.4 before it passes into the second region of the small intestine, the jejunum.

The jejunum and ileum are the second and third segments of the intestine. Jejunum means empty, as this section was usually empty in cadavers; while ileum means twisted. There is not an anatomical border between these sections, but rather a gradual change in cell population types as the small intestine reaches towards the large intestine. The small intestine is about 285 cm (about 9 feet) in length in living adults, but about 700 cm long (23 feet) in cadavers.
Most of the nutrients in food are absorbed in the jejunum and ileum. Except for the very distal area of the ileum, the healthy small intestine has few bacteria or other microbes. The small intestine is not adapted to house fermentation.

The large intestine also has three regions: the cecum, colon, and rectum. Residue from the chyme from the small intestine empties into the large intestine at the cecum. The appendix, a small appendage to the cecum, is a lymphatic organ that is part of the intestinal immune defenses.

The colon is the longest section of the large intestine. The colon extracts water and salts from the digestive slurry. It does not play a major role in the absorption of preformed nutrients as occurs in the small intestine. It is highly colonized, housing around 10^{13} bacteria; ten times more bacteria than there are human cells in the body. The human colon is normally colonized by a mix of about 150 different species of bacteria and other microbes. These bacteria ferment fiber and other non-absorbed food components which remain in the chyme. This aids in the final breakdown of food components, which have not been digested. The breakdown products of fiber include the formation of short-chain fatty acids, which are absorbed and used as fuel by the cells lining the colon and by the brain. Other bacteria break down other undigested food components which have escaped digestion and absorption. Not all bacteria housed in the colon are beneficial. For example, undigested proteins may be broken down and result in the production of carbon dioxide gas, ammonia, and toxins.

The colon also absorbs some fat-soluble vitamins. The bacteria living in the colon may also produce some vitamin compounds which may contribute to health. The final section of the large intestine is the rectum, which acts as a temporary storage site for the stool.

The GI tract has multiple hormonal functions that control energy balance and digestion. These hormones are outlined in Table 2-8 at the end of this chapter.

Detailed Structure of the Intestine

The lining of the intestine is called the mucosa. The mucosa is folded forming *plica* that expand the absorptive surface area of the intestine. Plica also helps churn the chyme as it moves through the intestine, assuring better absorption of nutrients. The mucosa is covered with tiny fingerlike projections *(villi)*, which greatly increase the surface area of the lumen of the intestines. The villi are from 0.2 to about 2 mm tall and give the mucosa a terrycloth-like appearance.

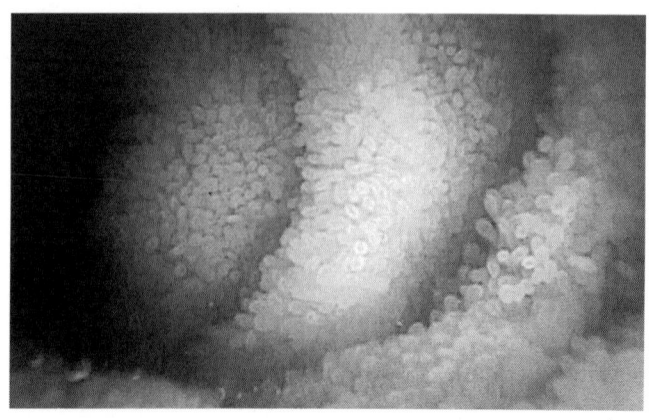

Figure 2-1: Endoscopic view of healthy duodenal mucosa[4].

Figure 2-4 illustrates the general organization of the wall of the small intestine. Within the outer serosa layer, there are two muscular layers. Loops of arterial (A) and venous (V) capillaries are shown extending into the villi. Also shown are lacteals (L), which are lymphatic capillaries that absorb lymph and chylomicron particles. Nerve fibers that innervate the muscles are marked N.

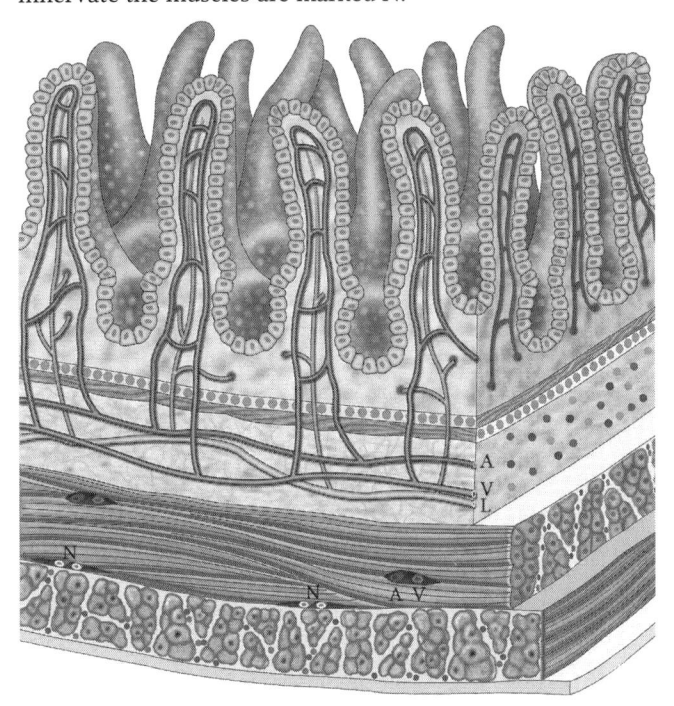

Figure 2-2: View of the Wall of the Small Intestine[5].

Cells of the Villi

Epithelial cells line the mucosa of the intestines from the lower esophageal sphincter to the anus. These cells form a continuous barrier that extends this span that separates the lumen of the GI tract from the inside of the body; separating the potentially contaminated outside of the body from the sterile inside.

The surfaces of the villi are covered with several types of epithelial cells that perform specialized functions. At the base of each villus is a crypt of Lieberkuhn (Figure 2-5).

Stem cells at the base of the crypts of Lieberkuhn provide for continual replacement of epithelial cells for the villi. These stem cells divide, creating new stem cells or daughter cells which differentiate into other intestinal epithelial cells. These cells differentiate along two different pathways: one pathway leads to the development of absorptive enterocytes and *Immune M cells*; the other lineage produces of endocrine cells and exocrine cells; the Paneth and goblet cells.

Enterocytes are the predominant cells which line the intestine along the exposed areas of the villi. These are absorptive cells that take up most nutrients and help control the absorption of other nutrients.

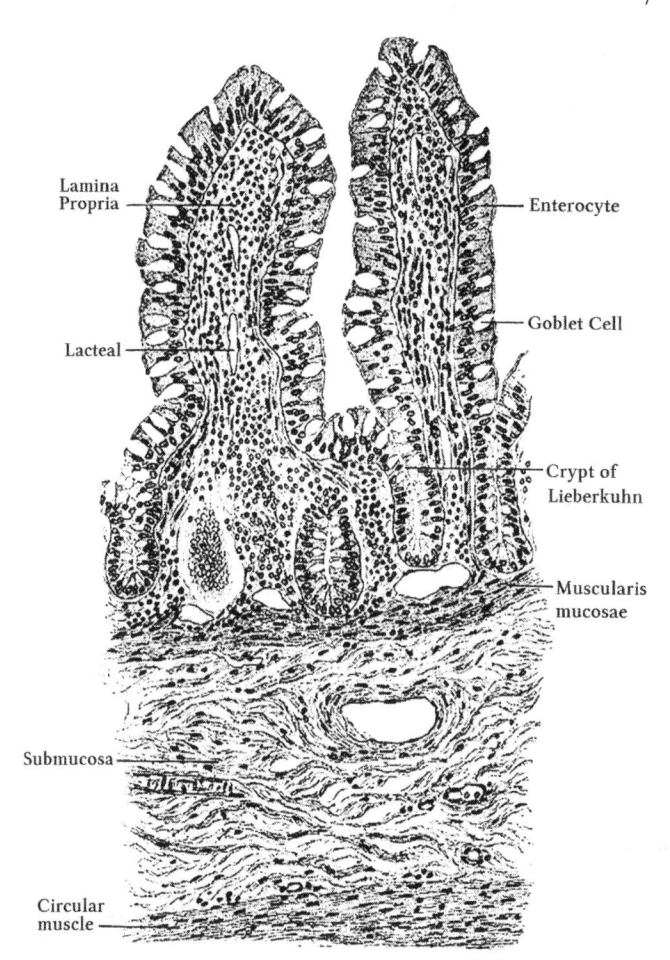

Figure 2-3: A cross-sectional microscopic illustration of two villi from the small intestine. Tall columnar enterocytes crowd the surface along with goblet cells, which appear empty in this preparation. In contrast to the cartoon image in Figure 2-4, it can be seen that the lamina propria is densely populated with cells. These comprise support cells and a large population of immune cells.

Enteroendocrine cells produce a variety of hormones. There are at least 15 different cell types. Enteroendocrine cells in the intestinal epithelium include I cells, K cells, L cells, endocrine M cells, N cells and S cells. Several of the cells bear receptors for free fatty acids, n-3 fatty acids and other receptors that act as taste receptors which help signal the presence of nutrients in the small intestine.

A subset of enteroendocrine cells are known as *enterochromaffin (EC) cells*. EC cells are also found in the epithelial lining of respiratory mucosa. Although usually thought of as a neurotransmitter in the brain, 90 percent of the body's serotonin is produced in mucosal EC cells of the intestine. Serotonin is released under the influence of various stimuli, including taste receptors for bitter compounds. Release of serotonin from these cells promotes secretory and peristaltic reflexes that increase intestinal motility. Serotonin secretion also acts on 5-HT$_3$ receptors, stimulating vagal afferents to the brain, and with sufficient stimulus, can trigger nausea. Some anti-emetic medications act by blocking 5-HT$_3$ receptors in the intestine. Most of the body's production of melatonin occurs in these cells.

M cells (Immune M Cells) aid in mediation of the immune response to microbes in the intestine. M cells are specialized antigen-capturing cells in the ileum that can take up antigens, through endocytosis or phagocytosis, including macromolecules and bacteria, and present these antigens to dendritic cells in the lamina propria of the villus[6]. These cells are concentrated over the Peyer's patches, which are lymph node-like thickenings in the ileum. Humans have about 30 of these areas, each a few centimeters in diameter.

Goblet cells secrete mucin, which dissolves in water and forms mucus. The mucus protects the cells from physical abrasion while allowing nutrients to diffuse into the absorptive cells.

Paneth Cells are found in the basal part of the intestinal crypts of Lieberkuhn. These cells secrete lysozyme and various α-defensins when exposed to bacteria. Defensins are proteins that can attach to the cell membranes of many microbes and form a pore. This pore causes loss of ions required for microbial survival. Defensins are active against many bacteria, fungi, and viruses. β-defensins are found in the saliva, esophageal mucosa, and respiratory mucosa; while α-defensins are found in the intestines, stomach, and neutrophils. Low levels of α-defensins have been found in inflammatory bowel disease though this is likely a result of the disease process rather than the cause[7]. Paneth cells also secrete lysozyme and phospholipase A2, both of which have antimicrobial activity. Paneth cells also produce growth factors. The principal function of the Paneth cells is the defense of the stem cells, which are essential for the maintenance of the intestinal epithelium.

Enterocytes

Enterocytes are the principal epithelial cells of the intestine, accounting for 90 percent of the crypt cells and 95 percent of the villus cells. Structurally, they are tall, thin cells. Enterocytes are responsible for absorption of nutrients. Colonic enterocytes are called colonocytes.

The apices of the endothelial cells, which face the lumen of the intestine, are covered with *microvilli*. These tiny projections further increase interaction with the contents of the intestine and expand the exposed surface area of the mucosa.

Epithelial Cell Lifecycle

Epithelial cells migrate from the crypts where they are formed as daughter cells of progenitor stem cells. They move out of the crypt and along the villus at a rate of about 3 micrometers an hour, equivalent to about an inch per year. The villi are about 0.2 to 2 millimeters long, generally shorter in the proximal intestines and longer in the distal intestines. The epithelial cells thus make their journey from the base to the apex of the villus in about four to ten days depending on the height of the villus[8]. These are very metabolically active and short-lived cells. Paneth cells are the only cells which migrate downwards into the crypts.

Epithelial cells have a high turnover rate; about 20 to 50 million epithelial cells are shed per minute in the small intestine. Two to five million cells are shed per minute in the colon[9].

When enterocytes have migrated to the area near the shoulder of the villus, lymphocytes from the lamina propria migrate into the epithelium and induce cell death of the enterocyte via apoptosis[10]. Apoptosis is likely triggered by cytokines that induce production of oxygen radicals that activate signaling of apoptosis[11]. The enterocyte shrinks while surrounding enterocytes squeeze the remnants of the dead cell to the surface where it is exfoliated, while maintaining the integrity of the epithelial barrier until the remnants of the cell are pinched off by the surrounding enterocytes[12]. Enterocyte remnants may be observed as small, white, inverted mushroom shapes near the tip of the villi in Figures 2-7 and 2-8. The rapid turnover of these cells, which are exposed to numerous toxins, greatly reduces the risk of malignant transformation. Certain toxins, such as phytohemagglutinin, increase the maturation and loss of these cells. Some disease states, celiac disease, for example, accelerate the lymphocytic-induced apoptotic loss of enterocytes[13].

Microvilli

The main function of the microvilli, which cover the apical surface of enterocytes, is the absorption of nutrients. The membranes of the microvilli hold enzymes for breaking down carbohydrates and proteins. The exposed membranes of the microvilli have embedded proteins that are specific transporter proteins for nutrients, such as amino acids, glucose, sodium, and certain vitamins. Lipids, such as short chain fatty acids, can pass easily through the lipid bilayer of the microvilli for absorption down a concentration gradient.

Special receptors are also present on the luminal microvilli membrane surface which can bind to certain molecules. Microvilli are not just a static surface, but each is attached to an actin filament, which acts like a tiny muscle fiber, which can cause the microvilli to evaginate. Through this process, proteins, protein fragments, pathogens, or other immunologically active molecules can be pulled into the enterocytes. Immune M-cells, which are also present on the villi, are also covered with microvilli, which capture proteins and pathogens and act as immune-presenting cells. Many of these molecules are subjected to lysosomal degradation in the cell, converting them into nonimmunogenic peptides or simple amino acids.

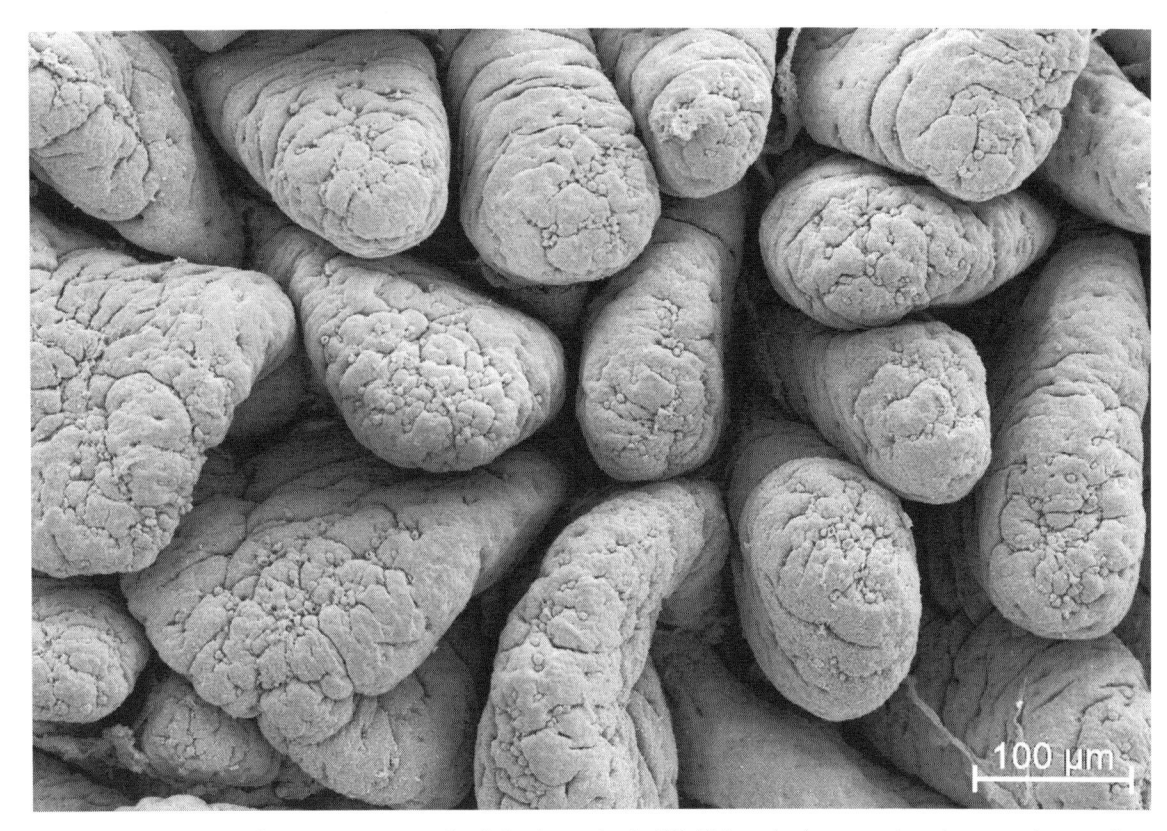

Figure 2-4: **Scanning electron micrograph of the intestinal villi.** This and other scanning electron micrographs in this chapter are provided courtesy of Tomsz Skrzypek, Ph.D., of the John Paul II Catholic University of Lublin, Poland.

The typical adult has about 300 million enterocytes. Each cell has hundreds of microvilli. The microvilli amplify the surface area of the enterocytes; the surface area of the microvilli is about 250 square meters, about the size of one-half of a tennis court. The microvilli are so fine that they cannot be individually seen under a light microscope; they appear as a fuzzy "brush border." Blue light has a wavelength of about 450 nm, but the villi only have a diameter of about 100 nm, which is too small to be measured with visible light, and thus, requires electron microscopy for visualization.

Figures 2-6 through 2-11 show various scanning electron micrographs of the villi and microvilli. Individual cells can be seen to "pave" the surface of the microvilli, usually with four or five sides as best seen in figure 2.9. Small round senescent cells can be seen, especially at the top of the villi. Figure 2-8 shows a few senescent cells in various stages of shrinkage and shedding. Individual microvilli can be seen in figures 2-9 and 2-10.

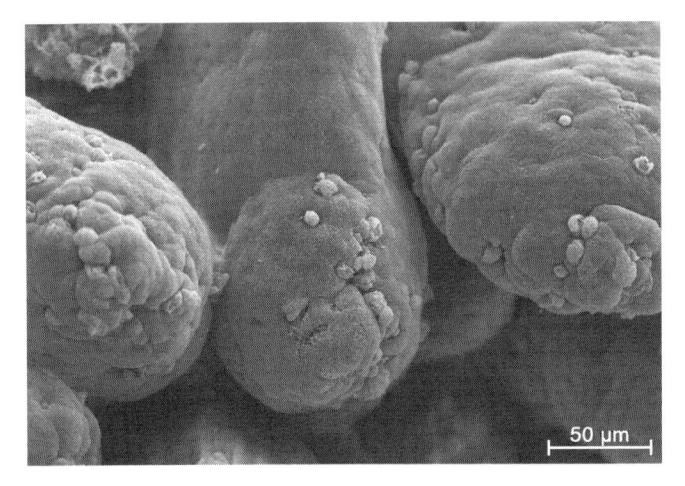

Figure 2-5: **A scanning electron micrograph (SEM) of several villi from the ileum.** Several small, round, exfoliating enterocytes which have completed their 4 to 10-day life cycle can be seen.

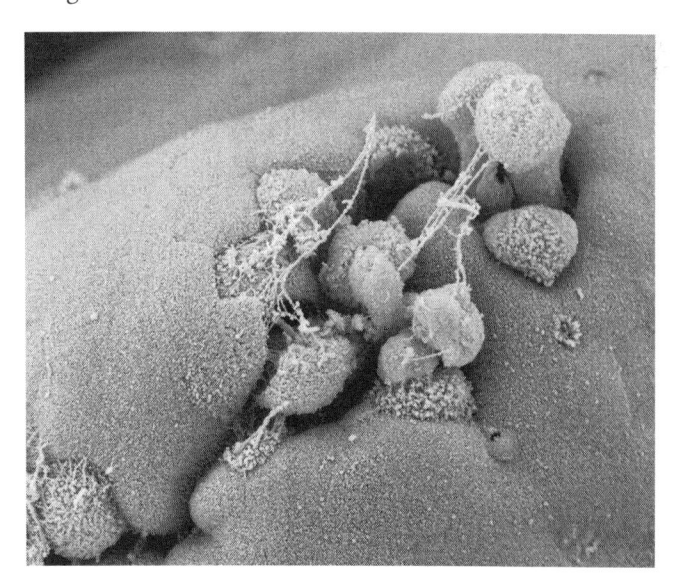

Figure 2-6: **SEM showing detail of shedding epithelial cells on villi.** A mushroom-shaped cell can be seen, detaching from surrounding cells and being pushed out.

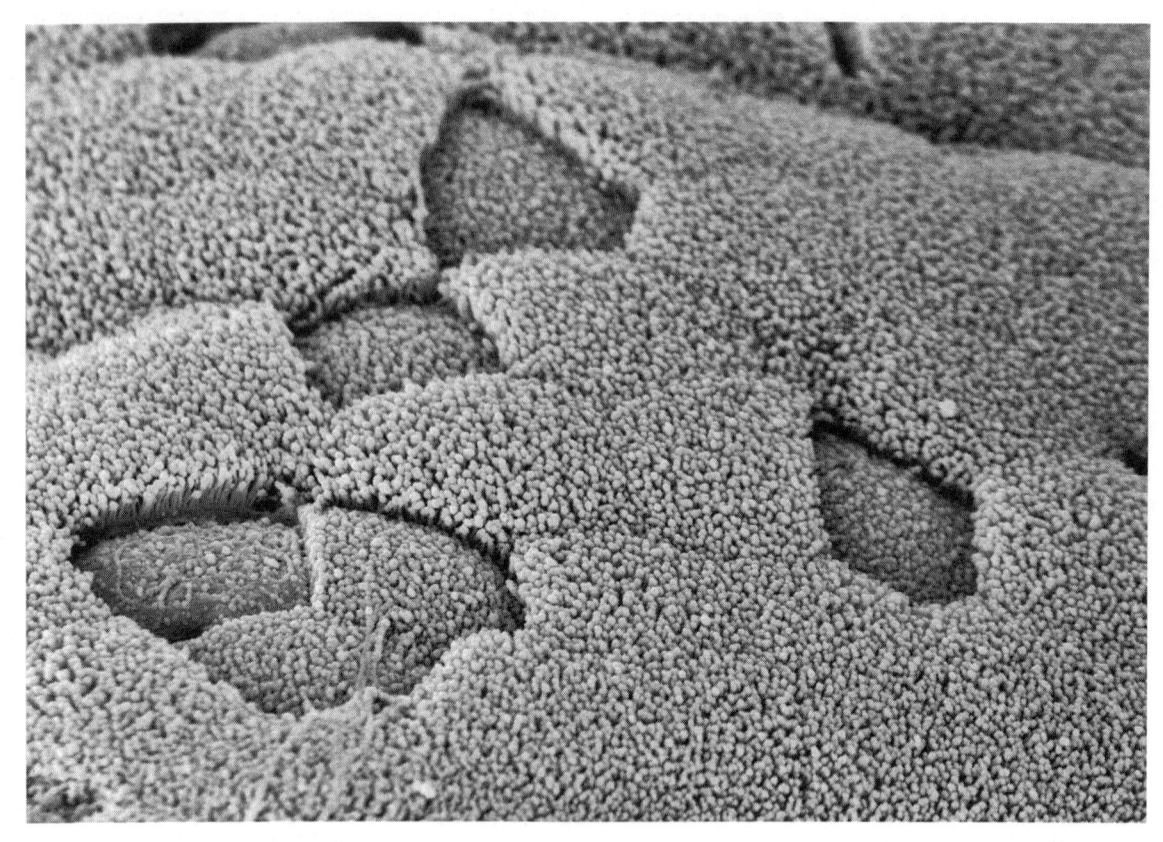

Figure 2-7: Microvilli on intestinal enterocytes. The cells that are depressed are those nearing the end of their life cycles.

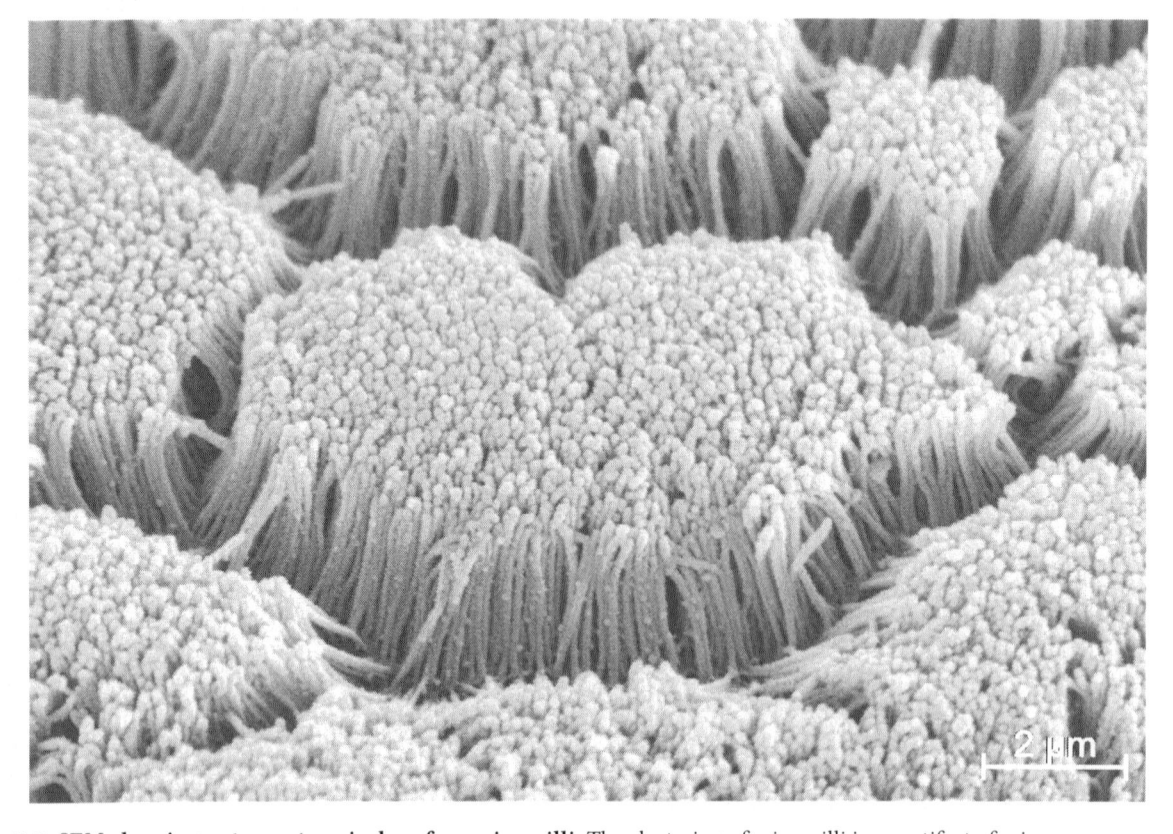

Figure 2-8: SEM showing enterocyte apical surface microvilli. The clustering of microvilli is an artifact of microscopy preparation.

The microvilli membrane is embedded with numerous proteins. Some of these proteins are channels and pumps for moving ions, sugar molecules, and other nutrients. The membrane also contains numerous glycoproteins that form the glycocalyx. The glycocalyx is a 300 nm thick meshwork of glycoprotein molecules that are made up neutral amino acids and sugars.

This layer of glycoproteins binds to mucus, largely composed of mucopolysaccharides produced by goblet cells. The luminal side of the mucous layer also adheres to a very thin layer of water, the unstirred water layer.

The glycocalyx and the mucus form a flexible coat which provides the cells protection from mechanical and chemical damage and help prevent the adherence of bacteria to the microvilli of the enterocytes. These glycoproteins also aid in digestion and absorption of nutrients.

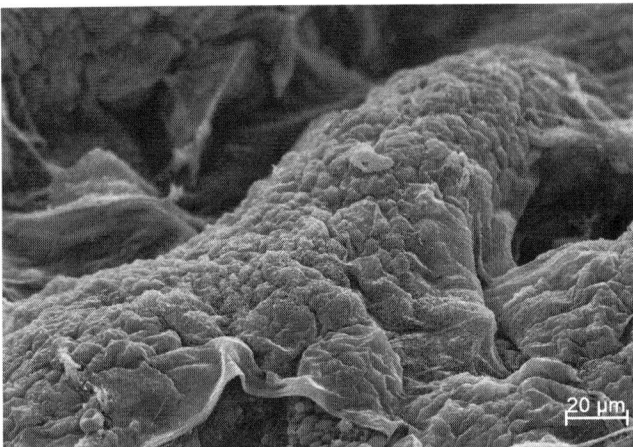

Figure 2-9: SEM showing the mucus layer overlying the enterocytes. This layer is usually removed in SEM of the cells for viewing of the cell surface.

The glycocalyx also contains digestive enzymes. Nutrients can diffuse into the mucus, be acted upon by the enzymes in the glycocalyx, and create an area of high concentration of the enzymatic products, such as simple sugars, fatty acids and amino acids, which are more easily absorbed when there is a high concentration gradient. Neutralizing immunoglobulins are also held in the mucous layer, which help prevent bacterial infection.

The unstirred water layer, which lays above the mucous layer of brush border, is 100-400 μm thick, (about a thousand times thicker than the glycocalyx). This layer helps increase the concentration of water-soluble nutrients and other compounds and helps with their absorption. It also slows the absorption of lipid-soluble molecules.

In the large intestine, an additional mucous layer protects the colonic endothelial cells. This inner and denser layer of mucin (Mucin2) acts as a physical barrier which excludes bacterial contact with the colonic epithelium[14]. Mucin2 forms a large protein complex that cross-links to form a membrane that tightly adheres to the epithelium. This is in contrast to the mucous layer of the small intestine, which is not a hospitable environment for colonization by bacteria. In experimental models where the mucus layer is disrupted by dextran sulfate or carrageen, bacteria are taken up by the colonocytes, and even normally commensal bacteria provoke inflammatory colitis[15].

Enterocytes produce several enzymes, including disaccharidases, endopeptidases, and aminopeptidase. These enzymes migrate into the glycocalyx layer overlaying the enterocytes in the upper villi. These enzymes include disaccharidases that cleave disaccharides into simple sugars (i.e., glucose and fructose) which can be absorbed by the enterocytes.

Table 2-4: Enzymes of the Intestinal Mucosa

Enteropeptidase	Produced in the jejunum, probably by Brunner's glands. Cleaves trypsinogen into the active form of the enzyme trypsin and procarboxypeptidase into carboxypeptidase.
Alanine amino-peptidase	Aminopeptidase is a brush border enzyme that cleaves amino acids from the amino end of a peptide and thus, is an exopeptidase. It acts in the final digestion of peptides generated by hydrolysis of proteins by gastric and pancreatic proteases. This enzyme is also produced in the kidney.
Dipeptidase	Cleaves pairs of amino acids (dipeptides) into single amino acids.
Alpha-glucosidase	Cleaves alpha-D-glucose bonds into polysaccharides
Lysozyme	Secreted by Paneth cells; has antibiotic activity
Phospholipase A2	Secreted by Paneth cells; promotes proinflammatory activity
Isomaltase, also called Sucrase	Disaccharidase; cleaves sucrose into glucose and fructose, and isomaltose into two glucose molecules.
Maltase	Disaccharidase; cleaves maltose into two glucose molecules
Lactase	Disaccharidase; cleaves lactose into glucose and galactose
Trehalase	Disaccharidase; cleaves trehalose into two glucose molecules

The continuous lining of epithelial cells in the stomach and intestines keeps most large, polar molecules (such as peptides, proteins and polysaccharides) outside of the epithelial barrier and inside of the lumen of the stomach and intestine. Similarly, the epithelial lining functions as a continuous barrier, preventing access of bacteria, fungi, and viruses to the body. Certain proteins, however, are recognized and taken into cells through endocytosis.

The enterocytes are packed and sealed together with special proteins that form a series of *tight junctions* between the cells. This is not a static barrier, but rather actively modulates the ability of certain molecules to pass.

Defects in epithelial permeability, caused by alterations of the tight junctions, are seen in celiac disease, inflammatory bowel disease, autism and type 1 diabetes[16]. These defects are often present in healthy family members of individuals with these conditions and precede the development of the diseases. Tight junctions and mucosal paracellular hyperpermeability are discussed in further detail in Chapter 25 (Leaky Gut).

Citrulline: Citrulline is a non-essential amino acid and metabolic intermediate in the urea cycle. There is very little citrulline in the diet; citrulline is synthesized almost exclusively by the enterocytes of the small intestine, mostly from dietary glutamine. It is absorbed into the portal vein, ignored by the liver, and carried into the blood stream. About 80% of the citrulline is converted to arginine by the kidneys. Citrulline takes part in the arginine-citrulline cycle for the formation of nitric oxide as well as the urea cycle, in which ammonia is converted to urea. By first creating citrulline and only later converting it to arginine, the body prevents first pass degradation of arginine into urea by the liver during absorption. The liver is the only organ that can convert ammonia into urea.

Citrulline level in the blood thus reflects the production by small intestinal epithelial cells. As long a person has normal kidney function (which prevents this conversion, raising levels), *the level of citrulline reflects the mass of small intestinal enterocytes*. The normal range for citrulline is 30 – 50 µmol/L. Citrulline less than 20 µmol/L thus indicates a severe compromise of small intestine enterocyte function.

Low plasma citrulline level is found and can be used in the diagnosis and management of diseases of the small intestine including, celiac disease, Crohn's disease, short-bowel syndrome, tropical sprue, and to assess damage from radiation or chemotherapy. It is useful for monitoring the efficacy of treatment. Patient on parenteral nutrition can usually tolerate a return to an oral diet when citrulline levels rise above 20 µmol/L[17]. Low citrulline level not only indicates a loss of absorptive function (Table 2-7) and integrity, but also a loss of mucosa enzymatic activity (Table 2-5), and increased colonic nutrient fermentation.

Endocrine Functions of the GI Tract

The GI tract has multiple hormonal functions which aid in energy balance and digestion. These hormones are outlined in Table 2-6, below.

Table 2-5: Enterocyte Absorptive Functions

Water Absorption	Transported as a result of an osmotic gradient resulting from Na^+/K^+ ATPase at the basal membrane of the enterocyte. Also, small amounts of water move between the cells.
Ion Uptake	Sodium, calcium, magnesium, and iron are taken up through active transport by specific membrane transport proteins.
Carbohydrates and Sugar Uptake	Polysaccharidases and disaccharidases in the glycocalyx break carbohydrates into simple sugars (glucose, fructose, and galactose), which are transported via protein pumps and channels.
Lipids	Lipids digested by pancreatic lipase bile can diffuse across the microvilli membranes. Short-chain fatty acids can be transported to the capillaries. Larger lipid molecules are processed within the enterocytes to form chylomicrons, which are exported through exocytosis into the lamina propria and taken up into the lacteals.
Proteins, Peptides, Amino Acids	Enteropeptidase in the glycocalyx activates pancreatic trypsinogen into trypsin. Trypsin in turn activates other pancreatic enzymes. These proteolytic endopeptidases cleave proteins into peptides. Pancreatic carboxypeptidases and amino-peptidase from the enterocytes cleave single amino acids from peptides small enough to be absorbed. Enterocytes also engulf proteins. Some are transported into lysosomes in the cell, where they are digested. Other proteins may be transported into the Golgi apparatus and used intact, such as immunoglobulins and enzymes.
Vitamin B_{12} Uptake	Enterocytes absorb vitamin B12 bound to gastric intrinsic factor in the ileum.
Unconjugated Bile Salts	Bile salts not emulsified by fats are normally reabsorbed in the terminal ileum.
Immunoglobulin A Secretion (IgA)	IgA from plasma cells in lamina propria of the villi are taken up through endocytosis at the enterocyte basal membrane and transported to the microvilli. Some may be released into the intestinal lumen, especially when attached to pathogenic bacteria. Secretory IgA can act as a neutralizing antibody, so that bacteria cannot adhere to the enterocyte membrane, and are dumped into the colon where the IgA and the bacteria are metabolized by other bacteria. Other IgA-bacteria conjugates are taken up by immune cells for processing.
Cytoprotection and Detoxification	The enterocytes produce alkaline phosphatase that removes phosphate groups from nucleotides, proteins, alkaloids, and other molecules.
Mucosal Barrier	Tight junctions near the apex of the enterocytes form a seal that acts as a barrier to the absorption of large molecules.

Table 2-6: Hormones of the GI Tract

GI Hormone	Function
Gastrin	Produced by *G cells* in the antrum of the stomach, stimulated by stomach distension and dietary protein. Also made by duodenal and pancreatic cells. Stimulates the production of gastric juice and the proteolytic enzyme pepsin. Gastrin acts synergistically with histamine on parietal cells to stimulate the production of stomach acid.
Histamine	Produced by *ECL cells* in the stomach. Released under activation by the vagus nerve and inhibited by somatostatin. Acts via histamine-2 receptors to augment gastrin-induced acid production.
Serotonin	Serotonin is present as a neurotransmitter in nerve endings in the intestine. It is also released as a hormone by *Enterochromaffin cells*. Serotonin is released into the lamina propria by the presence of food, which stimulates segmental contraction of the intestinal muscles – holding the food in place for digestion. Irritants cause release of high levels of serotonin, which triggers peristalsis and rapid emptying of the intestine (diarrhea). Systemic absorption of these high levels stimulates $5HT_3$ receptors in the CNS causing nausea and vomiting.
Melatonin	Most of the body's melatonin is made by enterochromaffin cells. Melatonin delays gastric emptying, reinforces peristaltic clearing of the small intestine[18] during the night, decreases appetite and supports endothelial cell growth.
Secretin	Produced by *S cells* in the duodenum. Regulates pH in the gut by controlling bicarbonate secretion from the pancreas and inhibiting gastrin production.
Cholecysto-kinin (CCK)	CCK, produced by *I cells* in the small intestine, stimulates pancreatic digestive enzymes production, bile release from the gallbladder, and slows gastric emptying. CCK acts on afferent vagal nerve fibers to the brain stem, which signals satiety and suppress hunger. CCK release is inhibited by trypsin, acting as a feedback control loop. Further detail in Chapter 8.
Grehlin	Grehlin is produced by *P/D1 cells* lining the fundus of stomach and pancreas. Grehlin stimulates hunger by acting on the hypothalamus and by counteracting the effects of leptin and PYY_{3-36}.
Gastric Inhibitory Peptide (GIP)	GIP is an incretin, produced by *K cells* of the duodenum and jejunum with GRP120 fatty acid sensors. GIP increases insulin production, stimulates lipoprotein lipase in fat cells.
Somatostatin	Produced by *Delta cells (D cells)* of the stomach and pancreas, intestine and brain. It inhibits the release of gastrin from the stomach, inhibits the release of secretin and CCK in the duodenum, and inhibits the release of glucagon from the pancreas. In the intestine, it inhibits the release of motilin, VIP, GIP, and enteroglucagon. In the pituitary, it inhibits the release of growth hormone and TSH.
Glucagon-like peptide-1 (GPL-1)	GPL-1 is an incretin, produced by *L cells* in the ileum. GPL-1 increases insulin secretion from the pancreas and decreases glucagon release.
Glucagon-like peptide 2 (GLP-2)	GLP-2 is produced by the *L cells* and various neurons in the CNS. GLP-2 is secreted along with GLP-1. It helps maintain the mucosal barrier.
PYY_{3-36}	PPY is produced by *L cells* in the intestines after meals. It inhibits feeding through action on the hypothalamus. It also increases the release of pancreatic enzymes and bile.
Motilin	Produced by *endocrine M cells* in the proximal small intestine. This hormone increases gastric emptying and peristalsis between meals[*]. It increases production of somatostatin and pancreatic polypeptide.
Neurotensin	Neurotensin is produced by *N cells* in the jejunum and ileum. N cells also produce GIP, which stimulates gastrin release from G cells. Neurotensin is released by the presence of fat in the chyme and stimulates the release of bile from the gallbladder and promotes the uptake of bile from the proximal small intestine[19].
Guanylin	Produced by *Paneth cells* in the colon, and to a lesser degree in the small intestine. It activates guanylate cyclase, which increases chloride secretion, decreases intestinal fluid absorption, and can cause diarrhea. An enterotoxin from certain strains of *E. coli* produces an analog of guanylin which causes diarrhea.
Vasoactive intestinal peptide (VIP)	VIP is produced in the small intestine, appendix, and colon, as well as in the heart and brain. This is a neuropeptide hormone which induces relaxation of smooth muscle, such as the lower esophageal sphincter, and the sphincter of Oddi. It stimulates the secretion of water into pancreatic fluid and bile, and the secretion of water and electrolytes in the intestine. It also inhibits the secretion of gastric acid.

---

[*] The antibiotic erythromycin is a motilin agonist. The utility of erythromycin is limited by its GI side effects (diarrhea, nausea, abdominal pain, and vomiting), as a result of its motilin-like action. IV erythromycin is sometimes used to promote GI peristalsis.

Table 2-7: Pancreatic Hormones, α to ε

Glucagon: Alpha Cells	Released by the pancreas when blood glucose levels get too low. Promotes glycolysis of glycogen stored in the liver into glucose. Stimulates insulin release so that insulin-dependent tissues can utilize the released glucose.
Insulin: Beta Cells	Regulates carbohydrate and fat metabolism. Causes the liver, muscle, and fat cells to take up glucose from the blood and store it as glycogen or fat. Insulin inhibits the utilization of glucagon and fat for energy.
Amylin: Beta Cells	Released with insulin from β-cells. Slows gastric emptying and interacts with leptin to promote satiety; thus, helps prevent post-prandial spikes in blood glucose levels and over-eating.
Pancreatic polypeptide: Gamma (PP) Cells	Secreted mainly by cells around the periphery of the islets of Langerhans. When administered, pancreatic polypeptide (PP) suppresses gastric secretion, gastric emptying, pancreatic enzyme secretion, and appetite. In experimental animals, lack of PP has been associated with obesity. Patients found to have PP-secreting tumors stay thin with little ill effect.
Somatostatin: Delta cells	Inhibitory effects on the GI system: Reduces stomach acid secretion, CCK, VIP, GIP, secretin, and thus, pancreatic exocrine output. Suppresses motilin and GI motility. Inhibits insulin dn glucagon release. In the pituitary somatostatin inhibits growth hormone, TSH and prolactin
Grehlin: Epsilon Cells	Pancreatic ε-cells are progenitor cells that can become α, β, or γ cells. Grehlin cells are found in several organs, See Table 8-2.

---

[1] Importance of lipolysis in oral cavity for orosensory detection of fat. Kawai T, Fushiki T. Am J Physiol Regul Integr Comp Physiol. 2003 Aug;285(2):R447-54. Epub 2003 Apr 17.PMID: 12702486

[2] Fat digestion in the newborn. Characterization of lipase in gastric aspirates of premature and term infants. Hamosh M, Scanlon JW, Ganot D, Likel M, Scanlon KB, Hamosh P. J Clin Invest. 1981 Mar;67(3):838-46.PMID: 7204558

[3] http://biogps.org/#goto=genereport&id=4069 BioGPS gene expression for LYZ

[4] Fluid filled endoscopic view of the duodenal mucosa. Courtesy of Dr. Peter Kelsey, Harvard Univ.

[5] Illustration of the walls of the small intestine. Alex Luengo

[6] Intestinal villous M cells: an antigen entry site in the mucosal epithelium. Jang MH, Kweon MN, Iwatani K, Yamamoto M, Terahara K, Sasakawa C, Suzuki T, Nochi T, Yokota Y, Rennert PD, Hiroi T, Tamagawa H, Iijima H, Kunisawa J, Yuki Y, Kiyono H. Proc Natl Acad Sci U S A. 2004 Apr 20;101(16):6110-5. Epub 2004 Apr 7.PMID: 15071180

[7] Defensins and inflammation: the role of defensins in inflammatory bowel disease. Ramasundara M, Leach ST, Lemberg DA, Day AS. J Gastroenterol Hepatol. 2009 Feb;24(2):202-8. PMID: 19215333

[8] Enterocyte digestive enzyme activity along the crypt-villus and longitudinal axes in the neonatal pig small intestine. Fan MZ, Stoll B, Jiang R, Burrin DG. J Anim Sci. 2001 Feb;79(2):371-81.PMID: 11219446

[9] Honor thy symbionts. Xu J, Gordon JI. Proc Natl Acad Sci U S A. 2003 Sep 2;100(18):10452-9. PMID:12923294

[10] The involvement of macrophages and lymphocytes in the apoptosis of enterocytes. Iwanaga T. Arch Histol Cytol. 1995 Jun;58(2):151-9. PMID:7576867

[11] REDOX regulation of IL-13 signaling in intestinal epithelial cells: usage of alternate pathways mediates distinct gene expression patterns. Mandal D, Fu P, Levine AD. Cell Signal. 2010 Oct;22(10):1485-94. PMID:20570727

[12] The fate of effete epithelial cells at the villus tips of the human small intestine. Shibahara T, Sato N, Waguri S, Iwanaga T, Nakahara A, Fukutomi H, Uchiyama Y. Arch Histol Cytol. 1995 Jun;58(2):205-19. PMID:7576872

[13] Intraepithelial and lamina propria lymphocytes show distinct patterns of apoptosis whereas both populations are active in Fas based cytotoxicity in coeliac disease. Di Sabatino A, Ciccocioppo R, D'Alò S, Parroni R, Millimaggi D, Cifone MG, Corazza GR. Gut. 2001 Sep;49(3):380-6.PMID:11511560

[14] The inner of the two Muc2 mucin-dependent mucus layers in colon is devoid of bacteria. Johansson ME, Phillipson M, Petersson J, Velcich A, Holm L, Hansson GC. Proc Natl Acad Sci U S A. 2008 Sep 30;105(39):15064-9. Epub 2008 Sep 19.PMID: 18806221

[15] Bacteria penetrate the inner mucus layer before inflammation in the dextran sulfate colitis model. Johansson ME, Gustafsson JK, Sjöberg KE, Petersson J, Holm L, Sjövall H, Hansson GC. PLoS One. 2010 Aug 18;5(8):e12238.PMID: 20805871

[16] The "perfect storm" for type 1 diabetes: the complex interplay between intestinal microbiota, gut permeability, and mucosal immunity. Vaarala O, Atkinson MA, Neu J. Diabetes. 2008 Oct;57(10):2555-62. Review.PMID: 18820210

[17] Plasma citrulline level as a biomarker for cancer therapy-induced small bowel mucosal damage. Barzał JA, Szczylik C, Rzepecki P, Jaworska M, Anuszewska E. Acta Biochim Pol. 2014;61(4):615-31. PMID:25473654

[18] Melatonin and serotonin effects on gastrointestinal motility. Thor PJ, Krolczyk G, Gil K, Zurowski D, Nowak L. J Physiol Pharmacol. 2007 Dec;58 Suppl 6:97-103.PMID:18212403

[19] Involvement of mast cells in basal and neurotensin-induced intestinal absorption of taurocholate in rats. Gui X, Carraway RE. Am J Physiol Gastrointest Liver Physiol. 2004 Aug;287(2):G408-16. Epub 2003 Dec 23. PMID:14693504

3. CARBOHYDRATES

The vast majority of caloric energy from food comes from three sources: fats, proteins, and carbohydrates. Both carbohydrates and protein provide four calories per gram while fat provides nine calories per gram.

- Carbohydrates: 4 calories/gram
- Protein: 4 calories/gram
- Fat: 9 calories/gram
- Alcohol: 7 calories/gram

Most of the carbohydrates in foods are either sugars or complexes of sugars (polysaccharides) that are used by plants and animals for energy storage and which may also be used for structure.

When carbohydrates are used for storage of energy, they are usually in the form of polysaccharides. The most common storage polysaccharide in animals is glycogen. In plants, polysaccharides are mostly stored as starch or pectin. Carbohydrates are also used for structure. Plants use cellulose as a structural element while arthropods and fungi use chitin in this capacity.

When energy is needed, the polysaccharides are cleaved by enzymes into smaller pieces (oligosaccharides), usually three to ten sugars long. These are then typically cut by other enzymes into disaccharides for transport as solutes. Another set of enzymes (disaccharidases) cleave the disaccharides into single sugars for use as energy by the cells.

Table 3-1: Sugar Types

Term	Description
Monosaccharide	Single sugar
Disaccharide	Sugar composed of two simple sugars
Oligosaccharide	Chain of a few sugars
Polysaccharide	Chain of many sugars

Digestion of Carbohydrates

During digestion, complex carbohydrates are broken down into monosaccharides (single sugar molecules) which can be directly absorbed by the cells lining the small intestines.

The breakdown of starch begins in the mouth. Starch is composed of amylose and amylopectin. Amylose is a simple chain of glucose molecules with α-(1,4) linkages as shown in Figure 3-1. Amylopectin (and glycogen) are also chains of α-(1,4)-linked glucose molecules, but also have α-(1,6)-linked side branches. Saliva contains the enzyme α-amylase which splits the α-(1,4) linkages of amylose and amylopectin. This enzyme is inactivated in the acid environment of the stomach, halting the process.

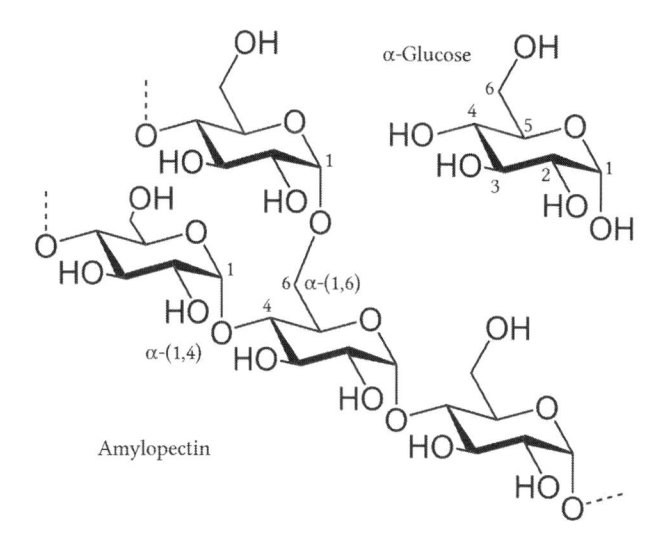

Figure 3-1: Diagram of amylopectin showing α-(1,4) and α-(1,6) linkages and a free, hydrolyzed α-glucose molecule.

Digestion of the α-(1,4) linkages continues in the small intestine with the addition of pancreatic α-amylase. Here, oligosaccharides are further split into glucose, maltose, and limit-dextrins. Limit-dextrins are short-chain remnants from amylopectin that contain both α-(1,4) and α-(1,6) links.

The absorptive cells of the small intestine (enterocytes) are covered with a brush border, with each cell having thousands of microvilli. These tiny finger-shaped projections are shown in Chapter 2; Figures 2-9 and 2-10. Microvilli greatly increase the surface area for absorption and contact of enzymes with the chyme (the digesting food slurry mixed with enzymes, saliva, and gastric fluids).

The surface of the microvilli presents many digestive enzymes, including glucan 1,4-alpha-glucosidase and glucan 1,6-alpha-glucosidase. These enzymes further cleave the limit-dextrins into glucose, maltose, and isomaltose. Additional brush border enzymes include the disaccharidases maltase, sucrase (isomaltase), trehalase, and lactase, which cleave the disaccharides into two simple sugars. Thus, the maltose and isomaltose from starch are ultimately cleaved into glucose. Similarly, sucrose is cleaved into glucose and fructose, and lactose is cleaved into glucose and galactose.

Table 3-2: Intestinal Brush Border Disaccharides

Enzyme	Substrate	Monosaccharide Products	Common Dietary Sources
Maltase	Maltose	glucose and glucose (α1-4)	Cereals, Barley, Starch
Sucrase (Isomaltase)	Sucrose and Isomaltose	glucose and fructose / glucose and glucose (α 1-6)	Cane and Beet Sugar / Fermentation products, Starch
Trehalase	Trehalose	glucose and glucose (α 1-1)	Mushrooms, Shrimp
Lactase	Lactose	glucose and galactose	Milk

The oligosaccharides and disaccharides are cleaved into the three main, simple sugars (glucose, fructose, and galactose) at the brush border and remain in the mucous/unstirred water layer, where they are in high concentration. They can then be transported into the absorbing cell, and then into the bloodstream where they can be used for energy or stored for later use. Glucose and galactose are transported across the brush border membrane by active transport or facilitated diffusion while fructose is transported across the membrane only by facilitated diffusion.

Table 3-3: Some Enterocyte Membrane Hexose Transfer Proteins

Transfer Protein	Symbol	Transport	Main Substrate
Sodium Glucose Transfer Protein-1	SGLT-1	Active	Glucose, Galactose
Glucose Transfer Protein 2	GLUT2	Facilitated	Glucose, Galactose, Fructose
Glucose Transfer Protein 5	GLUT5	Facilitated	Fructose

The two modes of hexose transport in the small intestine are:
1. Active transport of glucose and galactose, with facilitated diffusion of fructose (Figure 3-2);
2. Facilitated diffusion of glucose, fructose and galactose (Figure 3-3).

Active transport takes energy. Facilitated diffusion is free. Active transport is like pumping water uphill; facilitated diffusion is like water running downhill.

Active transport proteins pump a relatively low concentration of glucose to an area of higher concentration within the enterocyte and from there to the lamina propria, where it then diffuses into the blood stream. Active transport requires energy. In contrast, facilitated diffusion occurs when molecules move through membrane protein channels from a compartment of higher concentrations to one with a lower concentration. There is no active transport mechanism for fructose.

Active Transport: The membrane protein SGLT-1 can grab a glucose molecule from the unstirred water layer, flip over, and release the glucose into the enterocyte, along with a sodium ion (Na$^+$). The sodium pump (at the base of the enterocyte) uses energy to pump sodium out of the basal-lateral membrane into the extracellular fluid and from here it can enter the bloodstream. This results in a lower concentration of sodium in the cell than in the unstirred water layer. Thus, sodium is moving down a concentration gradient which drives this action, allowing glucose to be pumped from a low concentration to a higher concentration inside of the cell. Galactose is pumped into the bloodstream by the same transport protein. Once in the cell, glucose and galactose move into the bloodstream by facilitated transport by the GLUT2 transporter proteins, moving from a higher concentration in the extracellular space of the lamina propria of the villus to a lower concentration in the blood.

The active transport of glucose supports facilitated transport of fructose to enter the cell through the GLUT5 fructose transfer protein. Fructose flows down a gradient from a higher concentration in the unstirred water layer to a lower concentration in the enterocyte. The GLUT2 membrane protein then facilitates diffusion of glucose to the lesser concentration in the extracellular fluid.

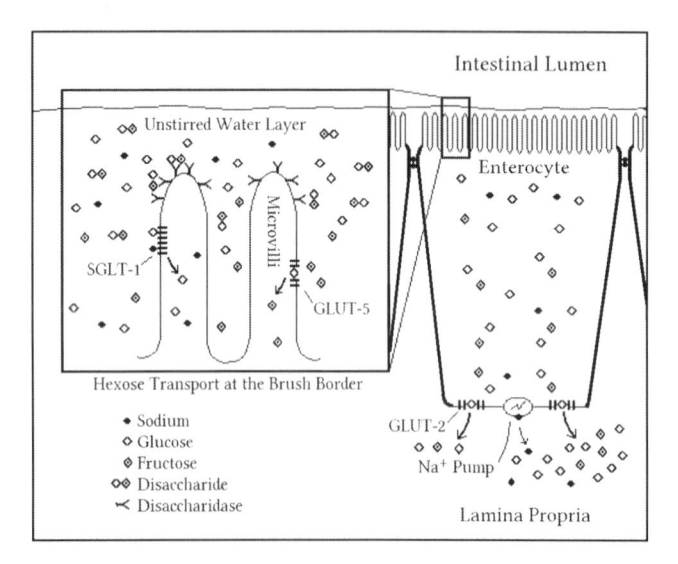

Figure 3-2: Cartoon of an enterocyte: showing the unstirred water layer in the lumen of the intestine and extracellular space of the lamina propria of the villi at its base. Microvilli are shown in the inset. Active transport membrane protein SGLT-1 drives glucose uptake while fructose passively diffuses through GLUT-5.

Facilitated Mode: When glucose concentration in the unstirred water level is high, glucose can be transported into the enterocyte down a concentration gradient without using the cell's energy. Within five minutes of having a high glucose concentration present in the unstirred water layer, the facilitated transport mode becomes activated.

GLUT2 proteins become active on the brush border, allowing glucose and galactose to move into the brush border cells, and for fructose to enter via GLUT5. GLUT2 and GLUT5 proteins on the basal-lateral membrane of the enterocyte also allow these sugars to move from the cell into the extracellular fluid of the villi, where it can then diffuse into the blood stream. During the facilitated mode, SGLT-1 transport is not active because a higher concentration of glucose in the enterocyte would move glucose backward into the unstirred water layer via the GLUT2 transporter.

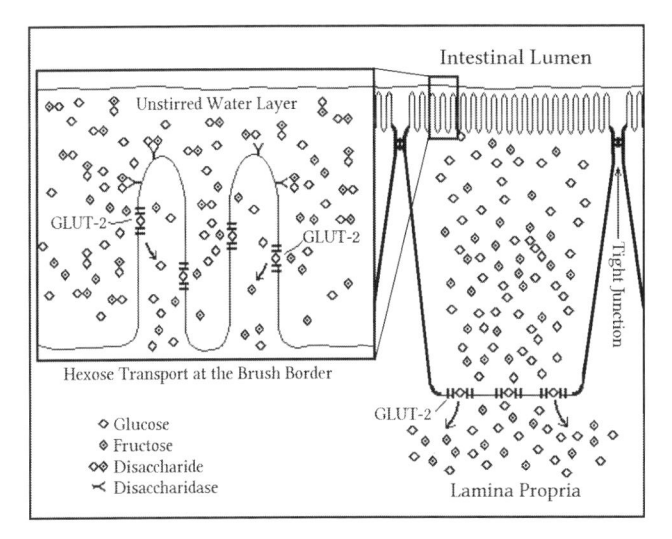

Figure 3-3: Cartoon of an enterocyte: showing the unstirred water layer in the lumen of the intestine and extracellular space of the lamina propria of the villi at its base. At high concentrations, GLUT-2 is active, allowing passive absorption of glucose, galactose, and fructose down a concentration gradient.

A key feature of carbohydrate digestion is that the disaccharidase enzymes are located at the brush border of the cells that absorb monosaccharides. These single sugar molecules are mainly produced only after entering the unstirred water layer at the brush border. The limited breakdown of oligosaccharides in the chyme makes it easier to control the water content in the intestine, which would have a greater osmotic force pulling water into it if there were higher concentrations of monosaccharides in the chyme. Producing simple sugars within the unstirred water layer at the brush border creates high concentrations of these sugars right at the absorptive surface. This allows for a gradient, where nutrients enter the bloodstream with little work, going from a higher concentration to a lower one.

Paracellular Absorption: There is an additional mechanism by which sugars and other small molecules are absorbed. Tight junctions, made up of specialized proteins that surround the enterocytes, seal these cells with their neighbors, linking the enterocytes together and forming a continuous barrier. These junctions are under the active control of the cells and can form a passageway for very small, water-soluble molecules to pass between the cells into the intercellular space. Under response to certain stimuli, the brush border cells unzip these proteins and pull these junctions open, allowing an increased passage of nutrients[1], including peptides, sugars, and perhaps some minerals. This active process occurs with stimulation of receptors, including taste receptors on the brush border membrane in respond to sweet and umami flavors[2]. Umami flavor is associated with certain amino acids and nucleic acids, usually found in foods high in protein.

The area of the intestinal surface composed of tight junctions accounts for only about 1/100 of a percent of the area covered by the brush border. Under normal conditions, only a limited number of compounds can pass these junctions. Usually, disaccharides are too large to pass through these channels, but monosaccharides can pass through. The epithelial tight junctions get progressively smaller along the course of the small intestine, decreasing permeability as nutrients move from the duodenum to the colon[3]. The junctions at the tip of the villi are small (<0.6 nm) but the junction in the crypts, a more protected area, are considerably larger (5-6 nm). The junctions in the crypts are large enough to allow passage of peptides, which are short chains of amino acids.

The tight junctions may also open in response to certain inflammatory mediators and to certain microbial and viral pathogen proteins. Opening the tight junction space can allow the passage of antigens, which provoke autoimmune disorders, including celiac disease, inflammatory bowel disease, type 1 diabetes, and other diseases. This will be discussed in more detail in later chapters.

---

[1] Alterations in intestinal permeability. M C Arrieta, L Bistritz, J B Meddings. Gut 2006;55:1512-1520

[2] An energy supply network of nutrient absorption coordinated by calcium and T1R taste receptors in rat small intestine. Mace OJ, Lister N, Morgan E, et al.. J Physiol 587.1 (2009) pp 195-210

[3] Dietary Reference Intakes for Energy, Carbohydrate, Fiber, Fat, Fatty Acids, Cholesterol, Protein, and Amino Acids (Macronutrients) (2005) National Academy of Science

4. THE COLON AND ITS INHABITANTS

The body of an adult human body is composed of around 50 trillion somatic cells; each built according to DNA coding that came as a birthday gift from the individual's parents. There are an additional 100 trillion cells in your body with DNA that did not come from your parents. These are alien cells that do not have human DNA and most do not even have animal or plant DNA.

These alien cells invaded and colonized your body soon after birth. "Invaded" is actually misleading. It was an intentional act of sabotage. You invited them in. As a newborn, your perfectly intact, healthy immune system, began producing CD71[+] cells that dialed back the immune system, risking dangerous infections from E. coli, Listeria, and other gram-negative bacteria, just to let these aliens take root and colonize your innards[1].

The average person plays host to 150 different species of microorganisms living in their gut, in addition to those occupying the mouth, the nasal pharynx, and residing on the skin. Ninety-nine percent of the commensal microbial species are bacterial species, and about one percent are Archae. In terms of mass, this microbial population is comprised almost entirely (over 99.9%) of obligate anaerobes, which only grow in low-oxygen environments.

What are Archae?

Life can be divided into three domains: Eukaryota, which includes ameba, plants, animals, and fungi; the other two domains are Archaea and Bacteria.

Archaea are about the size and shape of bacteria but are genetically closer to us than to bacteria. Archaea represent about 20% of the biomass on the planet. Many extremophiles that survive in extreme heat, such as deep-sea volcanic vents, extreme cold, or concentrated saline conditions are Archaea. They have been around for over 3 billion years and are not known to act as parasites or pathogens.

Although Archae are usually represented by a single species in the human colon, most commonly *Methanobrevibacter smithii*, they often make up 10 percent of the biomass of intestinal microbiota.

The colonic bacteria contain numerous species, some of which are commensal, some pathologic, and several which can become pathologic under certain stimuli. (This is discussed in more detail, in Chapter 23; Biofilms.) Commensal microbes are integral to health. Yeast can also live among the colonic microorganisms. They, however, are not known to contribute to health, but can contribute to disease.

Determinants of Bacterial Populations

About a thousand bacteria species commonly colonize the human colon[11]. The 150 or so, which thrive in a particular individual's colon, depend not only on exposure to those microbes, but just as importantly, on the local environment. Just as different plants grow in different areas depending on soil, terrain, climate, rainfall pattern, competing plants and pests; various bacteria thrive or fail to thrive in the colon depending on its environment and the mix of other species present. The microbial community depends on the resources available to them.

Table 4-1: Examples of Genera of Commensal Bacteria that Commonly Colonize the Colon

Anaerobes:	
Bacteroides	*Psuedoflavonifractor*
Bifidobacterium	*Odoribacter*
Clostridium	*Porphyromonas*
Desulfovibrio	*Ruminococcus*
Butyribvibrio	*Rosburia*
Coprococcus	*Veillonella*
Facultative Anaerobes:	
Enterococcus	*Enterobacteriaceae*
Staphylococcus	*Lactobacillus*

Commensal microbial community clusters, within various species of animals, have been linked to the animals' diets. Animals of different species share similar microbial community clusters depending on their diets, according to whether they are carnivores, omnivores or vegetarian[2].

What we eat, and more specifically what does not get digested and absorbed, affects the population of bacteria that live in the colon. These microbes feed and are nourished by the leftovers of digestion, sloughed cells from the intestine, IgA and killed bacteria, digestive enzymes, bile, and other residuals that make their way into the cecum and colon.

The materials that enter the large intestine are fermented by the microbes inhabiting it. The populations of the various species of microbes are highly influenced by the nutrients available to them. A change in diet can be accompanied within a couple of weeks by a bloom of new bacteria, and a fall-off of other bacteria[3]. This results in changing the populations of dominant species of bacteria. It is not the nutrients that are absorbed by our bodies, but what is left over for the bacteria to ferment that affects which populations of bacteria thrive in the large intestine.

Dietary fiber is composed of edible plant materials that are resistance to digestive enzymes, and thus, not broken down into sugars or other absorbable compounds in the small intestine. These materials end up in the colon where they are fermented. Different species of microbes are capable of processing different compounds; those that find food and a favorable environment, and are not out-competed by other organisms, feed and multiply.

The community of bacteria present may be influenced by the genetics of the host, and by which bacteria are first established in the previously sterile colon of an infant. Some pioneering species of bacteria modulate genetic expression of the host, making the environment more suitable for themselves, thus limiting the proliferation of other bacteria. Bacteria, further, are symbiotic; many depend on the products of other bacteria for nutrients.

Life in the Colon

Colonic microbes are more than just passengers. They help us survive. Commensal bacteria normally protect us from disease, help digest our food, and may help heal our wounds. In a very real way, they are part of our body, acting like an extra organ. They help feed our brain and affect our personality and mood. Thus, they affect who we are and how we think and feel. And, like other organs, things can go wrong; the microbes can cause disease. Not just belly aches, but mental illness, heart disease, obesity, dermatologic, dental and other disorders. Bacteria affect the growth and vascularity of the mucosa, and may help prevent infection and allergic reactions to foods[4].

Our bacteria are somewhat of an invading alien infestation. The influence of bacteria has been demonstrated in experiments with mice. Mice raised in a germ-free environment showed increased motor activity and decreased anxiety compared to mice with normal gut microflora. This may be due to the 280 percent increase in the plasma serotonin level seen when the gut is colonized by normal gut bacteria[5]. The germ-free mice showed a different expression of genes in the amygdala of the brain, with higher levels of brain-derived neurotrophic factor (BDNF) expression and a decreased number of serotonin$_{1A}$ receptors on neurons[6]. These effects could be reversed with the introduction of specific species of bacteria at an early age. If the introduction were delayed, the decreased response to stress stayed with the mice for the rest of their lives[7]. In this experiment, mice may have epigenetically adapted to low serotonin levels early on, and then required less throughout life.

Certain bacteria promote intestinal inflammation that causes obesity in mice[8]. The inflammatory signaling is exacerbated by a high-fat diet[9]. Gut microbiota can cause anxiety and depression[10] as a result the toxins and inflammatory cytokines induced by some gut bacteria.

Higher animals, such as humans, are complex and adaptive, yet we have a smaller genome than of a tomato. The ameba, *Amoeba dubia* has a genome more than 200 times larger than ours. Genes are susceptible to mutation and damage. DNA damage in independently living cells of species that reproduce by the billions per cubic centimeter every few hours is not a critical problem for that species' survival. Higher animals, however, benefit from a safer and more efficient strategy; we hire out much of the metabolic work to the microbes that do the job best for us. We change colonic bacteria when we change our diets. The human genome contains about 23,000 protein-coding genes; the species living within the average individual's gut have an aggregate of about 536,000 different genes[11]. Many of these are genes for proteins and enzymes that can do things that human cells cannot. A single common commensal colonic species, *Bacteroides thetaiotaomicron,* produces 172 different enzymes for the catabolism of various polysaccharides[4]. Our colonic biome adjusts to our state in life, in part, under hormonal control; the greatest biome diversity occurs during the third trimester of pregnancy when there is an increased population of *Actinobacteria* and *Proteobacteria* bacteria[12].

Micronutrient cofactors: Although few animal enzymes require molybdenum, and no animal enzymes are known to require boron or tungsten; this cannot be said for our commensal bacteria. Even though we may not use some trace minerals in our metabolism, our bacteria may require them for their activity. They may thus be needed for health.

Intestinal bacteria can affect steroid hormone levels. A large portion of the circulating sex hormones is excreted into the bile as glucuronide or sulfated conjugates. Once they reach the large intestine, they are deconjugated by bacterial β-glucuronidase and sulfatase enzymes and then reabsorbed. Without the bacteria, these hormones are eliminated in the feces. β-glucuronidase also increase the bioavailability phytoestrogens, and the flavonoids genistein and daidzein, that help prevent breast and prostate cancers.

Nevertheless, excessive levels of β-glucuronidase in the stool can be used as a marker for overgrowth (biofilm formation) of pathogenic bacteria in the colon.

Digestible dietary carbohydrates yield four Calories of energy per gram to the body. NDC, however, typically provide between 1.25 and 2 Calories per gram. This energy derived is from short-chain fatty acids (SCFA) formed by fermentation of NDC by microbes in the colon. The balance of the four Calories of energy from carbohydrates is consumed by bacteria, spent in heat production, remains as non-processed biomass, or goes up in smoke: as gasses, such as methane and hydrogen.

Not all products of intestinal bacterial fermentation are benign. Lactose intolerance is a common source of fermentable sugars in adults consuming milk or milk products. Most adults make very little "lactase." When milk is consumed, individuals with lactose intolerance are unable to digest the milk sugar, and thus, it is not absorbed. Instead, it ferments in the large intestine. Fermentation of lactose can produce toxic metabolites including alcohols, diols, ketones, acids and aldehydes, such as methylglyoxal[13] that causes glycation and is atherogenic[14].

Fermented amino acids may produce biogenic amines that are metabolically active and affect not only the gut, but also affect the central and peripheral nervous system. Fermentation of proteins can also produce ammonia. While carbohydrates are mostly fermented in the cecum and the right side of the colon, protein fermentation occurs mainly on the left side of the colon.

One theory for the development of autism proposes that the antibiotic Augmentin causes the formation of ammonia, which is a neurotoxin[15]. This theory cites the reported appearance of regressive autism in small children following ear infections that have been treated with this antibiotic. Rather than the antibiotic being the source of ammonia production, however, it is more likely the effect the antibiotic is the elimination of commensal gut bacteria and a shift to pathogenic bacteria that produce ammonia and other toxins. (Chapter 35)

Bacteria capable of proteolysis can ferment unabsorbed protein in the large intestine. Some bacteria incorporate the amino acids from protein for their own growth, while others use amino acids as an energy source, with ammonia and other toxins being produced as metabolic by-products.

Small amounts of colonic ammonia production are not a problem for healthy adults, as the liver can efficiently metabolize ammonia into non-toxic compounds. Infants, however, do not process ammonia well. Ammonia absorbed from the colon enters the bloodstream and can cross the blood-brain barrier. Here it is easily toxic, especially to astrocytes, which serve as support cells for neurons.

Ammonia can easily reach toxic levels and cause hepatic encephalopathy (HE) in those with liver cirrhosis. In HE, hyperammonemia causes irritability, memory loss, difficulty with concentration and tremor, and can result in death. Patients with liver cirrhosis and HE, and those with liver cirrhosis but without HE, have very different populations of bacteria living in their colons[16].

Hyperammonemia in HE can be treated, often reversing its symptoms. A well-accepted treatment is the use of lactulose, a disaccharide for which human do not have a disaccharidase. This disaccharide is taken orally and passes through the small intestine unabsorbed. In the colon, it is metabolized by colonic bacteria that incorporate nitrogen. This nitrogen then is passed in the feces, rather than being turned into ammonia[17]. HE can also be effectively treated with the use of probiotics[18]. Here, bacterial cultures are given in a capsule as a medication to seed the colon and change the population of microbes to ones that incorporate nitrogen. Yet another approach is to treat with prebiotics, which consists of dietary fiber that encourages the growth of different populations of bacteria[19]. A nonabsorbable antibiotic, such as rifaximin, which kills bacteria including those associated with ammonia production, is another treatment[20]. There is a risk, however, with antibiotics of relapse after treatment with potential bacterial resistance to these and other antibiotic medications.

Colonic bacteria can also produce toxins that can be absorbed from the colon, causing disease. *Clostridium bolteae* have been found in concentrations 46 times higher in children with autism than in control children[21]. *Clostridia* are well known for the formation of neurotoxins. *Clostridium difficile* causes pseudomembranous colitis, with frequent watery stools, abdominal pain, and fever, and is seen in patients after the use of broad-spectrum antibiotics. Thes kill many species of commensal bacteria and favor proliferation of spore-forming bacteria, such as *Clostridia*, as the spore can survive antibiotic treatment.

Prebiotics and Probiotics

Prebiotics have not enjoyed the notoriety of probiotics; however, they play a more important role in health.

Probiotics are cultures of bacteria that are consumed in an effort to seed the large intestine with beneficial, commensal organisms. Most commonly, *Lactobacillus* and *Bifidobacterium* species are utilized. These genera are nonpathogenic, as they are not known to cause human disease. Yogurt, which contains these bacteria, is promoted for this purpose. Probiotics have been shown to be helpful in many disease conditions, especially, but not exclusively, those of the GI tract, such as irritable bowel syndrome (IBS). The utility of probiotics is limited, however, as *Lactobacillus* and *Bifidobacterium* species, the most commonly used probiotics, compose only a tiny proportion of the commensal organisms in the large intestine, and many commensal organisms cannot be cultured.

Using probiotics is similar to tossing some seeds into an untended field. If you toss tomatoes into a vacant lot, some of their seeds might grow, but farming is rarely that easy. Depending on sun, soil, water, nutrients and pests, the plants best suited to the conditions in that field will dominate, and crowd out the rest. The environment, which supports the growth of the microbes currently thriving the intestine, will likely continue to support a similar mix of microbes. Using probiotics alone should not be expected to have more than short term benefits.

Prebiotics are food components, or other agents such as lactulose, which are not digested and absorbed in the small intestines. Once planted, the bacteria need to be feed with prebiotics to thrive. Prebiotics provide food for the growth of bacteria in the colon. Usually, the term prebiotic is used for commercial food supplements consumed for this purpose; however, the prebiotic effect of foods is part of normal nutrition. Prebiotics are more effective than probiotics in altering the microbial population of the gut. The diversity and population mass of colonic bacterial species is highly correlated with the diversity and amount of vegetables consumed in the diet. Rather, probiotics are more effective if used in combinations with prebiotics[22].

Chronic Fatigue Syndrome patients have been found to have an increased number of *enterococci* in their colon and lower population of *Escherichia coli* and *Bifidobacterium* species than control patients. Most irritable bowel syndrome (IBS) patients also have lower populations of commensal bacterial species[23].

Colonic bacteria can influence susceptibility to allergies. Infants who are colonized early with commensal bacteria, such as *Lactobacillus* and *Bifidobacterium*, are less likely to develop food allergies[24].

The bacterial mix inhabiting the colon may even influence obesity. If colonic bacteria from obese mice are planted in germ-free mice, these mice become obese[25]. These bacteria may cause slight increases in energy production from fiber that are sufficient to cause weight gain over time or may produce metabolites that increase appetite. Obese individuals have a different distribution of large intestinal bacterial species than do lean individuals.

Not all the bacteria living in the colon are commensal. Some bacteria that are usually benign may cause disease under certain stimuli (See Chapter 23: Biofilms). Some colonic bacteria process pre-carcinogenic compounds into active carcinogens, produce toxins, and trigger an inflammatory response; meanwhile, others impede immune hypersensitivity, inflammation, and the production of carcinogens.

Postbiotics?

In cases of severe, treatment-resistant pseudomembranous colitis, fecal transplants from healthy donors have had a 70 to 80 percent cure rate[26]. The patient's colon is inoculated with a normal colonic biome that displaces *C. difficile* and allows the establishment of a healthy commensal biome. In the future, diseases such as obesity or autism may be treated with fecal transplants or specifically cultured blends of bacteria along with selected prebiotics, to normalize the colonic biome and restore health.

Fiber

In humans, most of the nutritional components of food are absorbed in the small intestine. The leftover effluent moves into the cecum and colon, where it undergoes fermentation. Fermentation allows for further recovery of energy as well as absorption of water, some vitamins, hormones and some other compounds.

The human cecum contains a few ounces of fermenting biomass. Elephants, Earth's largest land animals, consume large amounts of poorly digestible leaves and tree bark. This requires a large volume for bacterial fermentation to supply the animal's nutritional requirements. The contents of an adult elephant's cecum comprise about 12 percent of the elephant's body weight, and thus contains about 1200 pounds of fermenting vegetable matter.

Most of the biomass from diet that remains unabsorbed at the end of the small intestine is comprised of complex carbohydrates. The amount of unabsorbed proteins is usually small. These components undergo fermentation in the large intestine. In healthy individuals, very little fat passes to the large intestine.

Table 4-2 gives the results of a study of undigested nutrients in patients with ileostomies[1] consuming a Western diet[27]. The study investigated the fate of low- and high-resistant starches that remain at the end of the small intestine. The treatment arm of this study used a high-resistant starch (RS) diet. As can be seen in Table 4-2, virtually all non-resistant starch is absorbed, while non-starch polysaccharides and resistant starches were not.

Table 4-2: Undigested Nutrients at the Terminal Ileum

Dietary Component	Grams Intake	Grams Undigested
Total starch (normal Western) diet	61 g (Low RS diet)	0.8
Non-starch Polysaccharides	15 g	15
Protein	101 g	16
Fat	69 g	1
High resistant starch (treatment) diet	164 g Total starch 35 g Resistant starch	35

In this study, nearly all dietary fat was absorbed. A considerable amount of protein remained in the ileal effluent, but some of this protein may not be dietary protein, but rather from endogenous sources, such as mucin, desquamated enterocytes and digestive enzymes. Sugars are completely absorbed in normal individuals. This study reveals that only small amounts of carbohydrates remain in the ileal effluent for entry into the colon, for persons consuming a Western Diet.

Resistant starches and non-starch polysaccharides make up most of the undigested food matter in the effluent of the small intestine that enters the cecum in healthy individuals. Starches are polysaccharides made up of chains of sugar molecules linked together. The enzyme amylase, present in saliva or produced by the pancreas, cleaves starches into disaccharides or trisaccharides (two- and three-sugar chains). The disaccharides and trisaccharides can then be cut into simple sugars by brush border enzymes and absorbed in the small intestine.

Other non-starch polysaccharides are resistant to amylase and do not get broken down into disaccharides or trisaccharides. These nondigestible carbohydrates (NDC) are often referred to as fiber.

NDC are not just byproducts of consumption, which simply pass through the gut, or just "roughage," which adds bulk to the stool. NDC are important to nutrition and disease prevention. They are a source of caloric nutrition, including the preferred source of energy for the cells lining the large intestine. We rely on the bacteria in the large intestine to digest these nutrients. Humans and other animals lack the

---

[1] An ileostomy is a surgically created opening of the end of the ileum at the skin, allowing discharge of the effluent from small intestine, so that the effluent is not required to enter the colon.

Ileostomies are used in patients with severe colon diseases, often as a temporary treatment until the colon can heal.

necessary enzymes to process many compounds that enter the colon, but bacteria and Archae, that specialize in these functions have the required enzymes for breaking down various carbohydrates and other compounds. Similarly, termites rely on commensal organisms to digest cellulose from wood and cattle rely on bacteria for digestion of grass.

Fermentation results in the formation of short chain fatty acids (SCFA) and gasses. The principal SCFA are acetate, propionate, and butyrate. Since bacteria tend to be specialists, the balance of SCFA production depends on the population distributions of bacteria in the large intestine, and this in turn depends on the food supply (type of fiber or nutrient) available to those organisms.

In the proximal small intestine, the enterocytes have glucose as a ready source of energy. By the time the chyme reaches the distal ileum, sugars are no longer available, and the enterocytes of the ileum depend on the amino acid glycine for energy. The colonocytes, the predominant cells lining the large intestine, also need a fuel source. The short-chain fatty acid butyrate, formed by the bacterial fermentation of NDC, is the major source of energy for these cells. These short chain fatty acids are also used as fuel for the brain and may decrease hunger between meals.

Table 4-3: Short Chain Fatty Acids Formed in the Colon

SCFA	Role and Effects[28]
Acetate	Enters peripheral circulation. Used as fuel by the brain. May increase cholesterol synthesis.
Propionate	Absorbed by the liver. Very little is measurable in the blood. Used to make glucose. Inhibits cholesterol synthesis.
Butyrate	The major energy source for the colonocytes. Decreases risk of colon cancer.

Non-Digestible Carbohydrates

Fiber (NDC) can be classified into the following groups:
- Fructans
- Pectin
- Cellulose and Hemicellulose
- Chitin
- Resistant Starches
- Certain Oligosaccharides

Fructans: While starch, formed of chains of glucose, is the most common carbohydrate for energy storage in plants, about 15 percent of flowering plants store energy as chains of fructose in polysaccharides called fructans[29]. Fructans, unlike starches, are water-soluble. Smaller fructans give a sweet flavor, but larger fructans have a neutral flavor and have a fat-like texture. Similar to cellulose, humans do not make digestive enzymes that breakdown fructans. Thus, they pass through the small intestine into the cecum where they may be degraded by bacteria.

Fructo-Oligosaccharides (FOS) are short segments of fructans that are either occur naturally or that have been created by enzyme degradation for use as food additives. Most plants that contain fructans have about half of their fructan content as short chains (FOS) and about half as longer, branch-chained polysaccharides. FOS and fructans are used as food additives because of their low caloric content, sweetness (up to 60 percent that of sucrose), and fat-like texture which can be used to replace fat content in the food.

> *Streptococcus mutans* can produce fructooligosaccharides from fructose. This is integral to the production of plaque formation on teeth that promotes dental caries.

Fructans and FOS pass through the small intestine unchanged. Once in the colon, bacteria ferment them and release gas (hydrogen, carbon dioxide, and methane) and short chain fatty acids. The colon absorbs these fatty acids and thus, allowing the body energy use from these carbohydrates. It is estimated that about 50 percent of the energy from these carbohydrates, about 2 Calories per gram, is absorbed as short chain fatty acids; the rest is lost as heat and gas, or passes unchanged into the stool.

Many health claims have been made about fructans and FOS as prebiotics that support the growth of beneficial bacteria in the colon. These beneficial bacteria may decrease the risk of colon cancer, lower cholesterol levels, and decrease inflammation. The diversity of dietary fructans is important; each type of molecular bond between these sugars requires a different enzyme for its breakdown. Different microbial species have specific enzymes for processing NDC's from various food sources. Thus, the various NDC's support different populations of microbes. Benefit or harm may be associated with these microbes. Some microbes cause gas and increase bloating. Some bacteria produce toxins, and some can cause disease.

There are five main families of fructans polysaccharides. Most fructans are formed around a single sucrose molecule attached to many chains of fructose molecules, as shown in gray in Figure 4-1. Thus, fructans include a single glucose molecule.

Inulins are a form of fructan produced by dicots; flowering plants with two embryonic leaves; (i.e., beans). Monocots (including grains and lilies) make other fructans known as **graminan** and **leven**. These fructans differ from each other by the types of bonds between the fructose units. The **neoseries fructans** differ as they have fructose chains attached to glucose at two different positions so that the glucose is in the middle.

Since these fructans differ from each other, they have differing effects on the proliferation of the intestinal microbiota. The largest source of fructans in the American diet is wheat. Onions are another significant source[30]. Other important sources are bananas and garlic. These pants are all monocotyledons.

When first introduced to the diet, NDC often promote flatulence, but as the make up of the microbiota adapts to species capable of utilizing more of the energy in the NDC, the amount of flatulence usually decreases. Thus, slow introduction of a particular NDC may cause less discomfort.

Table 4-4: Fructans

Fructan:	Fructose Links	Source	Example
Inulin	β(2→1) glycosidic bonds	Dicotyledons	Jerusalem artichoke
Levan	β(2→6) glycosidic bonds	Monocotyledons	Orchard grass
Graminan Mixed Leven	β(2→1) glycosidic bonds and β(2→6) glycosidic bonds	Monocotyledons	Wheat, barley
Inulin neoseries	β(2→1) glycosidic bonds (mF2-1F2-6G1-2F1-2Fn Fructose on both sides of glucose	Monocotyledons: Lily	Onions, garlic, asparagus
Levan neoseries	β(2→6) glycosidic bonds (mF6-1F2-6G1-2F1-6Fn) Fructose on both sides of glucose	Monocotyledons: grain	Oats
Fructose-Oligosaccharides (FOS)	Depends on plant source	Multiple Fructans	Jerusalem artichoke, banana, asparagus, garlic, onions, artichoke[31], jicama, wheat, barley

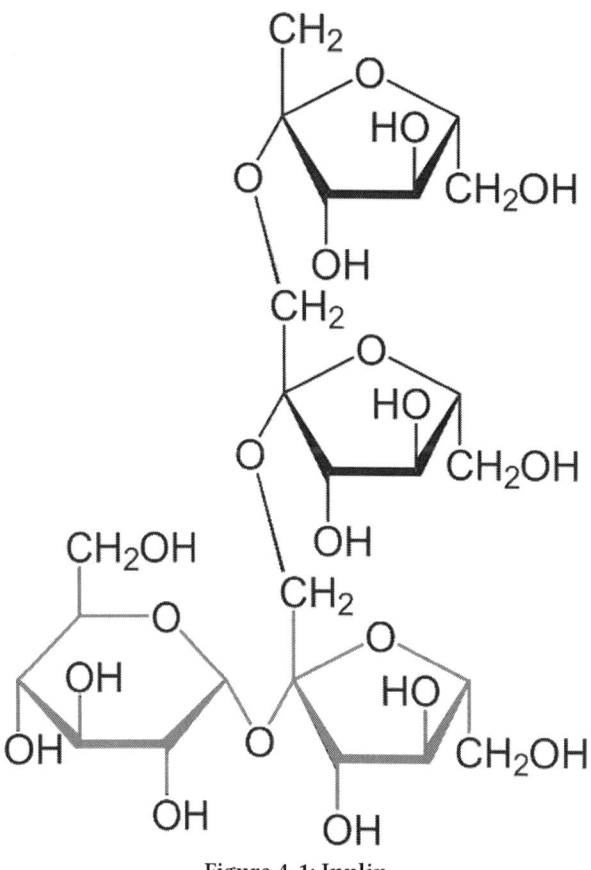

Figure 4-1: Inulin

Jerusalem artichokes (sunchokes), a dicotyledon, are high in the fructan inulin. English botanist John Goodyer, who introduced Jerusalem artichokes to England, noted in 1621:

"Which way soever they be dressed and eaten, they stir and cause a filthy loathsome stinking wind within the body, thereby causing the belly to be pained and tormented[32]."

Pectin: About one percent of the mass of fruits and vegetable in the diet is pectin. Pectins are a soluble fiber which are not digested in the ileum, but rather fermented by colonic bacteria. Pectin are made up of D-galactosyl uronic acid linked with other sugars, including D-galactose, L-arabinose, D-xylose, and L-rhamnose. Pectins from different sources are composed of different sugars.

Cellulose and β-glucans: Cellulose is the most common organic molecule on Earth, but there is little cellulose in human food. It is one component of non-soluble fiber. β-glucans are small chains of β-linked glucose molecules. Only a tiny fraction of the cellulose in the diet is broken down and utilized by bacteria in the human colon.

In addition to cellulose, methylcellulose, carboxymethyl-cellulose, and other cellulose derivatives are used as thickening agents in foods and treatments for constipation. These add bulk and pull moisture into the stool, making it larger and softer.

Hemicellulose: Hemicellulose is an amorphous matrix polysaccharide that is part of the cell wall of plants along with cellulose and pectin. Hemicellulose contains xylose and glucose, and can include rhamnose, arabinose, galactose, and mannose. Mannuronic acid and galacturonic acid are also often present in hemicellulose.

Chitin: Chitin forms the shells of insects, shrimp, and lobsters, but humans usually avoid consumption of these non-digestible carbohydrates. The small amounts of chitin found in the human diet come mostly from mushrooms.

> **Fun Fact:** Mushrooms are not plants but are more closely related to animals. Fungi produce both structural and storage polysaccharides in common with crustaceans and insects. Because of their similarities, there can be allergic cross-reactions between dust mites, cockroaches, shrimp, lobster, and mushrooms.

Table 4-5: Non-Digestible Polysaccharides

NDC	Sugar Links	Source	Example
Pectin	α (1→4) D-galactosyl uronic acid, mixed sugars	Fruit	Orange, apple, pear, okra
Hemi-cellulose	Mixed sugars, links	Plant cell walls	Vegetables
Cellulose β-glucans	Chains of cellobiose β(1→4) Glucose Disaccharide[33]	Most plants: Structural	Wood, cotton, corn seed coat
Chitin	B(1→4) glucose chains	Fungi, crustaceans	Mushrooms
Resistant Starch	α-(1→4) and α-(1→6) Glucose glycosidic bonds	Most plants: storage	Wheat, rice
Stachyose	gal(α1→6) gal(α1→6) glc(α1↔2β)fru	Plants	Beans
Raffinose	gal(α1→6) glc(α1↔2β)fru	Plants	Beans, Cabbage
Fructans	See Table 4-4		

Resistant Starches are an important source of SCFA, and one of the most important fibers for maintaining health. Starch is stored in granules that are resistant to enzymatic degradation. Milling and mastication help to break up these microscopic granules and cooking helps gelatinize them. These processes improve the starch's exposure to enzymatic degradation. Additionally, starch from different food sources has different availability. For example, milled (white) rice served warm is almost completely absorbed, with almost no resistant starch. If refrigerated, rice becomes hard, and its starch becomes resistant starch. Other starchy foods, such as potatoes, may contain as much as 30 percent resistant starches; these resist enzymatic degradation and thus become fodder for bacteria in the large intestine. Resistant starches are sometimes categorized as RS$_1$ to RS$_4$:

- RS$_1$: Partly milled grains and seeds.
- RS$_2$: Resistant granules, as found in potatoes, green bananas, some beans and legumes.
- RS$_3$: Cooked and cooled starches; bread, cold potato salad, cornflakes.
- RS$_4$: Chemically modified starches, as found in processed foods.

During cooking, starch granules absorb water and gelatinize. This is one reason that cooking is important; it allows a higher absorption of energy from many foods.

When gelatinized starches cool, the starches crystallize and harden, forming an RS$_3$ starch, which is non-digestible. RS$_2$ starches are the most completely fermented and produce more butyrate, compared to other RS types. RS$_3$ starch tends to produce more hydrogen and methane than other forms[34].

> Black (turtle) beans have unusually small starch granules as compared to other bean varieties, making them more easily digestible than most other beans. Their small size also makes them cook more readily.

Oligosaccharides: Two important non-digestible dietary oligosaccharides are *Raffinose* and *Stachyose*. Raffinose is a trisaccharide, and stachyose is a tetrasaccharide; both contain (α1→6) galactoside bonds. Humans lack the enzymes needed to digest to digest these bonds. These sugars are present in beans and cruciferous vegetables, such as cabbage and broccoli. Fermentation of these foods results in the formation of gas and flatulence, for which these vegetables are infamous. The product "Beano" contains the enzyme α-galactosidase, which helps in the digestion of these sugars, allowing them to be digested in the small intestine and thus avoid fermentation and production of gas.

It is not only the type of food that is important, but also its preparation. In a study using barley made into porridge, propionate was produced, but when barley kernels were ingested, butyrate was formed[35], suggesting that RS$_1$ and RS$_2$ starches are processed by different species of bacteria. Different NDC cause the formation of different SCFA and promote the growth of different populations of bacteria.

Polyphenolic Compounds

In addition to non-digestible carbohydrates, dietary fiber also includes polyphenolic compounds. The phenolic polymer *lignin* is the second most common organic polymer on earth. It comprises much of the cell walls of plants and makes up one-third of the mass of wood. Tannin is another large branched-chain phenolic polymer found in food.

Polyphenols are not absorbable, but first must be digested, in part by gastrointestinal enzymes, but more significantly by colonic bacteria[36]. Some *lignans* (not to be confused with lignin) are metabolized by gut bacteria to the enterolignans, enterodiol (a phytoestrogen) and enterolactone, which have anticarcinogenic and anti-inflammatory properties[37].

Foods also contain many smaller phenolic compounds, including monomers, dimers, and trimeric phenols. Many dietary phenols have physiologic effects, including reducing the risk of many chronic inflammatory diseases, such as heart disease and cancer[38].

Polyphenolic compounds that are absorbed are rapidly removed from the circulation, and thus have limited metabolic activity. The antioxidant activity associated with polyphenols in the blood may be limited to the creation of uric acid[39]. Uric acid is an antioxidant; however, it becomes a pro-oxidant when blood levels are elevated (Chapter 9; Syndrome X). Many mono-phenolic compounds, however, are well absorbed. Many of these have anti-inflammatory, antiproliferative, and antibiotic properties. Several phenolic compounds block the induction of protein synthesis for inflammatory mediators.

The lack of systemic absorption of polyphenols does not negate them from having health benefits. Smaller phenolic compounds with antioxidant activity may help keep food fresh and prevent the formation of lipid peroxides in foods. Polyphenols present in marinades prevent the formation of carcinogenic heterocyclic amines during the cooking of meats (See Chapter 40: Cancer Prevention). Phenolic compounds may protect the intestines from oxidative stress and pathogen overgrowth, even without being absorbed.

Health benefits associated with the consumption of small quantities of red wine are due to polyphenols. During the fermentation of wine, tannins from the grapes are broken down into smaller phenolic compounds that can be absorbed. Thus, red wine has more absorbable phenols than red grape juice. Colonic fermentation of polyphenols also increases their availability, thus, adding health benefits. This fermentation process alters the balance of microbes proliferating in the colon. These phenolic and polyphenolic compounds have antimicrobial activity[40] that decreases the pathogenicity of many intestinal microbes. (See Chapter 23: Biofilms.) These polyphenols increase the diversity of the colonic biome by decreasing the dominance of biofilm forming genera, that crowd out many others.

Non-Carbohydrate, Non-Absorbed Nutrients

Non-digested Proteinaceous Biomass: As noted in Table 4-2, an adult with a typical western diet may pass about 16 grams of protein into the large intestine a day. These proteins include some ingested proteins that have not been hydrolyzed by proteolytic enzymes. In health, most of this protein comes from endogenous sources from desquamated, retired enterocytes, mucin, antibodies and a small portion of the digestive enzymes used in digestion.

When there is inadequate protein digestion because of pancreatic exocrine insufficiency (PEI), damage to the cells lining the small intestine, or malabsorption caused rapid intestinal transit that precludes effective protein digestion and amino acid absorption, the amino acids and proteins passes into the colon and is fermented.

Proteins are passed into the colon are predominantly fermented in the left side of the colon. If the commensal biome is fed excessive proteinaceous biomass, it grows more of the bacteria that can ferment it, and they feed it back to us. The products of protein fermentation include hydrogen and carbon dioxide gas; ammonia, bioamines, and phenols; some SCFA and some branch-chained fatty acids. Butyrate, and some propionate, is used by the colonocytes, and the other fatty acids are absorbed. Hydrogen and carbon dioxide gasses may be absorbed and released in the breath, used by other bacteria, or form flatus that is released during flatulence. The ammonia, bioamines, and phenols are largely absorbed into the body and can have deleterious effects. Some bioamines can provoke migraine and may affect behavior. Biogenic amines are discussed in Chapter 13. Ammonia is toxic and a carcinogenic for the colon and may help explain the high frequency of colon cancers found in the distal colon and rectum where it is produced. Ammonia is absorbed and is can be converted to urea in the liver, and then eliminated from the body in the urine. In infants and individuals with liver cirrhosis, however, the liver does not convert ammonia efficiently to urea, and ammonia levels can rise, cross the blood-brain barrier and cause toxic encephalopathy.

Ammonia can be a substrate for growth of certain bacteria. Prebiotics, which support the growth of these bacteria, decrease the availability of ammonia to the colonic mucosa and decrease its absorption into the circulation. This has been suggested as a putative reason for low rates of colon cancer in populations with diets high in resistant starches[41]. When resistant starches are added to the diet, fermentation of ileal effluent provides a higher production of butyrate and decreases the production of ammonia by two-thirds[42]. In a study using the prebiotic lactulose, production of nitrogenous compounds was halved[10].

Patients with proteolytic enzyme deficiencies benefit from digestive enzyme supplements. Pancreatic exocrine function can be tested by measuring Fecal Elastase. Brush border proteolytic enzymes (peptidases) may also be deficient if there is injury to the enterocytes lining the small intestine, as occurs in celiac disease. Patients may also benefit from supplementation with these enzymes as well. Enzyme supplements aid absorption of amino acids for nutrition, but also prevent steatorrhea (lipase) dysbiosis, and help normalize colonic biome diversity. The benefit provided by enzyme supplements may be augmented by prebiotics and probiotics.

Non-Digested Fats: In normal individuals, very little fat escapes digestion and absorption in the small intestine. Dietary fats are mostly triglycerides and phospholipids. These are resistant to fermentation by colonic bacteria. Dietary fats that are not absorbed, as occurs in some malabsorption syndromes, pass through the colon into the stool, and may result in steatorrhea; fatty stools, which may float; be foul smelling; pale, if bile pigments are lacking; and accompanied with orange-colored fat droplets, which may float in the toilet water.

Steatorrhea can occur with pancreatic enzyme insufficiency (lipase), lack of bile salts, intestinal mucosal damage, and the use of the weight loss medication Orlistat, which blocks the activity of lipases. Additionally, Olestra, jojoba oil and some oily waxes in butterfish and escolar are not digestible, and they pass into the stool.

Belching, Gas, and Flatulence

Cattle are not the only greenhouse-gas producing animals. The human gut has large numbers and diverse populations of bacteria that break down complex carbohydrates and produce the greenhouse gasses methane and carbon dioxide, as well as the secondary greenhouse gas, hydrogen. Flatulence is normal, and most people fart 14 to 23 times in a 24-hour period, including during their sleep.

Most of the volume of intestinal gas, however, is not from fermentation, but from swallowing air. Air is swallowed during fast eating, as a result of anxiety, and during speech. Rapid drinking, smoking, chewing gum or use of poorly fitting dentures increases aerophagia, the swallowing of air. Frequent belching soon after a meal suggests aerophagia. Most of the volume of flatulence that is not from ingested air is formed by fermentation of NDC. Protein fermentation does not produce high volumes of gas, but that which is produced from protein can have a very foul odor.

The intestines usually contain about 200 ml of gas, some resulting from aerophagia. Air is composed of 78 percent nitrogen, 21 percent oxygen and about 1 percent other gasses, such as argon. Nitrogen is poorly absorbed by the tissues, so nitrogen that is swallowed must be expelled either through belching or flatulence. The tissues can absorb oxygen, so the oxygen from swallowed air decreases to the partial pressure in the cells lining the intestines or slightly lower, as aerobic activity in some intestinal bacteria that can utilize O_2.

Carbon dioxide can be produced during digestion of food. CO_2 is produced when stomach acid is neutralized by bicarbonate in the jejunum and during the breakdown of triglycerides into fatty acids. CO_2 can also result from the consumption of carbonated beverages. Some CO_2 is absorbed by the small intestines, transferred into the blood and released through the lungs into exhaled breath. If high levels of carbon dioxide are present in flatus, it is a result of bacterial activity in the colon. *L. delbrueckii*, and *L. plantarum MB 456*, as probiotics, inhibit the growth of gas forming *E. coli*[43].

Table 4-6: Intestinal Gases

Gas	Symbol	Typical Proportion
Nitrogen	N_2	20 – 90%
Oxygen	O_2	Up to 10%
Carbon Dioxide	CO_2	10 – 30%
Hydrogen	H_2	Up to 50%
Methane	CH_4	Up to 10%
Other gases		About 1%

Anaerobic bacteria produce hydrogen in the intestine. Methane is not produced by bacteria but rather by the Archae, *Methanobrevibacter*.

> Individuals who produce larger amounts of intestinal methane, as a result of fermentation by *Methanobrevibacter*, tend to have stools that float in the water of the toilet bowl.

Unpleasant Winds

Nitrogen, oxygen, carbon dioxide, hydrogen, and methane are all colorless, odorless gasses. They do not cause malodorous flatus or bad breath. Most of the foul odors in flatulence and some odors in halitosis come from sulfur-containing gasses, including hydrogen sulfide, allyl methyl sulfide, and methanethiol.

Some colonic microbes utilize CO_2, hydrogen, O_2 and methane. *Methanobrevibacter* utilizes CO_2 for the formation of methane. Other bacteria can metabolize methane during the fermentation of sulfur compounds, producing methanethiol, a gas with a rotten cabbage smell. Still other bacteria can utilize hydrogen and produce hydrogen sulfide that has a rotten egg odor. Hydrogen sulfide forms from the fermentation of sulfate, derived from the amino acids cysteine, found in mucin and methionine. Much of the foul odor of flatulence is derived from the fermentation of proteins.

Sulfur-containing foods include cruciferous vegetables and proteins. Eggs are an example of a food rich in the sulfur-containing amino acids, cysteine, and methionine.

While fructans in wheat ferment and create gas, rice starch digests well and is absorbed as glucose. Rice gives a very low production of gas[44].

Table 4-7: Foods Likely to Cause Gas Formation

High Gas Food	Non-Digested Carbohydrate
Beans	Oligosaccharides, Resistant Starch
Cruciferous Vegetables: Broccoli, Cabbage, Brussels Sprouts, Mustard Greens, Cauliflower, Water Cress, Arugula	Oligosaccharides (Sulfur -containing glucosinolates give odor)
Onions	Fructans
Pears, Plums	Fructose, Sorbitol
Wheat and whole grains	Fructans, Resistant starches
Soft Drinks, Fruit Juices	Fructose
Dairy (milk, fresh cheese; whey)	Lactose
Diet Sweets and gum	Sorbitol

Sugars that are not absorbed in the small intestine, usually due to disaccharidase deficiencies, cause an osmotic load in the small intestine and decrease the transit time; digestion, and absorption of other nutrients along with these sugars pass into the colon, where they are fermented.

Fermentation of sugars can cause gas production, but even more problematic is the loss of other nutrients, vitamins, hormones, and bile salts fats and proteins into the colon. Non-anaerobic bacteria produce hydrogen in the intestine. Methane is not produced by bacteria but rather by the Archae, *Methanobrevibacter*. Fermentation of non-absorbed protein from the meal ferments, causing putrid odor, ammonia and bioamine production. Passage of bile causes an increase in secondary bile acid formation and can cause diarrhea. Nutrients and hormonal imbalance may occur,

Retention of flatus, for example, in social situations, can cause bowel distention, cramping pain, and sensitization to bowel pain. Dry, mildly malodorous, tympanic flatus suggests healthy cecal fermentation with a normal transit time. Wet, and especially foul smelling flatus suggests malabsorption and rapid colonic transit, or fermentation in the distal colon associated with protein malabsorption.

Fiber and Disease

Dietary fiber has been demonstrated to decrease the risk for infection in hospitalized patients. For example, FOS supplements prevent recurrence of *Clostridium difficile* associated pseudomembranous colitis. Treatment of *C. difficile* disease with FOS with probiotics was shown to be more effective than using antibiotics. Dietary fructans and FOS have been shown to decrease the growth of *Candida, Listeria* and *Salmonella* in the colon. Inulin added to the diet stimulates the growth of *lactobacilli* and *bifidobacteria* in the colon, and is associated with deeper crypts, taller villi, increased goblet cell number, and a thicker mucus layer on the colonic epithelium[45].

In vitro fermentation of human colonic samples with β-glucans was associated with a four-fold increase in the number of bacteria from two families of bacteria that have a strong inverse association with obesity. Adding pectin to the diet decreased *Clostridiales* mass by half, caused a ten-fold decrease in *Bacterioidaceae*; a family often associated with disease conditions and raised the mass of beneficial *Bifidobacteriaceae* ten-fold[46].

FOS in the diet increases the production of protective IgA and decreases the production of IgG, suggesting that dietary FOS are associated with a lower inflammatory response by gastrointestinal mucosal immune cells[47]. Prebiotics may help prevent the development of immune hypersensitivity to foods[48]. Breast milk contains galacto-oligosaccharides (GOS) which promote the growth of beneficial commensal organisms in the colon. Similarly, fructose oligosaccharides promote the growth of beneficial organisms. Trials using GOS/FOS prebiotics have shown benefit in preventing atopic dermatitis in infants. Similar trials using probiotics have failed to show efficacy[49].

> Breastfed infants have very low levels of SCFA in their feces[50]. High levels of SCFA may be toxic to the immature intestinal mucosa and may contribute to the pathogenesis of neonatal necrotizing enterocolitis, a condition that leads to necrosis of the bowel and death in premature infants[51].

Fermentation of fiber, by *lactobacilli* and *bifidobacteria*, causes acidification of the colonic contents that enhance calcium, iron, magnesium, and zinc absorption[52], and thus, may help prevent osteoporosis, anemia, and other diseases. FOS supplements in animals fed a Western diet prevented accumulation of body fat, and thus, may prevent obesity[53].

Lactobacilli-induced acidification and production of H_2O_2 impairs the growth of the pathogens *Candida albicans, Escherichia coli* and *Gardnerella vaginalis* in the vagina[54]. Orally administered prebiotic strains of *lactobacilli* are recovered from the vagina[55], thus suggesting that probiotics, which enhance the growth of these bacteria, will also prevent the growth of vaginal pathogens.

Fiber and Cancer

For many years, there have been efforts to understand the role of fiber in preventing cancer, particularly colon cancer, and there have been many trials using fiber supplements in attempts to decrease the incidence of various cancers.

Studies of colon cancer, however, have shown that not just any fiber will do. Rather, it is the consumption of whole grains that is associated with decreased risk of colon cancer[56]. This risk reduction is greatest for the distal colon and rectum, and when consuming two servings of whole grains a day (1.25 servings per 1000 Calories of food intake)[57]. Eating more than one apple a day also decreased risk of colon cancer[58]. Fruit fiber (pectin) appears to only decrease the risk of distal colon and rectal cancers. This suggests that the fermentation of these fibers reduces exposure to carcinogenic products of protein fermentation. Fiber from grain binds to bile and lowers the fecal bile acid concentration of the stool[59]. The production of short-chain fatty acids (SCFA) by bacteria in the colon inhibits the production and absorption of secondary BA. This mechanism may help explain the anti-carcinogenic influences of SCFA in the colon[60], as secondary bile acids have been implicated in the pathogenesis of colon and rectal cancer. (See also Chapter 24: Small Intestinal Bacterial Overgrowth).

Diets with higher fiber levels have also been associated with a 13% reduction in breast cancer risk. The decreased risk was most clearly related to intake of soluble fiber from fruit[61] (pectin). Lignans, which are polyphenols and some of which are phytoestrogens, are associated with decreased risk of breast cancer[62]. (See Chapter 40: Cancer prevention)

Esophageal cancer risk is inversely associated with fiber, but only fiber from fruits and vegetables[63]. Caution, however, should be used when interpreting the relationships of individual dietary components with disease risk. Vegetable fiber may be associated with decreased risk, but vegetables also contain numerous other compounds. It may be other compounds present in fruits and vegetables, rather than the fiber that provides protection from the disease. Many phenolic compounds, found in vegetables have antiinflammatory and anticarcinogenic activities.

Supplements with wheat bran fiber have failed to reduce the risk of recurrent adenomas in patients with high risk of colon cancer[64]. This data should not be used to suggest that other NDC's, such as resistant starch from grain, do not lower the risk of colon cancer. It may not be one or the other component, but the effect the mix of fibers and other elements from whole foods, which affect the microbial biome, rather than effects of a single fiber. Single fiber supplements may cause excessive dominance of certain types of bacteria at the expense of other species.

> **Halitosis:** Malodorous compounds in breath are primarily volatile sulfurous compounds produced by fermentation by oral microorganisms. The source of sulfur is cysteine and methionine from proteins from exfoliated cells, leukocytes, saliva, blood, and food debris[65].

Colonic Transit Times

In health, and under normal conditions, the residuals of a meal appear in the stool, on average, about two days after eating. The non-digested contents spend a short time in the stomach, about 5 hours traversing the small intestine, and about 43 hours in the colon. Children, having a shorter colon, have a shorter colonic transit time; toddlers about 31 hours and elementary school aged children about 36 hours[66]. About two-thirds of the colonic transit time (CTT) is spent is spent in the rectosigmoid colon, where water is removed from the stool.

A CTT greater than 70 hours (>3 days from intake) is outside of the normal range. Long CTT time is common in irritable bowel syndrome with constipation and other forms of constipation. Short CTT is seen in irritable bowel syndrome with diarrhea, as well as in other forms of diarrhea. Both long and short CTT are associated with an increase in somatic symptoms, including headaches, back pain, insomnia, fatigue, palpitations, asthenia, anxiety, and depression[67].

Most adults are "regular," having one stool per day, at 24-hour intervals, usually occurs in the morning hours, soon after arising. For men, the most common stool-time is between 7 AM and 8 AM, and for women, it is an hour later. Nearly 90% of adults have five to 14 stools per week. About 60% of adults rate their stools as a "Type 3 or 4 stools" on the Bristol Stool Scale (Figure 4-1) [68].

The "Bristol Stool Scale" is a simple and helpful visual tool that approximates the CCT. The graphic can help identify abnormally long or short CTT's. The chart classifies stools from hard separate pellets to watery. Type 1 and 2 stools (hard pellets or a cluster of hard lumpy pellets) indicates an abnormally long CTT. Type 6 and 7 (fluffy, ragged, mushy stool or entirely liquid stool) indicate an abnormally short CTT. Most adults consider type 6 or 7 stools to be diarrhea; however the term actually refers to an increase in stool frequency. Many people do not, however, consider type 1 or 2, or infrequent stools as abnormal. Both long and short CCT indicate abnormal bowel function.

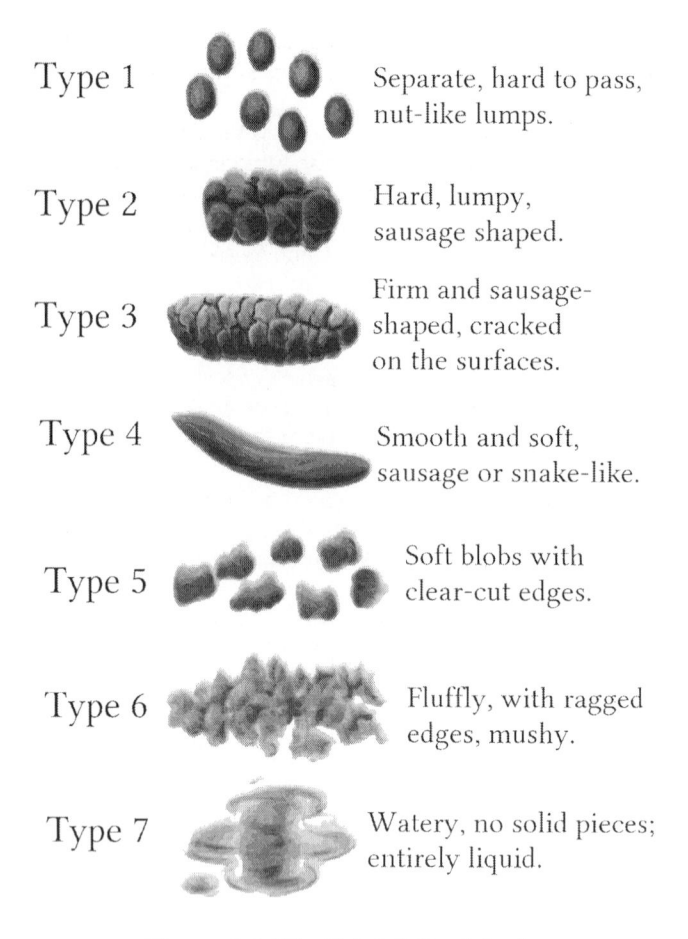

Type 1 — Separate, hard to pass, nut-like lumps.

Type 2 — Hard, lumpy, sausage shaped.

Type 3 — Firm and sausage-shaped, cracked on the surfaces.

Type 4 — Smooth and soft, sausage or snake-like.

Type 5 — Soft blobs with clear-cut edges.

Type 6 — Fluffly, with ragged edges, mushy.

Type 7 — Watery, no solid pieces; entirely liquid.

Figure 4-1: The Bristol Stool Scale.

Recommendations

Prebiotics: Fiber is an important part of nutrition. Dietary fiber may help maintain a normal weight by providing energy to the brain between meals, thus lowering appetite. Fiber may help prevent colon cancer by binding to bile acid.

1. There are multiple types of fiber, and different fibers are processed by different bacteria; a wide diversity of plant materials from eating a diversity of plants gives rise to a healthy and diverse bacterial biome. A diversified diet provides a milieu for amply diverse populations of bacteria; in effect providing a larger number of tools in the enzymatic toolbox and a lower chance dominion by a few species of bacteria.

2. FOS promote the growth of *lactobacilli* and *bifidobacteria* in the colon. Many studies find a beneficial response to the consumption of five to seven grams of FOS per day. Good dietary sources include onions, garlic, shallots, banana, and artichokes.

3. Some individuals may not tolerate large amounts of FOS or other NDC because they lack an intestinal microbiota ready to ferment NDC and their by-products. A slow, steady introduction of NDC may allow a more comfortable introduction of these nutrients.

4. Boron and other trace minerals may be prebiotic nutrients required for supporting a healthy biome.

5. Flatulence is normal, but excessive or foul-smelling flatulence can be a sign of disease or poorly digested foods. Foul-smelling flatulence may result from consumption of cruciferous vegetables or poor digestion of proteins. Inadequate digestion of proteins should be investigated.

Probiotics: We colonize our colon with bacteria in early childhood. Even *Helicobacter pylori*, bacteria that resist the effect of stomach acid that kills most other bacteria, usually colonizes the stomach before the age of ten. New interlopers are not easily welcomed. Stomach acids, pancreatic and other enzymes, bile acids, immunoglobulins and other defenses inhibit the survival of newly introduced bacteria. Established bacteria do their best to hold their ground, and often modify the environment to make it more suitable for themselves. *H. pylori* causes peptic ulcer disease and stomach cancer as a result of the modifications it makes to the stomach mucosa to make it more hospitable for its kind. Many bacteria that live in the colon modify the colonic environs to enhance their own survival over the survival of other species.

Antibiotic use often disrupts the colonic biome. A 2010 CDC study found that antibiotics were dispensed each year 83 times per 100 Americans. In Britain, the average person uses 70 courses of antibiotics over their lifetime. The use of broad-spectrum antibiotics creates a need to reestablish a healthy commensal biome. Replacing the biome is not as easy as is its destruction. Most probiotics include only a few species of culturable bacteria, and most bacteria do not survive the digestive transit.

A billion dehydrated *lactobacilli* in a gelatin capsule are likely to have a rough ride traversing the gantlet of hydrochloric acid, enzymes, and other defenses along their route to the cecum. Once there, the scant survivors have to compete against trillions of established bacteria, already embedded, already adapted to interact the hundred plus other species that comprise the local biome. Adding a significant presence of new commensal bacteria to the colon is not easy. Restoring populations containing dozens of interacting species, including many that have never been cultured in a lab, is a much greater hurdle.

Probiotics alone have transitory effects; the intestinal microbiota adapt to the environment created by the host and the nutrients available to them. Prebiotics from the diet sustain the population of bacteria. A combination of probiotics for the introduction of beneficial organisms, with a sustained diet containing prebiotic fiber, can give a quicker transition to a healthy intestinal biome.

Using Probiotics: To increase colonization by probiotics, I suggest taking the probiotic on an empty stomach with 1.7 grams sodium bicarbonate (about ¼ teaspoon of baking soda) dissolved in water. This neutralizes stomach acid for about 30 minutes. Then, fast for one hour to avoid the release of bile and digestive enzymes that destroy bacteria.

Phenolic Compounds: Phenolic compounds help increase the diversity of the intestinal microbiota and help promote the growth of bacteria needed for the absorption of phenolic compounds that lower the risk of chronic disease. Fruits, spices and other plant-based foods high in phenolic compounds are needed for the maintenance of a healthy colonic biome.

Digestive Enzymes: Lack of functioning digestive enzymes is likely to cause and maintain dysbiosis. Lack of proteolytic enzymes, especially, can increase the dominance of pathogenic bacteria. Digestive enzymes are often helpful for the recovery of a diverse and commensal colonic biome. These enzymes can help avoid excess entry of proteins and peptides from entering the colon, where they ferment and promote dysbiosis, ammonia, and other toxin formation.

Constipation and Slow CTT: Occasional hard stools or slow transit stools may be due to vagaries of diet and activity, and are not a concern, but chronic constipation and chronic slow CTT should be investigated and treated, as should new onset of sustained constipation or changing bowel habits in adults.

IBS with constipation (IBS-C) is common. IBS-C and simple constipation may respond to prebiotics and probiotics and digestive enzymes. Avoidance of foods causing immune sensitivities also helps in IBS. Chapter 26 discusses IBS and its treatment.

Glycine: The amino acid glycine is a required nutrient for ileal enterocytes. Trimethyl-glycine (betaine) supplement may help improve ileal function and uptake of bile acids, steroids and other compounds absorbed in the ileum.

---

[1] Immunosuppressive CD71+ erythroid cells compromise neonatal host defence against infection. Elahi S, Ertelt JM, Kinder JM, et al. Nature. 2013 Dec 5;504(7478):158-62. PMID:24196717

[2] Diet drives convergence in gut microbiome functions across mammalian phylogeny and within humans. Muegge BD, Kuczynski J, Knights D, et al. Science. 2011 May 20;332(6032):970-4. PMID:21596990

[3] Dominant and diet-responsive groups of bacteria within the human colonic microbiota. Walker AW, Ince J, Duncan SH, et al. ISME J. 2011 Feb;5(2):220-30. PMID: 20686513

[4] Honor thy symbionts. Xu J, Gordon JI. Proc Natl Acad Sci U S A. 2003 Sep 2;100(18):10452-9. PMID:12923294

[5] Normal gut microbiota modulates brain development and behavior. Heijtz RD, Wang S, Anuar F, et al. Proc Natl Acad Sci U S A. 2011 Jan 31. PMID:21282636

[6] Reduced anxiety-like behavior and central neurochemical change in germ-free mice. Neufeld KM, Kang N, Bienenstock J, Foster JA. Neurogastroenterol Motil. 2011 Mar;23(3):255-e119. PMID: 21054680

[7] Postnatal microbial colonization programs the hypothalamic-pituitary-adrenal system for stress response in mice. Sudo N, Chida Y, Aiba Y, Sonoda J, Oyama N, Yu XN, Kubo C, Koga Y. J Physiol. 2004 Jul 1;558(Pt 1):263-75. PMID: 15133062

[8] Replication of obesity and associated signaling pathways through transfer of microbiota from obese-prone rats. Duca FA, Sakar Y, Lepage P, et al. Diabetes. 2014 May;63(5):1624-36. PMID:24430437

[9] High fat diet-induced gut microbiota exacerbates inflammation and obesity in mice via the TLR4 signaling pathway. Kim KA, Gu W, Lee IA, et al. PLoS One. 2012;7(10):e47713. PMID:23091640

[10] Gut-brain axis: how the microbiome influences anxiety and depression. Foster JA, McVey Neufeld KA.Trends Neurosci. 2013 May;36(5):305-12. PMID:23384445

[11] A human gut microbial gene catalogue established by metagenomic sequencing. Qin J, Li R, Raes J, Arumugam M, et al. Nature. 2010 Mar 4;464(7285):59-65. PMID: 20203603

[12] Exploring host-microbiota interactions in animal models and humans. Kostic AD, Howitt MR, Garrett WS. Genes Dev. 2013 Apr 1;27(7):701-18. PMID:23592793

[13] Bacterial metabolic 'toxins': a new mechanism for lactose and food intolerance, and irritable bowel syndrome. Campbell AK, Matthews SB, Vassel N, et al. Toxicology. 2010 Dec 30;278(3):268-76. PMID: 20851732

[14] Glycation of LDL by methylglyoxal increases arterial atherogenicity: a possible contributor to increased risk of cardiovascular disease in diabetes. Rabbani N, Godfrey L, Xue M, et al. Diabetes. 2011 Jul;60(7):1973-80. PMID:21617182

[15] Could one of the most widely prescribed antibiotics amoxicillin/clavulanate "augmentin" be a risk factor for autism? Fallon J. Med Hypotheses. 2005;64(2):312-5. PMID: 15607562

[16] Linkage of Gut Microbiome with Cognition in Hepatic Encephalopathy. Bajaj JS, Ridlon JM, Hylemon PB, et al. Am J Physiol Gastrointest Liver Physiol. 2011 Sep 22. PMID:21940902

[17] Effects of lactulose on nitrogen metabolism. Weber FL Jr.Scand J Gastroenterol Suppl. 1997;222:83-7. PMID:9145455

[18] An open-label randomized controlled trial of lactulose and probiotics in the treatment of minimal hepatic encephalopathy. Sharma P, Sharma BC, Puri V, Sarin SK. Eur J Gastroenterol Hepatol. 2008 Jun;20(6):506-11. PMID:18467909

[19] Bifidobacterium combined with fructo-oligosaccharide versus lactulose in the treatment of patients with hepatic encephalopathy. Malaguarnera M, Gargante MP, Malaguarnera G, et al. Eur J Gastroenterol Hepatol. 2010 Feb;22(2):199-206. PMID:19730107

[20] Rifaximin treatment for reduction of risk of overt hepatic encephalopathy recurrence. Flamm SL. Therap Adv Gastroenterol. 2011 May;4(3):199-206. PMID:21694804

[21] Real-time PCR quantitation of clostridia in feces of autistic children. Song Y, Liu C, Finegold SM. Appl Environ Microbiol. 2004 Nov;70(11):6459-65. PMID: 15528506

[22] Effects of Lactobacillus casei Shirota, Bifidobacterium breve, and oligofructose-enriched inulin on colonic nitrogen-protein metabolism in healthy humans. De Preter V, Vanhoutte T, Huys G, et al. Am J Physiol Gastrointest Liver Physiol. 2007 Jan;292(1):G358-68. PMID: 16990449

[23] Luminal and mucosal-associated intestinal microbiota in patients with diarrhea-predominant irritable bowel syndrome. Carroll IM, Chang YH, Park J, Sartor RB, Ringel Y. Gut Pathog. 2010 Dec 9;2(1):19. PMID: 21143915

[24] Altered early infant gut microbiota in children developing allergy up to 5 years of age. Sjögren YM, Jenmalm MC, Böttcher MF, Björkstén B, Sverremark-Ekström E. Clin Exp Allergy. 2009 Apr;39(4):518-26.. PMID:19220322

[25] Obesity, metabolic syndrome, and microbiota: multiple interactions. Tilg H. J Clin Gastroenterol. 2010 Sep;44 Suppl 1:S16-8. PMID: 20535027

[26] Fecal transplant against relapsing Clostridium difficile-associated diarrhea in 32 patients. Jorup-Rönström C, Håkanson A, Sandell S, et al. Scand J Gastroenterol. 2012 May;47(5):548-52. PMID:22468996

[27] Ileal recovery of starch from whole diets containing resistant starch measured in vitro and fermentation of ileal effluent. Silvester KR, Englyst HN, Cummings JH. Am J Clin Nutr. 1995 Aug;62(2):403-11. PMID: 7625349

[28] Colonic health: fermentation and short chain fatty acids. Wong JM, de Souza R, Kendall CW, Emam A, Jenkins DJ. J Clin Gastroenterol. 2006 Mar;40(3):235-43. PMID: 16633129

[29] Fructan: more than a reserve carbohydrate? Vijn I, Smeekens S. Plant Physiol. 1999 Jun;120(2):351-60. PMID: 10364386

[30] Presence of inulin and oligofructose in the diets of Americans. Moshfegh AJ, Friday JE, Goldman JP, Ahuja JK. J Nutr. 1999 Jul;129(7 Suppl):1407S-11S. PMID: 10395608

[31] Fructan and free fructose content of common Australian vegetables and fruit. Muir JG, Shepherd SJ, Rosella O, Rose R, Barrett JS, Gibson PR. J Agric Food Chem. 2007 Aug 8;55(16):6619-27. PMID:17625872

[32] Gerard's Herbal, cited in Davidson A. (1999). The Oxford Companion to Food, first edition. Oxford University Press ISBN 0-19-211579-0.

[33] Cellulose biosynthesis. Delmer DP, Amor Y. Plant Cell. 1995 Jul;7(7):987-1000. PMID: 7640530

[34] Short-chain fatty acids and human colonic function: roles of resistant starch and nonstarch polysaccharides. Topping DL, Clifton PM. Physiol Rev. 2001 Jul;81(3):1031-64. PMID: 11427691

[35] Influence of the type of indigestible carbohydrate on plasma and urine short-chain fatty acid profiles in healthy human volunteers. Verbeke K, Ferchaud-Roucher V, Preston T, et al. Eur J Clin Nutr. 2010 Jul;64(7):678-84.. PMID: 20502475

[36] Digestion and absorption of phenolic compounds assessed by in vitro simulation methods. A review. Tarko T, Duda-Chodak A, Zajac N. Rocz Panstw Zakl Hig. 2013;64(2):79-84. PMID:23987074

[37] Enterolignan-producing phenotypes are associated with increased gut microbial diversity and altered composition in premenopausal women in the United States. Hullar MA, Lancaster SM, Li F, et al. Cancer Epidemiol Biomarkers Prev. 2015 Mar;24(3):546-54. PMID:25542830

[38] Update on uses and properties of citrus flavonoids: new findings in anticancer, cardiovascular, and anti-inflammatory activity. Benavente-García O, Castillo J. J Agric Food Chem. 2008 Aug 13;56(15):6185-205. PMID:18593176

[39] The biological relevance of direct antioxidant effects of polyphenols for cardiovascular health in humans is not established. Hollman PC, Cassidy A, Comte B, et al. J Nutr. 2011 May;141(5):989S-1009S. PMID:21451125

[40] Antimicrobial activity of flavonoids. Cushnie TP, Lamb AJ. Int J Antimicrob Agents. 2005 Nov;26(5):343-56. Feb;27(2):181. PMID:16323269

[41] Effect of lactulose and Saccharomyces boulardii administration on the colonic urea-nitrogen metabolism and the bifidobacteria concentration in healthy human subjects. De Preter V, Vanhoutte T, Huys G, Swings J, Rutgeerts P, Verbeke K. Aliment Pharmacol Ther. 2006 Apr 1;23(7):963-74. PMID: 16573799

[42] Ileal recovery of starch from whole diets containing resistant starch measured in vitro and fermentation of ileal effluent. Silvester KR, Englyst HN, Cummings JH. Am J Clin Nutr. 1995 Aug;62(2):403-11. Erratum in: Am J Clin Nutr 1996 Mar;63(3):407. PMID: 7625349

[43] Antagonistic effect of Lactobacillus strains against gas-producing coliforms isolated from colicky infants. Savino F, Cordisco L, Tarasco V, Locatelli E, Di Gioia D, Oggero R, Matteuzzi D. BMC Microbiol. 2011 Jun 30;11:157. PMID:21718486

[44] Are rice and spicy diet good for functional gastrointestinal disorders? Gonlachanvit S. J Neurogastroenterol Motil. 2010 Apr;16(2):131-8. PMID:20535343

[45] Studies with inulin-type fructans on intestinal infections, permeability, and inflammation. Guarner F. J Nutr. 2007 Nov;137(11 Suppl):2568S-2571S. PMID:17951504

[46] Influence of dietary fibers and whole grains on fecal mitrobiora during in vitro fermentation. Yang, J. 2012 http://digitalcommons.unl.edu/foodscidiss/24/

[47] Dietary fructooligosaccharides induce immunoregulation of intestinal IgA secretion by murine Peyer's patch cells. Hosono A, Ozawa A, Kato R, Ohnishi Y, Nakanishi Y, Kimura T, Nakamura R. Biosci Biotechnol Biochem. 2003 Apr;67(4):758-64. PMID:12784615

[48] Strategies to prevent or reduce allergic disease. Prescott S, Nowak-Węgrzyn A. Ann Nutr Metab. 2011;59 Suppl 1:28-42. PMID:22189254

[49] Probiotics and prebiotics in allergy prevention and treatment: future prospects. Grüber C. Expert Rev Clin Immunol. 2012 Jan;8(1):17-9. PMID:22149335

[50] Short-chain fatty acids and human colonic function: roles of resistant starch and nonstarch polysaccharides. Topping DL, Clifton PM. Physiol Rev. 2001 Jul;81(3):1031-64. PMID: 11427691

[51] Review article: the role of butyrate on colonic function. Hamer HM, Jonkers D, Venema K, et al. Aliment Pharmacol Ther. 2008 Jan 15;27(2):104-19.. PMID: 17973645

[52] Fructo-oligosaccharides enhance the mineral absorption and counteract the adverse effects of phytic acid in mice. Wang Y, Zeng T, Wang SE, Wang W, Wang Q, Yu HX. Nutrition. 2010 Mar;26(3):305-11. PMID:19665870

[53] Fructooligosaccharides suppress high-fat diet-induced fat accumulation in C57BL/6J mice. Nakamura Y, Natsume M, Yasuda A, et a;. Biofactors. 2011 Jun 14. PMID:21674638

[54] Prebiotic effects of oligosaccharides on selected vaginal lactobacilli and pathogenic microorganisms. Rousseau V, Lepargneur JP, Roques C, Remaud-Simeon M, Paul F. Anaerobe. 2005 Jun;11(3):145-53. PMID:16701545

[55] Randomized, double-blind, placebo-controlled study of oral lactobacilli to improve the vaginal flora of postmenopausal women. Petricevic L, Unger FM, Viernstein H, Kiss H. Eur J Obstet Gynecol Reprod Biol. 2008 Nov;141(1):54-7. PMID:18701205

[56] Intake of dietary fiber, especially from cereal foods, is associated with lower incidence of colon cancer in the HELGA cohort. Hansen L, Skeie G, Landberg R, et al. Int J Cancer. 2011 Aug 22. PMID:21866547

[57] Dietary fiber and whole-grain consumption in relation to colorectal cancer in the NIH-AARP Diet and Health Study. Schatzkin A, Mouw T, Park Y, Subar AF, Kipnis V, Hollenbeck A, Leitzmann MF, Thompson FE. Am J Clin Nutr. 2007 May;85(5):1353-60. PMID:17490973

[58] An apple a day may hold colorectal cancer at bay: recent evidence from a case-control study. Jedrychowski W, Maugeri U. Rev Environ Health. 2009 Jan-Mar;24(1):59-74. PMID:19476292

[59] Randomized, double-blinded, placebo-controlled study of effect of wheat bran fiber and calcium on fecal bile acids in patients with resected adenomatous colon polyps. Alberts DS, Ritenbaugh C, Story JA, Aickin et al. J Natl Cancer Inst. 1996 Jan 17;88(2):81-92. PMID:8537982

[60] Short-chain fatty acids and human colonic function: roles of resistant starch and nonstarch polysaccharides. Topping DL, Clifton PM. Physiol Rev. 2001 Jul;81(3):1031-64. PMID: 11427691

[61] Dietary fiber intake and risk of breast cancer in postmenopausal women: the National Institutes of Health-AARP Diet and Health Study. Park Y, Brinton LA, Subar AF, Hollenbeck A, Schatzkin A. Am J Clin Nutr. 2009 Sep;90(3):664-71. PMID:19625685

[62] Estimated enterolignans, lignan-rich foods, and fibre in relation to survival after postmenopausal breast cancer. Buck K, Zaineddin AK, Vrieling A, et al. Br J Cancer. 2011 Oct 11;105(8):1151-7. PMID:21915130

[63] Dietary factors and the risks of oesophageal adenocarcinoma and Barrett's oesophagus. Kubo A, Corley DA, Jensen CD, Kaur R. Nutr Res Rev. 2010 Dec;23(2):230-46. PMID:20624335

[64] Fecal bile acid concentrations in a subpopulation of the wheat bran fiber colon polyp trial. Alberts DS, Einspahr JG, Earnest DL, et al. Cancer Epidemiol Biomarkers Prev. 2003 Mar;12(3):197-200. PMID:12646507

[65] Correlation between the BANA test and oral malodor parameters. Kozlovsky A, Gordon D, Gelernter I, Loesche WJ, Rosenberg M. J Dent Res. 1994 May;73(5):1036-42. PMID:8006229

[66] Colon transit time in healthy children and adolescents. Velde SV, Notebaert A, Meersschaut V, et al. Int J Colorectal Dis. 2013 Dec;28(12):1721-4. PMID:23887805

[67] Epidemiology of slow and fast colonic transit using a scale of stool form in a community. Choung RS, Locke GR 3rd, Zinsmeister AR, et al. Aliment Pharmacol Ther. 2007 Oct 1;26(7):1043-50. PMID:17877511

[68] Defecation frequency and timing, and stool form in the general population: a prospective study. Heaton KW, Radvan J, Cripps H, et al. Gut. 1992 Jun;33(6):818-24. PMID:1624166

5. Meteorism, Trots, and Foul Winds

Sugar Malabsorption and its Consequences

One long weekend, back in the days when I was doing post-graduate work in nutritional epidemiology, I was invited with a friend to New Orleans for the St. Patrick's Day celebration. We caught a ride with one of her dorm buddies. The young woman was quite fetching, so I was well disposed to sit up front while she drove, and my friend slept in the back seat. My friend had told me that the girl had an unresolved medical problem and that I should see if I could help her. The girl was pretty, blond and svelte, with a sparkling personality and a great smile. This, of course, has little bearing on the story, but it did help engrave the trip into my memory.

When I first sat down, the young woman offered me a stick of gum. I thought that maybe my breath was off, so I took it. But it was really just that she was a smacker. She chewed gum constantly while we drove the 7-hour trip, frequently renewing her gum as we passed farms, forests towns and pit stops, and she told me about her life. When I mentioned that our friend asked me to talk to her about her health problem, she filled me in. She told me that she was planning to take a break from school. Her doctors had concluded that her health problems were caused by the stresses of her graduate program and had advised her to take a year off to see if that would help. She had been doing well in school and liked what she was doing, but she wanted to get better, so she was going to take their advice and put her health first.

She had had chronic diarrhea, abdominal pain, and bloating for over a year, and she had unintentionally lost over 15 pounds. She had been to multiple specialists, off and on-campus, which was at the time rated as the second best medical center in the United States. She had numerous lab tests, imaging studies as had upper and lower endoscopies with biopsies of her pancreas, duodenum, and colon. She had spent well over a year's wages trying to get a diagnosis without the doctors finding any cause for her problem.

I did not say much, and just lent a sympathetic ear. At the end of the journey, I thanked her for driving, and then told her the etiology of her condition and how to cure it. You might think that she would be pleased, but as often happens, she seemed vexed at me. How could I have figured it out without a single test or physical exam, when some of the best-qualified specialists in the country had not?! She had already made plans to leave her career program, and I was upsetting the apple cart.

It was not that I was so clever. Doctors usually make diagnoses in a few minutes, and I had plenty of time to contemplate a differential diagnosis. The other doctors had already ruled out metabolic, infectious, parasitic, inflammatory, and endocrine disorders. Moreover, I had the advantage of several hours of observation, something the other doctors had not. Plus, I had seen this condition before.

She just needed quit chewing gum.

It likely seemed a frivolous diagnosis, but she was suffering from sorbitol overload from her sugarless gum. In 2008, the British Medical Journal reported cases of severe diarrhea, bloating and weight loss from sorbitol-sweetened chewing gum[1]. One patient (similar to my traveling companion) was a 21-year-old woman who had diarrhea and abdominal pain for eight months, a 24-pound weight loss, and had fallen to a weight of about 90 pounds. She chewed about 15 sticks of gum a day. Another patient was a middle-aged man who had been hospitalized for chronic diarrhea and had an unexplained weight loss of 48 pounds over a year. He had been consuming about 30 grams of sorbitol a day through 20 sticks of gum and other sorbitol sweets. Both these individuals' problems resolved once off sorbitol.

Sugar Malabsorption Syndromes

Sorbitol is just one of several dietary carbohydrates which can cause disease conditions, some which can be incapacitating. Some very rare forms can be fatal. The problems occur, not from the toxicity of the carbohydrate, but from malabsorption and fermentation of these sugars in the gut. In contrast to the poorly absorbed oligo- and polysaccharides in our diets, most of the sugar (mono and disaccharides) we consume is well absorbed. Some sugars, especially in processed foods, are not, but these are generally present in limited amounts.

When sugars and small sugar complexes are not absorbed from the small intestine, they enter the large intestine where they are fermented by bacteria in the cecum and colon, producing carbon dioxide, hydrogen, and methane that can cause bloating, cramping, abdominal pain, and flatulence. These carbohydrates also decrease intestinal transit time and exert osmotic pressure, drawing water into the colon, causing diarrhea. Especially with chronic sugar malabsorption, other nutrients and bile enter the colon and are fermented, causing even more problems.

When the gas distends the belly so that it becomes drum-like and hollow sounding to percussion, it is colorfully referred to as meteorism, tympani, or tympanites. While these may represent a serious medical condition[*], most bloating and flatulence is caused by foods; these foods may also cause diarrhea. The most common cause of meteorism, bloating, and disturbing flatulence is malabsorption of sugars and other carbohydrates.

Sugar malabsorption often causes:

Nausea
Cramping
Flatulence
Loose, watery stools
Abdominal cramping pain
Bloating or abdominal distension
Poor weight gain or weight loss

Sugar malabsorption syndromes, Small Intestinal Bacterial Overgrowth (SIBO) and irritable bowel syndrome (IBS) have nearly identical symptoms[2]. Although these conditions may exist independently of each other, they very often overlap. Sugar malabsorption syndrome can impair pancreatic enzyme output (Chapter 8), support SIBO (Chapter 24), and contribute to IBS symptoms[3] (Chapter 26). Hydrogen breath tests (also in Chapter 24) may be useful to help differentiate these conditions sugar malabsorption from SIBO.

Normally it takes about five hours for food to reach the cecum after a meal. Sugar malabsorption can greatly decrease this time. In excess, unabsorbed sugars result in an osmotic load in the small intestine, inducing fluid secretion and preventing fluid absorption. This fluid load often results in rapid small intestinal transit of the chyme into the cecum. Fermentation in the colon results in the production of organic acids. These acids add to the osmotic load and pull water into the colon. This causes increased stool volume; the acids can stimulate intestinal motility, cause uncoordinated peristalsis, cramping pain, and diarrhea. There is also increased production of carbon dioxide, hydrogen, and other gasses; fueling bloating and flatulence. The rapid transit and acidic environment can lead to malabsorption of fat and other nutrients.

With SIBO, the first symptoms of carbohydrate intolerance (bloating and cramping) can occur within a half hour of ingestion because fermentation of the sugars occurs in the small intestine. Diarrhea may follow within minutes to hours. Fermentation in the small intestine may also increase the formation of secondary bile acids that further act as intestinal irritants. Rapid transit of the small intestines content also brings proteins into the large intestine where they ferment and can form ammonia and biogenic amines. Diarrhea caused by poorly absorbed sugars can be associated with loss of calcium and zinc into the stool and poor absorption of tryptophan[4], folic acid, and vitamins D and K. Sugar malabsorption syndrome promotes osteoporosis due to loss of vitamin K[5]. It can provoke Irritable Bowel Syndrome (IBS) and can cause depression[6]. Thus, malabsorption can cause secondary disease conditions and comorbidities.

The Folate Enterohepatic Cycle

Folic acid (Vitamin B_9) needs to be absorbed twice. First, it is absorbed as a mix of folate compounds from the diet. It is then converted in the liver to the active coenzyme forms, including 5-MTHF and excreted in the bile into the small intestine. There, it is again absorbed and distributed by the bloodstream to the rest of the body[7]. Folate is an essential cofactor for many enzymes including those required for the production of monoamine neurotransmitters. This may at least partially explain the high incidence of depression[8] associated with malabsorption syndromes.

Sugar malabsorption may also promote bile acid malabsorption through decreased small intestine transit time, worsen diarrhea, and promote the formation, through fermentation, of excessive secondary bile acids. These secondary bile acids may worsen Irritable Bowel Syndrome (IBS) and increase the risk of colon cancer.

Eating speed affects satiation and likely affects absorption. During a metabolic study, a test meal was eaten either over 5 minutes or 30 minutes. Polypeptide YY (PYY) and Glucagon-like peptide-1 (GPL-1) levels (see Chapter 2) were higher and lasted longer when a meal was eaten slowly. A relaxed pace of eating allows time for cholecystokinin (CCK) to close the gastroduodenal sphincter; this permits the stomach to retain food and give a sense of fullness. A leisurely meal provides a greater sense of fullness and relieves hunger better than the same meal consumed quickly. Insulin levels were found to be slightly higher, as were blood glucose, for meals eaten slowly[9]. This suggests that absorption is greater with a slowly eaten meal. When chyme arrives in the intestines in a large bolus, especially before CCK has an opportunity promote the release of pancreatic enzymes and bile acids, more nutrients are likely to reach the lower intestine undigested. This undigested food becomes fodder for intestinal bacteria. This mild malabsorption can promote intestinal gas formation, but can also increase the formation of bioactive amines and ammonia from bacterial fermentation of unabsorbed proteins and amino acids.

Beverage: In a study, subjects were given a meal in solid, semi-solid, or liquid form that was similar in palatability and macronutrient composition. Subjects were allowed to eat until they felt satisfied. The volunteers consumed about 15 percent more calories for the semi-liquid meal, and 30 percent more calories for the liquid meal, compared to the eating a solid meal[10]. In a different study, a test meal with the same nutritional and caloric content was given either as

---

[*] Tympani accompanied by unusually large, painful, bloating; high pitched tinkling bowel sounds; or a silent belly and lack of flatulence may be a sign of a severe condition requiring urgent medical care.

a liquid or a solid. When compared with the solid meal, the liquid meal gave less sense of fullness, lower blood sugar, lower insulin level and lower (des-acyl) ghrelin level[11]. Liquid meals stimulate less CCK release, are retained less time in the stomach, so the food passes into the intestines more quickly. Once in the small intestine these sugars stimulate rapid intestinal transport to the colon where they ferment, and these, along with other nutrients in the meal, are lost.

Consumption of caloric beverages can increase weight gain by circumventing appetite control. In individuals with sugar malabsorption, liquid forms are more likely to cause problems.

Major Dietary Sugars

There are four principal natural sugars present in fruit and fruit juices: sucrose, glucose, fructose, and sorbitol. Sucrose, a disaccharide, is made up of glucose and fructose. An additional sugar, lactose, is found in milk.

Table 5-1: Common Sugars in Foods

Sugar	Structure	Common Sources	Relative Sweetness
Glucose (Dextrose)	Glucose	Fruits, honey, corn syrup	0.74
Fructose (Levulose)	Fructose	Fruits, honey, corn syrup	1.73
Galactose	Galactose	From lactose	0.33
Lactose	Glucose + Galactose	Milk and milk products	0.16
Sucrose	Glucose + Fructose	Beet and cane sugars, molasses, maple syrup	1.0
Maltose	Glucose + Glucose	Malt products, from starch	0.33

During digestion in the small intestine, sucrose is split into glucose and fructose by brush border enzymes of the enterocytes: sucrose alpha-glucosidase and oligo-1, 6-glucosidase. Milk contains lactose; another disaccharide made up of glucose and galactose. Dietary starches are broken down by amylase into the disaccharides maltose and isomaltose, which are further cleaved into glucose. Sorbitol, a poorly absorbed sugar alcohol, is discussed later in this chapter.

Brush Border Enzyme-Related Malabsorption Syndromes

Lactose Intolerance

A common cause of meteorism and flatulence is lactose intolerance from the ingestion of milk or milk products. The enzyme lactase is usually present in the brush border of the intestine in children and other young mammals. Lactase cleaves milk sugar into glucose and galactose, which are transported into the cells and then into the bloodstream.

Table 5-2: Common Sugar Malabsorption Conditions

Sugar Malabsorption Conditions:	
Lactose Intolerance (Lactase-phlorizin hydrolase non-persistence)	Common; normal in almost all adult mammals. Affects 75% of adults worldwide, as many as 90% of African adults, and, in some areas, 100% of Asian adults. Universal in cats and dogs. Uncommon in some populations; as low as 2% in Denmark and the Punjab area of India. Congenital Lactose Deficiency is a rare disease of infancy. It causes colicky pain, meteorism, diarrhea, and malnutrition, and may be fatal.
Sucrose Intolerance (Congenital Oligo-1,6-glucosidase Deficiency; Sucrase-Isomaltase Deficiency	Rare, except among the Inupiat people of northwest Alaska. Also occurs as a secondary disorder from inflammatory damage of the mucosa of the small intestine. Isomaltose, a sugar made during the breakdown of certain starches, is "non-fermentable" (poorly fermentable), and thus does not produce gas. Isomaltose also has little osmotic effects.
Trehalase deficiency	This deficiency is rare in most areas but common among the population of Greenland (affecting about 10% of that population)[12]. It is uncommon as a primary (inherited) disorder in most populations, however; it often occurs in celiac disease. The sugar trehalose is also known as trechalose.
Fructose Malabsorption	Common; affecting about 30% of northern Europeans.
Hereditary Fructose Intolerance	A rare, potentially fatal, condition in which the liver enzymes that metabolize fructose are deficient.
Sorbitol Intolerance	Sorbitol is not well absorbed. Some individuals are intolerant to relatively small amounts of this sugar.
Other sugars	**Xylitol, Mannitol,** and other poorly absorbed sugars may be present in natural and processed foods.

There are three types of lactose intolerance:

- Congenital alactasia,
- Adult lactase non-persistence, and
- Secondary lactase deficiency.

Congenital alactasia is a rare condition inherited as an autosomal recessive condition. Babies with this condition have loose stools from the first days of life.

Adult lactase non-persistence: While most children digest lactose easily, this ability declines during childhood as lactase production declines, and by adulthood most adults lose most of this ability. This is usually referred to as Lactose Intolerance.

> Humans (some, not all) are the only adult mammal that produces sufficient lactase to be able to consume milk. It is only in the last 6000 years that a point mutation on chromosome 2 occurred, allowing lactase persistence into adulthood to become common in some human populations. This mutation persisted in populations whose survival depended on cattle, and for whom this mutation gave a survival advantage. These populations lived in climates favorable to cattle, reindeer, yaks, sheep or goat production and unfavorable to a year-round supply of other foods. These areas included northern Europe and some areas of North Africa and the Middle East, where nomadic herders could survive, and also an area in India.
>
> Lactose is made from and digested into glucose and galactose. Galactose is made from and converted back into glucose. The process of producing, packaging, absorbing and utilizing lactose involves numerous enzymes and at a considerable metabolic cost. Why add the complexity and risk, and not just put glucose into milk? Galactose stimulates growth in children. After bone growth ends, it is not needed. In areas where cattle carried disease, such as tuberculosis or brucellosis, which can be transmitted through milk, lactase persistence could be a disadvantage, endangering survival.
>
> Lactase *non-persistence* is the normal genetic phenotype. About 12 percent of European-Americans, 75 percent of African Americans and rural Mexicans, about 90 percent of Asian Americans, and nearly 100 percent of Native Americans have lactase non-persistence. Lactase-phlorizin hydrolase (LCT) non-persistence can be tested using genotype testing of the C/T-13910 LCT promoter region[13].

Many adults may not realize that they are lactose intolerant, but just avoid dairy products and the gastric discomfort and social embarrassment that can result from its consumption. Lactase activity is poorly inducible. This means that drinking milk will not increase the amount of lactase produced by the enterocytes. Bacterial fermentation of lactose, however, can be induced.

Adult lactase non-persistence generally allows consumption of limited amounts of lactose and dairy products without symptoms. Some lactase activity is preserved in all healthy adults as this enzyme also acts upon other substrates. Many adults with lactose intolerance may have symptoms with the consumption of 8 oz. of milk, which contains 12.3 grams of lactose, while others can consume this much with impunity, but will have symptoms when higher amounts are consumed[14]. Each individual has their own level of tolerance, and this can be affected by whether the milk is consumed with a meal or contains milk fat, which slows gastric emptying time. Thus, most lactose intolerant adults can consume a small amounts of milk with cereal, a scoop of ice cream, or milk in coffee without suffering gastric distress of excess flatulence. In normal adult lactose intolerance, it takes a minimum of 70 to 100 minutes for food to reach the cecum where fermentation begins. Symptoms are usually delayed for over an hour after consumption of the dairy product containing lactose. (See Chapter 24 on SIBO.)

Secondary lactose deficiency occurs, as a result of damage to the brush border and loss of enterocytes that produce lactase enzymes. This can cause a severe form of lactose intolerance even in children and lactase persistent adults. Here, a small amount of lactose can provoke cramping, meteorism, flatulence and diarrhea. Since lactase is often only marginally sufficient for the dietary load of lactose, secondary lactose deficiency is often the first enzyme deficiency to manifest, and one of the last disaccharidase to recover from brush border injury.

> One of the most common causes of diarrheal diseases in infants is rotavirus infection. In this condition, the stool is notably foul smelling. Rotavirus infects the enterocytes, thus, impairing brush border lactase activity and can cause secondary lactose intolerance in infected infants that can persist for weeks[15]. Sucrase (sucrase-isomaltase) activity can also be impaired, as a result of this infection[16]. Older children and adults can be infected with rotavirus, although protective immunity usually develops, and the disease is often asymptomatic.

New onset of lactose intolerance (other than the typical decline during childhood and adolescence) should be considered a sentinel event for epithelial injury in the small intestine. Damage to these cells allows access of partially digested proteins to immune cells that can then trigger the development of food allergies and antergies (Chapter 19).

Common causes of injury to the brush border cells are intestinal infections (viral or bacterial enteritis), parasites (*Giardia*), and immune reactions (gluten enteropathy or other food immunopathy). Recovery of damage to the enterocytes from infection allows recovery from lactose intolerance. Most patients with gluten enteropathy (GE) will develop secondary lactose intolerance if they eat wheat products, but many may be able to digest lactose again if they avoid gluten and recover a normal brush border.

Giardiasis

Parasitic infection with *Giardia* sometimes causes an abrupt onset of abdominal cramps, watery diarrhea, vomiting, foul flatus, and fever for a few days, before settling into a sub-acute disease. However, many infected persons only gradually develop symptoms. About 3 percent of those diagnosed with Irritable Bowel Syndrome (IBS) have *Giardia*.

In persistent *Giardia* disease, a person has greasy, foul-smelling stools that may fluctuate from diarrhea to constipation. GI symptoms include nausea, early satiety, bloating, substernal burning, sulfur breath, and acid indigestion. Weight loss is common. There is often a loss of appetite, malaise, and fatigue. Malabsorption may be accompanied by weight loss in adults; failure to thrive and growth retardation can occur in children.

Giardia can damage the intestinal epithelia leading to flattening of the villi, loss of intestinal brush border surface area, and loss of disaccharidase activity; causing lactose and other disaccharide intolerance; promoting the overgrowth of enteric bacterial flora[17]. Loss of other endothelial enzymes, such as diamine oxidase, which break down biogenic amines, may cause pseudoallergic reactions. The infection inhibits enterocyte barrier function[18], promoting increased absorption of allergens, immunoreactivity to foods, and mast cell infiltration[19]. Thus, giardiasis may provoke allergic manifestations such as bronchospasm (asthma), urticaria (hives), and erythema nodosum.

Testing: Lactose intolerance is often suspected from symptoms associated with consumption of milk or other dairy products. It is most commonly tested using hydrogen breath testing. (See Chapter 24: SIBO). An inexpensive method to test for lactose malabsorption is the failure of blood sugar to rise at least 20 mg/dL from a fasting blood glucose level within 30 minutes of a 25-gram oral test dose of lactose. Genotyping for C/T-13910 variants can also be done[20]; however, this will not diagnose secondary lactose intolerance from small intestinal endothelial damage.

Other sources of hidden lactose include prepared foods containing milk and milk products, including:

- Baked goods: cakes, cookies, biscuits, pancakes, waffles
- Cream soups
- Mashed potatoes, potato chips, snack foods
- Beverages: protein drinks, breakfast drinks, smoothies
- Non-dairy coffee creamer and whipped toppings
- Margarine and some salad dressings
- Filler in medications

Checking the ingredients on food labels is helpful in finding unexpected lactose in prepared foods. Any of the following words listed on a food label indicates that the product contains lactose: lactose, milk, whey, milk by-products, milk powder, and curds. Lactose is used as filler in some over-the-counter and prescription medications. Carefully read labels, especially for products used to treat stomach acid, as many of these contain lactose.

Management of Lactose Intolerance

1. Severe lactose intolerance should be investigated, especially after an acute, unexplained onset. If gluten enteropathy causes secondary lactose intolerance, gluten should be eliminated from the diet. Other causes of secondary lactose intolerance should be treated. Many individuals with gluten enteropathy will regain lactose tolerance with a gluten-free diet, but recovery often requires 6 to 12 months[21].

2. Lactose is contained in the whey component of milk; thus, hard cheese, made from the casein, does not usually cause symptoms of lactose intolerance. Soft cheeses; cottage cheese, cream cheese, and ricotta cheese; ice cream; and milk contain lactose. The lactose content of various dairy products is given in Table 5-3.

Table 5-3: Lactose content in some dairy products[22]:

Enfamil Ready to Feed	4 oz.	8.76 g
Low-fat milk; 1% milk fat	8 oz.	12.69
Whole milk 3.25% milk fat	8 oz.	12.83
Yogurt; unsweetened, whole milk	8 oz.	11.42
Ice cream	4 oz.	4.0
Dulce de Leche	100g	4.92
Cream, sour, cultured	100g	3.50
Cream cheese	100g	3.21
Cheese, cottage, low fat, 2%	100g	2.90
Cheese, Cheddar	100g	0.32
Cheese, mozzarella, whole milk	100g	0.07
Cheese, Swiss	100g	0.06
Butter	1 Tbsp	0.01

3. Adults may be able to rebuild some "tolerance" to lactose by slowly increasing and maintaining a daily intake of lactose. An individual can begin with a small amount of yogurt and increase from a spoonful to a serving over a couple of weeks. Then, they can try small amounts of milk or ice cream. If a person cannot tolerate even a couple of teaspoons of milk, there is likely a secondary problem in the gut causing the problem. Since lactase activity is poorly inducible, this increase in lactose "tolerance" most likely represents a promotion of commensal bacteria that help digest lactose.

4. Lactose in yogurt is better tolerated than lactose in milk. Although yogurt has considerable remaining lactose after it is cultured from milk, lactase, present in the living bacterial culture in yogurt, aids in the digestion of lactose. The lactose in yogurt produces about one-third as much hydrogen as the same amount of lactose in milk[23]. Frozen yogurt is not made from a live culture and does not provide this benefit. Lactase tablets (i.e., Lactaid) may be used when eating milk products, allowing lactose-intolerant individuals to enjoy milk products. Milk pre-treated with lactase may be tolerated. Lactase tablets do not allow persons with milk allergy to consume milk products safely.

Soy, rice, coconut or other vegetarian "milks" do not contain lactose, and may be a better choice for adults.

Note: Dairy is an important source of calcium in the diet. If lactose is being avoided, hard cheese may be tolerated. In the United States, milk is treated to provide vitamin D, and it can be an important source of this vitamin. Individuals who avoid milk need to be even more concerned to make sure they are getting sufficient vitamin D from sunlight exposure or supplements. See Chapter 20.

Fructose Malabsorption

About a third of the Caucasian population has some degree of fructose intolerance that can cause meteorism, flatulence, and diarrhea. Fructose is absorbed from the intestines in two ways. The first is facilitated transport associated with active glucose transport, and the second is passive transport by the fructose carrier, GLUT-5, on the cell membrane (Chapter 3). Thirty to forty percent of the population of central Europe has a low level of GLUT-5, and about half of these individuals get symptomatic fructose malabsorption[†]. Even for fructose-tolerant individuals, the amount of fructose that can be transported by this mechanism is limited to about 25 to 50 grams of fructose at one meal. About 80 percent of American adults have been found to have positive hydrogen breath tests, and 55 percent had symptomatic malabsorption with ingestion of 50 grams of fructose[24]. In another study, ingestion of 25 grams of fructose produced a positive hydrogen breath test in more than half of adults but did not give symptoms of bloating or abdominal distress[25]. Hydrogen from bacterial fermentation of sugars in the intestine gets absorbed into the blood and released in the exhaled breath from the lungs. A positive hydrogen breath test demonstrates that fermentation is occurring.

Fructose intolerance is a common cause of abdominal pain in children. In one trial of fructose intolerance in children with abdominal pain, 30 percent of those given 15 grams of fructose and 60 percent of those given 45 grams of fructose in a test meal had gastrointestinal symptoms and a positive hydrogen breath test[26]. Fructose has also been found to trigger worsening of IBS symptoms[27].

Sucrose, common table sugar, is a disaccharide made up of one molecule of glucose attached to one molecule of fructose. Brush border disaccharidases cleave sucrose into glucose and fructose. Since there is a one-to-one relationship, the glucose transporter GLUT-2 will transport a molecule of fructose into the cells along with each molecule of glucose, and thus, there is usually no fructose malabsorption. When fructose is not balanced by glucose, its absorption depends on passive, rather inefficient, absorption by GLUT5. When fructose exceeds the GLUT-5 capacity, it becomes fodder for bacteria in the gut. The bacteria readily consume it, producing carbon dioxide and hydrogen gas as a by-product, causing bloating and flatulence. In individuals with low GLUT-5 activity especially, fructose decreases intestinal transit time and pulls water into the intestine, and thus, diarrhea may result.

High fructose corn syrup used in soft drinks (HFCS-55) has about 40 percent glucose and 55 percent fructose (and about 5% oligosaccharides). Other forms of HFCS can have up to 90 percent fructose. This has many advantages for the food industry. Fructose has low water activity, which gives processed foods a long shelf life, by preventing microbial growth. Fructose also is sweeter than most other sugars and helps make low water content foods, such as cookies, softer. Additionally, it is less expensive to produce and to purchase than sucrose as a result of farm subsidies for corn.

High fructose-to-glucose containing foods, such as those with high fructose corn syrup, may thus cause symptoms in individuals with fructose malabsorption. A 16-ounce serving of soda pop has about 200 Calories (kcal) from corn syrup. That is equivalent to about 50 grams of HFCS-55 with 30 grams of fructose and 22 grams of glucose; there are 8 more grams of fructose than glucose. Alone, this may not cause problems, but serving sizes for soda pop are often larger and may be consumed with other foods containing fructose or other poorly absorbed sugars. This can result in malabsorption in individuals with fructose intolerance.

Fructose was obviously named after its main natural source: fruit. Table 5-6 gives the relative fructose to glucose content of various foods. Fruits with fructose to glucose ratio (FGR) greater than 1.0 have fructose in excess of glucose, and thus, are more likely to cause malabsorption problems. A simple test for fructose malabsorption can be performed by taking a test dose of 10 to 15 grams excess fructose as a tablespoon of agave nectar or drinking 12 ounces of natural apple juice. Many have tried this as an unwitting experiment with apple juice, and already are aware of the results.

Management of fructose malabsorption consists of avoiding dietary fructose, specifically when there is more fructose than glucose in a meal, and treating diseases that damage the brush border of the small intestine. When fructose is consumed with starch, the glucose made available from the digestion of starch helps with fructose absorption. Eating, rather than drinking fruit, allows improved absorption.

Sucrose Intolerance

Primary sucrose intolerance is rare, other than in the native populations of the Arctic. About 10 percent of the Inuit populations of Greenland and Canada have a congenital sucrase-isomaltase deficiency, causing sucrose intolerance. Symptoms usually first appear in sucrose-intolerant children if fruit juice is introduced into their diet.

The enzyme sucrase-isomaltase is also responsible for breaking isomaltose down into two glucose molecules. Isomaltose formed during the breakdown of starch is usually tolerated, as maltose only has about 10 to 20 percent of the osmotic activity of sucrose. Thus, less fluid is drawn into the intestine. Additionally, isomaltose is poorly fermentable.

Secondary sucrase deficiency can occur with injury or damage to the brush border of the small intestine and loss of sucrase-isomaltase activity, along with the loss of other enzyme activity.

[†] While fructose malabsorption is common, Hereditary Fructose Intolerance is a rare genetic condition, affecting about 1 in 10,000 persons, in which fructose must be avoided to prevent severe liver damage.

Sugar Alcohols

The sugar alcohols are hydrogenated sugars. Many occur in natural food, and they are also used as sweeteners in manufactured foods. The caloric effect of sugar alcohols is not the same as their caloric content. Since most sugar alcohols are poorly absorbed and may be poorly metabolized, the energy the body extracts from them is less than the combustion energy from their molecular bonds. Their energy is less efficiently captured than it is for glucose, fats, and most other foods.

Much of the energy from the sugar alcohols comes from the absorption of short-chain fatty acids (acetic, butyric, and capric acids) which are products during fermentation of these sugars by bacteria in the large intestine. The resulting fatty acids are absorbed by the colon and used by the colonocytes and other cells for energy. In general, most sugar alcohols provide about two Calories per gram; about half the caloric energy of other carbohydrates.

Most sugar alcohols, like sorbitol, can cause diarrhea and flatulence if consumed in excess. Sorbitol or xylitol excess may occasionally occur if large quantities of fruits containing them are consumed. Diarrhea and flatulence can also occur from consumption of sugar alcohols in manufactured foods, including sugarless (or "diabetic") cookies, candies, baked goods, and ice cream.

Sorbitol

Sorbitol is sweet-tasting alcohol sugar (a polyol) that is poorly absorbed by the intestine. Like many non-absorbed sugars, its presence has an osmotic effect, pulling water into the intestine, which can cause diarrhea. Consumption of large amounts of sorbitol can result in fermentation products, resulting in meteorism, flatulence, and abdominal pain, as well as an osmotic load, causing diarrhea.

Sorbitol is found in some fruits such as prunes (Table 5-5). It is for this reason that prunes and prune juice are used as laxatives. The FDA requires that sorbitol levels be labeled in foods if it is expected that 50 grams of sorbitol would be consumed in a day. A quantity of 50 grams of sorbitol is considered by the FDA to be the laxative threshold. One cup of dried, pitted prunes (132 grams) contains about 19.4 grams of sorbitol, a quantity that would send most adults to the restroom.

The Center for Science in the Public Interest has petitioned the FDA to change labeling on food, stating: "Numerous clinical studies show that the 50-gram threshold that triggers the label notice is too high, because susceptible adults can experience diarrhea and other symptoms at doses as low as 10 grams." They cite clinical research in which 70 percent of subjects had symptoms after only 10 grams of sorbitol ingestion.

Sorbitol is one of many small molecule fermentable carbohydrates that cause IBS. Combinations of various poorly absorbed sugars have been found to accentuate symptoms. When sorbitol was mixed with fructose, symptoms were accentuated[28].

The sugar alcohol erythritol is an exception, as it is well absorbed by the small intestine, but excreted by the kidneys, and thus, has a low caloric impact. Since it is absorbed, it does not cause diarrhea and is not subject to fermentation in the lower intestine as are most alcohol sugar sweeteners. Glycerol, which forms the backbone of triglycerides (dietary fats), is also, usually well absorbed.

Trehalose

Trehalose is a disaccharide made up of two glucose molecules joined by an α, α-1,1 glucoside bond. It is not a common dietary sugar, but it is the main blood sugar of flying insects. It is also found in most yeast and fungi. Trehalose is present in the diet in mushrooms, shrimp, lobsters, and sunflower seeds. It is the sugar that gives shrimp its mild sweet flavor. Trehalose is cleaved by the enzyme glycoside hydrolase.

Trehalose has a very cool property: it allows cells to dehydrate, and to rehydrate and come back to life. This is how sea monkeys can be dried out, shipped in envelopes, and then swim around when put in water. It also allows shitake mushrooms to rehydrate nicely after being dried.

Primary trehalase deficiency is very rare except in Greenland. In Europe, about 0.5 to 2% of the population is affected, and most of these are probably secondary trehalase deficiencies, usually resulting from gluten enteropathy. In many of these individuals, the deficiency of trehalase may resolve on a gluten-free diet.

PET WARNING

Xylitol is used as a sweetener, and dentists encourage its use as it decreases dental caries. Apparently, xylitol fools the bacteria into thinking it is food and starves the bacteria that cause dental caries.

Xylitol, however, is extremely toxic to dogs, with toxic effects occurring with 100 mg/kg of body weight. It can cause hypoglycemia-induced seizures and liver failure[29]. In dogs, xylitol causes the release of insulin from the pancreas. Drops in blood sugar occur within 30 minutes of ingestion[30]. As little as 1 gram, the amount in one piece of Epic chewing gum or in 2 Tic-Tacs, can poison a 22 pound dog. Ingestion of three grams of xylitol has been reported to kill a 65-pound dog.

Xylitol mostly occurs in the diet in artificially sweetened foods; however, it is a natural product present in certain foods, including strawberries and onions. Strawberries contain about 44 mg/100 grams, and onions contain about 13 mg/100 grams of fresh produce[31]. A pound of strawberries would thus contain only about 200 mg of xylitol. Xylitol toxicity in dogs is thus very unlikely to occur as a result of eating natural human foods.

Table 5-4: Sugar Alcohols in Foods

Sugar Alcohol	Structure	Common Dietary Sources	(Kcal) per gram	Sweetness compared to sucrose	Sweetness: calorie ratio to sucrose
Sorbitol (Glucitol)		Stone fruit, Sugarless gum, Sugarless candy and baked goods.	2.6	0.6	0.92
Xylitol		Berries, oats, plums Mushrooms, sugar-free gum, diabetic products.	2.4	1.0	1.67
Erythritol		Product of fermentation of glucose; used as an artificial sweetener.	0.213	0.812	15.25
Glycerol		From triglycerides	4.3	0.6	0.56
Isomalt		Beets, used in manufactured foods. Disaccharide composed of glucose and mannitol	2.0	0.5	1
Maltitol		Artificial Sweetener; disaccharide made by hydrogenation of maltose. Used in sugarless hard candies, chewing gum, baked goods, and ice cream.	2.1	0.9	1.71
Lactitol		Artificial Sweetener; disaccharide used in sugarless candy, ice cream, baked goods, and as a laxative.	2.0	0.4	0.80

> **Lactulose** is a synthetic disaccharide formed from fructose and galactose that is used as a medication. It is not digested and is used for the treatment of constipation and hepatic encephalopathy. It acts as an osmotic agent and is fermented in the lower intestines.

Management of Sugar Malabsorption

Sugar malabsorption is managed by limiting the dietary intake of the sugars which the patient does not absorb. Malabsorption of one sugar does not necessarily indicate that the patient has malabsorption of other sugars[32], especially if the problem is a primary intolerance.

Management of secondary sugar malabsorption, which has resulted from disease or injury, requires treatment of the underlying cause. Immune reactions to dietary proteins may damage the brush border of the enterocytes, as is the case in gluten enteropathy. Infections may also damage the enterocytes. With secondary sugar malabsorption, malabsorption of multiple sugars is more likely, as it results from loss of brush border surface area, accompanied by the diminution of several enzymes. Lactase is usually the enzyme most sensitive to damage as it is usually in short supply. Thus, it is usually the first deficit to be noticed and last to recover. Therefore, lactase intolerance may signal an underlying problem.

Sugar malabsorption can lead to rapid small intestinal transit and cecal fermentation of the sugars. Treatment with antibiotics can give temporary relief of the overgrowth, but the condition usually returns if sugars continue to enter the terminal ileum. By the time the chyme has reached the distal ileum, there should be little or no sugar left as a substrate for sugar fermenting bacteria.

Sugar malabsorption may also cause bile acid malabsorption through decreased small intestine transit time. This worsens diarrhea and results in the formation, through fermentation, of excessive secondary bile acids, which contribute to the symptoms of Irritable Bowel Syndrome, and may increase the risk of colon cancer.

Small intestinal bacterial overgrowth is discussed in Chapter 26, bile acid diarrhea in Chapter 26

Treatment of Sugar Malabsorption

1. Avoid consumption of poorly absorbed sugars. Avoid consuming food as a beverage, especially foods with sugars. There are fewer problems with eating fruit than drinking their juices.

2. Eat at a relaxed pace. Food should be eaten in a relaxed setting with sufficient time to eat and enjoy the meal, and allow time for CCK to slow gastric emptying. This is especially true for individuals with SIBO, poor digestion, borborygmi (noisy rumbling of the belly), or excess gas.

3. Remove foods from the diet that cause immune reactions which injure the intestinal mucosa, for example, wheat in patients with gluten enteropathy (See Chapters 19 and 22).

4. Whole milk may be better tolerated than skim milk as the fat may help slow gastric emptying, and provide a lower lactose load. Lactose may be less of a problem when part of a meal, for the same reasons. Lactose intolerance treatment is further discussed earlier in this chapter.

5. Treat infections, such as *Giardia*, that damage the intestinal mucosa.

> **Note:** In the past, The FODMAP diet was recommended for the treatment of inflammatory bowel disease and irritable bowel syndrome. It limited fermentable carbohydrates. FODMAP is an acronym for Fermentable Oligo-, Di- and Mono-saccharides and Polyols.
>
> These include:
> - fructose
> - lactose
> - polyols (sugar alcohols)
> - other sweeteners like polydextrose and isomalt
> - galacto-oligosaccharides (legumes & beans, Brussels sprouts, onions)
> - fructans (wheat, onions)
>
> Fructans and galacto-oligosaccharides are discussed in Chapter 4. Sugars that are poorly absorbed can act as osmotic agents and stimulate rapid intestinal transits, These should be avoided.
>
> Oligosaccharides and non-digestible fiber, however, are essential in the diet to maintain a healthful population of colonic bacteria. If these NDC cause digestive problems for an individual, they should be curtailed for a time, and then slowly reintroduced. Probiotics may be helpful. Commensal bacterial populations should adapt to the diet with time.
>
> Sugars that are poorly absorbed by an individual should not be reintroduced into the diet unless the malabsorption was secondary to a condition that has been treated successfully.

Table 5-5: Sorbitol Content of Foods:

Sorbitol content in grams/100 grams of fruit or juice[33]	
Dried Prunes	14.7
Prune Juice	6.1
Fresh Plums	2.7
Pear	2.1
Sweet Cherry	1.4
Peaches	0.9
Nectarines	0.6
Apricots	0.3
Apples (Winesap)	0.6
Apples (Golden Delicious)	0.2
Grapes (Black)	0.2
Grape (Red, white)	trace

Table 5-6: Fructose Loads in Various Foods:

Item	Serving	Grams glucose	Grams fructose	Excess Fructose	F:G ratio
Agave, cooked	100 grams	1.58	17.57	**15.99**	11.1
Agave Nectar	1 Tbsp.	1.14	12.65	**11.51**	11.0
Applesauce, unsweetened	1 cup	5.61	14.35	**8.74**	2.76
Apple Juice	8 oz	6.52	14.21	**7.69**	2.2
Sprite	12 oz.	11.55	19.15	**7.6**	1.7
Pear Juice	8 oz.	4.41	11.86	**7.45**	2.7
Apple, 3" diameter	1	4.42	10.74	**6.32**	2.4
Cola	12 oz.	16.94	22.45	**5.51**	1.3
Burger King Double Whopper, no Cheese	1	0	5.35	**5.35**	100%
Watermelon (about 1/16 melon)	280 grams	4.42	9.41	**4.99**	2.1
Baby food, apple and sweet potato	4 oz. jar	3.53	7.98	**4.45**	2.3
Baby food, apples and chicken	4 oz. jar	1.87	5.1	**3.23**	2.7
Wine, sweet, dessert	4 oz.	3.07	6.08	**3.01**	2.0
Chocolate power bar 2.4 oz.	2.4 oz.	8.12	10.85	**2.73**	1.3
Cinnamon Toast Crunch Cereal	1 cup	0.44	2.25	**1.81**	5.1
McDonald's Big Mac (without sauce)	1	1.92	3.48	**1.56**	1.8
Table Grapes	1 cup	10.87	12.28	**1.41**	1.1
Salad Dressing, Italian, Fat-free	3 Tbsp.	1.18	2.35	**1.17**	2.0
Honey	1 Tbsp.	7.51	8.6	**1.09**	1.1
Raisins (small box: 1.5 oz)	43 grams	11.93	12.76	**.83**	1.1
Raspberries	1 cup	3.16	3.95	**0.79**	1.3
Pineapple, Extra sweet variety	1 cup	2.81	3.55	**0.74**	1.3
Blackberries	150 grams	2.54	2.92	**0.38**	1.1
Orange Juice	1 cup	5.18	5.55	**0.37**	1.1
Green onion (tops)	1/2 cup	0.73	0.95	**0.22**	1.3
Gatorade (1 gram lactose)	16 oz	10.69	8.88	**-1.81**	0.8

Data from the USDA[22].

Table 5-7: Fruits without Sorbitol[3]

Strawberry	Raspberry	Lemons
Blackberry	Bananas	Limes
Cranberries	Figs	Dates
Raisins	Oranges	Pineapple

Table 5-8: Sorbitol in Sugar Free Foods

Sugar-Free Sorbitol-Sweetened Product	Serving Size	Sorbitol (grams per serving)
Hard Candies (Baskin Robbins)	17g (4 candies)	15 g
Chocolate Brownie Mix (Bernard Foods)	Two 5-square inch brownies	7g
Oatmeal Cookie Mix (Bernard Foods)	4 cookies	8g
Pancake Mix (Sweet 'N Low)	5 pancakes 3 inch diameter	9g
Low Calorie Strawberry Spread (Fifty 50)	1 Tsp. (17g)	3g
Lemon Sandwich Cookies (Murray)	3 cookies (28g)	6g
Wrigley Sugar-free Gum	1 stick	1.32g

---

[1] Severe weight loss caused by chewing gum. Bauditz et al. BMJ.2008; 336: 96-97

[2] Breath test for differential diagnosis between small intestinal bacterial overgrowth and irritable bowel disease: an observation on non-absorbable antibiotics. Esposito I, de Leone A, Di Gregorio G, Giaquinto S, de Magistris L, Ferrieri A, Riegler G. World J Gastroenterol. 2007 Dec 7;13(45):6016-21. PMID:18023092

[3] Self-reported milk intolerance in irritable bowel syndrome: what should we believe? Vernia P, Marinaro V, Argnani F, Di Camillo M, Caprilli R. Clin Nutr. 2004 Oct;23(5):996-1000. PMID:15380888

[4] Fructose malabsorption is associated with decreased plasma tryptophan. Ledochowski M, Widner B, Murr C, et al. Scand J Gastroenterol. 2001 Apr;36(4):367-71. PMID: 11336160

[5] Vitamin K2. Monograph. Altern Med Rev. 2009 Sep;14(3):284-93. PMID:19803553

[6] Fructose- and sorbitol-reduced diet improves mood and gastrointestinal disturbances in fructose malabsorbers. Ledochowski M, Widner B, Bair H, Probst T, Fuchs D. Scand J Gastroenterol. 2000 Oct;35(10):1048-52. PMID: 11099057

[7] 5-methyltetrahydrofolate. (Monograph) Altern Med Rev. 2006 Dec;11(4):330-7. PMID:17176169

[8] The methylation, neurotransmitter, and antioxidant connections between folate and depression. Miller AL. Altern Med Rev. 2008 Sep;13(3):216-26. PMID:18950248

[9] Eating slowly increases the postprandial response of the anorexigenic gut hormones, peptide YY and glucagon-like peptide-1. Kokkinos A, le Roux CW, Alexiadou K, et al. J Clin Endocrinol Metab. 2010 Jan;95(1):333-7. PMID:19875483

[10] The effect of viscosity on ad libitum food intake. Zijlstra N, Mars M, de Wijk RA, Westerterp-Plantenga MS, de Graaf C. Int J Obes (Lond). 2008 Apr;32(4):676-83. PMID:18071342

[11] Food form and portion size affect postprandial appetite sensations and hormonal responses in healthy, nonobese, older adults. Leidy HJ, Apolzan JW, Mattes RD, Campbell WW. Obesity (Silver Spring). 2010 Feb;18(2):293-9. PMID:19629055

[12] Activity of disaccharidases in arctic populations: evolutionary aspects disaccharidases in arctic populations. Kozlov A, Vershubsky G, Borinskaya S, Sokolova M, Nuvano V. J Physiol Anthropol Appl Human Sci. 2005 Jul;24(4):473-6.PMID: 16079601

[13] Correlation between lactose absorption and the C/T-13910 and G/A-22018 mutations of the lactase-phlorizin hydrolase (LCT) gene in adult-type hypolactasia. Bulhões AC, Goldani HA, Oliveira FS, Matte US, Mazzuca RB, Silveira TR. Braz J Med Biol Res. 2007 Nov;40(11):1441-6. PMID:17934640

[14] Hydrogen breath test for the diagnosis of lactose intolerance, is the routine sugar load the best one? Argnani F, Di Camillo M, Marinaro V, Foglietta T, Avallone V, Cannella C, Vernia P. World J Gastroenterol. 2008 Oct 28;14(40):6204-7. PMID:18985811

[15] An NSP4-dependant mechanism by which rotavirus impairs lactase enzymatic activity in brush border of human enterocyte-like Caco-2 cells. Beau I, Cotte-Laffitte J, Géniteau-Legendre M, Estes MK, Servin AL. Cell Microbiol. 2007 Sep;9(9):2254-66. Epub 2007 May 15. PMID: 17506819

[16] A cyclic AMP protein kinase A-dependent mechanism by which rotavirus impairs the expression and enzyme activity of brush border-associated sucrase-isomaltase in differentiated intestinal Caco-2 cells. Martin-Latil S, Cotte-Laffitte J, Beau I, et al. Cell Microbiol. 2004 Aug;6(8):719-31. PMID: 15236639

[17] Recent insights into the mucosal reactions associated with Giardia lamblia infections. Müller N, von Allmen N. Int J Parasitol. 2005 Nov;35(13):1339-47. Epub 2005 Aug 24. PMID:16182298

[18] Effect of chronic Giardia lamblia infection on epithelial transport and barrier function in human duodenum. Troeger H, Epple HJ, Schneider T, et al. Gut. 2007 Mar;56(3):328-35. PMID:16935925

[19] Mast cell hyperplasia and increased macromolecular uptake in an animal model of giardiasis. Hardin JA, Buret AG, Olson ME, Kimm MH, Gall DG. J Parasitol. 1997 Oct;83(5):908-12. PMID:9379297

[20] Frequency of lactose malabsorption among healthy southern and northern Indian populations by genetic analysis and lactose hydrogen breath and tolerance tests. Babu J, Kumar S, Babu P, Prasad JH, Ghoshal UC. Am J Clin Nutr. 2010 Jan;91(1):140-6. PMID:19889824

[21] Regression of lactose malabsorption in coeliac patients after receiving a gluten-free diet. Ojetti V, Gabrielli M, Migneco A, et al. Scand J Gastroenterol. 2008;43(2):174-7.PMID:17917999

[22] U.S. Department of Agriculture Nutrient Data Base, Nutrient Data Laboratory, Beltsville MD. Human Nutrition Research Center of the Agricultural Research Service, USDA.

[23] Yogurt--an autodigesting source of lactose. Kolars JC, Levitt MD, Aouji M, Savaiano DA. N Engl J Med. 1984 Jan 5;310(1):1-3. PMID: 6417539

[24] Ability of the normal human small intestine to absorb fructose: evaluation by breath testing. Rao SS, Attaluri A, Anderson L, Stumbo P. Clin Gastroenterol Hepatol. 2007 Aug;5(8):959-63.. PMID: 17625977

[25] Fructose intake at current levels in the United States may cause gastrointestinal distress in normal adults. Beyer PL, Caviar EM, McCallum RW. J Am Diet Assoc. 2005 Oct;105(10):1559-66. PMID:16183355

[26] Fructose intolerance in children presenting with abdominal pain. Gomara RE, Halata MS, Newman LJ, et al. J Pediatr Gastroenterol Nutr. 2008 Sep;47(3):303-8. PMID: 18728526

[27] Dietary triggers of abdominal symptoms in patients with irritable bowel syndrome: randomized placebo-controlled evidence. Shepherd SJ, Parker FC, Muir JG, Gibson PR. Clin Gastroenterol Hepatol. 2008 Jul;6(7):765-71. PMID: 18456565

[28] Malabsorption of Fructose-Sorbitol Mixtures Interactions Causing Abdominal Distress. J. J. Rumessen and E. Gudmand-Høyer. Scandinavian Journal of Gastroenterology 1987, Vol. 22, No. 4, Pages 431-436

[29] Acute hepatic failure and coagulopathy associated with xylitol ingestion in eight dogs. Dunayer EK, Gwaltney-Brant SM. J Am Vet Med Assoc. 2006 Oct 1;229(7):1113-7. PMID: 17014359

[30] Experimental acute toxicity of xylitol in dogs. Xia Z, He Y, Yu J. J Vet Pharmacol Ther. 2009 Oct;32(5):465-9. PMID:19754913

[31] Quantification of xylitol in foods by an indirect competitive immunoassay. Sreenath K, Venkatesh YP. J Agric Food Chem. 2010 Jan 27;58(2):1240-6. PMID:20030329

[32] Coincidental malabsorption of lactose, fructose, and sorbitol ingested at low doses is not common in normal adults. Ladas SD, Grammenos I, Tassios PS, Raptis SA. Dig Dis Sci. 2000 Dec;45(12):2357-62. PMID: 11258556

[33] Sources for sorbitol content of fruit: Quality Determination of Sugars, G. L. C. Separations of Derivatives; Kline, Davis, A., et al; Journal of AOAC, Vol. 53, No. 6, 1970, PP1198-1202

6. Fats: Essential to Health

I grew up in a town surrounded by farms. There were orchards and vineyards and cows grazing on wild oats in rolling green pastures, plenty of sunshine, room to roam, and giant, spreading oak trees providing shade on warm summer days. When I was in high school, my girl friend's father worked for a dairy that advertised that happy cows make better tasting milk. Unfortunately, there are now few cattle raised in this bucolic bliss, as, during the latter half of the 20th century, people and cattle became urbanized.

For a glimpse of a nightmarish and dysphoric future, look no further than a feedlot today. Most cattle in the U.S. live in crowded, squalid conditions, eat industrialized fast food, and get no exercise. In a typical feedlot operation, calves are brought in and fed a diet that is about 90% grain, (mostly corn) for about 140 days before being shipped off to slaughter for meat. During their time in the feedlot, they are kept confined; with less exercise, they gain weight faster and have more "marbled" (fatty) muscle.

These are not especially healthy animals. In fact, 70% of all antibiotics used in the United States are given to livestock as part of their feed. Without the antibiotics, they would not gain weight as fast, and most would not survive long enough to get to market. These animals are obese, and their flesh is high in saturated fats. One reason for the 140 days to slaughter is that if they are kept even a few weeks longer, even with all the antibiotics they are given, they get sick, cannot be sold, and would soon die.

> **Disclaimer:**
>
> I am not trying to compare cattle fed in feedlots to urbanized humans. Americans who consume the western diet do not get 90 percent of their calories from corn. No, they only get about 70% of their calories from corn.
>
> Posh! How could that possibly be?
>
> Calories come from carbon-hydrogen bonds in fats, carbohydrates, proteins and alcohol. Carbon comes from atmospheric carbon dioxide that is fixed during photosynthesis. Seventy percent of the carbon in the average American's body came from corn.
>
> Corn is used to feed farm animals: cows, pigs, chickens, turkeys, ducks and farmed fish. We eat meat, cheese, milk, butter and eggs. Almost all those calories started with corn fed to animals. We also eat sweets and ketchup and drink colas, all containing corn syrup as a sweetener or stabilizer. Corn oil is also used in preparing foods. The American diet is based on invisible corn that does not look anything like a vegetable (corn on the cob) and only slightly resembles grain (corn flakes, popcorn, corn chips, and cornstarch).
>
> Another 10 to 20 percent of the U.S. dietary carbon intake comes from another vegetable most Americans have never tasted in its natural form: soybeans, which are used mostly as animal feed, vegetable oil, shortening, and protein filler.

Food is inexpensive in the United States because of corn. A calf gets to market as beef in just five months while it takes several years to get grass-fed cattle to market. Grass-fed animals get exercise, are healthier and non-obese. Their meat has a much lower content of saturated fats and a higher percentage of n-3 polyunsaturated fats. Corn is very low in n-3 fats, and that is reflected in the cells of animals that consume it as the main staple of their diet.

Before the 20th century, meat was the major source of dietary fats and the major source of essential fatty acids in the diet. Since then, the ratio of n-6 to n-3 fats in the American diet has changed, mainly due to the way we feed our farm animals and the addition of vegetable oils to the diet. The consequences to our health have been profound.

Biochem 101

Dietary fats are tri-glycerides: three fatty acids chains connected to a three carbon glycerol molecule.

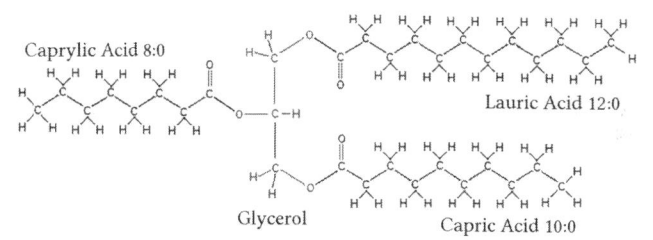

Figure 6-1: Triglyceride

The fatty acids are made up of chains of carbon molecules. Each carbon atom forms four bonds; each oxygen atom, two bonds; and each hydrogen atom, a single covalent bond to another atom. In the fatty acid chain, most carbon atoms hold onto a carbon on each side, leaving two bonds for two hydrogen atoms. If there are two hydrogen atoms for each carbon, this is a *saturated fatty acid* as shown Figure 6-2.

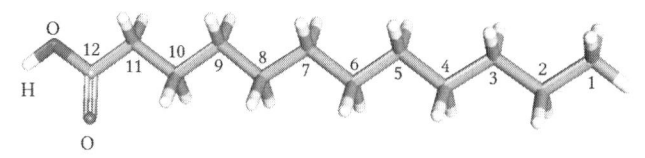

Figure 6-2: Lauric Acid. A 12 carbon saturated fat. White tips represent hydrogen and O: oxygen.

If there is at least one pair of carbon atoms where instead of a hydrogen atom there is a double carbon bond, it is an *unsaturated fatty acid* because not all the hydrogen positions are filled. This is illustrated in Figure 6-3.

Omega (ω) is the last letter of the Greek alphabet. The terms ω-3, ω-6, and ω-9 refer to the position of the first unsaturated carbon on a fatty acid chain. The terms n-3, n-6, and n-9 are also used to describe the position of the first unsaturated carbon atom. In Figure 6-3, two unsaturated bonds can be seen between the sixth and seventh carbon atoms, and between the ninth and tenth carbon atoms. Linoleic acid is thus an 18 carbon fatty acid, with 2 unsaturated bonds, with the first at the sixth carbon; this can be represented as 18:2 n-6.

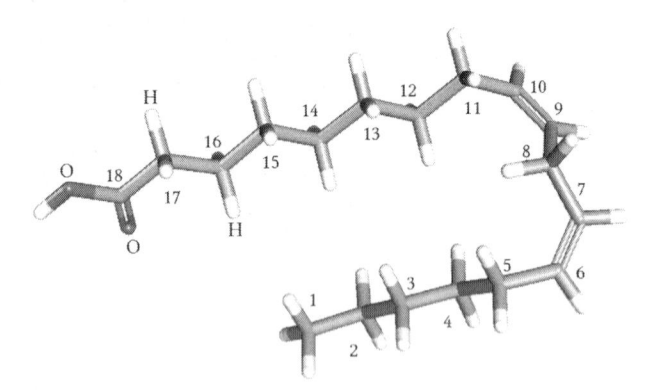

Figure 6-3: Linoleic Acid: 18:2 n-6

The unsaturated bonds cause bends in fatty acid molecules while saturated fats are straight. The straight molecules pack together better, and this gives a higher melting temperature. The longer the fatty acid chain and the more unsaturated the fatty acid is, the lower its melting temperature is. Butter and chocolate have mainly short chain saturated fats; they are solid at room temperature, but melt in your mouth at body temperature. Some animal fats (lard from sheep and cattle) are longer and mostly saturated. They melt at a temperature bit lower than chocolate does. Polyunsaturated fats are even longer and can be liquid even when refrigerated. Fish are cold-blooded animals, but can swim in very cold arctic waters because they have fat with very long unsaturated fatty acids which do not harden even at these near freezing, arctic temperatures.

Two fatty acids are referred to as essential fatty acids as animals are unable to synthesize them from other nutrients, and they are required in for health: linoleic acid (LA), an n-6 fatty acid (Figure 6-3), and α-linolenic acid (ALA), an n-3 fatty acid. Our bodies can transform these fatty acids into other polyunsaturated fatty acids required by the body. A third fatty acid, docosahexaenoic acid (DHA), should be considered as a semi-essential fatty acid because the conversion of DHA from eicosapentaenoic acid (EPA) is limited[1].

Table 6-1: n-3 and n-6 Fatty Acids

Fatty acid	Carbons in chain	Unsaturated bonds	1st double bond
Linoleic acid (LA)	18	2	6
Dihomo γ-linolenic acid (DGLA)	20	3	6
Arachidonic acid (AA)	20	4	6
α-Linolenic acid (ALA)	18	3	3
Eicosapentaenoic Acid (EPA)	20	5	3
Docosahexaenoic Acid (DHA)	22	6	3

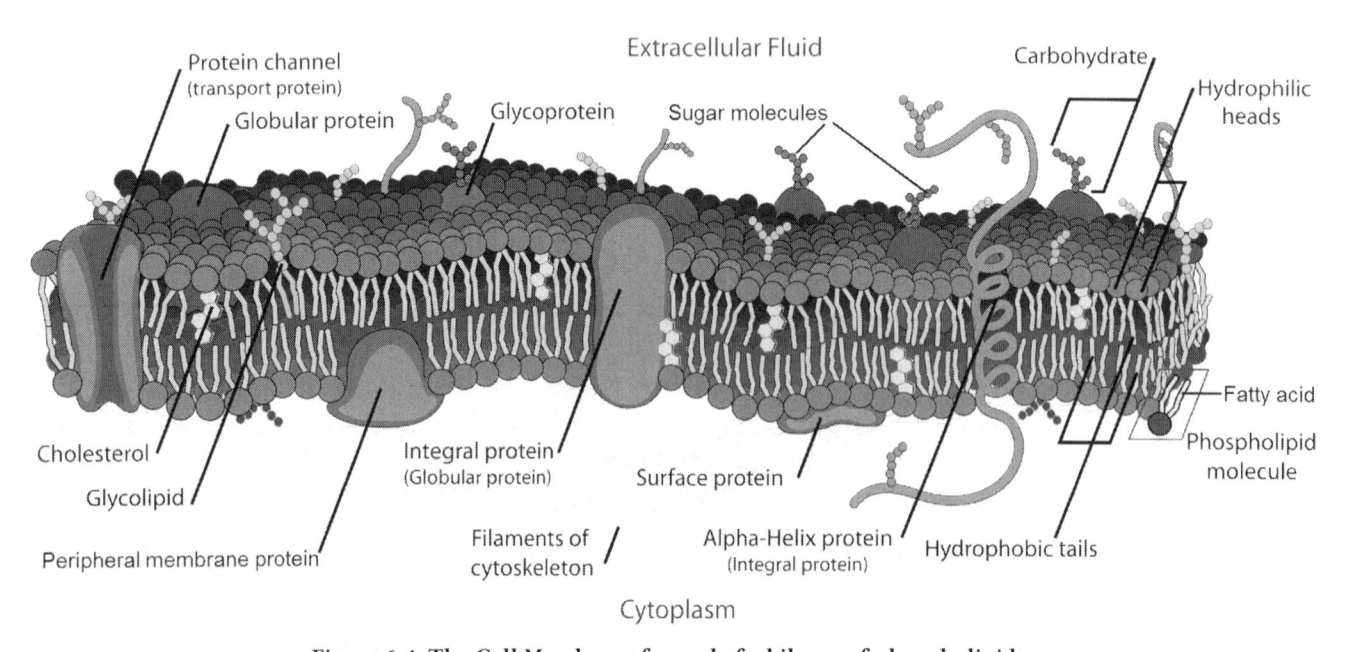

Figure 6-4: The Cell Membrane formed of a bilayer of phospholipids

Terrestrial plants mostly produce n-6 fatty acids, but also some n-3 and n-9 fatty acids, while aquatic plants produce predominantly n-3 fatty acids. These unsaturated fatty acids accumulate in the food chain. Thus, when cattle are fed plants with mostly n-6 fatty acids, such as found in corn and soy, their meat and fat will contain mostly n-6 fat. Corn has 45 times as much LA as ALA.

Fatty acids are stored as fat in adipocytes (fat cells) as triglycerides, for energy storage, insulation, and padding. However, the role of fatty acids is much more than fat. Fatty acids are also components of phospholipids. Most phospholipids are diacylglycerols; they contain phosphate, glycerol, and two fatty acids. Figure 6-4 illustrates the bilipid membrane which forms the cell membrane. On the left, a phospholipid molecule is shown illustrating the two hydrophobic, fatty acids attached to the hydrophilic phosphate head. The bulk of our cellular membranes is composed of phospholipids, and much of our brain's mass is phospholipids. Another phospholipid, sphingomyelin, which has only one fatty acid, makes up much of the insulation around nerves.

The fatty acids in phospholipids are not simply cell membrane components that impede movement of compounds in and out of the cell. These long-chain polyunsaturated fatty acids are used by the cells as a source of fatty acids for the production of eicosanoids: molecules that act as local hormones for nearby cells, and are essential signals in the control of inflammation and immune defense. The products of the polyunsaturated fatty acids are among the most potent immune modulators.

Eicosanoids are a group of compounds formed from 20-carbon essential fatty acids. They include prostaglandins, prostacyclin, leukotrienes, thromboxanes, isofurans, and resolvins. (Figure 6-6) These compounds are critical mediators of inflammation and immunity, and have potent effects on the central nervous system.

The two essential fatty acids, linoleic and α-linolenic acids, form two lines of eicosanoid products; in general, the products of the linoleic acid line; n-6 fatty acids, are proinflammatory and the products of the linolenic acid line; n-3 fatty acids, are mostly either anti-inflammatory or help to limit and resolve inflammatory processes. Inflammation from inflammatory prostaglandins triggers immune activity. Many of the diseases associated with a high n-6: n-3 ratio result from eicosanoid mediated inflammation or by oxidative damage caused by this activity.

The 20-carbon fatty acid made into an eicosanoid impacts which prostaglandin is formed and its resulting effects (Figure 6-5). Arachidonic acid (AA), the predominant 20-chain fatty acid, forms series-2 prostaglandins that are generally inflammatory, although they are also involved in the resolution of inflammation. Eicosapentaenoic acid (EPA), an n-3 fatty acid, forms series-3 prostaglandins that are anti-inflammatory. DGLA, formed from γ-linolenic acid, forms series-1 anti-inflammatory prostaglandins.

Table 6-2: Twenty-Carbon Eicosanoids

Eicosanoids	Main Actions
Prostaglandins	Multiple regulatory effects are mediated through several prostaglandins and at least 10 prostaglandin receptors. They affect smooth muscle, regulation of inflammation, calcium movement, cell growth, temperature control, affect blood flow and filtration in the kidney, and protection of the gastric mucosa.
Prostacyclins	Non-inflammatory vasodilator, antithrombotic; prevents intravascular clot formation. 6-keto $PGF_{1\alpha}$ is a weak vasodilator.
Thromboxanes	Vasoconstrictor, prothrombotic; facilitates platelet activation and aggregation.
Leukotrienes	Increase secretion of mucus, bronchoconstriction, inflammation, increased vascular permeability. Chemotaxis, white blood cell (WBC) aggregations, enzyme release from WBCs and mast cells, generation of superoxide in neutrophils. Stimulate antigen presentation and immune activation.

Eicosanoids are formed in cells after the release of 20-chain fatty acids from the cell's membrane inner surface phospholipids through the action of the enzyme phospholipase A2. Phospholipase A2, cyclooxygenase, and lipoxygenase are released under the influence of inflammatory mediators. Figure 6-6 diagrams the formation of several eicosanoids from arachidonic acid most of which are inflammatory in nature. Aspirin, naproxen, and similar anti-inflammatory medications act, in part, by blocking prostaglandin synthesis. Prostaglandins are designated as PG, the leukotrienes as LT and the thromboxanes as TX.

Diet and Eicosanoids

In the meat from grass-fed beef, the ratio of n-6 to n-3 fatty acids is about 3:2. In the meat from grain-fed beef from feedlots, the ratio of n-6 to n-3 fatty acids is about 15:2. Switching from grass to grain increases the availability of proinflammatory precursors of eicosanoids five-fold in the cattle and their meat. The typical Western human diet contains 11 to 30 times more n-6 than n-3 fatty acids[2].

The shift in the fatty acids composition of cell membranes to one composed with a high ratio of n-6 fats to n-3 fats provides a predominance of inflammatory precursors but supplies fewer precursors for eicosanoids that act in the resolution of inflammation. This is what has occurred as the diet has shifted over the last century. This shift is thought to go a long way in explaining the prevalence of many of the chronic diseases which plague our society. It has long been observed that Eskimos and Japanese, who have high consumption of the fatty acids EPA and DHA from seafood, have very low rates for coronary artery disease and lower rates of breast and colon cancers.

Figure 6-5: The Eicosanoid Pathway

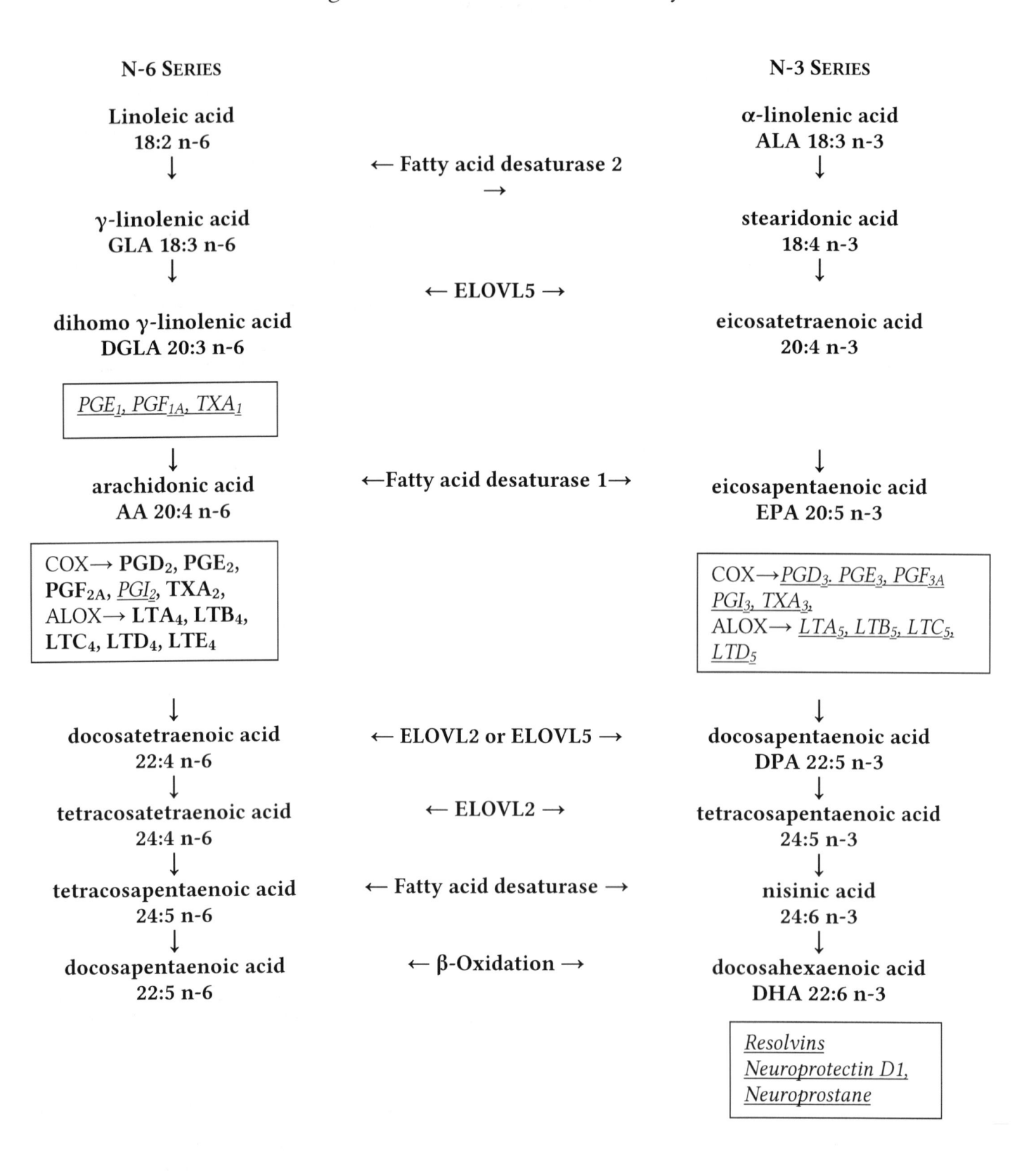

N-6 SERIES

Linoleic acid
18:2 n-6
↓

← Fatty acid desaturase 2 →

γ-linolenic acid
GLA 18:3 n-6
↓

← ELOVL5 →

dihomo γ-linolenic acid
DGLA 20:3 n-6

| _PGE$_1$, PGF$_{1A}$, TXA$_1$_ |

↓

arachidonic acid
AA 20:4 n-6

←Fatty acid desaturase 1→

| COX→ **PGD$_2$, PGE$_2$, PGF$_{2A}$,** _PGI$_2$_, **TXA$_2$,** ALOX→ **LTA$_4$, LTB$_4$, LTC$_4$, LTD$_4$, LTE$_4$** |

↓

docosatetraenoic acid
22:4 n-6
↓

← ELOVL2 or ELOVL5 →

tetracosatetraenoic acid
24:4 n-6
↓

← ELOVL2 →

tetracosapentaenoic acid
24:5 n-6
↓

← Fatty acid desaturase →

docosapentaenoic acid
22:5 n-6

← β-Oxidation →

N-3 SERIES

α-linolenic acid
ALA 18:3 n-3
↓

stearidonic acid
18:4 n-3
↓

eicosatetraenoic acid
20:4 n-3
↓

eicosapentaenoic acid
EPA 20:5 n-3

| COX→_PGD$_3$. PGE$_3$, PGF$_{3A}$ PGI$_3$, TXA$_3$,_ ALOX→ _LTA$_5$, LTB$_5$, LTC$_5$, LTD$_5$_ |

↓

docosapentaenoic acid
DPA 22:5 n-3
↓

tetracosapentaenoic acid
24:5 n-3
↓

nisinic acid
24:6 n-3
↓

docosahexaenoic acid
DHA 22:6 n-3

| _Resolvins_
Neuroprotectin D1,
Neuroprostane |

Key for Eicosanoids:
BOLD: Inflammatory
UNDERLINED   _ITALICS:_
antiinflammatory

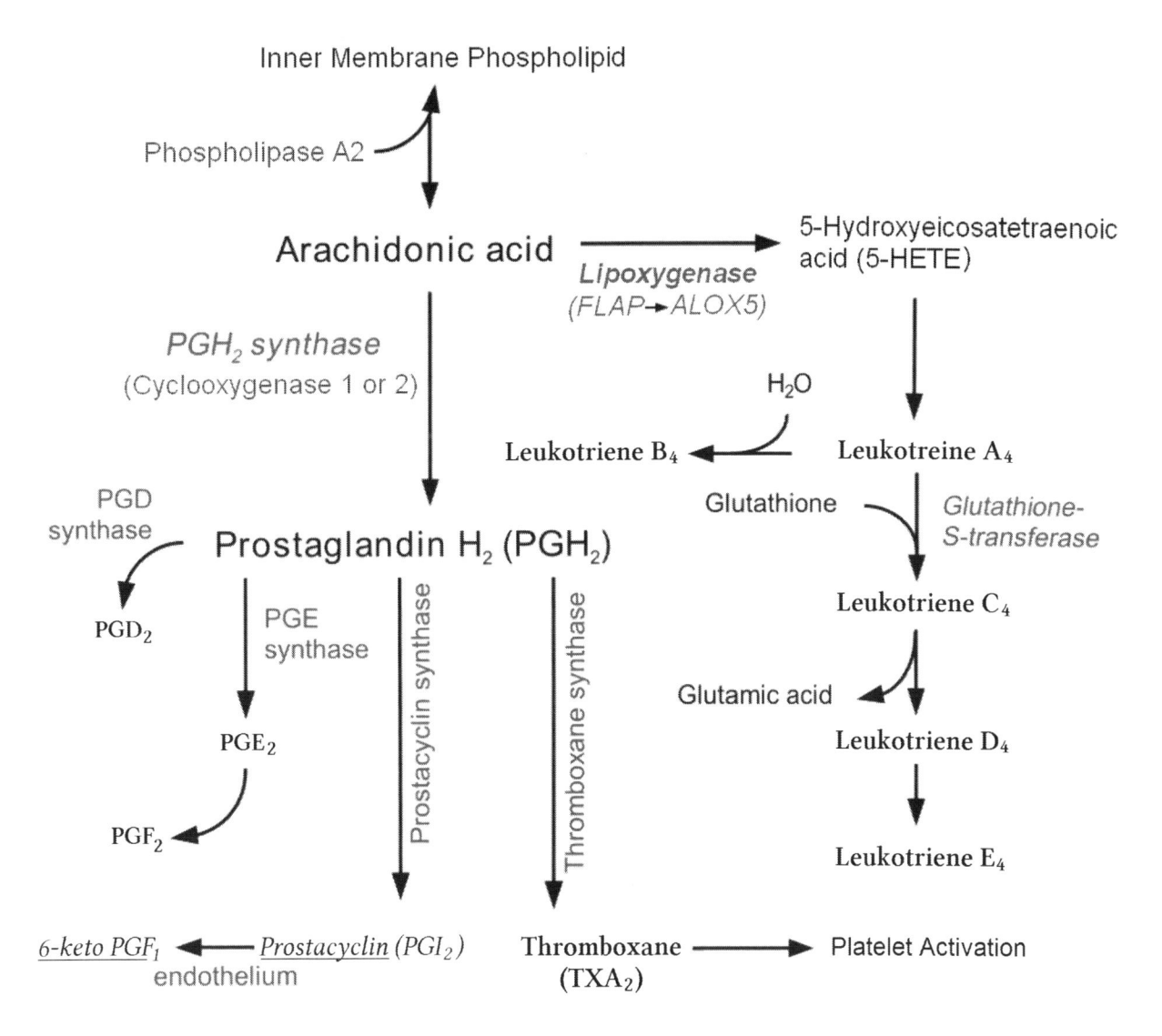

Figure 6-6: Arachidonic Acid Eicosanoid Biosynthesis
Underlined eicosanoids are antiinflammatory

Arachidonic acid (AA), EPA and DHA are constituents of the phospholipids which constitute much of the cell membrane mass. When these fatty acids are released from membrane phospholipids by the enzyme phospholipase A2, the EPA and DHA compete with AA for processing by the enzyme cyclooxygenase, a second step in the conversion of fatty acids to prostaglandins, thromboxanes and leukotrienes.

As an example, AA can be converted to thromboxane$_{A2}$, which activates platelets and clot formation; while the EPA produces thromboxane$_{A3}$, which is inactive, or at least much less active. Additionally, DHA (but not EPA) helps to stabilize myocardial mitochondrial membranes[3], and thus, to lower risk of cardiac dysrhythmias.

Although DHA may be directly converted through β-oxidation of nisinic acid in some animals, this has not been shown to occur in humans. In man, DHA production occurs through the "Sprecher's shunt," wherein EPA (20:5 n-3) is converted by elongase (EVOVL5) to form 22:5 n-3, and again to 24:5 n-3. (Figure 6-5) This fatty acid is then desaturated to 24:6 n-3 and then shortened to DHA (22:6 n-3) through beta-oxidation[4]. The enzyme "delta-4-desaturase," previously thought to convert EPA to DHA, does not appear to be an active enzyme in humans.

DHA is especially abundant in the cerebral cortex, sperm, and retinal tissue[5]. Low levels of dietary DHA have been associated with cerebral dysfunction and infertility.

N-3 deficiencies in lab animals provoke anxiety-like behavior that can be reversed by restoring DHA to the diet. Some deficiencies, however, do not respond. Infant animals with DHA deficiencies during lactation suffer irreversible damage to specific brain functions, including some related to dopaminergic function[6]. This may result in lifelong impacts, affecting reward-seeking behavior and impulsivity. DHA helps prevent inappropriate methylation of DNA[7], which can impact gene expression (Chapter 30).

DHA appears to reduce neuronal excitability, likely through the action of neuroprotectin D1 (NPD1), formed from DHA[8]. DHA may be helpful for migraine, seizures, anxiety, and aggressive behavior. It has been clinically demonstrated to be helpful for bipolar disorder and learning disabilities[9]. This effect may in part be secondary to the beneficial effect of DHA on sleep[10, 11]. Neuroprotectin D1 also protects human retinal pigment epithelial cells from oxidative stress and apoptosis[12], and may thus protect against macular degeneration and neuronal loss.

N-3 fatty acids (abundant in fish oils) tend to suppress T helper cell (T_H) activity and reduce T_H1 cytokine production, favoring T_H2 activity[13]. Generally, T_H1 cells help the body eliminate viruses and some bacteria; while T_H2 activity is directed at protecting the body from extracellular bacteria and parasites. (See Chapter 10.)

Table 6-3: N6: N3 Ratio Association with Disease

Elevated n6:n3 Ratio	Disease Association
AA: EPA	Positive association with Depression
AA: DHA	Positive association with Neuroticism
N-6:N-3 > 4.5:1	Increased risk of Coronary Artery[14]
AA:(EPA+DHA) > 1.4:2	Increased risk of Coronary Artery
N6: DHA	Positive association with Alzheimer's disease[15]
EPA: AA	Inhibits platelet aggregation[15]

Limitations of Supplementation

There is abundant epidemiologic data demonstrating increased disease risk associated with diets with high n-6: n-3 ratios, with high AA: EPA-DHA ratios and lack of certain n-3 fatty acids in the diet. There are supporting studies that correlate the amounts of these fatty acids in the tissues with disease. Yet, the numerous clinical trials using ALA or EPA/DHA supplements to prevent disease have demonstrated only limited clinical efficacy[16].

For example, fish oil does reduce heart disease death, but only by about 13 percent; mainly by preventing arrhythmia-associated deaths[17]. The levels of fish oil supplement needed for prevention of arrhythmias (about 1.5 grams/day) appears to be lower than that required to prevent inflammation (2 – 4 grams/day)[18], and ALA supplements are not helpful in the prevention of heart disease[19]. Adding supplemental EPA and DHA may help some as it decreases the conversion of LA to AA at high doses, and thus, reduces the formation of inflammatory eicosanoids. Aspirin Induced Asthma has been successfully treated with EPA/DHA supplements but requires 10 grams of fish oil a day[20] (Chapter 15). Disease treatment and prevention with EPA/DHA works, but it takes high doses to overcome the effect of excess LA in the diet.

ALA is not as avidly converted into the longer chain fatty acids as is LA, and thus, in the presence of excessive LA, more AA and less EPA is formed in the cell membrane phospholipids. The reason that adding n-3 fatty acids has been less effective than hoped in clinical trials for disease prevention is that, for many inflammatory conditions (such as listed in Table 6-4), it is not a deficiency of these essential fatty acids which need to be corrected, but rather there is excessive LA in the diet. For success in disease prevention, it is not just the ratio of n-6 to n-3 fats that needs to be modified, but also the total amount of n-6 and n-3 fats in the diet. This requires not just taking fish oil capsules, but actually changing the diet and limiting the intake of LA, the precursor of inflammatory eicosanoids.

Table 6-4: Diseases Associated with High N-6 Fatty Acid Levels

Disease	Chapter
Rage[21]	36
Bipolar disorder and major depression[9, 22]	31
Coronary artery disease[14]	9
Asthma	15
Alzheimer's disease[15] Parkinson's disease	31
Rheumatoid arthritis	33
Chronic headache[23]	28
Epilepsy[7]	
Obesity	9
Sleep disorders[9]	43
Neuro-oxidative stress[11]	30 - 31
Learning disorders[10] Anxiety	
Acne vulgaris[24]	37
Cancer	41

Improving the Diet

LA (Figure 6-2) is a precursor for AA; the main fatty acid for forming inflammatory eicosanoids. The amount of LA in the diet required for AA production is low, and the activity of the enzyme Fatty Acid Desaturase-2 appears to be easily saturated. Thus, when dietary consumption of LA is high, ALA is not efficiently converted to EPA[25]. Adding additional ALA to a diet high in LA does not help as the enzymes are already occupied. Using ALA supplements to increase an LA to ALA ratio, thus, does not provide benefit[26]. To augment the formation of n-3 eicosanoid precursors, the amount of LA in the diet must be limited at the same time as sufficient ALA is supplied. This does not occur while eating the standard Western diet.

Although the metabolic pathways exist, the amount EPA converted to DHA is inconsequential for much of the population. In fact, it is more common for dietary DHA to be converted to EPA[27]. Thus, DHA should be considered a nutritional requirement.

Some EPA is converted to DHA in women under the influence of reproductive hormones. DHA is essential for fetal brain and infant development, and DHA is present breast milk. Female hormones also decrease the conversion of DHA to EPA. Most natural food sources of EPA also contain DHA. In studies of depression, only fish oil supplements with an EPA to DHA ratio of 1.5:1 (60%:40%) or above were helpful[5]. An EPA: DHA ratio of 2:1 or greater is a desirable goal.

DHA appears to help prevent arrhythmias and epilepsy[28]; while EPA has more effect on lowering inflammation. EPA helps in depression; while DHA does not[29]. DHA is a component of cellular membranes in the mitochondria and neurons, and it influences signaling events in the neuron essential to nerve cell differentiation and survival[30]. Both EPA and DHA prevent the formation of AA, and thus, prevent excessive inflammation. ALA only minimally decreases AA levels. Additionally, DHA stimulates the formation of PPARγ, which down-regulates the production of inflammatory cytokines and immune growth factors (see Chapter 31).

The typical adult Japanese diet has about 25 percent of its caloric intake as fats but still confers a lower risk for inflammatory and heart disease than the American diet. A typical, Japanese, 2000-calorie diet contains about 10.9 grams of LA, 1.8 grams of ALA, and about 1.2 grams of EPA and DHA combined[31]. The major difference in fat intake between the Japanese diet and the Western diet is that the Japanese diet contains about five times as much EPA and DHA as the American diet because Japanese consume large quantities of fish.

A pure terrestrial plant vegan diet contains very limited amounts of EPA or DHA. Additionally, a high LA-content vegan diet would be healthy as it would prevent the conversion of ALA to EPA. For a vegetarian diet, LA intake should probably be limited to less than 5 grams per day, with at least 3 grams of ALA.

The amount of DHA that can be absorbed from the diet appears to be limited[32]. With a DHA supplement alone, plasma levels rise quickly with doses up to 2 grams of DHA a day, but plateau after about 3 grams a day. Using a combined EPA/DHA source raises EPA more than DHA and limits DHA absorption. This is usually desirable, as less DHA than EPA is required. Both EPA and DHA lower AA levels.

After raising the dietary intake of DHA and EPA, it takes time to get these fats incorporated into the cell membranes as phospholipids. It takes about 30 days for myocardial phospholipid DHA to reach their new steady state levels and greater than 60 days for EPA to do so. DHA may react more quickly, as it is incorporated into mitochondrial membranes, which have a faster metabolic turnover than cell membranes. AA levels in cell membrane phospholipids fall with increased consumption of DHA and EPA and reach a new steady state in around 60 days[33].

Food Sources of ALA

The Omega-3 fatty acid ALA is present in flaxseed oil, walnuts, soybeans, wheat and in low erucic acid rapeseed oil (Canola oil), whereas omega-6 fatty acids predominate in corn, sunflower, safflower and sesame seed oils.

Choices are limited when trying to increase ALA intake while maintaining limiting LA intake using commercial vegetable oils. An ideal oil for culinary use would give an n-3:n-6 ratio of greater than 0.5 to help balance fats in other foods, but as can be seen in Table 6-5, there are few good candidate oils.

Table 6-5: N-3 to N-6 Ratios of Various Dietary Fats

100g of Fat	LA Grams	ALA Grams	n3:n6 Ratio	Trans fat Grams
Flaxseed oil	12.7	53.3	4.2	
Butter	1.244	0.802	.64	
Canola oil	18.64	9.137	.49	0.395
Walnut oil	52.9	10.4	.20	
Soybean oil	50.418	6.789	.135	0.533
SDA Soy oil*	15 – 30	9 – 12	1.0	
Wheat germ oil	54.8	6.9	.126	
Olive oil	9.762	0.761	.078	
Avocado oil	12.53	0.975	.078	
Palm oil	9.1	0.2	0.22	
Corn oil	53.23	1.161	.022	0.286
Sesame seed oil	41.3	0.3	.007	
Almond oil	17.4	0	0	
Apricot oil	29.3	0	0	
Coconut oil	1.8	0	0	
Palm kernel oil	1.6	0	0	
Peanut oil	32	0	0	
Safflower oil	14.35	0	0	
Sunflower oil	65.7	0	0	
Animal Fats				
Sheep Tallow†	5.5	2.3	.42	
Cattle Tallow†	3.1	0.6	.19	
Lard (Pork)†	10.2	1.0	0.1	

Data from the U.S.D.A.[34] *Genetically modified SDA soy oil. See below for discussion. †: Solid at room temperature.

Flaxseed oil is used as an ALA supplement but is quickly oxidized even when refrigerated, making it a poor choice. Walnuts and pecans can be eaten, but walnut oil, too, is rapidly oxidized. Dairy cows are usually raised with at least some grass, so butter still has a good n-6:n-3 ratio; nevertheless, butter is composed mainly of shorter chain saturated fats, and thus, provides only small amounts of ALA. The n-6:n-3 ratio of lard and tallow reflect its source from the animals and their diet. The ratio may be worse than shown in USDA data if the lard comes from feedlot animals. Sheep are still usually raised, grazing on open land, and their meat, thus, has a more natural n-6: n-3 ratio.

Canola oil is the only grocery store shelf oil with a low n6:n3 ratio. However, it contains trans fatty acids, probably as a result of the high-temperature refining process. Soybean and corn oil also contain trans fatty acids (see Table 6-5) created during processing. When possible, cold-pressed oils are preferred, and should be kept refrigerated to prevent oxidation and rancidity. It would appear that refined vegetable oils are not what nature intended for our diet. Appendix I describes the production of soy oil.

The U.S. FDA has given genetically modified stearidonic acid enriched (SDA) soy oil GRAS (generally recognized as safe) status. At the time of this writing, however, it has not yet cleared by the US Department of Agriculture for planting, and SDA soy oil is not yet available on the market. Two genes, Δ6-desaturase from a primrose plant and Δ15-desaturase from the bread mold *Neurospora crassa*, have been transplanted into soybeans. This allows these soy plants to produce higher amounts of α-linolenic acid, and to produce γ-linolenic acid and stearidonic acid[35]. Consumption of SDA soy oil increases the amount of eicosapentaenoic acid in the red blood cells in human volunteers[36], and thus, may provide some health benefits similar to fish oil.

Food Sources of DHA

There are tiny amounts of DHA in poultry and eggs, but none in beef or pork[34]. Unlike humans, cows do not have DHA in their milk. For this reason, DHA has been added to infant formula. Terrestrial plants do not contain DHA.

Fish get EPA and DHA from eating algae. Vegans require dietary DHA, and algae are the only vegan source available. Not only microalgae, but also seaweed, such as kelp, wakame, and laver contain DHA and EPA. In fish, the richest sources of DHA and EPA are the muscle cell membranes.

Table 6-6: EPA and DHA Content of Various Fish[37]

Fish	Milligrams of EPA+DHA per Ounce	Ounces of Fish to get 1 gram of EPA+DHA	Mercury per 1000 mg EPA+DHA
Salmon	608.3	1.6	0.005
Herring	595	1.68	0.002
Sardines	274	3.7	0.004
Tuna: canned, light	244.3	4.1	0.164
Tuna: canned albacore	244.3	4.1	0.477
Flatfish	166	6.0	0.100
Pollock	153.3	6.5	0.130
Flounder	142	7.0	0.117
Shrimp	89	11.2	Not detected
Clams	80.3	12.4	Not detected
Haddock	67.7	14.8	0.148
Catfish	50.3	19.9	0.331
Cod	44.7	22.4	0.821

The n-3 fatty acid distribution in fish depends on what they have eaten. Since many of the fish we eat are predators, their fatty acid content depends on the fish they eat. Big fish eat smaller fish that eat zooplankton that consume phytoplankton and algae. The fatty acid content of fish depends upon where they feed, the type of algae they eat, and the time of year. Different algae have different amounts and ratios of fatty acids. Algae can have extremely different EPA: DHA ratios. For example, the algae *Skeltonema costatum* has 41 percent of its fatty acids as EPA and 7 percent as DHA; while *Thraustochytrium aureum* has 52 percent of its fatty acids as DHA and almost no EPA[38].

The fish with the most EPA per serving are herring, shad, salmon, mackerel, sardines, whitefish and oysters. These fish also contain a favorable EPA: DHA ratio. These fish have high amounts of EPA while being low in mercury.

The Mercury Hazard

Animals with large brains, and especially children and females who are pregnant or breastfeeding, or who plan to become pregnant, should avoid mercury in food. Mercury is a neurotoxin that is especially dangerous to developing fetuses and to young children.

Big fish eating little fish also concentrates some toxins. Shark, swordfish, king mackerel and tilefish are top predators and have very high levels of mercury in their flesh. Consumption of these fish should be avoided. Table 6-6 lists how much fish needs to be consumed to get one gram of EPA and DHA combined, and the mercury content associated with this amount of n-3 fatty acid.

Albacore, catfish, and cod should be avoided as a source of DHA because of the mercury content of these fish. Salmon is a great source of these fats and is low in mercury. Shrimp and clams do not have significant amounts of mercury; however, they are not especially rich in DHA and EPA. It requires eating 12 ounces of shrimp to get the same amount of DHA as found in two ounces of salmon. Light tuna is a better choice than albacore, as the level of mercury is much lower. Farmed salmon may contain high amounts of toxic polychlorinated biphenyls (PCBs).

The location where the fish feed determines the mercury content in the fish. Winds usually carry mercury in air pollution eastward from coal-burning power plants; the fallout deposits from dust and rain. High levels of mercury deposition along the Gulf coast of the U.S. reflect poorly regulated coal-powered electrical plants in Texas and other southern states as well as the high rainfall levels in this region. New mercury deposition has been reduced considerably in most of North America, especially in the northeast, over the last 20 years, as a result of legislative control of mercury pollution. Mercury, however, is cumulative in the environment, as it is in the body, and each year levels rise in the soil and in lake and river bottoms with this deposition.

China produces about half of the global atmospheric mercury pollution and North America about 6 percent of it. Almost half of the mercury that enters the atmosphere comes from fossil fuels used for heating and electricity (mostly from coal). Another 24 percent of the mercury results from gold mining and production and ten percent from other metal production. Cement production adds about 10 percent, and 6.5 percent comes from burning garbage. Ashes to ashes and dust to dust; cremation of our dearly departed accounts for 1.3 percent of global atmospheric mercury emissions; produced by incineration of teeth with mercury amalgam dental fillings[39].

Table 6-7: Mercury Content Levels of Various Fish

Least Mercury < 0.09 ppm Safe to Eat	Moderate Mercury 0.09 to 0.29 ppm O.K. to eat Occasionally	High Mercury 0.3 to 0.49 ppm Eat Rarely	Highest Mercury >0.5 ppm AVOID
Anchovies Butterfish Catfish Clam Crab (Domestic) Crawfish Crayfish Croaker (Atlantic) Flounder* Haddock (Atlantic)* Hake Herring Mackerel (N. Atlantic, Chub) Mullet Oyster Perch (Ocean) Plaice Pollock Salmon-Canned Salmon (Fresh) Sardine Scallop* Shad (American) Shrimp* Sole (Pacific) Squid (Calamari) Tilapia Trout Whitefish Whiting	Bass (Striped, Black) Carp Alaskan Cod* Croaker (White Pacific) Halibut (Atlantic)* Halibut (Pacific) Jacksmelt (Silverside) Lobster Mahi Mahi Monkfish* Perch (Freshwater) Sablefish Skate* Snapper* Tuna (Canned chunk light) Tuna: Skipjack* Weakfish (Sea Trout)	Bluefish Grouper* Spanish Mackerel Chilean Sea Bass * Tuna: Canned Albacore Tuna: Yellowfin*	King Mackerel Marlin* Orange Roughy* Shark* Swordfish Tilefish* Tuna: Bigeye, Ahi*

Table 6-7 lists typical mercury concentration levels in various fish eaten for food. Fish marked with asterisks are species that are being harvested in unsustainable numbers according to the Monterey Bay Aquarium. They recommended that consumption of these fish be limited as their use contributes to the depletion of these species and eventual loss of this resource.

Sphingolipids and Diet

The diet contains sphingolipids of plant, animal, and fungal sources. Depending on the source, these can contain very different sphingosine long chain bases and different ceramide fatty acid chains. Sphingolipids may undergo variable hydrolysis in the small intestine. Humans produce an alkaline sphingomyelinase in the bile and neutral sphingomyelinase as a pancreatic digestive enzyme. Even so, some sphingolipids pass into the large intestine where they may be hydrolyzed by intestinal bacteria, and some pass into the stool.

The sphingolipid that is absorbed is limited mostly to sphingosine, with perhaps some ceramide, and these are further degraded in the enterocyte. Some of the component molecules from these are recycled into sphingolipids used by the intestinal cells. At most, a very small amount of dietary sphingosine and ceramide survive intact and be transported chylomicrons.

Glycosphingolipids, such as cerebrosides and gangliosides contain a sugar molecule. Most of the sphingolipids from plant sources are cerebrosides. Glycosphingolipids remain mostly undigested. Unlike other fats that enter the colon, sphingolipids, and especially glycosphingolipids, behave much more like fiber; they can be processed by some bacteria into components molecules, some of which are absorbed, and used by the colonocytes.

Dietary sphingolipids from both plant and animals reduce the incidence of colon epithelial cell proliferation, and their consumption is associated with reduced incidence of colon cancer.

Many bacteria, bacterial toxins, and viruses bind to sugar residues on the cell membrane (figure 6-4) is a means for the pathogens or their toxins to enter their target cells. Bacteria, bacterial toxins, and viruses also adhere to glycosphingolipids in the intestine. Thus, dietary glycosphingolipids, bind to and prevent absorption of toxins such as cholera and botulism toxins, and to bacteria, preventing bacteria such as *E. coli* and *Pseudomonas aeruginosa* from adhering to colonocytes[40].

Phytosphingosine, a sphingolipid from plants, is a lipid similar to sphingosine, but has two fewer carbon atoms in the long chain base carbon chain, and contrary to sphingosine does not have an unsaturated bond. Phytosphingosine and phytoceramide, however, stimulated PPARγ and thus, have anti-inflammatory and antidiabetic effects[41]. Additionally, phytosphingosine has been found to reduce both serum cholesterol and triacylglycerol levels in mice[42]. Soybeans, sweet potatoes and wheat are foods particularly high in cerebrosides.

In plants, as in animals, sphingolipids participate in the immune defenses. A common mechanism for fungal attack of plants is through toxins which impair the plants sphingolipid metabolism. An example of these toxins is fumonisin B1 from the *Fusarium* mold that attacks corn and other grains. Fumonisin B1 has a molecular structure resembling a ceramide, and it inhibits the enzyme ceramide synthase in both plants and animals. In animals, this toxin increases oxidative stress, apoptosis and cytotoxicity. This toxin is neurotoxic, nephrotoxic, causes neural tube defects and is a carcinogen[43]. Fumonisins and another similar fungal toxin, AAL, promote programmed cell death through DNA fragmentation and caspase activation[44]. Humans and farm animals are exposed to this toxin mainly through the consumption of corn and sorghum infected with the *Fusarium* mold. AAL is produced by a strain of *Alternaria alternata*; a mold that caused disease in nearly 400 plant species, and whose spores are a common allergen in the home that triggers asthma[45].

Diet has profound effects the production of sphingolipids in our bodies. An early step in forming sphingolipids is the production of sphingosine. In humans, sphingosine is made from the amino acid serine and the fatty acid, palmitic acid. Dietary palmitic acid and fructose, whose calories are stored largely as palmitic acid, augment the production of sphingosine.

The second step is the formation of ceramide, which involves the addition of a second fatty acid. In mammals, the fatty acids that are most prevalent in ceramide are C24:1, followed by C24:0, with smaller amounts of C22:1 and C22:0. In individuals on a western diet high in palmitic acid and fructose, however, palmitic acid (C16:0) and other medium chain fatty acids become common or even predominate as the fatty acid moiety in ceramide.

Sphingomyelin (SPM), illustrated below, is a phospholipid found in cell membranes. Structurally, it is similar to other membrane phospholipids in that it has two nonpolar carbon chains and a polar, phosphate head. Also similar to phospholipids, in that sphingomyelin is a source of bioactive molecules that mediate inflammation. There is a high concentration of SM in the myelin sheath; here it acts as insulator and speeds nerve conduction.

Both high levels of sphingolipids and with sphingolipids with a lower percentage of long chain fatty acids are risk factors for obesity, diabetes, and heart disease (Chapter 9).

Trans Fatty Acids

Trans fatty acids occur in small amounts in nature, mostly as a result of rumination in cattle; however, almost all trans-fatty acids in the Western diet are created during processing of long chain unsaturated fats. Some trans fat content is unintentional, as in the case of refining vegetable oil, but most is intentional. Vegetable fats are treated with hydrogen; a process not surprisingly called hydrogenation, to raise the melting temperature and improve shelf life. This makes a cheap butter substitute (margarine), and a lard substitute (shortening) that offers processed foods a long shelf-life.

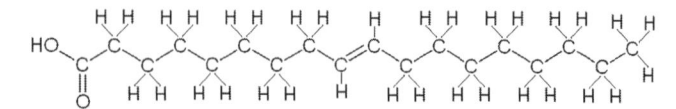

Figure 6-7. A Trans-Fatty Acid: Note the straight conformation

In natural fatty acids from plants, the two hydrogen atoms connected to the carbon atom are on the same side. During hydrogenation, hydrogen atoms get placed randomly; when some double bonds are hydrogenated, a hydrogen atom can get placed on each side. This causes a straight, rigid molecule, as illustrated in Figure 6-7, which packs densely and provides a higher melting temperature.

Shortening can be composed of ten to over 30 percent trans-fats. In some human populations, a similar amount of the body fat is trans fats. When women eat trans fats and breastfeed, trans fats end up in their breast milk; in North America, 7% of the fat in mother's milk is trans fat[46]. Unfortunately, humans do not have enzymes for breaking trans fats down. Thus, these fats are not food. Instead, they can be thought of as a slow poison disguised as food, which accumulates in the body.

Consumption of trans fatty acids is associated with increased risks of several disease conditions, including heart disease, dementia, breast cancer, and diabetes. Studies cited by the U.S. FDA estimate that between 30,000 and 100,000 Americans die from heart disease in the U.S. each year, as a result of dietary trans fats[47,48]. Trans fats also increase the risk of colon cancer[49] and infertility[50].

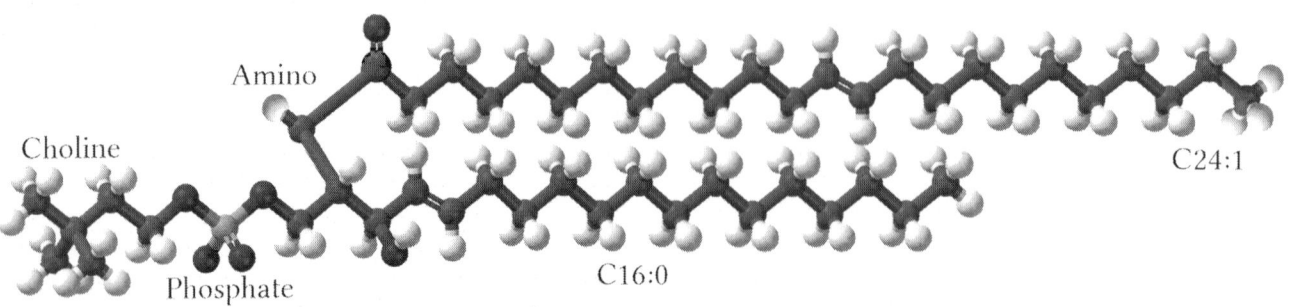

Figure 6-8: Sphingomyelin: The most common human form, with a C24:1 fatty acid, is illustrated.

In 2007, with the prospect of an outright ban by the FDA, manufacturers of food products voluntarily began lowering the amounts of trans-fats in their products. U.S. law now mandates labeling of the amount of trans-fats per serving. Many prepared foods now have "zero" trans fats. This is not your ordinary zero, but rather, a political zero.

As long as a serving contains less than 0.5 grams of trans-fats, it can be rounded down to zero on the product label. Thus, four hundred milligrams of trans fat per serving can be legally labeled as zero. A serving can be one cookie, a teaspoon of margarine, or a few potato chips. Each serving can be stated as having zero trans fats if it contains less than 0.5 grams, regardless of the number of servings or the total amount of trans fat likely to be consumed. Thus, eating foods labeled as having zero grams trans fats per serving can still allow the consumption of several grams of trans fats per day. If this neither seems a significant quantity nor provokes concern, then consider that the average American consumes only about 1.5 grams of the essential fatty acid linolenic acid a day, with most of that burned as calories. The average American consumes only 0.07 grams of DHA in their diet per day[51].

In November of 2013, the FDA issued a preliminary determination that partially hydrogenated oils (PHOs), the major dietary source of trans fat in processed food, are no longer "generally recognized as safe." If finalized, food containing PHOs will no longer be legal for sale in the United States[52].

Table 6-8: Trans fats still present prepared foods

Food	Serving size	Grams of Trans Fat[53]*
French fries	147 grams	8
Potato chips	Small bag 42 grams	2
Corn Chips	1 oz	1.5
Doughnut	1	5
Cookies (commercial)	3 (30 grams total)	2
Pound Cake (commercial)	1 slice, 80 grams	4.5
Candy Bar	40 grams (1.4 oz)	3
Shortening	1 Tbsp	4
Margarine (Tub)	1 Tbsp	0.5
Margarine (Stick)	1 Tbsp	3
Butter	1 Tbsp	0
Milk (whole)	1 cup	0
Mayonnaise	1 Tbsp	0

*Amounts vary significantly among food manufacturers.

Cooking in Oil

Different oils tolerate heating to different temperatures. Above an oil's smoke temperature, it will begin to smoke and can burst into flame. Oils with high smoke temperatures are easier to cook with, as they take less care in making sure that the cooking temperature is not excessive; they can get hotter without smoking. However, cooking food at high temperature comes other risks. When meat is cooked at high temperatures, several carcinogenic compounds are formed. The amount of the carcinogens formed increases quickly with temperatures between 300°C to 600°C. Heterocyclic amines[54] (HCA), polycyclic aromatic hydrocarbons (PAH), such as benz(a)pyrenes and nitrosamines, are chemicals which are formed when cooking meats at high temperatures. The formation of HCA accelerates at temperatures over 200°C (392°F). Nitrosamines, which also form at high temperatures, are potent oxidants. (See Chapter 40 on cancer prevention.)

PAH form when fat drips onto coals, a burner, or flame, and creates smoke. Many HCAs and PAH are carcinogenic and have been linked to prostate, pancreatic and colon cancers. They have been found to increase inflammatory cytokines IL-1β and TNF-α in the intestines. They reduce GLP-1 and thus may promote obesity and type 2 diabetes[55]. The highest concentration of these toxic compounds is found in the drippings and oil that remain in the pan. When meat is cooked at high temperatures, the drippings should not be eaten or used for gravy. Charred areas on meat should be trimmed and discarded. (See Chapter 40.)

The recommended temperature for frying food is 185°C (365°F). Temperatures lower than this are used for sautéing. Since virgin olive oil has a smoke point of about 200°C (392°F), it can be used as a temperature indicator, letting the cook know if smoking occurs that the cooking temperature is too high. This allows for safer food; although, more cautious use of heat is required to avoid smoking the oil. Virgin olive oil has a lower smoke point, than do the less desirable, more highly refined olive oils.

Table 6-9: Smoke Temperature for Some Cooking Oils

Fat	Degrees C	Degrees F
Butter	150	302
Coconut oil	177	351
Virgin olive oil	207	406
Corn oil	236	457
Soy oil	241	466
Canola oil	242	468

Another option for cooking meats is to use a covered electric pan that maintains the proper temperature for the food. Stewing meat, by simmering it at 70°C to 75°C (158°F to 167°F) improves digestibility and satiation better than frying (See Chapter 8).

Frying fish may undo any benefits imparted by the DHA and EPA content in fish. Fried fish consumption has been associated with the increased risk of stroke in the deep-fried South of the United States[56].

Eggs also should be cooked at temperatures no higher than the boiling point, and browning (lacing) of the egg white should be avoided. Eggs are best cooked to be tender rather than hard and rubbery. At a temperature of 65°C (150°F), egg whites will solidify, and they get much firmer at 82°C (180°F). The egg yolk solidifies at about 70°C (158°F).

Scrambled eggs set at around 165°F. The recommended grill or pan temperature for cooking a fried egg is 120°C (250°F) since only the surface is heated[57], and cooking must be achieved through conductance of heat through the egg. If the butter browns, the temperature has risen to over 150°C (300°F), a pan temperature that is excessive. Lower temperatures can be used if the pan is covered, so that the eggs cook in heated air, resulting in a more tender egg with better flavor. The secret to cooking eggs is patience; cooking at the correct temperature takes longer.

Summary of Dietary Recommendations

1. Limit Linoleic Acid Intake: Although adding supplements of n-3 fatty acids to raise the n-3:n-6 ratio may seem simpler than changing diet; it may not overcome the pro-inflammatory effects of excessive dietary LA consumption. Excess production of AA and the resultant promotion of inflammation can be better avoided by limiting LA intake. This may be most easily achieved by limiting the amount of fat in the diet.

2. Avoid Trans Fatty Acids: Limit the amount of manufactured foods consumed. Read labels. Recently the FDA has moved to greatly curtail trans fat content in foods. Approach manufactured foods created to have a long shelf-life with caution.

3. Consume a Diet High in EPA and DHA: DHA should be considered to be an essential fatty acid, as the body has quite limited capacity for its production. Several grams of EPA and DHA combined should be consumed each week. Japanese, who have lower rates of inflammatory diseases, consume about 8.5 grams per week of these fats. A four-ounce serving of salmon contains about 2 grams of these fats. Cold water fish tend to be better sources of these fats.

Fish oil supplements, preferably made from small fish such as sardines (herring), can be used to help to meet this goal. Stearidonic acid-rich foods may soon be available for replacing the requirement for marine oils, by allowing endogenous EPA production.

4. Avoid Consumption of Top Predator Fish: These fish are high in mercury, and their wild populations cannot be sustained for commercial harvest.

5. For Prevention of Inflammation Use More EPA than DHA: EPA is more anti-inflammatory than DHA. When EPA and DHA are used as a supplement, a source with a two-EPA to one-DHA ratio should provide the most favorable anti-inflammatory response.

Generally, EPA acts peripherally while DHA acts centrally (brain, retina) and acts on electrical conduction. Thus, EPA lowers peripheral inflammation, prevents hyper-coagulability and helps prevent and treat depression.

6. For Central Activity and Cardiac Arrhythmia, Start with More DHA: If the goal is to raise DHA levels quickly, as might be desired for treatment of diseases such as bipolar disorder, brain injury or cardiac arrhythmia, DHA supplements with lower EPA:DHA ratios allow quicker DHA absorption and may be more efficacious. After 30 days of supplementation, when tissue levels of DHA have risen, supplements with a higher ratio of EPA to DHA is recommended. It takes about one month to get tissue levels of DHA to steady state with supplementation, and over 60 days for EPA to get to steady state levels.

7. Split EPA/DHA Supplements: If large doses of EPA/DHA are used, the dose should be split to at least twice daily to maximize absorption. Three grams per day of EPA and DHA combined is likely the practical maximum utilizable dose. Supplements should be taken with meals.

8. Vegans: Algae-based EPA/DHA supplements are available for vegans and others who do not to consume fish. Vegans should also limit their intake of LA to avoid competition for ALA processing into EPA. One study found that vegans have very adequate EPA levels, but lower DHA than other dietary groups[58]. Vegans can increase their intake of ALA with the consumption of walnuts and flax seed. A goal of 3 grams of ALA a day is a ballpark estimate for dietary intake for vegans. Vegans should consider DHA to be an essential fatty acid, and use algae-derived or other DHA supplements to ensure adequate intake.

9. Ensure Adequate Vitamin D$_3$: Vitamin D enhances the anti-inflammatory effect of EPA and DHA by decreasing the conversion of AA to prostaglandins[59]. Assure that Vitamin D levels are sufficient. (See Chapter 20)

10. Ensure Adequate Levels of Vitamin B$_6$: Pyridoxal-5 phosphate deficiency can prevent the conversion of EPA to DHA[60]. Thus, Vitamin B$_6$ supplements may be helpful if levels are low.

11. Select the best oil for salads and cooking: If using salad oils, one with a higher n-3: n-6 fat ratio should be chosen for salad and cooking when possible. There are few high n-3 choices; thus, vegetable oil should be minimized in the diet. Oils with lower smoke points can be used as indicators to prevent cooking at excessive temperatures.

12. Don't Overheat Oils or Fats: Cooking at correct temperatures results in tastier, healthier foods. Use of lower frying temperatures decrease the risk of fire, reduce aerosols and odors in the home, and most importantly, decrease the creation of carcinogens in food. Cooking thermometers are inexpensive, and their use should be encouraged for the preparation of healthier food.

If cooking eggs in a pan, use butter and cover, keeping the pan temperature below 260°F. Avoid eating fried foods. If sautéing in oil, use a temperature-controlled heat source or use butter or olive oil, and cook at a temperature below the fat's smoke point. Drippings from cooking fried foods should be discarded as they likely contain carcinogens and potent oxidative compounds.

[1] Distribution, interconversion, and dose response of n-3 fatty acids in humans. Arterburn LM, Hall EB, Oken H. Am J Clin Nutr. 2006 Jun;83(6 Suppl):1467S-1476S. Review.PMID: 16841856

[2] A review of fatty acid profiles and antioxidant content in grass-fed and grain-fed beef. Daley CA, Abbott A, Doyle PS, Nader GA, Larson S. Nutr J. 2010 Mar 10;9:10. PMID: 20219103

[3] Dietary supplementation with docosahexaenoic acid, but not eicosapentaenoic acid, dramatically alters cardiac mitochondrial phospholipid fatty acid composition and prevents permeability transition. Khairallah RJ, Sparagna GC, Khanna N, rt al. Biochim Biophys Acta. 2010 Aug;1797(8):1555-1562. PMID: 20471951

[4] ELOVL1 production of C24 acyl-CoAs is linked to C24 sphingolipid synthesis. Ohno Y, Suto S, Yamanaka M, et al. Proc Natl Acad Sci U S A. 2010 Oct 26;107(43):18439-44. PMID:20937905

[5] Distribution, interconversion, and dose response of n-3 fatty acids in humans. Arterburn LM, Hall EB, et al. Oken H. Am J Clin Nutr. 2006 Jun;83(6 Suppl):1467S-1476S..PMID:16841856

[6] Therapeutic use of omega-3 fatty acids in bipolar disorder. Balanzá-Martínez V, Fries GR, Colpo GD, et al. Expert Rev Neurother. 2011 Jul;11(7):1029-47. PMID:21721919

[7] Effects of altered maternal folic acid, vitamin B12 and docosahexaenoic acid on placental global DNA methylation patterns in Wistar rats. Kulkarni A, Dangat K, Kale A, et al. PLoS One. 2011 Mar 10;6(3):e17706. PMID:21423696

[8] The omega-3 fatty acid-derived neuroprotectin D1 limits hippocampal hyperexcitability and seizure susceptibility in kindling epileptogenesis. Musto AE, Gjorstrup P, Bazan NG. Epilepsia. 2011 May 13. PMID:21569016

[9] Omega-3 fatty acids as treatments for mental illness: which disorder and which fatty acid? Ross BM, Seguin J, Sieswerda LE. Lipids Health Dis. 2007 Sep 18;6:21. PMID:17877810

[10] Supplementation of polyunsaturated fatty acids, magnesium and zinc in children seeking medical advice for attention-deficit/hyperactivity problems. Huss M, Völp A, Stauss-Grabo M. Lipids Health Dis. 2010 Sep 24;9:105. PMID:20868469

[11] Higher maternal plasma docosahexaenoic acid during pregnancy is associated with more mature neonatal sleep-state patterning. Cheruku SR, Montgomery-Downs HE, Farkas SL, et al. Am J Clin Nutr. 2002 Sep;76(3):608-13. PMID:12198007

[12] Neurotrophins induce neuroprotective signaling in the retinal pigment epithelial cell by activating the synthesis of the anti-inflammatory and anti-apoptotic neuroprotectin D1. Bazan NG. Adv Exp Med Biol. 2008;613:39-44. PMID:18188926

[13] Dietary fish oil decreases secretion of T helper (Th) 1-type cytokines by a direct effect on murine splenic T cells but enhances secretion of a Th2-type cytokine by an effect on accessory cells. Petursdottir DH, Hardardottir I. Br J Nutr. 2009 Apr;101(7):1040-6. PMID: 18680632

[14] Correlation of omega-3 levels in serum phospholipid from 2053 human blood samples with key fatty acid ratios. Holub BJ, Wlodek M, Rowe W, Piekarski J. Nutr J. 2009 Dec 24;8:58. PMID:20034401

[15] Omega-3 fatty acids: potential role in the management of early Alzheimer's disease. Jicha GA, Markesbery WR. Clin Interv Aging. 2010 Apr 7;5:45-61. PMID:20396634

[16] Omega-3 fatty acids as treatments for mental illness: which disorder and which fatty acid? Ross BM, Seguin J, Sieswerda LE. Lipids Health Dis. 2007 Sep 18;6:21. PMID:17877810

[17] Effect of fish oil on arrhythmias and mortality: systematic review. León H, Shibata MC, Sivakumaran S, et al. BMJ. 2008 Dec 23;337:a2931. PMID:19106137

[18] Risk stratification by the "EPA+DHA level" and the "EPA/AA ratio" focus on anti-inflammatory and antiarrhythmogenic effects of long-chain omega-3 fatty acids. Rupp H, Wagner D, Rupp T, et al. Herz. 2004 Nov;29(7):673-85. PMID:15580322

[19] n-3 Fatty acids from fish or fish-oil supplements, but not alpha-linolenic acid, benefit cardiovascular disease outcomes in primary- and secondary-prevention studies: a systematic review. Wang C, Harris WS, Chung M, et al. Am J Clin Nutr. 2006 Jul;84(1):5-17. PMID:16825676

[20] Control of salicylate intolerance with fish oils. Healy E, Newell L, Howarth P, Friedmann PS. Br J Dermatol. 2008 Dec;159(6):1368-9. PMID: 18795922

[21] Essential fatty acids and their role in conditions characterised by impulsivity. Garland MR, Hallahan B. Int Rev Psychiatry. 2006 Apr;18(2):99-105. PMID: 16777664

[22] Omega-3 polyunsaturated essential fatty acids are associated with depression in adolescents with eating disorders and weight loss. Swenne I, Rosling A, Tengblad S, Vessby B. Acta Paediatr. 2011 Jul 6. PMID:21732977

[23] Low omega-6 vs. low omega-6 plus high omega-3 dietary intervention for chronic daily headache: protocol for a randomized clinical trial. Ramsden CE, Mann JD, Faurot KR, et al. Trials. 2011 Apr 15;12:97. PMID:21496264

[24] The relationship of diet and acne: A review. Pappas A. Dermatoendocrinol. 2009 Sep;1(5):262-7. PMID:20808513

[25] Dietary linoleic acid has no effect on arachidonic acid, but increases n-6 eicosadienoic acid, and lowers dihomo-gamma-linolenic and eicosapentaenoic acid in plasma of adult men. Angela Liou Y, Innis SM. Prostaglandins Leukot Essent Fatty Acids. 2009 Apr;80(4):201-6. PMID: 19356914

[26] Conversion of alpha-linolenic acid in humans is influenced by the absolute amounts of alpha-linolenic acid and linoleic acid in the diet and not by their ratio. Goyens PL, Spilker ME, Zock PL, et al. Am J Clin Nutr. 2006 Jul;84(1):44-53.PMID: 16825680

[27] Distribution, interconversion, and dose response of n-3 fatty acids in humans. Arterburn LM, Hall EB, Oken H. Am J Clin Nutr. 2006 Jun;83(6 Suppl):1467S-1476S. PMID: 16841856

[28] Endogenous Signaling by Omega-3 Docosahexaenoic Acid-derived Mediators Sustains Homeostatic Synaptic and Circuitry Integrity. Bazan NG, Musto AE, Knott EJ. Mol Neurobiol. 2011 Oct;44(2):216-22. PMID:21918832

[29] EPA but not DHA appears to be responsible for the efficacy of omega-3 long chain polyunsaturated fatty acid supplementation in depression: evidence from a meta-analysis of randomized

[30] Therapeutic use of omega-3 fatty acids in bipolar disorder. Balanzá-Martínez V, Fries GR, Colpo GD, et al. Expert Rev Neurother. 2011 Jul;11(7):1029-47. PMID:21721919

[31] Dietary long-chain n-3 fatty acids of marine origin and serum C-reactive protein concentrations are associated in a population with a diet rich in marine products. Niu K, Hozawa A, Kuriyama S, et al. Am J Clin Nutr. 2006 Jul;84(1):223-9.PMID: 16825699

[32] Distribution, interconversion, and dose response of n-3 fatty acids in humans. Arterburn LM, Hall EB, Oken H. Am J Clin Nutr. 2006 Jun;83(6 Suppl):1467S-1476S. PMID: 16841856

[33] Effects of fish-oil supplementation on myocardial fatty acids in humans. Metcalf RG, James MJ, Gibson RA, et al. Am J Clin Nutr. 2007 May;85(5):1222-8.PMID: 17490956

34 US Department of Agriculture, national nutrient data base.

[35] GRAS Notice for Stearidonic (SDA) Omega-3 Soybean Oil. Food and Drug Administration. February 2009 http://www.accessdata.fda.gov/scripts/fcn/gras_notices/grn000283.pdf

[36] Dietary intake of stearidonic acid-enriched soybean oil increases the omega-3 index: randomized, double-blind clinical study of efficacy and safety. Lemke SL, Vicini JL, Su H, et al. Am J Clin Nutr. 2010 Oct;92(4):766-75. PMID:20739419

[37] n-3 fatty acid dietary recommendations and food sources to achieve essentiality and cardiovascular benefits. Gebauer SK, Psota TL, Harris WS, Kris-Etherton PM. Am J Clin Nutr. 2006 Jun;83(6 Suppl):1526S-1535S. PMID: 16841863

[38] Marine Nutraceuticals and Functional Foods Colin J. Barrow, Fereidoon Shahidi. CRC Press; August 2007. Table 2.7.

[39] AMAP/UNEP, 2008. Technical Background Report to the Global Atmospheric Mercury Assessment. Arctic Monitoring and Assessment Programme / UNEP Chemicals Branch. 159 pp.

[40] Sphingolipids in food and the emerging importance of sphingolipids to nutrition. Vesper H, Schmelz EM, Nikolova-Karakashian MN, et al. J Nutr. 1999 Jul;129(7):1239-50. PMID: 10395583

[41] Improved high-fat diet-induced glucose intolerance by an oral administration of phytosphingosine. Murakami I, Mitsutake S, Kobayashi N, et al. Biosci Biotechnol Biochem. 2013;77(1):194-7. PMID:23291756

[42] Dietary sphingolipids lower plasma cholesterol and triacylglycerol and prevent liver steatosis in APOE*3Leiden mice. Duivenvoorden I, Voshol PJ, Rensen PC, et al. Am J Clin Nutr. 2006 Aug;84(2):312-21. PMID:16895877

[43] A review of the toxic effects and mechanisms of action of fumonisin B1. Stockmann-Juvala H, Savolainen K. Hum Exp Toxicol. 2008 Nov;27(11):799-809. PMID:19244287

[44] Sphingolipids and plant defense/disease: the "death" connection and beyond. Berkey R, Bendigeri D, Xiao S. Front Plant Sci. 2012 Apr 10;3:68. PMID:22639658

[45] Exposure to Alternaria alternata in US homes is associated with asthma symptoms. Salo PM, Arbes SJ Jr, Sever M, et al. J Allergy Clin Immunol. 2006 Oct;118(4):892-8. PMID:17030243

[46] trans Fatty acids in milk produced by women in the United States. Mosley EE, Wright AL, McGuire MK, McGuire MA. Am J Clin Nutr. 2005 Dec;82(6):1292-7. PMID:16332663

[47] Trans fatty acids and cardiovascular disease. Mozaffarian D, Katan MB, Ascherio A, Stampfer MJ, Willett WC. N Engl J Med. 2006 Apr 13;354(15):1601-13. PMID:16611951

[48] Trans fatty acids and coronary heart disease. Zaloga GP, Harvey KA, Stillwell W, Siddiqui R. Nutr Clin Pract. 2006 Oct;21(5):505-12. PMID:16998148

[49] Consumption of trans-fatty acid and its association with colorectal adenomas. Vinikoor LC, Schroeder JC, Millikan RC, et al. Am J Epidemiol. 2008 Aug 1;168(3):289-97. PMID:1858713

[50] Dietary fatty acid intakes and the risk of ovulatory infertility. Chavarro JE, Rich-Edwards JW, Rosner BA, Willett WC. Am J Clin Nutr. 2007 Jan;85(1):231-7. PMID:17209201

[51] n-3 fatty acid dietary recommendations and food sources to achieve essentiality and cardiovascular benefits. Gebauer SK, Psota TL, Harris WS, Kris-Etherton PM. Am J Clin Nutr. 2006 Jun;83(6 Suppl):1526S-1535S. PMID: 16841863

[52] http://www.fda.gov/ForConsumers/ConsumerUpdates/ucm372915.htm FDA website accessed December 11, 2013

[53] Revealing Trans Fats Article U.S. Food and Drug Administration Revealing Trans Fats. Article Reprint 05-1329C

[54] Screening for heterocyclic amines in chicken cooked in various ways. Solyakov A, Skog K. Food Chem Toxicol. 2002 Aug;40(8):1205-11.PMID: 12067585

[55] Polycyclic aromatic hydrocarbons potentiate high-fat diet effects on intestinal inflammation. Khalil A, Villard PH, Dao MA, et al. Toxicol Lett. 2010 Jul 15;196(3):161-7. PMID: 20412841

[56] Racial and geographic differences in fish consumption: the REGARDS study. Nahab F, Le A, Judd S, et al. Neurology. 2011 Jan 11;76(2):154-8. PMID:21178096

[57] On Food and Cooking; The Science and Lore of the Kitchen. Harlold McKee. Scribner, New York 2004

[58] Dietary intake and status of n-3 polyunsaturated fatty acids in a population of fish-eating and non-fish-eating meat-eaters, vegetarians, and vegans and the product-precursor ratio [corrected] of α-linolenic acid to long-chain n-3 polyunsaturated fatty acids: results from the EPIC-Norfolk cohort. Welch AA, Shakya-Shrestha S, Lentjes MA, Wareham NJ, Khaw KT. Am J Clin Nutr. 2010 Nov;92(5):1040-51.. PMID:20861171

[59] Mechanisms of vitamin D-mediated growth inhibition in prostate cancer cells: inhibition of the prostaglandin pathway. Moreno J, Krishnan AV, Peehl DM, Feldman D. Anticancer Res. 2006 Jul-Aug;26(4A):2525-30. PMID:1688666

[60] Effects of vitamin B-6 on (n-3) polyunsaturated fatty acid metabolism. Tsuge H, Hotta N, Hayakawa T. J Nutr. 2000 Feb;130(2S Suppl):333S-334S. PMID:10721899

7. Proteins

The purpose of DNA and the genetic code is to code for proteins. Proteins are the machinery of life; understanding their function is a requirement for understanding health and disease.

Proteins are made up of chains of amino acids. About 500 amino acids (AA) have been identified, but we only employ a limited number of them. Only 22 amino acids are incorporated into the proteins of plants animal and fungi. Achaea utilize an extra one; pyrrolysine, and mitochondria and some bacteria make and use N-formylmethionine. The AA form all peptides and proteins, similar to how only 26 letters, plus a few Greek ones, are used to convey the myriad ideas express in this and other English language books. In addition to the proteinogenic α-amino acids, we also use a few other AA's as metabolic intermediaries and other uses.

Animals cannot synthesize AA's; however, we have the capacity to modify many amino acids from our diets into other AA's, using enzymes to perform this task. Nine amino acids, listed in Table 7-1, are considered essential; we require them preformed in our diet, as we cannot make them. Additionally, children have insufficient capacity to convert other essential amino acids into arginine, cysteine, and tyrosine; thus, these are essential for young children.

Table 7-1: Protein Forming Amino Acids

Essential	Nonessential	
Histidine	Alanine	Glutamine
Isoleucine	Arginine*	Glycine
Leucine	Asparagine	Proline
Lysine	Aspartic acid	Serine
Methionine	Cysteine*	Tyrosine*
Phenylalanine	Glutamic acid	
Threonine	*Essential in children	
Tryptophan	Post-translational	
Valine	Citrulline	Selenocysteine

Amino acids have an amino group (N) on one end of the molecule and a carboxy group (O:C:OH) on the other end. The proteinogenic AA are linked together by peptide bonds into chains that form the primary structure of peptides and proteins. Amino acids form chains, with the carboxy group covalently linked to the amino group. The term peptide refers to smaller molecules, generally less than 50-amino acids long, and may refer to molecules that are active hormones or functional proteins, as well as to fragments of proteins undergoing proteolytic breakdown. When peptides and proteins are formed, the carboxy end of one amino acid gives up a hydroxyl group (OH) and forms a covalent peptide bond to the nitrogen end (replacing a hydrogen) of the next amino acid. A water molecule (HOH) is formed, as a result. The arrow in Figure 7-1 points to a peptide bond between two amino acids.

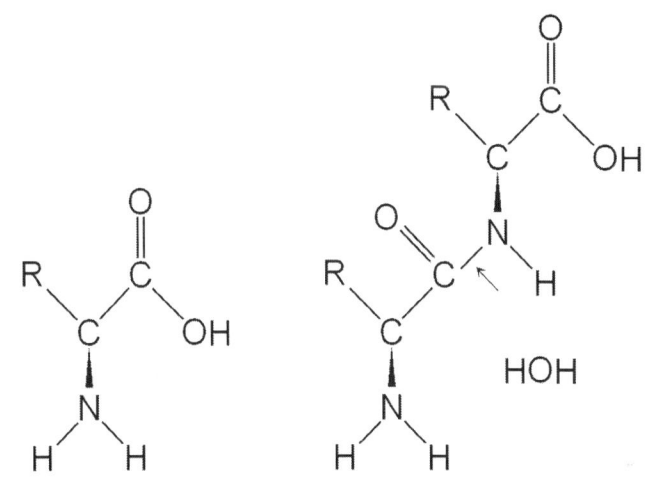

Fig. 7-1: An amino acid and a dipeptide. A molecule of water is formed during the formation of a dipeptide bond, and water is replaced during the hydrolysis of proteins.

In the simple amino acid structure shown in Figure 7-1, with two carbon atoms, R represents the location where various side chains may be attached, forming various AA's. Glycine, the smallest AA, has no side chain and has a pair of hydrogen atoms where the R is shown. Alanine has a single carbon and three hydrogen atoms. Other amino acids are more complex.

Nonprotein Roles of Amino Acids

In addition to the role of forming protein, AA's have other functions. As a few examples: Glutamate, also known as glutamic acid, is the principal excitatory neurotransmitter. Serotonin and melatonin are formed from tryptophan. The nucleotides are formed from aspartate, glycine, and glutamine. Glycine is used in the formation of porphyrins in the formation of heme. Histidine and several others form biogenic amines (Chapter 13) such as histamine; The catecholamines are formed from tyrosine. Tyrosine also forms the pigment melanin. Methionine forms the methyl donor S-adenosylmethionine (SAMe).

Non-protein forming AA's are also used by the body. Ornithine is an intermediary in the urea cycle, essential for ridding the body of ammonia and is a precursor for polyamines. Homocysteine is a metabolic intermediary. Gamma amino butyric acid (GABA, a γ-AA rather than an α-AA), is an inhibitory neurotransmitter, as is D-serine.

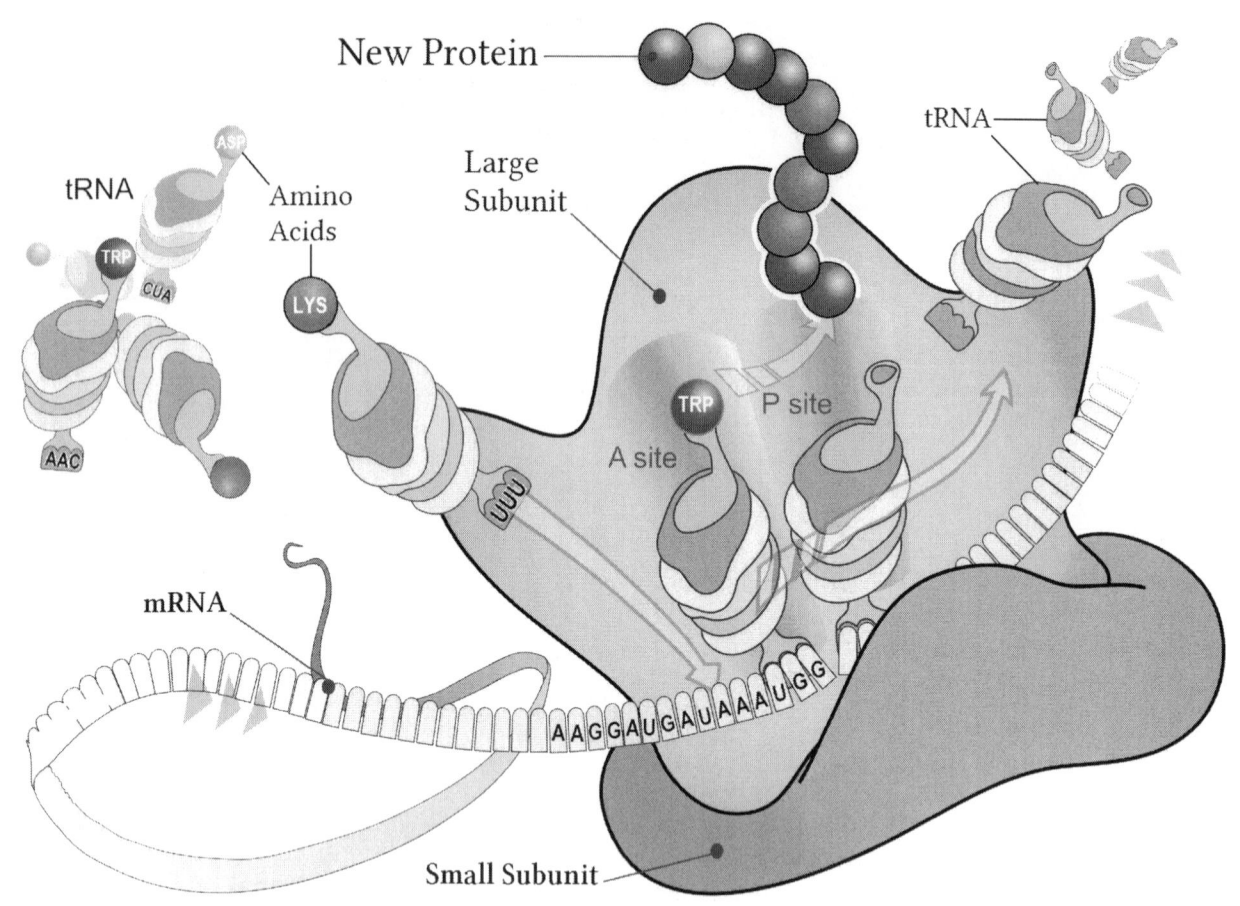

Figure 7-2: The Ribosome and Protein Synthesis

Building Proteins

In the cell, ribosomes read the messenger RNA (mRNA) transcript for a protein that has been copied from the DNA. Each AA has a unique transfer RNA (tRNA) which delivers it to the ribosome to sequentially build the primary protein structure. Triplets of nucleic acids called codons, code for the various tRNA; controlling the correct sequential assembly of the protein. The four nucleic acids in RNA are Adenine (A), Cytosine (C), Guanine (G), and Uracil (U). Since there are three nucleic acids per codon, there are 4^3 permutations; thus, there are 64 codons. There is a single codon for some AA's, while there are multiple codons for others. Three of the codons are stop codons.

The assembly begins with the start codon that codes for methionine in eukaryotes, and which may be preceded by an untranslated region, the 5'UTR. The messenger RNA terminates the protein-building process with one of three stop-codons that cause the protein chain to be released from the ribosome. One of these stop codons also acts to insert the amino acid selenocysteine into the protein chain. After transcription, further posttranslational modifications may be made to a protein. The amino acid hydroxyproline, a major component of collagen, is formed by hydroxylation of proline after translation. Arginine can be converted into citrulline. Most posttranslational modifications do not create new AA, but rather add functional groups, such as lipids or sugars to form lipoproteins and glycoproteins.

Ubiquitination is a post-translational modification.

As illustrated in Figure 7-4, proteins have primary, secondary, tertiary and quaternary structures. The primary structure of a protein is the order of the amino acids, held together by strong covalent bonds. The secondary protein structure results from weak hydrogen bonds. These weak bonds cause the proteins to fold-up into three-dimensional shapes. The sequence of the various amino acids and the hydrogen bonds cause the proteins to form α-helixes, β-sheets, and curves, in very specific conformations. Additionally, pairs of sulfur-containing amino acids (cysteine and methionine) can form disulfide bonds that also help to shape proteins. These S:S bonds have about 40 percent the binding energy of a covalent bond, and thus are easier to break and reform than covalent bonds, but are several times stronger than hydrogen bonds.

Since a protein may have several secondary conformational areas, including both α-helixes and β-sheets and curves, the overall structure is referred to as the tertiary structure. If a protein is made up of more than one protein chain, the combined protein structure is the quaternary structure. The tertiary and quaternary structures are important to the function of proteins. Figure 7-4 shows the quaternary structure of hemoglobin, the protein that carries oxygen in the blood. Normal adult hemoglobin is made up of two α-hemoglobin chains and two β-hemoglobin chains.

PRIMARY STRUCTURE:
Amino Acid Sequence

SECONDARY STRUCTURES

Beta Sheet

Alpha Helix

P13 Protein

TERTIARY STRUCTURE

Hemoglobin

QUARTERNARY STRUCTURE

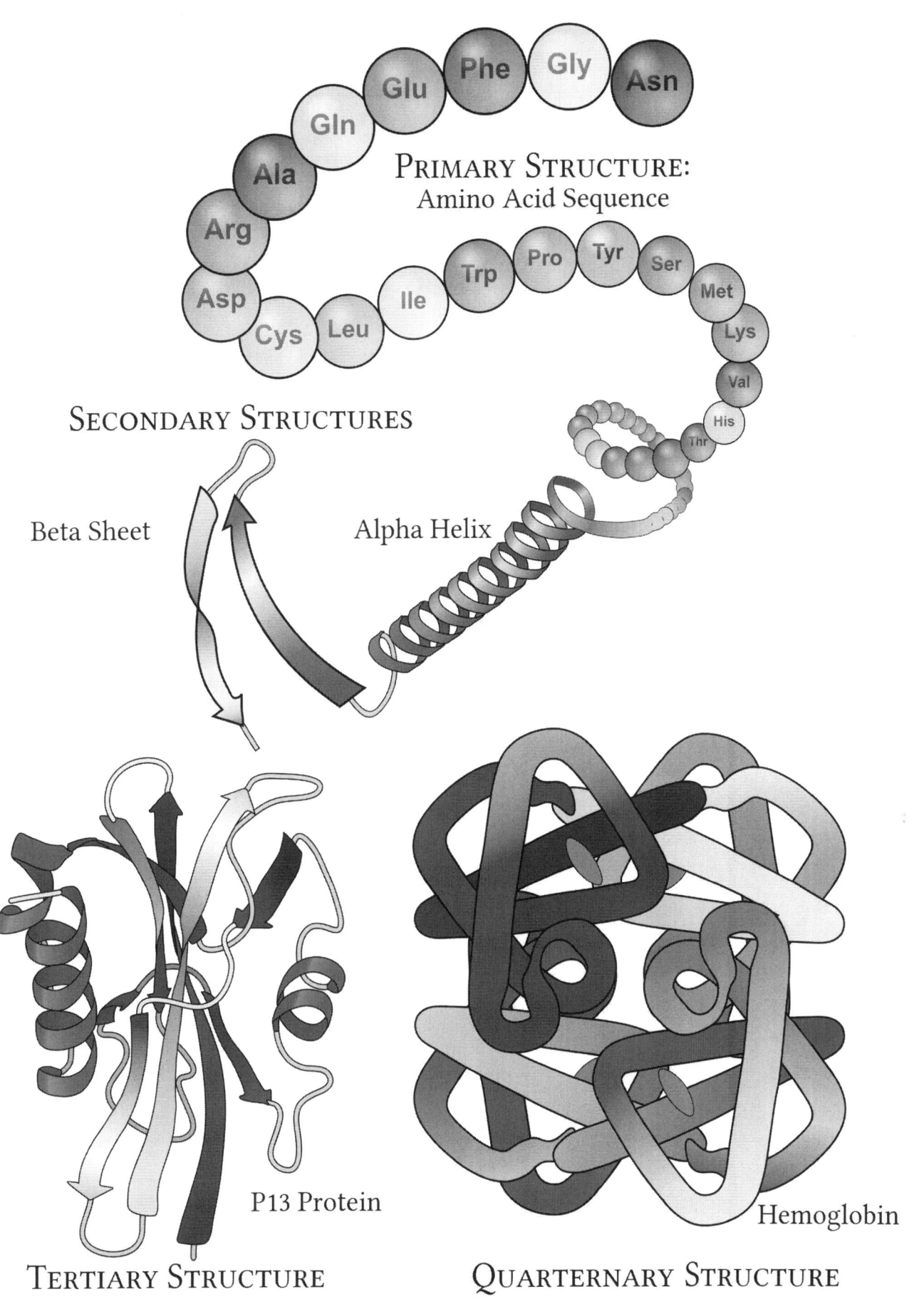

Figure 7-3: **Protein Structure:** Showing a simple tertiary protein and hemoglobin made up of four protein units.

Proteins Function

Proteins are capable of numerous specific functions. For example, collagen is a structural protein; lipases are enzymes that catalyze reactions; insulin is a hormone. Proteins function as transmembrane portals, such as sodium channels and glucose transporters; as ligands, such as immunoglobulins; movers such as myosin and actin in muscle; builders such as ribosomes which build the proteins, and editors, such as DNA repair proteins.

Proteins can serve these functions by acting as simple nanomachines. For example, a protein may grab a molecule, and hold it in a particular position. The protein may then change its conformation, effecting a change to the molecule, release the molecule, and then the protein may change back to its original conformation so that it can perform the action again.

Enzymes have very precise affinities for latching onto one or more specific chemicals substrates. This can be a single ion, a small molecule, a sugar, a fat, a molecule of ATP, or another protein or group of proteins. Enzymes function by grabbing substrate and holding it in place so that it will be in close proximity to another chemical. This allows exposure of substrates with the intended reactant, to occur much more intensely than would occur with random encounters.

Most proteins that have enzymatic activity function by breaking and reforming disulfide (S:S) bonds, and thereby, changing the conformation of the protein. S:S bonds are important in many proteins, as the bond can be broken and reformed, allowing it to have a toggle-like action. Muscles work by having one protein grab a second protein, change conformation, release, and grab again further along the second protein chain; in this repetitive reaction, the first protein ratchets along as second protein, like a farm-jack or ladder.

By linking several simple nanomachines together, complex nanomachines can be assembled. An example of such a nanomachine is the flagellum of a bacterium. The protein nanomachines form a tail that acts like a propeller spinning at high speed and propelling the bacteria through fluid.

Protein Malfunction

Substituting one AA for another within the primary structure of a protein occasionally causes alterations in the folding pattern or change the affinity of the protein for its ligand, causing dysfunction or disease. This is the basis of most inherited genetic diseases. Most single-gene genetic diseases are caused by alterations in a single DNA base pair which causes a nucleic acid in the mRNA to change. This alteration causes substitution of one amino acid during the synthesis of the protein for another causing a mis-sense mutation. While many modifications do not affect protein function, some changes can cause the protein to behave very differently. This occurs, especially when the character of the AA has been switched from acidic, basic, polar or nonpolar (hydrophobic) to a different type.

In sickle cell anemia, for example, the codon for the acidic AA, glutamic acid: GAG, is substituted by the codon for the hydrophobic AA, valine: GUG in the mRNA for the beta chain of the hemoglobin protein. This single-nucleic acid substitution causes oxygen-depleted hemoglobin to stick to itself and polymerize into stacks of rod-like fibers. These fibers stick to each other and form bundles that deform the red blood cell into stiff, elongated cells. These sickle-shaped RBC's aren't pliable enough to squeeze through the small venules; they and back up like a traffic jam; clogging and impeding blood flow to the area, causing painful ischemia.

In another example, a mis-sense mutation in one of the genes for the enzyme 5-α reductase causes a switch from nonpolar alanine (GCx) to the polar AA threonine (ACx). This raises 5-α reductase enzymatic activity that converts testosterone to dihydrotestosterone, a stronger androgen, thereby, increases the risk of prostate cancer[1].

DNA mutations also cause nucleotide substitutions that that result in a stop-codon or added or deleted nucleotides. β-thalassemia and McArdle's disease are caused by the early termination of transcription by mutations resulting in stop codons. In Huntington's disease, a string of CAG insertions adds a string of glutamines to a protein involved in microtubule function.

Cystic fibrosis (CF) is caused by an alteration in CFTR, a gene, that codes for a chloride ion transporter. The CFTR protein helps moves water out of cells and regulate the production of fluid in mucus secretions, digestive juices, and sweat. Without this function, the secretions are thick, and the individual is more susceptible to mucus plugging and respiratory infections, as well as other problems.

Many different mutations in the CFTR gene have been found that cause CF. In the most common mutation causing CF, there is a deletion of the trinucleotide, UUU; this missing phenylalanine at the 508th AA position of the CFTR protein causes CFTR to fold incorrectly. This mutation does not keep the protein from functioning, but rather, causes it to be degraded more quickly. As a result, CF patients have deficits of this type of chloride ion transporter. In other forms of CF, the mutation causes the ion channel to function less effectively or not at all. In some other forms of CF, there is an inadequate production of the ion channel[2].

Individuals who are carriers of sickle cell hemoglobin are less susceptible to malaria, and this gives them a survival advantage in regions where this disease has been endemic for millennia and a major cause of death. Carriers of recessive forms or CF are less susceptible than normal individuals to certain bacterial infections and to secretory diarrhea, a major killer of infants. Thus, these alterations can give unaffected disease carriers a significant survival advantage, even though the trait may be deadly when inherited from both parents.

Genetic diversity present in a gene coding for a protein is called polymorphism. An allele is a form of a gene that has variations in is sequence various forms within a population. Most allelic forms have no functional impact or only impact survival under unusual conditions. Polymorphisms can be seen in the phenotypic differences in hair and eye color and numerous other traits in a population. Some alleles give a survival advantage under certain conditions; people with lighter skin color produce vitamin D with less intense sunlight, and thus can thrive in northern latitudes. An allele of MAO causes a wider variance in aggressive behavior, allowing a child with this allele to better adapt to environmental conditions (Chapter 37). Many alleles are not phenotypically apparent and have no apparent impact.

Some alleles that are benign under most circumstances may, however, increase susceptibility to disease under physiologic or environmental stress. Alleles can affect how avidly an enzyme binds to its substrate, to vitamins, or to other cofactors for the enzyme. Thus, some individuals may have higher requirements for nutritional components or higher susceptibility to toxins or environmental stressors.

Protein Synthesis and Demise

Proteins are built upon demand. Humans have no storage proteins or warehouses for amino acids comparable to those for lipids (fat) and carbohydrates (glycogen). When a cell needs amino acids, there is not a set of 20 AA storage bins ready for use. Nevertheless, the absence of even one required amino acid required for forming a protein will prevent it from being produced. If requisite amino acids are not available, the cell sacrifices organelles and other proteins; scavenging amino acids from them. The cells contain proteases that break up and disassemble proteins. This process is also critical for removing old, worn-out organelles and forming new, efficient ones. Amino acids scavenged from muscle can also be utilized as a source of energy when energy supplies are low. During extended starvation, there can be muscle loss, which is difficult to replace, especially in older individuals.

Cofactors: In addition to requiring immediate availability of various amino acids for protein construction, most enzymes, and many other proteins require co-factors to perform their required functions. Most co-factors are metal ions and vitamins. For example, the electron transport chain proteins in the mitochondria requires the cofactors NAD and FAD which contain the B vitamins nicotinamide and riboflavin, and Coenzyme Q10 needs iron and copper. Hemoglobin requires an iron ion to transport and release oxygen to the tissues. Disease conditions that respond to an increased supply of enzyme cofactors are not rare. It has been estimated that about one-third of genetic diseases resulting from polymorphisms result from changes in affinity to enzyme cofactors.

Looking in the mirror, flexing your muscles, and seeing your skin with its collagen and elastin (both structural proteins), you might conclude that proteins last for months or even years. However, most proteins are quite ephemeral. In yeast, the average half-life of the 3,751 different proteins studied was 43 minutes[3]. Of these, 161 proteins had a half-life of under four minutes. Most of these are regulatory proteins. They do their jobs, and they are then retired. They are attacked by proteases and broken down into amino acids for recycling. In mammals, the average half-life of proteins is longer but probably still under two hours. It is important to realize that proteins are constructed and dismantled continuously, according to the demands of the cell's metabolism, the mitochondria, and hormonal action. A deficit of even one amino acid can impair protein transcription by the ribosomes. Some of the most potent and fast-acting toxins act by binding to the ribosome, in a way that stops protein synthesis. The cell needs a constant supply of each of the 21 proteinaceous amino acids, every minute of the day.

Survival cannot rely on having access to a balanced diet supplying sufficient essential amino acids every day of the year. So, when free amino acid levels in a cell grow low, the cell starts scavenging and recycling proteins. In adults, about three-quarters of the amino acids utilized to make protein in a day are supplied through recycling, and only about one-quarter of the supply is derived from the diet[4].

A factory manager would not wait until the production line stopped due to lack of materials to send a signal to look for supplies. A good factory manager has an inventory alert system, notifying them when supplies are low so that supplies can be timely ordered to prevent shutdowns in the production line. The cell does this, as well. When methionine supplies (manifest as SAMe) begin to get low, the cell turns up the recycling rate of old proteins. The cells know which proteins are old, as it continuously tags proteins in a process call ubiquitination, the longer the chain of ubiquitin, the older the protein.

Oxidative damage of proteins occurs as the result of reactive oxygen species (ROS) or reactive nitrogen species (RNS), that pull the protein into a different shape than would occur under normal environmental conditions. New hydrogen and disulfide bonds can form which would not have occurred during natural protein folding. The reactive oxygen species then releases, leaving the protein with an incorrect conformation that may be retained. Other oxidative reactions bind molecules to amino acids within a protein or crosslink proteins. The protein becomes dysfunctional. The ROS or RNS moves on to damage other targets of oxidation. One superoxide anion can damage millions of protein molecules per second.

These damaged proteins are usually eliminated by the normal protein turnover process, but sometimes the proteins are deformed into shapes that defy proteasomal degradation. This damage and similar oxidative damage to the DNA contribute to the process of aging. Oxidative damage to proteins, for example, causes accumulation of protein plaques in Alzheimer's disease. Oxidation injury is further discussed in Chapter 21.

Denaturing and Digesting Food Proteins

Heating proteins can break the hydrogen bonds that give proteins their three-dimensional structure; disabling their functions. Different proteins are denatured at different temperatures. When cooking eggs, ovotransferrin, a protein in the egg white, denatures at a temperature of about 65°C (150°F); ovalbumin in the yolk is denatured and coagulates around 80°C (180°F). Thus, it takes a higher temperature to cook the yolk of the egg than the white. Eggs can be cooked to have a solid white but a liquid yolk by controlling the cooking temperature and time. When eggs are cooked, some of the protein's hydrogen bonds are disrupted by the heat; when the bonds reform, random cross-linking occurs and the egg white becomes opaque and solid. With further cooking time, more crosslinking occurs; this can result in a dense, rubbery-textured egg, unfit for fine dining.

Cooking temperatures can disrupt the secondary, tertiary of quaternary structure of some, but not all proteins. Stomach acid, which is high in hydrogen protons (H^+), also denatures many proteins by disrupting hydrogen bonds. Denaturing the protein not only inhibits their function, but also may cause the primary protein structure to be more accessible to proteolytic enzymatic cleavage.

Many food proteins, especially animal proteins, can also be at least partially hydrolyzed by cooking in water; heating proteins in water or steam can hydrolyze proteins and break the covalent bonds. Stewing meat allows some of the collagen protein in tough cuts of meat to hydrolyze and turn into gelatin. This best occurs at a temperature of about 70° to 75°C (158° to 167°F) but takes several hours of cooking in a moist environment. Cow's milk is often hydrolyzed in infant formula, to decrease antigenicity. Food protein is also partially digested by fermentation processes. Many proteins are resistant to stomach acid and thus, cooking allows humans (and the animals we cook for) to digest a wider variety of foods. Cooking also denatures proteins in bacteria and most other pathogens, inactivating them and preventing infection. Some intact proteins inhibit digestion are or toxins. Some plant proteins, such as lectins and trypsin inhibitors, can be denatured or hydrolyzed through normal cooking; while others are more resistant. Legumes contain trypsin inhibitors, which are mostly inactivated by cooking at boiling temperature and are completely inactivated by cooking in a pressure cooker[5]. Nevertheless, some proteins found in foods are resistant to being denatured by heat or stomach acid and cannot be degraded sufficiently through cooking to avoid toxicity or immunogenicity. Potato trypsin inhibitors are only marginally degraded at boiling temperature.

Proteolytic Enzymes: Cooking and stomach acid help unfold proteins; this allows better access for proteolytic enzymes to act on them. Proteases digest proteins into small peptides and individual amino acids that can be absorbed and used as building blocks for new proteins. The enzyme pepsin in the stomach efficiently cleaves peptide bonds between hydrophobic aromatic amino acids such as tryptophan, tyrosine, and phenylalanine. Thus, pepsin could cleave the peptide at the open arrow shown in Figure 7-4. Later, in the small intestine, trypsin cleaves peptide bonds at the carboxyl side of arginine and lysine, as shown by the solid arrows, and thus cuts the protein chain into smaller peptides; chymotrypsin cleaves carboxyl peptide bonds on tyrosine, phenylalanine, tryptophan, methionine, and leucine. Other enzymes further disassemble the protein into its component amino acids.

Exopeptidases are enzymes that cut a single AA at a time from the end of a peptide chain. Endopeptidases cut proteins into peptides. The most active digestive proteases are pepsin from the stomach and trypsin and chymotrypsin from the pancreas. In addition to pancreatic proteolytic enzymes (Table 8-4), the intestinal mucosa has several enzymes that further disassemble peptides into individual AA's for absorption.

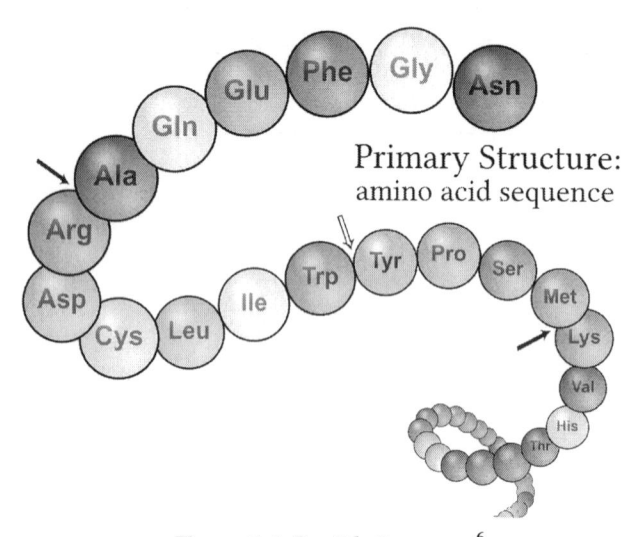

Figure 7-4: Peptide Sequence[6]

Dietary Lectins

Mannose-binding lectin (MBL) is a protein formed in the liver that is part of our innate immune system. One side of MBL binds to sugars on the surface of certain yeasts, such as *Candida albicans*, some viruses, bacteria, and parasites. The other side of the MBL protein can bind to a serine protease. When MBL binds to a target pathogen, it activates serine protease, triggering the complement cascade and the formation of a Membrane Attack Complex that creates a pore in the cell wall of the bacteria or other pathogen, leading to the cell's destruction.

Unlike immunoglobulins that can also bind specific sugars, lectins are not part of the adaptive immune system that learns to respond to pathogens in the environment. These proteins are coded in the DNA. Invertebrates, which do not have an adaptive immune system, use lectin as a major part of their innate immune response. Lectins are found in the slime covering slugs, snails, and eels[7]. We, superior beings are built outside-in; we keep our antimicrobial slime on the inside. **RegIII proteins** are formed by enterocytes and even moreso by colonocytes. These lectins bind to bacteria in the intestine prevent them from adhering to cells lining the intestine and thus preventing invasion and infection[8].

Lectins are proteins or glycoproteins (proteins with sugar complexes) capable of binding to one or more specific sugar residues. Glycoproteins are a type protein present on the surfaces of cells that the body uses to identify its own cells and differentiate them from foreign biologic matter. Glycoproteins are the reason that organ transplants are rejected if not genetically matched and that there are different and incompatible blood types. Cell membrane glycoproteins are illustrated in Figure 6-4.

Table 7-2: Examples of Human Glycoproteins

Function	Example
Structural	Collagen
Protective	Mucin produced in the intestine
Immune	Immunoglobulins (Antibodies), Histocompatibility antigens
Cell Membrane Receptors	Immunoglobulin E Receptor (Fcε)
Hormones	TSH, FSH, LH, Erythropoietin, HCG

Lectins are also common in plants. Lectins make up less than 5 percent of the proteins in most plant tissues but can make up as much as 20 to 50 percent of the proteins tubers, underground stems, and in seeds. Lectins act as protein storage units in tubers and seeds that support later growth. Since we and other animals consume many seeds and tubers, lectin proteins from plants are an important component of the diet. These typically globular proteins are resistant to digestion in the gastrointestinal tract. Lectins also serve as toxins to insects and animals, which prevent the plant from being heavily grazed upon.

Lectins bind to specific sugar chains, such as the sugar complexes that are part of cell membrane glycoproteins. Lectins can be grouped into several classes: as listed in Table 7-3. Chimeroproteins are common in plants and foods. Hololectins are of interest as they bind more than one glycoprotein, which allows them to agglutinate glycoproteins. For example, certain hololectins can bind red cells together. Some of these lectins are used for blood typing, as they will cause red blood cell types that have sugar chains which match the lectin to clump together. Hololectins are uncommon in food, as they are often toxic.

Table 7-3: Lectin Classes

Lectin	Action
Merolectins	Bind to a single glycoprotein site
Hololectins	Bind to two or more identical glycoproteins
Superlectins	Bind to two or more dissimilar glycoproteins
Chimeroproteins	A protein that is both a lectin and an enzyme; these lectins have the capacity to bind to a glycoprotein and then can act as an enzymatic.

Over one hundred food plants contain lectins; some are quite toxic if not denatured by cooking, however, cooking does not denature all lectins[9]. Most legumes; a family that includes edible peas, beans, peanuts, carob, and tamarind; are toxic. Even legumes we eat, such as kidney beans, are surprisingly toxic – when not properly prepared.

Kidney Bean Poisoning: Phytohemagglutinin (PHA) (phyto: plant; heme: blood; agglutinin: sticks together) is a plant product which causes red blood cells to stick to each other, forming clumps. PHA can activate mast cell degranulation, adding to the acute toxic reaction of PHA in the intestine. PHA is also a mitogen that activates cell division, and in sufficient doses causes toxic reactions.

Five uncooked kidney beans can be sufficient for acute toxicity in adults. The effects include extreme nausea, vomiting, and abdominal pain followed by diarrhea that begins about one to three hours after eating the beans. While effects can be severe, it generally lasts only a few hours. The immediate toxic effects of PHA are likely mediated through a combination of promoting the release of CCK[10] and provoking mast cell degranulation in the intestine.

The toxin, PHA, is destroyed by cooking the beans at boiling temperatures. Cooking at lower temperatures, as used for slow cookers, crock pots and most solar cookers, does not denature the lectin, but rather increases the bioavailability of the toxin. Cooking kidney beans at 80° C can increase their toxicity five-fold. Soaked and sprouted kidney beans are also toxic[11].

Broad beans and many other beans, also contain PHA, although in lower concentrations than in kidney beans. Cooking beans in boiling water for 10 minutes denatures the PHA and decreases its activity to non-toxic levels.

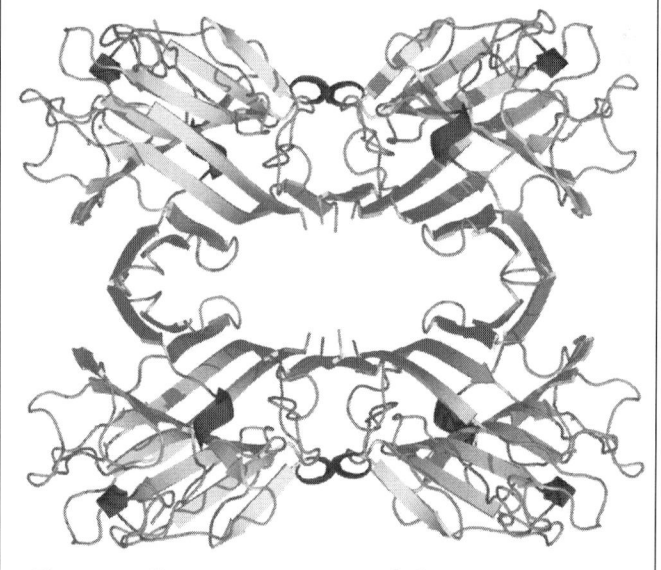

Figure 7-3: Quaternary structure of phytohemagglutinin

Rest in Peace: Type 2 RIPs (ribosome inactivating proteins) such as abrin (from the legume rosary pea) ricin (from castor oil plant), and modeccin (from various *Adenia species*) are lectins which irreversibly inactivate ribosomes, thus stopping protein synthesis and leading to cell death. These are the most potent known plant toxins. The lethal dose of abrin is 0.1 to 1.0 μg/kg orally, and many times less toxin is required to kill if injected[12]. For reference, the mass of a single, 0.3 mm, grain of table salt is about 60 to 100 μg.

Negative Health Effects of Lectins

1. Many lectins are directly toxic. Cooking reduces or eliminates the toxicity of most of the toxic lectins that are found in food items. Some other toxic plant lectins resist being denatured by cooking; thus, cannot be used as foods.

2. Lectins can induce basophils and mast cell activation. In a study of 16 lectins common in foods, five lectins including lentil lectin; phytohemagglutinin; *Pisum sativum* agglutinin from peas; and *Sambucus nigra* agglutinin from elderberries induce basophil production and the release of IL-4 and IL-13[13]. These cytokines induce T_H2 immunity and enhance immune reactivity to food; not just to these foods, but potentially to any food consumed while the immune system is primed for reactivity. Canavalin A, from jack beans; and *Solanum tuberosum* agglutinins, from potatoes, can cause mast cells to release histamine in patients with allergies[14]. Lentil, pea, wheat, and PHA lectins can induce histamine release in anergic patients[15].

3. Lectins are immunogenic: Lectins are common allergens in the diet. Lectins can induce the formation of IgA, IgE, IgG and IgM[16]. The anti-lectin IgA production, however, has been shown to be ineffective in preventing systemic absorption of dietary lectins[17]. Many food allergies are immune reactions to lectins that have been absorbed; including peanut, avocado, banana, chestnut, kiwi, peach, tomato, potato and bell pepper lectins[18].

IgG to lectins causes many food sensitivities. The immune system readily forms IgG_1 to lectins but also forms IgG_2 and IgG_4 immunoglobulins to lectins[19,20]. IgG formation to lectins can promote diverse systemic reactions (see Chapter 18; Immune Hypersensitivity Reactions). Some lectins bind to sIgA, and thus may deplete sIgA[21].

4. Lectins can act as adjuvants: Lectins can increase the immune response not only to themselves but also to other antigens. This may be useful in the development of vaccines[20] and immunity, but also may increase the antigenicity of foods, including to non-lectin proteins.

5. Lectins can impair mucosal integrity: Many lectins are absorbed intact; some lectins adhere to glycoproteins on the brush border membrane and stimulate endocytosis into the enterocyte. Once in the cell, some lectins stimulate cell growth. Different lectins bind to different populations of enterocytes at different parts of the intestine and thereby have different effects depending on the location and age of the enterocyte along the villus.

PHA and lectins in soy, wheat, and other foods stimulate and speed the growth of enterocytes and pancreatic beta cells. PHA can increase the rate of enterocyte migration on intestinal villi, decreasing the turnover from 72 hours to 12 hours. The metabolism of the cells, however, does not keep pace; enterocyte surface enzyme production levels fall, leading to maldigestion and lack of absorption of proteins and other nutrients. The integrity of the tight junctions can be lost; leading to the absorption of intact lectin proteins and other antigens[9]. Thus, lectins can increase absorption of antigens, contribute to leaky gut, increasing the risk of immune reactivity to foods.

6. Lectins can promote dysbiosis: Potatoes and soy lectins inhibit trypsin, and thus, inhibit the activity of proteases, lowering the digestion and absorption of proteins. The immaturity of enterocytes it causes further decreases nutrient digestion and absorption. Lectins that disrupt the mucosal barrier may allow bacteria to enter the body from the lumen of the intestine[6]. Malabsorption of nutrients alters the population of bacteria and promotes bacterial overgrowth and dysbiosis (Chapters 23 and 24). These proteins are then available for fermentation by gut bacteria and thus increase the growth and proliferation of toxin-producing *Clostridium* bacteria[22]. Both lectins from potatoes and soy have been shown to induce the intestinal growth of *Clostridium perfringens* and development of pseudomembranous colitis in animals[23,24]. PHA promotes the overgrowth of *E coli*[25].

7. Lectins that are absorbed have systemic effects: Lectins that bind to receptors on the surface of the microvilli may then be absorbed by endocytosis. These proteins may then be exported into the lamina propria where they can be presented as antigens, or they may also gain access to the circulation.

Additionally, lectins can have a direct action on the pancreas and other organs. High oral intakes of PHA (over 500 mg per kg body weight) resulted in the loss of about 30 percent of skeletal muscle mass in rats fed kidney bean diets for ten days. Cardiac muscle may also be affected. PHA decreases the rate of muscle protein synthesis. Peanut lectin increased the growth of smooth muscle and pulmonary arterial cells in animals. Lectins can also cause atrophy of the thymus and spleen[6].

8. Airborne Lectins: Lectins from grain dust (oats, barley, wheat, and corn) can induce baker's asthma and hypersensitivity pneumonitis[26].

Beneficial Health Effects of Lectins

At very low doses, some toxic lectins may have beneficial effects; while other lectins appear to be non-toxic. Lectins from tomatoes, garlic, and peas, have either low toxicity or are non-toxic.

1. Some lectins bind to bacteria and viruses: Many plant lectins adhere to glycoproteins on the surface of bacteria and may prevent the formation of biofilms. Lectins that bind to *Streptococcus mutans*, for example, may prevent dental plaque formation. Similarly, lectins that bind to bacteria in the intestine can act similarly to IgA, preventing bacterial overgrowth. These are usually non-toxic lectins, which do not bind to human cell glycoproteins, but rather, bind to bacterial glycoproteins. Merolectins that are not absorbed may prevent infections. Lectins in bananas increase T cell growth and adhere to the gp120 glycoprotein of the HIV virus, preventing its entry into the cell and inhibiting HIV replication[27].

2. Some lectins promote enterocyte development: Lectins from garlic increase the production of enterocyte disaccharidases and other digestive enzymes. Other lectins may aid in the regrowth of the intestinal mucosa[18] without being toxic, as is PHA that causes excessive proliferation of immature enterocytes.

3. Some lectins promote pancreatic islet cell development: Diets high in the consumption of bean proteins are associated with lower blood lipid levels. Low levels of PHA, as those levels found in properly cooked beans, may improve glucose tolerance.

Nevertheless, while some lectins are beneficial, as with any protein, idiosyncratic immune responses may develop to them, causing allergy or antergy (Chapter 19).

Table 7-5: A Sample of Edible Foods Containing Lectins

Common Name	Latin Name	Notes
Legumes		
Garden pea, split pea, snow pea	*Pisum sativum*	Promotes T_H2 response[11] Agglutinates bacteria
Horse bean, fava bean	*Vicia faba*	In G6PD deficiency, non-lectin toxin provokes hemolytic anemia.
Horse gram	*Macrotyloma uniflorum*	Toxic if not cooked properly. Eaten and fed cooked to animals in India.
Hyacinth bean	*Lablab purpureus*	Toxic if not cooked properly.
Jack bean	*Canavalia ensiformis*	Toxic if not cooked properly.
Kidney bean	*Phaseolus vulgaris*	Toxic if not cooked properly, Mast cell degranulation (uncooked)
Lentil	*Lens culinaris*	Promotes T_H2 response
Lima bean	*Phaseolus lunatus*	Toxic if not cooked properly.
Mung bean	*Phaseolus aureus*	Sprouts, eaten raw.
Peanut	*Arachis hypogaea*	Allergen, Mitogen
Scarlet runner bean	*Phaseolus coccineus*	
Soyabean	*Glycine max*	Toxic if not cooked properly. Contains a lectin that is a trypsin inhibitor.
Winged bean	*Lotus tetragonolobus*	
Monocotyledons		
Barley	*Hordeum vulgare*	
Rice	*Oryza sativa*	
Wheat	*Triticum vulgaris*	Toxic to enterocytes, an immune adjuvant.
Garlic	*Allium sativum*	
Banana	*Musa acuminata × balbisiana*	T cell mitogen, Anti-HIV
Other Plants		
Tomato	*Solanum lycopersicum*	Agglutinates bacteria
Potato	*Solanum tuberosum*	Lectin can cause mast cell degranulation. This lectin inhibits trypsin.
Elderberry	*Sambucus nigra*	Five different lectins have been identified from the bark, fruit, and seeds. SNA-II in the bark is quite toxic. SNA-V in the fruit may have anti-proliferative properties[28].
Avocado	*Persea americana*	Allergen
Bell Pepper	*Capsicum*	Allergen
Peach	*Prunus persica*	Allergen
Carrot	*Daccus carota*	Agglutinates bacteria

Other Dietary Proteins

Dietary proteins from animal sources can be immunogenic. Most animal protein is cooked before eating to kill pathogens. This process also inactivates most enzymes, makes the amino acids more available for digestion, and often improves flavor. Fish is sometimes prepared as ceviche; rather than cooking with heat, the muscle tissue is pickled in acidic vegetable juice which denatures the proteins. This process may not kill some pathogens that may be present. Raw milk is sometimes consumed, or only briefly heated in the pasteurization process. Pasteurization kills most pathogenic bacteria but does not denature the proteins in milk. Boiling milk changes its flavor, denaturing some of the proteins.

Although not usually eaten raw, egg yolks contain IgY. These are immunoglobulins passed from the hen to the chick and help prevent susceptibility to diseases to which the hen has been exposed. Oral treatment using IgY from hen eggs can provide passive immunity to other animals, protecting them and helping them recover from enteric diseases and bacterial toxins[29,30]. Protein from raw eggs is poorly digested and absorbed in humans.

Some protein function may remain even after cooking. Avidin, a protein in egg whites, binds the B vitamin biotin and prevents its absorption and availability. Consumption of raw egg whites can cause biotin deficiency[31]. Avidin retains much of its ability to bind biotin even after common methods of preparing eggs for consumption[32].

Proteins in milk, eggs, pork, fish, and shellfish are common allergens. Some fish allergies are actually immune reactions to parasites infesting the fish, rather than to the fish's own proteins. (See Chapter 11)

Enzymes are another group of proteins that may be consumed. Animal enzymes are usually denatured by cooking. Plants also contain enzymes, however, unlike meat; fruits are commonly consumed raw. Enzymes in fruit are usually denatured by stomach acidity but may be active in the mouth and throat, where they may act on local tissue. This enzyme activity is discussed in Chapter 16.

Protein Malabsorption

If protein is not absorbed in the small intestine, it passes into the large intestine where most of it is fermented by bacteria. Since fermentation is specialized by the substrate, these proteins alter the balance of microbiota in the intestine. Protein fermentation favors the growth of *Clostridia* species and the formation of toxins.

When amino acids are fermented in the colon, most are converted to ammonia, although some are converted into bioamines, and tryptophan is converted into indolamines. (See Table 13-3) Ammonia is toxic to the colonocytes and can disrupt the mucus protecting these cells from bacteria. Ammonia is easily metabolized by the liver, but in susceptible individuals, such as adults with liver disease, ammonia levels can rise and are toxic to the brain, causing hepatic encephalopathy. Infants have limited capacity to detoxify ammonia and can have neurologic damage from ammonia production that arises from intestinal fermentation of protein. (Chapter 35 has further discussion of the effects of ammonia on the brain).

Cysteine and methionine are sulfur-containing amino acids, and intestinal fermentation of these amino acids produces foul smelling, sulfurous flatulence.

Plant proteins are more likely to resist digestion than animal proteins. As noted above, many lectins resist digestion. Plants produce antinutritional proteins to prevent insects and other animals from feeding upon them, preventing the enzymatic degradation of nutrients. Many of these are trypsin inhibitors, and several of these also inhibit chymotrypsin activity. Table 23-3 list several foods with trypsin/chymotrypsin inhibitory activity. It has been proposed that chymotrypsin inhibitors may act as anti-carcinogenic agents, and thereby explain the lower incidence of cancer in populations that consume tofu made from soybean[33].

Inhibition of trypsin also allows for increased release of cholecystokinin (CCK) from the I cells of the intestine. This can cause early satiety. CCK acts in a feedback loop with digestive enzyme production in the pancreas. CCK stimulates the production of pancreatic enzymes, including trypsin. Animals fed unprocessed soy protein fail to grow but have enlarged pancreases, as a result of a trypsin inhibitors in soy protein[34]. Trypsin is essential to digesting as it activates several other digestive enzymes.

[1] Identification and characterization of somatic steroid 5alpha-reductase (SRD5A2) mutations in human prostate cancer tissue. Makridakis N, Akalu A, Reichardt JK. Oncogene. 2004 Sep 23;23(44):7399-405. PMID:15326487

[2] Cystic fibrosis. Rowe SM, Miller S, Sorscher EJ. N Engl J Med. 2005 May 12;352(19):1992-2001. PMID:15888700

[3] Quantification of protein half-lives in the budding yeast proteome. Belle A, Tanay A, Bitincka L, Shamir R, O'Shea EK. Proc Natl Acad Sci U S A. 2006 Aug 29;103(35): 13004-9. PMID:16916930

[4] Metabolic demands for amino acids and the human dietary requirement: Millward and Rivers (1988) revisited. Millward DJ. J Nutr. 1998 Dec;128(12 Suppl):2563S-2576S. PMID:9868206

[5] Thermal inactivation of lectins and trypsin inhibitor activity during steam processing of dry beans (Phaseolus vulgaris) and effects on protein quality. Van Der Poel T, Blonk J, Van Oort MG. 53(2)215-28. 1990 J Sci Food Agric.

[6] Illustration by Mariana Ruiz Villarreal, adapted by Author.

[7] Reconstruction of a probable ancestral form of conger eel galectins revealed their rapid adaptive evolution process for specific carbohydrate recognition. Konno A, Ogawa T, Shirai T, Muramoto K. Mol Biol Evol. 2007 Nov;24(11):2504-14. PMID:17827170

[8] The antibacterial lectin RegIIIgamma promotes the spatial segregation of microbiota and host in the intestine. Vaishnava S, Yamamoto M, Severson KM, et al. Science. 2011 Oct 14;334(6053):255-8. PMID:21998396

[9] Biological Effects of Plant Lectins on the Gastrointestinal Tract:Metabolic Consequences and Applications. Pusztai, A., Bardocz, S. Trends Glycosci. Glycotechnol.8:149-165.

[10] Red kidney bean lectin is a potent cholecystokinin releasing stimulus in the rat inducing pancreatic growth. Herzig KH, Bardocz S, Grant G, etal. Gut. 1997 Sep;41(3):333-8. PMID:9378388

[11] Bad Bug Book: Foodborne Pathogenic Microorganisms and Natural Toxins Handbook. FDA. http://www.fda.gov/food/foodsafety/foodborneillness/foodborneillnes sfoodbornepathogensnaturaltoxins/badbugbook/ucm071092.htm

[12] Abrin poisoning. Dickers KJ, Bradberry SM, Rice P, Griffiths GD, Vale JA. Toxicol Rev. 2003;22(3):137-42. PMID:15181663

[13] Dietary lectins can induce in vitro release of IL-4 and IL-13 from human basophils. Haas H, Falcone FH, Schramm G, et al. Eur J Immunol. 1999 Mar;29(3):918-27. PMID:10092096

[14] Potato lectin activates basophils and mast cells of atopic subjects by its interaction with core chitobiose of cell-bound non-specific immunoglobulin E. Pramod SN, Venkatesh YP, Mahesh PA. Clin Exp Immunol. 2007 Jun;148(3):391-401. PMID:17362264

[15] Interaction of lectins with human IgE: IgE-binding property and histamine-releasing activity of twelve plant lectins. Shibasaki M, Sumazaki R, Isoyama S, Takita H. Int Arch Allergy Immunol. 1992;98(1):18-25. PMID:1378039

[16] Antinutritional properties of plant lectins. Vasconcelos IM, Oliveira JT. Toxicon. 2004 Sep 15;44(4):385-403. PMID:15302522

[17] Modulation of immune function by dietary lectins in rheumatoid arthritis. Cordain L, Toohey L, Smith MJ, Hickey MS. Br J Nutr. 2000 Mar;83(3):207-17. PMID:10884708

[18] The latex-fruit syndrome. Wagner S, Breiteneder H. Biochem Soc Trans. 2002 Nov;30(Pt 6):935-40. PMID:12440950

[19] The potent IgG4-inducing antigen in banana is a mannose-binding lectin, BanLec-I. Koshte VL, Aalbers M, Calkhoven PG, et al. Int Arch Allergy Immunol. 1992;97(1):17-24. PMID:1582693

[20] The identification of plant lectins with mucosal adjuvant activity. Lavelle EC, Grant G, Pusztai A, Pfüller U, O'Hagan DT. Immunology. 2001 Jan;102(1):77-86.PMID:11168640

[21] The high lectin-binding capacity of human secretory IgA protects nonspecifically mucosae against environmental antigens. Davin JC, Senterre J, Mahieu PR. Biol Neonate. 1991;59(3):121-5. PMID:2054423

[22] Effect of trypsin inhibitor activity in soya bean on growth performance, protein digestibility and incidence of sub-clinical necrotic enteritis in broiler chicken flocks. Palliyeguru MW, Rose SP, Mackenzie AM. Br Poult Sci. 2011 Jun 1;52(3):359-67. PMID:21732882

[23] Effect of diets containing potato protein or soya bean meal on the incidence of spontaneously-occurring subclinical necrotic enteritis and the physiological response in broiler chickens. Fernando PS, Rose SP, Mackenzie AM, Silva SS. Br Poult Sci. 2011 Feb;52(1):106-14. PMID:21337205

[24] Effect of dietary protein concentrates on the incidence of subclinical necrotic enteritis and growth performance of broiler chickens. Palliyeguru MW, Rose SP, Mackenzie AM. Poult Sci. 2010 Jan;89(1):34-43. PMID:20008800

[25] Antinutritional properties of plant lectins. Vasconcelos IM, Oliveira JT. Toxicon. 2004 Sep 15;44(4):385-403. PMID:15302522

[26] Composition of extracts of airborne grain dusts: lectins and lymphocyte mitogens. Olenchock SA, Lewis DM, Mull JC. Environ Health Perspect. 1986 Apr;66:119-23. PMID:3709474

[27] A lectin isolated from bananas is a potent inhibitor of HIV replication. Swanson MD, Winter HC, Goldstein IJ, Markovitz DM. J Biol Chem. 2010 Mar 19;285(12):8646-55. PMID:20080975

[28] Ambucus nigra Agglutinin II and related lectins and their potential contribution to medicinal benefits of the elder tree. Elrod S. http://susanme.myweb.uga.edu/bcmb8010/report.pdf

[29] Specific egg yolk immunoglobulin as a new preventive approach for Shiga-toxin-mediated diseases. Neri P, Tokoro S, Kobayashi R, et al. PLoS One. 2011;6(10):e26526. PMID:22028896

[30] Egg Yolk Antibodies for Passive Immunity. Kovacs-Nolan J, Mine Y. Annu Rev Food Sci Technol. 2011 Mar 2. PMID:22136128

[31] Marginal biotin deficiency can be induced experimentally in humans using a cost-effective outpatient design. Stratton SL, Henrich CL, Matthews NI, etal. J Nutr. 2012 Jan;142(1):22-6. PMID:22157538

[32] Kinetics of thermal inactivation of avidin. T.D. Durance, N.S. Wong. Food Research International. 1992 Vol.25(2):89-92.

[33] The Bowman-Birk inhibitor from soybeans as an anticarcinogenic agent. Kennedy AR. Am J Clin Nutr. 1998 Dec;68(6 Suppl):1406S-1412S. PMID:9848508

[34] Trypsin inhibitors: concern for human nutrition or not? Liener IE. J Nutr. 1986 May;116(5):920-3. PMID:3517253

8. Appetite, Satiation, Satiety, and Pancreatic Exocrine Function

Hunger is a central and primal behavioral force; a force that compels animals to take risks and expose themselves to danger. Even for predators, hunting is a hazardous enterprise. Hunger is the voice, perhaps, of our strongest instinctual imperative. Aversion, fear, or will power only offset this drive temporarily. Starvation endangers survival, and the brain has adapted to mitigate this risk; sexual behavior and fertility diminish as famine is a poor time for pregnancy and raising young offspring. Famine-induced behavior engages; promoting energy conservation, lower activity, and depression, especially among females. Under starvation stress, males tend to become more aggressive.

Nevertheless, for most of the last century, dieters have been admonished to limit their food intake, count calories, and go hungry to lose excess weight. This strategy has provided the outcome one might expect; hunger, depression, and irritability, but little long-term weight loss.

It is hard to persevere against hunger and avoid eating when food is at hand, and really, it is only a matter of time before we succumb to it. Hunger and satiation are controlled by neurohormonal mechanisms, and one needs to be a saint or a fool to attempt to overcome these basic, primal mandates. Even when some weight has been lost, it is almost always gained back, often with additional weight gain. The key to understanding the epidemic of obesity requires understanding of the neurohormonal system that controls appetite and satiation and how the Western diet upsets these signals.

A Delicate Balance

Satiation and satiety give the state or feeling that one has had enough to eat and puts hunger to rest. The mechanisms that make us feel satisfied, signaling that we have had enough to eat and which dispel hunger, are essential in balancing our food energy requirements to avoiding either energy deficits or over consumption. Thus, the appetite/satiety mechanism helps avoid malnutrition and obesity.

In nature, even in areas where food is plentiful, wild animals are rarely obese. The neurohormonal feedback system, controlled by the hypothalamus and enteric nervous system, helps balance energy requirements. In natural conditions and times of adequate food supply, an individual's adult weight can remain stable over a 50-year period. This seems remarkable when one considers that if an extra 10 calories of energy a day were stored, just one extra bite of food and well less than $1/100^{th}$ of the daily intake; 50 pounds of excess fat would be accumulated over those 50 years. The neurohormonal appetite/satiation system can closely regulate energy needs and utilization.

There are both short- and long-term mediators of appetite and satiation. *Satiation* response to a meal comes from a feeling of fullness and sense of having had enough to eat; it engages soon after a meal has started. There is also a longer-term brake limiting appetite, referred to as *Satiety*; the effects of which last over a period of days.

The short-term factors that regulate hunger and appetite control how much is eaten during a given meal, and affect which foods are most highly desired. The longer-term factors of satiety are like a thermostat that sets the level at which satiety is lost, and hunger appears. It is the longer-term factors that may have the most bearing on obesity and especially on metabolically dangerous abdominal obesity.

Feeding behavior and hunger are mostly controlled by hormonal actions in the hypothalamus; however, other hormones acting in the liver, pancreas, gastrointestinal tract, and adipocytes interact to affect this system. Over two dozen hormones, affecting hunger, satiation and satiety, have been identified that act on the gastrointestinal system. Table 8-1 lists some important hormones affecting appetite.

Satiation: Having Enough to Eat at a Meal

Ending a meal depends on the short-term signals of *satiation*. These signals include a central feeling of satisfaction from hormones, such as cholecystokinin (CCK), glucagon-like peptide 1 (GLP-1), gastrin-releasing peptide (GRP), and neuromedin B (NMB), and fullness from stomach distension.

CCK is the master orchestrator of satiation, although many of its effects are mediated through other hormones. For example, CCK inhibits ghrelin and stimulates PYY in humans[1]. CCK acts on the brain and on the vagus nerve to increase satiation. The vagus nerve helps retain food in the stomach by tightening the gastro-duodenal (pyloric) sphincter, helping to promote a sense of fullness. CCK also acts as a hormone; it increases peptic acid output and triggers the release of pancreatic enzymes and bile into the duodenum, thus helping with the digestion of proteins, carbohydrates, fats, and nucleic acids.

In a study in which CCK activity was blocked, the subjects consumed 22.5 percent more food during their meals. For an average adult, this would be similar to consuming an extra 82 days worth of food in a year; enough to add an extra 40 pounds in excess weight gain over a single year.

Table 8-1: Hunger, Satiation, and Satiety Hormones

Hormone	Promotes Satiation
Cholecystokinin (CCK)	Produced by *I cells* in the small intestine. Causes the release of digestive enzymes from the pancreas and bile from the gallbladder; acts on the vagal nerve to the brain stem to slow gastric emptying to help promote fullness and slow digestion; signal satiety and suppress hunger.
Gastrin Releasing Peptide (GRP)	GRP is produced by postganglionic fibers of the vagus nerve. Inhibits gastric emptying and increases peptic acid production through the release of gastrin. Acts on the hypothalamus to signal satiety. Also affects GI motility, circadian rhythm, and thermoregulation.
Neuromedin B (NMB)	Produced by adipocytes. Signals satiety at the hypothalamus and affects GI motility. NMB suppresses TSH output.
Glucagon-like peptide-1 (GLP-1)	GLP-1 is an incretin, produced by *L cells* in the ileum. It increases insulin secretion from the pancreas and decreases glucagon release. GLP-1 helps to signal satiety in the brain. GLP-1 increases insulin output and insulin sensitivity while decreasing glucagon output from the pancreas.
Peptide YY (PYY$_{3-36}$)	Produced by *L cells* in the ileum and large intestine after meals. Inhibits appetite through action on the hypothalamus. Also, inhibits the release of pancreatic enzymes and bile, and decreases gastric emptying, while inhibiting gastric motility and slows digestion. PYY increases water and electrolyte absorption from the colon.
Leptin	Produced primarily by adipocytes in the white adipose tissue, but also by ovaries, skeletal muscles, stomach, and other tissue. Leptin acts on the hypothalamus inhibiting appetite by counteracting the effect of neuropeptide Y (NPY). Leptin helps regulate *long-term* energy needs and appetite level.
Pancreatic polypeptide (PP)	Released from the pancreas under vagal stimulation. Inhibits food intake and stimulates energy expenditures. Released in response to chewing certain foods, especially sweet palatable foods, but not chewing sweet gum or drinking sweet drinks.
Des-acyl Ghrelin	Des-acyl Ghrelin is an anorexigenic peptide which is released in the fed state and response to low pH in the stomach[2], as occurs after a meal. Des-acyl ghrelin inhibits stomach motility in the fasted state. **Note:** Ghrelin, des-acyl ghrelin, and obestatin are derived from a common prohormone; preproghrelin, originating in gastric endocrine cells. These peptides have different and opposite actions. Many studies of ghrelin have used probes which did not differentiate between des-acyl ghrelin and acyl ghrelin, and thus, results from those studies can be confusing.

Table 8-2: Hormones which Promote Hunger

Hormone	Promotes Hunger and Feeding
Ghrelin (Acyl-Ghrelin)	Produced by *P/D1 cells* lining the fundus of stomach and pancreas. Stimulates hunger by acting on the hypothalamus and by counteracting the effects of leptin and *PYY$_{3-36}$*. Ghrelin stimulates gastroduodenal motility in both in the fed and fasted states[3].
Somatostatin	Somatostatin is produced by *Delta cells* in gastric glands in the stomach. It inhibits the release of gastrin from the stomach; secretin and cholecystokinin in the duodenum; and glucagon from the pancreas.
Neuropeptide Y (NPY)	NPY is produced in the arcuate nucleus of the hypothalamus. NPY is an important up-regulator of food intake. Increased production and release of NPY is associated with obesity. Leptin is an inverse agonist of NPY.
Agouti-related peptide (AgRP)	AgRP is produced in the arcuate nucleus of the hypothalamus, along with Neuropeptide Y. It increases appetite and decreases energy expenditures. AgRP is a potent and *long-lasting appetite stimulator*. It is inhibited by leptin and activated by ghrelin.

CCK release in high levels can induce anxiety[4]. Anxiety acts as a signal that can help to terminate meals. Vigilance is an adaptive advantage for wild animals that are at high risk of attack by predators or competitors for the same food. Animals become warier once they have eaten sufficient food. Thus, animals often leave areas where food is available after satisfying their hunger.

High levels of CCK can cause nausea. Bacterial fermentation of protein produces polyamines; this occurs in spoiling meat. These polyamines can increase the release of CCK[5], and thereby increase in stomach acid, prevent food from emptying into the duodenum giving a sense of fullness that limits the meal size, and can cause visceral pain and nausea. The increase in stomach acid and longer retention time helps to kill bacteria that may be in the meal. Nausea can induce vomiting of the contaminated food. CCK promotes pain transmission and conditioned place avoidance[6], causing animals to avoid food from the places where it made them ill.

Neuromedin B (NMB) from the adipose tissue[7] and gastrin-releasing peptide (GRP) are released during feeding. They act similarly to CCK and are likely secondary messengers of CCK in producing satiation. These two peptides stimulate the bombesin receptors (BB1 and BB2)[8] present in the brain. Both receptors regulate satiety and GI motility.

The BB1 receptor is most sensitive to NMB and also regulates TSH output. The BB2 receptor is most specific to GRP and helps regulate pancreatic output and gastric acid release through gastrin. GRP also mediates circadian rhythm response to light and thermoregulation. A third receptor, BB3, present in the enteric nervous system, helps regulate satiety, glucose and insulin regulation, GI motility, and energy homeostasis.

Glucagon-like peptide-1 (GLP-1) also promotes satiation. It inhibits acid secretion and gastric emptying in the stomach and decreases food intake by signaling the brain. GLP-1 promotes storage of glucose by promoting insulin release, inhibits glucagon release and improves insulin sensitivity. Medications that protect GLP-1 are used in the treatment of diabetes; dipeptidyl peptidase-4 (DDP-4) breaks down GLP-1; DDP-4 inhibitors extend the very short half-life of GLP-1.

GLP-1 is produced primarily and released from L cells in the ileum, in response to anticipation of a meal[9], and also released in the presence of carbohydrates and fat in the ileum. It stimulates the islet cells in the pancreas to secrete insulin, helping lower blood glucose concentrations after carbohydrate ingestion. GLP-1 is thought to reduce stomach and gut motility, slowing the release of food from the stomach into the intestines to avoid large boluses of nutrients that could cause large swings in blood sugar levels, but also to prevent malabsorption. A GLP-1 infusion given with a meal was found to reduce energy intake by about twelve percent as compared to placebo[10]. Treatment with prebiotics that promote the proliferation of beneficial bacteria reduce bacterial populations associated with GI mucosal inflammation and increase GLP-1 production[11].

CCK Response to Diet

Amino Acids: CCK promotes satiety when it is released in response to certain nutrients in the proximal small intestine (SI). The aromatic amino acids, tryptophan, phenylalanine stimulate the release of CCK[12] through a calcium-sensing receptor. The first proteolytic enzyme during digestion is pepsin, which specifically cleaves aromatic amino acids in proteins, allowing for the early release of CCK upon the entry of these AA into the duodenum.

Cooking denatures many proteins found in food. In general, this allows better access for enzymes to lyse them. Amino acids, released along with released nucleotides from DNA and RNA, are important in giving the umami (or savory) flavor[13] to stews and soups. These easily available amino acids allow for early satiation. Rapid cooking methods for meat do not hydrolyze the proteins, and thus a person is more likely to eat more before the sense of satiety occurs.

Long Chain Unsaturated Free Fatty Acids: Long-chain unsaturated and n-3 free fatty acids (FFA) stimulate the release of CCK via specific brush border receptors on I cells in the duodenum that then stimulates GLP-1[14]. Medium-chain FFA do not stimulate CCK release[15]. Both mono- and polyunsaturated fatty acids appear to be equally effective in eliciting release of CCK. These long-chain fatty acids also induce the release of secretin, which triggers the release of bicarbonate from the pancreas[16]. Some CCK is released when long-chain and n-3 FFA are absorbed through the oral mucosa; more is released when these FFA enter the ileum[17]. N-3 FFA are more effective in promoting satiation than are unsaturated or N-6 fatty acids[18].

The hydrolysis of fat (triglycerides) by lipase is a critical step for fat-induced release of CCK, inhibition of ghrelin, and stimulation of GLP-1 and PYY. CCK stimulates release of pancreatic lipase and other pancreatic enzymes as well as bicarbonate. Dietary fats are triglycerides and must be first broken down by lipase for them to affect the release of CCK. The chewing of food increases the release of lingual lipase and the absorption of FFA through the oral mucosa.

Proteins: CCK release can also be triggered by certain intact proteins. In one case, the protein is a protease inhibitor present in potatoes. In a study of satiation that compared several common foods, boiled potatoes gave the highest satiation index for a given caloric intake, yielding a score three times higher than expected for its caloric content[19]. The reason appears to be the result of a protease inhibitor in potatoes[20] that survives the cooking process and triggers CCK release. Raw potatoes, which contain several protease inhibitors, may prevent the utilization of dietary proteins and should not be eaten. Fried potatoes provide less satiation than boiled or mashed potatoes[21]. The potato protease inhibitor's effect may be specific to this protein (a carboxypeptidase inhibitor) rather than from its enzymatic nature, as some other intact proteins can also affect CCK release beyond the aromatic AA effect[22].

Polyamines: Some polyamines can trigger the release of CCK[5]. These are present not only in rotting meat (to be avoided), but also in foods in which bacterial fermentation is intentional, such as in several highly flavored types of cheese. (Polyamines are further discussed in Chapter 13)

Ghrelin

Ghrelin release rises before meals and falls in response to certain foods. Although ghrelin stimulates appetite, it does not seem to cause a significant increase in consumption, but rather affects which foods we crave. Ghrelin is associated with pleasure and reward in the brain. Blocking ghrelin receptors in the brain suppresses reward-seeking behavior, including the consumption of reward foods, alcohol, nicotine, and perhaps, drugs of abuse. Ghrelin promotes the selection of food indulgences: sweets and foods with high palatability, including those high in saturated fats, which tend to be associated with obesity[23, 24]. Elevated ghrelin levels put an individual at risk, not only of dietary excesses but also at risk for increased appetite for alcohol and other substances of abuse.

Insulin reduces ghrelin release while glucagon increases it; thus, ghrelin may help regulate blood sugar via its influence on appetite. Sugar and fats in a meal lower ghrelin levels, dependent upon the individual's insulin sensitivity[25]. Therefore, insulin resistance increases appetite for and decreases response to, sweets and fats.

Improving Satiation

To improve satiation, plan meals that stimulate early release of CCK. Use long chain unsaturated and n-3 fats, especially in the first part of the meal. Chewing is important to release lingual lipase so that FFA can be absorbed. Aromatic amino acids promote CCK release from cells in the intestines. Boiled and baked potatoes trigger CCK release as does spermidine from cheese, peas, and soy.

Saturated fats, especially short chain fatty acids, do not trigger CCK release, and thus, do not promote satiation. Hydrogenated fats are often used in the fast food industry and packaged foods, as they give a long shelf life and resist smoking when heated. These hydrogenated fats do not stimulate CCK, or aid in satiation but are easily stored as fats. Sweets and carbohydrates stimulate little if any, CCK release and thus do not promote satiation.

Ghrelin is released when blood sugar is low, and this stimulates hunger. Allowing hunger to persist too long increases the appetite for sweet, fatty, palatable foods; foods that quickly increase blood sugar, have less effect on satiation, and are more likely to lead to storage of fat. Skipping meals, or waiting until one feels famished to eat, is likely to induce consumption of highly palatable, reward foods that do not satisfy the appetite, provide low-quality nutrition, and increase caloric intake.

Satiety: Long-term Appetite Balance

Leptin: Leptin is a hormone, produced by fat cells, that signals the brain that the fat cells are full. Leptin is also produced by the placenta, ovaries, skeletal muscles, liver, pituitary, and bone marrow. Lab mice bred with a gene defect that prevents them from making leptin become grossly obese. The brain interprets low leptin levels as an indicator of depleted fat reserves. Leptin Injections to leptin-deficient rats allows them to return to a normal weight.

Leptin is the major long-term satiety hormone. Leptin acts on the hypothalamus where it inhibits appetite by displacing NPY, a potent signal of hunger. Leptin regulates energy requirements over longer time periods (days to weeks), unlike most other appetite regulators, which affect appetite over minutes to hours.

Leptin levels correlate to body fat mass: the more body fat, the higher the leptin levels. Conversely, ghrelin (which acts as a short-term appetite stimulant) has lower levels with obesity. Thus, high leptin levels normally lower appetite, while high ghrelin levels increase appetite, especially for foods associated with the replenishment of fat stores. Some obesity may be caused by leptin resistance.

AgRP: AgRP has a long-term stimulatory effect on appetite and decreases metabolic activity and energy expenditure. Injections of AgRP in rats have been shown to cause hyperphagia that persists for a week. Acute inflammatory response to cytokine IL-1β causes an increase in production of AgRP but delays its release. This causes a temporary anorexia during disease, followed by an increased appetite when the inflammation resolves[26]. Thus, an animal would eat less while acutely ill or after injury, but would have increased appetite when well enough to seek food, and then seek protein and energy required for tissue repair.

AgRP stimulates hypothalamic-pituitary-adrenocortical axis release of ACTH and cortisol. AgRP may promote fat storage obesity through its action as an inverse agonist for the melanocortin receptors, MC3R and MC4R.

NPY: Neuropeptide Y is produced in the same hypothalamic nuclease as AgRP. Repeated or chronic stress and high-fat, high-sugar diets stimulate the release of neuropeptide Y, causing fat storage and fat build-up in the abdomen. NPY production is down-regulated by corticotropin-releasing hormone (CRH). High levels of glucocorticoids inhibit CRH and thus promote NPY release. Elevated NPY is associated with obesity, especially with the metabolically active, abdominal obesity, associated with insulin resistance, type 2 diabetes, hypercholesterolemia, and hypertension. NPY release may be higher in those with insulin resistance.

Pancreatic polypeptide (PP) acts under central nervous system (CNS) control through the vagus nerve, in response to eating sweet foods. Although still poorly understood, sweet, palatable foods that are chewed elicit this response (even when using artificial sweeteners). If salty or excessively sweet (and thus unpalatable), the same test food does not cause PP release. Sweet drinks and sweet chewing gum also do not promote PP release. Sucking and salivation may be important for PP release. PP is thought to trigger the release of insulin, in preparation of the incoming load of glucose from a meal and decreases the desire for sweets[27]. Ghrelin levels may also be lowered by this mechanism, also acting to decrease the desire for sweets.

Thus, sweet beverages do not prepare the body for a glucose load and do not satisfy the appetite. A similar CNS mechanism may promote the release of des-acyl ghrelin when foods with umami or salty flavor are eaten. Des-acyl ghrelin stimulates gastric vagal activity and thus stimulates satiation, increases pyloric pressure, and thus fullness.

- Food with an umami flavor, typical of foods rich in protein, stimulates the activity of the pancreatic, gastric, and hepatic branches of the vagal nerve.
- Sweet taste also increases the activity of the pancreatic and hepatic branches of the vagal nerve but inhibits the gastric branch.
- Salty tastes stimulate vagal taste nerve activity but decrease pancreatic and hepatic vagal activity[28].
- Some FFA from fatty foods increase CCK release.

Thus, the taste of the food helps the digestive organs prepare for the work ahead.

Sleep and Appetite

Getting sufficient sleep is crucial to maintaining a healthy weight and controlling appetite, as sleep and appetite are interrelated. Food-seeking behavior, activity, and vigilance during the daylight are coordinated with wakefulness; while satiety and sleep are associated with darkness[29]. Not only is appetite suppressed at night, growth hormone, TSH, T3 and leptin peak during the first half of the night, accompanied by a decline in ghrelin. Melatonin, at night, slows intestinal activity. Cortisol output peaks in the morning, followed by low levels during the day.

Orexin A and B are neuroexcitatory hormones produced in the lateral and posterior hypothalamus. Orexin is important in maintaining wakefulness. Orexin stimulates wakefulness, energy utilization, activity, and increased body temperature. There are only a small number of orexin producing neurons in the brain; about 10,000 to 20,000. Narcolepsy appears to be caused by autoimmune injury these orexin producing neurons; individuals having the HLA-DQB1*0602 type are at highest risk. Leptin inhibits the production of orexin; while ghrelin activates it. Thus, satiation helps with sleep but hunger promotes wakefulness.

Leptin, the long-term satiety hormone, has a diurnal cycle with a morning minimum, and in normal circumstances, a peak output during the sleep cycle. Sleep deprivation decreases the serum leptin levels and insulin sensitivity[30].

Short sleep is also associated with a decline in leptin and an increase in ghrelin. A crossover study compared two nights of either four or ten hours in bed. After short-sleep nights, leptin levels were 18 percent lower, and ghrelin levels 28 percent higher than with long-sleep nights. Short-sleep nights were associated with increased appetite, with a 24 percent increase in caloric intake; carbohydrate consumption increased by a third[31]. Even moderate sleep deficits reduce leptin and raise ghrelin levels, and when chronic, are associated with an increase in body mass[32]. Children who sleep fewer hours have been found to be more obese in follow-up several years later. Less than 12 hours of sleep in infants is associated with a higher body mass index (BMI) at age 3; less than 10.5 hours of sleep a day at age 3 is associated with a higher BMI at ages 7 and 9. Third graders who get less sleep are more likely to be overweight in the 6th grade[33]. Delayed bedtime (late to bed, late to rise) is also associated with risk of obesity in adolescents, although, this risk may alternatively be attributed to spending more time in front of the TV and computer, thus curtailing physical activity[34].

The increase in appetite associated with sleep deficit and increased ghrelin should thus be expected to increase appetite for sweets and fats. Further, sleep deficits are associated with increases in inflammatory cytokines. Chronic inflammation and sleep deficits promote abdominal obesity and, thus, insulin resistance. A sleep deficit or a disrupted circadian rhythm may also cause weight gain because of an increase in daytime cortisol production that promotes storage of abdominal fat.

Not Just Caloric Intake

A large energy imbalance is not required for obesity. Excess storage of one percent of daily caloric intake could easily be associated with a 20-pound weight gain over a decade or a 60-pound weight gain between the ages of 20 and 50. Thus, even a small variance in appetite may disrupt the normal equilibrium. If the body depended solely on the amount of food consumed, even minor influences of food availability or desirability would destabilize weight.

The hormones that control metabolic activity; Neuromedin B, (NMB) signals satiation but acts in a feedback loop with thyroid production. Hypothyroid animals have low pituitary NMB levels; the weight gain that occurs in hypothyroidism may result in part from reduced satiation.

Gastrin-releasing peptide (GRP) helps regulated circadian rhythms, and thermoregulation; thus, small excesses in caloric intake could easily be spent on thermogenesis and increased motor activity, such as motor activity during sleep. Small excesses or deficits in caloric intake are likely balanced by these same hormones (NMB and GRP), as well as by orexin under the influence of ghrelin and leptin[35]. Thus, these hormones not only control appetite and satiation, but also fine tune the balance and storage of energy in the body.

Insulin resistance can destabilize appetite/satiation by its effect on ghrelin. Once out of balance, a vicious cycle of increased appetite, weight gain, and further insulin resistance is promoted. Leptin resistance likely contributes to obesity.

Certain foods and its manner of preparation can affect satiation. Sleep deprivation and stress can cause an increase in appetite, especially for sweet and fatty foods, and encourage the storage of fat in the abdomen. Ghrelin is associated not only with an appetite for sweet and fatty foods, but also for alcohol, nicotine, and other addictive substances.

GI Biome

Bacterial inhabitants of the colon interact with diet and hunger. FOS fermented in the cecum produces propionic acid that causes the release PYY and GLP-1 from L cells in the mucosa. These hormones suppress appetite. Leptin levels are higher when *Lactobacillus* and *Bifidobacterium* populations are thriving, and lower when there are large populations of *Clostridium* and *Bacteroides* in the colon. Ghrelin levels are also affected by the bacterial biome, thus, affecting short-term appetite as well appetite[36]. A bacterial biome with more diversity and including a substantial population of *Lactobacillus* and *Bifidobacterium* is associated with easier satiation and satiety. A gut biome associated with the production of LPS and other bacterial toxins stimulates inflammation, and this inflammation promotes appetite and obesity through TLR4 signaling[37].

High-fat diets promote the growth of pro-inflammatory bacteria such as *Clostridium* and *Bacteroides*[38] and increase the level of oxidative stress in the colon[39]. These bacteria also thrive on proteins that have by-passed digestion and absorption.

Diets with sufficient fiber such as FOS resistance starches and polyphenolic compounds curtail the proliferation and biofilm formation in the colon by these toxin-producing bacteria in the colon (Chapter 23).

Speed Eating

Rapid consumption of meals is also associated with obesity[40, 41]. This may occur because the food is eaten before neurohormonal mechanisms of satiation can act, thus, allowing larger amounts of food to be eaten before the individual feels satisfied or full. It may also be the result of eating more palatable, mechanically soft foods that are easier and quicker to eat. These fast-eaten foods are often higher in fat and sugars, and lower in fiber. With fast eating, there is less chewing, less pancreatic peptide release and less opportunity for lingual lipase to free fatty acids to promote CCK release. Washing food down and swallowing whole decrease the osmolarity of the chyme, and thus, decreases pancreatic bicarbonate output, which is needed for activation of pancreatic digestive enzymes. Poorer digestion alters absorption, the colonic biome, and appetite.

Avoid Obesity by Promoting Satiation and Satiety

1. Promote CCK output: Satiation can be promoted by avoiding foods that do not increase CCK, and thus encourage overeating. Foods that increase CCK output may be eaten early in the meal, and carbohydrates and sweets later in the meal. Appetizers can be prepared with olive oil (to supply long-chain fatty acids), or with walnuts (to supply long-chain n-3 fatty acids). Protein early in the meal may help. Boiled potatoes rather than fries increase CCK. Foods high in spermidine (aged cheddar, legumes,) may also help with satiation. If a fish oil supplement is used, it might be given early in a meal to help with satiation.

2. Include prebiotic fiber in the diet: Prebiotics (Chapter 5) increase production of GLP-1 and PYY and decrease growth of deleterious bacteria that support inflammation. GLP-1 supports satiation, while inflammatory cytokines increase AgRP, and thus, increase appetite. Prebiotics (fructans) may help normalize appetite by supporting commensal intestinal microbiota and prevent the growth of bacteria that produce inflammatory LPS[11]. Dietary phenolic compounds also decrease the growth of bacteria that promote LPS and inflammation (Chapter 23).

3. Avoid caloric beverages: Caloric beverages, especially sweet beverages, should be avoided. Fruit should be eaten rather made into beverages.

4. Get sufficient sleep: Getting sufficient sleep is important for long-term satiety. Sleep deficits increase the desire for sweet and fatty foods that promote obesity. (See Chapter 41 on sleep).

5. Take the time to enjoy meals: Relaxed meals, with conversation, enhance satiation with lower consumption. Avoid waiting to eat until feeling ravenous, as this encourages rapid eating and eating sweet and fatty pleasure foods. Mastication, sucking, and salivation increase the release of pancreatic peptide.

6. Avoid Stress: Stress increases the output of glucocorticoid hormones that inhibit CRH, and thus, promote NPY release, and increased appetite. Stress reduction is discussed in Chapter 29.

7. Avoid Inflammation: The inflammatory cytokine IL-1β causes an increase in the production of AgRP, and thus, an increase in appetite and a decrease in energy utilization that can result in weight gain.

8. Avoid Immunogens: Avoiding foods that an individual has immune reactions to may help normalize appetite and result in significant weight loss (Chapter 19).

9. Limit Fructose: Fructose is not recognized by the brain and does not provide satiation. It is more likely than other calories to be metabolized to fat. This is further discussed in Chapter 9.

Pancreatic Function

The pancreas has both endocrine and exocrine functions. Pancreatic hormonal function occurs in the islets of Langerhans, which constitutes only one to two percent of the pancreatic mass. Pancreatic endocrine functions are listed in Table 8-4, below. Pancreatic exocrine functions are performed by acinar cells in the pancreas. These glands secrete digestive enzymes and bicarbonate into the duodenum. The pancreatic enzymes are listed in Table 8-3. Several of the pancreatic enzymes are zymogens; inactive proenzymes that must be activated, often by cleavage of a segment of the protein.

Pancreatic Exocrine Output (PEO) is closely coordinated with meals and the delivery of chyme into the duodenum; there is low-level PEO between meals; PEO peaks within the first hour after the meal. PEO levels off at a somewhat lower rate for 3 – 4 hours and then returns to the inter-digestive output. The postprandial enzymatic output is from 3 to 10 times the basal PEO level.

The output of pancreatic enzymes is controlled largely by CCK from I cells. These and other enteroendocrine cells in the small intestine have brush border "taste" receptors that trigger an influx of calcium ions when in contact with their ligands. The I cells have receptors for long-chain fatty acids, n-3 fatty acids, and the aromatic amino acids phenylalanine and tryptophan. The influx of calcium causes a release of CCK from I cells. A meal composed predominantly of carbohydrates does not induce a PEO much above basal output, only inducing a PEO about a third that of a meal composed with 40% of the calories as fat, In response to a meals, the PEO increases by three to ten times. The brain also increases PEO; looking at a delicious cinnamon roll, smelling, and tasting its warm, gooey goodness all increase PEO output. CCK also stimulates the release of bile from the gallbladder. Low CCK output is associated with risk for cholelithiasis[42], as there is less regular emptying of the gallbladder.

PEO is maximized by at an output of 2 – 3 Calories/minute from the stomach into the duodenum; and from solid food rather than liquid meals; PEO is sustained, thus maximized by slow postprandial emptying. A meal of about 7 to 10 Calories per kilogram ideal body weight maximizes PEO; thus, a meal of about 600 Calories meal for a 70 Kg adult.

Generally the pancreatic enzymes are secreted in parallel; foods that stimulate lipase also stimulate amylase and trypsin output, however, more protein in a meal will increase the ratio of trypsin to amylase produced. The ratio of amylase to lipase is usually stable; however, obese individuals and diabetics have higher lipase to amylase ratios, and islet cell transplants that restore insulin production also restore amylase production[43].

On a normal diet, the combined amylase, lipase, and trypsin output is about 90 U/min/kg between meals and 210 – 250 U/min/kg after meals.

Table 8-3: Pancreatic Enzymes

Enzymes	Activity
Trypsinogen	Trypsinogen is secreted in the jejunum. Enteropeptidase, an enzyme produced in the mucosa of the duodenum, cleaves it into the active enzyme, trypsin. Trypsin in turn converts more trypsinogen into trypsin and also activates other pancreatic zymogens. Thus, only a small amount of enteropeptidase is required to activate the pancreatic enzymes. Trypsin is a proteolytic endopeptidase.
Chymo-trypsinogen	A proenzyme which is converted by trypsin into chymotrypsin; another proteolytic endopeptidase.
Proelastases	There are four pancreatic elastase zymogens which are activated by trypsin. These endopeptidases have the ability to cleave proteins at specific amino acid sites commonly found in collagen and elastin in meat.
Procarboxy-peptidases	Carboxypeptidases cleave a single amino acid at a time from the carboxyl end of a peptide and thus, are exopeptidases. Procarboxypeptidase is a zymogen which can be activated by enteropeptidase or trypsin.
Colipase	Colipase is a coenzyme for pancreatic lipase. Colipase requires activation in the intestinal lumen by trypsin.
Pancreatic lipases	While secreted in their active form, these enzymes require colipase for activity. These enzymes break triglycerides into two free fatty acid molecules and a monoacylglycerol. This lipase activity is dependent on bile to emulsify fat into small particles so that the fat is accessible to the enzyme.
Bile salt-dependent lipase	Similar to pancreatic lipase. Bile salts are required to stabilize this lipase, protecting it from proteolytic hydrolysis in the intestine.
Phospho-lipases	Phospholipases are released as zymogens. They hydrolyze phospholipids, releasing, a free fatty acid.
Sterol esterase	Sterol esterase cleaves sterol esters into a sterol and a free fatty acid.
Pancreatic α-amylase	Pancreatic α-amylase acts on starches, glycogen, and some other carbohydrates (excluding cellulose). It randomly cleaves α (1-4) glycosidic links of amylose to yield the sugars dextrin, maltose or maltotriose, which are two and three glucose chain fragments.
Pancreatic Ribonuclease	Endonucleolytic cleavage (cutting between nucleotides) of RNA.
Pancreatic Deoxyribo-nuclease I	Endonucleolytic cleavage of double-stranded DNA

Lipase is the most abundant enzyme in the PEO. There is generally 3 to 6 times as much lipase as amylase and more amylase than trypsin. Proteolytic enzyme output adapts to a high protein diet. The pancreatic enzymes are mostly inactivated by the time they reach the distal ileum, mostly by the enzyme chymotrypsin[44]. One study found that following a high carbohydrate meal, 74% of amylase activity, 22% of trypsin activity, and 1% of lipase activity survived the transit. The high susceptibility of lipase to inactivation may explain why steatorrhea is the most common presenting syndrome in pancreatic exocrine insufficiency[45]. With steatorrhea, there is also a loss of the lipid soluble vitamins A, D, E, and K. This decline in enzyme activity during transit, especially in lipase activity, may be accentuated by a high protein diet. Inactivation of enzymes may not indicate their proteolytic destruction, as significant immune reactivity to the enzymes is preserved. The presence of substrate helps preserve the activity of its corresponding enzyme.

PEO of bicarbonate is controlled by secretin from intestinal S cells. The S cells have chemoreceptors for food, but secretin is mostly secreted in response to acidic, high osmolar chyme entering the duodenum. Thus, liquid meals, those diluted with beverages, and chyme with low stomach acidity pass through the pylorus into the duodenum more quickly and produce less secretin and less bicarbonate response. Bicarbonate is needed to neutralize stomach acid. The average pH of the mouth is 6.8. The pH drops to 1.5 in the stomach with HCl production, and rises to 6.4 in the duodenum with the pancreatic secretion of bicarbonate, but may fall back to a pH of 5 to 5.5 in the second hour after a meal with decreased bicarbonate output. The pH gradually rises to 7.4 as the chyme reaches the distal small intestine (SI). The pH again falls in the cecum to 5.9 as a result of fermentation and the production of short-chain fatty acids and other organic acids, and then rises to 6.5 by the time the stool reaches the rectum[46].

While the gastric enzyme pepsin has its optimal enzymatic activity in an acidic environment with a pH of 1.5 – 2.5, pancreatic enzymes need a more neutral environment. In the presence of bile, pancreatic lipase is active at a wide range of pH's between 5.7 and 7.5, peaking at a pH of about 6.3[47]. Without bile, pancreatic lipase has a peak activity at a pH of 8.0 and is less active when the pH is less than 7. Thus, in patients without a gallbladder to concentrate bile, and release it at meal time, lipase activity may suffer. The optimal pH for pancreatic amylase is 7.0, for free trypsin it is 7.1 but higher for substrate bound trypsin.

> Cool, clear, water: Half the volume of water consumed while fasting is absorbed in only 12 minutes[48]. Water is not absorbed from the stomach but first must pass into the small intestine. When the stomach contents are hypotonic or isotonic to the blood (~300 mOs), the pyloric sphincter relaxes, allowing the contents to quickly pass into the small intestine (SI). In the proximal SI, chyme rapidly becomes isotonic[49], either by absorption of water or by secretion of water and pancreatic juices. The chyme remains isotonic as it moves through the SI, as salts, sugars, other solutes, and water are absorbed. It is only in the distal ileum and colon that water is absorbed against the osmotic gradient.
>
> Oral rehydration fluids and sports beverages are usually isotonic so that the water can be quickly absorbed.

Similar to the proximal SI, there are nutrient receptors in the distal ileum and colon. The propionic acid formed by fermentation of fiber such as FOS in the cecum is detected by free fatty acid receptor-2 on colonic L-cells. This stimulates the release of the hormones PYY and GLP-1[50]. These hormones decrease appetite, prevent weight gain[51], and inhibit PEO.

L-cells also release PYY and GLP-1 in response to the presence of undigested, unabsorbed carbohydrates and fats in the distal ileum and decrease PEO and bile output[52, 53, 54]. Thus, amino acids and long-chain fatty acids in the proximal small intestine increase CCK and PEO, nutrients, particularly sugars and fats, in the distal small intestine inhibit PEO. Thus, malabsorption suppresses appetite, but also suppresses PEO that further promotes malabsorption. Eating despite a lack of appetite, or appetite dysregulation, may worsen malabsorption.

Enzyme Recycling: PEO contains a significant mass of protein created at high metabolic cost. The total amount of protein in the PEO is about 14 grams per day[54], about half of the WHO recommended daily dietary protein intake. To conserve energy, and increase enzymatic activity, certain digestive enzymes are recycled intact. Lipases and amylase are internalized by enterocytes, taken up by the Golgi apparatus and transported through the basal membrane of the enterocyte into the lamina propria, where they reach the blood circulation[55]. This recirculation utilizes molecular chaperone proteins secreted in the PEO that adhere to the enterocytes their enzyme and guide endocytosis[56]. Amylase has enhanced activity when bound to the brush border by its chaperone[57], at least in part because of the advantage of releasing a high concentration of sugars in proximity to the brush border.

These enzymes are then taken up by the pancreas (and presumably salivary enzymes by the salivary glands), where they can be redeployed again for the same and later meals. Without recycling, PEO of proteins falls after the first hour following a meal; pancreatic enzyme synthesis cannot produce sufficient enzymes without this recycling[58]. Lipases and amylases are secreted in their active form and thus, these enzymes are unchanged and can be recycled. In contrast, most zymogens are activated after secretion to prevent autodigestion of the pancreas, often by cleavage of a segment of the protein. Thus, they cannot be restored. Lipase activity, however, requires the zymogen colipase. The fate of the zymogens in the intestine has not been clarified, but their activity is lost by the time the chyme reaches the large intestine.

Pancreatic Exocrine Insufficiency

Overt Pancreatic Exocrine Insufficiency (PEI) is most commonly caused by the destruction of the pancreatic parenchyma with the loss of ductal and acinar tissue. Common causes of parenchymal destruction are chronic pancreatitis (CP), cystic fibrosis, tumors, and surgical resection. The most common cause of chronic pancreatitis is alcohol abuse. PEI commonly develops within 5 – 6 years of alcoholic pancreatitis. In cystic fibrosis, highly concentrated, viscous pancreatic juices condense, blocking the pancreatic ducts, causing acinar atrophy, fibrosis, and fatty replacement. In cystic fibrosis, severe damage has usually already occurred by the time of birth. Severe PEI and malabsorption are found in 80-90% of pancreatic cancer patients. Tumors obstructing the pancreatic duct can cause PEI and eventual destruction of the pancreas.

Steatorrhea and creatorrhea (lack of digestion of meat) only occurs when more than 90% of pancreatic exocrine function has been lost. In patients that have essentially no pancreatic exocrine function, intra-duodenal delivery of even 5% of the normal lipase output can abolish steatorrhea. However, much higher levels of enzyme are required when delivered orally, in part, as orally dosed enzymes are destroyed by stomach acid, and because lipase is most efficient when coordinated with bile salts, colipase, and a neutral to alkaline environment.

Additionally, CP patients have an abnormal CCK and secretin response to amino acid stimulus and exhibit disordered intestinal motility. Pancreatic ductal damage in CP impairs bicarbonate secretion, preventing the neutralization of stomach acid; this acidity impairs enzyme activity. Pancreatic lipase is irreversibly inactivated by a pH of 4. Accelerated gastric emptying worsens the low pH dilemma. Most patients with CP have small intestinal bacterial overgrowth (SIBO). PEO and bile are bacteriocidal, and malabsorption disrupts normal intestinal motility. CP causes alterations in the intestinal mucosa and increases the risk of immune reactivity to foods as undigested proteins retain their antigenicity[59].

PEI also occurs from causes external to the pancreas. This can occur from "postcibal asynchrony". Postcibal synchrony refers to the coordination of the appropriate production, release and recycling of pancreatic enzymes; excretion of bicarbonate and bile; hormonal control by CCK, secretin, VIP, GLP-1, and amylin; peristalsis and appropriate output of chyme from the stomach into the duodenum; and the absorption of nutrients as the chyme moves through the SI. (See Gastrointestinal Motility in Chapter 24) In health, the concentration of trypsin in the PEO adapts to the protein load; secretin stimulates sufficient bicarbonate to drop the pH of the chyme to a level in which the enzymes are most active, and CCK stimulates sufficient bile excretion to maximize lipase activity. If these processes are disturbed it can result in postcibal asynchrony; where PEO is discordant to time and need.

When these processes do not coordinate, malabsorption can occur. Furthermore, malabsorption can cause postcibal asynchrony. This may be exacerbated by liquid meals[60], sugar malabsorption (such as lactose intolerance), poorly digestible proteins, such as those in raw eggs and meat, or other causes of malabsorption that result in the delivery of nutrients to the distal ileum and colon. Malabsorption, which causes rapid SI transit, can flush pancreatic enzymes along with nutrients into the colon, where they are fermented. The presence of unabsorbed nutrients in the ileum and cecum is sensed by L-cell receptors and colon that trigger the release of PPY and GPL-1, inhibiting PEO, bile excretion, gastric emptying, and decreasing appetite. This acts as a safety mechanism to decrease further enzymatic and nutrient wasting but decreases PEO.

The decrease in PEO and bile output decrease nutrient absorption, allow survival of ingested bacteria, and colonic dysbiosis as the gut bacteria are fed nutrients that would not be normally available to them. These factors also participate in the pathology of small intestinal bacterial overgrowth (SIBO; Chapter 24).

PEI is also common after gastric resection; there is loss of control over the synchrony between gastric emptying, the secretion of bile, bicarbonate, and pancreatic enzymes. With the removal of gastric mucosa, there is a loss of gastric lipase and pepsin, and their activity. This limits the digestion of triglycerides to the long chain and n-3 FFA that stimulate CCK. Pepsin specifically lyses the aromatic amino acids tryptophan and phenylalanine from dietary proteins that trigger the release of CCK. If the pylorus is removed, there is a loss of control of chyme secretion from the stomach, as well as loss of somatostatin production.

In atrophic gastritis, there is also decrease in these nutrients and acidity that explain the decrease in bicarbonate and pancreatic enzymes common in the elderly[61]. Fortunately, with the exception of decreased fat absorption, PEO is usually not clinically significant in gastric atrophy.

Most diabetic patients with disease severe enough to cause neuropathy have PEI. Although diabetes is a disease of the pancreas, it is an islet cell (endocrine) rather than acinar cell (exocrine) disease. While the causation of PEI in diabetes is not fully elucidated, neuropathy, gastroparesis, and acinar-islet hormonal interactions are likely causal. Low fecal chymotrypsin is a more sensitive test of PEI in diabetes than is low fecal elastase-1[54].

PEI also occurs during pathologic conditions of the small intestine. In celiac disease, there is damage and flattening of the mucosa, especially in the proximal small intestine. This loss includes the loss of I and S cell function; thus, there postcibal asynchrony, with a decline in CCK and secretin production, and PEO response, contributing to the malabsorption seen in this disease.

About 40 percent Crohn's disease (CrD) patients have PEI. CrD often causes large loss of small intestine absorptive surface area, resulting in malabsorption and delivery of nutrients to the distal ileum and colon. This is accompanied by an exaggerated release of PYY and GLP-1, hormones, which inhibit PEO. Loss of proximal SI mucosa impairs CCK and secretin output. Short bowel syndrome, after bowel resection also causes PEI, likely for similar reasons. Additionally, CrD patients often have increased levels of pancreatic enzymes in their blood and may have autoantibodies to pancreatic enzymes. On autopsy about half of CrD patients have pancreatic fibrosis[54].

Mild PEI is common irritable bowel syndrome, and about five percent of IBS patients have severe PEI. In IBS with diarrhea, there is a loss of I, K, S and delta cells in the duodenum, thus a loss of CCK, GIP, secretin, and somatostatin production. In IBS with constipation, there is a loss of I and S cells[62].

> There are only low concentrations of cholesterol in the bile, but in pathologic conditions, it can form accretions forming gallstones in the gallbladder. If these stones obstruct the opening of the gallbladder it can cause cholecystitis, or worse; they can pass down the common bile duct and obstruct the sphincter of Oddi. If this occurs, is can cause obstruction of the pancreatic duct and pancreatitis.

Management of Pancreatic Exocrine Insufficiency

Fecal elastase-1 is specific for PEI, but it is insensitive to mild or moderate PEI. A more sensitive test, the 13C-mixed triglyceride breath test, can be used to monitor pancreatic enzyme replacement therapy (PERT), but this test is not widely available[63]. Patients with suspect PEI should be tested for both fecal elastase-1 and chymotrypsin. Although elastase-1 is specific, fecal chymotrypsin testing adds a disease marker. Steatorrhea is diagnostic of PEI and stool fat can be measured. (See Appendix C.)

Where the pancreatic parenchyma has been destroyed, treatment requires PERT. In PEI, pancreatic enzyme replacement therapy, especially with acid suppression can give significant pain relief.

It is, of course, imperative to treat the underlying cause of the disease. In CP alcohol and tobacco should be avoided. In disease of the small intestine, malabsorption or SIBO, the underlying causes need to be addressed.

Where mucosal injury has occurred, as occurs in celiac, IBS, and Crohn's diseases, PERT helps with recovery and nutrition. PERT also help prevent delivery of undigested foods to distal ileum and colon and prevent further negative feedback of PEO.

Enzyme dosing is based on lipase the predominant enzyme. Five hundred units of lipase per kilogram of body weight per meal is a typical dose for older children and adults with PEI. Children 6 months to 3 years usually require 1000 units and infants less than 6 months 2000 units of lipase per kilogram of body weight[64]. A typical adult dose is 25,000 to 40,000 units of lipase per meal, with half this quantity taken with snacks. Excessive PERT can cause constipation, and fibrosing colonopathy at very high doses.

Pancreatic enzymes that are not protected from the acid environment of the stomach are little more than protein supplements and potential antigens. Most formations are enteric coated. Bacterial lipase, such as that from *Burkholderia plantarii*, is resistant to gastric acid and proteolytic enzymes, and thus may offer an advantage over that harvested from animals. Chymotrypsin inhibitors in food may help slow the degradation of lipase and be of benefit in steatorrhea.

Stool fat can be used as a metric for enzyme replacement success; with adequate PE treatment there should be less than is less than 15 grams of stool fat per day in adults, although 7 grams of stool fat is the upper limit in health.

When there is low PEO but adequate pancreatic exocrine function there are several strategies can be used to improve PEO, depending on the cause of the deficit.

1. Medium sized, less liquid, meals give a slower delivery of chyme to the SI, and maximize PEO. Small meals, of about 7 to 10 Calories/Kg give the most favorable PEO. Carbohydrates are weak inducers of PEO. Solid meals and slower gastric emptying times give a more sustained PEO.

2. If the proximal SI mucosa is normal, CCK output responds to long chain and n-3 free fatty acids (FFA). These FFA are released from triglycerides by lingual lipase when food is chewed, and some freed fatty acids are absorbed in the mouth. The stomach also produces lipase. The meal needs to include the n-3 and long chain fatty acids.

3. Pepsin, in an acid environment, releases tryptophan and phenylalanine form proteins. These amino acids trigger CCK release from I cells. If stomach acid or pepsin are not present, small supplements of these amino acids might be helpful. Spermidine may also release CCK[5]; high levels are present in aged cheddar, green peas, soy, pears, and lentils[65].

There are different brush border receptors for long chain FFA, n-3 FFA, and aromatic amino acids; the presence of all three nutrients may stimulate a more robust CCK response.

1 Effect of CCK-1 receptor blockade on ghrelin and PYY secretion in men. Degen L, Drewe J, Piccoli F, et al. Am J Physiol Regul Integr Comp Physiol. 2007 Apr;292(4):R1391-9. PMID: 17138722

[2] Localization of acyl ghrelin- and des-acyl ghrelin-immunoreactive cells in the rat stomach and their responses to intragastric pH. Mizutani M, Atsuchi K, Asakawa A, et al. Am J Physiol Gastrointest Liver Physiol. 2009 Nov;297(5):G974-80. PMID: 20501445

[3] Ghrelin, des-acyl ghrelin, and obestatin: regulatory roles on the gastrointestinal motility. Fujimiya M, Asakawa A, Ataka K, et al. Int J Pept. 2010;2010. pii: 305192. PMID: 20721292

[4] Anxiogenic effect of cholecystokinin in the dorsal periaqueductal gray. Netto CF, Guimarães FS. Neuropsychopharmacology. 2004 Jan;29(1):101-7. PMID: 14583742

[5] Induction of postprandial intestinal motility and release of cholecystokinin by polyamines in rats. Fioramonti J, Fargeas MJ, Bertrand V, Pradayrol L, Buéno L. Am J Physiol. 1994 Dec;267(6 Pt 1):G960-5. PMID: 7810663

[6] Cholecystokinin enhances visceral pain-related affective memory via vagal afferent pathway in rats. Cao B, Zhang X, Yan N, Chen S, Li Y. Mol Brain. 2012 Jun 9;5:19. PMID:22681758

[7] Expression of neuromedin B in adipose tissue and its regulation by changes in energy balance. Hoggard N, Bashir S, Cruickshank M, et al. J Mol Endocrinol. 2007 Sep;39(3):199-210. PMID: 17766645

[8] Bombesin-related peptides and their receptors: recent advances in their role in physiology and disease states. Gonzalez N, Moody TW, Igarashi H, Ito T, Jensen RT. Curr Opin Endocrinol Diabetes Obes. 2008 Feb;15(1):58-64. PMID: 18185064

[9] Meal-anticipatory glucagon-like peptide-1 secretion in rats. Vahl TP, Drazen DL, Seeley RJ, D'Alessio DA, Woods SC. Endocrinology. 2010 Feb;151(2):569-75.. PMID: 19915164

[10] Glucagon-like peptide 1 promotes satiety and suppresses energy intake in humans. Flint A, Raben A, Astrup A, Holst J. J Clin Invest 1998; 101:515–20.

[11] Changes in gut microbiota control inflammation in obese mice through a mechanism involving GLP-2-driven improvement of gut permeability. Cani PD, Possemiers S, Van de Wiele T et al. Gut. 2009 Aug;58(8):1091-103. PMID:19240062

[12] Amino Acids Stimulate Cholecystokinin Release Through the Calcium-Sensing Receptor. Wang Y, Chandra R, Samsa LA, et al. Am J Physiol Gastrointest Liver Physiol. 2010 Dec 23. PMID: 21183662

[13] Taste enhancements between various amino acids and IMP. Kawai M, Okiyama A, Ueda Y. Chem Senses. 2002 Oct;27(8):739-45. PMID: 12379598

[14] Role of fat hydrolysis in regulating glucagon-like Peptide-1 secretion. Beglinger S, Drewe J, Schirra J, et al. J Clin Endocrinol Metab. 2010 Feb;95(2):879-86. PMID: 19837920

[15] Effect of CCK-1 receptor blockade on ghrelin and PYY secretion in men. Degen L, Drewe J, Piccoli F, et al. Am J Physiol Regul Integr Comp Physiol. 2007 Apr;292(4):R1391-9. PMID: 17138722

[16] Cellular mechanism of sodium oleate-stimulated secretion of cholecystokinin and secretin. Chang CH, Chey WY, Chang TM. Am J Physiol Gastrointest Liver Physiol. 2000 Aug;279(2):G295-303. PMID: 10915637

[17] Effect of fat saturation on satiety, hormone release, and food intake. Maljaars J, Romeyn EA, Haddeman E, Peters HP, Masclee AA. Am J Clin Nutr. 2009 Apr;89(4):1019-24. PMID:19225118

[18] A diet rich in long chain omega-3 fatty acids modulates satiety in overweight and obese volunteers during weight loss. Parra D, Ramel A, Bandarra N, Kiely M, Martínez JA, Thorsdottir I. Appetite. 2008 Nov;51(3):676-80. PMID:18602429

[19] A satiety index of common foods. Holt SH, Miller JC, Petocz P, et al. Eur J Clin Nutr. 1995 Sep;49(9):675-90. PMID: 7498104

[20] Potato protease inhibitors inhibit food intake and increase circulating cholecystokinin levels by a trypsin-dependent mechanism. Komarnytsky S, Cook A, Raskin I. Int J Obes (Lond). 2011 Feb;35(2):236-43. PMID: 20820171

[21] Glycaemic and satiating properties of potato products. Leeman M, Ostman E, Björck I. Eur J Clin Nutr. 2008 Jan;62(1):87-95.. PMID: 17327869

[22] Protein hydrolysates induce CCK release from enteroendocrine cells and act as partial agonists of the CCK1 receptor. Foltz M, Ansems P, Schwarz J, Tasker MC, Lourbakos A, Gerhardt CC. J Agric Food Chem. 2008 Feb 13;56(3):837-43. PMID: 18211011

[23] Hedonic and incentive signals for body weight control. Egecioglu E, Skibicka KP, Hansson C, et al. Rev Endocr Metab Disord. 2011 Feb 22. PMID: 21340584

[24] Ghrelin increases intake of rewarding food in rodents. Egecioglu E, Jerlhag E, Salomé N, et al. Addict Biol. 2010 Jul;15(3):304-11. PMID: 20477752

[25] Ghrelin secretion is modulated in a nutrient- and gender-specific manner. Greenman Y, Golani N, Gilad S, et al. Clin Endocrinol (Oxf). 2004 Mar;60(3):382-8. PMID: 15009005

[26] Regulation of agouti-related protein messenger ribonucleic acid transcription and peptide secretion by acute and chronic inflammation. Scarlett JM, Zhu X, Enriori PJ, et al. Endocrinology. 2008 Oct;149(10):4837-45.. PMID: 18583425

[27] Cephalic phase pancreatic polypeptide responses to liquid and solid stimuli in humans. Teff KL. Physiol Behav. 2010 Mar 3;99(3):317-23.. PMID:19944113

[28] Effect of umami taste stimulations on vagal efferent activity in the rat. Niijima A. Brain Res Bull. 1991 Sep-Oct;27(3-4):393-6. PMID:1959036

[29] Ghrelin, Sleep Reduction and Evening Preference: Relationships to CLOCK 3111 T/C SNP and Weight Loss. Garaulet M, Sánchez-Moreno C, Smith CE, Lee YC, Nicolás F, Ordovás JM. PLoS One. 2011 Feb 28;6(2):e17435. PMID: 21386998

[30] Role of sleep and sleep loss in hormonal release and metabolism. Leproult R, Van Cauter E. Endocr Dev. 2010;17:11-21. PMID: 19955752

[31] Brief communication: Sleep curtailment in healthy young men is associated with decreased leptin levels, elevated ghrelin levels, and increased hunger and appetite. Spiegel K, Tasali E, Penev P, Van Cauter E. Ann Intern Med. 2004 Dec 7;141(11):846-50. PMID: 15583226

[32] Short sleep duration is associated with reduced leptin, elevated ghrelin, and increased body mass index. Taheri S, Lin L, Austin D, Young T, Mignot E. PLoS Med. 2004 Dec;1(3):e62. PMID: 15602591

[33] Shorter sleep duration is associated with increased risk for being overweight at ages 9 to 12 years. Lumeng JC, Somashekar

D, Appugliese D, Kaciroti N, Corwyn RF, Bradley RH. Pediatrics. 2007 Nov;120(5):1020-9. PMID: 17974739

[34] Sleep duration or bedtime? Exploring the relationship between sleep habits and weight status and activity patterns. Olds TS, Maher CA, Matricciani L. Sleep. 2011 Oct ;34(10):1299-307. PMID:21966061

[35] The role of leptin and orexins in the dysfunction of hypothalamo-pituitary-gonadal regulation and in the mechanism of hyperactivity in patients with anorexia nervosa. Baranowska B, Baranowska-Bik A, Bik W, Martynska L. Neuro Endocrinol Lett. 2008 Feb;29(1):37-40. PMID: 18283238

[36] Gut microbiota composition in male rat models under different nutritional status and physical activity and its association with serum leptin and ghrelin levels. Queipo-Ortuño MI, Seoane LM, Murri M et al. PLoS One. 2013 May 28;8(5):e65465. PMID:23724144

[37] High fat diet-induced gut microbiota exacerbates inflammation and obesity in mice via the TLR4 signaling pathway. Kim KA, Gu W, Lee IA, Joh EH, Kim DH. PLoS One. 2012;7(10):e47713. PMID:23091640

[38] Propensity to high-fat diet-induced obesity in rats is associated with changes in the gut microbiota and gut inflammation. de La Serre CB, Ellis CL, Lee J, et al. Am J Physiol Gastrointest Liver Physiol. 2010 Aug;299(2):G440-8. PMID:20508158

[39] Alterations of the gut microbiota in high-fat diet mice is strongly linked to oxidative stress. Qiao Y, Sun J, Ding Y, Le G, Shi Y. Appl Microbiol Biotechnol. 2013 Feb;97(4):1689-97. PMID:22948953

[40] Retrospective longitudinal study on the relationship between 8-year weight change and current eating speed. Tanihara S, Imatoh T, Miyazaki M, e. Appetite. 2011 Aug;57(1):179-83. PMID:21565235

[41] Faster self-reported speed of eating is related to higher body mass index in a nationwide survey of middle-aged women. Leong SL, Madden C, Gray A, Waters D, Horwath C. J Am Diet Assoc. 2011 Aug;111(8):1192-7. PMID:21802566

[42] Cholelithiasis as a possible manifestation of systemic digestive diseases. Vakhrushev IaM, Gorbunov AIu, Tronina DV, et al. Ter Arkh. 2015;87(2):54-8. PMID:25864350

[43] Islet transplantation restores normal serum amylase levels in diabetic rats. Barneo L, Esteban MM, Garcia-Pravia C, et al. Eur Surg Res. 1990;22(3):143-50. PMID:1702386

[44] Fate of pancreatic enzymes in the human intestinal lumen in health and pancreatic insufficiency. Layer P, Gröger G. Digestion. 1993;54 Suppl 2:10-4. PMID:7693530

[45] Fate of pancreatic enzymes during small intestinal aboral transit in humans. Layer P, Go VL, DiMagno EP. Am J Physiol. 1986 Oct;251(4 Pt 1):G475-80. PMID:2429560

[46] Measurement of gastrointestinal pH and regional transit times in normal children. Fallingborg J, Christensen LA, Ingeman-Nielsen M, et al. J Pediatr Gastroenterol Nutr. 1990 Aug;11(2):211-4. PMID:2395061

[47] Influence of bile salt, pH, and time on the action of pancreatic lipase; physiological implications. Borgstroem B. J Lipid Res. 1964 Oct;5:522-31. PMID:14221095

[48] Pharmacokinetic analysis of absorption, distribution and disappearance of ingested water labeled with D_2O in humans. Péronnet F, Mignault D, du Souich P, et al. Eur J Appl Physiol. 2012 Jun;112(6):2213-22. PMID:21997675

[49] Effect of beverage osmolality on intestinal fluid absorption during exercise. Gisolfi CV, Summers RW, Lambert GP, Xia T. J Appl Physiol (1985). 1998 Nov;85(5):1941-8. PMID:9804602

[50] The short chain fatty acid propionate stimulates GLP-1 and PYY secretion via free fatty acid receptor 2 in rodents. Psichas A, Sleeth ML, Murphy KG, et al. Int J Obes (Lond). 2015 Mar;39(3):424-9. PMID:25109781

[51] Weight loss during oligofructose supplementation is associated with decreased ghrelin and increased peptide YY in overweight and obese adults. Parnell JA, Reimer RA. Am J Clin Nutr. 2009 Jun;89(6):1751-9. PMID:19386741

[52] Inhibition of human pancreatic and biliary output but not intestinal motility by physiological intraileal lipid loads. Keller J, Holst JJ, Layer P. Am J Physiol Gastrointest Liver Physiol. 2006 Apr;290(4):G704-9. PMID:16322090

[53] Human pancreatic secretion and intestinal motility: effects of ileal nutrient perfusion. Layer P, Peschel S, Schlesinger T, Goebell H. Am J Physiol. 1990 Feb;258(2 Pt 1):G196-201. PMID:1689548

[54] Human pancreatic exocrine response to nutrients in health and disease. Keller J, Layer P. Gut. 2005 Jul;54 Suppl 6:vi1-28. PMID:15951527

[55] Internalization and transcytosis of pancreatic enzymes by the intestinal mucosa. Cloutier M, Gingras D, Bendayan M. J Histochem Cytochem. 2006 Jul;54(7):781-94. 2006 Mar 3.PMID: 16517974

[56] Roles of molecular chaperones in pancreatic secretion and their involvement in intestinal absorption. Bruneau N, Lombardo D, Levy E, Bendayan M. Microsc Res Tech. 2000 May 15;49(4):329-45. PMID: 10820517

[57] Pancreatic α-Amylase Controls Glucose Assimilation by Duodenal Retrieval through N-Glycan-specific Binding, Endocytosis, and Degradation. Date K, Satoh A, Iida K, Ogawa H. J Biol Chem. 2015 May 28. PMID:26023238

[58] Conservation of digestive enzymes. Rothman S, Liebow C, Isenman L. Physiol Rev. 2002 Jan;82(1):1-18. PMID:11773607

[59] Morphological and functional alterations of small intestine in chronic pancreatitis. Gubergrits NB, Linevskiy YV, Lukashevich GM, et al. JOP. 2012 Sep 10;13(5):519-28. PMID:22964959

[60] Human pancreatic secretion and intestinal motility: effects of ileal nutrient perfusion. Layer P, Peschel S, Schlesinger T, Goebell H. Am J Physiol. 1990 Feb;258(2 Pt 1):G196-201. PMID:1689548

[61] Changes, functional disorders, and diseases in the gastrointestinal tract of elderly. Grassi M, Petraccia L, Mennuni G, et al. Nutr Hosp. 2011 Jul-Aug;26(4):659-68. PMID:22470008

[62] Is irritable bowel syndrome an organic disorder? El-Salhy M, Gundersen D, Gilja OH, et al. World J Gastroenterol. 2014 Jan 14;20(2):384-400. PMID:24574708

[63] Synopsis of recent guidelines on pancreatic exocrine insufficiency. Löhr JM, Oliver MR, Frulloni L. United European Gastroenterol J. 2013 Apr;1(2):79-83. PMID:24917944

[64] Management of pancreatic exocrine insufficiency: Australasian Pancreatic Club recommendations. Toouli J, Biankin AV, Oliver MR, et al; Med J Aust. 2010 Oct 18;193(8):461-7. PMID:20955123

[65] Polyamines in foods: development of a food database. Atiya Ali M, Poortvliet E, Strömberg R, Yngve A. Food Nutr Res. 2011 Jan 14;55. PMID:21249159

9. Obesity, Syndrome X and the Company it Keeps

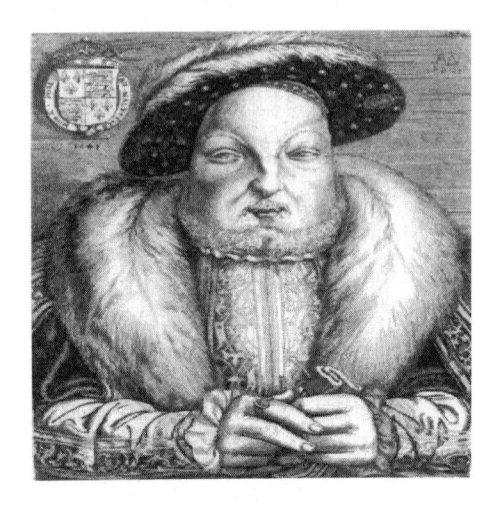

KING HENRY VIII IN HIS LATER YEARS

Life was ever so simple during medical school and my doctoral studies in chronic disease epidemiology. Back then, obesity was the result of the combined effect of two deadly sins: gluttony and sloth - too many calories in, too lazy to work them off. We were taught to entreat our patients to eat less and get more exercise, and that obesity and its related diseases resulted from gluttony and chronic couch "potation".

While most of us have been taught the piggy bank theory of obesity (Savings = coins in minus coins out), it turns out not to be helpful, and the paradigm actually encourages harmful dietary manipulations. Sixty years of calorie counting and deprivation, clearly, have not worked. Nevertheless, understanding of obesity can be illuminated with a wee bit of metabolic history.

A tad more than fourteen million years ago, a pair of fireballs streaked through the atmosphere and exploded into the European land mass at a speed of 45,000 miles per hour. The larger asteroid's diameter was 1.5 kilometers and left the Nördlinger Ries crater in southwestern Germany as evidence of the event. The smaller asteroid, a mere 150 meters across, caused the Steinheim crater 26 miles away. The tremendous explosions had a force 1.8 million times that of the atomic bomb detonated over Hiroshima.

This event appears to have caused the Middle Miocene Extinction. The massive amount of dust lifted into the upper atmosphere blocked enough sunlight to cause a "nuclear" winter that persisted several hundred thousand years.

Before this meteor blast, there had been about 100 different species of apes. Most, however, could not survive the ensuing ice age. Those that were able to survive did so as a result of metabolic adaptations that helped them store energy.

The series of genetic mutations, which aided survival through that cold spell, progressively reduced and then silenced the enzyme, urate oxidase (a.k.a. uricase), in certain ape lineages. This enzyme, present in most mammals, degrades uric acid[1]. This mutation increased uric acid levels, giving a survival advantage to the distant ancestors of the great apes. Those with the mutation were able to survive a very long, cold winter, while those without the extra bit of uric acid did not.

During times of prolonged fasting or starvation, birds and mammals first undergo a period of rapid weight loss followed by a slower and longer period of fat depletion. When the fat stores are exhausted, the body begins to break down protein. A degradation product of this protein is xanthine, which then is metabolized to uric acid. Uric acid has some properties similar to its chemical cousin caffeine. It wakes up hibernating animals so that they go out and forage. When migrating birds or nesting male penguin's fat stores are depleted, uric acid rises, and they go looking for food.

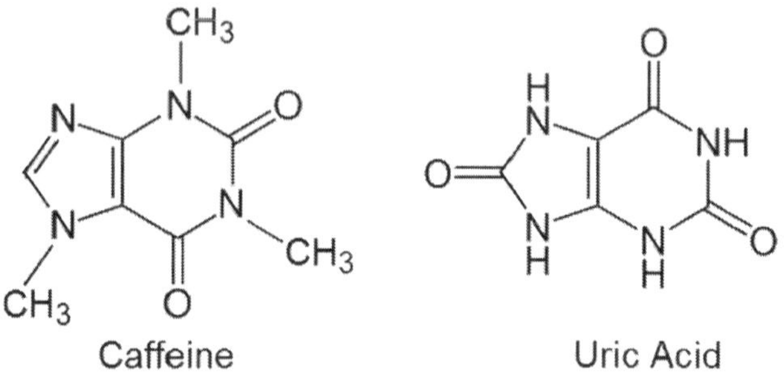

Figure 9-2: Methylxanthines

Uric acid helps with the recovery of depleted adiposity by increasing triglyceride levels in the blood and helping to store energy as fat. Uric acid also protects the body from hypotension associated with low serum protein levels. Additionally, it helps protect from dehydration by making the body more sensitive to sodium. Uric acid further acts as an important antioxidant and may protect the brain[2] and other organs from oxidative damage. These adaptations provide a considerable advantage for animals facing starvation and trying to get through a long cold winter, and needing a stimulus to go out into the cold and forage for food.

Elevated blood uric acid, however, has a significant dark side; it is the underlying cause of Syndrome X. SYNDROME X. It sounds like something from 1960's science fiction film; a perfect name for a cosmic cataclysm that killed off most of the simian species on the planet of the apes 14.4 million years ago.

The name Syndrome X, as this set of disturbances was originally known, has fallen out of favor and been supplanted with the bland moniker Metabolic Syndrome, which while not as colorful, is more descriptive. It is also referred to as insulin resistance. Insulin resistance, however, is a secondary result of this condition; thus, Metabolic Syndrome (MetS) is a preferable name.

In bygone days, peasants were unlikely to get MetS. It was rare for even the wealthy. One needed to be king, like Henry VIII, to get MetS. However, the world has grown more democratic. You too can have the disease of kings!!!! You do not even need to be rich. In fact, in the U.S., having a low income gives an advantage to getting it.

What are the benefits and privileges of MetS? It is the direct or indirect cause of the following ever-popular pastimes:

> Stroke
> Obesity
> Dementia
> Sleep Apnea
> Hypertension
> Osteoarthritis
> Type 2 Diabetes
> Hypercholesterolemia
> Ischemic Heart disease
> Congestive Heart Failure
> Increased risk of colon cancer
> Increased risk of breast cancer

The list is likely longer; nevertheless, these are sufficient to demonstrate that there are better ways to spend retirement.

It has been long appreciated that high levels of uric acid in the blood can precipitate in the joints and cause painful gouty arthritis. Patients with gout describe the joint pain, typically in the great toe, as being so intense that they cannot bear the weight of a sheet over their feet at night. What was not widely recognized until the last decade was that high uric acid levels were associated with elevated risk for[3]:

> Stroke
> Obesity
> Hypertension
> Preeclampsia
> Type 2 diabetes
> Metabolic syndrome
> Cardiovascular events
> Chronic kidney disease

In a study of over 14,000 American adults, uric acid (UA) was linearly correlated with insulin production, fasting insulin levels, insulin resistance and body mass index[4]. Uric acid was also correlated with fasting blood sugar in non-diabetics. (UA is inversely related to blood sugar and HgA1c in diabetics, perhaps due to lower production, or more rapid clearance). Elevated uric acid is also associated with increased inflammation and inflammatory cytokines[5].

Although UA is an antioxidant, when UA levels are elevated, UA can act as a pro-oxidant.

It is not necessary to wait a long time to see the effects of elevated UA. These changes are seen in children under the age of ten[6]. The youngest patient I have diagnosed with Type 2 (adult onset type) diabetes was six years old. The United States is currently witnessing an epidemic of obese 6-month-old infants. Obesity in children is now so common that the excess estrogen production by fat cells has caused an alarming rise in early breast development in girls in the U.S. Ten percent of Caucasian girls, and nearly a quarter of African American girls begin breast development by age 7[7]! Early puberty puts them at higher risk of teenage pregnancy and higher lifetime risk for breast cancer.

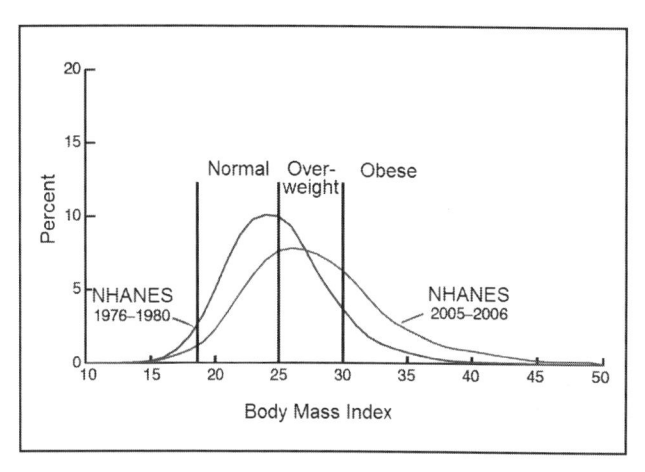

Figure 9-3: Population Distribution of Overweight and Obesity. Data from the NHANES Studies[8]

Since 1980, the average overweight person has gotten progressively heavier, and the prevalence of obesity has more than tripled, and the obese population is far more obese than it previously had been. As of 2010, 36% of adults and 17% of adolescents in the United States were obese[9].

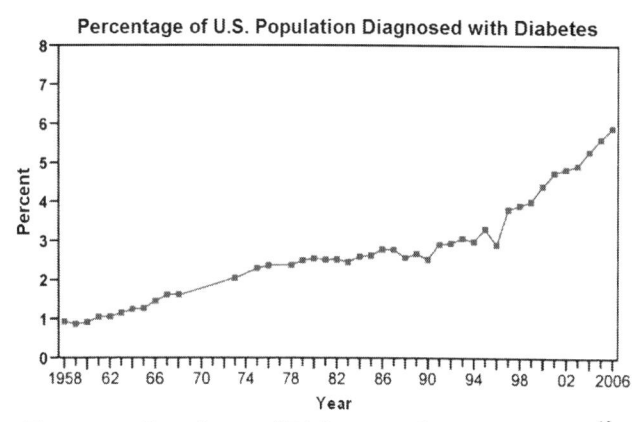

Figure 9-4: Prevalence of Diabetes in the U.S. over time[10].

Part of the rise in diabetes prevalence seen prior to 1980 can be attributed to an increase in diagnostic awareness and earlier diagnosis. Only 2% of healthy weight adults become diabetic compared to 12% of the very obese. The increase since 1990 is associated with epidemic obesity.

Table 9-1: Metabolic Effects of Elevated Uric Acid

Metabolic Effect	Result
Reduces nitric oxide availability to endothelial cells, fat cells, and vascular smooth muscle cells	Vasoconstriction and elevated blood pressure. Hypertension, kidney damage, increased risk of heart disease, erectile dysfunction, and stroke. Impaired insulin response in skeletal muscles, resulting in insulin resistance and storage of energy as fat.
Elevates triglycerides	Fatty liver, fat storage, weight gain. Increases risk of atherogenesis and ischemic heart disease, stroke, dementia.
Activates the Renin-Angiotensin System	Fluid retention and salt retention, leading to hypertension
Decreases adiponectin	Weight gain, insulin resistance, obesity, metabolic syndrome
Increases oxidative stress and inflammation	Lipid oxidation, atherosclerosis Decreases nitric oxide activity
Hyperuricemia and/or elevated xanthine oxidase activity	Increases platelet adhesion, leading to thrombogenesis Vascular damage, smooth muscle proliferation Inflammation
Stimulates vascular smooth muscle cells, enters cells via a specific organic anion transport pathway, with the stimulation of mitogen-activated kinases (p38 and ERK) and nuclear transcription factors (nuclear factor-B (NF-κB) and activator protein-1 (AP-1)	Platelet-derived growth factor-dependent proliferation Cyclooxygenase-2-dependent thromboxane production MCP-1 and C-reactive protein synthesis Stimulation of angiotensin II, leading to inflammation, platelet activation and hypertension, increased IL-6
Elevates small dense LDL cholesterol Decreases HDL cholesterol	Increases risk of atherogenesis and ischemic heart disease, stroke, and dementia
Inhibits endothelial cell proliferation and migration	Slows healing
Uric acid has potent effects on proximal tubular cells (stimulating MCP-1 production) as well as adipocytes	Induces oxidative stress, stimulating oxidization of lipids, and lowering NO levels
Increases C-reactive protein (CRP)	Inflammation and heart disease
Increases Tumor Necrosis Factor (TNF-α)	Increases inflammation, increases appetite, apoptosis (cell death)
Increases Interleukin-6 (IL-6)	Inflammation
Decreases Ghrelin	Delays satiation, increases consumption of sweets and fat, decreases insulin output
Increases Leptin	Decreases food intake, however, effect is antagonized by TNF-α.
Adenosine antagonist in the CNS	Impairs homeostatic (time awake) sleep drive, increasing dopamine and glutamate; may increase the risk of excitotoxicity.

But why now? Why did humans wait until 1980 to have an explosive epidemic of obesity, hyperuricemia, and MetS?

Certain individuals have hereditary conditions that make them more susceptible to hyperuricemia and more likely to get gout, but these are not common, and this did not suddenly become epidemic in the last 40 years. There are drugs that block the excretion of uric acid; unfortunately, this includes medications meant to treat some of the conditions associated with MetS, thus making it worse, but these did not start the fire. To understand the epidemic, it is helpful to understand how the body makes uric acid. There are three main metabolic pathways for the formation of UA.

One metabolic pathway that creates uric acid is starvation, as discussed above. During starvation, the body can start degrading proteins, which make up muscles and organelles in cells. When protein breaks down into its component amino acids, the amino acid glutamate can be broken down into ammonia, converted to glutamine, then to xanthine and then to uric acid. Since starvation does not lead to obesity, it can be ruled out as the cause of pandemic MetS.

Overeating and maldigestion of proteins can result in bacterial degradation of unabsorbed amino acids in the colon. Bacteria in the colon convert some amino acid to ammonia, which is absorbed and converted to urea or glutamine in the liver. This ammonia is quite toxic to the brain in infants and in individuals with liver disease (see Chapter 35). Urea is normally expelled in the urine, so this is not a problem for individuals with normal liver function.

A second pathway for the formation of UA is the breakdown of purines (guanine and adenine), which are nucleic acids. This can occur when there is a massive die-off of cells, and DNA and RNA are released. This can occur with necrotic injuries, cancer, and hemolytic anemia. Again, these events fail to explain the epidemic of obesity.

The third pathway for the production of uric acid is depletion of ATP. ATP is the basic energy unit for cell function. Depletion of ATP not only robs energy from the cells, but it can also activate JNKs (mitogen-activated protein kinases) that can trigger inflammation or even apoptosis. What could cause ATP depletion, and redirect energy to be stored as fat?

The answer is the sugar fructose.

Most cells cannot transport fructose across their membranes, and thus, cannot use fructose as an energy source. The hepatocytes, the main cells of the liver, are able to use fructose, so most of the fructose consumed is concentrated here. Once in the liver, phosphate from ATP (adenosine triphosphate) is rapidly transferred to the sugar by fructokinase, forming fructose-1-phosphate, and ATP is downgraded to ADP (adenosine diphosphate). In contrast to glucose phosphorylation, there is no negative feedback in fructose phosphorylation. As long as ATP and fructose are present the depletion continues. A large load of fructose will deplete hepatic ATP, resulting in intracellular phosphate depletion. ADP is then degraded to AMP (adenosine monophosphate), and then to IMP, xanthine and then to uric acid[11].

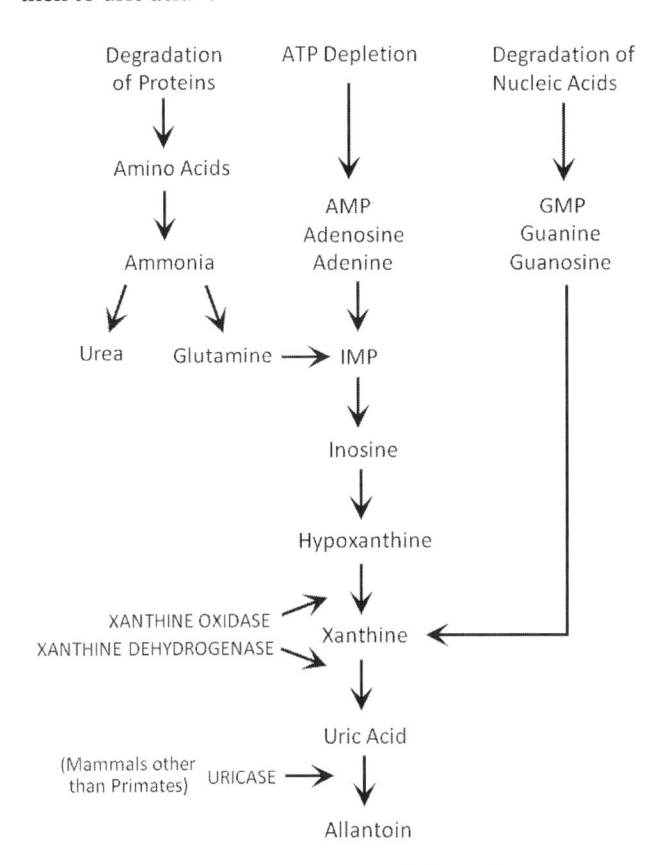

Figure 9-5: Uric Acid Metabolic Pathway

The more fructose consumed, the more the body adapts, and the more fructose-1-phosphate the liver makes. It is as if the body sees fructose as a toxin, and fructose induces the production of more enzymes to eliminate it, as the liver does for many other toxins.

Within an hour of drinking a refreshing lemon-lime soda, uric acids level can rise 40 percent. Transient but consistently increased UA levels can be achieved within weeks on a high fructose diet. Data from the Third National Health and Nutrition Examination Survey involving over 14,000 people showed a linear increase in uric acid levels with the number of high fructose corn syrup (HFCS) soft drinks consumed per day, while there was no correlation between uric acids level and sugar-free soft drinks[12].

Furthermore, the causal relation between fructose and MetS does not stop with the formation of uric acid. Uric acid may stimulate feeding and storage of fat, but the calories have to come from somewhere. Fructose is a calorie source with special effects.

Most of the energy from glucose is stored as glycogen that acts as ready fuel for muscles and other organs. When the liver has had its fill of glycogen, blood sugar begins to rise, the beta cells of the pancreas release insulin in response to glucose, which helps cells store it away, and the hunger signal (acyl-ghrelin) is switched off. The brain responds to glucose by modulating hunger and taste. When blood sugar goes up, food does not taste as good, and we stop eating.

In the 1960's, NASA was experimenting with elemental diets. A diet with 89% of its calories from glucose did not seem to cause problems, and, in fact, it was associated with lower cholesterol levels. When sucrose was substituted, so that about 12% of the calories were derived from fructose, cholesterol levels rose[13].

Fructose is like a stealthy invader. Since the brain cannot use fructose, it does not detect it as a fuel source. There is no down-regulation of hunger in response to increased blood fructose levels. The pancreas does not react to fructose, and insulin is not released in response to high fructose levels.

Thus, fructose is somewhat invisible, but at the same time it is sweet. It is about 2.3 times sweeter than glucose. When acyl-ghrelin levels are high, it makes us want to eat more sweets and fats to get blood sugars up, but this sweetness alone does not suppress appetite[14]. Isotonic fructose-water solutions (a.k.a.: soda pop) don't stimulate CCK release, do not close the pyloric sphincter, and quickly pass from the stomach into the small intestine where they are absorbed; the CO_2 release neutralizes stomach acid and gives a short-term fullness, but without providing satiation.

Table 9-2: Use of Glucose and Fructose

	Glucose	Fructose
Acyl-Ghrelin: Hunger signal for sweets and fats	Suppresses	No Suppression
Leptin: Long-term full signal	Stimulates	No stimulation
Insulin: Full signal	Stimulates	No stimulation
Brain	Can use	Can't use

Modern Fruit – Not so Natural

When Johnny Appleseed sold apple trees to the settlers in the Ohio Valley in the early 1800's, they were tart apples for making cider, unlike modern, sweet cultivars such as Red Delicious apples now found in grocery stores. Wild fruit typically is much less sweet than modern cultivars. Additionally, to beat the animals to the fruit, humans likely gathered them before they had sugared completely and while they were higher in vitamin C.

When you think of fructose, do you think of fruit sugar, the sweet, succulent juice of a navel orange that pours juice down your chin as you bite into it? A medium size orange has about 3 grams of fructose.

Hunter-gatherers, consuming a "caveman diet," probably consumed less than seven grams of fructose per day. Small amounts of wild berries are produced throughout the growing season, but the big harvest of fruit from trees is in the fall. This works our well for putting on a thick layer of fat in preparation for winter, which is great for hibernation; if you sleep in a cave or are a bear.

By 1900, Americans were eating about 15 grams of fructose a day. By the beginning of World War II, before sugar rationing, fructose consumption had risen to about 20 grams a day. That is equivalent to 80 calories, a significant 4 to 5 percent of caloric intake. Obesity was still uncommon even though the average total caloric intake for Americans changed little from 1900 to 1960.

In the early 1970's, farm subsidies made growing corn profitable, made corn cheap, and high fructose corn syrup was invented. The HFCS now commonly used in food, with 55% fructose, 42% glucose, and 3% starch fragments, was not available on the market until 1977. Prior to that, HFCS was 42% fructose and 58% glucose[15], less fructose than table sugar. Between 1960 and 1984 the average per capita added fructose (from sugars and syrups) fluctuated between 49 and 51 grams a day; about 200 calories from added sugars. Then it began to ramp up. By 1999, when it peaked, the average per capita added fructose consumption was 65.6 grams a day. As of 2008, the average daily consumption had dropped to a mere 60 grams of fructose a day.

Fructose has about 4 Calories per gram. It takes 3500 calories to make a pound of fat, so it takes 875 grams of fructose to make a pound of fat.

Just for fun, let's pretend for a moment that the average adult gets a "free no consequence" 50 grams of consumption of fructose a day without weight gain. If this were true, this average American over the twenty-year period from 1960 to the end of 1979 would have gained an extra 1.5 pounds of weight from excess fructose. If this was true, and fructose was the only bad player, the average mythical adult, starting at age 20 in 1960, would reach middle age (40) weighing 1.5 pounds more than they had 20 years earlier.

Next, let's examine a mythical American child of our mythical person. This person was age 20 in 1985 and reached the age of 40 at the end of 2004 eating the average American dietary content of fructose. Such a person, consuming the average American fructose intake, would have gained 83 pounds over those 20 years. Today, the average person in America is getting 10 more grams of fructose a day than Americans did from 1960 to 1984. That is enough calories to add 4 extra pounds each year; 80 pounds in 20 years. That is for the *average* American; half of all American consume more!

Compare this to the prevalence trends for obesity in the U.S. In 1960, the prevalence of obesity in adults was 13.4%. By the late 1970's, 15% of adults were obese. By 1999, 31% of adults were obese, and by 2005, 35% of Americans were obese[16].

If weight gain were the only thing these extra calories did, it would not be pretty. But the metabolism of fructose is unique.

Most of the energy from glucose gets stored as glycogen in the liver, kidneys and muscles. Fructose, however, is not stored as "frycogen." It is turned into fat. Fructose can be used in the citric acid cycle for energy, but when excess fructose is consumed, as in the high amounts found in western diets, there is nowhere else for it to go. Fructose-1-phosphate is metabolized into free fatty acids. Fructose exposure induces the production of lipogenic proteins, which increases the efficiency of creating fats. Some of these triglycerides are packed into VLDL cholesterol particles for transport. VLDL carries fat to the adipose cells for storage, and what is left become small-dense-LDL cholesterol particles; the type that confers risk for atherosclerosis and ischemic heart disease. Not all of the fat is transported out of the liver and thus fructose, like alcohol, causes fatty liver disease.

Fatty liver is associated with abdominal obesity, insulin resistance, oxidative pathways, inflammation and mitochondrial dysfunction; the liver becomes less sensitive to insulin, thus, causing insulin resistance. High-fat diets add to the problem. High-fat diets can cause increased inflammation and induce the production of the inflammatory cytokines IL-1β and TNF-α in the GI system[17].

Fructose also causes a negative feedback loop that prevents glucose from being stored as glycogen. While fructose does not directly increase insulin production, it causes insulin resistance and thus, higher blood sugar levels.

The hallmark of type 2 diabetes is insulin resistance. This disease is initiated by a decline in adipose and other cell's sensitivity to insulin. To compensate, the pancreas produces more insulin. As the cells become progressively less sensitive to insulin, eventually, the overworked pancreas gives out; no longer able to ratchet up the production of sufficient insulin. The individual's blood sugar rises and the person becomes diabetic.

Leptin resistance is the hallmark of most obesity. The hormone leptin, produced in the adipose cells, tells the brain there is plenty of food in the pantry, and that the fat cells do not need additional fuel. In experiments with young animals bred for leptin resistance, high-fat diets cause obesity. In older animal models with leptin resistance, any diet will cause increased feeding and obesity[18].

Diets high in fructose also cause leptin resistance[19]. A high fructose diet induces the production of the inflammatory cytokine Tumor Necrosis Factor-alpha (TNF-α)[20], and this cytokine causes leptin and insulin resistance in the hypothalamus, fat cells and muscle cells[21, 22].

Dietary sorbitol is very poorly absorbed, and very little enters the blood stream. This is a good, as sorbitol damages cells. In hyperglycemic conditions, glucose is taken up by cells some is turned into fat. However, if there is excess glucose taken up by the cell, the enzyme aldose reductase converts glucose into sorbitol, which is then converted into fructose. This process consumes NADH, causing oxidative stress and the formation of advanced glycation end products (AGEs), which damage the cell. This is part of the process responsible for the formation of cataracts, diabetic retinopathy, vascular damage and renal disease, aging and cell death[23]. (See Chapter 21, section on Aging). Remember, most cells cannot import fructose; nor can they export it.

Table 9-3: Cells that can transfer Fructose[3]

Organ and cell type	Functions and Effects
Intestine (enterocytes)	Absorb fructose into the body
Kidney (tubular cells)	Reabsorb filtered sugars Kidney damage
Vascular (endothelial cells)	Epithelial dysfunction, vascular disease
Fat (adipocytes)	Storage as fat Central obesity
Liver (hepatocytes)	About 50 to 75% of all fructose is metabolized in the liver. Most fructose is converted into triglycerides (fat) Fatty liver

Renal damage from sweetened beverages can be seen even in thin persons. Two 12-ounce servings of sweetened drinks a day are enough to raise the risk of albuminuria, where the kidneys leak protein, a sign of damage to the kidneys[24]. This is more apparent in thin persons, perhaps because, for these individuals, the fructose in just 24 ounces of soda pop can represent 10% of their caloric intake. Many adolescent boys in America now consume as much as 17% of their daily caloric intake as fructose!

With insulin resistance, the body does not respond normally to insulin; more insulin is needed to move glucose out of the blood and into the cells where it can be stored or used for energy. A normal, healthy adult probably makes about 10 to 15 units of insulin a day. With insulin resistance, it takes more. One of my professors joked about the "300 Club": Type 2 diabetics who weighed 300 pounds, used 300 units of insulin a day and whose blood sugars still ran around 300 mg/dl. (Normal fasting range: 60 to 105 mg)

As an individual becomes insulin resistant, the pancreas works harder to make more insulin to try to keep blood sugar normal. Only about 1 to 2 percent of the cells in the pancreas are insulin-producing beta cells. After awhile the pancreas cannot keep up with the demand; it simply wears out. When it cannot keep up with the demand, the person's blood sugar goes out of control, and they are considered pre-diabetic or diabetic.

Healthy Serum Uric Acid (SUA) Levels

Where is the cutoff for normal and high SUA levels? Women have lower SUA levels than men and seem to more sensitive to its effects. Elevated cytokines can be used as an indicator of safe SUA levels. UA levels above 250 µmol/liter (4.2 mg/L) are associated with elevated C-reactive protein, TNF-a, and IL-6 in women, while levels above 400 µmol/L (6.7 mg/L) are required to increase levels of these cytokines in men[5].

Using currently available data, optimal serum uric acid level ranges are:

- 200 to 250 µmol/L (3.4 to 4.2 mg/dl) for adult women;
- 310 to 400 µmol/L (5.2 to 6.7 mg/dl) for adult men[25].

Low uric acid levels are also associated with disease; the effects of low levels are discussed at the end of this chapter.

Soft drinks:

It should go without saying, but just in case: soft drinks are not food. They are perhaps the single, major contributor to obesity and metabolic syndrome. They contain a lot of fructose. A 12-ounce can of Sprite has the same fructose content as 10 teaspoons of sugar. Additionally, the sugars and acids in sports drinks, energy drinks, and soft drinks dissolve the enamel on teeth. It softens the enamel, making it easy to get dental caries. Fructose is a favored food for the cariogenic bacteria *Streptococcus mutans* to form dental plaque.

The average American drinks 50 gallons of soda pop a year. That is 219 calories a day. However, as I don't consume my share, someone else must be. Two 16-ounce servings of soda pop contain about 400 calories. That is sufficient calories to gain an extra pound of fat every 9 days. Even if only the calories from fructose are counted, adding two 16-ounce servings of soda pop to the diet is enough to add a pound of fat every 16 days; an ounce of body fat for each quart of soda pop; 23 pounds of ugly and dangerous fat per year.

Calories per 12-Ounce Serving	
Gatorade Original	75
Gatorade Energy	110
Coca-Cola Classic	144
Sprite	150
Pepsi	150
Mug Root Beer	150
A&W Root Beer	180
Jones Energy	210

Many energy drinks and sports drinks are no longer even available in 12-ounce sizes. More typical are half liter (16.9 oz) to 22-ounce sizes.

Individuals in the Framingham study who drank more than 12 ounces of soda pop a day were 30 percent more likely to be obese (BMI > 30) and 62% more likely to develop metabolic syndrome[26]. Drinking sweets trains the palate for sweet, high-caloric foods. Fructose gives sweetness and calories that do not provide satiation so that the person remains unsatisfied and eats and drinks more.

What about Gatorade for rehydration, for example, after working out or when dehydrated? The World Health Organization, after many studies of dehydrated patients, recommends an oral rehydration fluid with 13.5 grams of carbohydrates per liter as being effective for rapid oral rehydration[27]. The typical soft drink contains about 100 grams of sugars per liter, over seven times as much. Modern Gatorade has much more fructose than the original beverage designed for athletes. Moreover, while glucose assists in water uptake by the intestine, fructose is not a good sugar for rehydration. It is more difficult to absorb, especially if it is present in higher concentration than glucose as it is in high fructose corn syrup. Further, about 30 percent of Caucasians have fructose malabsorption – where a large fructose load pulls water from the body into the intestine, worsening dehydration.

The sports medicine community no longer recommends forcing hydration, and now recommends drinking to your thirst, the amount that feels good.

Dietary Fructose Recommendations

Earlier in this chapter, a fiction was used, as an illustration, wherein a daily intake of 50 grams of fructose was used an upper safe limit. So what is a reasonably safe consumption of fructose for a healthy adult with a normal metabolism?

1. Meals with high in fructose and saturated fat should be avoided. It is no surprise that a juicy burger, with fries, washed down with a super-sized soda pop is not an ideal meal. The mid-length saturated fats along with the fructose raise plasma triglyceride levels and almost ensure fat deposition[13]. Not only will fructose turn to fat, it will help dietary fat be stored, rather than be burned as energy. It only takes half the amount of fructose to raise triglycerides when saturated fats are combined with a meal.

2. Avoid sweet beverages. Whether soda pop or fruit juice, don't drink the Kool-Aid. First, beverages do not trigger the cephalic phase hormone release of pancreatic polypeptide as do solid foods to prepare the body for the sugar load, and beverages do not suppress appetite, as do solid foods. Later, once absorbed, blood fructose does not suppress hunger, so more calories will be consumed. When a large bolus of fructose hits the liver, no good comes of it.

Fruit that is chewed and contains fiber helps satisfy the appetite[28]. The same fruit, when eaten as apple sauce has less effect on satiation, and the juice of the apple even less. Fiber acts as a slow release mechanism for sugars, including sucrose and glucose. This helps prevent insulin rebound; where insulin response is brisk enough to lower blood sugar sufficiently to provoke more hunger.

Orange juice drinkers in the U.S., however, are healthier and leaner than their non-OJ consuming peers; however, OJ indulgers, have better diets, overall[29]. When OJ was provided freely in one study, those drinking OJ consumed on average 16 ounces of OJ a day. After 12 months, OJ consumers has lower LDL cholesterol and apolipoprotein B[30]. OJ has a 1.1:1 F: G ratio (Table 5-7), and if unfiltered contains beneficial fiber. It takes 24 ounces of OJ a day to raise HDL and apoA[31] but drinking this much OJ every day sounds more like a chore than a pleasure.

3. Fructose should make up no more than ten percent of the caloric intake. Based on the typical pre-1980 American diet, I recommend that fructose should constitute no more than 10 percent of daily caloric intake. Fifty grams of fructose provide 194 calories. There are about 22 grams of fructose in 12 ounces of a typical soda; about the same amount as in 4 medium oranges or two medium apples. I see people drinking 18 oz. of cola frequently; I rarely see anyone eat 11 oranges in a sitting*. For reference, a half cup of sugar contains 50 grams of fructose.

Individuals with high triglyceride levels, type 2 diabetes, or waist circumference greater than 36 inches should keep fructose levels even lower.

*When I was in the Peace Corps, during mango season, it was not uncommon to see people eat 10 mangos in a sitting, and there were delightful occasions when 20 mangos a day would easily pass my lips. Another natural fructose binge is watermelon; a quarter of a sweet 10-pound watermelon can have nearly 40 grams of fructose. Pear, apple and grape juice have very high fructose contents, comparable to soda pop, and should be avoided; they cause obesity in children.

Alcohol

Fructose is not the only agent of uric acid trolls. Alcohol also raises uric acid levels and causes fatty liver. Ironically, beer actually does cause beer-belly[32,33]. And who would have guessed that alcohol increases leptin resistance[34]?

The Beer Institute, in Washington, D.C., reports that nearly 6.5 billion gallons of beer were consumed in the U.S in 2009. That is about 21.8 gallons for every man, woman and child residing in the country. However, since on average men consume 10 times as much beer as women and children drink even less, it can be estimated that the average man in the U.S. consumes about 60 gallons of beer a year in the U.S. Over a gallon a week! (Again, I am failing to do my part, leaving the burden of this beverage on others.)

Beer has about 13 calories per ounce; about 4 calories from carbohydrates and most of the rest from alcohol. If a man consumes 60 gallons of beer a year, that is only about 21 ounces of beer a day and 273 calories, a bit more than 10 percent of the dietary caloric intake of the average Joe. This is a significant number of calories; enough to add a pound of fat to the belly in 2 weeks.

However, beer (and liquor) does not just add calories. Alcohol is a toxin to the liver, and like fructose, it raises uric acid levels[35], plasma triglyceride levels and can cause fatty liver. When beer adds fat, it increases waist circumference; adding visceral fat, the type is associated with increased risk of diabetes, inflammation, and metabolic syndrome.

What about wine?

For the average person, wine does not increase uric acid levels[35] nor does it cause obesity[32]. Wine drinkers have smaller waists and lower uric acid levels than abstainers or beer or liquor drinkers. Most, if not all health benefits attributed to alcohol can be attributed to red wine.

Part of this effect may be that wine drinkers are less prone to binge drinking. The healthful effects of drinking a glass of wine a day, however, does not translate to consumption of seven glasses of wine on a Friday evening[36]. Even with beer and liquor, the pattern of alcohol consumption is important. While the volume of beer and liquor are associated with abdominal obesity, for a given amount of alcohol, the more evenly distributed throughout the week, the lower the risk of obesity. Thus drinking three beers a day is less fattening than saving up three and a half six packs of beer and drinking them over the weekend.

Wine also contains phenolic antioxidants, such as resveratrol; it is not the alcohol, but these factors in wine that are health-friendly. The health effects of alcohol are further discussed in Chapters 17 and 41.

Salt

It is generally recognized that diets high in salt are associated with high blood pressure. It is also recognized that salts added to foods make you thirstier; the salt added to colas encourages the consumer to drink more. When foods are salty, you tend to eat more of the food, as well. Salted foods raise blood sugar and insulin output more than unsalted foods. Salt (sodium chloride) is thought to accelerate the digestion of starches to glucose in the gut because chloride increases the activity of amylase, and sodium facilitates the uptake of glucose[37] (See facilitated transport in Chapter 3.)

In effect, salt raises the glycemic index of starchy foods, so that, for the same number of calories, blood sugar rises higher, gets there faster, requires more insulin output, turns more calories into fat, and gets you hungrier again, sooner.

Sphingolipids and Syndrome X

Sphingolipids are a diverse class of lipids based on sphingosine, an amino alcohol with an unsaturated hydrocarbon chain. Sphingosine is synthesized in the liver in humans from the amino acid serine and palmitoyl CoA. By adding a second fatty acid chain to sphingosine, ceramide is formed. Sphingomyelin, an important component of cell membranes and nerve sheaths is formed from ceramide by adding a phosphocholine or phosphoethanolamine polar head to the molecule.

Palmitoyl-CoA is formed from palmitic acid, a 16-carbon, saturated fatty acid (16:0). Palmitic acid (PA) is found in the diet from various sources, which include palm oil, but most of that found in the diet comes from meat, especially poultry, and dairy products. Palmitic acid is also formed in the liver from excess carbohydrates; *especially from fructose*. (PA) is atherogenic, and not coincidentally, is the most abundant fatty acid in the pro-atherogenic, Western diet.

PA is the fatty acid used exclusively by serine-palmitoyl transferase for the formation of sphingosine; increasing the supply of PA increases the production of sphingosine, ceramide, and sphingomyelin, and other sphingolipids in the liver, muscle fat tissues, and lipoproteins.

It is likely that ceramide is the element that puts the bad into "bad" LDL-cholesterol. In health, LDL-cholesterol is a transport vehicle for lipids. Lipids, including sphingolipids are needed to build and maintain healthy cells. LDL is just a delivery truck for raw materials; there is nothing inherently evil about it. In atherogenic diets, however, rich in PA or fructose there is a greater production of sphingosine and ceramide to be transported. Serum sphingolipid levels are directly correlated with insulin resistance, obesity, LDL levels and the proinflammatory cytokine TNF-α[38,39].

Moreover, the second fatty acid chain in ceramide is also affected by diet. The fatty acid attached to sphingosine to form ceramide is generally a long chain, predominantly C24:1, (Figure 6-8), followed by C24:0, but is can also include medium chain, monounsaturated or saturated fats. Individuals consuming diets high in PA and fructose have a significantly higher percentage of C16:0 as the second fatty acid moiety in the ceramide and sphingomyelin they form, and a lower percentage of long-chain fatty acids.

Sphingolipids are immune modulators greatly impact immune cell activity and survival. LDL or VLDL very rich in 16:0 ceramide as the second chain causes acid-SMase activity to decline in favor of serum-SMase activity in macrophages. This enhances uptake of LDL by macrophages and promotes their migration into the walls of the arteries, where they transform into inflammatory foam cells, causing atherosclerosis. The inflammatory cytokines IL-1β and INF-γ also stimulate serum-SMase in macrophages[40]. Minimally oxidized LDL or exposure to certain bacterial toxins, such as LPS, enhances the immune cascade in foam cells[41]. Ceramide with a lower percentage of long chained fatty acids is associated with cognitive decline in coronary artery disease patients[42].

It may also be a sphingolipid that imbues HDL with virtue. "Good" cholesterol (HDL) is also a lipid transport vehicle. About five percent of HDL particles contain the apoprotein, ApoM, that transports and makes delivery of sphingosine-1-phosphate (S1P). HDL, thus, transports and delivers S1P, which can have an anti-inflammatory, lipid-signaling activity when oxidative stress is low. About 65% of the S1P is transported through the blood is via HDL. The remaining 35% is transported via albumin[43], although when transported by this carrier, it may not be delivered to the same set of cells.

Ceramide is a risk factor for coronary artery disease (CAD) death[44]. Homocysteine, a risk factor for CAD, may exert its toxicity through its activation of acid-SMase activity and the resultant intracellular ceramide accumulation[45]. Secretory-SMase is upregulated in congestive heart failure[46], which may further damage the already weakened myocardium.

Sphingolipids are also involved in the pathogenesis of both type 1 and type 2 diabetes. Ceramide increases insulin resistance, decreases the production of insulin and induces the apoptosis of pancreatic β-cells[47].

Avoiding Metabolic Syndrome

1. Avoid Excess fructose: Avoid corn syrup sweetened soft drinks and fruit juices. Limit fructose to less than 10 percent of the daily caloric intake. Avoid fruit juice, even natural juice, with high fructose to glucose ratios.

2. Get Sufficient Magnesium: See Chapter 31.

3. Avoid Alcohol: Especially beer and distilled spirits.

4. Salt: Avoid salty, fatty snack foods.

5. Fatty foods: Avoid fatty meals, especially in combination with sweets, especially fructose. Limit the amount of palmitic acid in the diet.

6. Keep Uric acid levels in the normal range:
- Women: 200 to 250 μmol/L (3.4 to 4.2 mg/dl)
- Men: 310 to 400 μmol/L (5.2 to 6.7 mg/dl)

> **Cherries**: A couple of serving of cherries a day can keep the gout away. Gout patients that eat cherries have a third fewer attacks of gout[48]. Cherries have been shown to lower uric acid levels[49], raise urine urate levels, decrease levels of several markers of inflammation[50], and lower the activity of xanthine oxidase[51]. Cherries are high in phenolic acids and anthocyanin flavonoids[52]. Other fruits tested did not have a hyperuricemic effect.
>
> **Purines**: Diets high in purines can increase uric as purines are metabolized to uric acid. Dietary purines from animal flesh, (including seafood) however, appear to raise uric acid levels most potently; purines from vegetable[53] or dairy sources have much less impact[54].

7. Avoid the production of TNF-α: TNF-α increases insulin and leptin resistance that cause type 2 diabetes and obesity. TNF-α increases the apoptotic potential of ceramide and other sphingolipids. High fructose diets increase TNF-α. Melatonin may help avert TNF-α induced insulin resistance[55].

Anthocyanin, a phenol from fruit, appears to protect against the inflammatory effects of fructose[56], as do the polyphenolic compounds in green tea[57]. Curcumin also prevents inflammatory signaling, prevents the inflammatory cascade that promotes obesity, increases the production of the anti-inflammatory protein adiponectin by fats cells, and inhibits adipocyte differentiation[58]. Flavonoids and other related compounds in ginger, cinnamon, cloves, red chili and black pepper have similar capacities[59]. Whole foods and spices contain these phenolic compounds. Soda pop does not.

TNF-α is also strongly stimulated by lipopolysaccharide (LPS) from intestinal dysbiosis; the overgrowth of pathogenic bacteria in the gut is usually the major source of LPS in the body. LPS and dysbiosis are further discussed in Chapter 23. The phenolic compound chlorogenic acid, found in high concentrations in green coffee and plums, has been associated with weight loss[60].

Other phenolic compounds, including other hydroxy-cinnamic acids, also reduce dysbiosis and inflammation, thereby reducing inflammatory cytokines and obesity. Some phenolic compounds demonstrated to reduce TNF-α are listed in Table 31-2.

8. Eliminate antergens from the diet: Elimination of foods for which an individual has IgG immune reactivity has been found to cause weight loss of about one pound per week, accompanied by a reduction in waist circumference of nearly 3 inches over 90 days, without restricting caloric intake[61]. The mechanism of action is likely the reduction of inflammatory cytokines, as evidenced by the preferential loss of abdominal obesity. Food antergies are discussed in Chapter 19.

9. Avoid wheat: While fructose and alcohol are two of the principal causes of obesity and metabolic syndrome, wheat may also be an important contributor. When the Mediterranean diet was compared with a Paleolithic diet in patients with diabetes, the later was associated with improved insulin sensitivity and weight loss, with a loss of abdominal girth. The main difference between the diets was consumption of less wheat and dairy in the Paleolithic diet[62]. In heart disease patients, the Paleolithic diet was also found to be more satiating than the Mediterranean diet[63]. The health effects of wheat are discussed in more detail in Chapter 22.

10. Get Sufficient Sleep: Sleep deprivation promotes inflammation, hunger and weight gain. See Chapter 41.

11. Ensure Vitamin D levels are adequate: Low levels of vitamin D are associated with obesity, insulin resistance, diabetes, CAD, and inflammation. Vitamin D increases the metabolism of inflammatory ceramide to anti-inflammatory S1P. Vitamin D is discussed in Chapter 20.

12. Magnesium and Vitamin B$_6$: Magnesium and vitamin B$_6$ are essential cofactors for the SphK enzymes which convert ceramide to S1P. Magnesium is discussed in Chapter 31. Vitamin B6 is discussed in Chapter 40.

13. Alpha Lipoic Acid: The nutritional supplement ALA prevents non-enzymatic glycation of proteins and prevents the extensive cross-linking of collagen in the skin of animals fed high levels of fructose[64], and prevents insulin resistance in fructose-fed rats[65] and glomerular damage in diabetic animals[66]. It reduces established atherosclerotic plaques in rabbits[67] and restores the activity of the citric acid cycle in metabolizing glucose. Lipoic acid may prevent organ damage and curtail the aging effects of metabolic syndrome. ALA is discussed in Chapter 40.

14. Avoid Stress: Stress is associated with increased levels of TNF-α and cortisol, abdominal obesity, and insulin resistance. Stress is discussed in Chapter 29.

15. Evaluate for Mast Cell Activation Disorders: Rapid onset obesity, which occurs during adulthood, may result from mast cell activation disorders, and at times, it is easily treatable. See Chapter 12.

Insulin Resistance Syndrome Cluster[68]

Resistance to insulin-stimulated glucose uptake
Glucose intolerance
Hyperinsulinemia
Hypertension
Dyslipidemia with high triglyceride, small-dense-LDL and low concentrations of HDL
Central obesity
Increased uric acid concentrations
Higher circulating plasminogen activator inhibitor 1
Decreased circulating concentrations of adiponectin

Low Uric Acid Levels and Disease

Low uric acid levels (< 5.2 mg/dl, < 310 μmol/L in men or < 3.4 mg/dl, < 200 μmol/L in women) are a risk factor for mortality in hemodialysis patients. This may reflect protein malnutrition, oxidative stress, or other factors[69]. Both low and high uric acid levels are associated with increased mortality.

Reduced uric acid concentrations have been found in several neurological conditions, including multiple sclerosis, Parkinson's disease, Alzheimer's disease and optic neuritis[2]. Molybdenum deficiency may cause low UA levels due to impaired xanthine oxidase activity (Chapter 14). Additionally, uric acid induces astrocytes to produce a protein (EAAT-1) that protects neurons from glutamate toxicity.

Uric acid may act as an antioxidant that prevents the formation of the free radical peroxynitrite, which is formed by the reaction of nitric oxide (NO) with superoxide. Peroxynitrite is a strong oxidant, which selectively binds to the amino acid tyrosine in proteins; this can cause enzyme inactivation. Peroxynitrite can also inhibit the electron transport chain in the mitochondria by altering the permeability of the mitochondrial membrane, leading to cellular energy depletion and damage.

The inflammatory cytokines, IL-6 and IL-8, can induce increased urinary uric acid excretion and hypouricemia in patients with cancer or severe acute respiratory syndrome[70]. Fractional excretion of uric acid also becomes elevated in patients when blood oxygen saturation is low[71].

Numerous diseases are associated with elevated serum UA levels, and others are associated with low levels. High UA levels can cause gout, but high (or low) uric acid levels, do not in themselves, constitute a disease.

It is important to evaluate and understand the underlying condition and treat it. For example, about 80 percent of patients with elevated triglycerides have elevated serum UA levels; the goal should be to treat the cause of the lipid disorder. This hyperlipidemia may respond to dietary restrictions of fructose and alcohol.

Conversely, adding fructose and alcohol would not constitute a therapeutic approach to low serum UA levels in patients on dialysis. Oxidative and neurologic risk-associated low uric acid levels may be mitigated by supplementation with vitamin C as vitamin C supports the antioxidant activity of UA[72]. The underlying inflammatory disorder causing low uric acid levels needs to be investigated and treated.

Table 9-4 A (Mostly Humorous) History of Human Adaptations to Food

Adaptation	Time Occurred	Explanation
Metabolic Syndrome	1978	High fructose corn syrup and trans fats. Post reproductive age death – little survival pressure to effect evolution
Heart disease	1940	Trans fats, margarine, shortening. Lower fertility.
Dental Caries	1800	Refined sugar in the diet.
Lactose Tolerance	6000 B.C.	Punjab Indians and later Northern Europeans, become lactose tolerant to survive on milk (or die off)
Gluten Enteropathy	9000 B.C.	Wheat cultivated by the Syrians, becomes a staple. Allows greater storage of food, adaptation to dryer climates, the development of beer, and specialization away from hunter gathering to the development of trades and towns. Selects out individuals with HLA 2 and 8 alleles who do not tolerate it.
Pale faces	35,000 B.C.	Northward Migration, Clothing. Europeans lose skin pigmentation to adapt to less sunlight so they can make vitamin D more easily or die during childbirth as a result of pelvic deformation from rickets. Celts and Basques may have interbred with cold-adapted Neanderthals who had fair skin and red hair, providing an adaptive advantage. Asians and Inuits eat animal liver or die).
Loss of hair on face	1,000,000 B.C.	Loss of facial hair to better convey facial expression. Female primates lose their beards, to better convey facial expression to children. Disgusted facial expression to bitter substances (alkaloid toxins, conveys to others in the group not to eat it. Allows higher primates to experiment and eat wider array of plants. A sour facial expression reaction to acid substances – tells others in the group the fruit is not ripe and has little vitamin C.
Uricase Deficiency	Miocene Era 14 million B.C.	Allows upper primates to store fat more efficiently, and to survive the ice age, by increasing the storage of body fat from fructose in the diet.
Vitamin C recycling	20-25 million B.C.	Primates loose the ability to make vitamin C from glucose, and gain the ability to recylce it efficeintly[73], conserving the equivalent of 10 days worth of calories per year. Causes primates to select fruits that are ripe and higher in carbohydrates. Increased the consumption of vitamin C.
Scombroid Type Reaction	Jurassic Era	Disease from eating bacterial-infested flesh. 1. The smell of rotting flesh becomes unpleasant and foul. 2. Neuroreceptors (H3R) trigger fear memory, nausea and headache; gut receptors trigger vomiting and diarrhea, rapid heart and respiratory rate, dizziness. Think you're about to die. H2R increases stomach acid.

---

[1] Lessons from comparative physiology: could uric acid represent a physiologic alarm signal gone awry in western society? Johnson RJ, Sautin YY, Oliver WJ, et al.. J Comp Physiol B. 2009 Jan;179(1):67-76.. PMID: 18649082

[2] Altered uric acid levels and disease states. Kutzing MK, Firestein BL. J Pharmacol Exp Ther. 2008 Jan;324(1):1-7. PMID: 17890445

[3] Hypothesis: could excessive fructose intake and uric acid cause type 2 diabetes? Johnson RJ, Perez-Pozo SE, Sautin et al. Endocr Rev. 2009 Feb;30(1):96-116. PMID: 19151107

[4] Haemoglobin A1c, fasting glucose, serum C-peptide and insulin resistance in relation to serum uric acid levels--the Third National Health and Nutrition Examination Survey. Choi HK, Ford ES. Rheumatology (Oxford). 2008 May;47(5):713-7. PMID: 18390895

[5] Elevated serum uric Acid is associated with high circulating inflammatory cytokines in the population-based colaus study. Lyngdoh T, Marques-Vidal P, Paccaud F, et a;. PLoS One. 2011;6(5):e19901. PMID:21625475

[6] Uric acid is associated with features of insulin resistance syndrome in obese children at prepubertal stage. Gil-Campos M, Aguilera CM, Cañete R, Gil A. Nutr Hosp. 2009 Sep-Oct;24(5):607-13.PMID: 19893872

[7] Recent data on pubertal milestones in United States children: the secular trend toward earlier development. Herman-Giddens ME. Int J Androl. 2006 Feb;29(1):241-6; discussion 286-90. PMID:16466545

[8] Data from the National Health and Nutrition Examination Surveys. CDC.

[9] Prevalence of Obesity in the United States, 2009–2010. Ogden CL, Carroll MD. NCHS Data Brief No. 82 January 2012

[10] Data from the Centers for Disease Control and Prevention

[11] Hypothesis: could excessive fructose intake and uric acid cause type 2 diabetes? Johnson RJ, Perez-Pozo SE, Sautin et al. Endocr Rev. 2009 Feb;30(1):96-116..PMID: 19151107

[12] Sugar-sweetened soft drinks, diet soft drinks, and serum uric acid level: the Third National Health and Nutrition Examination Survey. Choi JW, Ford ES, Gao X, Choi HK. Arthritis Rheum. 2008 Jan 15;59(1):109-16.PMID: 18163396

13 Food carbohydrates and plasma lipids--an update. Truswell AS. Am J Clin Nutr. 1994 Mar;59(3 Suppl):710S-718S. PMID: 8116555

[14] Cephalic phase pancreatic polypeptide responses to liquid and solid stimuli in humans. Teff KL. Physiol Behav. 2010 Mar 3;99(3):317-23. Nov 26. PMID:19944113

[15] Data derived from USDA Economic Research Service: http://www.ers.usda.gov/Data/FoodConsumption/FoodAvailSpreadsheets.htm#sweets

[16] National Center for Health Statistics, NHANES data.

[17] Polycyclic aromatic hydrocarbons potentiate high-fat diet effects on intestinal inflammation. Khalil A, Villard PH, Dao MA, et al.. Toxicol Lett. 2010 Jul 15;196(3):161-7.. PMID: 20412841

[18] Leptin resistance: a prediposing factor for diet-induced obesity. Scarpace PJ, Zhang Y. Am J Physiol Regul Integr Comp Physiol. 2009 Mar;296(3):R493-500..PMID: 19091915

[19] Fructose-induced leptin resistance exacerbates weight gain in response to subsequent high-fat feeding. Shapiro A, Mu W, Roncal C, et al. Am J Physiol Regul Integr Comp Physiol. 2008 Nov;295(5):R1370-5..PMID: 18703413

[20] Anti-inflammatory effect of atorvastatin on vascular reactivity and insulin resistance in fructose fed rats. Mahmoud MF, El-Nagar M, El-Bassossy HM. Arch Pharm Res. 2012 Jan;35(1):155-62. PMID:22297754

[21] Modulation of hypothalamic PTP1B in the TNF-alpha-induced insulin and leptin resistance. Picardi PK, Caricilli AM, de Abreu LL, et al. FEBS Lett. 2010 Jul 16;584(14):3179-84. PMID: 20576518

[22] Insulin resistance induced by tumor necrosis factor-alpha in myocytes and brown adipocytes. Lorenzo M, Fernández-Veledo S, Vila-Bedmar R, et al. J Anim Sci. 2008 Apr;86(14 Suppl):E94-104. PMID:17940160

[23] The polyol pathway as a mechanism for diabetic retinopathy: attractive, elusive, and resilient. Lorenzi M. Exp Diabetes Res. 2007;2007:61038..PMID: 18224243

[24] Sugary soda consumption and albuminuria: results from the National Health and Nutrition Examination Survey, 1999-2004. Shoham DA, Durazo-Arvizu R, Kramer H et al. PLoS One. 2008;3(10):e3431..PMID: 18927611

[25] Serum uric acid and cardiovascular mortality the NHANES I epidemiologic follow-up study, 1971-1992. National Health and Nutrition Examination Survey. Fang J, Alderman MH. JAMA. 2000 May 10;283(18):2404-10. PMID:10815083

[26] Soft drink consumption and risk of developing cardiometabolic risk factors and the metabolic syndrome in middle-aged adults in the community. Dhingra R, Sullivan L, Jacques PF, et al. Circulation. 2007 Jul 31;116(5):480-8.. PMID: 17646581

[27] Recent Advances of Oral Rehydration Therapy (ORT). Suh JS, Hahn WH, Cho BS. Electrolyte Blood Press. 2010 Dec;8(2):82-6. PMID:21468201

[28] The effect of fruit in different forms on energy intake and satiety at a meal. Flood-Obbagy JE, Rolls BJ. Appetite. 2009 Apr;52(2):416-22. PMID:19110020

[29] 100% orange juice consumption is associated with better diet quality, improved nutrient adequacy, decreased risk for obesity, and improved biomarkers of health in adults: National Health and Nutrition Examination Survey, 2003-2006. O'Neil CE, Nicklas TA, Rampersaud GC, Fulgoni VL 3rd. Nutr J. 2012 Dec 12;11:107 PMID:23234248

[30] Long-term orange juice consumption is associated with low LDL-cholesterol and apolipoprotein B in normal and moderately hypercholesterolemic subjects. Aptekmann NP, Cesar TB. Lipids Health Dis. 2013 Aug 6;12(1):119. PMID:23919812

[31] HDL-cholesterol-raising effect of orange juice in subjects with hypercholesterolemia. Kurowska EM, Spence JD, Jordan J, et al. Am J Clin Nutr. 2000 Nov;72(5):1095-100. PMID:11063434

[32] Association of the waist-to-hip ratio is different with wine than with beer or hard liquor consumption. Atherosclerosis Risk in Communities Study Investigators. Duncan BB, Chambless LE, Schmidt MI, et al. Am J Epidemiol. 1995 Nov 15;142(10):1034-8.PMID: 7485048

[33] Waist circumference in relation to history of amount and type of alcohol: results from the Copenhagen City Heart Study. Vadstrup ES, Petersen L, Sørensen TI, Grønbaek M. Int J Obes Relat Metab Disord. 2003 Feb;27(2):238-46.PMID: 12587005

[34] Alcohol intake modifies leptin, adiponectin and resistin serum levels and their mRNA expressions in adipose tissue of rats. Pravdova E, Macho L, Fickova M. Endocr Regul. 2009 Jul;43(3):117-25. PMID:19817506

[35] Beer, liquor, and wine consumption and serum uric acid level: the Third National Health and Nutrition Examination Survey. Choi HK, Curhan G. Arthritis Rheum. 2004 Dec 15;51(6):1023-9.PMID: 15593346

[36] The relation between drinking pattern and body mass index and waist and hip circumference. Tolstrup JS, Heitmann BL, Tjønneland AM, Overvad OK, Sørensen TI, Grønbaek MN. Int J Obes (Lond). 2005 May;29(5):490-7.PMID: 15672114

[37] Salt and the glycaemic response. Thorburn AW, Brand JC, Truswell AS. Br Med J (Clin Res Ed). 1986 Jun 28;292(6537):1697-9. PMID: 3089360

[38] Serum sphingolipids and inflammatory mediators in adolescents at risk for metabolic syndrome. Majumdar I, Mastrandrea LD. Endocrine. 2012 Jun;41(3):442-9. PMID:22228496

[39] Plasma sphingosine-1-phosphate is elevated in obesity. Kowalski GM, Carey AL, Selathurai A, Kingwell BA, Bruce CR. PLoS One. 2013 Sep 6;8(9):e72449. PMID:24039766

[40] Characterization of secretory sphingomyelinase activity, lipoprotein sphingolipid content and LDL aggregation in ldlr-/- mice fed on a high-fat diet. Deevska GM, Sunkara M, Morris AJ, et al. Biosci Rep. 2012 Oct;32(5):479-90. PMID:22712892

[41] The SYK side of TLR4: signalling mechanisms in response to LPS and minimally oxidized LDL. Miller YI, Choi SH, Wiesner P, Bae YS. Br J Pharmacol. 2012 Nov;167(5):990-9. PMID:22776094

[42] Ceramides predict verbal memory performance in coronary artery disease patients undertaking exercise: a prospective cohort pilot study. Saleem M, Ratnam Bandaru VV, Herrmann N, et al. BMC Geriatr. 2013 Dec 12;13:135. PMID:24330446

[43] An update on the biology of sphingosine 1-phosphate receptors. Blaho VA, Hla T. J Lipid Res. 2014 Jan 23. PMID:24459205

[44] Molecular lipids identify cardiovascular risk and are efficiently lowered by simvastatin and PCSK9 deficiency. Tarasov K, Ekroos K, Suoniemi M, et al. J Clin Endocrinol Metab. 2014 Jan;99(1):E45-52. PMID:24243630

[45] Homocysteine induces cerebral endothelial cell death by activating the acid sphingomyelinase ceramide pathway. Lee JT, Peng GS, Chen SY, et al. Prog Neuropsychopharmacol Biol Psychiatry. 2013 Aug 1;45:21-7. PMID:23665108

[46] Secretory sphingomyelinase is upregulated in chronic heart failure: a second messenger system of immune activation relates to body composition, muscular functional capacity, and peripheral blood flow. Doehner W, Bunck AC, Rauchhaus M, et al. Eur Heart J. 2007 Apr;28(7):821-8. PMID:17353227

[47] Role of ceramide in diabetes mellitus: evidence and mechanisms. Galadari S, Rahman A, Pallichankandy S, Galadari A, Thayyullathil F. Lipids Health Dis. 2013 Jul 8;12:98. PMID:23835113

[48] Cherry consumption and decreased risk of recurrent gout attacks. Zhang Y, Neogi T, Chen C, Chaisson C, Hunter DJ, Choi HK. Arthritis Rheum. 2012 Dec;64(12):4004-11. PMID:23023818

[49] Consumption of cherries lowers plasma urate in healthy women. Jacob RA, Spinozzi GM, Simon VA, et al. J Nutr. 2003 Jun;133(6):1826-9. PMID:12771324

[50] Sweet bing cherries lower circulating concentrations of markers for chronic inflammatory diseases in healthy humans. Kelley DS, Adkins Y, Reddy A, Woodhouse LR, Mackey BE, Erickson KL. J Nutr. 2013 Mar;143(3):340-4. PMID:23343675

[51] Hypouricemic effect of the methanol extract from Prunus mume fruit in mice. Yi LT, Li J, Su DX, Dong JF, Li CF. Pharm Biol. 2012 Nov;50(11):1423-7. PMID:22856880

[52] http://www.phenol-explorer.eu/contents/food/47 Accessed December 2013.

[53] Purine-rich foods intake and recurrent gout attacks. Zhang Y, Chen C, Choi H, Chaisson C, Hunter D, Niu J, Neogi T. Ann Rheum Dis. 2012 Sep;71(9):1448-53. PMID: 22648933

[54] Purine-rich foods, dairy and protein intake, and the risk of gout in men. Choi HK, Atkinson K, Karlson EW, Willett W, Curhan G. N Engl J Med. 2004 Mar 11;350(11):1093-103. PMID:15014182

[55] Melatonin improves metabolic syndrome induced by high fructose intake in rats. Kitagawa A, Ohta Y, Ohashi K. J Pineal Res. 2011 Dec 7. PMID:22220562

[56] An extract of chokeberry attenuates weight gain and modulates insulin, adipogenic and inflammatory signaling pathways in epididymal adipose tissue of rats fed a fructose-rich diet. Qin B, Anderson RA. Br J Nutr. 2011 Dec 6:1-7. PMID:22142480

[57] Green tea polyphenol extract regulates the expression of genes involved in glucose uptake and insulin signaling in rats fed a high fructose diet. Cao H, Hininger-Favier I, Kelly MA, et al. J Agric Food Chem. 2007 Jul 25;55(15):6372-8. PMID:17616136

[58] Curcumin and obesity. Bradford PG. Biofactors. 2013 Jan;39(1):78-87. PMID:23339049

[59] Targeting inflammation-induced obesity and metabolic diseases by curcumin and other nutraceuticals. Aggarwal BB. Annu Rev Nutr. 2010 Aug 21;30:173-99. PMID:20420526

[60] The use of green coffee extract as a weight loss supplement: a systematic review and meta-analysis of randomised clinical trials. Onakpoya I, Terry R, Ernst E. Gastroenterol Res Pract. 2011;2011. pii: 382852. PMID:20871849

[61] Eliminating Immunologically-Reactive Foods from the Diet and its Effect on Body Composition and Quality of Life in Overweight Persons. Lewis JE, Woolger JM, Melillo A, et al. J Obes Weig los Ther. (2012) 2:112.

[62] Beneficial effects of a Paleolithic diet on cardiovascular risk factors in type 2 diabetes: a randomized cross-over pilot study. Jönsson T, Granfeldt Y, Ahrén B, et al. Cardiovasc Diabetol. 2009 Jul 16;8:35. PMID:19604407

[63] A paleolithic diet is more satiating per calorie than a Mediterranean-like diet in individuals with ischemic heart disease. Jönsson T, Granfeldt Y, Erlanson-Albertsson C, Ahrén B, Lindeberg S. Nutr Metab (Lond). 2010 Nov 30;7:85. PMID:21118562

[64] Fructose diet-induced skin collagen abnormalities are prevented by lipoic acid. Thirunavukkarasu V, Nandhini AT, Anuradha CV. Exp Diabesity Res. 2004 Oct-Dec;5(4):237-44. PMID:15763937

[65] Lipoic acid prevents liver metabolic changes induced by administration of a fructose-rich diet. Castro MC, Massa ML, Schinella G, Gagliardino JJ, Francini F. Biochim Biophys Acta. 2013 Jan;1830(1):2226-32. PMID:23085069

[66] Effects of dietary supplementation of alpha-lipoic acid on early glomerular injury in diabetes mellitus. Melhem MF, Craven PA, Derubertis FR. J Am Soc Nephrol. 2001 Jan;12(1):124-33. PMID:11134258

[67] Lipoic acid effects on established atherosclerosis. Ying Z, Kherada N, Farrar B, et al. Life Sci. 2010 Jan 16;86(3-4):95-102. PMID:19944706

[68] Fructose, weight gain, and the insulin resistance syndrome. Elliott SS, Keim NL, Stern JS, Teff K, Havel PJ. Am J Clin Nutr. 2002 Nov;76(5):911-22. Review.PMID: 12399260

[69] Low serum uric acid level is a risk factor for death in incident hemodialysis patients. Lee SM, Lee AL, Winters TJ, et alJ. Am J Nephrol. 2009;29(2):79-85. PMID:18689987

[70] Hyponatremia, hypophosphatemia, and hypouricemia in a girl with macrophage activation syndrome. Yamazawa K, Kodo K, Maeda J, Omori S, Hida M, Mori T, Awazu M. Pediatrics. 2006 Dec;118(6):2557-60. PMID:17142545

[71] Renal hypouricemia is an ominous sign in patients with severe acute respiratory syndrome. Wu VC, Huang JW, Hsueh PR, et al. Am J Kidney Dis. 2005 Jan;45(1):88-95. PMID:15696447

[72] Uric acid as a CNS antioxidant. Bowman GL, Shannon J, Frei B, Kaye JA, Quinn JF. J Alzheimers Dis. 2010;19(4):1331-6. PMID:20061611

[73] Erythrocyte Glut1 triggers dehydroascorbic acid uptake in mammals unable to synthesize vitamin C. Montel-Hagen A, Kinet S, Manel N, Mongellaz C, et al. Cell. 2008 Mar 21;132(6):1039-48. PMID:18358815

10. Immune Cells

It's a dangerous life. There are the great predators: lions, tigers and bears, wolves and sharks. There are storms with lightning, mudslides, and tornadoes. There are pesky humans that delight in waging wars or break into homes at night. But the most dangerous of threats are the ones too small to see: the microbes. We protect ourselves with clubs and teeth, walls, fighter jets and guns, but our most important defense for survival is an immune system which can destroy the really tiny and most dangerous things. But like most weapons, the immune system is dangerous, can backfire, and cause injury and disease.

Hematopoiesis

Hematopoiesis is the development of blood cells and immune cells from stem cells which mostly reside in the bone marrow. Long-term hematopoietic stem cells (**LT-HSC**) reproduce themselves and also create short-term hematopoietic stem cells (**ST-HSC**). These ST-HSCs are the source for red blood cells and platelets as well as for white blood cells, which comprise much of the immune system. The LT-HSC reproduce to create a large number of ST-HSC in the bone marrow which supply the various immune and blood cells needed for the body. The various hematopoietic cells are produced under the influence of signaling cytokines and hormones.

Table 10-1: Blood Cell Derivation

Precursor Cell Type	Cells Produced	Stimulating Cytokine/Hormone
Short-term hematopoietic stem cells (ST-HSC)	Common Myeloid Progenitor	Interleukin-3 (**IL-3**)
	Common Lymphocytic Progenitor	Interleukin-7 (**IL-7**)
	Tissue Mast Cells	Stem Cell Factor (**SCF**) Interleukin-6 (**IL-6**), Others
Common myeloid progenitor (**CMP**) (CFU-GEMM)	Granulocyte-macrophage progenitor (**GMP**)	SCF, Granulocyte-macrophage colony-stimulating factor (**GM-CSF**)
	Megakaryocyte-erythroid progenitor (**MEP**)	GM-CSF
Granulocyte-macrophage progenitor (**GMP**)	Monocytes → Macrophages, microglia	Macrophage colony-stimulating factor (**M-CSF**), IL-6
	Myeloid Dendritic Cells	M-CSF, FMS-like tyrosine kinase 3 ligand (**FLT3-L**)
	Granulocytes	Granulocyte colony-stimulating factor (**G-CSF**)
Granulocytes	Neutrophils	IL-6
	Basophils	IL-6
	Eosinophils	Interleukin-5 (**IL-5**)
Megakaryocyte-erythroid progenitor (**MEP**)	Red Blood Cells (**RBCs**)	Erythropoietin (**EPO**)
	Megakaryocyte → Platelets	Thrombopoietin (**TPO**) Interleukin-11 (**IL-11**)
Common lymphocytic progenitor (**CLP**)	T Cells → T helper cells, Memory cells, and Cytotoxic T cells	IL-7
	B Cells → Plasma Cells	IL-7, FLT3-L
	Natural Killer Cells	
	Lymphoid Dendritic Cells	FLT3-L
T Helper Cells	T helper 1 (**T$_H$1**) cell	Interleukin-2 (**IL-2**), Interferon Gamma (IFN-γ) Interleukin-27 (**IL-27**)
	T helper 2 (**T$_H$2**)	IL-2, IL-4, Notch
	T helper 17 (**T$_H$17**)	IL-6, IL-17, IL-17, Transforming Growth Factor Beta (**TGF-β**)
	Regulatory T Cell (**T$_{REG}$**)	Interleukin-10 (**IL-10**), TGF-β

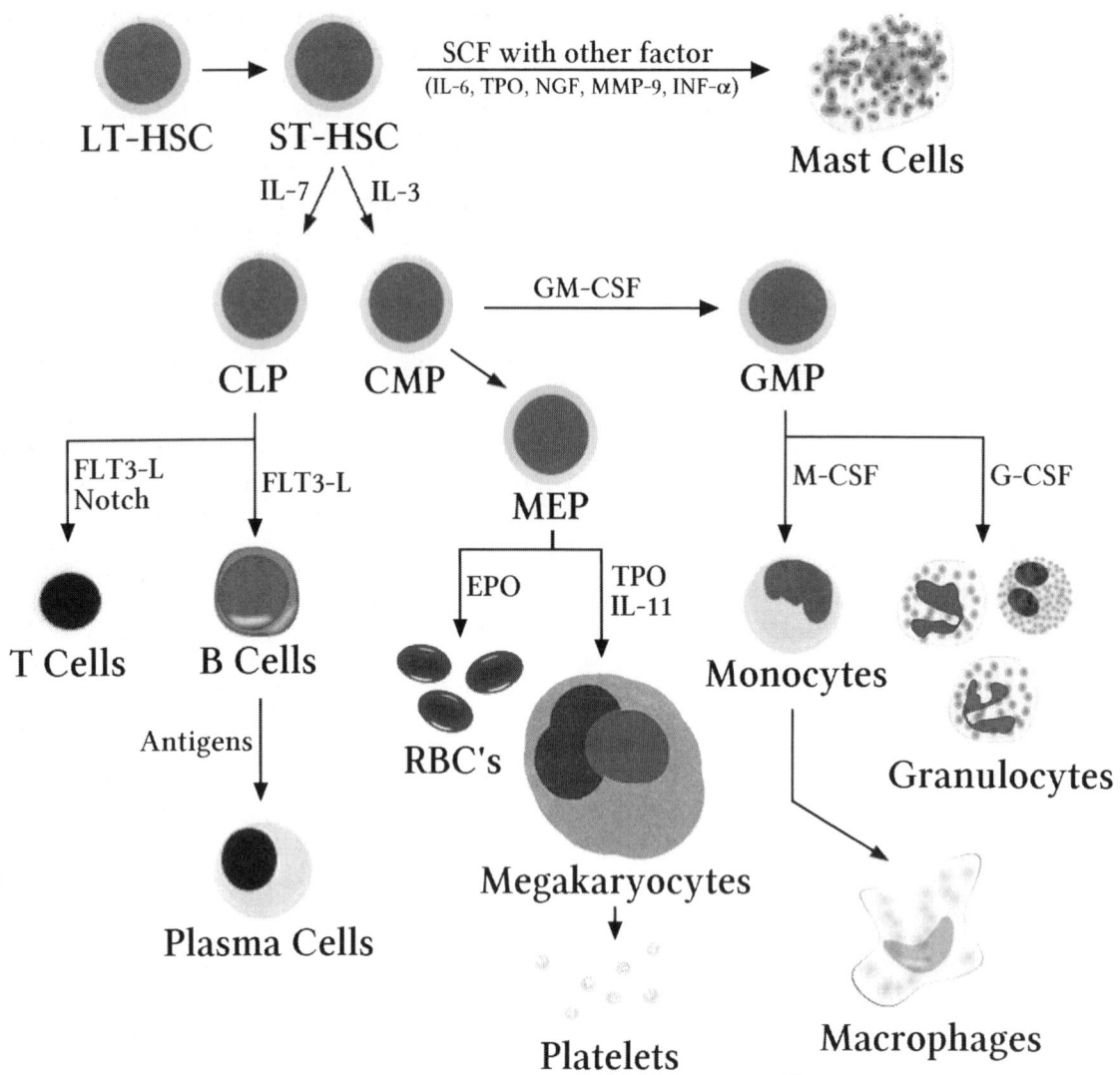

Figure 10-1: Hematopoietic Differentiation[1,2]

Granulocytes

If the white blood cells were an army, the granulocytes would be soldiers; they have weapons, attack in mass, and often create a mess. There are three forms of granulocytes: neutrophils, basophils, and eosinophils.

Neutrophils, the most prevalent white blood cell (WBC), usually comprise about 70 percent of the circulating WBC population. Neutrophils are the principal WBCs attacking infections. At the site of injury or infection, TNF-α promotes adhesion molecules that allow WBC's to stick to the blood vessel endothelium and then migrate into the tissue. They are attracted to the site of injury or infection by chemotaxis, a process of traveling up a concentration gradient of signaling cytokines: IL-8, INF-γ, C5a, and leukotriene B_4. Once at the site of the infection or injury, neutrophils phagocytize bacteria and cellular debris. Armed with superoxide, a powerful reactive oxygen species, and lytic enzymes, they kill and degrade the material they phagocytize. Neutrophils can releases granules with antibacterial and proteolytic enzymes, and proteins that act like a web that traps bacteria.

Basophils mostly migrate into the tissue and recognize foreign proteins. When activated, basophils release granules with proteolytic enzymes, cytokines, heparin, and histamine. They help fight parasitic infections. Basophils secrete IL-4 and likely play a role in the development of allergies.

Eosinophils, like basophils, help fight parasitic infections and also trigger allergic reactions. They contain numerous inflammatory mediators, including cytokines, inflammatory eicosanoids, and reactive oxygen species.

Monocytes: Monocytes are WBC's that circulated for one to three days, and then migrate into the tissue where they differentiate into either macrophages or dendritic cells. Monocytes and their progeny act principally in phagocytosis, antigen presentation, and cytokine production. Cytokines produced by monocytes include TNF, IL-1, and IL-12. Monocytes respond to inflammatory signals, move to the area of inflammation and then transform into tissue macrophages.

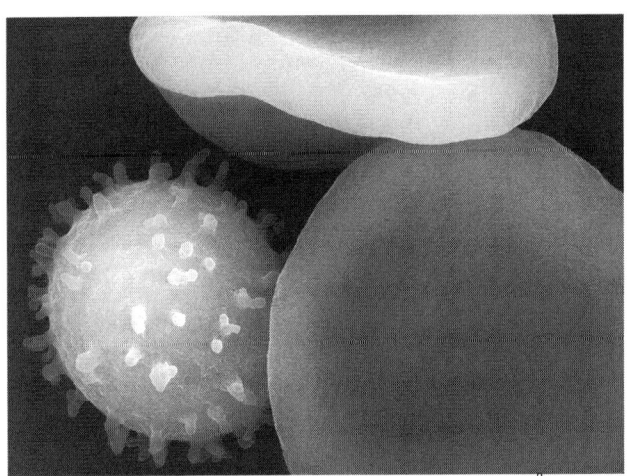

Figure 10-3: Monocyte with red blood cells[3]

Macrophages are large phagocytic cells and immune surveillance cells. They consume microorganisms, such as bacteria and yeast and digest cellular debris. Macrophages can also act as antigen-presenting cells. They deliver proteins, usually from the surface of pathogens they have digested, to T-helper cells. They thus aid in developing immune recognition.

Some tissues have macrophages that are differentiated sufficiently to be recognized as specific cell types. These include osteoclasts, in the bone; Kupffer cells, in the liver; Dust cells, in the pulmonary alveoli; histiocytes, in the connective tissue; Hofbauer cells, in the placenta; and microglia, in the brain and spinal cord.

Macrophages differentiate into specialized subpopulations within the organs they develop in. One subpopulation of macrophages clean up tissue damage in muscles, and other acts in tissue repair after injury, for example. There are eight named subpopulations of microglia in the brain, each with specialized abilities.

Microglia: Microglial cells develop from a unique form of monocyte that can enter across the blood-brain barrier. Microglia are specialized phagocytic cells in the brain and spinal cord which act like police patrolling the central nervous system (CNS) and looking for intruders. They can recognize and avidly phagocytize foreign matter, and clean up dead or damaged cells. They can also trigger inflammatory reactions in the brain.

Since most immunoglobulins are too large to enter through the blood-brain barrier, microglia are endowed with the ability to identify and react to infections without the benefit of antibodies. They are extremely sensitive to and become activated by perturbations in extracellular calcium levels, which occur at the site of nerve injury[4]. They act largely as part of the innate immune system. The innate (inborn) immune system acts by recognizing self from non-self, rather than adaptive immune response which recognize foreign materials it has had experience with. Microglia are also activated by LPS and other bacterial products. Brain trauma can easily active the microglia (Chapter 30).

Mast cells: Mast cell progenitor cells are developed in the bone marrow, and then migrate to the tissue depending on exposure chemotactic factors. For example, mast cells expressing chemokine receptor 2 (CXCR2) migrate to the intestinal mucosa under the influence of interleukin-8[5]. Mast cell growth and differentiation depend on Stem Cell Factor (SCF) binding to c-kit ligand, which is present on the mast cell surface. Many other progenitor cells carry c-kit ligand, but mast cells are the only terminally differentiated cell with this receptor. SCF for mast cell development is produced by endothelial cells, epithelial cells, and fibroblasts. Thus, mast cells congregate in the mucosa, skin, and blood vessels. The mast cell population can grow locally, under the influence of several cytokine cofactors. These cofactors include IL-6, Nerve Growth Factor (NGF), TPO, Interferon-α (INF-α), and matrix metallopeptidase 9 (MMP-9)[6].

Mast cells are like sentries with guns loaded, ready to shoot. Mast cells are similar to basophils; they develop from hematopoietic stem cells directly in the tissue rather than in the bone marrow. They form granules that contain over 200 different mediators, many of which are ready to be released upon activation. Like eosinophils and basophils, the mast cell surface has many FcεRI receptors that bind to the Fc (base) portion of IgE antibodies. When two or more IgE antibody Fab recognition surfaces bind to a pathogen or allergen, it triggers degranulation of the mast cell with the release of histamine and numerous other inflammatory mediators.

Lymphocytes

If granulocytes are the ground troops, the lymphocytes are commanders, scouts, spies, and snipers. It is the lymphocytes that coordinate the immune system and the defense against aliens and foreign agents. The lymphocytes use signaling molecules (cytokines) that give instructions to other white blood cells.

B-cell lymphocytes that have been activated become **Plasma Cells** that produce antibodies that target specific antigens or cells which bear those antigens. Plasma cells are committed to producing antibodies to a single antigen; however antibody class can change. The antibodies are exported from the plasma cells and act as ligands for linking antigens to white blood cells.

Antibodies are immunoglobulins (immune proteins). Most have a site for attaching to immune cells; the fixed region, at one end of the molecule, and areas configured to adhere to specific antigens; the antigen binding sites, on the other end. Antibodies are produced by B-cells that have developed into plasma cells in response to activation by T helper cells. Immunoglobulins have specific receptors on the granulocytes, macrophages, and mast cells. For example, immunoglobulin receptors on neutrophils and macrophages allow recognition of antibodies that have adhered to antigens on bacteria, and thus, allow the phagocytosis of those bacteria.

Depending on the conformation of the immunoglobulins and the type of cells they attach to, immunoglobulins are grouped into various classifications.

Table 10-2: Antibodies

Immunoglobulin	Principal Actions
IgA	Protects the respiratory, urogenital, and gastrointestinal mucosa. No fixed region: IgA neutralizes bacteria, preventing their adhesion and endocytosis.
IgD	Antigen receptor on B cells prior to immune activation by T cells.
IgE	IgE is associated with reactions to parasites and also allergic reactions. It first adheres to the mast cell, basophil or eosinophil and later to antigens the cells come into contact with. IgE triggers release of inflammatory mediators from mast cells and basophils.
IgG	The major antibodies providing protection against invading pathogens
IgM	Associated with new infections – Eliminates pathogens while IgG reactivity is under development.

T Cells

Natural Killer T (NKT) cells recognize glycolipid antigens and can eliminate some tumor cells and cells infected by some viruses. When activated, NKT cells rapidly produce stimulating cytokines that can promote the induction of various T helper cells.

T cells originate in the bone marrow and move to the thymus where they specialize. T cells are a large class of lymphocytes integral to the immune system. T cells differ from other lymphocytes, such as B cells and natural killer cells, in that they mature in the thymus and have special T cell receptors (TCR). Initially, they do not express CD4 or CD8 antigens; later in their development, they express both. Still later, they lose one antigen and become CD4+/CD8- bearing cells or CD4-/CD8+ bearing cells.

Only about 2 percent of T cells mature and leave the thymus as immunocompetent T cells. Most are selected out and are consumed by macrophages because of failure to recognize major histocompatibility complexes/ self-antigens. T cells need to be able to recognize the MHC/self-antigens in order to affect an immune response. At the same time, cells that are capable of binding too strongly with self-antigens are eliminated as they could cause autoimmunity and attack healthy organs. T cells that survive and recognize MCH class I antibodies become CD8+ T cells and those which recognize MCH class II antibodies become CD4+ T cells.

Cytotoxic T cells are CD8+ T cells that have CD8 glycoproteins on their surface. These cells recognize antigens associated with MHC class I molecules that are present on the surface of all cells of the body other than red blood cells. The MHC class I molecules are surface antigens that act like a flag that lets the CD8+ T cells know that the cell is not a foreign invader; the cytotoxic T cells thus leave these cells alone. If a cell is hijacked by viruses or becomes a tumor cell, it will usually not produce the MCH class I antigen or not present them correctly; the cytotoxic T cell will then attack and destroy the cell.

As cytotoxic T cells attack cells, they do not recognize as self, they act in transplant rejection. IL-10 and adenosine can down-regulate (decrease the production of) cytotoxic T cells and cause anergy: the lack of immune response.

Memory T cells are a subset of antigen-specific T cells (either CD4+ or CD8+) that persist long after the infection has resolved. They remember antigens that have attacked the body in the past, and can quickly expand the number of effector T cells if the antigen they recognize reappears. This provides long-term immunity to many infectious agents that we have experienced. These cells are the reason that we usually only get a specific viral illness, such as measles or chicken pox, once during our lifetime as the body can recognize the invaders and deal with them quickly.

Dendritic cells (DC) are specialized surveillance cells acting like spies embedded in the tissues. Tissue dendritic cells can develop from common lymphocytic progenitor cells or originate from monocytes. They are embedded in tissues and have many long thin arms which project between cells so that they can monitor for foreign antigens. They phagocytize materials and recognize non-self antigens. When they have gathered sufficient foreign antigens, they migrate back into the blood stream or lymphatic drainage, and then to the lymph nodes or spleen, where they present the antigens to T cells for further processing.

The dendritic cells are professional antigen presenting cells (APC) that can induce T-cell immune response to class I and II MHC antigens. In the lymph nodes or spleen, they present class I antigens to CD8+ T cells, and class II antigens to CD4+ T cells. The binding of the T-cell receptor to the APC MHC and antigen is called signal 1. If the APC does not react to the antigen, it stops there, and the T cell assumes that the antigen is not a problem. If the APC does react to the antigen, it produces another surface protein, B7-1 (CD80) or B7-2 (CD86) which bind to CD28 on the T cell. This signal 2 activates the production of IL-2, which stimulates activation and proliferation of T cells that respond to that antigen.

The activated T helper cell, still bound to the APC, produces an immunoglobulin, CTLA-4, which binds CD28 on the T cell, blocking adhesion to B7 molecules on the

APC. This acts as a stop signal for T cell proliferation and keeps the immune system from over activity. Mutations in CTLA-4 that prevent its activity have been found in some cases of autoimmune diseases, including multiple sclerosis, type 1 diabetes, systemic lupus erythematosus, (SLE), and Grave's disease. Conversely, CTLA-4 binding antibodies, such as ipilimumab, which prevent CTLA-4 activity, have been found to be useful in treating some cancers, as they inhibit immune tolerance and allow continued immune stimulation.

T Helper Cells: T helper cells are a special type of white blood cells derived from Naïve CD4+ cells, which are neither cytotoxic nor phagocytic; they do not attack bacteria or other cells. Instead, they activate and direct other cells in the immune system. In a way, these cells have the most critical job among the immune cells. If they do their job correctly, the body is usually well protected from infectious disease and cancer. If they do not, we are in trouble.

The T helper cells help promote B cells into plasma cells and direct the switching of antibody classes. They also help in the activation and reproduction of cytotoxic T cells. Once activated, T helper cells divide rapidly and produce cytokines that regulate the immune response.

Naïve CD4 T cells in the lymph nodes can differentiate into at least three different classes of CD4 effector T cells during their initial response to an antigen. They either become T_H1, T_H2 or T_H17 cells; cells with very different activities. Exposure of naïve T4+ helper cells to various cytokines determines the type of the T4+ cell they differentiate into. These differentiated T helper then produce more cytokines which promote the development of more of the same type of T helper cell, and suppress the development of other classes of T helper cells; allowing the immune system to dedicate its resource to one type of injury or infection at a time.

T_H1 Lymphocytes: T_H1 lymphocytes specialize in the regulation of the immune response to intracellular infections. Viruses are obligate intracellular pathogens. Some bacteria and fungi are capable living and reproducing either inside or outside of host cells, as facultative intracellular parasites while others are obligate intracellular parasites. Table 10-4 shows some of the important intracellular microbial pathogens which cause human disease. T_H1 cells also help to eliminate tumor cells through the formation of IFN-γ.

T_H2 Lymphocytes: T_H2 lymphocytes defend the body from extracellular infections. When extracellular parasites are identified by the immune system, for example, by dendritic cells carrying their antigens to lymph nodes, T_H2 cell production is up-regulated. More T_H2 cells capable of interacting with parasites such as eosinophils are produced. T_H2 cells are also responsible for chronic rhinitis and chronic asthma.

Table 10-3: T Helper Cell Immune Function

T Helper	CD4+ Naïve Cell Products
T_H1 Cells: Intracellular pathogens	Dendritic cells collect antigens from viruses and some classes of bacteria, and in response, release interleukin-12 (IL-12) and induce NK cells to produce interferon-γ (IFN-γ). Naïve CD4 T cells (T_H0 cells) exposed to IL-12 and IFN-γ become T_H1 cells that help the body eliminate host cells infected by viruses or intracellular bacteria. When the T_H1 cells are activated by exposure to these antigens, they release more IFN-γ; promoting more T_H1 cell production and down-regulation of the conversion of T_H0 to T_H2 or T_H17 cells.
T_H2 Cells: Extracellular pathogens	Other pathogens, such as helminths, cause NK1.1 T cells to produce and release interleukin-4 (IL-4). T_H0 cells activated in the presence of IL-4, become T_H2 cells. When T_H2 cells are activated by exposure their antigen, they release more IL-4 and IL-13, which promotes more T_H2 cells.
T_H17 Cells: Enteric bacteria, fungi	T_H17 cells are common in the lamina propria of the distal small intestine and large intestine. They are important in protecting the body from gram-negative bacterial and fungal infections[7]. A combination of the cytokines IL-6 and transforming growth factor-β (TGF-β) promote differentiation of naïve T_H0 cells into T_H17 cells.
T_H22 Cells: Candida	May be active in the defense against fungal infection. Elevated in psoriasis and systemic sclerosis. Produce IL-22.
T_{REG} Cells	T_{REG} cells down-regulate the immune response and return the system to a normal baseline. T_{REG} cells are induced (iT_{REG} cells) following antigenic stimulation in the presence of related antigen and specialized immunoregulatory cytokines, such as TGF-β, IL-10, and IL-4. Inducible T_{REG} cells express CD25 and FoxP3. Induction of T_{REG} cells is inhibited by IL-6.

The release of IL-4 from T_H2 cells induces production of IgE that is responsible for allergic reactions. IL-4 also inhibits IFN-γ, decreasing T_H1 cell production. Thus, the more exposure a person has to allergens they react to, the more likely it is that the person will develop other allergies. Additionally, an immune system focusing on allergic hypersensitivity reactions is less able to control viral and some bacterial infections. IL-25, also produced by T_H2 cells, antagonizes differentiation into T_H17 cells.

Conversely, IFN-γ from T_H1 cells inhibits IgE production. IFN-γ inhibits the development of T_H2 cells, and both IL-4 from T_H2 cells and IFN-γ from T_H1 cells inhibit the development of T_H17 cells.

Table 10-4: Examples of Intracellular Parasites Causing Human Disease

Type of Infection	Obligate Intracellular Parasites	Facultative Intracellular Parasites
Viruses	All viruses	
Bacteria	*Chlamydia*, and closely related species *Rickettsia* (Typhus, Spotted Fever) *Coxiella* (Q fever) Certain species of *Mycobacterium* such as *Mycobacterium leprae* (Leprosy)	*Brucella* (Brucellosis) *Legionella* (Legionnaire's disease) *Mycobacterium* (Tuberculosis) *Yersinia* (Plague) *Neisseria meningitides* (Meningitis) *Francisella tularensis* (Tularemia) *Listeria monocytogenes*
Fungus		*Candida albicans* *Histoplasma capsulatum* (Histoplasmosis)
Protozoa	*Plasmodia species* (Malaria) *Leishmania spp.* *Toxoplasma gondii* (Toxoplasmosis) *Trypanosoma cruzi* (Chagas disease)	

Another cytokine, IL-27, important for the differentiation of T_H1 cells acts as a potent inhibitor of T_H17 differentiation. IL-2, which is a growth factor for most T cells and T cell subsets, appears to have inhibitory effects on the expansion of T_H17 cells[8].

Once T helper cells are committed, they produce cytokines that induce replication of more T helper cells of the same lineage and suppress the development of other T helper cell lineages.

Interleukin-6 inhibits the induction of naïve CD4 lymphocytes into T_{REG} cells. Thus, IL-6 prevents down regulation of the immune system after infection. Additionally, IL-6 helps transform naïve T_H0 cells into T_H17 cells, essential for protecting the body from pathogenic microbes that cross the colonic mucosa membrane into the lamina propria. T_H17 cells take part in autoimmune reactions, including diseases that affect organs having few resident T_H17 cells.

Infectious Disease and Immune Subversion: Acute exacerbations of chronic bronchitis are the stairway to heaven for many smokers. Each exacerbation causes an irreversible loss of lung capacity and another step down into respiratory insufficiency. Trypsin, heparin, and other proteases and immune products damage the lung tissue. Between exacerbations, there is little decline in lung function.

Initially, asthma is triggered by specific antigens, usually IgE allergens that the patient has become sensitized to. However, with continued exposure, the lungs become hyperreactive and react to exposure to non-specific irritants, such as smoke and environmental pollutants, triggering T_H2-dominant inflammatory reactions.

The large majority of exacerbations of COPD are caused by rhinoviruses, the common cold virus. This virus does not cause lung disease in healthy individuals. In chronic asthmatics and patients with chronic bronchitis, where T_H2 cells predominate, T_H1 antiviral defenses are suppressed, and they cannot mount a normal antiviral defense. The T_H2-dominated response is adapted for the destruction of multicellular parasites, large and small, rather than the precision elimination of infected cells as that is accomplished by T_H1 activation.

Smooth muscle contraction, increased vascular permeability, and mucus secretion may be helpful in fighting parasites, but does not help fight viral infection. Mast cell degranulation releases chymase, tryptase, serine esterases, and metalloproteinases which can easily cause the destruction of lung tissue.

Similarly, patients chronically exposed to IgG food sensitivities (antergens; see Chapter 19) may be at greatly increased susceptibility to recurrent or chronic intracellular infections as these antergies divert immune activation, supporting T_H17 cells response at the expense of T_H1 cell activity. Recurrent Herpes simplex and Herpes zoster, for example, may be an indication of a subverted immune response, and may go into remission with avoidance of T_H17 antigenic stimulation by foods to which the patient has IgG sensitivities.

Patients with inflammatory conditions should avoid allergens and other immunogens they react to in order minimize the predominance of the immune system by T_H2 or T_H17 cells.

T_H17 Lymphocytes: T_H17 cells are unusual, in that a supermajority of the body's population of them is limited to the lamina propria of distal ileum and the large intestine. Here they protect the body from gram-negative bacteria in the intestine and additionally from fungal infections. These cells help to maintain the endothelial barrier by supporting the tight junctions. In disease conditions, however, they produce cytokines that promote autoimmune disease activations. T_H17 activity is elevated in as rheumatoid arthritis, Crohn's disease, psoriasis and multiple sclerosis. Although cytokines usually act locally, these cells do not need to be present in the end organs being damaged in these diseases.

Table 10-5: Roles of T Helper Cells

T_H1 Cells	T_H2 Cells	T_H17 Cells[9]
Intracellular microbes and viruses. Directs cell-mediated immune responses against intracellular parasites. T_H1 cells produce IFN-γ and lymphotoxin (TNFβ)	Extracellular: Helminths, parasites, and extracellular bacteria. Involved in eosinophilic inflammation. T_H2 cells secrete IL-4, IL-13, and IL-25	Gram Negative Bacteria and fungi. T_H17 cells secrete IL-17, IL-17F, and IL-23, and have significant roles in protecting the host from bacterial and fungal infections, particularly at mucosal surfaces of the intestines.
Induce B cells mainly into IgG production; particularly IgG2a and IgG3. IgG2 is adapted to carbohydrate antigens found on cell surfaces and has limited complement activating abilities.	Induces B cells mainly into IgE production.	Induces B cells mainly into IgA production. Secretory IgA (sIgA) is associated with mucosa.
Cytotoxicity, eliminating tumor cells.	Allergic Reactions	Potent inflammatory potential; key mediators of autoimmune disease.

T_H17 cells recruitment appears to require symbiotic microbiota of very specific commensal intestinal bacteria: segmented filamentous bacterium[10] (SFB) along with other antigens[11]. SFB colonization results in the production of Serum Amyloid Antigen that acts on dendritic cells, inducing T_H0 cell transformation into T_H17 cells. A combination of the cytokines IL-6 and transforming growth factor-β (TGF-β) promote differentiation of naïve T cells into T_H17 cells. TGF-β without IL-6 tends to promote T_{REG} cells that down-regulate immune function. IL-23 can promote the proliferation of T_H17 cells that may cause destructive inflammatory reactions[12].

The presence of T_H17 cells in the intestinal mucosa presents the potential for contact with antigenic materials in the diet, particularly with incompletely digested proteins. Immunoglobulins to foods has been linked to rheumatoid arthritis[13], multiple sclerosis[14], and Crohn's disease[15], as well as other autoimmune diseases. Bacterial overgrowth in the small intestine also stimulates T_H17 activity.

T_H22 Lymphocytes: T_H22 cells are very rare in healthy individuals; they comprise fewer than 0.05 to 0.11% of circulating CD4 cells. Levels may be twice this in patients with psoriasis[16] and are also elevated in systemic sclerosis[17]. These cells produce IL-22 and are thought to be active in the defense against fungal infections.

T_{REG} Lymphocytes: Regulatory T (T_{REG}) cells have an essential role in maintaining immune homeostasis. T_{REG} cells suppress the development of other T cells, limit the immune response, and help maintain immunologic tolerance. These cells are essential in shutting down T cell-mediated immunity towards the end of an immune response and they suppress auto-reactive T cells which have escaped from the thymus.

There are both CD4+ and CD8+ derived T_{REG} cells. About five to ten percent of CD4+ cells become natural T_{REG} cells. These are T cells with high affinity for self-antigens. These cells down-regulate the immune system and help prevent autoimmune reactions. They do not require external cytokines for development.

Inducible T regulatory (iT_{REG}) cells: When an infection has been successfully overcome, the immune system needs to stand down. The iT_{REG} cells participate in this function. In the presence of specialized immunoregulatory cytokines, such as TGF-β, IL-10, and IL-4, iT_{REG} cells are formed that down-regulate the immune response. This helps to reverse the positive feedback loop that occurs during the mounting of an immune response.

Excessive iT_{REG} activity may prevent an antitumor immune response. Elevated numbers of T_{REG} cells have been found in several malignant disorders including cancers of the breast, pancreas, and lungs.

The immune system acts more powerfully by dedicating resources to eliminate one type of threat at a time. The more action T_H1, T_H2 or T_H17 cells get, the more the immune system becomes committed to that particular line of defense. As these cells become activated by encountering antigens they are keyed to, they release chemical mediators that signal for the development of more T_H0 cells to differentiate into their own type. Thus, the more viral infections one is exposed to, the more likely the T_H0 lymphocytes are to become T_H1 cells, capable of stimulating antiviral immune function; the more action T_H2 cells see, the more likely T_H0 lymphocytes will become T_H2 cells, capable of allergic response. The immune system moves resources around in infections to fight the disease agent. This, however, can lead to lower immune competence in other areas. Inappropriate immune reactions, such as chronic allergy, can lower the body's ability to react to some infections.

Paracytic infections and allergies increase T_H2 cell activity. The more exposure to allergens, the more likely that the body will aggressively view food, pollen or other foreign substances as dangerous foreign agents, and thus, the more likely new allergies will develop.

Cytokines

Cytokines are signaling molecules that help control inflammation. They help direct the immune response by signaling activation and growth of certain populations of immune cells in response to specific stimuli; act as chemoattractants; suppress the growth of other immune cells; signal when it is time for the inflammatory response to switch to a repair and regrowth response and for inflammatory cells to undergo apoptosis. These small proteins are produced by most nucleated cells; however among their most significant roles is their activity in the immune cells, including lymphocytes, macrophages, and mast cells. Cytokines also are produced by endothelial cells lining the blood vessels, fibroblasts, and muscles. They are produced in response to infection, trauma, and cancer, but also to exercise. They signal reproduction and growth; apoptosis of immune and nonimmune cells; and help regulate metabolism.

Cytokines include interleukins (IL), chemokines (CCL, CXCL), tumor necrosis factor (TNF), interferons (INF), transforming growth factors (TGF) and colony stimulating factors (CSF). Cytokine names do not always represent clearly distinct molecular or functional groups; their name may be derived from the cell type or function in which they were first identified. For example, the IL-10 cytokine subfamily includes interferons. The term lymphokine refers to cytokines produced by lymphocytes and myokines to those produced by muscles, although the same cytokine might be produced by either cell type.

While many cytokines are pro-inflammatory, others help resolve inflammation. Cytokines function through their stimulus of specific cell surface cytokine receptors but may also have nuclear receptors. One cytokine may activate more than one cytokine receptor, and a given cytokine receptor may react to more than one cytokine. The activity promoted by a cytokine depends on the cell type, the receptors currently manifested on the cell at the time, and by which other cytokines are also influencing the cell.

IL-6, for example; which is elevated by chronic stress, obesity, and sleep deprivation; helps maintain active production of T helper cells, especially T_H17 cells, and prevents the formation of T_{REG} cells. TH17 cells also produce IL-6. IL-6 can thereby maintain an inappropriate immune response, especially in the intestinal mucosa where the T_H17 cells are mostly situated. Excessive activity of T_H17 cells can lead to an inappropriate immune response to foods (Chapter 19) and can promote inflammatory and autoimmune disease. IL-6, however, is also formed and released by muscles during exercise, which can raise circulating IL-6 levels up to 100 times the resting levels. As a myokine, IL-6 induces lipolysis and oxidation of fat. It is released with dozens of other myokines after exercise[18] that together, have an anti-inflammatory effect. IL-15, another myokine, is an anabolic cytokine which increases muscle growth[19].

Table 10-6: Examples of Cytokine Activity

Cytokine	Activity
CCL5	This chemokine recruits T cells, eosinophils, and basophils into the site of inflammation
IL-1β	Proinflammatory; induces prostaglandin synthesis
IL-2	Induces T cell proliferation and promotes T cell immune memory.
IL-4	Transformation of T_H0 to T_H2 cells. Increases production of IgE
IL-5	Promotes eosinophils.
IL-6	Crosses blood-brain barrier. It raises body temperature, is proinflammatory in the presence of TNF-α, and anti-inflammatory when not. It is anti-inflammatory as a myokine released after exercise[19].
IL-10	Anti-inflammatory activity; less T_H0 to T_H1
IL-13	Promotes T_H0 to T_H2 cells in response to parasites. Active in asthma.
INF-γ	Immune response against viral and other intracellular infections. Induces NK cells, IgG2a, and IgG3 production, macrophage activity, chemotaxis, and other functions. Interferons have antitumor activity.
TNF-α	Antitumor activity; induces apoptosis.

Toll-like Receptors

The toll-like receptors are a family of membrane receptors that bind to and respond to pathogen-associated molecular patterns (PAMPs), such as some molecules found bacterial cell walls. These proteins are highly conserved in nature; humans have ten of them. They play a major part in immune recognition by white blood cells and other cells. Most are surface receptors, but some are intracellular; TLR3, TLR7, TLR8, and TLR9 are located on endosomes in immune cells and recognize viral DNA or RNA.

Table 10-7: Human Toll-Like Receptors and Ligands

TLR	Ligand
TLR1	Bacterial Lipopeptides
TLR2	Lipoteichoic acid: Gram-positive bacteria Glycolipids: Bacteria Zymosan: Fungi Heat shock proteins: From damaged host cells
TLR2/10	Peptidoglycans: Gram-positive bacteria
TLR3	Double-Stranded RNA: Viruses
TLR4	Lipopolysaccharides: Gram-negative bacteria Heat shock proteins, Fibrinogen, Heparin sulfate and Hyaluronic acid fragments: from host cells. Nickel, oxidized LDL, and certain opioid drugs
TLR5	Flagellin: Bacteria
TLR6	Diacyl-lipopeptides: Mycoplasma
TLR7	Single-Stranded RNA: RNA viruses
TLR8	Single-Stranded RNA: RNA viruses
TLR9	CpG oligodeoxynucleotides: Bacterial and DNA virus DNA

TLR's act in pairs, forming dimers. Some are homodimers, such as TLR4/4, while others may form mixed pairs. Heterodimers, such as TLR1/6, TLR1/2 or TLR2/10, have different ligand specificity. When the TLR binds its ligand, it can be pulled into the cell by endocytosis, where it activates a response cascade. There are two TLR signaling pathways; via MyD88 or TRIF. Other than TLR3, all TLRs use MyD88; several TLR's use both pathways.

TLR's inflammatory signal is mediated by the intracellular protein MyD88. Activation of MyD88 indirectly promotes the phosphorylation of Iκ-Ba, which frees NF-κB. NF-κB can then diffuse into the nucleus of the cell. MyD88 also activates MAPK (Mitogen-activate protein kinase). MAPK, depending upon the cells other influences, may promote cellular proliferation, cellular arrest, and even apoptosis via the transcription factor AP-1. In the TRIF pathway, inactive IRF3 is phosphorylated and forms a complex with CREBBP that is then translocated to the nucleus. TLR1 and TLR2 activation causes TRIF phosphorylation that also activates the TRAF6 → RIP → P13K → Akt → Iκ-Ba pathway, releasing NF-κB.

NF-κB, AP-1, and IRF3/CREBBP are nuclear transcription factors. They bind to specific DNA areas and transcribe RNA for inflammatory response peptides and proteins. NFκB also promotes ubiquitin-mediated proteolysis; thus providing materials for new inflammatory proteins.

The cytokines shown in Figure 10-4 show only some of the proteins produced. CD80, for example, stimulates T cells. CXCL9 is a T cell chemokine, and CCL5 is a chemokine for neutrophils, immature dendritic, and NK cells. CASP8 activation does not necessarily lead to apoptosis; rather it is influenced by the activation or inhibition of other elements in the apoptotic cascade.

Various inflammatory cells, and cells in different organs, not only express different TLRs, or different amounts of TLRs, they also express differing amounts of the proteins that control inflammatory signaling. NFκB and TRIF activation, thus, produces differing amounts of cytokines and different inflammatory, proliferative, or apoptotic actions, depending on the TLR ligand, the cell, and the cellular milieu at the time of activation.

TLR4 is activated by LPS from the cell walls of most anaerobic gram-negative bacteria. LPS is transported in the blood, bound to LPS binding protein (LBP), which binds to CD14. Activation of CD14 dimerizes two MD2-TLR4 complexes in the cell membrane, binding them together and activating the TLR4 inflammatory cascade that helps fight the bacterial infection. This inflammatory process can also cause disease. Minimally-oxidized LDL cholesterol can also dimerized and activate TLR4 on macrophages, especially in synergy with LPS. This TLR4 activation of macrophages induces foam cell production in the walls of arteries and is an essential step in the pathogenesis of atherosclerosis[20]. Many opiates are also TLR4 agonists, but naloxone is a TLR4 antagonist.

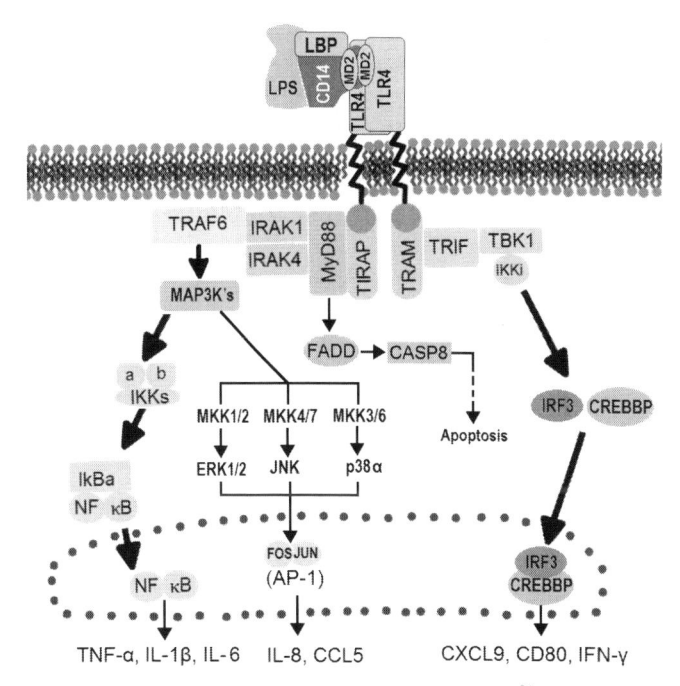

Figure 10-4: TLR activation cascade[21].

TLRs in the GI Tract: Toll-like receptors also play and essential role in the protecting the gastrointestinal epithelium from microbia. TLR4 and TLR5 are present on intestinal epithelial cells. Additionally, the immune cells of the GI tract use TLRs for recognition and immune defenses against pathogens.

Most of the colonic biome is composed of gram-negative rods; lipopolysaccharide (LPS) is part of the outer coat of the cell wall in these bacteria. TLR4 recognizes LPS. Clostridia are gram-positive bacteria. TLR5 on the enterocyte is activated by the ligand flagellin on these bacteria[22]. In the small intestine, intraepithelial T-lymphocyte in the villi are activated by enterocyte MyD88 signaling from the TLR's; this stimulates the production of antimicrobial peptides such as RegIIIγ. RegIIIγ is an antibacterial lectin which binds to bacteria in the mucus, preventing them from adhering to the enterocytes, and forming biofilms[23]. Thus, TLR's are integral to maintaining a physical barrier that separates the microbiota of the intestines from contacting its cells.

The TLRs induce or suppress thousands of genes that participate in growth, differentiation, the inflammatory response, and cell death.

Lipid Rafts

Many immune functions depend on recognition of foreign proteins. This process involves the binding of an antigen to a recognitions site, such as an antigen receptor, such as the IgE receptor Fcε, or the dimerization of TLR4's. Perhaps as a precaution against activation by innocuous debris, many immune receptors must react as pairs. Thus, for these reactions, binding of the peptide to a single receptor does not trigger immune activation. It requires an antigen with at least two binding sites in close proximity, or sufficient concentration to activate two receptors, which when activated, must link to each other to trigger the immune event. This helps prevent pieces of proteins from food or from pathogens that have already been killed from triggering immune processes. The requirement for receptor pair activation can be found in both innate and adaptive immune processes. It is seen in IgE activation of mast cells, for antigen presentation to T-cells for the MHC, and in B-cell receptor signaling. Toll-like receptors function in pairs that are located within lipid rafts[24].

If the receptors were randomly distributed, floating about in the cell membrane, it would require a huge number of receptors to cover the immune cell surface; otherwise, reactions would be slow and rare. The very efficient solution to this is that these receptors are thus clustered into lipid rafts within the cell membrane.

The lipid rafts are regions of the cell membrane that contain three to five times as much cholesterol and have a fifty percent higher concentration of sphingolipids, such as sphingomyelin, and lower levels of glycerophospholipids, such as phosphatidylcholine, than other areas. These sphingolipid/cholesterol-rich regions self-assemble within the lipid bi-layer.

Sphingomyelin (SPM) is a phospholipid found in cell membranes. Structurally, it is similar to other membrane phospholipids in that it has two nonpolar carbon chains and a polar, phosphate head. One of its carbon chains is based on C16:0 saturated palmitic acid, and the second is usually a long monounsaturated or unsaturated fatty acids, as shown in Figure 6-8. SPM is narrower and stiffer than most other phospholipids in the membrane, and it densely clusters with cholesterol in the membrane. This forms a locus where the membrane is unusually thick, rigid, and hydrophobic. The diacylglycerophospholipids that are more common in cell membranes usually have fatty acid moieties with multiple, double bonds that are kinked, causing the molecules to be shorter and wider and less dense.

SPM is found in high concentrations in the interior "leaf" of lipid rafts within the cell membrane and in the outer leaf of the nuclear, bilipid membrane. Thus, SPM tends to be found in high concentrations in membranes facing the cytosol, where intracellular enzymes can interact with it. Lipid rafts are also found on some organelle membranes, such as on lysosomes membranes.

Only proteins matching this thick hydrophobic/hydrophilic domain on the lipid raft side of the membrane can aggregate or anchor within the raft; meanwhile proteins with narrower hydrophobic domains are excluded. This provides increased stability of the raft structure; receptors within the raft may also be less susceptible to proteasomal degradation, and thus, these proteins tend to have longer-term activity than other cell surface proteins.

Sphingolipids and Immune Function

The lipid rafts also serve as sphingolipid storage areas. Just as phosphodiesterase A2 releases long-chain fatty acids from the cell membrane as a source for eicosanoids, sphingomyelinase (a.k.a. sphingomyelin phosphodiesterase) releases ceramide from sphingomyelin in the lipid raft.

Ceramide, sphingosine, sphingosine-1-phosphate (S1P) and ceramide-1-phosphate (C1P) are bioactive lipids that mediate apoptosis, cell proliferation, differentiation, adhesion, and migration, principally through their activity as signaling molecules. They help regulate immune activity, angiogenesis, growth, nociception, and apoptosis. They are integral to the regulation of immune cell activity and for protection and growth of the nervous system. Dysfunction in the regulation of these sphingolipid metabolites is seen in and may be the cause of various cancers, autoimmune diseases, and mood disorders. Ceramide promotes atherosclerosis and the damage during ischemic events. Sphingolipids mediate various opposing actions; for example, ceramide promotes arrest of growth and apoptosis; while S1P and C1P promote cell proliferation and survival.

As shown in Figure 10-5, sphingosine is formed from the amino acid serine and palmitoyl-CoA. Palmitoyl-CoA is formed from palmitic acid, a 16-carbon, saturated fatty acid (16:0). Most sphingolipids are formed de novo in the liver and enterocytes, as little if any sphingolipid from the diet is absorbed intact.

Serine + palmitoyl-CoA
↓
Sphingosine
↓
Sphingomyelin ⇌ (SMase / SM Synthase) Ceramide ⇌ (Ceramide Kinase / Phosphatase) Ceramide-1-phosphate
↕ (Ceramidase / Ceramide Synthase)
Sphingosine
↕ (SphK1 SphK2 / Phosphatase)
Sphingosine-1-phosphate
↓ S1P Lyase
Phosphoethanolamine + Palmitaldehyde

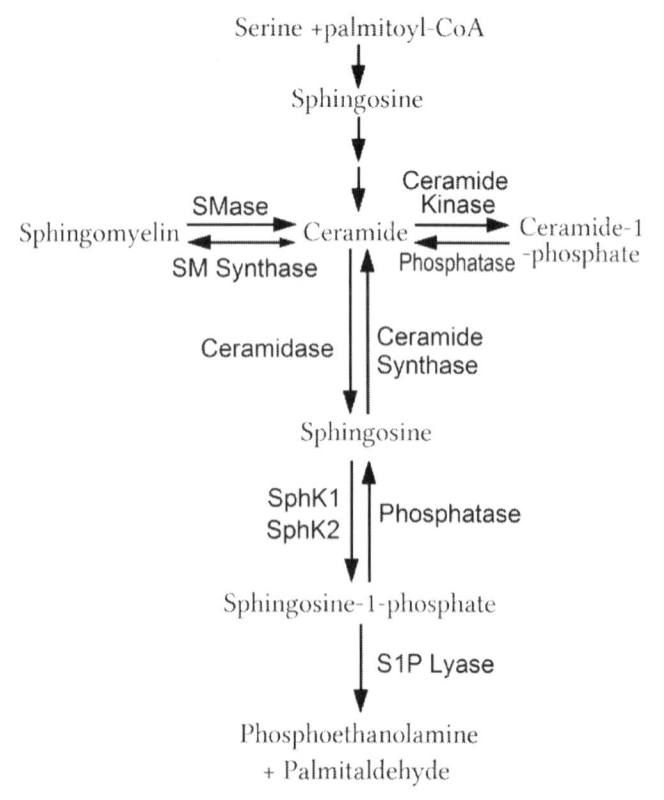

Figure 10-5: Sphingolipid Pathway

Sphingomyelin synthase can work bidirectionally; nevertheless, its dominant action is the transfer of phosphorylcholine from phosphatidylcholine to ceramide, to create sphingomyelin. Sphingomyelin synthase helps remove ceramide from the local environment, and thus, protect cells from ceramide induced death.

There are at least five human sphingomyelinases (SMase) isoenzymes and perhaps two dozen other enzymes with sphingomyelinase activity. The most relevant of these are classified as acid, neutral and alkaline sphingomyelinases, classified by the pH of the environment in which they are most active. Even though they have similar functions, the various SMases may be structurally diverse. There are seven human ceramidases. Ceramidases, decrease the presence of ceramide and thus tend to decrease the impact of inflammatory cytokines; thus, these enzymes are essential for cell proliferation and survival.

Sphingolipids are involved in a wide range of diseases. During cellular stress, enzymatic lysis of sphingomyelin occurs via one of several SMase isoenzymes, releasing ceramide or its metabolites that exert their effects as signaling molecules. Thus, local hydrogen peroxide production, elevated temperature, alcohol-related toxicity[25], or osmotic stress can increase the formation of ceramide and its products. Extracellular TNF-α activates SMase through membrane TNF receptors and thus, acts as a secondary messenger for inflammation.

SMase converts sphingomyelin from the lipid membrane into ceramide, which can then be can converted to sphingosine-1-phosphate (S1P). Although having very different effects, ceramide and S1P are both part of the inflammatory process. Ceramide inhibits cell growth induces oxidative stress and promotes apoptosis. In contrast, SIP induces proliferation and survival of inflammatory cells.

SMase is an important mediator of sickness behavior. Activation of the TNF-R1 receptor activates the cascade of SMase → Ceramide → MAPK's → and the NF-κB transcription of inflammatory mediators. Ceramide also downregulates cystathionine β-synthase (CβS; Figure 31-4), causing an elevation of homocysteine (HCY) that triggers production ROS via NADPH oxidase activity[26]. This induces sickness behavior, neurotoxicity, impairs muscular strength, and causes fatigue[27]. LPS induced oxidative stress in the endoplasmic reticulum can be inhibited by blocking acid SMase[28]. Thus, TLR4 also participates in SMase activation.

Ceramide can cause injury in the heart, lungs, liver, kidneys and brain. Secretory SMase levels are elevated in congestive heart failure, and their level is correlated with sTNF-R1[29], the receptor for TNF-α. SMase induces muscular fatigue and impairs the function of the diaphragm by promoting reactive oxygen species (ROS) mediated stress[30]. In cystic fibrosis, ceramide increases the death of epithelial cells; the release of DNA from these cells triggers further inflammation and susceptibility to infection. Ceramide also induces fibrosis in this disease[31]. Ceramide induces HCY mediated oxidative damage that underlies glomerular injury in many forms of kidney disease[32]. Glomerular damage can be inhibited either by inhibiting acid SMase[33]. Alcoholic liver damage and can be mitigated using SMase inhibitors, or by reducing HCY level production. Ceramide-1-phosphate (C1P) prevents apoptosis and promotes survival of inflammatory cells.

Alcohol induces SMase, resulting in S1P activity that causes anxiety-like behavior and nociception in animals, followed by neurodegeneration[34]. Acid SMase, leading to the production of ceramide and COX2, causes astrocyte cell death[35]. In strokes, ceramide induced HCY causes cerebral endothelial cell dysfunction and death[36]. Spinal cord injury may be ameliorated by inhibiting SMase[37].

Some of the most effective antidepressant medications are functional inhibitors of acid SMase (FIASMA). Amitriptyline, a strong FIASMA has been found useful in the treatment of cystic fibrosis as it prevents ceramide production. (See Appendix M)

Intervention at various levels of the SMase → Ceramide → HCY → oxidative injury cascade can intervene to prevent injury. First, prevention of activation of SMase, be preventing TNF-α, TLR4, or other inflammatory signal receptor activation. SMase can be inhibited by FIASMA medications. IKK disassociation from NF-κB can be prevented by quercetin, resveratrol or by several other phenolic compounds. HCY production can be mitigated by betaine. Alcohol can be avoided. By preventing ROS production, N-acetyl cysteine (NAC), can block the weakness and fatigue induced by SMase and the production of HCY[38] by helping to replenish glutathione.

Sphingosine kinases 1 (SphK1) and 2 (SphK2) transfer a phosphate group from ATP to sphingosine, forming S1P and ADP. SphK1, SphK2, and ceramide kinase require magnesium as a cofactor. In general, magnesium facilitates several sphingosine enzyme pathways that decrease inflammation and increase cell survival; while copper, zinc, and iron tend to increase the accumulation of ceramide.

Giving a simplified explanation; these kinases require energy; healthy cells have sufficient energy reserves to phosphorylate sphingosine into S1P that support growth and repair, meanwhile, in debilitated or severely injured cells ceramide is more likely to remain unphosphorylated, and thus, promote cell destruction.

SphK1 and SphK2 are the enzymes that exert the most influence in controlling the balance in sphingolipids, and thus, in the control of growth or elimination of cells. Cell growth and survival are usually a good thing; however, it can also mean the proliferation of cancer. High levels of S1P are seen in ovarian cancer, where it promotes not only cell proliferation, but also adhesion, angiogenesis, and metastasis[39].

Sphingosine-1-phosphate helps mediate inflammation and repair. There are five S1P receptors, and depending on the cell type and the cell's current status, it may express different amounts of the various S1P receptors, and thus, respond accordingly. For example, S1P$_1$R and S1P$_3$R activate macrophage and monocyte chemotaxis and migration to the site of injury; while S1P$_2$R blocks chemotaxis so that these cells stay in place and work. Thus, S1P can promote apoptosis, destruction and removal of hopefully fatally injured of unneeded cells, or support repair and growth. Its actual function is dependent upon the cytokine milieu. Exposure to high TNF-α levels tends to put S1P on the warpath.

S1P lyase (aka S1P aldolase) deactivates S1P by cleaving it into phosphoethanolamine and palmitaldehyde. The vitamin B$_6$ compound, pyridoxine-5-phosphate, is a required cofactor for this enzyme reaction. S1P lyase is generally present and active in cells.

Sphingomyelin is also found in high concentration in the myelin sheath, where it provides electrical insulation to axons, isolating and facilitating nerve conduction. Sphingolipids are key regulators of immune cells, neurons, and neuroglia, and greatly impact enteroimmune, autoimmune and neuroinflammatory diseases.

Elevations in acid-SMase (aSMase) levels have been found in patients suffering from major depression, and many antidepressant medications have been found to be effective inhibitors of aSMase activity[40]. ASMase also mediates the ceramide-induced lung damage that occurs in patients with cystic fibrosis (CF)[41]. Inhalation of nebulized amitriptyline, fluoxetine, or sertraline; antidepressants with aSMase inhibiting activity, were effective in preventing *Pseudomonas aeruginosa* infection in an animal model of CF[42]. Mast cell calcium channel activation is inhibited through aSMase inhibition by amitriptyline[43], and several anti-histamine medications, including desloratadine, clemastine, and hydroxyzine, inhibit aSMase[44].

Sphingolipids act as both intracellular and extracellular signaling molecules. Ceramide is proapoptotic as an intracellular signal, via BAX activation.

S1P likely has intracellular functions; however, its extracellular autocrine and paracrine activities are those best characterized. S1P activity is largely mediated through sphingosine-1-phosphate, G-protein-coupled receptors. The five S1PRs have varying distribution according to the cell type and state of activation. S1P4R is found specifically on hematopoietic and immune cells while S1PR5 is expressed primarily in the white matter of the CNS and spleen.

S1P mediates many aspects of immune cell biology, including differentiation, trafficking, proliferation, and migration. Like an S-O-S distress signal, during infection or injury, stressed tissue produces S1P that acts as a signal, calling for immune cell activity. The chemokine receptor CCR7 prevents immune cell migration from the lymph nodes (LN); S1P counteracts this signal, allowing their egress. S1P induces B-cell migration into the mantle zone of the lymph nodes where dendritic cells, whose migration to the LN was stimulated through S1P, present antigens to the B cells, allowing for antibody production. Table 10-7 outlines some of S1P's effects on immune cells.

While S1P generally enhances cell survival, in the presence of TNF-α, induces expression of Receptor Activator of Nuclear Factor κB (RANK), and thus, increases inflammation and apoptotic signaling. S1P1R induces T cells to differentiate into T$_H$17 cells and decreases the number of T$_{REG}$ cells. In general, S1P increases the survival and activity of immune cells, and regulate the selection and survival of activated B-cells as plasma cells or allow their apoptosis. S1P1R and S1P3R promote macrophage migration towards the source of S1P; while S1P2 receptors induce repulsion of these cells away from S1P.

Table 10-7: S1P Receptor Activity on Immune Cells[45]

	Immune Cell Response
S1P1R	T Cells: ↑ T$_H$17 and T$_H$1, ↓ T$_{REG}$ Migration: ↑ Egress of B cells from bone marrow; B cells, T cells and NK cell egress from the LN. ↑ E/M migration; ↑ M/M chemotaxis. ↑ DC migration *to* LN and B cell migration to mantel zone where antigen presentation occurs.
S1P2R	Activation of IgE receptor Fcε on E/M cells. M/M: ↑ Survival, ↑ Fc mediated phagocytosis, ↓ migration from the area.
S1P3R	B cells: bone marrow and LN positioning. Neutrophil: migration, proinflammatory cytokines M/M: ↑ Chemotaxis and proliferation. E/M: ↑ Chemotaxis. Dendritic Cells: ↑ Maturation and ↑ endocytosis.
S1P4R	T Cells: ↓ T$_H$17 polarization ↓ chemotaxis Neutrophil: ↑ migration DC: ↓ Migration to LN, ↑ T$_H$17 polarization
S1P5R	NK: Bone marrow egress

M/M: Macrophages and monocytes; NK: natural Killer cells; DC: Dendritic cells, E/M: Eosinophils and mast cells.

Sphingolipids and the Intestinal Mucosa

S1P regulates B cell trafficking in Peyer's patches (PP). M cells in the PP take up and transport antigens from the intestinal lumen to dendritic cells. The DC then processes and presents the antigens to T cells that differentiate into follicular helper cells that help the B cells switch antibody class; usually from IgM to IgA. Once the B cells have switched to IgA, they further differentiate into IgA plasmablasts that can self-replicate. These cells migrate out of the PP and spread out into the intestinal lamina propria where they continue the committed production of targeted IgA for a specific antigen. IgA binds to intestinal bacteria, preventing the bacteria from adhering to the mucosa, forming biofilms (Chapter 23) or transmigrating across the enterocyte membrane (Chapter 25). S1P1 receptors are present on B cells but are downregulated during certain phases of their differentiation. Suppression of S1P1 causes the retention and accumulation of plasmablast in the PP and impairs the production of IgA from the intestinal mucosa. The trafficking and migration of peritoneal B1 cells into the intestinal mucosa also requires S1P mediated signaling[46]. B1 cells are specialized B cells that produce IgA to bacterial cell wall antigens, such as lipopolysaccharides, and other evolutionarily stable antigens. Even though these cells are part of the innate immune response, their trafficking is under the direction of S1P receptors.

Sphingolipid activity is enhanced by cytokines and growth factors, which regulate the immune response. TNF-α induces S1P production in endothelial cells, hepatocytes, neutrophils, monocytes, fibroblasts and other cells by the induction of sphingosine kinase[47]. S1P activates NFκB and the transcription of inflammatory cytokines and induces the production of PGE2, NO, free radicals, chemoattractants and adhesion molecules that promote neutrophil migrating to the tissue. S1P further enhances the survival of neutrophils by preventing their apoptosis. Ceramide has nearly the opposite effect; it promotes apoptosis and autophagy; nevertheless, it is also involved in growth regulation.

S1P also mediates T cell trafficking to the intestinal epithelium. The intestinal intraepithelial lymphocyte (IEL) population is composed predominantly of T cells; however, unlike those in other lymphoid organs, this population has an abundance of T cells with γδ T cell receptors (γδTCR) in addition to the usual αβ T cell receptors (αβTCR). In contrast to the more common αβTCR T cells, γδTCR T cells produce IL-17, a cytokine that promotes the development of T_H17 T-cells[48]. αβTCR T cells are dependent upon S1P for their migration from the thymus to the intestines; γδTCR T cells migrate to the intestinal epithelium independently of S1P; thus, T_H17 activity can be seen as part innate immune defense of the intestine.

αβTCR T cells activity is modulated by S1P. Inhibition of S1P1R inhibits the formation of IL-4 and IL-5 by T_H2 cells. Blocking S1P1 also prevents mast cell migration to the lamina propria of the intestine, indirectly; by impeding the production of T_H2 cell cytokines for mast cells (IL-4 and IL-5), and directly; as mast cells bear S1P1 receptors. S1P is thus involved in the development of food allergies and mast cell activation disorders[49].

Although γδTCR T cells do not need S1P stimulus to migrate to the IEL, it does not mean that these cells do not respond to it. TH17 cell development and proliferation is mitigated by SIP1 receptor blockade[50]. These cells also express S1P4R that is activated by S1P[51] activation. S1P and its receptors are, thus, involved in the pathogenesis of diseases mediated by TH17 cells; thus, S1P and its receptors are targets for the treatment of autoimmune diseases such as multiple sclerosis[52] (Chapter 33).

---

1 Images by FujiMan Production (Japan), modified by author

2 Hematopoiesis. Ivan Maillard, 2011, University of Michigan School of Medicine. 010311.imaillard.hematopoiesisteaching-im0.pdf

3 SEM Image by Louisa Howard, Darmouth University

4 Activation of KCNN3/SK3/K(Ca)2.3 channels attenuates enhanced calcium influx and inflammatory cytokine production in activated microglia. Dolga AM, Letsche T, Gold M, , et al. Glia. 2012 Dec;60(12):2050-64. PMID:23002008

5 Mast cell migratory response to interleukin-8 is mediated through interaction with chemokine receptor CXCR2/Interleukin-8RB. Nilsson G, Mikovits JA, Metcalfe DD, Taub DD. Blood. 1999 May 1;93(9):2791-7. PMID:10216072

6 Wintrobe's Clinical Hematology 12 ed. John P. Greer editor, 2008

7 Th17: the third member of the effector T cell trilogy. Bettelli E, Korn T, Kuchroo VK. Curr Opin Immunol. 2007 Dec;19(6):652-7. Epub 2007 Sep 4. .PMID: 17766098

8 Th17: the third member of the effector T cell trilogy. Bettelli E, Korn T, Kuchroo VK. Curr Opin Immunol. 2007 Dec;19(6):652-7. Epub 2007 Sep 4. PMID: 17766098

9 Potential role of Th17 cells in the pathogenesis of inflammatory bowel disease. Liu ZJ, Yadav PK, Su JL, Wang JS, Fei K. World J Gastroenterol. 2009 Dec 14;15(46):5784-8. PMID: 19998498

10 Induction of intestinal Th17 cells by segmented filamentous bacteria. Ivanov II, Atarashi K, Manel N, et al. Cell. 2009 Oct 30;139(3):485-98. PMID: 19836068

11 Restricted microbiota and absence of cognate TCR antigen leads to an unbalanced generation of Th17 cells. Lochner M, Bérard M, Sawa S, et al. J Immunol. 2011 Feb 1;186(3):1531-7. Epub 2010 Dec 22. PMID: 21178008

12 The increased expression of IL-23 in inflammatory bowel disease promotes intraepithelial and lamina propria lymphocyte inflammatory responses and cytotoxicity. Liu Z, Yadav PK, Xu X, et al. J Leukoc Biol. 2011 Jan 7. PMID: 21227898

13 The gut-joint axis: cross reactive food antibodies in rheumatoid arthritis. Hvatum M, Kanerud L, Hällgren R, Brandtzaeg P. Gut. 2006 Sep;55(9):1240-7. Epub 2006 Feb 16. PMID: 16484508

14 IgA antibodies against gliadin and gluten in multiple sclerosis. Reichelt KL, Jensen D. Acta Neurol Scand. 2004 Oct;110(4):239-41. PMID: 15355487

15 Clinical relevance of IgG antibodies against food antigens in Crohn's disease: a double-blind cross-over diet intervention study. Bentz S, Hausmann M, Piberger H, et al. Digestion. 2010;81(4):252-64. PMID: 20130407

16 Circulating Th17, Th22, and Th1 cells are increased in psoriasis. Kagami S, Rizzo HL, Lee JJ, Koguchi Y, Blauvelt A. J Invest Dermatol. 2010 May;130(5):1373-83. PMID:20032993

17 Increased frequency of circulating Th22 in addition to Th17 and Th2 lymphocytes in systemic sclerosis: association with interstitial lung disease. Truchetet ME, Brembilla NC, Montanari E, et al. Arthritis Res Ther. 2011;13(5):R166. PMID:21996293

18 Identification and validation of novel contraction-regulated myokines released from primary human skeletal muscle cells. Raschke S, Eckardt K, Bjørklund Holven K, Jensen J, Eckel J. PLoS One. 2013 Apr 24;8(4):e62008. PMID:23637948

19 The role of exercise-induced myokines in muscle homeostasis and the defense against chronic diseases. Brandt C, Pedersen BK. J Biomed Biotechnol. 2010;2010:520258. PMID:20224659

20 The SYK side of TLR4: signalling mechanisms in response to LPS and minimally oxidized LDL. Miller YI, Choi SH, Wiesner P, Bae YS. Br J Pharmacol. 2012 Nov;167(5):990-9. PMID:22776094

21 Image by Niels Olsen, modified by author

22 Toll-like receptor 5 stimulation protects mice from acute Clostridium difficile colitis. Jarchum I, Liu M, Lipuma L, Pamer EG. Infect Immun. 2011 Apr;79(4):1498-503. PMID:21245274

23 Innate immunity in the small intestine. Santaolalla R, Abreu MT. Curr Opin Gastroenterol. 2012 Mar;28(2):124-9. PMID: 22241076

24 Fatty acids modulate Toll-like receptor 4 activation through regulation of receptor dimerization and recruitment into lipid rafts in a reactive oxygen species-dependent manner. Wong SW, Kwon MJ, Choi AM, Kim HP, Nakahira K, Hwang DH. J Biol Chem. 2009 Oct 2;284(40):27384-92. PMID:19648648

25 ASMase is required for chronic alcohol induced hepatic endoplasmic reticulum stress and mitochondrial cholesterol loading. Fernandez A, Matias N, Fucho R, et al. J Hepatol. 2013 Oct;59(4):805-13. PMID:23707365

26 Inhibition of ceramide-redox signaling pathway blocks glomerular injury in hyperhomocysteinemic rats. Yi F, Zhang AY, Li N, Muh RW, Fillet M, Renert AF, Li PL. Kidney Int. 2006 Jul;70(1):88-96. PMID:16688115

27 Sphingomyelinase stimulates oxidant signaling to weaken skeletal muscle and promote fatigue. Ferreira LF, Moylan JS, Gilliam LA, et al. Am J Physiol Cell Physiol. 2010 Sep;299(3):C552-60. PMID:20519448

28 ASMase is required for chronic alcohol induced hepatic endoplasmic reticulum stress and mitochondrial cholesterol loading. Fernandez A, Matias N, Fucho R, et al. J Hepatol. 2013 Oct;59(4):805-13. PMID:23707365

29 Secretory sphingomyelinase is upregulated in chronic heart failure: a second messenger system of immune activation relates to body composition, muscular functional capacity, and peripheral blood flow. Doehner W, Bunck AC, Rauchhaus M, et al. Eur Heart J. 2007 Apr;28(7):821-8. PMID:17353227

30 Sphingomyelinase promotes oxidant production and skeletal muscle contractile dysfunction through activation of NADPH oxidase. Loehr JA, Abo-Zahrah R, Pal R, Rodney GG. Front Physiol. 2015 Jan 21;5:530. PMID:25653619

31 Ceramide mediates lung fibrosis in cystic fibrosis. Ziobro R, Henry B, Edwards MJ, Lentsch AB, Gulbins E. Biochem Biophys Res Commun. 2013 May 17;434(4):705-9. PMID:23523785

32 Inhibition of ceramide-redox signaling pathway blocks glomerular injury in hyperhomocysteinemic rats. Yi F, Zhang AY, Li N et al. Kidney Int. 2006 Jul;70(1):88-96. PMID:16688115

33 Acid sphingomyelinase gene knockout ameliorates hyperhomocysteinemic glomerular injury in mice lacking cystathionine-β-synthase. Boini KM, Xia M, Abais JM, Xu M, Li CX, Li PL. PLoS One. 2012;7(9):e45020. PMID:23024785

34 Sphingolipids in psychiatric disorders and pain syndromes. Mühle C, Reichel M, Gulbins E, Kornhuber J. Handb Exp Pharmacol. 2013;(216):431-56. PMID:23563670

35 Ceramide pathways modulate ethanol-induced cell death in astrocytes. Pascual M, Valles SL, Renau-Piqueras J, Guerri C. J Neurochem. 2003 Dec;87(6):1535-45. PMID:14713309

36 Homocysteine induces cerebral endothelial cell death by activating the acid sphingomyelinase ceramide pathway. Lee JT, Peng GS, Chen SY, et al. Prog Neuropsychopharmacol Biol Psychiatry. 2013 Aug 1;45:21-7. PMID:23665108

37 Inhibition of ceramide biosynthesis ameliorates pathological consequences of spinal cord injury. Cuzzocrea S, Deigner HP, Genovese T, et al. Shock. 2009 Jun;31(6):634-44. PMID:18838947

38 Sphingomyelinase stimulates oxidant signaling to weaken skeletal muscle and promote fatigue. Ferreira LF, Moylan JS, Gilliam LA, Smith JD, Nikolova-Karakashian M, Reid MB. Am J Physiol Cell Physiol. 2010 Sep;299(3):C552-60. PMID:20519448

39 Sphingosine 1-phosphate signalling in cancer. Pyne NJ, Tonelli F, Lim KG, Long JS, Edwards J, Pyne S. Biochem Soc Trans. 2012 Feb;40(1):94-100. PMID:22260672

40 Acid sphingomyelinase-ceramide system mediates effects of antidepressant drugs. Gulbins E, Palmada M, Reichel M, et al. Nat Med. 2013 Jul;19(7):934-8. PMID:23770692

41 Ceramide accumulation mediates inflammation, cell death and infection susceptibility in cystic fibrosis. Teichgräber V, Ulrich M, Endlich N, et al. Nat Med. 2008 Apr;14(4):382-91. PMID:18376404

42 Acid sphingomyelinase inhibitors normalize pulmonary ceramide and inflammation in cystic fibrosis. Becker KA, Riethmüller J, Lüth A, Döring G, Kleuser B, Gulbins E. Am J Respir Cell Mol Biol. 2010 Jun;42(6):716-24. PMID:19635928

43 Role of acid sphingomyelinase in the regulation of mast cell function. Yang W, Schmid E, Nurbaeva MK, Set al. Clin Exp Allergy. 2014 Jan;44(1):79-90. PMID:24164338

44 Identification of novel functional inhibitors of acid sphingomyelinase. Kornhuber J, Muehlbacher M, Trapp S, et al. PLoS One. 2011;6(8):e23852. PMID:21909365

45 An update on the biology of sphingosine 1-phosphate receptors. Blaho VA, Hla T. J Lipid Res. 2014 Jan 23. PMID:24459205

46 The immunosuppressant FTY720 down-regulates sphingosine 1-phosphate G-protein-coupled receptors. Gräler MH, Goetzl EJ. FASEB J. 2004 Mar;18(3):551-3. PMID:14715694

47 Activation of sphingosine kinase by tumor necrosis factor-alpha inhibits apoptosis in human endothelial cells. Xia P, Wang L, Gamble JR, Vadas MA. J Biol Chem. 1999 Nov 26;274(48):34499-505. PMID:10567432

48 Unexpected role for the B cell-specific Src family kinase B lymphoid kinase in the development of IL-17-producing γδ T cells. Laird RM, Laky K, Hayes SM. J Immunol. 2010 Dec 1;185(11):6518-27. PMID:20974990

49 Immunological function of sphingosine 1-phosphate in the intestine. Kunisawa J, Kiyono H. Nutrients. 2012 Mar;4(3):154-66. PMID:22666543

50 Cutting edge: Alternative signaling of Th17 cell development by sphingosine 1-phosphate. Liao JJ, Huang MC, Goetzl EJ. J Immunol. 2007 May 1;178(9):5425-8. PMID:17442922

51 Sphingosine-1-phospate receptor 4 (S1P₄) deficiency profoundly affects dendritic cell function and TH17-cell differentiation in a murine model. Schulze T, Golfier S, Tabeling C, et al. FASEB J. 2011 Nov;25(11):4024-36. PMID:21825036

52 Sphingosine 1-phosphate receptor 1 as a useful target for treatment of multiple sclerosis. Chiba K, Adachi K. Pharmaceuticals (Basel). 2012 May 18;5(5):514-28. PMID:24281561

11. Type I Hypersensitivity and IgE Food Allergies

An allergy is a maladaptive immune response to a substance that an individual has become sensitized to. The most common environmental allergies are to airborne substances, such as pollen or animal dander. Airborne exposure to these substances commonly causes hay fever allergic rhinitis, (hay fever), allergic conjunctivitis, and can trigger asthma. Another environmental allergy is allergic reactions to insect envenomation. These reactions can be notoriously life-threatening, systemic reactions. Common, non-allergic reactions to insect envenomation are localized swelling, heat, itching and inflammation. In allergic reactions, the response can be greatly exaggerated, may become generalized, and may cause anaphylaxis.

Food allergies can also cause localized or generalized reactions that can range from mild to fatal. These reactions can have a near immediate response with hives, itching, swelling, and difficulty breathing, occurring within minutes of exposure. In anaphylaxis, there is widespread mast cell degranulation and release of histamine, leukotrienes, and many other mediators; in multiple organs including the skin, intestines and lungs. Mast cells release numerous inflammatory mediators, most famously histamine.

Histamine, in concert with other mediators, triggers vasodilation, which allows fluid from the blood to leak into the tissue. When this happens in the skin, it causes urticaria (hives). The stretching of the skin causes itching. When fluid leaks into the tissue around the larynx, it can cause difficulty breathing and if severe, asphyxiation. Vasodilation causes fluid to leak into the lungs, and along with leukotrienes that cause delayed, long-lasting broncho-constriction, wheezing and a fall in oxygenation can occur. Leaking of fluid from the vasculature can also occur in the intestine, causing abdominal discomfort and borborygmi. The rapid loss of fluid from the blood stream may cause a fall in blood pressure, resulting in dizziness, syncope, or if severe, shock and even death. Emergency treatment for severe allergic reactions includes histamine blockers, epinephrine, IV fluids, and corticosteroids.

Although immunopathic sensitization involves other types of immunoglobulins, the term "allergy" is synonymous with immunoglobulin E (IgE); mast cells and basophils; the rapid release of histamine, and other immune mediators. For this reason, the term allergy is reserved for IgE related, Type I immune hypersensitivity. IgG sensitization reactions are discussed in Chapter 19 and have been dubbed "anterigies" to distinguish them from allergies.

In allergy, preformed IgE immunoglobulins are attached to receptors on mast cells prior to the reaction. Histamine and many other preformed immune mediators are also located in mast cells granules. Contact with the allergen acts as a triggering mechanism causing an immediate release of these immune mediators, and thus, can cause an immediate reaction. Some food reactions may be delayed according to exposure time delay: an allergic reaction to food may occur quickly if the mouth or stomach are involved, and more slowly, if the allergic reaction is due to a peptide which is only made present after partial digestion of a protein.

T_H2 lymphocytes help defend the body from extracellular organisms, including parasites. T_H2 cells produce IL-4, which stimulates B lymphocytes to produce IgE antibodies. These antibodies bind to Fcε receptors on mast cells and basophils, where they act as armed sentries waiting for intruders. Mast cells concentrate mainly in the skin and mucous membranes, and thus, protect entrances into the body through the skin, intestinal mucosa and the airways. They are also present in the tissue around small blood vessels. Thus, inhaled allergens cause hay fever symptoms when the nasal mucosa is exposed and asthma when the bronchial mucosa is exposed.

IgE-mediated food reaction occurs after a food allergen is ingested. When two or more adjacent IgE immunoglobulin proteins that are attached to Fcε receptors the on a mast cell bind to an allergen, they cross-link and activate a calcium channel, allowing an influx of extracellular calcium into the mast cell. This calcium influx triggers an all-or-none mast cell activation and degranulation process. The release of immune mediators from mast cell granules causes vascular permeability, and outflow of fluid into the gut may cause diarrhea. Contraction of intestinal smooth muscles can cause cramping and diarrhea. As the allergen diffuses into the blood vessels, it can go to the skin where tissue mast cells degranulate causing hives. Allergens may also be transported through the blood to the lungs and causing asthma. A severe systemic reaction may cause anaphylaxis.

Basophils are similar to mast cells and also participate in allergic reactions. When activated, basophils degranulate, releasing histamine; the proteoglycans, heparin and chondroitin; and the proteolytic enzymes, elastase, and lysophospholipase. Like mast cells, basophils also secrete eicosanoids, inflammatory mediates and cytokines.

Activation of the mast cells and basophils, additionally, induces the new production of inflammatory cytokines, prostaglandins, leukotrienes, and thromboxane. These agents are responsible for the late-phase response which may occur two to 24 hours after exposure to the antigen. The chemokines provoke the migration of neutrophils, lymphocytes, eosinophils and macrophages to the area. In the case of a parasite, these cells would continue the attack on the invader and help with the clean up of cellular debris.

Table 11-1: Examples of Mast Cells Mediators

Preformed Mediators	Activity
Histamine:	Bioamine, vasodilator, increases WBC movement to the area
Tumor Necrosis Factor-α (TNF-α)	Activates inflammation and apoptosis
Serotonin	Bioamine; slows parasite movement, vasoconstrictor, tissue repair
Tryptase and other serine proteases	Digest parasites and proteins
Heparin	Anti-adhesion to prevent parasite defense and increase the immune response. Releases DAO from cells membranes, causing its inactivation in strong reactions.
Lipid Mediators (Eicosanoids)	These are formed at time of mast cells activation
Thromboxane	Vasoconstriction, platelet aggregation
Prostaglandin D2	Bronchoconstriction and vasoconstriction
Leukotriene C4	Bronchoconstriction and vasoconstriction
Platelet-activating factor (PAF)	Bronchoconstriction, platelet aggregation
Cytokines	
Eosinophil chemotactic factor	Recruits more eosinophils to the area
Interleukin-4 (IL-4)	Stimulates T_H2 cells and formation of IgE and further allergic activation

When mast cells degranulate, they release histamine and other preformed mediators from granules. Mast cells activation also promotes the formation of inflammatory eicosanoids and cytokines. Table 11-1 has a few examples of the over 200 mediators formed by mast cells.

IgE likely evolved as the body's defense mechanism against parasites. Parasites are large targets for an immune system that usually combats bacteria and viruses, and or single aberrant cells. While parasites can be unicellular, they can also be multicellular organisms; parasitic worms may be microscopic, to several feet long.

In order to penetrate the mucosa of the host's intestines, the parasite needs to disrupt the cell barrier lining the gut. They do this using enzymes. Our immune system reacts to the enzymes that parasites use to get across our skin or mucosa as well as other proteins on the surface of the parasite. *Most allergens are proteins, and many of these proteins are enzymes.* Enzymes that are on the surface of the parasites bind to specific IgE immunoglobulins that are bound to mast cells. When two IgE molecules in close proximity are bound to an allergen and link to each other, the mast cell is activated and releases histamine and other agents which attack the worm to kill it. This may occur as soon as the parasite crosses the enterocyte membrane into the body.

The enzymes utilized by parasites have evolved over billions of years. Many of the proteins and enzymes in our bodies are little different from those in bacteria, yeasts, and worms. Humans share many DNA sequences with bakers yeast, and our mitochondria are quite similar. Thus, the enzymes that parasites have on their surfaces are not all that different than enzymes found in plants and their pollen, or insects and their venom. An immune function, geared to identify parasites, can also react to plants, insects, and arthropods.

Lectins are another class of proteins that are often allergenic. Lectins bind to proteins in the cell membrane or to other glycoproteins, similar to the manner in which some bacteria attach themselves to cells. Some lectins also bind non-specifically to IgE and can trigger mast cell activation (See Chapter 14).

Anisakis Sea Food Allergy

Although many people have allergies to shellfish and fish, one of the most common causes of IgE-mediated seafood allergy is not an allergy to fish or to other shellfish. It is an allergy to *Anisakis*, a parasite that lives in fish, squid, and mollusks[1]. These worms live in the flesh of the fish, and if eaten, can trigger an immune hypersensitivity reaction. The most common reaction is urticaria, but abdominal pain is not uncommon, and anaphylaxis may occur. Fish are variably infested with these nematodes, for example, about 10% of tuna are infested. This may explain why eating one type of fish may cause a reaction on one occasion but not on another; it can depend on whether the fish was infected.

Far grosser than eating well seasoned and cooked worms hidden in a fish filet, is eating live worms and having them eat you back! Allergy to *Anisakis* is most likely the result of a previous infection by this worm. Consumption of raw (e.g., sushi), pickled (e.g., ceviche), or inadequately cooked fish allows live *Anisakis* larvae to invade the intestinal wall. A few hours after consumption of live *Anisakis* larvae, nausea, abdominal pain, and vomiting may occur. If the larvae are successful at burrowing into the stomach or intestinal wall, an inflammatory granuloma will form over the next several days, which can give symptoms similar to inflammatory bowel disease[2]. In rare cases, this can cause bowel obstruction. In contrast to fish, the human immune system is usually able to rid itself of this parasite, but the immune reaction sets the stage for IgE-mediated allergic reactions to *Anisakis* proteins in the future.

Anisakis larvae live in crustaceans, and in the fish and squid that consume them. Freezing seafood and storing at/or below -4°F (-20°C) for 7 days will kill the *Anisakis* larva, as well as those of *Pseudoterranova* (cod worm) and *Diphyllobothrium* (fish tapeworms)[3]; other parasites that humans can acquire from eating fish. Home freezers are not made to get this cold and may allow survival of these parasites. Cooking fish to an internal temperature of over 160° will also kill the parasites.

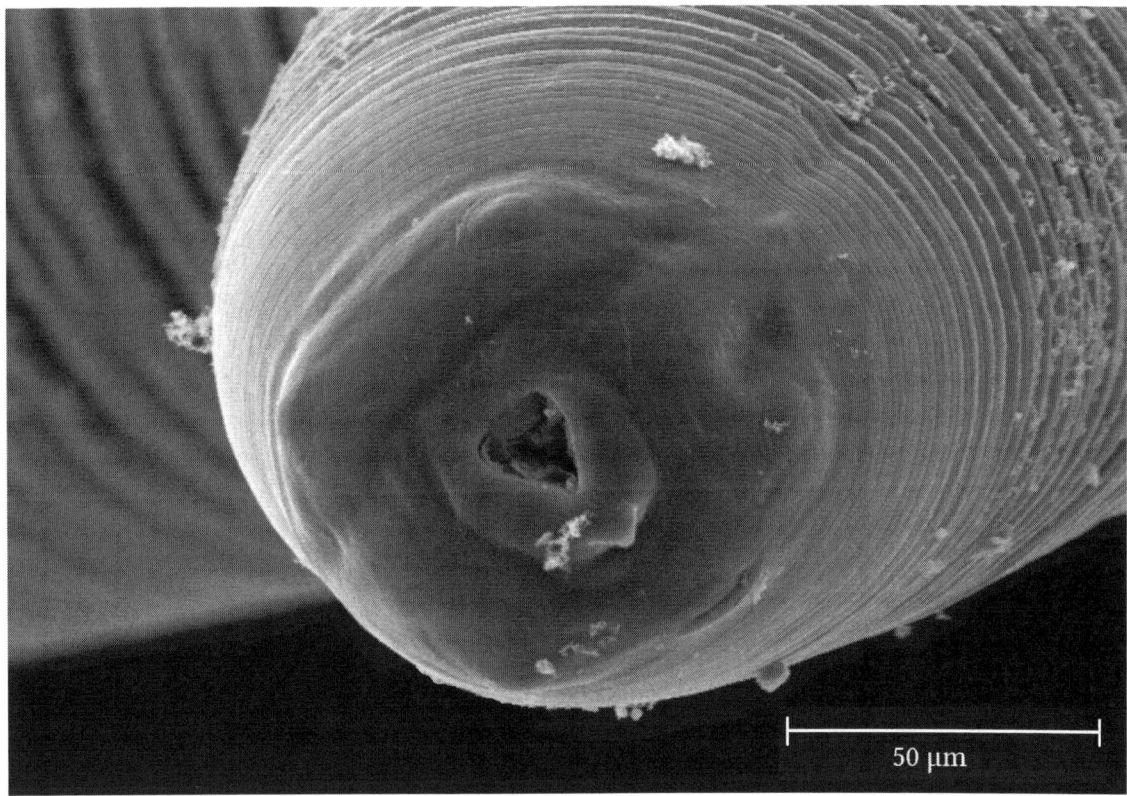

Figure 11-1: Scanning electron micrograph of the mouthparts of *Anisakis simplex*

Cooking may decrease allergenicity somewhat but does not eliminate the allergic reactions[4]. The best way to avoid developing allergy to *Anisakis* is to avoid the brief infestation by this parasite by eating properly prepared seafood. Ceviche, sushi, and other uncooked seafood should only be prepared with fish that have been frozen for at least seven days in a commercial freezer; never fresh.

> Fraudulent Fish
>
> Fish fakery flourishes in the U.S. A 2013 study, using DNA fingerprinting, determined that about one-third of fish purchases in the U.S. was not "as labeled." In Sushi restaurants, 74% of fish was misrepresented; 38% of fish in restaurants and 18% at grocers were also mislabeled. Red snapper was severely overfished, perhaps as a result of the blackened redfish craze of the 1980's, and while still popular, the fish is hard to come by. Sushi represented as having red snapper is usually tilapia on the East coast and rockfish in the West but almost never red snapper[5]. White tuna is mislabeled 59% of the time; 84% of this is actually escolar, a.k.a., snake mackerel; a fish banned from sale in Japan and Italy because of its high concentration of gempylotoxin. This fish, like oilfish, accumulates toxic wax esters, and if consumed in sufficient quantity causes cramping and keiorrhea; diarrhea or anal leakage with orange, oily, greasy stools, usually a few hours, but up to 4 days after consumption[6]. Most salmon sold as wild-caught is actually farm-raised. Other fish are also frequently mislabeled. This can be a problem for individuals with allergies or of IgG reactions to certain fish as they may be served a species of fish that they were trying to avoid.

Cheating on Allergies: Exposure to foods that cause even mild IgE-type reactions should be avoided. Food that gives mild hives on one occasion can give a severe reaction on another. The immune system learns to react to these allergens, and repeated lessons tend to increase the immune system's reactivity to the allergen.

People often assume that eating only a small serving or eating food with only a tiny amount of an allergen will not cause, or only cause a mild allergic reaction. However, it does not take much allergen to trigger allergic hypersensitivity; in fact, small amounts can favor the development of immune reactions.

> How much antigen is required to cause an immune reaction? Imagine the cumulative suffering caused by a severe ragweed allergy over an entire season for someone with asthma in response to this allergen. A person living in an area where ragweed is common would be expected to be exposed to less than one microgram of ragweed pollen during an entire year. This amount is equivalent to about one one-hundredth the mass of a single grain of table salt.

Even a tiny exposure to allergens can trigger a dangerous reaction. Trace amounts of peanut allergen present in foods not containing peanuts, but only processed in equipment previously used to process other foods containing peanuts, can provoke allergic reactions. Similarly, many schools do not serve peanut butter in their cafeterias as cross contamination can be sufficient to cause allergic reactions. I had a patient who after becoming despondent, nearly succeeded in suicide by shrimp-allergy.

Foods known to trigger allergic reactions in an individual should be carefully avoided. Known allergens should be avoided as each exposure can increase the T_H2 response, and increase the likelihood of developing more intense and numerous allergies.

Young children are at much higher risk than are older children and adults to develop IgE reactions to food. Using caution in the introduction of highly allergenic food may help avoid the development of allergies. Allergy to egg white affects one to two percent of young children, and this rate is typical for several other common food allergies.

Susceptibility to food allergies is, at least in part, genetically mediated. Fraternal twin pairs are much more likely to react to the same food than are unrelated individuals, and identical twins are more likely to share specific food or environmental allergies in common than are fraternal twins[7]. Thus, care should be used to avoid development of allergies in the younger siblings and children of anergic persons.

The most common food allergies occurring in children are to milk, peanuts, tree nuts, eggs, soy, and wheat. Children usually develop tolerance to most allergic reactions, (other than peanut and tree nuts); often by the age of five and usually before the age of 10. The most common IgE reactions in adults are to peanuts, tree nuts, fish, shellfish, citrus fruit, and wheat. The U.S. Food and Drug Administration (FDA) require labeling for the eight most common ingredients that trigger food allergies. The eight foods requiring food allergy labeling are estimated to provoke 90% of all IgE allergic reactions.

Table 11-2: Common Food Allergens

- **Milk**
- **Eggs**
- **Peanuts**
- **Tree Nuts**   (e.g., Walnuts, Hazelnuts, Almonds, Pecans, Brazil nuts, Pine nuts)
- **Fish**   (e.g., Bass, Cod, Salmon)
- **Shellfish**   (e.g., Crab, Mussels, Shrimp)
- **Soy**
- **Wheat**

Another common allergen is plant lipid transfer protein, a highly conserved protein found in peaches and several related species[8]. Plant lipid transfer protein was found to be the most common food allergen to provoke anaphylaxis in a European study.

Food Allergy and Autoimmune Disease Prevention in Infants and Children

Prenatal risk factors for the development of allergies include exposure to tobacco smoke, environmental pollutants, lack of sunlight (low vitamin D levels; see Chapter 20), and abnormal intestinal microbiota in the mother (see Chapters 4 and 23). Prenatal factors that reduce the risk for development of allergies include a healthy balanced diet, prebiotics and probiotics, sufficient sunlight or vitamin D supplements, and a diet rich in n-3 fats (Chapter 6). Factors which reduce the risk for development of allergies in infants are similar, with the addition that breastfeeding for 6 months or more, and the introduction of a wide variety of foods between 4 and 6 months of age, lowers risk[9, 10, 11].

American Academy of Pediatrics' current advice for reducing the risk of developing allergies is to:

- Breastfeed for a minimum of 4 – 6 months
- Delay introduction of supplementary foods until the age of 4 – 6 months
- Hydrolyzed cow milk formulas may offer benefit[12].

The period between the beginning of the 4th and the end of the 6th month (120 to 180 days of age) is a time during which the immune system seems particularly able to develop immune tolerance to foods. The transplacental IgG from the mother is diminishing during these months, and breastfeeding is no longer adequate for the growing infant. Thus, this is the natural time for the gut to meet the culinary world. The introduction of cow's milk during this time is associated with decreased risk of type 1 diabetes, in contrast to when it is introduced at other ages.

What did I do with my own children? I encouraged my wife to breastfeed for at least nine months. Breast milk contains galactose oligosaccharides that act as a prebiotic, encouraging the growth of beneficial commensal bacteria in the gut. Mother's milk also contains spermidine that helps the intestinal mucosa mature.

If infant formula is needed before the age of four months, it should be made from hydrolyzed milk to reduce the mill's antigenicity. Infant formula can be purchased that contains probiotics, and that is fortified with the n-3 fatty acid DHA.

At around four months of age, foods should be introduced in small amounts; various foods can be given, each food about once a week. Cooked foods are less allergenic, as many proteins are denatured. Rice is not especially allergenic and may be given more frequently.

Foods given to infants should be well-cooked and mixed in small amounts with other well-tolerated foods. Some examples might include: a small amount of cow's milk cooked into rice cereal which has been allowed to boil, a small piece of an oatmeal cookie to introduce egg and wheat, and if this is tolerated, a small piece of peanut butter cookie; thus, cooked peanut butter. Fish, wheat, corn, cow's milk, peanut butter, and other high-risk allergenic foods should be limited to about once a week each during this period. The amounts and frequency can be increased with time, watching and avoiding any foods that give adverse reactions. By seven months, the infant should eat a well-rounded diet of foods they are ready for while continuing breastfeeding if possible.

Wheat and oats introduced between 120 and 210 days of age gave the lowest risk of later development of celiac disease in children[13]. When wheat and other gluten grains are introduced between 120 and 210 days of age, the risk of developing islet cell antibodies, associated with Type 1 diabetes, is several times lower than if introduced earlier or later[14]. Fruits and vegetables, especially root vegetables, should not be introduced until the age of four months[15].

Introduction of food between four and six months does not eliminate the risk of autoimmune disease but is does lowers it. Nor does it eliminate the risk of allergic reactions to these foods. Families with a history allergic sensitivity need to exercise added vigilance in recognizing and eliminating foods triggering allergic reactions in their infants.

Peanuts consumed during the last trimester of pregnancy increases the risk of developing peanut allergy in an infant[16], while eating potatoes during this period of pregnancy lowers the risk of a child developing islet cell antibodies[17], perhaps by inducing IgG to a potato protein. Early introduction of root vegetables (such as potatoes) also increases the risk for Type 1 diabetes in children[12]. Fried potatoes should be avoided in pregnant women[18, 19]. Since potatoes are not especially allergenic, but appear to amplify immune sensitivity, and contain several toxins, I suggest avoiding potatoes before the age of 2.

Note: *Allergenic foods should not be introduced when a child has colic, gastroenteritis, or diarrhea, as the intestinal mucosa may be disrupted, and thus, food antigens have more access to the immune system. Highly allergenic foods should be avoided for about three weeks after gastroenteritis to give time for the mucosa to heal completely.*

Allergen Clusters

Many children with strong allergic reaction to cow's milk are also allergic to eggs[20]. The large majority of children allergic to soy are also allergic to another legume; peanuts[21]. Many individuals of any age who are allergic to peanuts become sensitized to tree nuts[22]. Children allergic to eggs and milk are also likely to be allergic to peanuts. These children have high levels of IL-4 and up-regulation of T_H2 lymphocytes[23]. Thus, reacting to one allergen puts them at higher risk of reacting to other allergens. Appendix A lists some common cross-reacting allergens

Recovering from Allergies

Fortunately, children outgrow most food allergies and develop tolerance to foods. About half of children will develop tolerance to foods that have been avoided, over a three-year period from the onset of the allergy[24]. Some children stay allergic until adolescence, and a small percentage never develop a tolerance to the allergen.

Tolerance to eggs develops in about half of children between the ages of 4 and 6[25]. Tolerance to wheat allergy develops in about half of children by the age of six and a half[26]. Tolerance to soy develops in about half of children with soy allergy by the age of seven[21].

Peanut and tree nut allergies do not resolve so easily. Only 10 to 20 percent of individuals who develop antigenicity to peanuts become tolerant and some, (about eight percent) of those who develop tolerance, latter suffer recurrences of allergic reactions to peanuts[27]. Only about nine percent of individuals who develop IgE sensitivity to tree nuts develop tolerance[28].

Several treatments for food allergy have been shown to help; most involve immunotherapy, in which extremely small amounts of the antigen are given in a controlled situation, and the amounts are sequentially increased. This process promotes the development of IgG_4 antibodies to the food, which is believed to preempt the binding of allergens to IgE. This desensitization process may not suppress IgE production to the antigen and does not eliminate T_H2 cells dedicated to this antigen. For many foods, the allergic response may reoccur if the IgG4 levels are not maintained by a continued challenge by consuming the food or cross-reacting allergens. Further, not all patients tolerate or respond to this treatment. Also, it may be that children who do respond to this treatment would have outgrown the allergy on their own while non-responders are those who would not have outgrown the allergy[29]. Allergy desensitization shots bypass the digestive process.

The development of immune tolerance may depend on the resistance of the allergen to enzymatic degradation in the stomach and proximal intestine. Peanuts and Brazil nut allergenic proteins are rapidly degraded during digestion, so they do not survive in the intestines long enough to provoke allergenic tolerance. In an experimental model in mice, however, prevention of the digestion of these proteins, by inactivating pepsin using bicarbonate, allowed induction of tolerance[30]. Conversely, reminding the immune system of a threat can amplify the immune response, making it worse on subsequent exposures. Thus, exposures to allergens to which the body reacts should be avoided.

Avoiding allergens that stimulate the T_H2 cell development and maintenance may help with recovery from allergies. If a food allergen is completely avoided for a couple of years, the food can sometimes be reintroduced without adverse reaction. Sometimes this works, sometimes not. Environmental allergens the person reacts to should also be avoided, especially those which cross-react with the food allergens (Appendix A).

Extracellular pathogens and parasites also stimulate T_H2 cell dominance of the immune system, and thus, should be avoided or treated. Nevertheless, deliberate infestation with the *Trichuris suis* (Pig Whipworm) has been used to treat immune hypersensitivity. This intestinal parasite produces the cytokine IL-10 in sufficient amounts to down-regulate the intestinal immune defenses against parasites, and thereby, down-regulates the T_H2 response to allergens.

Environmental allergies are also treated through a "desensitization" process using allergy shots containing extremely diluted allergens, and progressively increasing the concentration with time. This can be a life-saving preventive treatment for severe allergic reactions to environmental allergens that cannot be easily avoided, such as insect stings, pollen, and mold.

Food allergens may be hidden in foods, and children may not understand, or may not control which foods they eat. Even in adults, over one in five allergic reactions to food resulted from an allergen that was not expected to be in the food[31]. For patients with severe, potentially life-threatening food allergies, desensitization is highly recommended. For more mild reactions, avoidance is preferable, as allergy desensitization is a trade for IgG_4 sensitization, which may have longer-term costs.

Some children may outgrow food allergies through incidental desensitization. This may occur as children ingest very small quantities of the denatured antigen or cross-reacting antigens in their food or environment. For example, very small amounts of egg cooked into baked goods might not cause an overt reaction. Baking may help by denaturing some proteins, making them less allergenic. Denaturing may also promote the proteolysis of allergenic proteins by digestive enzymes into peptides that the immune system recognizes as food rather than foe, and thus, down-regulate its response to. Although this might occur incidentally, it is not recommended as an intentional method of treatment as the attempt could result in result in a severe allergic reaction.

My Personal Bias for Allergy Testing for IgE[32]

ImmunoCAP fluorescent enzyme immunoassays have good sensitivity and specificity in determining allergen-specific IgE food allergies and have cut-off values that correlate well with clinical allergies. A low percentage of food allergens can be missed, however. CAP testing has largely supplanted the older RAST tests.

Skin prick testing (SPT) gives immediate results, but a high rate of false positives. Negative results, however, are highly predictive that the individual will not have an IgE-mediated reaction to the food. SPT is best done with fresh food. Commercial reagents age and may have lower antigenicity than food that would usually be consumed.

Intradermal testing gives very high rates of false positives and has low specificity. They are also associated with higher risk of severe allergic reactions than are SPT. Intradermal allergy testing should be avoided.

Here is my bias: Test the blood. Allergists usually want to start with provocative SPT testing. Allergists are trained and comfortable doing SPT testing. I consider blood testing to be a wiser first choice. It can be done by the primary care provider and poses no risk of an allergic reaction. It also tests the organ where the reaction takes place: the blood.

Numerous allergens can be tested quickly and cost effectively. The blood test gives a quantitative value to the degree of the immune response which can be reevaluated over time. Since part of the goal is to tone down T_H2 immune response, it is better to eliminate even mild immune responses that may show up on this test.

Some foods are very difficult to eliminate, and hunger, deprivation and malnutrition from an unnecessarily restricted diet are not the goal of therapy. It is reasonable to do specific SPT testing for results that are borderline on CAP testing, for which there is a low suspicion of reaction if they are important to a person's diet. SPT testing can be used to determine if these borderline positive tests are likely to cause clinically relevant allergic reactions. It may be easy to eliminate buckwheat from the diet, and the patient may not care. The same may not be true for corn and milk.

In my opinion, foods that test positive to IgE should be avoided if possible, even when the skin test is minimally reactive (1 to 4 mm). Even subclinical reactions may keep the immune system dominated by T_H2 lymphocytes. Thus, not only should food allergens be avoided, but also environmental allergens.

Provocative SPT can also be useful for testing prior to the reintroduction of foods that were eliminated as a result of a severe reaction, or which showed up on blood testing.

Gastrointestinal Allergies

In a study of patients reporting abdominal symptoms (nausea, abdominal pain, vomiting and/or diarrhea) after eating certain foods, blinded, placebo-controlled food challenges were used to establish a set of foods which caused histamine-type reactions for the patients. Only about a third of the patients had extra-intestinal signs of allergy (e.g., skin reactions, asthma, or rhinoconjunctivitis). The patients underwent skin prick tests, serum IgE test (RAST test), were interviewed about foods perceived to cause a reaction, and were tested for histamine response to the antigen in colonic biopsy samples. The following results were found[33]:

- Patient history   Sensitivity 30.8%
- Skin prick testing: Sensitivity 47.4%
- RAST IgE testing: Sensitivity 57.9%
- Colorectal mucosa testing: Sensitivity 63.1%

Patients, usually, were not aware of which foods caused their abdominal symptoms. Skin prick test was poorly sensitive for identifying isolated gastrointestinal allergic reactions. RAST blood tests for IgE were better, but still not especially sensitive. CAP testing was not performed for this study; however, it would be expected to be more sensitive than RAST testing. Even though colorectal mucosa testing was better, it only identified 2/3rds of the offending foods that patients were sensitive to on blinded challenge.

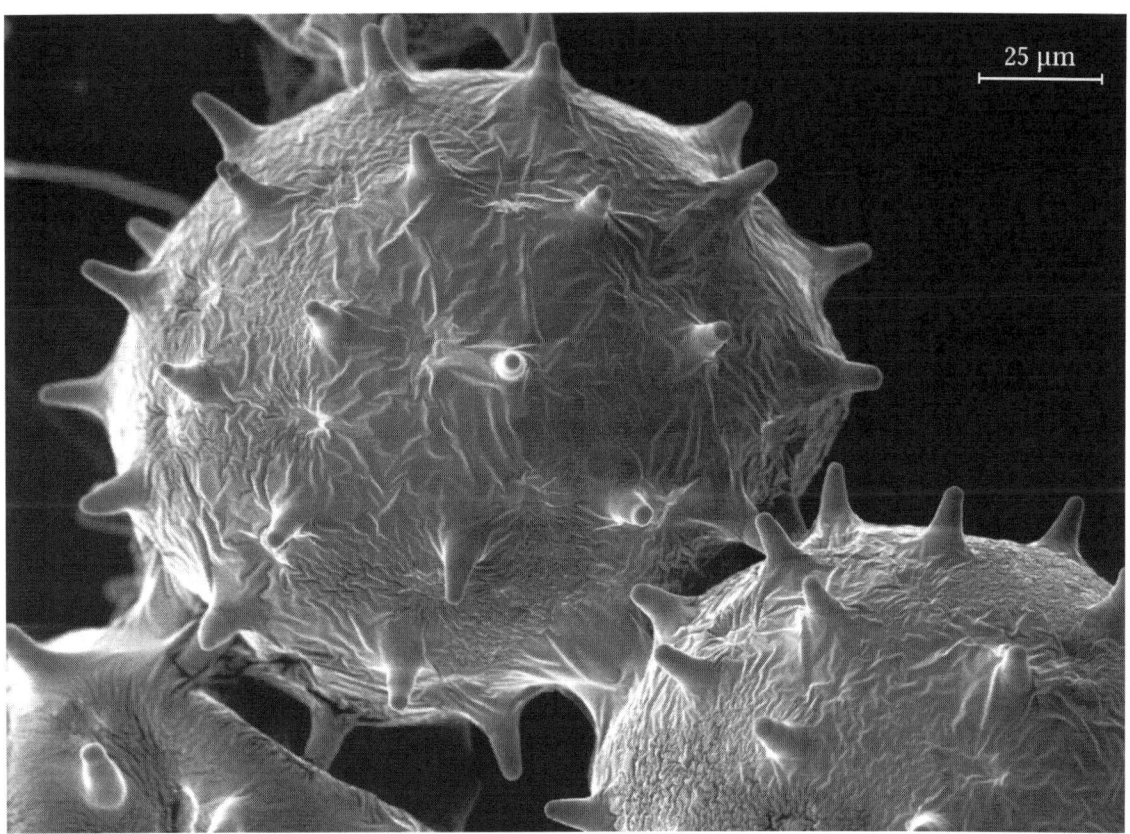

Figure 11-2: Scanning electron microscope image of *Hibiscus schizopetalus* pollen. By Louisa Howard

One limitation of testing mucosa from the intestine is that different areas can react while others will not. In one study of peptic ulcer disease, twenty-eight percent of patients were found to have IgE-bearing cells on biopsy of the stomach while only four percent of controls did. Mucosa from the duodenal bulb was the area where IgE was most frequently found[34] while other areas were less sensitive. Another study found duodenal biopsy for IgE-bearing cells correlated with food reactions better than skin reactions or total serum IgE[35]. SPT is poorly sensitive for identifying gastrointestinal allergies.

Pollinosis and Airborne Allergies

Allergy to pollen, called hay fever or pollinosis, manifests as allergic rhinitis (runny nose, nasal congestion) and itchy, watery eyes with conjunctival edema. Pollinosis can also trigger asthma. Pollinosis is often associated with food hypersensitivities because of dietary proteins that cross-react to the pollen. For example, allergy to birch pollen may be accompanied by an allergy to hazelnuts, walnuts, and kiwi fruits (Appendix A). About one in five to six persons suffers from hay fever. Since hay fever does not usually appear until the child is about six years old, this is suggestive that food allergy may develop first.

Pollens that are light weight and spread by the wind (anemophilous pollens) are typically responsible for hay fever. Showy flowers, plants that require insects, such as bees, for pollination, or those with large, heavy pollen such as pine trees, are much less likely to cause pollinosis. Early spring allergies are often caused by oaks, birch, hickory and pecan trees; followed in early summer by grasses, and then in late summer and fall, by ragweed. Patients often wrongly attribute their allergies to pollens that are large and easily visible, rather the actual culprits.

Table 11-3: Allergy Seasons

Common Airborne Allergens	Season
Hay fever:	
Oak, birch, pecan, hickory	February - May
Grasses	Early Summer
Ragweed	Late summer and Fall
Molds	Anytime: Depends on climatic region
Dust mites	Any time
Pet Dander	Any time
Fragrances (Perfumes, cosmetics, laundry detergent)	Any time
Cockroaches	Any time

Pollen-Food Allergy

Pollen food allergy (PFA) is common in adults with pollinosis. Also known as an oral allergy syndrome, the allergic reaction occurs when a person eats food with allergens similar to the pollen they are allergic to. The allergic reaction is usually limited to the mouth, lips tongue and throat, but may involve the nose and eyes and other areas. Like other IgE reactions, PFA reactions occur within minutes of exposure to the food.

Many proteins are denatured by cooking, and this may limit or destroy their antigenicity. Thus, PFA is most common with raw and uncooked foods. Stomach acids also denature many proteins, so this prevents intestinal reactions to some proteins which react in the mouth. Certain proteins are resistant to cooking and digestion and thus remain allergenic. For other allergens, it is the primary protein structure which is allergenic, and this not changed by cooking or exposure to stomach acid. Tree nuts and celery are examples of food proteins which remain allergenic after cooking.

Latex allergy can also trigger an oral allergy. Many fruits, especially tropical fruits, contain or cross-react with latex.

Other Allergy-like Conditions: Mechanisms other than allergy may also trigger mast cell degranulation. These include IgG anti-IgE antibodies, and some other proteins which can directly trigger mast cell degranulation. Pseudo allergic reactions are discussed in Chapters 13 through 17.

Summary

Diagnosis: Food allergies are often easily identified from clinical manifestations. CAP testing of the blood for both foods and environmental allergens (pollen, molds, animal dander, etc.) may be helpful to identify and eliminate less obvious allergens that help maintain allergic reactivity. Skin prick testing may be helpful to rule out false positive results, but has poor sensitivity to food allergies, especially those which only cause gastrointestinal symptoms.

Treatment: Avoidance is essential for successful treatment of food allergens. Desensitization is most useful for environmental allergens where control of exposure is difficult, especially when anaphylaxis is a risk. All allergens should be avoided to help down regulate the activated T_H2 immune response.

Food allergies are more likely to develop when the intestinal mucosa is inflamed or compromised. Testing for gluten intolerance may be appropriate for individuals with severe food or environmental allergies. Medical treatments include histamine blockers, medications which act on leukotrienes (montelukast, zileuton), corticosteroid, and other medications.

Primary Prevention: Breastfeeding for at least 6 months and careful introduction of foods to infants 4 through 6 months of age may help prevent the development of food and environmental allergies. Tobacco smoke and other pollutants increase the risk for development of allergies.

Secondary Prevention: Avoidance of allergens may allow down regulation of the T_H2 immune response and decrease the maintenance and development of allergies. Several steps for treating and secondary prevention of Mast Cell Activation Disorders (MCAD) also apply to the secondary prevention of allergies. These are items one through six in the summary section of Chapter 12 on MCAD.

---

[1] The clinical characteristics of Anisakis allergy in Korea. Choi SJ, Lee JC, Kim MJ, Hur GY, Shin SY, Park HS. Korean J Intern Med. 2009 Jun;24(2):160-3. Epub 2009 Jun 8.PMID: 19543498

[2] Anisakidosis: report of 25 cases and review of the literature. Bouree P, Paugam A, Petithory JC. Comp Immunol Microbiol Infect Dis. 1995 Feb;18(2):75-84. PMID: 7621671

[3] HACCP: Hazard Analysis Critical Control Point Training Curriculum (Blue) SGR 120 4th Edition. Appendix 3: Hazards Found in Seafood

[4] Immediate and cell-mediated reactions in parasitic infections by Anisakis simplex. Ventura MT, Tummolo RA, Di Leo E, D'Ersasmo M, Arsieni A. J Investig Allergol Clin Immunol. 2008;18(4):253-9.PMID: 18714532

[5] Oceana Study Reveals Seafood Fraud Nationwide. Warner K, Timme T, Lowel B, Hirhsfiled M.

[6] Bad Bug Book: Handbook of Foodborne Pathogenic Microorganisms and Natural Toxins. FDA

[7] Genetic and environmental contributions to allergen sensitization in a Chinese twin study. Liu X, Zhang S, Tsai HJ, Hong X, Wang B, Fang Y, Liu X, Pongracic JA, Wang X. Clin Exp Allergy. 2009 Jul;39(7):991-8. Epub 2009 Mar 17. PMID:19302247

[8] Causes of food-induced anaphylaxis in Italian adults: a multi-centre study. Asero R, Antonicelli L, Arena A, et al. Int Arch Allergy Immunol. 2009;150(3):271-7. Epub 2009 Jun 4. PMID:19494524

[9] Strategies to prevent or reduce allergic disease. Prescott S, Nowak-Węgrzyn A. Ann Nutr Metab. 2011;59 Suppl 1:28-42. PMID:22189254

[10] Early consumption of peanuts in infancy is associated with a low prevalence of peanut allergy. Du Toit G, Katz Y, Sasieni P, et al. J Allergy Clin Immunol. 2008 Nov;122(5):984-91.PMID: 19000582

[11] Age at first introduction of cow milk products and other food products in relation to infant atopic manifestations in the first 2 years of life: the KOALA Birth Cohort Study. Snijders BE, Thijs C, van Ree R, van den Brandt PA. Pediatrics. 2008 Jul;122(1):e115-22.PMID: 18595956

[12] American Academy of Pediatrics recommendations on the effects of early nutritional interventions on the development of atopic disease. Thygarajan A, Burks AW. Curr Opin Pediatr. 2008 Dec;20(6):698-702. Review.PMID: 19005338

[13] Risk of celiac disease autoimmunity and timing of gluten introduction in the diet of infants at increased risk of disease. Norris JM, Barriga K, Hoffenberg EJ, Taki I, Miao D, Haas JE, Emery LM, Sokol RJ, Erlich HA, Eisenbarth GS, Rewers M. JAMA. 2005 May 18;293(19):2343-51. PMID:15900004

[14] Timing of initial cereal exposure in infancy and risk of islet autoimmunity. Norris JM, Barriga K, Klingensmith G, Hoffman M, Eisenbarth GS, Erlich HA, Rewers M. JAMA. 2003 Oct 1;290(13):1713-20. PMID:14519705

[15] Infant feeding and the risk of type 1 diabetes. Knip M, Virtanen SM, Akerblom HK. Am J Clin Nutr. 2010 May;91(5):1506S-1513S. PMID:20335552

[16] Maternal consumption of peanut during pregnancy is associated with peanut sensitization in atopic infants. Sicherer SH, Wood RA, Stablein D, Lindblad R, Burks AW, Liu AH, Jones SM, Fleischer DM, Leung DY, Sampson HA. J Allergy Clin Immunol. 2010 Dec;126(6):1191-7. Epub 2010 Oct 28. PubMed PMID: 21035177

[17] Maternal diet during pregnancy and islet autoimmunity in offspring. Lamb MM, Myers MA, Barriga K, Zimmet PZ, Rewers M, Norris JM. Pediatr Diabetes. 2008 Apr;9(2):135-41. PMID:18221424

[18] Effects of fried potato chip supplementation on mouse pregnancy and fetal development. El-Sayyad HI, Abou-Egla MH, El-Sayyad FI, El-Ghawet HA, Gaur RL, Fernando A, Raj MH, Ouhtit A. Nutrition. 2011 Mar;27(3):343-50.PMID:21329872

[19] Structural and ultrastructural evidence of neurotoxic effects of fried potato chips on rat postnatal development. El-Sayyad HI, El-Gammal HL, Habak LA, Abdel-Galil HM, Fernando A, Gaur RL, Ouhtit A. Nutrition. 2011 Oct;27(10):1066-75. PMID:21907898

[20] Specificity of IgE antibodies to sequential epitopes of hen's egg ovomucoid as a marker for persistence of egg allergy. Järvinen KM, Beyer K, Vila L, Bardina L, Mishoe M, Sampson HA. Allergy. 2007 Jul;62(7):758-65. PMID:17573723

[21] The natural history of soy allergy. Savage JH, Kaeding AJ, Matsui EC, Wood RA. J Allergy Clin Immunol. 2010 Mar;125(3):683-6. PMID:20226303

[22] Immunological analysis of allergenic cross-reactivity between peanut and tree nuts. de Leon MP, Glaspole IN, Drew AC, Rolland JM, O'Hehir RE, Suphioglu C. Clin Exp Allergy. 2003 Sep;33(9):1273-80. PMID:12956750

[23] Immunologic features of infants with milk or egg allergy enrolled in an observational study (Consortium of Food Allergy Research) of food allergy. Sicherer SH, Wood RA, Stablein D, et al. J Allergy Clin Immunol. 2010 May;125(5): 1077-1083.e8. PMID: 20451041

[24] Prediction of tolerance on the basis of quantification of egg white-specific IgE antibodies in children with egg allergy. Boyano-Martínez T, García-Ara C, Díaz-Pena JM, Martín-Esteban M. J Allergy Clin Immunol. 2002 Aug;110(2):304-9. PMID:12170273

[25] Prediction of tolerance on the basis of quantification of egg white-specific IgE antibodies in children with egg allergy. Boyano-Martínez T, García-Ara C, Díaz-Pena JM, Martín-Esteban M. J Allergy Clin Immunol. 2002 Aug;110(2):304-9. PMID: 12170273

[26] The natural history of wheat allergy. Keet CA, Matsui EC, Dhillon G, Lenehan P, Paterakis M, Wood RA. Ann Allergy Asthma Immunol. 2009 May;102(5):410-5. PMID:19492663

[27] How do we know when peanut and tree nut allergy have resolved, and how do we keep it resolved? Byrne AM, Malka-Rais J, Burks AW, Fleischer DM. Clin Exp Allergy. 2010 Sep;40(9):1303-11. Epub 2010 Jul 20. PMID: 20645999

[28] The natural history of tree nut allergy. Fleischer DM, Conover-Walker MK, Matsui EC, Wood RA. J Allergy Clin Immunol. 2005 Nov;116(5):1087-93. Epub 2005 Oct 10. PMID:16275381

[29] Future therapies for food allergies. Nowak-Węgrzyn A, Sampson HA. J Allergy Clin Immunol. 2011 Mar;127(3):558-73; quiz 574-5. Epub 2011 Jan 31. PMID:21277625

[30] Failure to induce oral tolerance in mice is predictive of dietary allergenic potency among foods with sensitizing capacity. Bowman CC, Selgrade MK. Toxicol Sci. 2008 Dec;106(2):435-43. Epub 2008 Sep 19. PMID:18806252

[31] Involvement of Hidden Allergens in Food Allergic Reactions. B Anibarro, FJ Seoane, MV Mugica. J Investig Allergol Clin Immunol 2007; Vol. 17(3): 168-172

[32] Diagnostic tests for food allergy. Gerez IF, Shek LP, Chng HH, Lee BW. Singapore Med J. 2010 Jan;51(1):4-9. PMID:20200768

[33] Colorectal mucosal histamine release by mucosa oxygenation in comparison with other established clinical tests in patients with gastrointestinally mediated allergy. Raithel M, Weidenhiller M, Abel R, Baenkler HW, Hahn EG. World J Gastroenterol. 2006 Aug 7;12(29):4699-705. PMID:16937442

[34] [Specific IgE in the gastric and duodenal mucosa. An epiphenomenon or pathogenetic mechanism of some forms of "peptic" ulcer?]. De Lazzari F, Venturi C, Fregona I, Galliani EA, Bortolami M, Violato D, Floreani AR, Plebani M, Naccarato R. Minerva Gastroenterol Dietol. 1994 Mar;40(1):1-9. Italian. PMID:8204699

[35] Local allergic reaction in food-hypersensitive adults despite a lack of systemic food-specific IgE. Lin XP, Magnusson J, Ahlstedt S, Dahlman-Höglund A, Hanson L LA, Magnusson O, Bengtsson U, Telemo E. J Allergy Clin Immunol. 2002 May;109(5):879-87. PMID:11994715

12. Mast Cell Activation Disorders

Mast cells are an essential part of the immune system. As noted in Chapter 10, mast cells act as sentries; they are stationed predominantly in the skin and mucous membranes where our body meets the environment, guarding the periphery and keeping out intruders. Mast cells are best recognized for their leading role in allergies and; however; they are also sentinel cells in mucosal defense against gram-negative bacteria; these multitalented cells can also phagocytize bacteria and present antigens[1].

Mast cells can also be villains; mast cells can mimic a wide array of disease conditions when their behavior becomes deranged and magnifies their response to normal stimuli. The conditions caused by mast cells with aberrant behavior are referred to as mast cell activation disorders (MCAD).

These diseases can be categorized into clonal and non-clonal mast cell disorders.

Clonal mast cell disorders:

- Mast Cell Leukemia
- Mast Cell Sarcoma
- Mastocytoma
- Systemic Mastocytosis
- Cutaneous Mastocytosis
- Monoclonal Mast Cell Activation Syndrome (MMAS)

Mast cell leukemia and sarcoma are rare, malignant diseases. Mast cell tumors, such as mastocytomas, while common in dogs and especially in some breeds, such as boxers, are less common in cats and horses, rare in cattle, and very rare in humans[2].

In mast cell diseases, mast cell clones have mutations that affect the clone's activity. Typically, it is not a single mutation, but rather multiple mutations that affect these clones. In MMAS, the mutations provide primarily for an increase in mast cell activity; increased sensitivity to release and/or increased production of inflammatory mediators. In mastocytosis, mast cell leukemia, mast cell sarcoma and mastocytoma, the mutations provoke mast cell proliferation and thus an increased number of mast cells.

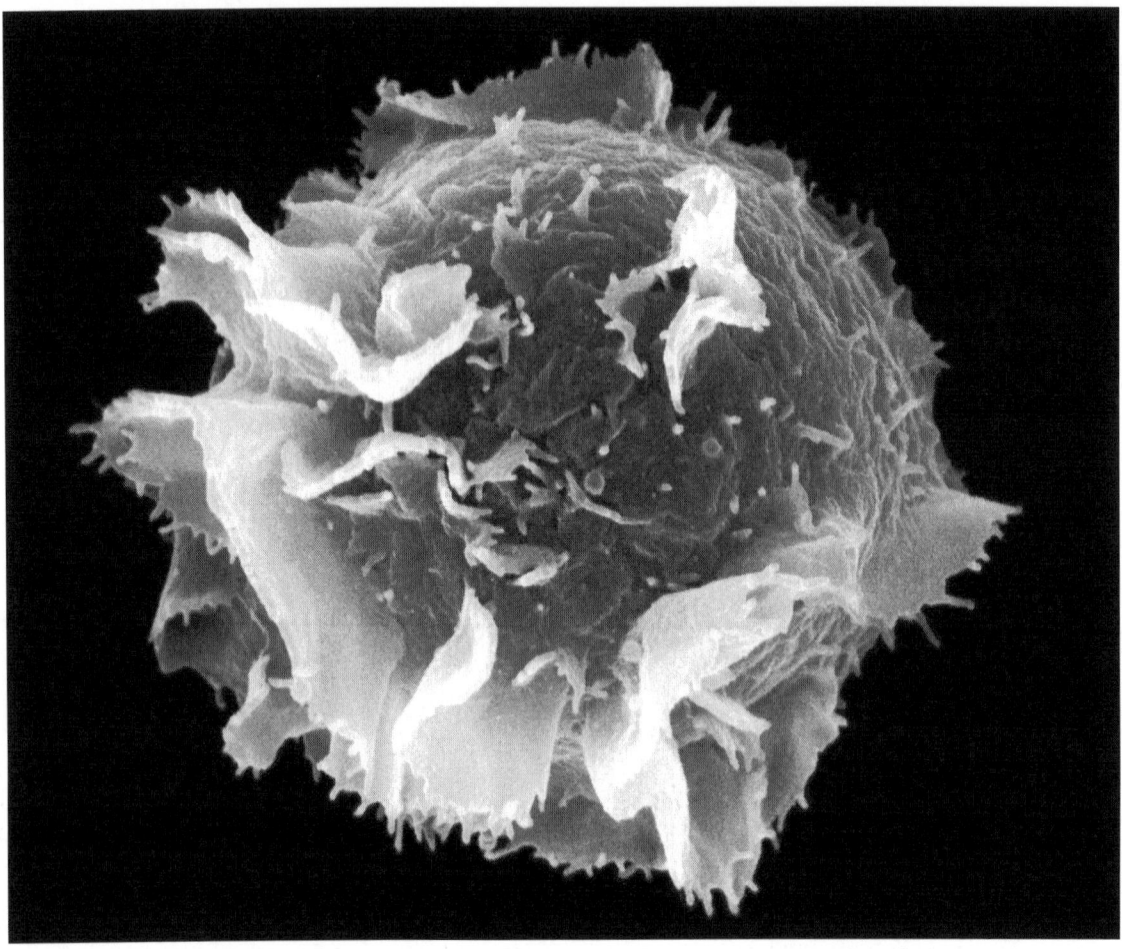

Figure 12-1: Activated mast cell. SEM. Micrograph by Janet M Oliver[3]

It is often difficult to distinguish between MMAS and systemic mastocytosis (SM). Many of the symptoms and signs are common to both conditions. There are often multiple mutations even in the same gene. These conditions may be regarded as varying presentations of a common root process of mast cell dysfunction, rather than distinct disease entities[12]. In 90% of cases of SM, the disease is caused by a specific codon mutation which is responsible for aberrant mast cell activity[4]. Mast cell proliferation is uncommon in SM; it is even more rarely if ever seen in Mast Cell Activation Syndrome (MCAS) a condition that portrays similar, but more diverse, aberrant mast cell behavior.

Cutaneous Mastocytosis

Cutaneous mastocytosis (CM) is primarily a pediatric disease. The most common forms of pediatric CM are maculopapular mastocytosis (formerly called urticaria pigmentosa), solitary mastocytoma of skin, and diffuse cutaneous mastocytosis[5]. In children, about 65 percent of patients have maculopapular mastocytosis, in a fifth of these, the lesion is present at birth, in the remainder, the lesions are present by the first birthday. Seventeen percent of these cases have family members with CM. Since pediatric CM usually resolves with time, on average by the age of 10, family incidence may actually be higher as many cases go undiagnosed. About one in three cases of CM present with mastocytoma; in about 40 percent of these children the lesions are present at birth, and the other have the lesion by one year of age[6]. In contrast, family history is not a risk factor for mastocytosis.

About 12 percent of children with CM experience flushing and about 10 percent have asthma, which can be triggered by activity, foods, or medications that trigger mast cell degranulation. Fewer than 2% of pediatric CM patients have associated abdominal pain or fever associated with mast cell degranulating exposures[6] above. Progression to systemic mastocytosis and malignant transformation after early childhood onset CM is extremely rare. Most children with CM do not require any treatment and require only annual follow-up visits to monitor for possible systemic progression[5]. If treatment is required, it usually consists of avoidance of triggers and use of antihistamines.

Less than 20 percent of cases of CM appear outside of the first years of life, and these delayed onset cases are generally diagnosed after the age of 15[7]. Adult onset CM has a high incidence of multisystem involvement, high risk of malignant transformation[8], and thus, delayed onset CM should be considered to be systemic mastocytosis with cutaneous manifestations.

Systemic Mastocytosis

Systemic Mastocytosis (SM) is an uncommon disease which usually presents after the age of 15. As in pediatric CM, the most common presentation is the result of the proliferation of mast cells that have migrated to the skin, causing maculopapular mastocytosis. Multiple fixed, red to brown patches usually are found on the chest, back, and/or forehead. Skin lesions can be aggravated by minor trauma, which causes degranulation, the release of histamine and other inflammatory mediators, and symptoms associated with these mediators: most often itching, edema of the skin, and flushing. Degranulation can also occur from exposure to certain foods and medications.

In SM, other forms of mast cell skin lesions also can occur, and other organs are often involved, especially the respiratory, GI tract, and vascular endothelium; other areas of mast cell concentration. For example, excessive histamine production in the stomach mucosa promotes excessive gastric acid production that can cause damage to the esophagus and severe dyspepsia. Asthmatic symptoms are also common and may be provoked by certain foods, drugs or even exercise. Anemia, hepatosplenomegaly, and thrombocytopenia may be present in SM, and bone marrow involvement is common[8]. Mast cell hyperplasia in these organs can result in nonspecific multi-organ symptoms which often cause diagnostic confusion when cutaneous lesions and the diagnosis of SM are missed.

Table 12-1: Mast Cell Disorder Manifestations[4, 12, 9]

Constitutional	Fatigue, asthenia, anaphylaxis, chills, sweats, environmental sensitivities,
Eyes	Conjunctivitis, difficulty in focusing
Nose, Mouth, Throat	Sinusitis, rhinitis, aphthae, burning mouth pain, globus sensation
Pulmonary	Dyspnea, cough, wheezing, increased production of viscous mucus and compulsive throat clearing,
Cardiac	Tachycardia, palpitations, postural hypotension, syncope, non-cardiac chest pain, coronary artery vasospasm
Gastrointestinal	Diarrhea, abdominal pain, obstipation, nausea, vomiting, gastroesophageal reflux, malabsorption, cramping, bloating, gastritis, hepatomegaly, splenomegaly, hyperbilirubinemia, elevation of liver transaminases, hypercholesterolemia, obesity
Urinary	Bladder pain; cystitis, prostatitis
Musculoskeletal	Osteoporosis, osteopenia, migratory arthritis, myalgia, joint laxity (Ehlers-Danlos Syndrome type III) degenerative disk disease
Dermatologic	Dermatographia, pruritus, flushing, rashes, itching hives maculopapular lesions, angioedema, slow healing sores
Neuropsychiatric	Headaches, depression, anhedonia, neuropathic pain, decreased attention span, cognitive difficulties; especially short-term memory and word finding problems, anxiety, sleeplessness, vertigo, tinnitus, polyneuropathy, paresthesias, organic brain syndrome
Hematologic	Coagulopathies, lymphadenopathy

In SM, degranulation occurs as a result of exposure to substances that trigger immune or non-immune-mediated degranulation. These include IgE, IgG, and substances including foods, medications or other exposures that directly provoke mast cell activation or degranulation.

The symptoms from degranulation in SM are most commonly itching, urticaria and flushing. Anaphylaxis may occur without IgE antibodies triggering the event. Systemic symptoms may appear to occur spontaneously or may be related to emotion, exposure to heat, exercise or to certain foods and drugs. Some of the foods and drugs which have been related to systemic reactions in SM are listed in Table 12-2. A more detailed discussion of foods and medications which commonly trigger nonimmune degranulation is given in Chapter 14.

Table 12-2: Examples of Food and Drugs Associated with Symptoms in Mastocytosis[10]

Foods	Medications
Anchovies, sardines	Salicylates,
Potatoes, tomato, green peas, spinach	Nonsteroidal anti-inflammatory drugs
Nuts, including peanuts and tree nuts	Polymyxin B, colimycin
Strawberry, banana, oranges	Morphine, codeine, opiates
	Scopolamine, quinine, thiamine
Spicy foods	Reserpine, pilocarpine, hydralazine
Hot beverages	Certain hormones
Fermented beverages and foods: i.e.: wine, beer, cheese, sauerkraut	(See Chapter 14 and 15 for others)

Although IgE is well known to induce mast cell degranulation, mast cells also bear FcγIIA receptors for IgG, and IgG can trigger mast cell degranulation resulting in inflammation and even anaphylaxis[11].

In normal hematopoiesis, mast cell population growth is regulated through stimulation by the growth factor Stem Cell Factor (SCF), which is produced by endothelial cells, epithelial cells, and fibroblasts. Thus, mast cell proliferation can occur in the skin and connective tissues, mucosa, and blood vessels. Other organs which can be affected in addition to the skin, are the lining of the gastrointestinal tract, the eyes, and the respiratory tract, as these are organs with endothelial cells, epithelial cells, and fibroblasts.

In SM, mastocytosis occurs as a result of one or more point mutations which cause proliferation of clonal mast cells. In the most common form of SM, the amino acid aspartate has been substituted for phenylalanine or valine at the 816th amino acid in the protein 'KIT' that codes for the CD117 receptor. Mast cells are the only mature cell in the body with CD117. When activated, the CD117 receptor signals cell division; the growth factor SCF is the ligand for CD117. When this mutation is present, excessive cell division of mast cells occurs. Other mutations in this and other genes that regulate mast cell growth and activity may more rarely cause this disease, but most commonly, the mast cell clone has multiple mutations. Furthermore, patients may have more than one mast cell clone. Mutations involving the H$_4$ receptor are among several mutations associated with mast cell proliferation[12].

Mast Cell Activation Disorders

Mast Cell Activation Disorders (MCAD) are diseases in which mast hyperactivity causes a disease syndrome with array of non-specific conditions included listed in Table 12-1, but which does not include Cutaneous Mastocytosis, Systemic Mastocytosis, or mast cell cancers. These disorders fall into three groups[4]:

- Primary:
  Monoclonal Mast Cell Activation Syndrome (MMAS) (Heritable)
- Secondary:
  Allergic
  Inflammatory
  Autoimmune
- Idiopathic:
  Mast Cell Activation Syndrome (MCAS) (Acquired)

The difference between these groups is etiologic rather than necessarily clinical. Alteration in mast cell activity may be due to heritable gene traits or monoclonal cell line mutations. More commonly, mast cell activation may result from epigenetic alterations. Inflammatory conditions can trigger both increases in mast cell number and local deposition, as well as epigenetic alterations in activity. Idiopathic cases, of course, are those that elude a clear understanding of their causation.

Typically, in MCAD there is not great increases in mast cell population as would be expected in proliferative disorders; rather, the mast cells may be more active (produce more inflammatory mediators), more easily activated (more easily triggered to degranulate) and more resistant to apoptosis; thus increasing the mast cell population in the affected tissue to up to a few times normal. Alternatively, there may be the aberrant release of variable subsets of mast cell mediators[12]. In MCAD, the mast cells can have abnormal expression of certain proteins, which alters their behavior.

Mast cells can be activated by IgE, as in the case of allergies, as well as by IgG against IgE (anti-IgE IgG), as seen in chronic urticaria. Mast cell IgE activation can also be triggered by dietary lectins; certain lectins can directly bind with, and activate the FcεRI IgE receptors. Anti-FcεRI-IgG can also activate mast cells[4] (Chapter 14). Mast cells have IgG receptors that can induce activation. These receptors are up-regulated by INF-γ.

Mast cells can also be activated independently of IgE and IgE receptors. Table 12-3 lists several additional factors which can activate mast cells[4]. Mast cells express numerous receptors that can trigger specific sets of activity.

Table 12-3: Some Non-IgE/IgE Receptor Mast Cell Activators

Cytokines	Stem Cell Factor: Binds to CD117 (*c-Kit*)
	Nerve Growth Factor: binds to tyrosine kinase receptor
	Chemokine ligand 3 (CCL3): a chemokine
Complement factors	C3a, C5a
Toll-Like Receptors Activators	Bacterial Compounds:
	TLR 2: Lipoteichoic acid: (see Table 42-4)
	TLR 4: LPS, opiates, amyloid β (Figure 31-4)
	TLR 5: Flagellin
Hormones	Progesterone, Estrogen, α-MSH, CRH
Physical Stimuli	Heat, cold, pressure
Drugs: Idiosyncratic	Muscle relaxants, radiocontrast material, adenosine, opiates (see Chapters 14 and 15)
Others	Certain neuropeptides
	Leukotriene C$_4$ (Chapter 15)
	fMLP: Activates neutrophils and mast cells.

Mast Cell Activation Syndrome

The systemic symptoms of MCAD are the same as those in SM listed in Table 12-1. While SM and MMAS are rare, Mast Cell Activation Syndrome (MCAS) an acquired condition, is very common. MCAS manifest as common, often syndromic diseases, such as interstitial cystitis or irritable bowel syndrome, often with accompanied by multiple non-specific, symptoms.

The varied presentations of mast cell disease result from mast cell's array of 200 to 300 immune mediators[13]. Depending on the trigger for degranulation and the aberrant behavior of the mast cell, activation may release an atypical set of immune modulators, and thus, result in specific disease manifestations. Reactions may be immediate or slow depending on the mediators released. Some mast cell activators are more specific than others; some may promote the release of a few immune modulators, and others a generalized release of mast cell factors. Thus, certain mast cell activators may cause a different set of symptom than other mast cell activators. Similarly, different clones of mast cells may cause different sets of symptoms. Symptoms also depend on the organ in which mast cells have been deposited.

The histamine H$_4$ receptor supports the formation of new mast cells in the bone marrow and acts as a chemoattractant for mast cell migration into the tissues from which histamine is released. Thus, the release of histamine recruits more mast cells into that tissue[14]. Any chronic stimulus for mast cell activation and degranulation which includes histamine supports a positive feedback loop for mast cell deposition. Allergies or parasites may promote mast cell chemotaxis. IgG immunoreactivity to foods also support reactive mast cell populations in the gut. IgG food immunogenicity is documented in patients with migraine and IBS, interstitial cystitis, and rheumatoid arthritis.

The more demand for mast cells production by the bone marrow under the stimulation of histamine, SCF and cytokines, the more likely it is that mutations will occur that can result in mast cell activation diseases. Exposure to mutagens also increases the risk. Mast cells may also become hosts for intracellular bacteria that modify mast cell gene expression, alter mast cell behavior and prevent mast cell apoptosis[15, 16].

MCAS explains the pathology of several somatic disease conditions; one example of MCAS is Burning Mouth Syndrome, a chronic disorder most often troubling older women[17] that had long been considered a psychosomatic disorder. Mastocytosis occurs about ten times more frequently in children with autism than in the general population of children[18] and mast cell activation disorders are also more common in autism[19], suggesting an etiologic role in autism. Some conditions that have been recognized to be associated with MCAD are listed in Table 12-4[12].

Table 12-4: Diseases Associated with Mast Cell Activation Disorders

- Fibromyalgia
- Irritable Bowel Syndrome[20, 21]
- Bladder Pain Syndrome/Interstitial Cystitis
- Chronic Prostatitis
- Burning Mouth Syndrome
- Unprovoked anaphylaxis
- Kounis syndrome (mast cell activated coronary angina)
- Inflammatory Arthritis
- Autism

Few MCAD are deadly. Kounis syndrome is one of the few that can directly cause death. However, neuropsychiatric morbidities and pain may provoke suicidal behavior. It has been observed that MCAS patients respond more poorly to cancer chemotherapy, but may improve with successful treatment for MCAS[22].

Diagnosis

MCAD resists detection as it does not cause abnormalities that are detected upon routine laboratory or radiologic testing. Thus, the multisystem morbidity associated with MCAD is often diagnosed as a "somatic" disorder. Confirmation of the diagnosis of MCAD is difficult even when clinically suspected.

Formal criteria for the diagnosis of MCAD were published in 2011[23]. The criteria include require a "constellation of clinical complaints as a result of a pathologically increased mast cell activity" (such as those listed in Table 12-1) and laboratory evidence of non-cutaneous mast cell hyperplasia, aberrant mast cell morphology or genetics, or an increase of mast cell mediators in the blood or urine.

Laboratory tests (see Appendix C) that may have elevated levels in mast cell activation disorders include:

- Serum tryptase
- Serum chromogranin A
- Plasma heparin
- Urinary N-methylhistamine
- Urinary prostaglandin D_2
- Urinary leukotriene E_4[24]

In many, perhaps in the majority of patients with MCAD and SM, these tests may give normal results. The idiopathic form, MCAS, the diagnosis is made when lab alterations are found, and at least two symptoms from Table 12-1 are present. Testing for dermatographia, which indicates cutaneous mast cell hyperreactivity, should be included in any standard comprehensive physical exam.

Testing

Diagnosis may require flow cytometry for CD25+ mast cells[25] or immunohistological staining of biopsied bone marrow. Stem Cell Factor receptor, (KIT/CD117 receptor), is a growth factor receptor found exclusively on mast cells (and stem cells), and specific CD117 staining can reveal an excessive population of mast cells in tissues affected by MCAS. Biopsy of an affected organ with tissue staining for CD117 may reveal an elevated number of mast cells. Biopsy of the intestinal mucosa, for example, may be stained for CD117 to help in the diagnosis of MCAS.

Serum tryptase reflects the population mass of mast cells in the body, rather than the level the mast cell activation. A significantly elevated serum tryptase, thus, is indicative of mast cell proliferation. When serum tryptase is not elevated, bone marrow biopsy is unlikely to show mast cells in the aspirate, and therefore bone marrow biopsy is not required. Mast cell proliferation is a possible precursor to mast cell leukemia or mast cell sarcoma. Bone marrow biopsy can be reserved for aggressive disease, elevated serum tryptase, the presence of splenomegaly in mast cell disease, or for an unusually high number of mast cells in the blood.

Urinary prostaglandin D_2 (PGD2) testing requires the urine to be chilled upon collection and remain refrigerated until testing has been completed. NSAIDs or aspirin can lower PGD2 and LTE4 levels, and proton pump inhibitors (PPI) increase chromogranin A. Patients should be off these medications for several days, if possible, for several days prior to the collection of blood or urine samples.

Treatment of MCAD

The mainstay of treatment for MCAD's is avoiding exacerbating factors, and controlling the disease with antihistamines and other medications. Since there is a significant risk of malignant transformation, SM should be closely followed, especially in aggressive disease where bone marrow biopsies may be required.

MCAD are complex diseases with significant morbidity. However, treatment of MCAD symptoms is sometimes surprisingly simple and effective; over-the-counter antihistamines and NSAIDs may give long-term benefits. In other cases, however, finding an effective treatment can be challenging.

Medications:

Antihistamines: For broader coverage, use both an H_1 and an H_2 blocker, preferably at bedtime. Splitting the dose to twice daily may minimize side effects while allowing higher dose. A sedating H_1 blocker may be used at bedtime.

H_1 antagonist: Loratadine (Claritin, 10 mg QD or BID) has a favorable side effect profile and fewer drug-to-drug interactions than most other non-sedating H_1 antagonists. Fexofenadine (Allegra, 180 mg) is excreted intact into the bile and thus may have favorable efficacy in mast cell conditions of the intestine. Cetirizine (Zyrtec) is excreted intact by the kidneys and has demonstrated efficacy in interstitial cystitis (Chapter 27).

H_2 antagonist: Tagamet (cimetidine), and to a lesser extent most other H_2 blockers, impair the enzyme ALDH, and thus may slow the breakdown of histamine. (See Chapter 13.) Famotidine (Pepcid) (20 to 40 mg BID) does not block this enzyme and thus is the preferred H_2 blocker. Ranitidine (Zantac) 75-150 mg or Nizatidine (Axid) 150-300 mg BID may be used as alternatives.

2. Other Meds: Aspirin and NSAIDS, such as naproxen may be helpful to decrease prostaglandin production. These medications, however, can trigger degranulation in some patients. (See below). Celecoxib, (100 mg BID) can sometimes be used when NSAIDS are not tolerated. Anti-leukotriene medications (cysteinyl leukotriene receptor blockers, montelukast and zafirlukast or 5-lipoxygenase inhibitor (zileuton), and mast cell stabilizers (cromolyn sodium) can at times be effective. Mast cells have GABA receptors. Especially for emergency management of MCAD, shorter-acting benzodiazepines can be helpful. Hydroxyurea is sometimes used.

MCAD patients resistant to treatment may require monoclonal antibody medications such as imatinib or omalizumab may be required[12]. The CD117 receptor acts through tyrosine kinase (TK) activity. Imatinib prevents CD117 TK from activating. However, in most SM patients, the DV816 mutation causes mast cell CD117 TK to pre-activated, without SCF stimulation, and thus, imatinib does not help for patients with this mutation. Imatinib is often helpful in other MCAD's.

Trials of medication should start with those best tolerated and with the lowest chance of side effects or harm. It should not be assumed that pricier or newer prescription medications will be any more effective than over-the-counter medications for a given patient. Additionally, symptomatic treatment may be helpful; for example, bronchodilators for asthmatic symptoms.

Secondary Preventive Treatment

1. Promote Histamine Disappearance: There are five enzymes utilized in the catabolism of histamine (including two forms of ALDH); each requires nutritional cofactors. Copper Containing Diamine Oxidase, for example, requires vitamin C in a reduced oxidative state. Serum histamine levels have been shown to be inversely associated with vitamin C levels, and histamine levels fall with vitamin C supplementation if vitamin C levels have been insufficient[26]. Table 13-6 in Chapter 13 lists the enzymes and cofactors required for the enzymes that metabolize histamine, and it gives recommended doses for the vitamin and mineral cofactor supplements to optimize the efficient catabolism of histamine. Table 13-11 lists agents that impair the function of the enzymes that catabolize histamine.

2. Avoid Immune-Mediated Mast Cell Activation: Mast cell degranulation can be activated by IgE crosslinking in the presence of specific antigens associated most frequently with allergies. Testing for allergens and immunoreactions to foods, and eliminating those provocations can not only give relief of symptoms, but can reduce the stimulus for mast cell chemotaxis and survival.

IgG immune reactions to food are a major source of cytokines and mast cell activators especially in adults; while IgE food allergies are more commonly seen in children. Many of the cytokines that act as mast cell growth factors result from inflammation. Allergic reactions are discussed in Chapter 11. IgG induced immune sensitivities to food (antergies), are a common activator of mast cells. These are covered in Chapter 19.

3. Avoid Non-immune Mast Cell Activators: Several medications act as direct mast cell activators. Opiates act directly on mast cells.

While NSAID's and aspirin are often effective additions to the treatment of MCAD, these medications, which block cyclooxygenase 1 (COX1), shift eicosanoid production towards the formation of leukotrienes. Leukotrienes in turn lower the threshold for degranulation of mast cells upon immunogenic stimulation[27]. Leukotriene induced reactions are covered in Chapter 15. Certain hormones, foods, sulfites, and several other medications which induce degranulation are covered in Chapter 14.

4. Prevent Mast Cell Stimulation: Without stimulation, mast cells eventually undergo apoptosis. Histamine, through H_4 receptors, serves to increase mast cell growth and proliferation. Histamine provides positive feedback on mast cell growth in the bone marrow and for chemotaxis via the H_4 receptors. Avoiding excess systemic histamine and local histamine production may help to down-regulated this process.

Preventing degranulation and lowering serum histamine level, should be expected to decrease mast cell production. Eliminating allergens and immunogens that stimulate mast cells helps to down-regulate their activity. Mast cells do not live forever; the typical life span of a mast cell is weeks to months. Thus, if left unstimulated, the mast cell mass may diminish with time. There are no H_4 receptor antagonist medications currently available.

Mast cell proliferation may also be impeded by preventing the production of SCF, the ligand for CD117 that stimulates cell reproduction. This growth factor is produced by fibroblasts, endothelial cells, and epithelial cells, likely during growth and repair. Avoiding injury may reduce mast cell growth.

Table 12-5: Mast cell growth cofactors[28]

Interleukin-6 (IL-6)
Interleukin-8 (IL-8)[29]
Nerve Growth Factor (NGF)
Thrombopoietin (TPO)
Interferon-α (INF-α)
Matrix metallopeptidase 9 (MMP-9)
Interleukin-2 (IL-2)
Tumor Necrosis Factor-α (TNF-α)

Mast cells also depend on cofactors for cell growth and survival. They will undergo apoptosis if deprived of the inflammatory cytokine stimulus on which act as growth cofactors[30].

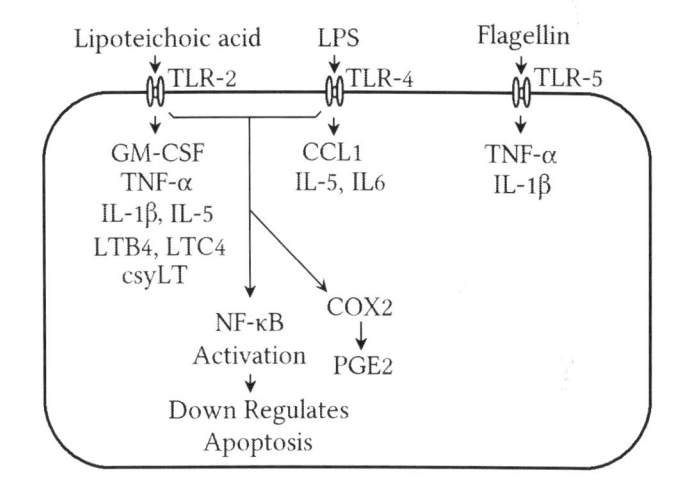

Figure 12-2: Toll-Like receptors on human mast cell surface and some of the mediators their activation induces[27].

Mast cells have Toll-like Receptors (TLR) for bacterial cell wall components, including lipoteichoic acid (LTA) from gram-positive bacteria, LPS from gram negative bacteria, and flagellin from flagella found on most motile bacteria; these compounds activate the mast cell immune response. These receptors may not, however, trigger degranulation, but rather act to increase immune response, increase cytokine production, and inhibit apoptosis[31]. Histamine increases the expression of TRL-2 and TLR-4 on mast cells and amplifies their sensitivity to LTA and LPS[32]. The H_1 blocker diphenhydramine, but not the H_2 blocker famotidine, was shown to prevent the increased production of IL-6 from mast cells stimulated with LTA or LPS[33].

Mast cells play an important role in protecting the mucosa from gram-negative bacteria[1]. Dysbiosis, such as SIBO and biofilms from bacterial overgrowth, increases the production of LPS, which thus increases mast cell activity and survival in enteroimmune disease. LTA may similarly contribute to asthma, chronic dermatitis, acne and other diseases involving gram-positive bacteria. Control of dysbiosis and LPS formation are discussed in Chapters 23 through 25. Acne is discussed in Chapter 37.

Chronic stress increases the production of IL-6 and IL-8[34]. Corticotropin Releasing Hormone (CRH) is also elevated in chronic stress and not only increases IL-6 and IL-8, but also directly induces mast cell degranulation. Chronic stress can be avoided (Chapter 29).

Sleep deprivation increases IL-6. Mast cells have MT1 and MT2 receptors for melatonin, and melatonin decreases mast cell activation[35]. Enterochromaffin cells produce most of the bodies melatonin in the lamina propria of the intestine, which is also a site of high concentrations of mast cells. Melatonin also has epigenetic effects through histone H3 acetylation, via MT1 receptors[36]. Melatonin decreases the hyper-reactivity and perhaps hyper-proliferation, of these cells[37]. Melatonin decreases NF-κB production[38] and thus, decreases mast cell survival. Regular sleeping and eating cycles, adequate vitamin B_6, avoidance of late evening meals and exposure to light at night, help assure normal production of melatonin.

Exercise decreases chronic stress and the production of inflammatory cytokines. Substance P also increases the production of IL-6 and IL-8. IL-6 is also produced by adipocytes and is increased in obesity. Elevated uric acid is associated with increased IL-6 levels. Diets high in fructose increase uric acid levels (Chapter 9). LPS toxins from enteric bacterial dysbiosis increase the production of TNF-α, IL-6, IL-8 and COX2. γ-tocotrienol and flavonoid compounds from foods mitigate this response to LPS[39]. The natural flavonoid quercetin blocks ALOX-5 has been found to be helpful in many MCAD patients. (See Table 15-4).

Diets high in n-6 fats and low in n-3 fats favor the production of arachidonic acid in the cell membrane, which is converted to pro-inflammatory prostaglandins and leukotrienes that participate in mast cell activation. A high n-3, low n-6 ratio diet is advised. (See Chapter 6).

5. Induce Apoptosis of Mast Cells: Bax (Bcl-2–associated X protein) is the major inducer of mast cell apoptosis[30]. Prostaglandin E_2 (PGE_2) has an anti-apoptotic effect, by preventing the formation of Bax. COX2-inhibiting medications prevent the formation of PGE_2 and may prevent inhibition of apoptosis. PGE_2 production can also be mitigated by vitamin D_3[40], vitamin E tocotrienols[41], and γ-tocopherol[42] through the inhibition of COX2 enzyme activity (Figure 41-1, in Chapter 41). Sulforaphane, available from broccoli, cabbage, and other cruciferous vegetables, also has pro-apoptotic effects. (See Chapter 41 on cancer prevention for more detail). PGE_2 production can also be avoided by a diet low in n-6 fats and with diets high in the long chain n-3 fats, EPA and DHA (Chapter 6). Resetting the epigenetic alterations causing MCAS may also be possible using these and similar agents (Chapter 19).

Sphingolipids mediate immune cell trafficking; apoptosis vs. proliferation; ceramide increases mast cell apoptosis; while S1P enhances immune cell proliferation and survival. S1P also promotes migration of mast cells to the intestinal lamina propria[43]. TNF-α promotes conversion of ceramide to S1P by inducing sphingosine kinase, preventing apoptosis. Functional inhibitors of acid SMase (FIASMA) inhibit ceramide formation. Mast cell calcium channel activation is inhibited through acid SMase inhibition[44] and several H1 blockers, including loratadine, clemastine, and amitriptyline, are FIASMA. Thus, while they may block H1 activity, they may also inhibit mast cell apoptosis. (See Appendix M) Vitamin B_6 is a cofactor for S1P lyase, which degrades S1P, and the metabolic products of this reaction may also induce apoptosis[45]. Alpha lipoic acid decreases the formation of S1P and promotes the production of ceramide.

LPS, IL-6, and IL-1β inhibit apoptosis[46] through activation of transcription factor NF-κB. Factors that activate the TLR2 and TLR4 also activate NF-κB. Nutritional factors, supplements and medications useful in the mediation of TLR-2, TLR-4, and NF-κB activation, are detailed in Chapters 31 and 42. Patients with MCAD should be tested for vitamin D and magnesium sufficiency.

Primary Prevention

With mast cell hyperplasia, there is increased risk for mutations that can give rise to mast cell proliferative disorders. Avoiding activation of allergies and parasitic infections may reduce the risk of mast cell activation diseases. Mutagens in the diet may increase the risk of developing aberrant mast cell clones.

Alcohol and heterocyclic amines are prominent examples of mutagens that may induce mast cell mutations. Adequate folate, vitamin B_{12}, pyridoxine, vitamin D_3 and the fatty acid DHA also help maintain normal levels of DNA methylation for adequate protein transcription, but limit excess DNA exposure that raises the risk of damage and mutation. Insufficiencies of these nutrients should be treated.

Hyperpermeability of the intestinal mucosa allows for increased contact of antigens with the immune cells in the lamina propria and increases the chemotaxis and development of mast cells into this and other areas of the body.

The same measures, used to prevent impairment of the enterocyte membrane and prevent cancer, are applicable to primary and secondary prevention of MCAD. These measures are discussed in Chapter 25 on "Leaky Gut Syndrome" and in Chapter 41 on cancer prevention.

Mast cell activation is responsible for much of the morbidity discussed in this book. The next several chapters discuss the role of histamine and factors which cause the release of histamine from mast cells. In subsequent chapters, several diseases are discussed in which mast cell activation may play a role. Treatment of MCAS is a means for decreasing the activity of these disease conditions.

Table 12-6: Some Additional Diseases with Evidence of Mast Cell Activation

- Atopic Dermatitis
- Autoimmune disease
- Drug Allergy
- Chronic Fatigue
- Depression
- Intractable Migraine
- Rage (Explosive Disorder)
- Chronic Urticaria
- Rosacea
- Exercise-induced anaphylaxis[47]
- Autism[18]
- Some seizure disorders
- Female sexual dysfunction
- Polycythemia[48]

---

[1] Mast cells as critical effectors of host immune defense against Gram-negative bacteria. Matsuguchi T. Curr Med Chem. 2012;19(10):1432-42. PMID:22360480

[2] Mast cell tumours and other skin neoplasia in Danish dogs--data from the Danish Veterinary Cancer Registry. Brønden LB, Eriksen T, Kristensen AT. Acta Vet Scand. 2010 Jan 22;52:6. PMID:20096110

[3] Janet M Oliver, New Mexico Spatiotemporal Modeling Center

[4] Mast cell activation syndrome: Proposed diagnostic criteria. Akin C, Valent P, Metcalfe DD. J Allergy Clin Immunol. 2010 Dec;126(6):1099-104.e4. PMID:21035176

[5] Mastocytosis in children: a protocol for management. Heide R, Beishuizen A, De Groot H, Den Hollander JC, Van Doormaal JJ, De Monchy JG, Pasmans SG, Van Gysel D, Oranje AP; Dutch National Mastocytosis Work Group. Pediatr Dermatol. 2008 Jul-Aug;25(4):493-500. PMID:18789103

[6] Pediatric cutaneous mastocytosis: a review of 180 patients. Ben-Amitai D, Metzker A, Cohen HA. Isr Med Assoc J. 2005 May;7(5):320-2. PMID:15909466

[7] Cutaneous mastocytosis: demographic aspects and clinical features of 55 patients. Akoglu G, Erkin G, Cakir B, Boztepe G, Sahin S, Karaduman A, Atakan N, Akan T, Kolemen F. J Eur Acad Dermatol Venereol. 2006 Sep;20(8):969-73. PMID:16922947

[8] Cutaneous mastocytosis in adults; evaluation of 14 patients with respect to systemic disease manifestations. Tebbe B, Stavropoulos PG, Krasagakis K, Orfanos CE. Dermatology. 1998;197(2):101-8. PMID:9732155

[9] Omalizumab treatment of systemic mast cell activation disease: experiences from four cases. Molderings GJ, Raithel M, Kratz F, Azemar M, Haenisch B, Harzer S, Homann J. Intern Med. 2011;50(6):611-5. PMID:21422688

[10] Multiple nodular lesions of upper limbs: nodular mastocytosis. Fenniche S, Marrak H, Zghal M, Khayat O, Debbiche A, Ben Ayed M, Mokhtar I. Dermatol Online J. 2002 Oct;8(2):20. PMID:12546775

[11] Human FcγRIIA induces anaphylactic and allergic reactions. Jönsson F, Mancardi DA, Zhao W, Kita Y, Iannascoli B, Khun H, van Rooijen N, Shimizu T, Schwartz LB, Daëron M, Bruhns P. Blood. 2011 Dec 2. PMID:22138510

[12] Mast cell activation disease: a concise practical guide for diagnostic workup and therapeutic options. Molderings GJ, Brettner S, Homann J, Afrin LB. J Hematol Oncol. 2011 Mar 22;4:10. PMID:21418662

[13] www.copewithcytokines.de/cope.cgi?key=mast%20cells Site accessed May 2012

[14] Histamine H4 receptor mediates chemotaxis and calcium mobilization of mast cells. Hofstra CL, Desai PJ, Thurmond RL, Fung-Leung WP. J Pharmacol Exp Ther. 2003 Jun;305(3):1212-21. PMID:12626656

[15] Anaplasma phagocytophilum infects mast cells via alpha1,3-fucosylated but not sialylated glycans and inhibits IgE-mediated cytokine production and histamine release. Ojogun N, Barnstein B, Huang B, et al. Infect Immun. 2011 Jul;79(7):2717-26. PMID:21536789

[16] Staphylococcus aureus evades the extracellular antimicrobial activity of mast cells by promoting its own uptake. Abel J, Goldmann O, Ziegler C, Höltje C, Smeltzer MS, Cheung AL, Bruhn D, Rohde M, Medina E. J Innate Immun. 2011;3(5):495-507. PMID:21654154

[17] Burning mouth syndrome and mast cell activation disorder. Afrin LB. Oral Surg Oral Med Oral Pathol Oral Radiol Endod. 2011 Apr;111(4):465-72. PMID:21420635

[18] Autism spectrum disorders and mastocytosis. Theoharides TC. Int J Immunopathol Pharmacol. 2009 Oct-Dec;22(4):859-65. PMID:20074449

[19] Mast cell activation and autism. Theoharides TC, Angelidou A, Alysandratos KD, Zhang B, Asadi S, Francis K, Toniato E, Kalogeromitros D. Biochim Biophys Acta. 2012 Jan;1822(1):34-41. PMID:21193035

[20] The shifting interface between IBS and IBD. Spiller R, Lam C. Curr Opin Pharmacol. 2011 Dec;11(6):586-92. PMID:22000604

[21] Evidence for mast cell activation in patients with therapy-resistant irritable bowel syndrome. Frieling T, Meis K, Kolck UW, Homann J, Hülsdonk A, Haars U, Hertfelder HJ, Oldenburg J, Seidel H, Molderings GJ. Z Gastroenterol. 2011 Feb;49(2):191-4. PMID:21298604

[22] Personal communication with Dr. Larry Afrin, Hematologist/Oncologist, University of Minnesota.

[23] Mast cell activation disease: a concise practical guide for diagnostic workup and therapeutic options. Molderings GJ,

Brettner S, Homann J, Afrin LB. J Hematol Oncol. 2011 Mar 22;4:10. PMID:21418662

[24] Increased leukotriene E4 excretion in systemic mastocytosis. Butterfield JH. Prostaglandins Other Lipid Mediat. 2010 Jun;92(1-4):73-6. PMID:20380889

[25] Primary role of multiparametric flow cytometry in the diagnostic work-up of indolent clonal mast cell disorders. Perbellini O, Zamò A, Colarossi S, Zampieri F, Zoppi F, Bonadonna P, Schena D, Artuso A, Martinelli G, Chilosi M, Pizzolo G, Zanotti R. Cytometry B Clin Cytom. 2011 Jun 8. PMID:21656905

[26] Vitamin C depletion is associated with alterations in blood histamine and plasma free carnitine in adults. Johnston CS, Solomon RE, Corte C. J Am Coll Nutr. 1996 Dec;15(6):586-91. PMID:8951736

[27] Cysteinyl leukotrienes enhance the degranulation of bone marrow-derived mast cells through the autocrine mechanism. Kaneko I, Suzuki K, Matsuo K, Kumagai H, Owada Y, Noguchi N, Hishinuma T, Ono M. Tohoku J Exp Med. 2009 Mar;217(3):185-91. PMID:19282653

[28] Wintrobe's Clinical Hematology 12 ed. John P. Greer editor, 2008

[29] Mast cell migratory response to interleukin-8 is mediated through interaction with chemokine receptor CXCR2/Interleukin-8RB. Nilsson G, Mikovits JA, Metcalfe DD, Taub DD. Blood. 1999 May 1;93(9):2791-7. PMID:10216072

[30] Pro-apoptotic Bax is the major and Bak an auxiliary effector in cytokine deprivation-induced mast cell apoptosis. Karlberg M, Ekoff M, Labi V, Strasser A, Huang D, Nilsson G. Cell Death Dis. 2010 May 13;1:e43. PMID:21364649

[31] TLR signaling in mast cells: common and unique features. Sandig H, Bulfone-Paus S. Front Immunol. 2012;3:185. PMID:22783258

[32] Histamine promotes the expression of receptors TLR2 and TLR4 and amplifies sensitivity to lipopolysaccharide and lipoteichoic acid treatment in human gingival fibroblasts. Gutiérrez-Venegas G, Cruz-Arrieta S, Villeda-Navarro M, Méndez-Mejía JA. Cell Biol Int. 2011 Oct;35(10):1009-17. PMID:21418040

[33] Histamine induces Toll-like receptor 2 and 4 expression in endothelial cells and enhances sensitivity to Gram-positive and Gram-negative bacterial cell wall components. Talreja J, Kabir MH, B Filla M, Stechschulte DJ, Dileepan KN. Immunology. 2004 Oct;113(2):224-33. PMID:15379983

[34] The sympathetic nerve--an integrative interface between two supersystems: the brain and the immune system. Elenkov IJ, Wilder RL, Chrousos GP, Vizi ES. Pharmacol Rev. 2000 Dec;52(4):595-638. PMID:11121511

[35] The protective effects of melatonin against water avoidance stress-induced mast cell degranulation in dermis. Cikler E, Ercan F, Cetinel S, Contuk G, Sener G. Acta Histochem. 2005;106(6):467-75. PMID:15707656

[36] Epigenetic targets for melatonin: induction of histone H3 hyperacetylation and gene expression in C17.2 neural stem cells. Sharma R, Ottenhof T, Rzeczkowska PA, Niles LP. J Pineal Res.2008 Oct;45(3):277-84.PMID:18373554

[37] Gene regulation by melatonin linked to epigenetic phenomena. Korkmaz A, Rosales-Corral S, Reiter RJ. Gene. 2012 Jul 15;503(1):1-11. PMID:22569208

[38] Melatonin protection against burn-induced hepatic injury by down-regulation of nuclear factor kappa B activation. Bekyarova G, Apostolova M, Kotzev I. Int J Immunopathol Pharmacol. 2012 Jul-Sep;25(3):591-6.PMID:23058009

[39] Inhibition of nitric oxide in LPS-stimulated macrophages of young and senescent mice by δ-tocotrienol and quercetin. Qureshi AA, Tan X, Reis JC, Badr MZ, Papasian CJ, Morrison DC, Qureshi N. Lipids Health Dis. 2011 Dec 20;10:239. PMID:22185406

[40] Selective inhibition of cyclooxygenase-2 (COX-2) by 1alpha,25-dihydroxy-16-ene-23-yne-vitamin D3, a less calcemic vitamin D analog. Aparna R, Subhashini J, Roy KR, Reddy GS, Robinson M, Uskokovic MR, Venkateswara Reddy G, Reddanna P. J Cell Biochem. 2008 Aug 1;104(5):1832-42. PMID:18348265

[41] Tocotrienols suppress proinflammatory markers and cyclooxygenase-2 expression in RAW264.7 macrophages. Yam ML, Abdul Hafid SR, Cheng HM, Nesaretnam K. Lipids. 2009 Sep;44(9):787-97. PMID:19655189

[42] gamma-tocopherol and its major metabolite, in contrast to alpha-tocopherol, inhibit cyclooxygenase activity in macrophages and epithelial cells. Jiang Q, Elson-Schwab I, Courtemanche C, Ames BN. Proc Natl Acad Sci U S A. 2000 Oct 10;97(21):11494-9. PMID:11005841

[43] Immunological function of sphingosine 1-phosphate in the intestine. Kunisawa J, Kiyono H. Nutrients. 2012 Mar;4(3):154-66. PMID:22666543

[44] Role of acid sphingomyelinase in the regulation of mast cell function. Yang W, Schmid E, Nurbaeva MK, Set al. Clin Exp Allergy. 2014 Jan;44(1):79-90. PMID:24164338

[45] Truth and consequences of sphingosine-1-phosphate lyase. Aguilar A, Saba JD.Adv Biol Regul. 2012 Jan;52(1):17-30. PMID:21946005

[46] Phosphorylation of CBP by IKKalpha promotes cell growth by switching the binding preference of CBP from p53 to NF-kappaB. Huang WC, Ju TK, Hung MC, Chen CC. Mol Cell. 2007 Apr 13;26(1):75-87. PMID:17434128

[47] Exercise-induced anaphylaxis: a serious but preventable disorder. Miller CW, Guha B, Krishnaswamy G. Phys Sportsmed. 2008 Dec;36(1):87-94. PMID:20048476

[48] Polycythemia from mast cell activation syndrome: lessons learned. Afrin LB. Am J Med Sci. 2011 Jul;342(1):44-9. PMID:21642812

13. Bioactive Amine Induced Pseudoallergy

One of our evolutionary imperatives is to avoid rotting flesh. Our sense of smell warns us not to get too close and certainly not to eat putrefying flesh from disease-infested carrion.

When animals die, bacteria from the animal's bowels migrate out into the abdominal cavity and then to other tissues where they digest the proteins in the animal's body. The bacteria ferment some of the amino acids from proteins into bioamines. These include *histamine* formed from the amino acid histidine; and the diamines *putrescine*, from ornithine and *cadaverine*, from lysine. As you may have guessed, the name putrescine is Latin for "essence of putrid" and cadaverine from "essence of cadaver." The amine compound, trimethylamine, provides the odor "essence of rotting fish."

If we happen to eat spoiled food, there usually a strong incentive not to repeat the behavior. At low levels, histamine increases stomach acid, which is bacteriocidal. At higher levels, histamine triggers nausea and provokes diarrhea which can quickly clear the contents of the stomach and bowels. Histamine causes tachycardia, perhaps as an adaptation to overcome the loss of fluids. At the same time, the brain is slowing down unneeded functionality other than to increase aversion memory to permanently embed: "I don't care how hungry I was and how good it tasted; I will never, ever eat at that restaurant again!!!" I can still see the face of that pleasant, elderly waiter who served me a plate of poison fish nearly 30 years ago. Anxiety and a sense of doom resulting from histamine reinforce this. The headache feels like the pounding of a hammer as if drives the message in. Other biogenic amines can promote other adverse reactions.

Table 13-1: Effects of Histamine Levels in the Blood

Level in ng/mL	Histamine Effect
0 - 1	Normal
1 - 2	Increased gastric acid secretion, increased heart rate
3 - 5	Further increase the heart rate, urticaria, itching, and headache
6 - 8	Fall in blood pressure from loss of blood volume
7 - 12	Bronchospasm

Scombroid Poisoning

Scombroid poisoning is most common after eating fish from the Scombroidea family (tuna, mackerel, skipjack, and bonito). However, it can occur after eating many types of fish or shellfish. If fish are stored at a temperature that is not cool enough, bacteria from the fish's digestive system escape into the flesh of the fish and grow. Fish are cold-blooded, and their commensal bacteria are adapted to grow in cooler temperatures that those of most land animals.

Several of these bacteria have enzymes that can convert amino acids from the protein in the fish flesh into biogenic amines. Although scombroid has long been considered to result from histamine toxicity, histamine is only one of the biogenic amines involved, and by itself, it is insufficient to cause scombroid toxicity. Putrescine, tyramine[1], and cadaverine are also produced by bacteria in decomposing fish. In combination, these amines can inhibit the brush border enzymes that under normal conditions breakdown bioamines, preventing their absorption and thus, toxicity.

When these biogenic amines are present in fish for consumption, a black pepper or spicy hot flavor and sensation may be noted. Then, sometimes in minutes, or up to a few hours later, a histamine type reaction occurs:

- Flushing of the face
- Nausea
- Headache
- Runny nose and congestion
- Dizziness
- Rapid pulse
- Anxiety

It then may proceed to add:

- Hives
- Generalized swelling
- Abdominal cramps and diarrhea

In severe cases there may be:

- Blurred vision,
- Bronchoconstriction/asthma,
- Laryngeal edema/ swelling of the tongue

Cooking the fish does not destroy or reduce levels of the biogenic amines. Rather, it can make them more toxic. Putrescine and cadaverine, under acid conditions; in the stomach, or heat; cooking at frying or barbecue temperatures, can be converted into nitrosamine compounds. Cadaverine is converted into nitrosopiperidine and putrescine into nitrosopyrrolidine[2]. Both are gastrointestinal and liver toxins and potent carcinogens.

Treatment of scombroid poisoning is supportive, and histamine blockers may help. Most cases last for several hours and resolve, but symptoms can last for a couple of days. It may take several days to feel well again. The memories can last a lifetime.

In scombroid toxicity, urocanic acid, another bacterial fermentation product of histidine that is produced under cooler bacterial growth conditions, can trigger mast cell degranulation[3] through its effect on Substance P or CGRP[4]. Thus, scombroid toxicity is, additionally, a degranulation syndrome.

The symptoms of scombroid poisoning are similar to a generalized allergic reaction because it works by the same mechanism; release of histamine into the blood stream. Scombroid gives the prototypic histamine reaction as a result of histamine formed by bacterial fermentation of the amino acid histidine in the fish's flesh. The FDA has established 10 mg /100 g of histamine in tuna as the hazard action level.

Urticaria is edema of the skin that results from histamine allowing fluid to pass between cells and leak out of the blood stream. The stretching of the skin increases itching. Fluid loss from the bloodstream into the tissues and the intestine provokes the loss of blood volume that can cause hypotension. Bronchospasm results in part from the effect of histamine on smooth muscle cells, but also from leaking of fluid into the respiratory mucosa.

Histamine and the other biogenic amines are responsible for migraine, anaphylaxis, stuffy nose, itchy eyes, wheezing and multiple other disease conditions. Histamine and the biogenic amines might be considered evil incarnate if only we did not need them for our survival.

The fertilized ova cannot implant in the endometrium without histamine. The placenta cannot grow and take nourishment and oxygen for a new life without this bioamine. The biogenic amines spermine and spermadine are in breast milk and are important for the maturation of the intestines to prepare the infant for other foods. They are growth factors for cell division. Putrescine and cadaverine are important for wound healing. And no one alive lacks mast cells; missing mast cells appears to be incompatible with life. Biogenic amines; they are important mediators in the immune system, and act as neurotransmitters and growth regulators; however, they need to present in appropriate amounts. Bioamine levels are largely controlled by enzymes that break down the amines.

Pseudo-allergy from Bioactive Amine Toxicity

In allergic reactions, mast cells and basophils degranulate in response to IgE antibody/antigen interactions, triggering the release of histamine and other amines. This provokes the well-known range of IgE-mediated allergic reactions; from mild sniffles and sneezes to wheezes and anaphylaxis from environmental allergens, and hives, stomach pain, nausea, diarrhea, and asthma from food IgE allergies. In pseudo-allergy, biogenic amines can provoke a similar array of reactions, but here, there are no triggering antigens, antibodies to the food, or degranulation of mast cells or basophils. Pseudo-allergy is not an immune response, but rather a toxic reaction from histamine and other biogenic amines in food.

Dietary biogenic amines are not limited to rotten meat and spoiled fish. They are present in aged cheese, fine red wines, and rich chocolate; all of which are common triggers for migraine. Bioamines are often present in fermented foods but are also found in some foods without fermentation. Fish, fowl, and beast are also not alone in having intestinal bacteria that produce these biogenic amines. We have them as well, and we don't have to wait until we are dead for these bacteria to produce biogenic amines.

Proteins that are not digested, and enzymes, peptides and amino acids which are not absorbed in the small intestine, pass into the large intestine undergo fermentation by bacteria. The same bacteria that rot flesh after death are there fermenting undigested amino acids while we live.

Table 13-2: Important Biogenic Amines[*]

Amine	Precursor	Blood Vessels[**]	Crosses Blood-Brain Barrier	Amine Groups[#]	Action
Synephrine	Tyrosine	VC		1	Nasal decongestant
Tyramine	Tyrosine	VC low VD high	?	1	Releases NE
Octopamine	Tyrosine			1	
Phenylethylamine	Phenylalanine	VD	Yes	1	
Tryptamine	Tryptophan	VC	Yes	1	Prostaglandin release
Serotonin	5 hydroxy-tryptophan	VC	Yes	1	Bronchoconstrictor
Histamine	Histidine	Capillary VD	Yes	2	Immune mediator
Putrescine	Ornithine			2	Cell growth
Cadaverine	Lysine			2	Cell growth
Spermidine	Putrescine			3	Cell growth
Spermine	Spermidine			4	Cell growth
Agmatine	Arginine			4	Cell growth, Anxiolytic[5]

[*]The neurotransmitters epinephrine, norepinephrine and dopamine, are biogenic monoamines but are not included here as they are not implicated in pseudoallergic reactions.   [**] VC: vasoconstrictor, VD: vasodilator.

[#] Monoamines have a single amine group; diamines, two; and polyamines, three or more amine groups.

One of these bacteria, *Morganella morganii*, (a common resident of the fish and human intestine) produces the enzyme histidine decarboxylase which converts the amino acid histidine, plentiful in the muscle of scombroid fish, into histamine. Other bacteria contain other enzymes that convert amino acids into bioamines and other substances. Table 13-3 lists the products of amino acid fermentation by bacteria in the gut.

Table 13-3: Products of Amino Acid Fermentation by Intestinal Bacterial

Amino Acid Substrate	Bioamine	Other Compounds
Histidine	Histamine	
Tyrosine	Tyramine	
Lysine	Cadaverine	
Ornithine	Putrescine	
Arginine	Agmatine	
Cysteine and Methionine		Hydrogen sulfide
All amino acids		Ammonia
Tryptophan		Indole and skatole

The bioamines produced by fermentation in the gut can be absorbed, and the results can be unpleasant. Amino acid fermentation not only forms bioamines; other compounds are also produced. Ammonia can be made from any dietary amino acid. It is absorbed from the intestine into the portal venous flow into the liver where it is converted mainly into urea or glutamine. Ammonia is toxic, especially to the brain and especially in infants; ammonia that escapes breakdown by the liver can cause disease (See Chapter 35). Hydrogen sulfide and ammonia are toxic to the colonocytes and disrupt the mucous layer in the colon, allowing for increased absorption of bioamines. Indole and skatole have strong fecal odors.

Histamine

Histamine has multiple actions on the body. These actions are specific to the tissue and are controlled by which types of histamine receptor are present in the cell membrane of that tissue. There are four histamine receptors recognized in humans, each with specific functions. Medications that block these receptors can be used to prevent some specific effects of histamine.

Histamine Absorption

If an equivalent oral dose of histamine to that consumed during scombroid intoxication is taken orally by itself, it does not cause toxicity. A dose of 0.1 mg of histamine given by I.V. will cause facial flushing within 20 seconds and a histamine headache within one minute. In normal individuals, an oral dose of 225 mg of histamine in water does not provoke any reaction. An oral dose of 100 to 180 mg of histamine, however, will cause symptoms if mixed with tuna. Thus, other factors are involved in histamine absorption.

Table 13-4: Effects of Histamine on Organ Systems

System	Effect
CNS	Causes headache through vasodilation, vertigo, nausea and vomiting. Histamine affects the circadian cycle, body temperature control, and memory.
Cardiovascular	Vasodilation, tachycardia. Can provoke arrhythmias, hypertension, and hypotension in anaphylaxis.
Respiratory	Bronchoconstriction, mucus production, nasal congestion, sneezing, coryza.
Gastrointestinal	Abdominal pain, increased acid secretion, edema, flatulence, diarrhea, and inflammation.
Skin and dermis	Flushing, urticaria, and itching.
Reproductive	Uterine cramping in dysmenorrhea, increased estrogen production.
Bone marrow	Increased production of mast cells

Normally, histamine is not absorbed from the lumen of the intestine, and even high luminal histamine concentrations do not elicit clinical histaminosis. The intestinal mucosa actively works to rid itself of histamine. Histamine which is absorbed or released by mast cells into the lamina propria of the intestine is actively taken up by an organic cation transporter protein at the basolateral membrane of the enterocytes where it is catabolized or exported to the intestinal lumen[6].

Two enterocyte enzymes are responsible for most of the catabolism of histamine: amine oxidase copper containing (AOC1) at the enterocyte brush border; and histamine N-methyl-transferase (HNMT), in the enterocyte cytoplasm. Very high doses of histamine are needed to exceed the cell's ability to eliminate histamine and allow absorption[7]. These two enzymes are equally active in the large intestine, but AOC1 activity is about nine times higher than that of HNMT in the jejunum[8]. AOC1 activity appears to be more important for the catabolism of dietary histamine in the small intestine while HNMT is mainly responsible for the catabolism of histamine derived during fermentation of amino acids in the colon.

Absorption of histamine can be greatly increased by the loss of enzymatic activity of HNMT or AOC1. Although usually adequate, these enzymes can be diminished by damage to the enterocytes, or if inhibited by drugs or other substances that impair the function of these enzymes.

It has been demonstrated that cadaverine and amino-guanidine greatly potentiate the uptake of histamine by the enterocytes[9] through inhibition of the enzymes that catabolize histamine. Putrescine also inhibits these enzymes. In addition to bioamines, which may be found in food, caffeine and theobromine, found in chocolate, can inhibit the activity of these enzymes.

Histamine is absorbed across the lamina propria and into the blood stream as a result of paracellular absorption down a concentration gradient across tight junction membranes between the enterocytes[10]. Thus, agents that open the tight junctions or otherwise increase intestinal paracellular permeability greatly enhance histamine absorption.

The gastrointestinal absorption of histamine and other bioactive amines also depends on the activity of the enzymes that catabolize them, and agents which inhibit those enzymes. Paracellular permeability and the factors which affect it are discussed in Chapter 24: Leaky Gut Syndrome. A list of bioamines, medications, and other substances, which inhibit the activity of AOC1 and HNMT, is given in Table 13-15, at the end of this chapter.

Table 13-5: Histamine Receptors and their Functions

Histamine Receptor	Effects [11,12]	Antagonist Effect
H_1R Smooth Muscle Endothelium Central Nervous System	Smooth muscle contraction Bronchoconstriction Mucous secretion Separation of endothelial cells: Itching Urticaria, Edema Flushing Motion sickness Vomiting Headache ↑ T-Helper 1 response Estrogen? ↑ Vigilance? ↑ Attention? ↓ Feeding?	Antiallergic Antipruritic Antiemetic
H_2R Stomach (Parietal cells) Lymphocytes Vascular smooth muscle cells	Gastric acid secretion ↑T_H1 and ↓T_H2 activity Vasodilatation	Anti-ulcer
H_1R, H_2R	Vasodilation Increased vascular permeability Tachycardia Dysrhythmias Alterations in blood pressure Cramping, bloating diarrhea Nasal congestion, coryza Bronchoconstriction Laryngeal edema	Anti-allergy
H_3R Central Nervous System Peripheral Nervous System	Decreases release of histamine, acetylcholine, norepinephrine, serotonin CNS: arousal, circadian rhythm ↑ aversion memory, anxiety and impulsivity ↓ learning, judgment, and memory acquisition ↓ Food intake? Neuropathic pain? Headache?	Clinical potential: Schizophrenia Dementia Narcolepsy ADHD Obesity
H_4R Basophils Bone Marrow Thymus	Mast cell, eosinophil and other WBC chemotaxis, chemokine production Endocytosis of antigens by dendritic cells (increased immune response to antigens[13].) Increase production of mast cells	Clinical potential: Anti-inflammatory Anti-mastocytosis

Histamine Catabolism

The primary intracellular enzyme responsible for the catabolism of endogenous histamine is histamine n-methyltransferase (HNMT), which usually accounts for 50 to 80% of histamine biotransformation[14]. This enzyme transfers a methyl group from s-adenosylmethionine (SAMe), onto histamine, resulting in the formation of N-methylhistamine. Methylhistamine exerts a negative feedback on HNMT; thus, the efficient removal of N-methylhistamine by monoamine oxidase (MAO) is essential for clearance of histamine. HNMT is an intracellular enzyme; so, histamine must be absorbed into cells from the blood for its catabolism.

Polymorphisms in HNMT, the most important enzyme for degradation of histamine in the bronchial epithelium, have been found in individuals with asthma[25].

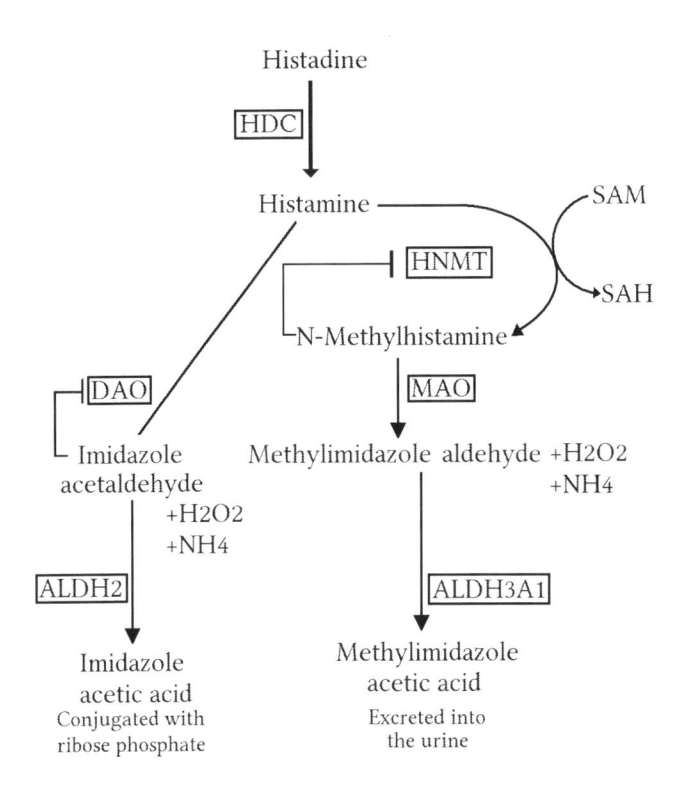

Figure 13-1: Histamine Metabolic Pathway

The other enzyme important for removal of histamine is amine oxidase copper containing 1 (AOC1), once known as diamine oxidase* (DAO) because of its preference for diamines as substrates. AOC1 is the main extracellular enzyme which degrades histamine. AOC1 also catabolizes other polyamines, such as putrescine and spermidine. It is a membrane glycoprotein that is stored in vesicles in the plasma membrane and is released to the cell surface upon stimulation. Thus, AOC1 acts on the surface of the cell.

*Amine oxidase copper-containing 1 changes name frequently. It has been officially dubbed diamine oxidase, histaminase, and amiloride-binding protein 1 (ABP1).

Table 13-6: Histamine Catabolism Enzymes and Cofactors

Enzyme	Cofactors	Dose
Histamine N-methyl transferase (HNMT)	S-adenosyl-methionine (SAMe) SAMe is recycled using folate as a methyl donor. Vitamin B_{12} is as cofactors for this. Betaine also acts as a methyl donor. Methionine + ATP form SAMe. Figures 31-4, 31-5	S-adenosyl-methionine* Folate 400 mcg to 600 mcg daily. 5-MTHF preferred. Cyanocobalamin if serum levels less than 500 ng/mL B_6 as pyridoxine HCl, 5 mg a day. Betaine (TMG)
Monoamine Oxidase B (MAOB)	FAD: Riboflavin (Vitamin B_2) Mg^{2+} Zn^{2+}	Riboflavin 5 mg per day. Magnesium oxide or magnesium citrate, 200 mg daily Zinc 10 mg daily
Amine oxidase, copper containing 1 (AOC1) (DAO) (ABP1)	FAD: Copper PQQ Vitamin C[15] Calcium	FAD – as above. Copper deficiency is rare[†]. Vitamin C 50mg each meal. Calcium deficiency: treat malabsorption, Vitamin D.
Aldehyde dehydrogenase ALDH	NAD (Niacin, Mg^{2+}) NADP (Niacin, Mg^{2+})	Magnesium as above Niacin or Niacinamide ALDH is inhibited by some H2 blockers, alcohol, and some mushrooms.

*Use of supporting vitamins is preferable over the use of S-adenosylmethionine supplements because of potential toxicity. Vitamin supplements are discussed in Chapter 40; vitamin D is discussed in chapter 20.

[†]Copper needs to be in a reduced state for the enzyme reaction, and adequate reduced vitamin C is required for that activity[16]. Copper should not be supplemented unless the deficiency is documented with testing as deficiency is unusual, and copper supplementation is associated with increased mortality.

There is negative feedback on the enzymatic activity of both AOC1 and HNMT by their catabolic products. This may occur as the products need to diffuse out of the area so that new substrate to get into position for catalysis. It may also be an adaptive advantage as the products of these enzymes are toxic. The oxidation reaction requires water and oxygen and results in an aldehyde, ammonia, and hydrogen peroxide. H2O2 is an oxidant, and ammonia and aldehydes are toxins. Aldehydes are removed by aldehyde dehydrogenase enzymes that are essential for preventing the buildup of histamine products that have negative feedback on the histamine catabolism enzymes.

Acetaldehyde can also be formed by the action of alcohol dehydrogenase (ADH) on ethanol acetaldehyde. Acetaldehyde is much more toxic to astrocytes[17], the support cells for neurons than is alcohol (ethanol) itself. It is acetaldehyde that causes alcohol-induced hangovers. Acetaldehyde is also carcinogenic. Acetaldehyde is catabolized by aldehyde dehydrogenase (ALDH), mainly by ALDH2.

About 10 percent of individuals of Asian descent (from Korea, Japan, and China) are homozygous for the ALDH2*2 allelic form of ALDH2. ALDH2 activity is extremely low in these individuals. When these people consume alcohol, acetaldehyde accumulates causing a flushing syndrome. These individuals rarely become alcoholics, as the alcohol experience is so unpleasant[18]. Disulfiram, a medication used to treat alcohol abuse, acts by inhibiting ALDH, causing the accumulation of aldehyde, resulting in hangover-like symptoms if even small amounts of alcohol are consumed. Symptoms include flushing of the skin, accelerated heart rate, nausea, vomiting, and a throbbing headache. With more severe aldehyde toxicity, there can be shortness of breath, visual disturbances, mental confusion and circulatory collapse.

In addition to alcohol and disulfiram, several H_2 antagonists also inhibit ALDH. Cimetidine inhibits the enzymes ALDH2 and ALDH3[19]. Ranitidine also inhibits ALDH; nizatidine does so to a lesser extent. Famotidine (Pepcid) does not suppress ALDH[20]. Thus, famotidine may have a therapeutic advantage over other H_2 antagonists as it does not impede the catabolism of histamine. Certain edible mushrooms also block ALDH.

Ammonia and aldehydes are toxic to astrocytes. These cells control blood flow to the brain, and dysregulation may contribute to vascular headache. There is considerable overlap of symptoms in hangovers and bioamine-induced headaches.

Monoamine oxidase (MAO)

Monoamine oxidase catabolizes of methylhistamine. MAO enzymes are out mitochondrial membrane enzymes, important in the catabolism of bioamine neurotransmitters.

There are two forms of MAO: MAO_A and MAO_B. MAO_A actively metabolizes tyramine, serotonin, norepinephrine and dopamine, while MAO_B is most active for dopamine and phenylethylamine. MAO_A inhibitors are effective in the treatment of depression while MAO_B is sometimes used for Parkinson's disease. Both isoforms are present in most tissues; however, their relative presence varies. The liver has both in about equal amounts while MAO_B is the dominant form in the brain; MAO_A is the dominant isoform in the intestines and peripheral neurons.

MAO is inhibited by alcohol, by some bioamines, and by some medications. MAO-inhibiting drugs, for depression (MAO_A inhibitors), have limited use because of side effects that can occur with ingestion of foods high in monoamines such as tyramine. A list of MAO- inhibiting medications is included in Table 13-14 at the end of this chapter.

Polymorphisms of MAO are associated with risk of several diseases. A polymorphism of MAO_A was found to confer risk of migraines[21], anger and suicide[22], and polymorphisms of MAO_B has been found to confer risk for ADHD[23] and negative emotions[24].

Amine Oxidase Copper Containing 1 (AOC1)

AOC1 is present in the lumen of the intestine at the brush border of the enterocytes. It is the primary enzyme responsible for the catabolism of histamine and diamines in the gut. AOC1 prevents most of the biogenic amines in food or produced by the intestinal bacteria from being absorbed. In addition to histamine, AOC1 also breaks down the diamines putrescine, spermadine, and cadaverine.

If AOC1 or its activity is reduced, ingestion of bioamine-rich food can provoke histamine reactions including diarrhea, headache, nasal congestion, urticaria, itching, bronchoconstriction and wheezing, hypotension, cardiac arrhythmias and other reactions.

AOC1 is expressed in highest amounts (by far) in the placenta, followed by the kidneys, colon, prostate, small intestine, and B cell lymphoblasts. AOC1 also degrades other biogenic amines, and its action can be greatly slowed by these other bioamines. Like HNMT, AOC1 activity is down-regulated by its product, so removal of imidazole acetaldehyde by the enzyme aldehyde dehydrogenase (ALDH) is critical for the removal of histamine. Acetaldehyde from alcohol metabolism inhibits AOC1 activity.

Polymorphisms of AOC1 are associated with food allergies, gluten enteropathy, and inflammatory bowel disease[25]. This suggests that allelic variations that reduce AOC1 activity may increase susceptibility to histamine. Histamine is directly active, but additionally, promotes mast cell chemotaxis to the exposed area and proliferation via H_4 receptors (Chapter 12). Colonic AOC1 activity is low in patients with ulcerative colitis (UC)[26]. UC patients who require immunosuppressive therapy are 2.4 times more likely to have a mutation in the gene that codes for AOC1[27]. Polymorphisms of AOC1 have also been associated with colon adenomas[25]. AOC1 acts as a negative feedback control of cell proliferation of the intestinal mucosa.

Damage or inflammation of the intestinal mucosa can cause loss of brush border enzymes including AOC1, lactase, and other enzymes. This occurs in inflammatory conditions such as gluten enteropathy, parasitic disease such as giardiasis, viral or bacterial gastroenteritis, and chemotherapy.

Regulation of Biogenic Amines

Biogenic amines in the blood are usually quickly broken down. Enzymes, specific for the amines, are found on the surface of the cells and in the plasma. AOC1 is present in high concentrations on the brush border membranes of epithelial cells in the kidneys and enterocytes in the intestine. These enzymes efficiently clear biogenic amines from the blood plasma. AOC1 on the surface of the enterocytes destroys bioamines in food, preventing its absorption from the intestine. Other enzymes inside of the cells also break down biogenic amines. Heparin causes the release of AOC1 from the brush border cell surface into the circulation, from which it is quickly removed[28], causing a loss of its activity. Heparin is released from mast cells during degranulation, and this helps prolong the histaminergic reaction.

Histamine in Pregnancy

The placenta produces high levels of histamine decarboxylase (HDC), the enzyme that converts the amino acid histidine into histamine. The maternal side of the placenta requires histamine in order to stay implanted in the wall of the uterus. Histamine acts as a vasodilator and insufficient histamine results in ischemia due to deficient angiogenesis and placental insufficiency. Pregnancies in which the placenta has an inadequate number of mast cells and lower than normal histamine production result in intrauterine growth retardation.

The placenta also produces AOC1, which breaks down the histamine, protecting mother and fetus. Plasma AOC1 levels are usually about 0 – 2 U/mL, but at the beginning of pregnancy levels begin to rise and increase to around 2000 U/mol by the 22nd week of pregnancy, and remain around that level throughout the rest of the pregnancy. If AOC1 levels do not rise, the pregnancy will be doomed. Pregnancies lacking sufficient AOC1 activity or having excessive HDC activity are at risk of hyperemesis gravidarum, spontaneous and threatened abortion and pre-eclampsia[29].

High AOC1 levels may explain why some women feel so much better while pregnant and also explain the reduction in the frequency of migraines and other histamine reactions during pregnancy. High AOC1 levels lower histamine levels through much of the pregnancy and protect pregnant women from histamine and other biogenic amines that would otherwise have them not feel as well.

Pseudoallergy

Pseudoallergy refers to non-immune reactions that mimic allergic reactions, usually through the action of biogenic amines. In a Type 1 allergic reaction, antigens bind to IgE on mast cells, initiating cross-linking of the IgE and triggering degranulation of mast cells and the release of histamine and other inflammatory mediators. In pseudoallergic reactions, there is not an immune reaction; there is no antigen-antibody interaction.

Histamine Intolerance: About one percent of the population suffers from histamine intolerance[29]. In this condition, ingestion of certain foods can provoke a histamine-like reaction, which may cause headache, diarrhea, wheezing, urticaria, flushing dysmenorrhea, premenstrual syndrome or other symptoms. The quantity of histamine in the food may have little correlation with the symptoms experienced by the patient. As with the scombroid reaction, other factors may influence the reaction.

Here, histamine may be the product of bacteria from the gut rather than being pre-formed in the food. Other bioamines may cause the reaction directly, or by blocking the breakdown of histamine by AOC1 or HNMT, or of their products by MAO and ALDH2. Spermadine and phenylethylamine have been shown to inhibit MAO$_B$[30]. Many individuals with histamine intolerance likely have decreased levels of AOC1 in the intestine. In other individuals, histamine intolerance-like symptoms may be the result of other types of pseudo allergies discussed other chapters. Table 13-8 lists various mechanisms for bioamine reactions from food due to histamine and other bioamines.

With direct mast cell degranulation, the pseudoallergic reaction may include activation of eicosanoids, or the release of inflammatory mediators and cytokines, in addition to the release of histamine and serotonin. Immune-mediated mast cell reactions are discussed in Chapters 11 and 19, and direct mast cell activation in Chapter 14. Other pseudoallergic reactions are discussed in this chapter and Chapters 12, 15 and 16.

Table 13-7: Loss of Amine Catabolic Enzyme Activity

Damage to the enterocytes and villi	Celiac disease, infections (e.g.; rotavirus, Giardia), secondary bile acids, SIBO, intestinal dysbiosis.
Enzyme inhibitors	AOC1 inhibitors, alcohol, other bioamines, enzyme products
Polymorphisms	Genetic variants with lower MAO, AOC1, HNMT, ALDH2 or other related enzyme pathway activity.
Cofactor Deficiencies	Most enzymes rely on cofactors, which may be deficient, especially in individuals with malabsorption.

Table 13-8: Adverse Bioamine Reactions from Food

Bioamine Reaction from Food	Source of Bioamines
Type 1 Immune Reaction (Allergy) (Chapter 11)	Food allergen binds to IgE on mast cells, triggering degranulation.
Direct mast cell activation (Chapter 14)	Some agents can cause direct degranulation of mast cells. These include certain hormones, sulfites, and some opiates. Some agents promote general mast cell activation; others release specific mast cell mediators, depending on the agent.
Loss of enzymatic degradation of bioamines	Loss of AOC1 and HNMT enzymatic activity or the accumulation of their waste products can prevent the destruction of bioactive amines from food or bioamines formed in the intestine. The can occurs in conditions where there is a loss of brush border enzymes from damage to the enterocytes. It may also occur in those with polymorphisms for genes for bioamine catabolism. Alcohol impairs AOC1 activity by generating acetyl-aldehyde. Lack of SAMe or inhibition of MAO may impair intracellular bioamine catabolism.
Preformed bioamines in food	Caused by bacterial fermentation of amino acids in the food, usually by enteric bacteria; e.g., scombroid in fish, tyramine in cheese.
Leaky Gut Syndrome	Increases absorption of bioamines between enterocyte tight junctions.
Loss of proteolytic enzymes or protease inhibitors, allowing fermentation of amino acids in the intestine	Loss of proteolytic enzymes from stomach and pancreas will allow proteins, peptides, and amino acids to pass the small intestine unabsorbed. Pancreatic enzyme deficiency from pancreatitis, cystic fibrosis, damage to the enterocyte brush border enzymes, and malabsorption syndromes can cause loss of proteolytic enzymes. Undigested protein and unabsorbed amino acids ferment in the colon can form bioactive amines (See Table 13-3 above), and can provoke immune hypersensitivity reactions.
Loss of mucin protection in colon	Histamine binds to mucin in the colon. Loss of the protection can increase absorption of histamine.
Mast Cell Activation Disorders	Hyperplasia of mast cells, or aberrant clones of mast cells that are hyperreactive to normal stimuli.

Bioamine Intoxication: Consumption of excessive amounts of bioamines can cause acute intoxication, as in scombroid poisoning. However, by far the most common cause of bioamine intoxication results from abnormally low enzyme activity for the catabolism of bioamines. Affected individuals are susceptible to symptomatic reactions after ingesting a level of biogenic amines that would not affect most people. Even in the case of scombroid poisoning, the histamine reaction probably only occurs when other bioamines are present that impair enzyme activity. The cause of the low enzyme activity may be a polymorphism of the enzyme causing lower activity, damage to the enteric mucosa with loss of these enzymes, use of medications or agents such as alcohol which inhibit the enzymes, lack of cofactors for the enzyme or a combination of these factors (Table 13-8).

Monoamines

Tyramine Intoxication: Dietary tyramine may provoke migraine, hypertension, schizophrenia, Parkinsonism, depression[31], atrial fibrillation[32], and eating disorders[33].

Food can contain large amounts of tyramine, with most of this tyramine being the result of bacterial fermentation. Depending on the strain of bacteria, the tyramine levels can range from non-detectable to nearly 40 mg/liter in red wines, ale, and stout. A wide range of tyramine content may be present in aged cheese; for a given variety, the tyramine content in cheese can range from non-detectable to over 250 mg/100 grams.

> The strain or strains of bacteria involved in the fermentation process (as well as growing conditions for the bacteria: temperature, moisture, and nutrients) can create large differences in the bioamine content of a given food. Thus, a given variety of cheese, sausage, wine, pickle, or other food prepared by fermentation, can have a wide variance in bioamine content.
>
> This variance in bioamine content can make it difficult to associate food exposure with symptoms provoked; the same food may cause symptoms on one occasion and not another. Further, many bioamines competitively inhibit the enzymes that degrade other bioamines; the mix of bioamines present adds to the complexity of the response. Mixing various foods can thus increase the complexity, as does the consumption of alcohol with a meal or other agents that inhibit bioamine breakdown.
>
> If the reaction to bioamines were immediate, as it is in IgE allergic reactions, it would make identification of the causative agent simpler. Many of the reactions to bioamines, migraine, and mood disturbances, for example, are delayed for up to 48 hours after a meal. Thus, the symptoms of bioamine-invoked pseudo allergies can be difficult to associate with the cause.

Some dietary tyramine is taken up by the brush border cells of the small intestine and converted into dopamine by tyrosine hydroxylase (TH). Dopamine is temporarily inactivated by sulfation, and then enters the circulation and is distributed to the cells that will utilize it. When there is excess dietary tyramine, it is deaminated by in the enterocyte by MAO. In the case of tyramine hydroxylase or MAO dysfunction, tyramine can be absorbed and enter the circulation unprocessed, and have systemic effects. Excess tyramine can also be absorbed in leaky gut syndrome (Chapter 24). Biopterin from tetrahydrobiopterin (THB) and iron are required cofactors for tyrosine hydroxylase. Tyrosine hydroxylase dysfunction can promote neurological diseases, including Parkinson's disease, dystonia, psychiatric disorders, such as affective disorders and schizophrenia, and cardiovascular disease[34]. THB is synthesized in the body utilizing three enzymes, zinc, magnesium and NAD (niacin) are cofactors for these enzymes.

The trace monoamines (tyramine, synephrine, octopamine, phenylethylamine and tryptamine) can function as "false neurotransmitters" by displacing the classic monoamine neurotransmitters from their storage pools in the extracellular space, via an amphetamine-like mechanism. Tyramine in the blood is taken up by the nerve terminals of the sympathetic nervous system. This stimulates the release of norepinephrine and impairs re-uptake of the NE back into the nerve terminals. Under normal situations, the amount of NE released from sympathetic nerves is tiny, the NE is transported back into the nerve, and α_2-receptors block further NE release, so very little gets into the bloodstream.

During cardiac ischemia, there can be an unregulated, pathological leakage of NE from sympathetic nerve terminals. Tyramine (and dextroamphetamine) can cause a similar the pathologic release of NE into the circulation[35]. This can provoke a severe reaction with vasoconstriction, an increase in heart rate, elevated blood pressure, and increased cardiac output, and may result in palpitations and dysrhythmias. Other symptoms may include pupillary dilation, widening of the eyelids, lacrimation, salivation, fever, vomiting, headache, increase in respiration and elevation of blood sugar.

The Cheese Reaction

MAO$_A$ inhibitors were an early and effective medicine for depression. Their use was abandoned, however, because of dangerous reactions that occasionally occurred in patients using these medications after eating aged cheese or other foods high in tyramine. The "Cheese Reaction" provoked a hypertensive crisis accompanied by a severe headache that lasted from several minutes to several hours. Patients had nausea, vomiting, muscle cramps, stiff neck, visual disturbances, and photophobia. Chest pain, heart failure, pulmonary edema, stroke, and even death occurred in patients as a result of the reaction from use of the MAO$_A$ inhibitors combined with food high in tyramine.

There are still medications that inhibit MAO used in medicine (see Table 13-14 at the end of this chapter). In 2005, eight of 386 patients in a Japanese hospital had pseudoallergic reactions, including flushing, palpitations, headache, itching, wheezing, and diarrhea, after eating fish paste that was served with a meal. All eight of the patients who had the reaction were in the tuberculosis ward and took isoniazid, which is a MAO inhibitor. The fermented saury paste was analyzed and found to have an elevated histamine content[36].

In normal individuals, 20 to 80 mg of I.V. tyramine will cause a marked elevation in blood pressure. In an average individual, it takes an oral dose of about 400 mg of tyramine to give a hypertensive reaction[37]. However, in patients on MAO-inhibiting medication, 6 mg orally can provoke a dangerous hypertensive reaction.

Table 13-9: Foods Potentially High in Tyramine or other Bioamine Content

Meats and Seafood	Pickled, aged, smoked, fermented, or marinated products; shrimp paste, salami pepperoni, prosciutto, any improperly stored or spoiled meat or seafood.
Fermented (alcoholic) Beverages	Wine, sake, beer, spirits, non-distilled alcoholic beverages
Fermented Diary Products	Cheese, especially aged cheeses such as blue, feta, brie, and Swiss cheese, sour cream, yogurt, Kefir, cultured buttermilk. Note: Fresh cheeses, i.e., cottage cheese, cream cheese, ricotta cheese are not fermented and are unlikely to have high bioamine contents.
Fermented Soy Products	Soy sauce, soybean condiments, teriyaki sauce, tofu, tempeh, miso soup
Chocolate	Cocoa beans are usually fermented
Fermented vegetables	Sauerkraut, pickles, capers, kimchi, Tabasco
Legumes	Broad (Fava) beans, Italian flat (Romano) beans, green bean pods, Chinese (snow) pea pods, peanuts
Fruits	Avocados, bananas, figs, red plums, pineapple, raspberries
Others foods	Brazil nuts, cacti, coconuts, vanilla, eggplants, overripe fruit and vegetables with bacterial breakdown.
Yeast	Yeast extracts, dietary supplements or flavorings such as Marmite, sourdough bread.

The tyramine content of a fermented food depends on the bacterial culture that was used in the foods preparation. One batch of blue cheese might have very high levels while another may have much lower levels; one bottle of capers may have low levels while another they may be high. Most Californian wines use commercially grown yeast and bacteria cultures which have been selected to produce wines with low biogenic amine levels. In Portugal, the tradition is to use wild yeast, accompanied by wild bacteria. Thus, some wines may have very high levels while others, made in the same style, may have low levels of bioactive amines.

In addition to the displacement of monoamines, there are trace amine receptors in the brain and other tissues. Typically, the cheese reaction does not manifest psychoactive effects. However, foods with high tyramine content are often associated with migraine headaches. In one blinded, placebo-controlled trial of patients, 100 mg of tyramine, given orally, were sufficient to trigger migraines on two separate occasions[38], while the placebo did not. The migraines began as early as 90 minutes after ingestion of tyramine and as late as 16 hours later. Tyramine did not provoke migraine in migraineurs without a dietary history of food-related migraines.

Headaches may be induced by tyramine, synephrine, and octopine, through a different mechanism than occurs in the cheese reaction. There are trace amine receptors for these monoamines in the CNS. Patients with migraine and cluster headaches have been found to have elevated circulating levels of tyramine and other trace amines[39].

> **Trace amine associated receptors (TAAR)**
>
> There are seven functioning trace amine associated receptors in humans, and most of them serve as receptors for serotonin as well as trace amines. TAAR RNA expression is widely distributed throughout the body, including brain areas associated with emotion and behavior. The trace amines tyramine, synephrine, and octopine may affect mood and behavior, promoting restlessness, anxiety, depression, and other stress reactions[40]. The amine that has the strongest reaction with TAAR$_1$ is β-phenylethylamine; tyramine has much lower TAAR$_1$ activity. Amphetamine (α-methyl-phenylethylamine) is also a strong ligand for TAAR$_1$.
>
> Amphetamines are used in the treatment of ADHD, and trace amines receptors are the target of research for the treatment of schizophrenia and bipolar disorder[41]. TAAR are encoded on the sixth chromosome at 6q23.2. One heritable form of schizophrenia, (SCZD5), has been mapped to this area. Additionally, amphetamines are known to unmask early subclinical schizophrenia.
>
> The mechanism for dietary bioamine-triggered migraines is not resolved; however, it may be associated with their effect on trace amine receptors in the brain and cerebral arteries. TAAR$_1$ is activated by, and binds to, the amines β-phenylethylamine and tyramine, and less so to octopamine and serotonin. Several other TAAR are also activated by tyramine, β-phenylethylamine, serotonin and other monoamines.
>
> Serotonin activity inhibits migraine, likely through its inhibition of dopamine release. Both ergotamine and triptan medications for migraine are thought to work via their effect on the 5-HT$_{1B}$ serotonin receptors.
>
> Tyramine, β-phenylethylamine, and other bioamines in foods may trigger migraines by antagonizing the action of serotonin or by mimicking the action of dopamine.

Phenylethylamine Intoxication: β-phenylethylamine (βPEA) can act as a neurotransmitter through the TAAR receptors or act by provoking the release of norepinephrine and dopamine. Dietary β-phenylethylamine may provoke migraine, and worsen phenylketonuria[31].

β-phenylethylamine, like tyramine, crosses the blood-brain barrier and avidly binds with TAAR$_1$ in the brain. It also acts similarly to tyramine in the release of NE and dopamine from the sympathetic nerves. Like tyramine, dietary βPEA can trigger migraine headaches; however, it can do so at lower doses. In a double-blinded, placebo-controlled trial, volunteers were given 25 mg of histamine, 25 mg of tyramine or 5 mg of βPEA in apple juice. Only the 5 mg of βPEA produced symptoms, and these included headache and dizziness[42].

β-phenylethylamine is found in chocolate, especially when the cocoa beans have been fermented. It is also found in meat and fish, wine, and other fermented foods. βPEA can act as a psychomotor stimulant when a MAO$_B$ inhibitor is used[43], but under normal conditions it is rapidly cleared from the system.

Chocolate is widely identified as a trigger for migraine and behavioral changes, especially in children. Chocolate provides an initial sense of energy and pleasant excitement, but can be followed by depression and moodiness hours to a day later. This effect has often been attributed to β-PEA. Chocolate, however, also contains high levels of theobromine, an isomer of caffeine. βPEA, theobromine, caffeine, and theophylline are all inhibitors of AOC1. βPEA, caffeine, and theophylline are also inhibitors of HNMT. Additionally, theobromine is toxic (see Chapter 17). The effects of chocolate likely result from the combination of its multiple compounds, with β-PEA playing a minor role.

Tryptamine, Octopamine, and Synephrine: Dietary tryptamine may provoke migraine, hypertension, schizophrenia, Parkinsonism, and depression[31]. Tryptamine can cause similar reactions to tyramine with headache and increased blood pressure. Elevated platelet octopamine levels have been found in patients with migraine without aura and elevated synephrine levels have been found in patients with migraine with aura[44].

Octopamine may provoke hypertension, hepatic encephalopathy, phenylketonuria, and depression[31]. Octopamine can be formed by microbes or converted from tyramine by tyramine β hydroxylase in the adrenal cortex. Octopamine can be further converted to synephrine in the adrenal medulla by the enzyme phenylethanolamine N-methyltransferase (PNMT). The base source for the manufacture of synephrine is certain varieties of oranges, and trace amounts of synephrine are almost certainly present in citrus fruit.

Putrescine and Cadaverine, Spermidine and Spermine: Putrescine and cadaverine are diamines. They have distinctive, foul odors after which they are named. Spermine and spermidine are polyamines and also have distinctive odors that earned them their names. Spermine and spermadine smell like semen or bleach. Uncooked shrimp, which has had bacterial growth, will sometimes have a bleach-like odor from these bioamines.

These polyamines act principally as growth factors, and also act as antioxidant free-radical scavengers. Agmatine, another polyamine, has similar actions plus anxiolytic effects[5]. Polyamines as growth factors are required for normal growth and development.

Spermidine, spermine, and putrescine are present in human and other mammalian milk, and act as growth and maturation factors for the GI system[45]. Polyamines help with the development of the mucosal barrier and thus may help prevent the development of food allergies[46]. Polyamines are essential for the implantation of the embryo in the uterus[47] and differentiation and proliferation of blood cells[48]. Depletion of pancreatic polyamines can induce acute pancreatitis[49]. Polyamines are produced by bacteria in the colon and absorbed for use by the body[50].

Cadaverine, putrescine, spermadine, and spermine are found in injured tissue and likely act as growth factors for tissue repair and healing and angiogenesis. Histamine is sometimes found in healing wounds and causes itching. This may be the result of bacterial enzymatic activity.

> PURE SPECULATION: Certain non-pathogenic commensal skin bacteria may produce polyamines in wounds that promote healing. Histamine production and itching likely result from undesirable bacterial growth.

Like histamine, which is required for life but dangerous in high levels, these polyamines can be toxic in high quantities. These growth factors are produced by, and support, the growth of tumors. They act by inhibiting apoptosis. Blocking the production of polyamines has been shown to decrease tumor growth in colon cancer. High dietary levels of polyamines theoretically could support tumor growth. Putrescine and cadaverine are transformed into carcinogenic nitrosamines by high-temperature cooking and acid in the stomach. Additionally, spermine and spermadine can also form nitrosamines in the presence of nitrites, commonly used as additives to preserve meat. The nitrosamines can be metabolized in the liver to nitrite and a secondary amine[51]. Nitrite (NO_2^-) can then form nitric oxide (NO), a vasodilator that may be a pathway for triggering a migraine.

In a study of chronic toxicity of bioamines, high levels of tyramine, cadaverine, putrescine, spermadine, and spermine were given in chow to Wistar rats. At toxic doses, there was aggressiveness, emaciation, convulsions and paralysis of the hind legs. The animals became anemic, and kidney function was impaired. Spermine was the most toxic, followed by spermadine[52]. In this study, the maximal daily dose of these bioamines which did not cause toxicity was 180 mg/kg body weight for tyramine, cadaverine and putrescine, 83 mg/kg for spermadine and 19 mg/kg for spermine, which would be equivalent to an allometrically corrected daily dose of 200 mg a day in a 70 Kg man. Thus, in chronic dietary exposure, the polyamines may have toxicity similar to or more toxic than tyramine though these chronic doses are unlikely to occur in a normal diet.

Dietary polyamines may impart their acute toxic effect, as seen in scombroid poisoning and perhaps in migraine, as a result of their inhibitory effect on AOC1, MAO, and HNMT, enzymes which catabolism histamine and monoamines.

Imbalances of polyamines may be involved in mental disorders. Schizophrenic patients have been found to have elevated levels of polyamines and decreased levels of plasma amine oxidase[5]. Nevertheless, polyamines should not be regarded as toxins to be avoided. Although they may be toxic at high levels, they are important for the maturation and growth of the intestinal mucosa and pancreas. Spermidine promotes autophagy of cellular organelles and promotes longevity[53].

Table 13-10: Polyamine Rich Foods

Polyamine	Foods
Spermine	Beef liver, green peas, pork, and chicken[54].
Spermidine	Soybeans, green peas, lentils, red beans, pears, mushrooms, broccoli, cauliflower, corn, chicken liver, aged cheddar cheese, potatoes, mango, hazelnuts, and mustard seeds[54]. Blue cheese and fermented sausage[55]. Fermented fish and shrimp may have very high levels.
Putrescine	Citrus fruits, mangoes, sauerkraut and crab.

Fermented fish can have high levels of spermidine and cause symptoms in some individuals; however, these symptoms may come from histamine or other bioamines that are also found in high levels in fermented products.

Serotonin: Mast cell degranulation releases serotonin (5-hydroxytryptamine; 5-HT) as one of numerous immune mediators. Serotonin slows the movement of parasitic worms, and thus, it helps keep parasites in the area of the inflammatory response mounted to destroy them. Serotonin may also help with wound repair after parasitic injury. There is, however, a downside to this; 5-HT can promote smooth muscle hypertrophy, vascular remodeling, and pulmonary hypertension when elevated in chronic inflammatory reactions[56].

There is little data to suggest that dietary serotonin promotes any disease condition. Serotonin does not cross the blood-brain barrier, so no direct psychotropic effect is expected. Diets high in serotonin have been shown to increase platelet serotonin by as much as 300 percent[57], and it is plausible that mast cell and basophil serotonin levels might also be higher in high serotonin diets. Dietary serotonin may have an effect on 5-HT receptors in the GI tract, where it may slow transit time; high levels of serotonin in the gut may cause intestinal discomfort in individuals with low MAO activity. Western diets may increase serotonin availability in the enterochromaffin cells of the GI mucosa[58], and this may slow GI transit. This increase in serotonin, however, is more likely from high levels of tryptophan in the diet than from serotonin content in the diet. Smokers have lower levels of MAO, the principal enzyme which degrades serotonin[56].

Although the serotonin levels in tree nuts, listed in Table 13-10, are high, only small amounts of these nuts are usually consumed; thus, bananas, pineapple, and tomatoes are the largest sources of serotonin in the Western diet. Serotonin levels were tested in 80 commonly consumed foods including meats, fish, chicken, grains, and other fruits and vegetables. Foods with serotonin levels over 0.1 µg/g of are listed in Table 13-11.

Table 13-11 Foods High in Serotonin[59]

Food	µg/g*
Butternuts	398
Black walnuts	304
English walnuts	87
Pecans	29
Plantains	30
Pineapple	17
Banana	15
Kiwi	5.8
Plums	4.7
Tomatoes	3.4
Avocados	1.5
Dates	1.3
Cantaloupe	0.9
Grapefruit	0.9
Honeydew	0.6
Black Olives	0.2
Broccoli	0.2
Eggplant	0.2
Figs	0.2
Spinach	0.1
Cauliflower	0.1

Serotonin Toxidrome: Serotonin toxicity, also called serotonin storm or syndrome, was once a rare condition but now occurs frequently in the U.S., the land where two-thirds of the world's antidepressants are consumed. Serotonin toxicity occurs when excessive serotonin is present in the brain, usually as a result of an unintentional overdose. In this toxic reaction, there may be headache, confusion, hallucinations, hypomania or coma; akathisia, tremor, clonus, hyperreflexia; tachycardia, sweating or shivering, nausea and diarrhea. Serotonin storm (SS) can be fatal.

The overdose can be from a single agent, but more commonly, it results from combining two or more agents. Several classes of antidepressants, opioids, CNS stimulants, migraine medications, lithium, or other medications, some herbs (St. John's wort, ginseng, nutmeg, yohimbine), and some psychedelics, such as LSD can interact to cause SS. For example, use of two serotonergic agents, use of a serotonergic agent with a MAO inhibitor, or use of a serotonergic agent with a medication that prevents the metabolism of a serotonergic agent being used (such as a combination of citalopram with fluconazole (Diflucan)) can cause the SS.

Table 13-12: Serotonin Syndrome Signs[60]

System	Minor Signs	Major Signs
Mental	Agitation Restlessness Insomnia Hyperactivity	Confusion Delirium Coma
Autonomic	↑Heart Rate ↑Respiratory Rate Shortness of breath Blood pressure change Flushing Diarrhea	Fever Sweating
Muscular	Incoordination Pupils Dilated	Akathisia (constant motion) Involuntary muscle clonus Tremor Shivering Hyperreflexia Rigidity

Pseudoallergy to Medications

Many medications can cause adverse reactions that mimic allergic reactions, but are not associated with IgE-mediated mast cell or basophil activity. Several medications inhibit AOC1 activity, and others that inhibit MAO or HNMT activity may have this effect. Tables 13-14 and 13-15 list several of these medications.

Individuals with marginal AOC1 activity may be at increased risk for bioaminergic reaction upon exposure to certain medications. History of pseudoallergy should serve as a warning for the use of medications that inhibit AOC1. Similar warnings are appropriate for MAO and HNMT inhibiting medications. H_2 blockers, although not strong inhibitors, are commonly used and available without a prescription. Nicotine inhibits HNMT. In combination, these may have additive or synergistic effects.

Similarly, foods high in bioamines have an increased risk of causing reactions when consumed together, with alcohol or other enzyme inhibitors. Other medications may cause pseudoallergy through direct non-immune mast cell degranulation. Table 14-5 lists such medications. Additionally, in some individuals, aspirin, and nonsteroidal anti-inflammatory medications may cause pseudoallergic reactions as discussed in Chapter 15.

Table 13-13: Bioamine Enzymes and Inhibitors

Enzyme	Favored Substrates	Cofactors	Inhibitors
Histidine decarboxylase (HDC)	Histidine (Histamine formation)	Pyridoxal phosphate	
Histamine N-methyl transferase (HNMT) (Present I myeloid cells, macrophages, ubiquitous at lower levels)	Histamine	S-adenosylmethionine	Inhibitors: N-methylhistamine S-adenosylhomocysteine
Monoamine oxidase Isoform B (MAO$_B$) (Present in the brain, small intestine, uterus, liver, kidneys)	Histamine Phenylethylamine Dopamine Tyramine Serotonin Tryptamine	FAD (Cofactors of FAD are Vitamin B$_2$: Riboflavin, Mg^{2+}, Zn^{2+})	Inhibitors: Alcohol, MAO$_B$ inhibitors (see Table 13-14)
Amine Oxidase Copper containing 1 (AOC1) AKA: Diamine oxidase (DAO) Amiloride-binding protein-1 (ABP1) or histaminase. (Present in the placenta, kidneys, colon, prostate, small intestine)	Histamine Tryptamine Putrescine Cadaverine N-methylhistamine Agmatine Spermidine	Copper FAD Vitamin C	Inhibitors: imidazole acetaldehyde and several medications. See Table 13-15
Aldehyde dehydrogenase (ALDH)		NAD (Cofactors of NAD are Niacin, Mg^{2+})	Inhibitors: Disulfiram, some medicines; H$_2$ blockers (cimetidine) some mushrooms.
Tyrosine hydroxylase (TH) (converts tyrosine into dopamine)	Tyrosine	Biopterin iron	Note: formation of biopterin requires zinc, magnesium and NAD as cofactors
Ornithine decarboxylase	Ornithine	Pyridoxal phosphate	
N^1-acetylpolyamine oxidase	Spermine Spermadine Agmatine	FAD*	
Spermadine/spermine N-1-acetyltransferase	Spermine-Spermadine (inter-conversion)	FAD*	
Spermidine synthase Spermine synthase	Putrescine Spermidine	S-adenosylmethionine	

Table 13-14: Food Related Bioamine Conditions

Bioamine Reaction from Food	Prevention and Treatment	Chapter
Type 1 Immune Reaction	Avoid food allergens. Perhaps allergy desensitization, especially for environmental (airborne) allergens.	Chapter 11
Direct mast cell activation	Avoidance of agents that directly trigger mast cell degranulation.	Chapter 14
Loss of enzymatic degradation of bioamines	Prevent or treat damage to the intestinal mucosa. Avoid alcohol and other enzyme inhibitors. Assure sufficient enzyme cofactor availability.	Chapter 25 Table 13-12 Table 13-12
Preformed bioamines in food	Avoid fermented foods and foods rich in bioamines. Use AOC1 supplement	
Avoid Absorption	Avoid and treat Leaky Gut Syndrome.	Chapter 25
Protease inhibitors or loss of proteolytic enzymes	Avoid raw food with protease inhibitors (e.g., legumes, potatoes). Supplement deficient trypsin and pancreatic enzymes. Avoid enzyme wasting.	Chapters 7 and 23
Fermentation of amino acids in the intestine	Avoid poorly absorbed sugars. Avoid protein and fat malabsorption. Treat small intestinal bowel overgrowth (SIBO).	Chapter 5 Chapter 24
Loss of mucin protection in colon	Treat malabsorption of protein. See. Assure sufficient sulfur compounds in the diet.	Chapters 7 and 23

Prevention and Treatment of Bioamine Intolerance

Histamine and most other biogenic amines preformed in foods are normally not sufficiently absorbed to provoke toxicity. However, inhibition or loss of the enterocyte enzymes which catabolize these compounds may allow high levels to be absorbed, especially if the enterocyte membrane is impaired. Bioamines can undergo paracellular absorption in pathological conditions. Factors that increase paracellular permeability can greatly increase the amount of bioamines absorbed. (See Chapter 25). Alcohol, some medications, methylxanthines such as caffeine, and other bioamines may inhibit the enzymes that catabolize histamine and other bioactive amines, increasing their availability. Genetic polymorphism may also affect the activity of these enzymes.

1. Prevent Inhibition of AOC1 and HNMT: Alcohol, certain medications, and damage to the intestinal mucosa can impair the action of the enzymes responsible for the destruction of histamine and other bioamines in the intestine; avoid these agents. Dietary bioamines also interfere with the catabolism of other bioamines. Individuals who are susceptible to pseudoallergic reactions to food should, thus, limit bioamines consumed by limiting fermented foods. Other bioamines in these foods compete for use with and slow the activity of these enzymes. Table 13-9 lists foods which may be high in tyramine, or other bioamines. The bioamine content of food depends on the strain of bacteria and conditions under which the food was prepared.

2. Ensure Optimal Enzymatic Activity: Supplementation with vitamins, mineral, and other co-factors for these enzymes may be helpful. Malabsorption can easily cofactor deficiencies. AOC1 function at the intestinal brush border is vulnerable as it requires vitamin C to be available and in its reduced form for the function of this enzyme. During bioamine deactivation by AOC1, vitamin C is oxidized. Thus, reduced vitamin C needs to be replenished to maintain AOC1 activity. The amount of vitamin C required is small but is best when part of each meal. Cofactors for the enzymes are listed in Table 13-6. Supplements are only helpful when there is a deficiency, however; individuals with some polymorphisms respond to supplementation of cofactors at levels higher than required by most individuals.

3. Prevent the Loss of these Enzymes: For most patients, the most important factor in avoiding bioamine intolerance is repair of the function of the intestinal mucosa. Diseases and conditions which damage the enterocytes will cause a loss of these enzymes.

Impaired mucosal function increases the risk of histamine or allergen absorption; thus, promoting the subsequent increased mast cell proliferation. Loss of enterocyte enzymes includes not only the loss of enzymes that catabolize bioamines, but also the loss of disaccharidases and peptidases which help absorb nutrients and prevent them from fermenting. Unabsorbed sugars can result in diarrhea, fast intestinal transit time, and dysbiosis. Rapid transit time increases the likelihood that amino acids and proteins pass through the ileum unabsorbed, and thus, are available for fermentation in the colon, where amino acids can be transformed into bioamines. This will also increase the fermentation of bile acids, forming secondary bile acids, which may further damage the intestinal mucosa, permitting increased absorption bioamines.

The enzyme AOC1 is available as a nutritional supplement (Histame) which may be helpful in the prevention of amine toxicity.

4. Prevent the Absorption of Bioamines: Bioamine absorption is increased when intracellular permeability in increased. Chapter 25 discusses the causes and prevention of hyperpermeability of the intestinal mucosa. Gluten enteropathy (Chapter 22), SIBO (Chapter 23), *Giardia*, and other infections of the intestine may damage the mucosa and increase intercellular permeability.

5. Look for and Treat the Underlying Conditions: If there is hypersensitivity to dietary bioamines, there is certainly at least one underlying cause. Mucosal damage from gluten enteropathy or other disease, increased permeability, bacterial overgrowth, and accumulation of secondary bile acids are some of the more common causes.

Absorption of histamine increases chemotaxis of mast cells to the lamina propria and with it increases the risk for mast cell activation diseases.

Table 13-15: MAO-Inhibiting Medications

Treated Condition	Medication
Depression: (MOA$_A$ Inhibitor)s	Tranylcypromine Moclobemide Iproniazid Isocarboxazid Phenelzine
(MAO$_B$ Inhibitors) Alzheimer's Disease Parkinson's Syndrome	Selegiline Rasagiline
Tuberculosis	Isoniazid (INH) isocarboxazid
Hypertension	Pargyline
Cancer	Procarbazine
Infection	Furazolidone

Table 13-16: AOC1 and HNMT Inhibition Jejunal Mucosa[61, 62]

Class	AOC1	HNMT
Bioamines Quantified Effects	Aminoguanidine 100% Anserine 100% Carnosine 100% Histamine 99% Agmatine 97% Thiamine 92% Cadaverine 87% Tyramine 77%	Tyramine 99% Phenylethylamine 98% Tryptamine 98% Octopamine 94% Agmatine 87% Aminoguanidine 81% Nicotine 78%
Bioamines and other compounds	Putrescine Phenylethylamine Indole 1-Methylhistamine Phenylethylamine Piperazine Spermine Spermidine Synephrine Tryptamine	Cadaverine Indole Tartrazine Trimethylamine Putrescine
Methyl-xanthines	Caffeine Theobromine Theophylline Xanthine Hypoxanthine Aminophylline	Theophylline
Medication	H₂ Blockers (Cimetidine) MAO inhibitors Alcohol (Ethanol) Barbiturate: Sodium thiopental Aspirin Prilocaine Dobutamine Verapamil, clonidine Propafenone Amiloride Metoclopramide Cefuroxime, cefotiam, isoniazid, pentamidine, clavulanic acid Chloroquine Acetylcysteine, ambroxol Amitriptyline	Quinacrine Chloroquine Amodiaquine Chloroquine Hydroxychloroquine Pyrimethamine Promethazine Chloroguanil Proguanil *Tripelennamine* *Metoclopramide* *Ranitidine* *Primaquine phosphate* *Cimetidine* *Trimethoprim*

* Medications in italics are unlikely to be used at high enough concentrations to inhibit HMT systemically, but may be high enough to inhibit the enterocyte enzymes during drug absorption.

[1] [Determination of nonvolatile amines in foods by liquid chromatography following excimer-forming fluorescence derivatization and solid-phase extraction]. Sakamoto T, Akaki K, Hiwaki H. Shokuhin Eiseigaku Zasshi. 2010;51(3):115-21. PMID:20595792

[2] Biogenic amines in fish: roles in intoxication, spoilage, and nitrosamine formation--a review. Al Bulushi I, Poole S, Deeth HC, Dykes GA. Crit Rev Food Sci Nutr. 2009 Apr;49(4):369-77. PMID: 19234946

[3] Histamine fish poisoning revisited. Lehane L, Olley J. Int J Food Microbiol. 2000 Jun 30;58(1-2):1-37. PMID:10898459

[4] cis-Urocanic acid stimulates neuropeptide release from peripheral sensory nerves. Khalil Z, Townley SL, Grimbaldeston MA, Finlay-Jones JJ, Hart PH. J Invest Dermatol. 2001 Oct;117(4):886-91. PMID:11676828

[5] Implication of the polyamine system in mental disorders. Fiori LM, Turecki G. J Psychiatry Neurosci. 2008 Mar;33(2):102-10. PMID:18330456

[6] Bioelimination of histamine in epithelia of the porcine proximal colon of pigs. Aschenbach JR, Honscha KU, von Vietinghoff V, Gäbel G. Inflamm Res. 2009 May;58(5):269-76. PMID:19184353

[7] Paracellular tightness and catabolism restrict histamine permeation in the proximal colon of pigs. Aschenbach JR, Ahrens F, Garz B, Gäbel G. Pflugers Arch. 2002 Oct;445(1):115-22. Epub 2002 Jul 16. PMID:12397395

[8] Histamine inactivation in the colon of pigs in relationship to abundance of catabolic enzymes. Aschenbach JR, Schwelberger HG, Ahrens F, Fürll B, Gäbel G. Scand J Gastroenterol. 2006 Jun;41(6):712-9. PMID:16716971

[9] Cadaverine and aminoguanidine potentiate the uptake of histamine in vitro in perfused intestinal segments of rats. Lyons DE, Beery JT, Lyons SA, Taylor SL. Toxicol Appl Pharmacol. 1983 Sep 30;70(3):445-58. PMID:6636174

[10] Paracellular tightness and catabolism restrict histamine permeation in the proximal colon of pigs. Aschenbach JR, Ahrens F, Garz B, Gäbel G. Pflugers Arch. 2002 Oct;445(1):115-22. PMID:12397395

[11] Histamine H3 receptor antagonists: preclinical promise for treating obesity and cognitive disorders. Esbenshade TA, Fox GB, Cowart MD. Mol Interv. 2006 Apr;6(2):77-88, 59. PMID: 16565470

[12] Histamine H3 receptor antagonists go to clinics. Sander K, Kottke T, Stark H. Biol Pharm Bull. 2008 Dec;31(12):2163-81. PMID: 19043195

[13] Histamine improves antigen uptake and cross-presentation by dendritic cells. Amaral MM, Davio C, Ceballos A, Salamone G, Cañones C, Geffner J, Vermeulen M. J Immunol. 2007 Sep 15;179(6):3425-33.PMID: 17785776

[14] Histamine: new thoughts about a familiar mediator. Jones BL, Kearns GL. Clin Pharmacol Ther. 2011 Feb;89(2):189-97. Epub 2010 Dec 22. PMID:21178984

[15] Effect of ascorbic acid nurniture on blood histamine and neutrophil chemotaxis in guinea pigs. Johnston CS, Huang SN. J Nutr. 1991 Jan;121(1):126-30.PMID:1992049

[16] Highly site-specific oxygenation of 1-methylhistidine and its analogue with a copper (II)/ascorbate-dependent redox system. Uchida K, Kawakishi S. Biochim Biophys Acta. 1990 Jun 20;1034(3):347-50. PMID:2364090

[17] Comparison of ethanol and acetaldehyde toxicity in rat astrocytes in primary culture. Sarc L, Lipnik-Stangelj M. Arh Hig Rada Toksikol. 2009 Sep;60(3):297-305. PMID: 19789159

[18] Acetaldehyde as an underestimated risk factor for cancer development: role of genetics in ethanol metabolism. Seitz HK, Stickel F. Genes Nutr. 2009 Oct 22. [Epub ahead of print] PMID:19847467

[19] Cimetidine and other H2-receptor antagonists as inhibitors of human E3 aldehyde dehydrogenase. Kikonyogo A, Pietruszko R. Mol Pharmacol. 1997 Aug;52(2):267-71. PMID: 9271349

[20] Effects of H2-receptor antagonists on gastric alcohol dehydrogenase activity. Caballería J, Baraona E, Deulofeu R, Hernández-Muñoz R, Rodés J, Lieber CS. Dig Dis Sci. 1991 Dec;36(12):1673-9. PMID:1684149

[21] Association study of the serotoninergic system in migraine in the Spanish population. Corominas R, Sobrido MJ, Ribasés M, Cuenca-León E, Blanco-Arias P, Narberhaus B, Roig M, Leira R, López-González J, Macaya A, Cormand B. Am J Med Genet B Neuropsychiatr Genet. 2010 Jan 5;153B(1):177-84. PMID:19455600

[22] MAOA and MAOB polymorphisms and anger-related traits in suicidal participants and controls. Antypa N, Giegling I, Calati R, et al. Eur Arch Psychiatry Clin Neurosci. 2013 Aug;263(5):393-403. PMID:23111930

[23] Exploration of 19 serotoninergic candidate genes in adults and children with attention-deficit/hyperactivity disorder identifies association for 5HT2A, DDC and MAOB. Ribasés M, Ramos-Quiroga JA, Hervás A, et al. Mol Psychiatry. 2009 Jan;14(1):71-85. Epub 2007 Oct 16. PMID:17938636

[24] Negative emotionality: monoamine oxidase B gene variants modulate personality traits in healthy humans. Dlugos AM, Palmer AA, de Wit H. J Neural Transm. 2009 Oct;116(10):1323-34. PMID:19657584

[25] Histamine and histamine intolerance. Maintz L, Novak N. Am J Clin Nutr. 2007 May;85(5):1185-96. PMID:17490952

[26] Diamine oxidase activities in the large bowel mucosa of ulcerative colitis patients. Mennigen R, Kusche J, Streffer C, Krakamp B. Agents Actions. 1990 Apr;30(1-2):264-6. PMID:2115242

[27] Severity of ulcerative colitis is associated with a polymorphism at diamine oxidase gene but not at histamine N-methyltransferase gene. García-Martin E, Mendoza JL, Martínez C, Taxonera C, Urcelay E, Ladero JM, de la Concha EG, Díaz-Rubio M, Agúndez JA. World J Gastroenterol. 2006 Jan 28;12(4):615-20. PMID:16489678

[28] Structure and inhibition of human diamine oxidase. McGrath AP, Hilmer KM, Collyer CA, Shepard EM, Elmore BO, Brown DE, Dooley DM, Guss JM. Biochemistry. 2009 Oct 20;48(41):9810-22. PMID:19764817

[29] Effects of histamine and diamine oxidase activities on pregnancy: a critical review. Maintz L, Schwarzer V, Bieber T, van der Ven K, Novak N. Hum Reprod Update. 2008 Sep-Oct;14(5):485-95. Epub 2008 May 22. PMID:18499706

[30] On the Hormetic Behaviour of Drugs Binding to Different Redox States of Amine Oxidase Enzymes. Deepak Narang, G. Reid McDonald, David J. Smith, Maria Luisa Di Paolo, Dale E. Edmondson and Andrew Holt. Am.J. Pharmacology and Toxicology 3 (1): 125-136, 2008

[31] Following the trace of elusive amines. Premont RT, Gainetdinov RR, Caron MG. Proc Natl Acad Sci U S A. 2001 Aug 14;98(17):9474-5. PMID:11504935

[32] Atrial fibrillation precipitated by tyramine containing foods. Jacob LH, Carron DB. Br Heart J. 1987 Feb;57(2):205-6. PMID:3814458

[33] Study of tyrosine metabolism in eating disorders. Possible correlation with migraine. D'Andrea G, Ostuzzi R, Bolner A, Francesconi F, Musco F, d'Onofrio F, Colavito D. Neurol Sci. 2008 May;29 Suppl 1:S88-92. PMID: 18545905

[34] Tyrosine hydroxylase: human isoforms, structure and regulation in physiology and pathology. Nagatsu T. Essays Biochem. 1995;30:15-35. PMID:8822146

[35] Sources and significance of plasma levels of catechols and their metabolites in humans. Goldstein DS, Eisenhofer G, Kopin IJ. J Pharmacol Exp Ther. 2003 Jun;305(3):800-11. PMID:12649306

[36] An outbreak of histamine poisoning after ingestion of the ground saury paste in eight patients taking isoniazid in tuberculous ward. Miki M, Ishikawa T, Okayama H. Intern Med. 2005 Nov;44(11):1133-6.PMID:16357449

[37] Monoamine oxidase inhibitors: a modern guide to an unrequited class of antidepressants. Stahl SM, Felker A. CNS Spectr. 2008 Oct;13(10):855-70. PMID:18955941

[38] Preliminary report on tyramine headache. Hannington E. Br Med J. 1967 May 27;2(5551):550-1. PMID: 5337268

[39] Elevated levels of circulating trace amines in primary headaches. D'Andrea G, Terrazzino S, Leon A, Fortin D, Perini F, Granella F, Bussone G. Neurology. 2004 May 25;62(10):1701-5. PMID:15159465

[40] Biochemistry of neuromodulation in primary headaches: focus on anomalies of tyrosine metabolism. D'Andrea G, Nordera GP, Perini F, Allais G, Granella F. Neurol Sci. 2007 May;28 Suppl 2:S94-6. PMID:17508188

[41] Trace amine-associated receptors as emerging therapeutic targets. Sotnikova TD, Caron MG, Gainetdinov RR. Mol Pharmacol. 2009 Aug;76(2):229-35. Epub 2009 Apr 23. PMID:19389919

[42] [Biogenic amines in food: effects of histamine, tyramine and phenylethylamine in the human] Lüthy J, Schlatter C. Z Lebensm Unters Forsch. 1983;177(6):439-43. German. PMID: 6364621

[43] Psychomotor stimulant effects of beta-phenylethylamine in monkeys treated with MAO-B inhibitors. Bergman J, Yasar S, Winger G. Psychopharmacology (Berl). 2001 Dec;159(1):21-30. Epub 2001 Sep 6. PMID:11797065

[44] Abnormal platelet trace amine profiles in migraine with and without aura. D'Andrea G, Granella F, Leone M, Perini F, Farruggio A, Bussone G. Cephalalgia. 2006 Aug;26(8):968-72. PMID:16886933

[45] Estimation of 24-hour polyamine intake from mature human milk. Dorhout B, van Beusekom CM, Huisman M, Kingma AW, de Hoog E, Boersma ER, Muskiet FA. J Pediatr Gastroenterol Nutr. 1996 Oct;23(3):298-302. PMID: 8890081

[46] Are milk polyamines preventive agents against food allergy? Dandrifosse G, Peulen O, El Khefif N, Deloyer P, Dandrifosse AC, Grandfils C. Proc Nutr Soc. 2000 Feb;59(1):81-6. PMID:10828177

[47] Polyamines are essential in embryo implantation: expression and function of polyamine-related genes in mouse uterus during peri-implantation period. Zhao YC, Chi YJ, Yu YS, Liu JL, Su RW, Ma XH, Shan CH, Yang ZM. Endocrinology. 2008 May;149(5):2325-32. Epub 2008 Jan 17. PMID:18202119

[48] Role of polyamines derived from arginine in differentiation and proliferation of human blood cells. Maeda T, Wakasawa T, Shima Y, Tsuboi I, Aizawa S, Tamai I. Biol Pharm Bull. 2006 Feb;29(2):234-9. PMID:16462024

[49] Activation of polyamine catabolism in transgenic rats induces acute pancreatitis. Alhonen L, Parkkinen JJ, Keinanen T, Sinervirta R, Herzig KH, Jänne J. Proc Natl Acad Sci U S A. 2000 Jul 18;97(15):8290-5. PMID:10880565

[50] The human gut bacteria Bacteroides thetaiotaomicron and Fusobacterium varium produce putrescine and spermidine in cecum of pectin-fed gnotobiotic rats. Noack J, Dongowski G, Hartmann L, Blaut M. J Nutr. 2000 May;130(5):1225-31. PMID:10801923

[51] Metabolic denitrosation of diphenylnitrosamine: a possible bioactivation pathway. K.E. Appel 1, S. Gfirsdorf 1, T. Scheper 1, H. H. Ruf 2, C. S. Rühl 1, and A. G. Hildebrandt J Cancer Res Clin Oncol (5987) 113:131-136

[52] Acute and subacute toxicity of tyramine, spermidine, spermine, putrescine and cadaverine in rats. Til HP, Falke HE, Prinsen MK, Willems MI. Food Chem Toxicol. 1997 Mar-Apr;35(3-4):337-48. PMID:9207896

[53] Spermidine: a novel autophagy inducer and longevity elixir. Madeo F, Eisenberg T, Büttner S, Ruckenstuhl C, Kroemer G. Autophagy. 2010 Jan;6(1):160-2. PMID:20110777

[54] Polyamines in foods: development of a food database. Atiya Ali M, Poortvliet E, Strömberg R, Yngve A. Food Nutr Res. 2011 Jan 14;55. PMID:21249159

[55] Biogenic amine contents in selected Egyptian fermented foods as determined by ion-exchange chromatography. Rabie MA, Elsaidy S, el-Badawy AA, Siliha H, Malcata FX. J Food Prot. 2011 Apr;74(4):681-5. PMID:21477488

[56] Smoking related diseases: the central role of monoamine oxidase. Rendu F, Peoc'h K, Berlin I, Thomas D, Launay JM. Int J Environ Res Public Health. 2011 Jan;8(1):136-47. Epub 2011 Jan 14. PMID:21318020

[57] Influence of a serotonin- and dopamine-rich diet on platelet serotonin content and urinary excretion of biogenic amines and their metabolites. Kema IP, Schellings AM, Meiborg G, Hoppenbrouwers CJ, Muskiet FA. Clin Chem. 1992 Sep;38(9):1730-6. PMID: 1382000

[58] A Western diet increases serotonin availability in rat small intestine. Bertrand RL, Senadheera S, Markus I, Liu L, Howitt L, Chen H, Murphy TV, Sandow SL, Bertrand PP. Endocrinology. 2011 Jan;152(1):36-47. PMID:21068163

[59] Serotonin content of foods: effect on urinary excretion of 5-hydroxyindoleacetic acid. Feldman JM, Lee EM. Am J Clin Nutr. 1985 Oct;42(4):639-43. PMID:2413754

[60] The serotonin syndrome. Bijl D. Neth J Med. 2004 Oct;62(9):309-13. PMID:15635814

[61] In vitro inhibition of rat intestinal histamine-metabolizing enzymes. Taylor SL, Lieber ER. Food Cosmet Toxicol. 1979 Jun;17(3):237-40. PMID:115771

[62] Histamine N-methyl transferase: inhibition by drugs. Pacifici GM, Donatelli P, Giuliani L. Br J Clin Pharmacol. 1992 Oct;34(4):322-7. PMID:1457266

14. Mast Cell Degranulation Induced Pseudoallergy

In allergic reactions, allergens adhere to IgE molecules bound to mast cells and basophils. Antigens with multiple binding sites for IgE can adhere to two or more IgE molecules, allowing for cross-linking of IgE; this triggers activation of the mast cell or basophils and release of preformed immune mediators from granules in these cells. It also triggers activation of nuclear transcription factors for the formation of inflammatory eicosanoids and other immune modifiers. IgG can also trigger mast cell activation.

Mast cell degranulation can also be triggered through non-immune mechanisms, including hormones, drugs, and other substances. These agents do not necessarily cause the all-or-none, generalized mast cell activation seen in an IgE response, but rather, may trigger specific elements of activation, such as a limited degranulation, or induce the formation of eicosanoids and chemokines. Mast cells can form hundreds of compounds that mediated inflammation[1]. The immune mediators released by this activation can vary according the stimulus, and do not necessarily utilize the full array of the cells armament. Thus, the effect of mast cell activity and related symptoms depend on the activating agent.

Some pseudoallergic reactions to foods can be explained by non-immune mast cell degranulation or other activation of these cells. Direct histamine release, for example, can result from the consumption of foods containing mast cell degranulating agents. These may give an allergic-like reaction, but do not involve immunoglobulin. Therefore, IgE testing for these reacting agents may be negative. The patient, however, may have IgE to other allergens they have become sensitized to.

Hormones Promoting Direct Mast Cell Activation

Several hormones can cause mast cell and basophil activation resulting in degranulation. While the activity of these hormones is usually very site-specific and well regulated, hormones can promote mast cell activity.

CGRP (Calcitonin Gene-Related Peptide) is the most potent peptide vasodilator known, and it acts in the transmission of pain. It acts, at least in part, by inducing mast cell degranulation. CGRP has a central role in the theoretical model that explains how NO (nitric oxide) triggers delayed onset migraine headaches[2]. The inflammatory cytokine IL-1β can induce CGRP promoting the expression of COX2, thereby stimulating the production of PGE$_2$. This inflammatory prostaglandin then activates neurons to release CGRP about 24 hours after stimulation by IL-1β[3]. When this occurs in the trigeminal nerve, it can trigger a migraine headache.

The neuro-enteric polypeptide hormone, neurotensin, mainly found in the hypothalamus and N cells of the small intestine, is a powerful mast cell degranulation agent. Mast cells have a specific receptor for neurotensin. Neurotensin stimulates the release of histamine as a physiologic mechanism that helps regulate feeding, GI motility, and other GI functions. Neurotensin has an anorexic effect in the hypothalamus via the release of histamine[4]. The anorexic effect of leptin likely acts via neurotensin and histamine[5,6]. This may explain the mechanism by which H$_1$ antihistamines and some antidepressant medications induce weight gain. Neurotensin release of histamine modulates GI motility and the uptake and release of bile[7].

Other hormones that trigger histamine release include thyroid releasing hormone (TRH), corticotropin-releasing hormone (CRH) and estrogen. These hormones help decrease appetite through histamine release[8,9]. TRH induced release of histamine stimulates sexual arousal in rats. CRH also induces histamine release from mast cells through a neurotensin-mediated reaction[10]. Substance P may also induce the activation and degranulation of mast cells[1], as does VIP. Gastrin mediates the release of histamine in the stomach to regulates the production of stomach acid.

Complement proteins C3a, C4a and C5a, that form during IgG-antigen reactions, also trigger histamine release from mast cells and basophils. Platelet Activating Factor (PAF), a phospholipid produced by neutrophils, basophils, platelets, and endothelial cells, can also trigger degranulation and histamine release.

Foods Promoting Direct Mast Cell Activation

Mast cells degranulate under the influence of IgE receptors (Fcϵ) on mast cells. In order to trigger degranulation, an Fcϵ pair must "cross-link," which causes a calcium channel to open in the mast cell. If there is sufficient release of calcium, it triggers an all-or-none degranulation response. Figure 14-1 illustrates how IgE in the Fcϵ can "cross-link" when the pairs of IgE bind to an antigen. Lectins that have an affinity for sugars in an IgE molecule or Fcϵ can also "cross-link" IgE or Fcϵ, and thereby, trigger degranulation. Degranulation of mast cells by lectins appears to occur only in patients with active immune hypersensitivity[11]. Anti-IgE IgG can also link IgE pairs.

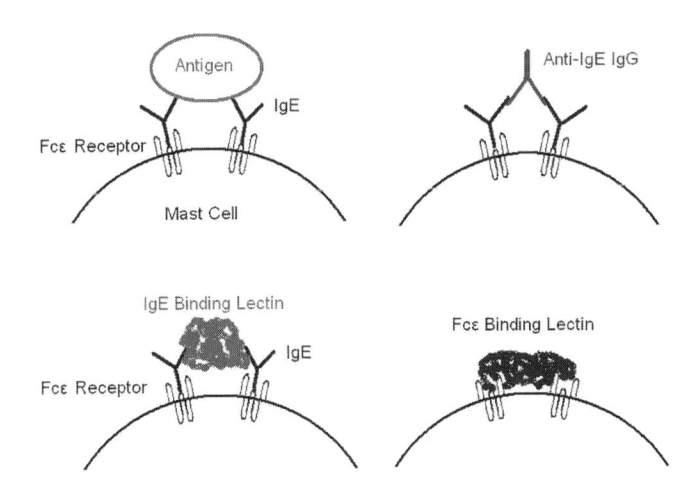

Figure 14-1: Mast Cell Activation by way of IgE Receptors[12]

Another food lectin with the capacity to provoke degranulation in anergic patients is Solanum tuberosa agglutinin lectin, from potatoes. In a study from India, nearly half of patients with asthma or allergic rhinitis avoided eating potatoes as they recognized that it worsened their symptoms within two hours of eating them. Many of these patients also had gastrointestinal symptoms with potato consumption, including stomach cramps, nausea, reflux, and borborygmi. Potatoes retain about half of their lectin activity after boiling for 20 minutes, which is about twice the typical cooking time. Lectin from tomatoes and concanavalin A lectin from jack beans can also cause mast cell degranulation. Wheat germ agglutinin lectin binds the same class of polysaccharides as do potato lectins, and thus, it can trigger mast cell degranulation without specific immunity to it[12]. Another close relative if potatoes, eggplant, also causes nonspecific-IgE histamine release[13].

Potatoes also contain glycoalkaloids which are toxic, and which can disrupt the intestinal mucosal barrier[14]. This may contribute to the ability of the lectins to gain access to the mast cells and the blood stream. Mucosal integrity is further discussed in Chapter 25.

Sulfites

Sulfites, a group of chemicals that are widely utilized as preservatives in the food and pharmaceutical industries, can cause hypersensitivity reactions in susceptible individuals. Skin and oral exposure to sulfites can induce adverse reactions in sensitive individuals; including dermatitis, urticaria, flushing, hypotension, abdominal pain, diarrhea, and asthma. Sulfite exposure can cause life-threatening anaphylactoid reactions[15]. Disease manifestations from sulfite exposure may be acute or chronic. Sulfite consumption is associated with inflammation that can be observed by sigmoidoscopy in patients with ulcerative colitis[16].

The most frequent source of exposure to sulfites is foods and beverages in which sulfites have been used as preservatives. Other sources of exposure include medications (including injected medications), cosmetics, and occupational exposure.

Sulfites can trigger mast cell and basophil degranulation, especially under conditions of oxidative stress[17]. Unlike IgE and CGRP, this process does not involve calcium flux into the cell.

Sulfite is the ionized form of sulfur dioxide (SO_2). Sulfur dioxide is a major air pollutant from volcanoes and coal and oil burning power plants. Breathing polluted air containing SO_2 can trigger asthma, apparently through direct degranulation of mast cells.

Low levels of sulfites are naturally occurring in some foods, especially fermented foods. During fermentation, a small amount is produced by yeast. Nevertheless, the principal source of exposure comes from sulfites added as antibacterial agents to foods, cosmetics, and medications. They are also used to maintain color in dried fruit; apricots, for example, and to stop the fermentation process in wine.

The human body also produces about one gram of sulfites a day. Consumption of food preserved with sulfites is not a problem for most people; however, some individuals are sensitive to them, and some of these individuals have anaphylactoid reactions from consumption of foods containing sulfites.

Reactions to sulfites predominantly affect the respiratory system, with asthmatic-type reactions that can be severe. Sulfite hypersensitivity is found in about five to ten percent of asthmatics[18]. These patients experience a greater than 20% decrease in FEV1 within 30 minutes of a challenge with an oral capsule of potassium metabisulfite[19]. Additional reactions to sulfites may include flushing, abdominal pain, nausea, angioedema, itching, hives, contact dermatitis, swelling of eyes, hands and feet, nausea and diarrhea, and anaphylactic shock[20]. Although migraine has often been attributed to sulfites in wine, there is no medical literature documenting that sulfites provoke migraine headache.

The reaction to sulfites seems to be variable and dependent on interactions with the environment. It has been difficult to reliably recreate reactions of sulfites in wine in double-blinded controlled trials. A smoky environment, high pollen count or other factors that provoke asthma, may play a critical role as to whether a meal with sulfites triggers asthma or not[21]. An individual's level of oxidative stress likely plays an essential role in provoking susceptibility to sulfite reactions[17].

Sulfites are metabolized in the body by the enzyme sulfite oxidase (SUOX) to sulfates plus the oxidative molecule hydrogen peroxide:

$$\text{Sulfite} + O_2 + H_2O = \text{sulfate} + H_2O_2$$

SUOX is a mitochondrial enzyme that is expressed in high levels in the liver, as well as in the kidney, adipocytes, and immune cells. SUOX is one of few mammalian enzymes that require metal molybdenum as a cofactor.

Table 14-1: Molybdenum Dependent Enzymes

Molybdenum cofactor sulfurtransferase (MoCo)	MoCo is required for enzymatic activity of XDH, AOX1, and SUOX. It requires pyridoxal-5-phosphate is a cofactor.
Aldehyde oxidase (AOX1)	Aldehyde catabolism, H2O2 production
Sulfite oxidase (SUOX)	Metabolizes cysteine and methionine requires MoCo1 and heme as cofactors
Xanthine oxidase /dehydrogenase (XDH)	Purine and aldehyde metabolism- uric acid formation, retinol.
mARC1	Reduces N-hydroxylated prodrugs

SUOX is required in the catabolism of excess sulfur-containing amino acids cysteine and methionine. Genetic defects in the SUOX enzyme can cause a rare, but fatal disease in newborns, sulfite oxidase deficiency, which causes mental retardation, neurological disorders, physical deformities, and brain damage.

Impairment of SUOX can occur in molybdenum deficiency, and sulfite sensitivity has been successfully treated with weekly intravenous molybdenum treatment[22]. Urinary sulfite is a marker of sulfite oxidase dysfunction; urine sulfite levels are normally zero, but may be 10 to 40 ppm in deficiency states. Urine samples need to be iced for accurate testing.

Normally, molybdenum is well absorbed from the stomach and small intestine. Foods rich in molybdenum include whole grains, legumes, nuts, meats, and yeast. Excessive molybdenum levels (from toxic exposure) may put individuals at risk for gout and copper deficiency. Deficiencies of molybdenum have occurred in patients on total parenteral nutrition.

Susceptibility to mast cell degranulation by sulfites is also dependent on the activation of the reduced form of nicotinamide adenine dinucleotide phosphate oxidase complex[17]. Thus, availability of reduced glutathione as a reactive oxygen species (ROS) acceptor should prevent oxidative stress in mast cells that participate in sulfate-induced degranulation. In healthy tissues, glutathione is about 90% in the reduced form and functions as an important intracellular antioxidant.

Glutathione is present in food but is not easily absorbed. However, cysteine, a precursor for glutathione, can be supplemented with N-acetylcysteine (NAC). Zinc is required as a coenzyme in the formation of glutathione from cysteine. S-adenosylmethionine (SAMe), alpha-lipoic acid, and melatonin may also increase the level of reduced glutathione. Vitamin D_3 promotes glutathione peroxidase (and superoxide dismutase) expression[23].

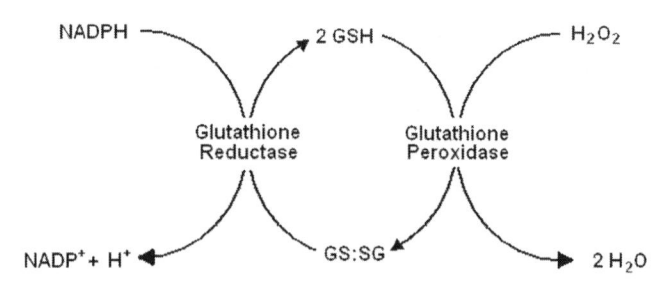

Figure 14-2: GSH: Reduced Glutathione GS: SG Oxidized Glutathione Disulfide

Table 14-2: Agents that may Decrease Sulfite Induced Mast Cell Degranulation

Enzyme or Agent	Nutritional Cofactor or Supplement
Sulfite Oxidase	Molybdenum, pyridoxal-5-phosphate (PLP; B_6)
Glutathione Peroxidase	Selenium, Vitamin D_3
Glutathione Reductase	FAD (Riboflavin), Copper
NADPH	Niacin
Glutathione	N-acetylcysteine, Zinc, SAMe[A]
Antioxidants	Alpha lipoic acid, Taurine[B], Melatonin
Taurine formation*	Niacin, iron, PLP, molybdenum

[A] Rather than using SAMe as a supplement, it is preferable to ensure adequate vitamins folate, B_6, B_{12}, and betaine, which the body uses to form SAMe and recycle SAMe. See Figure 31-4 and 31-5.

[B] Taurine is a sulfur-containing amino acid that acts as a sacrificial antioxidant. It is formed from cysteine by enzymes requiring NADH, NADPH, iron, pyridoxal phosphate[24] and which may require molybdenum.

Avoidance of Sulfites

Sulfites are used in manufactured foods as preservatives, but also occur naturally in some foods. *The key to avoiding sulfites is to read labels on all manufactured foods.* Table 14-3 gives sulfite-containing ingredients listed on food labels.

Table 14-3: Sulfite Containing Food Additives

Potassium bisulfite	Sodium bisulfite
Potassium metabisulfite	Sodium metabisulfite
Sulfur dioxide (E220 in Europe)	Sodium sulfite

Wines are an area of concern for individuals with sulfite intolerance. Almost all wines contain sulfites. Wines from the United States contain an average of about 80 mg/L sulfites, similar to European wines. In the U.S., wines that have more than 10 mg/liter must have a "Contains Sulfites" warning label. This labeling, however, is not very helpful, as 10 mg/liter would be equivalent to 1 mg in a four-ounce glass of wine; an amount unlikely to cause problems. However, the same labeling would be used for wine that could contain as much as 350 mg/L of sulfite, and thus contain 35 mg of sulfite in a four-ounce serving, a significant amount. One ounce (28 grams) of dried, sulfured apricots typically contains about 56 mg of sulfites.

Table 14-4: Foods Commonly Containing Sulfites

- Baked goods
- Soup mixes
- Jams
- Canned or frozen vegetables
- Frozen fruit juices
- Pickled foods, pickles, relishes
- Gravies
- Dried fruit (apricots, apples, yellow raisins, etc.)
- Potato chips
- Dehydrated potatoes
- Trail mix
- Bottled or canned beverages including teas,
- Bottled or canned fruit and vegetable beverages
- Many condiments
- Guacamole
- Maraschino cherries
- Glacéed fruit
- Molasses
- Hard cider
- Shrimp, lobster (may be added while on the fishing boat and not be labeled)
- Wine (especially white wines and dessert wines)

Treatment of Sulfite Sensitivity

The principal preventive treatments for sulfite sensitivity are mitigation of oxidative stress and avoidance of sulfites. Molybdenum supplements are recommended only after documentation of deficiency.

Medications and Mast Cell Degranulation

Certain medications can cause mast cell or basophil activation and degranulation. Many medications, especially injectable medications, contain a sulfite as a preservative.

Morphine and codeine trigger mast cell degranulation in some individuals, and presents as an allergic-type reaction. It appears that the degranulation acts through the delta opiate receptor[25] on the mast cells rather than through immune-mediated degranulation. It is also suggested that pseudoallergic reactions to contrast media used in radiology acts through mast cell degranulation. The mechanism for this has not been elucidated, but some contrast media contains sulfites. Many of the drugs listed in Table 14-5, which have been associated with mast cell degranulation, are from older references; degranulation may have been due to preservatives (sulfites) used those medications,

The mast cell stabilizer cromolyn is thought to act by inhibiting the release of chemical mediators from sensitized mast cells, by blocking the release of calcium from intracellular vesicles. More potent and specific mast cell stabilizing agents, however, have not been found to be as effective as cromolyn in preventing allergic response. Thus, although cromolyn is a mast cell stabilizer, its beneficial effect may operate through other mechanisms. There is no indication that mast cell stabilizers are more effective for preventing a reaction to sulfite or other mast cell activating agents than are other medications used in the treatment allergic-type responses.

Table 14-5: Drugs Associated with Mast Cell Degranulation[26, 27]

Drug Class	Details
Aspirin and NSAIDS	COX inhibitors: See Chapter 16
Alcohol	May not cause degranulation, but rather inhibits bioamine metabolism. See chapter 13
Radiographic Dyes	Contrast Media: may be secondary to sulfites in dyes used as preservatives. See above.
Opiates	Morphine and codeine: direct degranulation in some individuals.
Paralytic agents	Pancuronium, alcuronium, tubocurarine and decamethonium
Hormones	Chymotrypsin, ACTH, CRH, Neurotensin, CGRP, Substance P, VIP
Others drugs to which degranulation has been attributed	Benzodiazepines Sulfites: Used as a preservative in some medications Cytostatic: Cyclophosphamide Paralytics: Pancuronium, alcuronium, tubocurarine Cannabinoids: Marijuana, marinol Antibiotics: Polymyxin B, colimycin Others: Procaine, scopolamine, gallamine, quinine, reserpine, pilocarpine, hydralazine.

False Pseudo-Allergy

Pseudo-pseudoallergy refers here to some older medical literature which reported that some foods trigger the release of histamine through a direct non-immure mechanism. This is sometimes repeated in newer medical literature[28], often on internet food and health sites. This hypothesis suggests that certain foods have direct, nonimmune (no IgE binding and cross-linking) mast cell degranulation capacities, especially for mast cells in the GI tract. Foods commonly implicated are listed in Table 14-6.

Most noticeable about foods included in this list is that, with the exception of licorice and spinach, these are common food allergens. Much of the support for the non-immune mechanism dates from literature published prior to 1955[29]. IgE was not discovered until 1967 and testing for it was developed in 1974. A more likely explanation is that the observed reactions to these foods were simply immune mediated reactions for which skin prick testing had given false negative results. Licorice not only does not stimulate degranulation, but rather inhibits it[30].

Table 14-6: Foods Alleged to Release Histamine

Foods alleged to have direct (nonimmune) histamine-releasing capacities[28]		
Citrus fruits	Liquorice	Pork
Chocolate	Tree Nuts	Spices
Crustaceans	Papaya	Spinach
Egg White	Peanuts	Strawberries
Fish	Pineapple	Tomatoes

Hypersensitivity reactions to these foods are more likely immune-mediated than pseudo-allergic. Skin prick testing for food has poor sensitivity for gastrointestinal reactivity. Negative serum IgE testing may occur if the allergen is not identical to the one tested as may occur if the allergen is modified by digestion. Alternatively, the response may be an IgG reaction rather than an IgE reaction. Some lectins, however, can directly provoke degranulation.

Testing for Pseudo Allergy

Laboratory tests that may be helpful for diagnosing pseudoallergic reactions include testing of urinary sulfite, sulfite enzyme function, cofactors levels, and testing for oxidative stress.

Table 14-7: Lab Tests that may be useful in Sulfite Sensitivity

Urinary sulfite	The normal level is zero (not detectable). Higher levels indicate inadequate sulfite oxidase function.
Molybdenum	Low urine uric acid to xanthine ratio and urinary sulfite. Uric acid levels may be low due to the decreased xanthine oxidase activity with molybdenum deficiency.
Markers of Oxidative stress	4-Hydroxynonenal (4-HNE) 8-Hydroxy-2'-deoxyguanosine (8-OHdG)
Whole Blood for Metals	Inadequate cofactors (Cu, Zn, Se, Mg) Toxic elements (Arsenic, Cadmium)
Vitamin D	25-hydroxy vitamin D3

Summary: Treatment of Mast Cell Degranulation

1. Avoid Lectin-Containing Foods that Trigger Mast Cell Degranulation. Patients with allergies, food sensitivities or mast cell activation disorders should do a trial of avoiding potatoes, tomatoes, eggplant, and wheat to see if these foods are aggravating symptoms through direct degranulation of mast cells and basophils. Kidney beans and other sources of PHA can also induce degranulation; however, PHA is almost completely destroyed during adequate cooking. Jack beans and horse gram, rarely eaten in the U.S., may also cause problems.

Except for those in whom an allergic reaction would be dangerous, a trial can then be made with the lectin containing food to see if allergy or gastrointestinal symptoms worsen in the hours following ingestion of the food. If the provocative trial is positive, the aggravating food should be avoided. Foods suspected of causing delayed sensitivity reactions should be eliminated for a week, or more before a food challenge is done. Food challenges are most successful when the person is feeling well so that changes in symptoms are clearly defined. It is more difficult to identify triggers when symptoms are nonspecific.

Degranulation sensitivity to food lectins may indicate an abrogated mucosal membrane, discussed in Chapter 24.

2. Sulfites: Sulfites are present in food, cosmetics, and medications, and exposure to sulfites can also occur from air pollution and through industrial exposure. Exposure to sulfites can provoke mast cell and basophil degranulation, resulting in pseudoallergic reactions, most often affecting the respiratory system. Susceptibility may depend on the inadequate activity of sulfite oxidase and upon oxidative stress in mast cells and other granulocytes. Preventive treatment of sulfate intolerance may include avoidance of sulfites, by assuring sufficient sulfite oxidase cofactors, and by supporting the glutathione antioxidant system.

3. Medications: Opiates can trigger degranulation in some individuals in what appears to be an immune response. In other medications, the mechanism is less well understood, but often secondary to sulfite content used as a preservative in the medication. These medications should be avoided in patients who react to them.

4. Allergic Patients: Patients with mast cell activation are at higher risk for pseudo-allergic degranulation. Thus, exposure to allergens should be avoided. Patients may benefit testing and treatment for intestinal parasites.

Individuals who are susceptible to pseudo-allergies from idiopathic degranulation evoked by foods, sulfites or medication, should be considered for assessment for MCAS or other mast cell disorders (Chapter 12).

5. Supplements: Assure adequate nutrition of enzyme cofactors for sulfate degradation and to ensure adequate glutathione and other antioxidant activity. See Table 14-2.

6. Assure Efficient Histamine Catabolism: Avoid alcohol. Use enzyme cofactor supplements when needed for proper histamine catabolism (See Table 13-6 on pseudo allergies). Vitamin D supplement may be helpful if levels are less than optimal (Chapter 20).

7. Avoid Oxidative Stress: Testing for oxidative stress may be helpful. Foods high in polyphenols and other antioxidants are recommended. Antioxidant supplements such as tocotrienols, vitamin C, r-alpha lipoic acid, and melatonin may help reduce oxidative stress. Limit alcohol intake. See Chapters 17 and 40.

8. Use Appropriate Medications: Antihistamines and mast cell stabilizers may be helpful.

[1] Burning mouth syndrome and mast cell activation disorder. Afrin LB. Oral Surg Oral Med Oral Pathol Oral Radiol Endod. 2011 Apr;111(4):465-72. PMID:21420635

[2] Headache-type adverse effects of NO donors: vasodilation and beyond. Bagdy G, Riba P, Kecskeméti V, Chase D, Juhász G. Br J Pharmacol. 2010 May;160(1):20-35. Epub 2010 Mar 19. PMID:20331608

[3] IL-1β stimulates COX-2 dependent PGE2 synthesis and CGRP release in rat trigeminal ganglia cells. Neeb L, Hellen P, Boehnke C, Hoffmann J, Schuh-Hofer S, Dirnagl U, Reuter U. PLoS One. 2011 Mar 4;6(3):e17360. PMID:21394197

[4] The anorectic effect of neurotensin is mediated via a histamine H1 receptor in mice. Ohinata K, Shimano T, Yamauchi R, Sakurada S, Yanai K, Yoshikawa M. Peptides. 2004 Dec;25(12):2135-8. PMID:15572202

[5] Impaired anorectic effect of leptin in neurotensin receptor 1-deficient mice. Kim ER, Leckstrom A, Mizuno TM. Behav Brain Res. 2008 Dec 1;194(1):66-71. Epub 2008 Jul 1. PMID:18639588

[6] Involvement of the histaminergic system in leptin-induced suppression of food intake. Morimoto T, Yamamoto Y, Mobarakeh JI, Yanai K, Watanabe T, Watanabe T, Yamatodani A. Physiol Behav. 1999 Nov;67(5):679-83. PMID:10604837

[7] Involvement of mast cells in basal and neurotensin-induced intestinal absorption of taurocholate in rats. Gui X, Carraway RE. Am J Physiol Gastrointest Liver Physiol. 2004 Aug;287(2):G408-16. Epub 2003 Dec 23. PMID:14693504

[8] Hypothalamic neuronal histamine signaling in the estrogen deficiency-induced obesity. Gotoh K, Masaki T, Chiba S, Higuchi K, Kakuma T, Shimizu H, Mori M, Sakata T, Yoshimatsu H. J Neurochem. 2009 Sep;110(6):1796-805. Epub 2009 Jul 8. PMID:19619143

[9] Hypothalamic neuronal histamine mediates the thyrotropin-releasing hormone-induced suppression of food intake. Gotoh K, Fukagawa K, Fukagawa T, Noguchi H, Kakuma T, Sakata T, Yoshimatsu H. J Neurochem. 2007 Nov;103(3):1102-10. Epub 2007 Aug 30. PMID: 17760865

[10] Corticotropin-releasing hormone induces skin vascular permeability through a neurotensin-dependent process. Donelan J, Boucher W, Papadopoulou N, Lytinas M, Papaliodis D, Dobner P, Theoharides TC. Proc Natl Acad Sci U S A. 2006 May 16;103(20):7759-64. Epub 2006 May 8. PMID:16682628

[11] Studies on the modulatory aspects of certain Dietary Lectins in relation to Hypersensitivity and Immunogenecity. Pramod, S.N. (2007) PhD thesis, University of Mysore.

[12] Potato lectin activates basophils and mast cells of atopic subjects by its interaction with core chitobiose of cell-bound non-specific immunoglobulin E. Pramod SN, Venkatesh YP, Mahesh PA. Clin Exp Immunol. 2007 Jun;148(3):391-401. PMID:17362264

[13] A cross-sectional study on the prevalence of food allergy to eggplant (Solanum melongena L.) reveals female predominance. Harish Babu BN, Mahesh PA, Venkatesh YP. Clin Exp Allergy. 2008 Nov;38(11):1795-802. PMID:18681854

[14] Potato glycoalkaloids adversely affect intestinal permeability and aggravate inflammatory bowel disease. Patel B, Schutte R, Sporns P, Doyle J, Jewel L, Fedorak RN. Inflamm Bowel Dis. 2002 Sep;8(5):340-6. PMID:12479649

[15] Clinical effects of sulphite additives. Vally H, Misso NL, Madan V. Clin Exp Allergy. 2009 Nov;39(11):1643-51. Epub 2009 Sep 22. Review.PMID: 19775253

[16] Associations between diet and disease activity in ulcerative colitis patients using a novel method of data analysis. Magee EA, Edmond LM, Tasker SM, Kong SC, Curno R, Cummings JH. Nutr J. 2005 Feb 10;4:7. PMID:15705205

[17] Effect of sodium sulfite on mast cell degranulation and oxidant stress. Collaco CR, Hochman DJ, Goldblum RM, Brooks EG. Ann Allergy Asthma Immunol. 2006 Apr;96(4):550-6. PMID:16680925

[18] Histamine and histamine intolerance. Maintz L, Novak N. Am J Clin Nutr. 2007 May;85(5):1185-96. PMID:17490952

[19] Prevalence of sensitivity to sulfiting agents in asthmatic patients. Bush RK, Taylor SL, Holden K, Nordlee JA, Busse WW. Am J Med. 1986 Nov;81(5):816-20. PMID:3535492

[20] Molybdenum. Monograph. [No authors listed] Altern Med Rev. 2006 Jun;11(2):156-61. No abstract available. PMID:16813464

[21] Role of sulfite additives in wine induced asthma: single dose and cumulative dose studies. Vally H, Thompson PJ. Thorax. 2001 Oct;56(10):763-9. PMID:11562514

[22] Molybdenum. Monograph. Altern Med Rev. 2006 Jun;11(2):156-61. PMID: 16813464

[23] 1Alpha,25 dihydroxyvitamin D3: therapeutic and preventive effects against oxidative stress, hepatic, pancreatic and renal injury in alloxan-induced diabetes in rats. Hamden K, Carreau S, Jamoussi K, Miladi S, Lajmi S, Aloulou D, Ayadi F, Elfeki A. J Nutr Sci Vitaminol (Tokyo). 2009 Jun;55(3):215-22. PMID:19602829

[24] Ascorbic acid and pyridoxine in experimental anaphylaxis. Alvarez RG, Mesa MG. Agents Actions. 1981 Apr;11(1-2):89-93. PMID:6166175

[25] Codeine induces human mast cell chemokine and cytokine production: involvement of G-protein activation. Sheen CH, Schleimer RP, Kulka M. Allergy. 2007 May;62(5):532-8. PMID:17441793

[26] Multiple nodular lesions of upper limbs: nodular mastocytosis. Fenniche S, Marrak H, Zghal M, Khayat O, Debbiche A, Ben Ayed M, Mokhtar I. Dermatol Online J. 2002 Oct;8(2):20. PMID:12546775

[27] Pediatric cutaneous mastocytosis: a review of 180 patients. Ben-Amitai D, Metzker A, Cohen HA. Isr Med Assoc J. 2005 May;7(5):320-2. PMID:15909466

[28] Histamine and histamine intolerance. Maintz L, Novak N. Am J Clin Nutr. 2007 May;85(5):1185-96. PMID: 17490952

[29] Mastocytosis and adverse reactions to biogenic amines and histamine-releasing foods: what is the evidence? Vlieg-Boerstra BJ, van der Heide S, Oude Elberink JN, Kluin-Nelemans JC, Dubois AE. Neth J Med. 2005 Jul-Aug;63(7):244-9. PMID:16093574

[30] In vitro and in vivo antiallergic effects of Glycyrrhiza glabra and its components. Shin YW, Bae EA, Lee B, Lee SH, Kim JA, Kim YS, Kim DH. Planta Med. 2007 Mar;73(3):257-61. PMID:17327992

15. Leukotriene Associated Hypersensitivity

Aspirin sensitive asthma (ASA) is present in five to twenty percent of adult asthmatics and typically occurs as a triad of symptoms; *asthma, eosinophilic rhinosinusitis, nasal polyposis*[1]. In these patients, asthmatic exacerbations can be induced by exposure to aspirin, from as little as 5 mg to 500 mg. Exercise-Induced Asthma (EIA) is a related condition which is exacerbated by the use of aspirin. Another condition known as "Salicylate Sensitivity" provokes the same inflammatory conditions; however, salicylic acid, and related compounds from foods, condiments, toiletries, and medications provide the triggering agents. These are not an immune reaction to aspirin, but rather the result of its pharmacologic action, in an individual with an aberrant immune response. For reasons that will become clear in this chapter, these conditions are referred to in this document as Leukotriene Associated Hypersensitivity (LAH).

LAH is a progressive disease, unusual in children, which typically presents in the third or fourth decade of life. It usually manifests with nasal congestion and a chronic coryza (runny nose), and nasal polyps form in about 70% of LAH patients within a few years. Asthma and other reactions to aspirin, salicylate or other agents develop over 2 to 15 years. Once developed, the intolerance usually continues for life.

LAH can also present with cutaneous manifestations such as angioedema or urticaria. These are actually more common than the respiratory syndrome. Less frequently, individuals may have both respiratory and dermatologic manifestations of LAH[2].

Another cluster of LAH manifestations causes gastrointestinal disease, with meteorism, diarrhea, colitis, erosions, and ulcers[2]. A small percentage of patients with inflammatory bowel disease have LAH, and aspirin and salicylates can trigger disease exacerbations. Angina and myocardial infarction have been documented to occur as a result of LAH, even in patients with anatomically normal coronary arteries[3]. Table 15-1 lists other organ systems that can be affected by LAH, especially during anaphylactoid reactions that can occur with exposure to aspirin.

Part of the underlying mechanism for LAH may be a shift in inflammatory eicosanoid production. A key finding in patients with Aspirin Sensitive Asthma is an elevated production of the cysteinyl leukotrienes C_4, D_4, and E_4, which are sequentially synthesized from arachidonic acid (AA). LTC_4 and other cysteinyl leukotrienes provoke bronchoconstriction, increase vascular permeability, mucus secretion, and recruit eosinophils; and thus, can provoke asthma. LTE_4 is the principal metabolite of leukotrienes found in the urine, and its levels correlate well with the severity of asthma in ASA patients[4].

Eicosanoids are produced when the enzyme phospholipase A2 (PLA2) liberates arachidonic acid and other long chain essential fatty acids from the second fatty acid position of phospholipids from the inner leaf of the cell membrane. PLA2 is an intracellular enzyme that is induced by inflammatory cytokines; lipopolysaccharides (LPS), an endotoxin formed in the outer membrane of gram-negative bacteria; and other certain other inflammatory stimuli. These agents typically also induce the enzymes COX2 and microsomal prostaglandin E synthase-1 (mPGES-1). Figure 15-1 outlines the biosynthesis of the principal inflammatory eicosanoids. PLA2 is also present in snake and insect venoms[5]; the liberation of arachidonic acid and the formation of eicosanoids explain the venom's effects.

AA is converted to prostaglandin H_2 by cyclooxygenase (COX), which can then be converted to other prostanoids, or AA can be converted to leukotrienes, via a lipoxygenase enzyme. *In LAH, AA conversion into prostaglandins is inhibited, and excess substrate is converted into leukotrienes.*

While prostaglandin E_2 (PGE_2) initially acts as an inflammatory agent, it later participates in the down-regulation of inflammation. PGE_2 acts in negative feedback, by inhibiting lipolysis by phospholipase A2, and thus, it decreases the release of arachidonic acid from the cell membrane. PGE_2 thus limits the formation of leukotrienes[6] as well as limiting the formation of prostaglandins. If PGE_2 is blocked downstream of AA release, feedback is lost, and AA remains available for leukotriene production. This can occur if PGH_2 synthase is blocked, for example, by COX inhibitors, or by inhibition of PGE synthase.

The effects of PGE_2 also depend on the target tissue. For example, alveolar macrophages protect the lungs from bacteria. PGE_2 inhibits alveolar macrophage antimicrobial function, while LOX-derived leukotrienes, LTB_4, LTC_4, LTD_4, and LTE_4, enhance the macrophage activity[7], particularly when the IgG receptor, FcγR, is activated.

Aspirin, naproxen, ibuprofen and other non-steroidal anti-inflammatory medications (NSAIDs) inhibit PGH synthase (COX). COX_1 is constitutively active and provides for a baseline level of prostaglandin production, whereas COX_2 is only activated by inflammatory stimuli. NSAID medications can cause a shift in the production of eicosanoids from the prostaglandin pathway towards the leukotriene pathway.

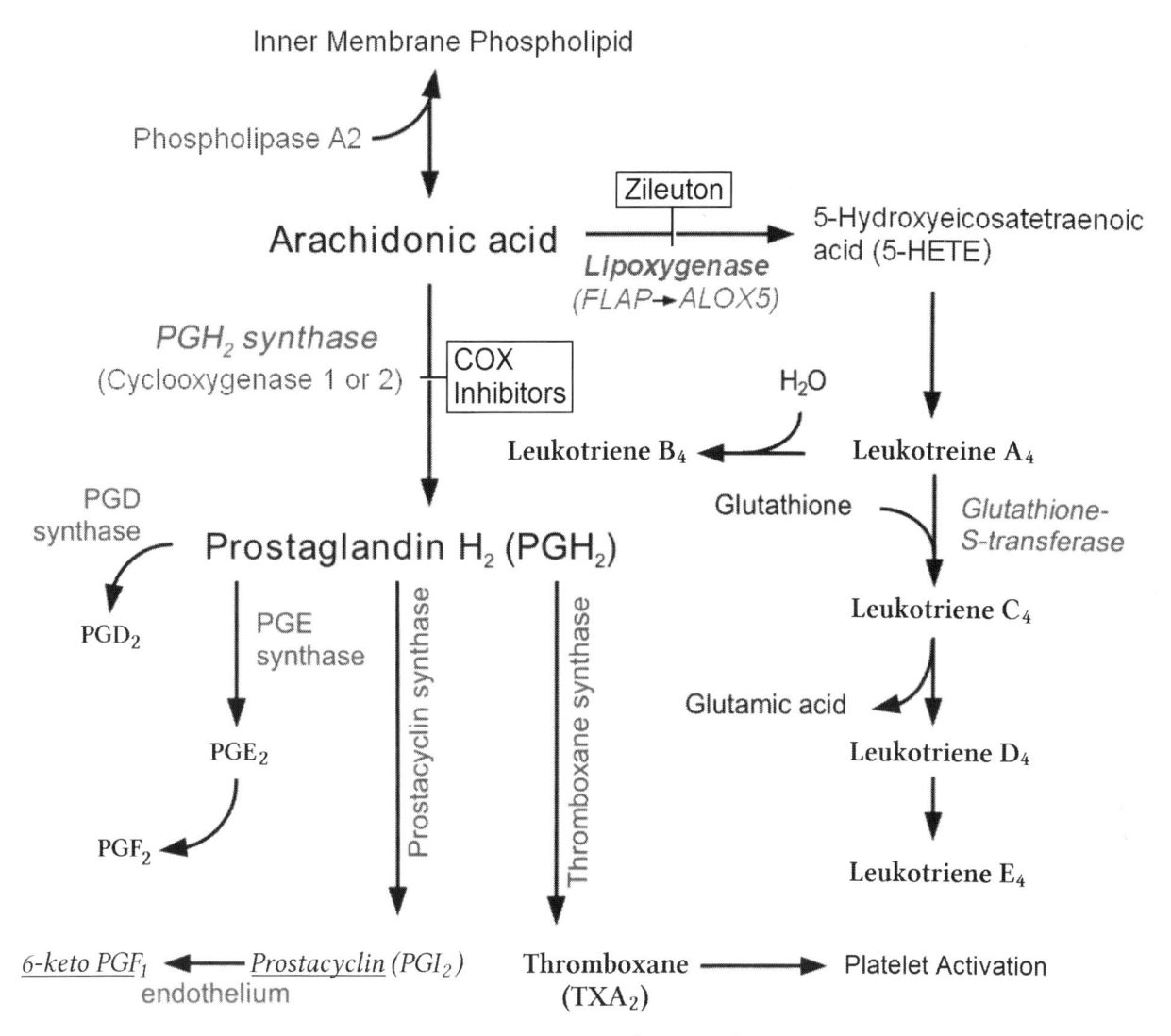

Figure 15-1: Eicosanoid Biosynthesis

Mast Cell Waves

While some NSAIDs provoke LAH, other COX₂ inhibitors do not. Aspirin, however, can provoke LAH reactions at doses far lower than those required for inhibition of COX enzymes. Low concentrations of aspirin (0.1 to 0.3 mM) can efficiently induce the release of LTC₄ from mast cells[8]. Low-dose aspirin can also induce the release of heat shock proteins, IL-6, and TNF-α from mast cells[9].

Mast cells have calcium channels that can be activated by exposure to low concentrations of aspirin. This can trigger calcium release within the mast cell, activating cytosolic phospholipase A2 and 5-lipoxygenase (ALOX-5). These enzymes promote the release of AA and formation and secretion of LTC₄ from mast cells. Calcium influx also triggers mast cell degranulation when activated by IgE. It appears that, at low concentrations, aspirin can potentiate mast cell activation by IgE or IgG through calcium-activated mechanisms. At higher levels (3.0 mM) of aspirin, however, calcium release is inhibited. Salicylic acid was found to have a similar effect to aspirin on LTC4 release[8].

A central feature in LAH is LTC₄, released from mast cells, acting as a signal for neighboring mast cell degranulation. This, too, is mediated through calcium-dependent channels. This can only occur, however, when other mast cells are in sufficiently close proximity for LTC₄ to induce propagation of waves of mast cell activation; LTC₄ induces release of LTC₄ from other nearby mast cells, and that LTC₄ subsequently activates other mast cells. This propagation of waves of degranulation has been demonstrated in nasal polyp tissue[10]. This action occurs through special CRAC calcium channels which have all-or-none reactions for triggering degranulation[11].

Propagation of LTC₄ dependent activation depends on mast cells being in close proximity to each other; perhaps less than 50 μm; half the width of an average human hair. *This limits these reactions to areas of mast cell hyperplasia;* tissues in which mast cells population density is abnormally high. Propagation of mast cell activation waves can occur in MCAS or other mast cell activation disorders (Chapter 12), but is not expected in normal tissue. In nasal polyps, a similar or coordination role is likely in eosinophils.

Genetic and Epigenetic Alterations

Low concentrations of aspirin and salicylate promote activity of CRAC calcium channels; while higher concentrations impede it[8]. Studies of patients with ASA have revealed numerous polymorphisms that may explain the altered immune activity in this condition[12]. Polymorphisms in over 20 different genes have been described in these patients. In a genome-wide analysis of *epigenetic* alterations, hypermethylation, limiting gene expression, was detected in 296 genes. Meanwhile, hypomethylation, which increases gene expression, was detected in 141 genes. These alterations suggest that patients with ASA have increased protein transcription of genes that promote lymphocyte proliferation, leukocyte activation, cytokine biosynthesis and secretion, immune responses, inflammation, and immunoglobulin binding; and have decreased transcription for genes involved in hemostasis, wound healing and calcium ion binding. The PGE synthase gene was hypermethylated, leading to a down-regulation of prostaglandin E synthesis. There was also hypomethylation, thus increased transcription, of the genes for PGD synthase, 5-lipoxygenase-activating protein (FLAP), and for the leukotriene B4 receptor. These alterations lead to lower PGE_2 production and increase in leukotriene production and activity[13]. Usually, this disease is not associated with more eosinophils in the tissue, but rather with increased reactivity of those cells[14].

> A diet that was originally developed by Feingold for ASA intolerance has been used for children with ADHD for over 30 years. About one in four children respond[15]. Several food additives can trigger LAH; sodium benzoate, tartrazine, and other artificial colorants have been shown to exacerbate hyperactivity in several clinical trials. Tartrazine and certain other yellow food colorants have been banned in several countries for this reason[16]. The hyperactivity effect of these food additives has been suggested to be provoked by the release of histamine by a non-IgE-mediated pathway[17]. The fact that LAH is unusual in children and that this is a neurological condition rather than asthma, suggests a different disease process for the salicylate effect in ADHD, nevertheless, they sharing some mechanism of action.

Disease Manifestations

In Europe, "Aspirin Intolerance"[18] is a common disorder affecting between 6 and 25 persons per thousand, and it is more commonly seen in women than in men. Salicylates and related compounds which are present in certain foods, toothpaste, and ointments can also have aspirin-like effects and can provoke LAH. The dose of aspirin required to elicit clinical symptoms can vary by a factor of as much as 100 (e.g., 5-500 mg)[19].

Table 15-1: LAH Manifestations

System	LAH Manifestations[20]
General	Angioedema
	Fevers
Respiratory	Sinusitis
	Secretions
	Nasal Congestion
	Nasal polyps
	Bronchoconstriction
	Larynx Edema
	Pulmonary Infiltrates
Gastrointestinal	Meteorism
	Erosions
	Abdominal Pain
	Edema, Swelling
	Ulcers
	Diarrhea,
	Colitis
	Fibrosis
	Strictures
Dermatologic	Chronic Urticaria
	Angioedema
	Itching
	Atopic dermatitis
Heart	Myocarditis
	Kounis syndrome*
Kidneys	Pericarditis
	Interstitial Nephritis
Neurologic	Hyperactivity?
	Irritability?

> * The **Kounis syndrome** is the provocation of coronary artery vasospasm by allergic or pseudoallergic reaction. This syndrome has been documented in children as young as two years of age[21], secondary to food allergies[22], insect envenomation[23], and most frequently, allergic-type reaction to medication. Although the coronary arteries may be normal, the presence of coronary artery atheroma increases the risk for ischemia and myocardial infarction resulting from allergic or pseudoallergic reactions.

Table 15-2 gives estimates from various studies of the portion of patients affected by LAH with various conditions. LAH is common, and a significant portion of patients with immune sensitivities respond to avoidance of aspirin and related compounds. In Europe, about ten percent of adult asthmatics are estimated to have LAH.

Testing for LAH

Testing for LAH can be done by measuring urinary cystyl-leukotriene or urinary LTE_4 after a challenge[24]. In LAH, no change in N-methylhistamine is observed; while LTE_4 is increased. Unfortunately, there is a 25 percent false negative rate for this test among affected persons.

Table 15-2: LAH Prevalence in Various Conditions

Condition	Percent of Adults with Condition having LAH	Percent of Adults with LAH having Condition
Sinusitis	15 to 20	76
Nasal Polyps	76	31
Asthma	6 – 34	16.4
Ulcerative Colitis	7.4	
Crohn's Disease	2.1	
Gastrointestinal Hypersensitivity[#]	5.9	
Carbohydrate Malabsorption	0.6	
Chronic Urticaria	2-3?	
General Population	0.6	

[#] Gastrointestinal Hypersensitivity occurs in about 1% of adults and refers to histamine-mediated abdominal symptoms, nausea, cramping, vomiting and/or diarrhea after exposure to certain foods. About 6% of patients with this condition also have LAH.

LAH Treatments

Treatment of LAH is explained more clearly by parsing the disease's mechanism of action into parts: the shift of eicosanoid production towards leukotriene production, and the triggering of mast cell degranulation waves by LTC_4, induced by low dose aspirin or related compounds. As long-term tertiary prevention, treatment to reverse of mast cell hyperplasia and restore of normal DNA methylation levels should be undertaken.

Avoid Agents which Trigger Degranulation

Low concentrations of aspirin or salicylic acid can trigger calcium channel mediated mast cell activation. In an effort to prevent degranulation in LAH, aspirin may be avoided, but similar compounds found in foods are more difficult to avoid. Table 15-3 shows some similar molecules found in foods.

A study published in 1985 by Swain analyzed the salicylate content of a wide variety of foods[25]. This study became and remained the primary source used in avoidance of foods that provoked "salicylate sensitivity." Salicylate, which is closely related to aspirin, is found in willow bark and has been used for millennia for fever and pain. Like aspirin, salicylate acts by inhibiting COX as well by other mechanisms. Unfortunately, however, the methodology used in Swain's study did not withstand the test of time.

Salicylate, also known as salicylic acid (SA), is a hydroxybenzoic acid, phenolic compound. Only tiny amounts are found in human food. On average, beer contains 0.6 mg of SA per 12 oz. serving, the highest amount of SA per serving of any food, and ten times higher than the second highest food per serving: red wine. It would take 9 servings of beer or 90 servings of wine to amount to 5 mg of dietary SA; comparing it to 5 mg of aspirin as the minimum dose required to exacerbate LAH.

Table 15-3: Aspirin and Related Compounds

Sources:[26]	Chemical Agent	Usage
Aspirin	Acetyl Salicylate aka: 2-acetyloxybenzoic acid	Analgesic
4-OH benzoic acid	4-Hydroxybenzoic acid	Antioxidant found in coconuts[27] strawberries[28] carrots[29]
Wintergreen	Methyl 2-hydroxybenzoate aka: methyl salicylate	Flavoring; mint flavor, used in topical heating rubs.
Salicylic acid	2-Hydroxybenzoic acid aka: salicylate	Medication (usually topical) Willow bark
Sodium benzoate	Sodium benzoic acid	Preservative

While SA is uncommon in food, there are several other related compounds that are common in food that may provoke food related "salicylate sensitivity." Of over 500 phenolic compounds identified in food, 29 of these are hydroxybenzoic compounds. These hydroxybenzoic acids are listed in the Phenol Explorer database[30], a comprehensive online compendium of phenolic compounds in foods.

The average French adult consumes about 41 mg of hydroxybenzoic acids a day. However, most of that (25 mg) comes from 5-O-Galloylquinic acid from tea (13 mg), and Gallic acid from tea (5 mg), red wine (4 mg), green chicory (2 mg), and other minor sources[31]. Not all hydroxybenzoic compounds, however, are suspected of triggering mast cell activity. The relative pharmacologic impact off the various individual hydroxybenzoic acid compounds on mast cell degranulation is also not known.

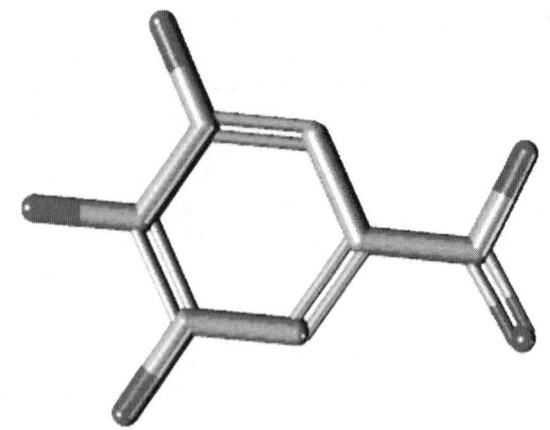

Figure 15-2: Gallic Acid, One of 29 Hydroxybenzoic Acids Found in Foods

Coconut, strawberries, carrots, loquats and olives contain high levels of 4-OH benzoic acid that may trigger LAH reactions. Cloves, chestnuts, chicory and black tea are high in gallic acid. Cherries, raspberries[32], celery seeds and carrot seeds have also been shown to inhibit COX_1 activity. Little is known as to which hydroxybenzoic acids present in foods trigger mast cell activity or inhibit COX.

Mint flavoring (wintergreen) is used in toothpaste and candy contains salicylates. Salicylate in rubbing creams with wintergreen may cause skin reactions. Sodium benzoate is used as a preservative in foods and cosmetics.

The FDA estimates daily intakes of dietary benzoic acid range from 0.9-34 mg a day and sodium benzoate intake ranges from 34-328 mg a day. In human testing, over one-third of an ingested carbon$_{13}$ labeled dose of ingested benzoic acid was recovered as salicyluric acid, the urinary metabolite of salicylic acid[33].

Aspirin and some related compounds inhibit the COX enzymes; this shifts eicosanoid synthesis to production of leukotrienes. Non-steroidal anti-inflammatory medications (NSAIDS) that inhibit COX may also worsen LAH.

Several studies have shown that the selective COX2 inhibitor celecoxib may be used in patients with aspirin or NSAID-induced asthma for the treatment of pain[34, 35], without triggering LAH reactions. Celecoxib (Celebrex) also inhibits the enzyme ALOX-5 and limits leukotriene production. Rofecoxib (Vioxx) and etoricoxib, another selective COX2 inhibitor, did not inhibit ALOX-5[36]. Thus, COX2 inhibitors that do not inhibit leukotriene production should also be avoided in individuals with LAH.

Hydroxybenzoates in foods do not only trigger degranulation, but some also inhibit COX enzymes. Hydroxybenzoates are not alone in this activity. Many other phenolic compounds, such as certain curcuminoids, also inhibit COX1 and thus may increase LTC_4 formation. The spice turmeric, which is found in curry, is about four percent curcuminoid by weight and at least one of these, curcumin, is a COX1 inhibitor[37].

Another group of phenolic compounds are the flavonoids. Many of these have been found to inhibit inflammation through their effects on COX1, COX2, and nitrous oxide synthetase. In a test of 26 naturally occurring flavonoids, 12 were found to inhibit LPS-induced PGE_2 production. COX1 and COX2 are inhibited by the flavonoids catechin and cyanidin-3-O-beta-galactopyranoside[38]. Table 15-4 lists some flavonoid phenols which affect prostaglandin biosynthesis by inhibiting COX2 and microsomal PGE synthase-1 (mPGES-1).

For most individuals, the anti-inflammatory effects of plant phenols are welcome. These compounds do not come isolated in foods, and many other compounds present in the foods may have various actions on prostaglandin and leukotriene metabolism.

Even in individuals with LAH, some of these foods may have beneficial, rather than harmful, effects. Curcumin inhibits both COX2 and ALOX-5 formation[39]. Luteolin-7-O-glucoside, a polyphenol found in Mexican oregano, celery seed, peppermint leaves and black olives inhibits LTC_4-induced degranulation of mast cells[40]. Genistein inhibits both COX2 and leukotriene synthesis[41]. Other flavonoids, including kaempferol, quercetin, morin and myricetin, inhibit ALOX-5. Hamamelitannin and galloylated proanthocyanidins are potent polyphenol ALOX-5 inhibitors[42].

Foods are not isolated compounds and are not eaten in isolation. Thus, they may have combined effects in promoting LAH and inhibit LAH reactions. Until research has better identified which compounds put individuals with LAH at risk, patients with LAH need to astutely watch their reactions to food and eliminate those that seem to be problematic.

The many different phenolic compounds in foods that may be capable of inhibiting COX1 or COX2 would not be expected to have equal bioavailability, nor equal activity in inhibiting COX1. Most dietary polyphenols are poorly absorbed by the body and rapidly eliminated. Many flavonoids inhibit the pathogenic effects of LPS, the induction of eNOS, and eicosanoid synthesis, and thus would be expected to decrease degranulation.

LAH Safe Foods: Fresh meat, fish, shellfish, poultry, eggs, and dairy do not contain LAH-inducing compounds. Grains, cereals, and bread contain mostly complex polyphenols that are large and poorly absorbed. These are not associated with LAH.

LAH Risk Foods: Foods rich in phenols, including but not limited to hydroxybenzoic acid may put individuals with LAH at risk of a reaction. Foods high in small phenolic compounds include fruits, vegetables, herbs, and spices.

Salicylic acid is a phenolic compound, produced by willow trees, which protects the tree from attack by bacteria. Similar compounds are often present in seeds, young fruit, root vegetables, and the skin and peel of fruits and vegetables that are highly exposed to bacteria. These are the same set of foods that have been associated with ASA and other forms LAH. Foods high in phenolic compounds are usually highly flavored, often have bitter flavors. Herbs and spices typically have high phenol content.

Other Foods: Certain wild edible mushrooms[43, 44] contain compounds that can inhibit COX1.

Table 15-4: Some Phenolic Compounds which Down-Regulate COX2 and mPGES-1 Expression and Leukotriene Activity[45]

Food Phenolic Compound	Foods Containing Flavonoid[46]
Inhibit COX$_2$ expression	
Isorhamnetin	Yellow onions, red onions, red wine
Daidzein	Soybean meal products
Genistein	Soybean meal products
Epicatechin	Chocolate, broad beans, green tea, blackberries, many other foods
Catechin	Chocolate, prune juice, broad beans, apple cider, black tea
Inhibit mPGES-1 expression	
Kaempferol	Black beans, capers, cumin, cloves, caraway, Loganberries
Isorhamnetin	Yellow onions, red onions, red wine
Resveratrol[47]	Loganberry, cranberry, muscadine grape wine
Curcumin[48]	Tumeric (curry)
Epigallocatechin-3-gallate[49]	Green tea, oolong tea, black tea, pecans
Inhibits ALOX-5	
Quercetin	Elderberries, capers, cloves, chocolate, Mexican oregano
Kaempferol	Black beans, capers, cumin, cloves, caraway, Loganberries
Curcumin[50]	Tumeric (curry)
Genistein	Soybean meal products

Table 15-5: Some foods high in hydroxybenzoic phenols:

Fruits	Loquats, cranberries, raspberries, dates, blackberries, pomegranate, strawberries, red currants, cloudberries
Nuts	Chestnuts, walnuts, coconut
Tea	Black tea, green tea, oolong tea
Spices	Cloves, star anise, Ceylon cinnamon
Herbs	Oregano, thyme, mint, sage, rosemary
Vegetables	Chicory, carrots
Olives	Green and black olives
Other	Oats, sorghum, beer

Nitrates can provoke aspirin-like reactions in individuals with aspirin hypersensitivity. Nitrites are used in processed meats. While nitrates do not inhibit prostaglandins, they increase the formation of leukotrienes[51].

Potatoes can also trigger inflammatory reactions in individuals with LAH, especially in patients with gastrointestinal LAH reactions; however, it does not appear to be caused by inhibition of COX or from hydroxybenzoate compounds in potatoes. The effect may be caused by 5-lipooxyenase in potatoes, which turns arachidonic acid into leukotriene A$_4$[52]. This reaction may be limited to the intestinal lumen. Alternatively, potato lectins can cause mast cell degranulation (Chapter 14).

Medical Treatment of LAH

One of the most successful treatments for LAH is Aspirin desensitization. DO NOT TRY THIS AT HOME. The method is simple: Put the patient in the hospital for six days and have a crash cart at the bedside; keep the person under close observation ready to resuscitate them if they go into anaphylactoid shock. Start with 25 mg intravenous lysine-aspirin, and slowly increase the dose twice daily over the week spent in the hospital to 500 mg I.V. If the patient tolerates this dose, they can go home, taking 325 mg of aspirin by mouth daily, every day for the rest of their lives[53]. If they miss one dose, it is not a problem. If they miss more than that, start the process over from the beginning to avoid a potentially fatal reaction to aspirin, which can occur using the same dose they had been taking daily.

Leukotriene Receptor Antagonists (LAR) (montelukast and zafirlukast) are a class of medication that do what their name states. They are useful for asthma and allergic rhinitis, and may be helpful in the prevention of other LAH reactions. These medications may allow these patients to discontinue the use of steroids[54]. Zileuton may be helpful for LAH as it blocks lipoxygenase-5 activity upstream of leukotriene formation. Montelukast, however, blocks LTD$_4$ receptors downstream from LTC$_4$-induced mast cell degranulation but remains helpful.

Histamine H$_1$ receptors (HRH$_1$) and Histamine H$_4$ receptors (H$_4$R) have been found to be elevated in nasal polyp tissue[55]. H$_4$R is associated with chemotaxis of mast cells[56] and mast cell development in the bone marrow. No H$_4$ antagonist medications are currently available; however, H$_1$ antagonist medications may be helpful for symptomatic relief of congestion from nasal polyps, and perhaps other symptoms.

> **Salicylates in IBD:** Mesalamine, also known as 5-aminosalicylic acid, is a medication used for the treatment of inflammatory bowel disease (IBD). About three percent of patients with IBD develop cramping, acute abdominal pain, and bloody diarrhea, and some, fever, headache, and rash, with the use of mesalamine[57]. This may be an LAH reaction.

Food-Dependent Exercise-Induced Anaphylaxis

Some individuals suffer exercise-induced anaphylaxis (EIA) after a combination of exposures that have additive or synergistic effects that trigger mast cell degranulation. In EIA, patients may have food allergies or sensitivity to aspirin, but typically require exercise to trigger an immune reaction, which may include urticaria, hives, and bronchoconstriction. Immune response to a food they have eaten within several hours, or the use of aspirin, other non-steroidal anti-inflammatory or other contributing factors, can set the stage for the reaction. Foods that trigger other allergies are commonly the same ones that act here. Wheat gluten is a particularly common contributing factor in EIA. Food allergy and testing is recommended for patients with EIA[58].

Preventive Treatment of LAH

1. Avoid Triggers: The first line of treatment of LAH is the avoidance of agents such as aspirin, NSAID's and hydroxybenzoate compounds that trigger degranulation.

2. Anti-leukotrienes: Medications that prevent degranulation or prevent the formation of series 4 leukotrienes may be helpful. Many dietary phenolic compounds down-regulate or inhibit enzymes promoting inflammatory leukotrienes. Table 15-6 lists some foods with high content of phenolic compounds that inhibit leukotriene formation.

Table 15-6: Dietary Sources of Leukotriene Inhibiting Phenolic Compounds

Black elderberries, Loganberries
Capers, Black olives
Tumeric (curry), Cloves
Soybean meal products (tofu, soy milk, soy burgers) Black beans
Chocolate
Mexican oregano Peppermint leaves
Cumin, Caraway, Celery seed

3. Reduce Inflammatory Reactivity: Large doses of fish oil are successful in the treatment of LAH as they decrease the ratio of arachidonic acid (AA) to eicosapentaenoic acid (EPA) in the phospholipids of the cell membrane.

In response to certain inflammatory signals, phospholipase A2 liberates AA, ETA or EPA from the membrane phospholipids. Lipoxygenase-5 (LOX5) converts AA into series-4 leukotrienes that are proinflammatory and promote waves of degranulation. LOX5, however, converts eicosatetraenoic acid (ETA) into series-5 leukotrienes that are inactive or mildly anti-inflammatory[59]. See Figure 6-5.

In a trial of patients with aspirin-sensitive asthma, ten grams of fish oil used taken daily. After six to eight weeks of treatment, symptoms were reported to be completely, or almost completely, resolved. When the treatment was stopped, however, the condition returned[60].

ETA is the preferred substrate of LOX5 over AA when sufficient EPA is present[61]. EPA acts not only as a precursor to ETA but also inhibits AA formation from linoleic acid. Olive oil contains oleic acid (18:1,n-9), which can be elongated by ELOVL5 and desaturated to mead acid (20:3,n-9), which also competitively inhibits the production of AA[62]. Thus, diets high in fish oil, α-linolenic acid, and oleic acid lower the endogenous production of AA from linoleic acid, and thus, have an anti-inflammatory influence on health.

The western diet has a high proportion of n-6 fatty acids LA and AA, which are pro-inflammatory. A diet low in n-6 and high in n-3 fatty acids can be used to treat LAH. Limiting dietary n-6 fatty acids intake is probably more effective than adding n-3 or n-9 fatty acids.

Antioxidants: Oxidative stress not only induces ALOX-5 in B lymphocyte, but also supports the conversion of 5-HETE into active inflammatory leukotriene products which act as potent eosinophil chemoattractants in asthma[63]. Antioxidant support is recommended in the treatment of LAH. Many dietary phenols are antioxidants. Environmental, oxidative stressors such as tobacco smoke, promote systemic inflammation and the development of nasal polyps[64], as in LAH. Antioxidants are discussed in Chapter 21.

Remove allergens and immunogens: The degranulation of mast cells is an all-or-none response mediated by calcium channels. Aspirin in LAH serves to lower the threshold for degranulation of mast cells that have IgE or IgG activation. Avoidance of antigens helps decrease mast cell activation. IgE testing for food and environmental allergens and IgG testing for food immunogens should be performed for affected individuals, and the reactive antigens avoided.

Patients with LAH may have other pseudo allergies as their immune response is highly up-regulated. Other triggers for degranulation also need to be avoided and treated. Other triggers for mast cell, basophil and eosinophil degranulation are covered in Chapters 11 through 14.

Treat the Underlying Condition

The essential goal of treatment is not to restrict the diet to vigilantly eliminate hydroxybenzoic acids, but rather to treat the underlying inflammatory disorder.

Treatment with fish oil successfully treats LAH after six to eight weeks. It requires this much time to adequately replace the proinflammatory n-6 dominated phospholipids in the cell membrane with less inflammatory ones that include a sufficient balance of n-3 fatty acids. The disease recurs, however if the treatment is stopped; this treatment is inadequate, at least in the short-term, to eliminate mast cell hyperplasia and the epigenetically aberrant, mast cell and eosinophil activation.

Mast cells and eosinophils have limited life spans; normally, it is in the order days to a few weeks. Eliminating the inflammatory milieu might be easy if these cells would just behave normally. These cells, however, have altered epigenetic, and occasionally genetic, adaptations that make them abnormally reactive to even minor inflammatory stimuli. This maintains inflammation and their survival. Stimuli that should be innocuous may promote the activation, chemotaxis, survival and proliferation of these Inflammatory cells.

Inflammation can be divided into two principal phases; destruction and repair. The first phase involves mounting a defense against invading microbes or invading or infected cells. The second part of the inflammatory process is eliminating inflammatory cells that are no longer required and repairing the tissue where the battle took place.

Inflammatory positive-feedback loops that support inappropriate immune activity and prevent apoptosis of inflammatory cells after an infection or injury are the basis of many chronic diseases. Successful treatment requires long-term, vigilant avoidance of inflammatory promotion and support for the transition to the second phase; repair. The repair stage of inflammation is guided by down-regulation of mediators such as NF-κB, an anti-apoptosis agent, and up-regulation of AP-1. Various combinations of cytokines greatly influence whether there is a continuation of destructive inflammation or the apoptosis and repair functions. TNF-α and IL-1β are pro-inflammatory cytokines that help maintain the destructive inflammation.

Epigenetic modification of inflammatory cells, such as mast cells and eosinophils, are stable and unlikely to revert during division and proliferation in the target tissues. New cell development from precursor cells, however, can supply new, inflammatory cells with normal behavior *if they develop in a healthy milieu.*

Many chronic diseases can be prevented and treated by avoiding inflammation, supporting apoptosis and repair, and promoting an epigenetic reset to normal activity. Elimination of aberrant inflammatory cells often requires a long-term, multifaceted approach to breaking the cycle of inflammation and complete their apoptosis.

Reverse Mast Cell and Eosinophil Hyperactivity: Mast cell hyperplasia is essential for propagation of LTC$_4$-induced waves of mast cell degranulation. LAH has similarities to mast cell activation disorder. Preventive treatment of mast cell and eosinophil hyperactivity and hyperplasia are the same as those described for promoting apoptosis is mast cell activation disorders discussed in Chapter 12.

Systemic and topical steroids nasal sprays have been shown to promote the regression of nasal polyps. Nasal steroids induce apoptosis of inflammatory cells and fibroblasts in the polyps[65],[66]. The corticosteroids suppress inflammatory cytokines, chemokines, including IL-5 that supports eosinophil development, and growth factors for polyp development, and induce pro-apoptotic factors[67],[68], and thus, withdraw support for inflammatory cell hyperplasia and survival.

Chronic inflammation is supported by activation of TLR's. LPS stimulates the activation of phospholipase A2, COX2 and ALOX-5 via TLR4. LPS levels become significant in intestinal bacterial biofilm formation (Chapters 23 and 24).

Sphingosine-1-Phosphate helps maintain inflammatory cells. Pyridoxine is a cofactor for S1P lyase (Chapter 10). Magnesium promotes the induction of inflammatory repair (Chapter 30).

Epigenetic Reset: LAH develops with age from exposure to an imbalanced immune milieu, which results in epigenetic changes that favor the survival of hyper-reactive immune cells and immune cell hyperplasia. Impaired apoptosis and inappropriate levels of methylation or acetylation of DNA may result from exposure to mutagens in the environment and diet, chronic inflammatory stress, and nutritional deficiencies.

Epigenetic reset of inflammatory cells, such as mast cells and eosinophils, likely does not occur much during division and proliferation in the tissues. Nevertheless, avoidance of mutagens and adequate levels of nutrients, including folate, vitamin B$_{12}$, Vitamin D$_3$, pyridoxine and DHA, are likely to reduce the risk of aberrant methylation and provide an environment in which new, inflammatory cells from hemopoietic precursor cells have normal methylation and acetylation and behave normally. "Epigenetic Reset" is discussed in Chapter 29 and mutagens and their prevention is discussed in Chapter 41.

[1] Aspirin-induced asthma: advances in pathogenesis, diagnosis, and management. Szczeklik A, Stevenson DD. J Allergy Clin Immunol. 2003 May;111(5):913-21; quiz 922. PMID:12743549

[2] Significance of salicylate intolerance in diseases of the lower gastrointestinal tract. Raithel M, Baenkler HW, Naegel A, et al. J Physiol Pharmacol. 2005 Sep;56 Suppl 5:89-102.PMID: 16247191

[3] The Kounis-Zavras syndrome with the Samter-Beer triad. Schwartz BG, Daulat S, Kuiper J. Proc (Bayl Univ Med Cent). 2011 Apr;24(2):107-9. PMID: 21566756

[4] Increase in salivary cysteinyl-leukotriene concentration in patients with aspirin-intolerant asthma. Ono E, Taniguchi M, Higashi N, Mita H, Yamaguchi H, Tatsuno S, Fukutomi Y, Tanimoto H, Sekiya K, Oshikata C, Tsuburai T, Tsurikisawa N, Otomo M, Maeda Y, Hasegawa M, Miyazaki E, Kumamoto T, Akiyama K. Allergol Int. 2011 Mar;60(1):37-43. PMID:21099251

[5] Honeybee venom secretory phospholipase A2 induces leukotriene production but not histamine release from human basophils. Mustafa FB, Ng FS, Nguyen TH, Lim LH. Clin Exp Immunol. 2008 Jan;151(1):94-100. Epub 2007 Nov 14. PMID:18005261

[6] Effects of non-steroidal anti-inflammatory drugs on cyclo-oxygenase and lipoxygenase activity in whole blood from aspirin-sensitive asthmatics vs healthy donors. Gray PA, Warner TD, Vojnovic I, Del Soldato P, Parikh A, Scadding GK, Mitchell JA. Br J Pharmacol. 2002 Dec;137(7):1031-8. PMID:12429575

[7] Crosstalk between prostaglandin E2 and leukotriene B4 regulates phagocytosis in alveolar macrophages via combinatorial effects on cyclic AMP. Lee SP, Serezani CH, Medeiros AI, Ballinger MN, Peters-Golden M. J Immunol. 2009 Jan 1;182(1):530-7.PMID: 19109185

[8] Analysis of the mechanism for the development of allergic skin inflammation and the application for its treatment: aspirin modulation of IgE-dependent mast cell activation: role of aspirin-induced exacerbation of immediate allergy. Suzuki Y, Ra C. J Pharmacol Sci. 2009 Jul;110(3):237-44. PMID:19609060

[9] Stimulation of cysteinyl leukotriene production in mast cells by heat shock and acetylsalicylic acid. Mortaz E, Redegeld FA, Dunsmore K, Odoms K, Wong HR, Nijkamp FP, Engels F. Eur J Pharmacol. 2007 Apr 30;561(1-3):214-9. PMID:17306251

[10] Intercellular Ca2+ wave propagation involving positive feedback between CRAC channels and cysteinyl leukotrienes. Di Capite J, Shirley A, Nelson C, Bates G, Parekh AB. FASEB J. 2009 Mar;23(3):894-905. PMID:18978154

[11] All-or-none activation of CRAC channels by agonist elicits graded responses in populations of mast cells. Chang WC, Di Capite J, Nelson C, Parekh AB. J Immunol. 2007 Oct 15;179(8):5255-63. PMID:17911611

[12] Genetic mechanisms in aspirin-exacerbated respiratory disease. Shrestha Palikhe N, Kim SH, Jin HJ, Hwang EK, Nam YH, Park HS. J Allergy (Cairo). 2012;2012:794890. PMID:21837245

[13] Genome-wide methylation profile of nasal polyps: relation to aspirin hypersensitivity in asthmatics. Cheong HS, Park SM, Kim MO, Park JS, Lee JY, Byun JY, Park BL, Shin HD, Park CS. Allergy. 2011 May;66(5):637-44. PMID:21121930

[14] Degranulation patterns of eosinophil granulocytes as determinants of eosinophil driven disease. Erjefält JS, Greiff L, Andersson M, Adelroth E, Jeffery PK, Persson CG. Thorax. 2001 May;56(5):341-4. PMID:11312400

[15] Relative effects of drugs and diet on hyperactive behaviors: an experimental study. Williams JI, Cram DM, Tausig FT, Webster E. Pediatrics. 1978 Jun;61(6):811-7. PMID: 353680

[16] Committee on Toxicity of Chemicals in Food, Consumer Products and the Environment. Statement on Research Project (T07040) Investigating the Effect of Mixtures of Certain Food Colours and a Preservative on Behavior in Children Food Standards Agency (UK) Committee on Toxicity.

[17] The effects of a double blind, placebo controlled, artificial food colourings and benzoate preservative challenge on hyperactivity in a general population sample of preschool children. Bateman B, Warner JO, Hutchinson E, Dean T, Rowlandson P, Gant C, Grundy J, Fitzgerald C, Stevenson J. Arch Dis Child. 2004 Jun;89(6):506-11. PMID: 15155391

[18] Aspirin desensitization in aspirin intolerance: update on current standards and recent improvements. Pfaar O, Klimek L. Curr Opin Allergy Clin Immunol. 2006 Jun;6(3):161-6. PMID: 16670507

[19] Nonsteroidal anti-inflammatory drug hypersensitivity syndrome. A multicenter study. I. Clinical findings and in vitro diagnosis. De Weck AL, Sanz ML, Gamboa PM, et al. J Investig Allergol Clin Immunol. 2009;19(5):355-69.PMID: 19862935

[20] Significance of salicylate intolerance in diseases of the lower gastrointestinal tract. Raithel M, Baenkler HW, Naegel A, Buchwald F, Schultis HW, Backhaus B, Kimpel S, Koch H, Mach K, Hahn EG, Konturek PC. J Physiol Pharmacol. 2005 Sep;56 Suppl 5:89-102.PMID: 16247191

[21] Kounis Syndrome or Allergic Coronary Vasospasm in a Two-year-old. Parent B, Wearden P, Kounis NG, Chrysostomou C. Congenit Heart Dis. 2011 Mar 21. PMID:21418536

[22] Coronary vasospasm secondary to allergic reaction following food ingestion: a case of type I variant Kounis syndrome. Wada T, Abe M, Yagi N, Kokubu N, Kasahara Y, Kataoka Y, Otsuka Y, Goto Y, Nonogi H. Heart Vessels. 2010 May;25(3):263-6. Epub 2010 May 29. PMID:20512455

[23] Kounis syndrome associated with hypersensitivity to hymenoptera stings. Kogias JS, Sideris SK, Anifadis SK. Int J Cardiol. 2007 Jan 8;114(2):252-5. Epub 2006 May 2. PMID:16647768

[24] Urinary metabolites of histamine and leukotrienes before and after placebo-controlled challenge with ASA and food additives in chronic urticaria patients. Di Lorenzo G, Pacor ML, Vignola AM, Profita M, Esposito-Pellitteri M, Biasi D, Corrocher R, Caruso C. Allergy. 2002 Dec;57(12):1180-6. PMID:12464047

[25] Salicylates in foods. Swain AR, Dutton SP, Truswell AS. J Am Diet Assoc. 1985 Aug;85(8):950-60. PMID:4019987

[26] The aspirin disease. Schiavino D, Nucera E, Milani A, Del Ninno M, Buonomo A, Sun J, Patriarca G. Thorax. 2000 Oct;55 Suppl 2:S66-9. PMID:10992564

²⁷ Profiling C6-C3 and C6-C1 phenolic metabolites in Cocos nucifera. Dey G, Chakraborty M, Mitra A. J Plant Physiol. 2005 Apr;162(4):375-81. PMID:15900879

²⁸ Bioavailability of strawberry antioxidants in human subjects. Azzini E, Vitaglione P, Intorre F, Napolitano A, Durazzo A, Foddai MS, Fumagalli A, Catasta G, Rossi L, Venneria E, Raguzzini A, Palomba L, Fogliano V, Maiani G. Br J Nutr. 2010 Oct;104(8):1165-73. Epub 2010 May 21. PMID:20487578

²⁹ Characterization and distribution of phenolics in carrot cell walls. Kang YH, Parker CC, Smith AC, Waldron KW. J Agric Food Chem. 2008 Sep 24;56(18):8558-64. PMID:18759449

³⁰ Databases on food phytochemicals and their health-promoting effects. Scalbert A, Andres-Lacueva C, Arita M, Kroon P, Manach C, Urpi-Sarda M, Wishart D. J Agric Food Chem. 2011 May 11;59(9):4331-48. Epub 2011 Apr 12. PMID:21438636

³¹ Dietary intake of 337 polyphenols in French adults. Pérez-Jiménez J, Fezeu L, Touvier M, Arnault N, Manach C, Hercberg S, Galan P, Scalbert A. Am J Clin Nutr. 2011 Jun;93(6):1220-8. PMID:21490142

³² Cyclooxygenase inhibitory and antioxidant cyanidin glycosides in cherries and berries. Seeram NP, Momin RA, Nair MG, Bourquin LD. Phytomedicine. 2001 Sep;8(5):362-9. PMID:11695879

³³ Salicylic acid sans aspirin in animals and man: persistence in fasting and biosynthesis from benzoic acid. Paterson JR, Baxter G, Dreyer JS, Halket JM, Flynn R, Lawrence JR. J Agric Food Chem. 2008 Dec 24;56(24):11648-52. PMID:19053387

³⁴ Biochemical and clinical evidence that aspirin-intolerant asthmatic subjects tolerate the cyclooxygenase 2-selective analgetic drug celecoxib. Gyllfors P, Bochenek G, Overholt J, et al. J Allergy Clin Immunol. 2003 May;111(5):1116-21.PMID: 12743579

³⁵ Tolerability of selective cyclooxygenase inhibitor, celecoxib, in patients with analgesic intolerance. Celik G, Paşaoğlu G, Bavbek S, Abadoğlu O, Dursun B, Mungan D, Misirligil Z. J Asthma. 2005 Mar;42(2):127-31.PMID: 15871445

³⁶ Celecoxib inhibits 5-lipoxygenase. Maier TJ, Tausch L, Hoernig M, Coste O, Schmidt R, Angioni C, Metzner J, Groesch S, Pergola C, Steinhilber D, Werz O, Geisslinger G. Biochem Pharmacol. 2008 Oct 1;76(7):862-72. PMID:1869202

³⁷ Curcumin blocks prostaglandin E2 biosynthesis through direct inhibition of the microsomal prostaglandin E2 synthase-1. Koeberle A, Northoff H, Werz O. Mol Cancer Ther. 2009 Aug;8(8):2348-55. PMID:19671757

³⁸ Cyclooxygenase inhibitory and antioxidant compounds from crabapple fruits. Seeram NP, Cichewicz RH, Chandra A, Nair MG. J Agric Food Chem. 2003 Mar 26;51(7):1948-51. PMID:12643656

³⁹ Curcumin, an atoxic antioxidant and natural NFkappaB, cyclooxygenase-2, lipooxygenase, and inducible nitric oxide synthase inhibitor: a shield against acute and chronic diseases. Bengmark S. JPEN J Parenter Enteral Nutr. 2006 Jan-Feb;30(1):45-51. PMID:16387899

⁴⁰ Luteolin-7-O-glucoside suppresses leukotriene C(4) production and degranulation by inhibiting the phosphorylation of mitogen activated protein kinases and phospholipase Cγ1 in activated mouse bone marrow-derived mast cells. Jin M, Son KH, Chang HW. Biol Pharm Bull. 2011;34(7):1032-6. PMID:21720009

⁴¹ A mechanism of benefit of soy genistein in asthma: inhibition of eosinophil p38-dependent leukotriene synthesis. Kalhan R, Smith LJ, Nlend MC, Nair A, Hixon JL, Sporn PH. Clin Exp Allergy. 2008 Jan;38(1):103-12. PMID:17979994

⁴² Molecular targets of dietary polyphenols with anti-inflammatory properties. Yoon JH, Baek SJ. Yonsei Med J. 2005 Oct 31;46(5):585-96. PMID:16259055

⁴³ Cyclooxygenase inhibitory and antioxidant compounds from the mycelia of the edible mushroom Grifola frondosa. Zhang Y, Mills GL, Nair MG. J Agric Food Chem. 2002 Dec 18;50(26):7581-5. PMID:12475274

⁴⁴ Cyclooxygenase inhibitory and antioxidant compounds from the fruiting body of an edible mushroom, Agrocybe aegerita. Zhang Y, Mills GL, Nair MG. Phytomedicine. 2003;10(5):386-90. PMID:12834003

⁴⁵ Effects of flavonoids on prostaglandin E2 production and on COX-2 and mPGES-1 expressions in activated macrophages. Hämäläinen M, Nieminen R, Asmawi MZ, Vuorela P, Vapaatalo H, Moilanen E. Planta Med. 2011 Sep;77(13):1504-11. PMID:21341175

⁴⁶ Phenol-Explorer Database. Accessed December 2011 http://www.phenol-explorer.eu/foods

⁴⁷ Resveratrol potently reduces prostaglandin E2 production and free radical formation in lipopolysaccharide-activated primary rat microglia. Candelario-Jalil E, de Oliveira AC, Gräf S, Bhatia HS, Hüll M, Muñoz E, Fiebich BL. J Neuroinflammation. 2007 Oct 10;4:25. PMID:17927823

⁴⁸ Curcumin blocks prostaglandin E2 biosynthesis through direct inhibition of the microsomal prostaglandin E2 synthase-1. Koeberle A, Northoff H, Werz O. Mol Cancer Ther. 2009 Aug;8(8):2348-55. PMID:19671757

⁴⁹ Green tea epigallocatechin-3-gallate inhibits microsomal prostaglandin E(2) synthase-1. Koeberle A, Bauer J, Verhoff M, Hoffmann M, Northoff H, Werz O. Biochem Biophys Res Commun. 2009 Oct 16;388(2):350-4. PMID:19665000

⁵⁰ Curcumin blocks prostaglandin E2 biosynthesis through direct inhibition of the microsomal prostaglandin E2 synthase-1. Koeberle A, Northoff H, Werz O. Mol Cancer Ther. 2009 Aug;8(8):2348-55. PMID:19671757

⁵¹ Increased leukotriene production by food additives in patients with atopic dermatitis and proven food intolerance. Worm M, Vieth W, Ehlers I, Sterry W, Zuberbier T. Clin Exp Allergy. 2001 Feb;31(2):265-73.PMID: 11251628

⁵² Novel study on the elicitation of hypersensitive response by polyunsaturated fatty acids in potato tuber. Fanelli C, Castoria R, Fabbri AA, Passi S. Nat Toxins. 1992;1(2):136-46. PMID:1344908

⁵³ Eicosanoids, aspirin-intolerance and the upper airways—current standards and recent improvements of the desensitization therapy. Pfaar O, Klimek L. J Physiol Pharmacol. 2006 Dec;57 Suppl 12:5-13. PMID:17244950

⁵⁴ Improvement of aspirin-intolerant asthma by montelukast, a leukotriene antagonist: a randomized, double-blind, placebo-

controlled trial. Dahlén SE, Malmström K, Nizankowska E, et al. Am J Respir Crit Care Med. 2002 Jan 1;165(1):9-14.PMID: 11779723

[55] Histamine H4 receptor expression is elevated in human nasal polyp tissue. Jókúti A, Hellinger E, Hellinger A, Darvas Z, Falus A, Thurmond RL, Hirschberg A. Cell Biol Int. 2007 Nov;31(11):1367-70. PMID:17611128

[56] Histamine H4 receptor mediates chemotaxis and calcium mobilization of mast cells. Hofstra CL, Desai PJ, Thurmond RL, Fung-Leung WP. J Pharmacol Exp Ther. 2003 Jun;305(3):1212-21. PMID:12626656

[57] Pentasa package insert prescribing information, June 2008

[58] Food-dependent exercise-induced anaphylaxis. Morita E, Kunie K, Matsuo H. J Dermatol Sci. 2007 Aug;47(2):109-17. PMID:17507204

[59] Omega-3 fatty acids suppress the enhanced production of 5-lipoxygenase products from polymorph neutrophil granulocytes in cystic fibrosis. Keicher U, Koletzko B, Reinhardt D. Eur J Clin Invest. 1995 Dec;25(12):915-9. PMID:8719931

[60] Control of salicylate intolerance with fish oils. Healy E, Newell L, Howarth P, Friedmann PS. Br J Dermatol. 2008 Dec;159(6):1368-9. Epub 2008 Sep 15.PMID: 18795922

[61] Ligand-operated synthesis of 4-series and 5-series leukotrienes in human neutrophils: critical dependence on exogenous free fatty acid supply. Grimminger F, Dürr U, Seeger W. Mol Pharmacol. 1992 Apr;41(4):757-66. PMID:1569925

[62] Tissue-specific, nutritional, and developmental regulation of rat fatty acid elongases. Wang Y, Botolin D, Christian B, Busik J, Xu J, Jump DB. J Lipid Res. 2005 Apr;46(4):706-15. Epub 2005 Jan 16. PMID:15654130

[63] 5-Oxo-ETE is a major oxidative stress-induced arachidonate metabolite in B lymphocytes. Grant GE, Gravel S, Guay J, Patel P, Mazer BD, Rokach J, Powell WS. Free Radic Biol Med. 2011 May 15;50(10):1297-304. Epub 2011 Feb 18. PMID:21334434

[64] Analysis of the roles of smoking and allergy in nasal polyposis. Görgülü O, Ozdemir S, Canbolat EP, Sayar C, Olgun MK, Akbaş Y. Ann Otol Rhinol Laryngol. 2012 Sep;121(9):615-9. PMID:23012901

[65] Do corticosteroids induce apoptosis in nasal polyp inflammatory cells? In vivo and in vitro studies. Saunders MW, Wheatley AH, George SJ, Lai T, Birchall MA. Laryngoscope. 1999 May;109(5):785-90. PMID:10334231

[66] Induction of apoptosis in nasal polyp fibroblasts by glucocorticoids in vitro. Hirano S, Asano K, Namba M, Kanai K, Hisamitsu T, Suzaki H. Acta Otolaryngol. 2003 Dec;123(9):1075-9. PMID:14710911

[67] Mechanism of action of glucocorticoids in nasal polyposis. Fernandes AM, Valera FC, Anselmo-Lima WT. Braz J Otorhinolaryngol. 2008 Mar-Apr;74(2):279-83. PMID:18568209

[68] Regression of polypoid nasal mucosa after systemic corticosteroid therapy: a proteomics study. Farajzadeh Deroee A, Oweinah J, Naraghi M, Hosemann W, Athari B, Völker U, Scharf C. Am J Rhinol Allergy. 2009 Sep-Oct;23(5):480-5. PMID:19723368

16. Reactions to Enzymes in Food and Effects of Cooking

Plant Enzyme Reactions

A food reaction that is sometimes mistaken for an allergic reaction can result from the enzymatic activity of the food. Enzymes are great allergens; parasites use enzymes to help invade our bodies; thus, our immune system tends to be suspicious and will often form antibodies to enzymes. It is enzymes in pollen that people become highly sensitized to. Many immune reactions to food allergens are due to enzymes, but enzymes also have direct, non-immunogenic actions, which cause adverse reactions.

Meat tenderizers, which usually contain papain, from papaya; or bromelain, from pineapple, act as proteolytic enzymes that help break down proteins in meat. This occurs in living flesh, as well and likely has happened to you. The most notable example is pineapple, especially when harvested before it has completely ripened. This fruit contains the enzymes bromelain, ananain, and comosain[1], which are proteolytic; they break down protein, including those that make up the mucous membranes of the mouth. When in high concentrations, these enzymes irritate, burn, and even cause bleeding in the mouth and throat. Caution should be exercised in giving fresh pineapple to small children who may suck on it and get "burns" in their mouths. Another example is melons, which contain enzymes that can cause an irritated or itchy throat.

Smoothies prepared with certain fresh fruits (pineapple, papaya, cantaloupe, kiwi or fig) with milk curdle and turn bitter after a few minutes of making them. This is the effect of proteolytic enzymes acting on the proteins in the milk, and exposing bitter-tasting amino acids. The label on a box of gelatin warns that these fruits will prevent the gel from setting. This results from proteolytic enzymes in the fruit breaking down collagen proteins in gelatin.

Heating fruit to above 60° C (140° F) will denature most proteolytic enzymes found in them. Fruits are heated during canning; thus, enzymes in canned fruits are usually inactivated. Fresh fruit can be heated in a microwave to denature the proteolytic enzymes, before making smoothies or gelatin desserts.

Note: True allergic reactions to the fruits listed in Table 16-1 are common, and heating the fruit is very unlikely to prevent those reactions. The direct, local effect of these enzymes on mucous membranes of the mouth often occurs as a result of direct contact with these enzymes rather than as an immune response. Non-local reactions (i.e.; hives, rhinitis, asthma, and anaphylaxis) suggest an immune-mediated response. Pineapple and figs are also high in tryptamine, and thus could also contribute to a pseudoallergic reaction.

Table 16-1: Fruits with Proteolytic Enzymes

• Papaya
• Pineapple
• Figs
• Melons
• Kiwi Fruit

Cooked Food Allergenicity and Toxicity

Some individuals may find that they have immune reactivity to a raw foods, but not if the food is cooked. Recall that the primary structure of a protein is the amino acid order in the chain forms the protein. The secondary structure is the folded shape the protein takes. When protein is heated, its secondary, tertiary or quaternary structure may be denatured. Cooking (in water) can also hydrolyze some proteins. Cooking eggs, which causes cross-linking, makes them more digestible; only 6% of the proteins in a cooked egg escaped digestion and absorption in the small intestine of healthy volunteers, while 35% of the protein in raw eggs escaped digestion. Much of the undigested proteins showed up in the urine as products of bacterial fermentation[2], and many of these are toxic.

If an individual has an immune response to the protein structure of a raw food, cooking, especially pressure cooking in water (higher temperature and longer time in water promote hydrolysis of proteins) it may decrease of eliminate the protein's immunogenicity.

Papayas, cantaloupes, and pineapples are common food immunogens. In some individuals, cooked or canned pineapple does not provoke an immune reaction while raw pineapple does. This is the result of having some of its enzymes denatured. Melons and papaya are not usually served cooked.

The immune system can also react to peptides from partially disassembled proteins. The primary structure of the protein usually does not change with most cooking methods. Digestion may cut the proteins into peptide fragments that are more immunogenic. The immune response to the primary structure or to one of its fragments may remain immunogenic. Cooking may occasionally make proteins more antigenic as the immune-reacting portion of the proteins may become more exposed[3].

Fruits are not the only foods that containing proteins with metabolic effects. Potatoes contain several proteins that prevent protein digestion. These include including a trypsin inhibitor, a kallikrein inhibitor, and an enterokinase inhibitor. Potatoes also contain hemagglutinin; which can cause red blood cells to clump. Animals given raw potatoes in their feed grow more slowly and have poor utilization of protein in their feed. Most, but not all of these proteins, are inactivated by cooking the potatoes[4]. Potatoes should not be eaten raw.

Potatoes also contain carboxypeptidase inhibitor, a protein which is not denatured by cooking. The carboxypeptidase inhibitor causes the release of CCK in the intestine, slowing gastric emptying, increasing satiation and decreasing appetite, thus making meals with boiled or baked (but not fried) potatoes[5] helpful for weight loss[6]. Carboxypeptidase inhibitor may, however, inhibit the digestion of certain proteins. Potatoes also contain lipoxygenase-5, which may help form leukotrienes in the intestinal lumen. Potatoes also contain a lectin which can trigger mast cell degranulation (Chapter 14).

Recommendations

1. Localized reaction to raw fruit: Some fruits, especially when not completely ripe, contain proteolytic enzymes that can cause local irritation in the mouth and mucous membranes. Heating fruit to 60-70°C (160°F) denatures most of these enzymes. This can prevent irritation of the oral mucous membranes and prevent smoothies containing milk from turning bitter.

2. Cooking foods may make proteins more or less allergenic: Cooking foods in an attempt to make them less immunogenic is not a safe strategy for foods to which a person is highly allergic; the temperature at which the allergen may be denatured is different for different proteins and may be well above cooking temperatures. Thus, while it may be effective for some foods, it may not be for others. It is possible that eating a food that is usually served and does not cause an immune reaction when cooked, may provoke an unexpected reaction if consumed raw. Allergy tests that use cooked foods to prepare antigens may give false-negative results for the food if it is consumed raw.

3. Not all foods are safe raw: There are many reasons to cook food. These include killing bacteria and parasites, denaturing proteins, and hydrating starches to make them more digestible. Foods which are traditionally eaten only after cooking usually have good reason for it.

While many fruits evolved as bait, to increase dispersion of their seeds, tubers serve as energy storage areas for plants. Tubers often contain toxins to prevent them from being eaten by insects and animals. Potatoes contain proteins which are anti-nutritive when eaten raw and prevent protein digestion. Cassava (yucca) contains cyanogenic glycosides, which are metabolized into cyanide. Large fractions of these toxins are destroyed or removed during cooking. Kidney beans and some other edible beans contain phytohemagglutinin which is toxic if not destroyed by cooking at boiling temperature.

Proteins and starches that are consumed raw may be poorly digested. Undigested proteins ferment in the colon, forming bioactive, often toxic compounds including ammonia. Foods that are traditionally only consumed after cooking should not be assumed to be safely consumed as a raw food.

---

[1] Purification and characterization of multiple forms of the pineapple-stem-derived cysteine proteinases ananain and comosain. Napper AD, Bennett SP, Borowski M, Holdridge MB, Leonard MJ, Rogers EE, Duan Y, Laursen RA, Reinhold B, Shames SL. Biochem J. 1994 Aug 1;301 (Pt 3):727-35. PMID: 8053898

[2] Amount and fate of egg protein escaping assimilation in the small intestine of humans. Evenepoel P, Claus D, Geypens B, et al. Am J Physiol. 1999 Nov;277(5 Pt 1):G935-43. PMID:10564098

[3] Allergic reactions during allergy skin testing with food allergens. Pitsios C, Dimitriou A, Kontou-Fili K. Eur Ann Allergy Clin Immunol. 2009 Aug;41(4):126-8. PMID:19877567

[4] Handbook of Vegetable Science and Technology (Food Science and Technology) by D. K. Salunkhe and S. S. Kadam (Mar 1, 1998) CRC Press

[5] A satiety index of common foods. Holt SH, Miller JC, Petocz P, Farmakalidis E. Eur J Clin Nutr. 1995 Sep;49(9):675-90. PMID: 7498104

[6] Potato protease inhibitors inhibit food intake and increase circulating cholecystokinin levels by a trypsin-dependent mechanism. Komarnytsky S, Cook A, Raskin I. Int J Obes (Lond). 2011 Feb;35(2):236-43. Epub 2010 Sep 7. PMID: 20820171

17. CHOCOLATE AND WINE: THE DARK SIDE

Chocolate and Sleep: Chocolate can disturb sleep. Chocolate contains caffeine; less than coffee, but depending on the individual and the amount consumed, there may be sufficient caffeine to prevent sleep. Chocolate also contains the alkaloid theobromine, a methylxanthine compound similar to caffeine, but at a level several times higher than its caffeine content. Like caffeine, theobromine binds to adenosine receptors, stimulates wakefulness and may cause insomnia. Theobromine's effect on wakefulness, however, is milder than that of caffeine. Caffeine is partially metabolized into theobromine. Black and green tea, cola, and guarana also contain caffeine and theobromine.

Caffeine   Theobromine

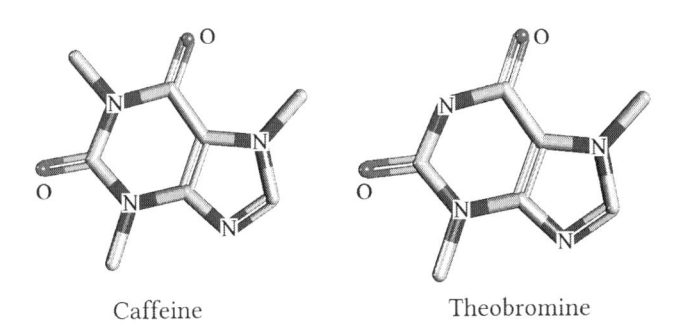

Figure 17-1: Structural Similarity of Caffeine and Theobromine

For most individuals, the half-life of theobromine (TBr) is from five to nine hours[1]. This means that 25% of the TBr is still present in their system 14 hours after the ingestion of chocolate. For someone who metabolizes TBr slowly, the TBr can accumulate from one day to the next. Most people can enjoy small amounts of dark chocolate early in the day to give an energy boost. However, consuming dark chocolate late in the day may provoke insomnia and irritability. Sleep disturbances from chocolate may be avoided by limiting the amounts of dark chocolate consumed, and having milk or white chocolate in the afternoon or early evening. Even small amounts of milk chocolate may be too much for children.

Death by Chocolate

The toxicity of chocolate to pets from theobromine in is well documented and occasionally featured as dark humor in popular media. When pets eat chocolate, the effects of TBr toxicity include nausea, vomiting, diarrhea, and increased urination. Poisoning can also cause seizures, cardiac arrhythmia, and death.

Less well known is that TBr poisoning from ingestion of chocolate also occurs in humans. Theobromine toxicity is rarely recognized, but it can present in the emergency department, usually as smaller women, with confusion and difficulty in walking. It looks like what it is: drug overdose or poisoning.

Chocolate poisoning, assumed to be caused by excessive TBr, causes hyperventilation, which may trigger panic attack symptoms; confusion, anxiety, agitation, emotional lability, increased urination, hypotension, and tachycardia. Ataxia (difficulty walking) and slurring of the speech have also been reported. Seizures and cardiac dysrhythmias can occur from TBr toxicity[1].

The usual minimal toxic dose of TBr in humans is about 10 mg per pound (25 mg/kg) of body weight. At this dose, the toxic effects may include sweating, nausea, anorexia, trembling and severe headache. This may occur in adults consuming 800 to 1500 mg of TBr in a day. White chocolate has very low levels of TBr, and a 1½ ounce Hershey milk chocolate bar only has about 75 mg of theobromine. Dark chocolate, however, has much higher levels; an extra dark chocolate bar can have five times the TBr content per ounce as milk chocolate. A three-ounce extra dark 82% cacao bar has 733 mg of theobromine (plus 113 mg of caffeine). Spread over several hours, most adults might enjoy a pleasant pharmacologic stimulus without ill effect. Consumption of two dark chocolate bars or its equivalent in brownies, fudge, cake, ice cream and beverages in a small adult in less than a couple of hours can be sufficient to win a siren award; with flashing lights, a gurney, a bag of saline, and a mad dash to hospital.

Theobromine is metabolized by cytochrome P450 enzymes in the liver. Two different enzymes' CYP2E1 and CYP1A2, appear to be responsible for this process; however, there is genetic variability, and CYP1A2 does not process TBr in some individuals[2]. Further, these enzymes can be inhibited by certain medications, such as Tagamet, ciprofloxacin, contraceptives, and caffeine; or foods, such as certain mushrooms and grapefruit. Enzyme activity is genetically and epigenetically determined, and less active in some people. CYP2E1 and CYP1A2 activity are often lower in the elderly, because of slower metabolism, and from use of medications. Children may be at risk because of their smaller body mass. Like alcohol, where consumption of two drinks over several hours is unlikely to cause intoxication, but a couple of shots, over a few minutes, can have a potent effect, larger amounts of chocolate over a short time raise blood levels of TBr higher, and induce more risk of toxicity, especially on an empty stomach.

Chocolate and Behavior: Chocolate consumption can trigger hyperactivity, emotional lability and irritability. This is especially evident in children who are susceptible as they are likely to consume more chocolate, in relation to their body mass.

When my children were small, chocolate was banished from the home; not because of the great highs, with my kids bouncing on the bed, the singing, silliness and laughter, but because of the terrible tears and fits that followed, lasting longer than the bliss. This response to chocolate is likely the combined effects of caffeine, theobromine, β-phenylethylamine (βPEA) and sugar. Children's frontal lobes are less developed giving them less control over their emotions and behavior. Thus, children's behavior is more strongly affected by chocolate than is adult behavior.

β-PEA and tyramine are strong agonists for the trace amine receptors TAAR1 and TAAR2. βPEA has been described as the body's endogenous amphetamine[3]. The hyperactivity and pleasure derived chocolate may result from an amphetamine-like effect of βPEA and release of NE from nerve terminals. Some chocolate preparations also contain food coloring that may provoke hyperactivity (See Chapters 39).

Chocolate Headaches: In addition to the toxic effects of TBr, other natural compounds in chocolate can trigger headaches, even at low doses. βPEA from food is usually metabolized quickly by monoamine oxidase (MAO), and thus, has a half-life of only several minutes. MAO-inhibiting medications, however, can cause great increases in the amount of tyramine and βPEA reaching the brain. Amine oxidase, copper containing 1 (AOC1), which breaks down histamine and other bioamines, is inhibited by theobromine, caffeine, βPEA and TBr, all found in chocolate. Thus, chocolate may trigger migraine in part by inhibiting enzymes that break down histamine and other bioamines.

When chocolate provokes migraine, it usually occurs 10 or more hours after consuming the chocolate. This suggests a secondary reaction, rather than the direct action of βPEA. βPEA is a preferred ligand for trace amine receptors in the brain, and the delayed onset of migraine suggests action via the calcitonin gene-related peptide (CGRP). The role of CGRP on migraines is discussed in Chapter 28, on headaches. Caffeine withdrawal can also trigger rebound headaches, and this may also occur with theobromine.

Immune Reactions: The delayed adverse reaction to chocolate which results in migraine suggests the induction of protein synthesis, as occurs with CGRP and migraine, or may be secondary to delayed (IgG) hypersensitivity reaction requiring the formation of leukotrienes or other secondary responses. Immunologic reactions can also affect sleep and cause irritability and fatigue. Chocolate can also trigger immediate (IgE) allergic reactions. Individuals with immune reactions to chocolate should avoid it completely.

Osteoporosis: Daily chocolate consumption has been found to lower bone density in women[4]. Consumption of high levels of caffeine, more than 3 cups of coffee a day, is also associated with an increased risk of osteoporosis.

Osteoporosis and its prevention and treatment are discussed in Chapter 43.

Benefits of Chocolate

Having rained on one of life's pleasures, casting it as a potentially malevolent toxin and immuno-villain, it is only fair to note the positive aspects chocolate merits.

Excuses for loving chocolate:

It tastes great.
It makes you feel good.
Gifts of chocolate can promote positive relationships with women.
It makes you feel good.
It tastes great.

Aside from the pleasure of chocolate, dark chocolate is rich in polyphenols with health benefits.

- It lowers blood pressure in persons with hypertension[5].
- Flavanoid-rich chocolate increases blood flow to the coronary arteries[6].
- It improves insulin sensitivity and beta cell function in persons with insulin resistance[7].
- It may prevent LDL cholesterol from becoming oxidized and may increase HDL cholesterol[8].
- It may improve symptoms in patients with chronic fatigue syndrome[9].
- Several studies have failed to find any increase in body weight associated with dark chocolate consumption.
- It has anti-inflammatory properties[10] and may decrease the formation of TNF-α in response to LPS (See Chapter 23).

Most of the health benefits of chocolate, including its antioxidant activity, results from chocolate's content of phenolic compounds, which is higher than those of black or green tea or red wine[11]. The phenolic compounds are richest in dark chocolate, such as bittersweet dark chocolate. In general, the phenolic content of chocolate is: cocoa powder > baking chocolate > dark chocolate or bittersweet baking chips > milk chocolate > chocolate syrup[12].

It appears that there may be a sweet spot for the health effects of dark chocolate. For blood pressure control, 20 grams of dark chocolate daily were found to be equally effective as 40 grams[13]. In another study[10], the most beneficial anti-inflammatory effect appeared to be associated with consuming one to three servings of dark chocolate a week, with a serving size of about twenty grams.

Therefore, I submit for use the "Dark Chocolate Serving Equivalent" in which one serving is equivalent to 20 grams of 70 – 75% dark chocolate, as provided in Table 17-1, as an appropriate adult serving size for healthful consumption.

Table 17-1: Dark Chocolate Serving Equivalents

Chocolate	Serving Equivalents
Cocoa powder	1 tablespoon
Baking chocolate	1 tablespoon
Dark chocolate or baking chips	20 grams – 0.7 ounces
70-75% Dark chocolate bar	@ ¼ of a 3-oz. bar or 1/5 of a 3.5-oz. bar

If the health benefits are the excuse to justify eating chocolate, then dark chocolate high in polyphenols should be selected, and the amount consumed should be limited to about one "dark chocolate serving equivalent" per day, best dosed at 1 to 3 times a week. A tablespoon of cocoa is about the amount that might be used in a cup of mild hot chocolate, or a thin slice of chocolate cake.

New methods of preparing chocolate are being developed to help preserve and enhance polyphenol content. The bioavailability of these phenolic compounds will determine the optimal daily content for health.

Phenols are a large class of chemical compounds found in foods, and science is just beginning to ask the questions as to which phenolic compounds contribute to health and how they act. Various phenolic compounds in foods have antioxidant, anti-inflammatory, and antibiotic effects. Although generally considered healthful and benign, some dietary phenolic compounds may induce disease reactions in some individuals, as discussed in chapter 15, and some may not be safe in high doses during pregnancy for the developing fetus. Thus, it is prudent to consume phenols from a variety of healthy food sources, including spices, herbs, olives, capers, citrus fruits, dark grapes wine and berries. Use of refined phenolic compounds, such as found in supplements, should be avoided during pregnancy unless they have been approved for that use.

Just to be complete: There may be another adverse effect to chocoholism; Jeanne Calment, who regularly ate 7 ounces of chocolate a day, died soon after her doctor convinced her to cut back on sweets, at the age of 122 [14].

Summary for Chocolate

1. Chocolate is a source of phenolic compounds: Chocolate is a healthful food high in phenolic compounds. Consuming one chocolate equivalent a day (0.7 oz. of dark chocolate) three times a week appears to be sufficient to provide the optimal health benefits from chocolate.

2. Chocolate can be toxic in high doses Enjoy it in moderation. The pharmacologic effects of chocolate can cause behavioral effects, especially in children. Keep it away from animals.

3. Chocolate is a stimulant and can cause insomnia.

4. Chocolate can cause both immune and pseudoallergic reactions.

5. Chocolate is a common trigger for migraine headaches. See chapter 28.

Wine

WARNING: Alcohol is a toxin, and toxic amounts should be avoided. Even small amounts of alcohol should be considered toxic in children. Alcohol can also lead to dependence in many individuals. Alcohol is a teratogen and causes fetal alcohol syndrome and thus should be avoided in women who are or may be pregnant. Alcohol is a carcinogen at levels which cause intoxication.

Wine is another food consumed for pleasure, which can cause idiosyncratic disease even when used in the small amounts that promote health in most individuals. While most alcoholic beverages are associated with obesity, consumption of moderate amounts of red wine (three to four ounces a day) is associated with a lower body mass index in women. Red wine contains phenolic compounds that are thought to have health benefits, including lowered risk for cardiovascular disease.

Nevertheless, many individuals have adverse reactions to wine, including flushing, shortness of breath and headaches following its consumption. To understand these reactions, it is helpful to understand how wine is made.

Winemaking 101:

In making wine, the grapes are crushed to form "must": grape juice with the pulp, skin, and seeds are included. The winemaker determines how long the must sits before separating out the juice and adding the yeast. During this first stage, putrescine, cadaverine, and phenylethylamine can be formed by wild bacteria and wild yeast. Wine yeast is then added for the alcoholic fermentation, and low levels of ethylamine and phenylethylamine may be formed.

Next, the winemaker usually adds a *Lactobacillus* culture for malolactic fermentation. Grapes grown in cooler regions have higher levels of malic acid, which makes them tart and gives the wine a green apple flavor. The malolactic fermentation step turns some of the tart malic acid into the milder, and more buttery tasting, lactic acid.

The malolactic fermentation process is the main mechanism of biogenic amine formation in wine, especially of histamine, tyramine, and putrescine[15]. The strain of bacteria used has a large effect on the amount of bioamines produced. Thus, some wines have less biogenic amine content than others. Red wines often have higher tyramine levels and sake (rice wine) often has high histamine levels[16].

Commercially cultured bacteria used in wine making are usually selected to avoid strains of bacteria that produce high levels of biogenic amines. More traditional methods of wine making, however, use wild yeast and bacteria that permit less control over the taste of the wine and the levels of bioamines formed in it.

Sulfites are then added to stop the fermentation process before bottling, but they also halt the further conversion of amino acids into bioamines. Without sulfites, fermentation would continue in the bottle, causing cloudiness, CO_2 production, and spoiling the wine's flavor.

Port wine is produced by adding distilled wine alcohol to the grape must, thereby stopping the fermentation process at a point where only about half of the grape sugars have been fermented into alcohol. The port is then aged. This gives a sweet wine with higher alcohol content.

Wine Allergy and Pseudo Allergic Reactions

Alcoholic beverages, and wine especially, can trigger flushing, sneezing, migraine, asthmatic attack, or even anaphylactoid reactions. These histamine-like reactions do not necessarily correlate with the amount of histamine in the wine, and higher levels of plasma histamine are sometimes found after the reaction than can be attributed to the amount consumed[15]. These effects from wine may be caused by:

1. Allergic reaction to wine or to a contaminant in the wine.
2. A reaction to biogenic amines such as tyramine and phenylethylamine in the wine.
3. The inhibition of AOC1 by alcohol and inhibition of AOC1 and HNMT by bioamines in the wine. This is especially problematic for individuals with marginal MAO, AOC1, or ALDH2 activity.
4. Histamine or tyramine in food or formed in the gut by other foods consumed at the same time as wine, with the alcohol decreasing AOC1 activity.
5. Sulfites in the wine can cause mast cell degranulation in some individuals.
6. The combination of these factors.

Wine Allergy: Immediate type 1 allergic reaction to wines are not common but do occur. Allergic reactions to wine, including oral allergy syndrome (local burning or itching of the mucosa of the mouth), flushing, and asthma; anaphylaxis can occur.

IgE testing for wine allergy, however, is not straightforward. A large percentage of heavy drinkers of alcohol test positive to Cross-reactive Carbohydrate Determinants (CCD)[17]. CCD are n-glycans present in plants and insects. These n-glycans cross-react with hymenoptera (bee/wasp) venom, latex, and peanuts. Thus, heavy drinkers will show positive IgE results, but not have allergic reactions to these allergens.

There are enzymes in wine that some individuals are allergic to; however, heavy drinkers may have IgE which binds to these proteins, but which does not provoke allergic reaction to them[18], perhaps, as a result of desensitization by IgG_4. Individuals who have an allergic reaction to wine tend to react to young wine and red wines[19]. Lighter drinkers may react with hymenoptera venom, even when having no history of exposure to stings. Hymenoptera venom may be present in wine from wasps or bees which get crushed along with the grapes during harvest.

Bioamine Reactions: Biogenic amines in the wine inhibit AOC1, thus blocking the breakdown of histamine, which can provoke migraine or other histamine reactions. For example, an individual prone to migraines may eat a meal that would usually produce some histamine, but not enough to reach a migraine-triggering threshold. The accompanying acetaldehyde formed from alcohol can decrease the breakdown of histamine, tyramine, and phenylethylamine. Adding, even small amounts of putrescine or other polyamines that inhibit AOC1 can raise the levels enough to trigger a migraine. As little as 6 mg of tyramine or as little as 2.5 mg of histamine in half a liter of wine can provoke a migraine, levels not unusual in wine. The bioamines also prevent the catabolism of acetaldehyde by ALDH2, which is a major factor causing hangover headaches. (Bioamines are discussed in Chapter 13)

Sulfites: Almost all wine contains sulfites, especially white wines and dessert wines. In addition to the sulfite used to stop fermentation, there are some naturally occurring sulfites in grapes. Sulfites can trigger anaphylactoid reactions through mast cell degranulation, but do not cause migraines. (See Chapter 14 for more details).

Wine During Pregnancy

South African mothers of children with *partial* fetal alcohol syndrome reported drinking five drinks a week, but mostly on weekends, and three drinks at a time[20]. Partial fetal alcohol syndrome is a severe condition in which there are cranial deformities and large losses in IQ levels, associated with peak blood alcohol content of 0.102 during the third trimester (the period of highest susceptibility to damage)[21]. This level of blood alcohol may be associated with disinhibition, impairment in reasoning and depth perception, staggering and slurring of the speech. Clearly this level is toxic and not moderate intake. It is peak alcohol level that appears to be most damaging.

One drink (5 ounces of wine) contains 0.6 ounces of alcohol; enough to raise the blood alcohol to 0.05% in a 100-pound woman. Driving with this blood level or higher is considered "driving under the influence" in most countries. Children with prenatal exposure to even light alcohol consumption [more than zero, but less than 0.3 ounces of alcohol a day (2.5 ounces of wine; half a drink)] are more than three times more likely to with have elevated scores on externalizing behavior (aggressive and delinquent) and internalizing behavior (anxious/depressed and withdrawn) syndrome scales[22]. In utero exposure to alcohol also likely increases the risk of breast cancer in the offspring[23].

Alcohol up-regulates the expression of TLR4 and TLR2 on microglial cells in the brain, activating an inflammatory response and inducing the production of inflammatory cytokines and reactive oxygen species. This causes apoptosis of neurons[24], in a similar mechanism to that which promotes chronic inflammatory brain damage after traumatic brain injury. Resveratrol, in red wine, may impede the inflammatory cascade initiated by TLR activation. Alcohol also impedes production of nerve growth factors.

Alcohol should be completely avoided during pregnancy. If a woman is pregnant and can feel the effects of alcohol – she has achieved a level toxic to the fetal brain. There is no benefit, and no justification for exposing a child to severe, lifelong harm.

> Men: Paternal alcohol consumption prior to conception can have detrimental effects on the physical and mental development of offspring, even when there is no alcohol exposure during pregnancy. Alcohol reduces the activity of DNA methyltransferase enzymes, causing hypomethylation of DNA, and aberrant expression of normally silent genes in the sperm[25]. Paternal fetal alcohol syndrome not only affects the child's development, but also decreases the offspring's fertility, and may even affect subsequent generations[26].
>
> It takes about 90 days for sperm to develop from stem cells. It is prudent for men planning on fathering a child to avoid more than limited alcohol intake (more than one drink on any day) for three months prior to expected conception.

For adults, outside of pregnancy, a limit of one ounce of red wine per day, for every 30 pounds of body weight, consumed with a meal is probably insufficient to cause mood disorders, and may have health benefits. Other forms of alcohol, such as beer and spirits, do not offer health benefits.

> Alcohol as a Sexual Lubricant
>
> Even in marital relationships, alcohol is often employed, especially by women, to lower sexual inhibition or reluctance. Alcohol, however, suppresses the release of oxytocin, which is normally released during gentle touch, physical intimacy, and orgasm. Thus, alcohol prevents oxytocin-induced promotion of emotional bonding, the experience of intimacy, and romance. Use of alcohol during intimate contact can reduce the appetite for future sexual pairing and thus reinforce the requirement for alcohol as a sexual lubrication. Without oxytocin to reinforce bonding, sexual activity is dry and can lead to the failure of intimacy.

Excuses for Enjoying Red Wine

Red wines (consumed in moderation: three or four ounces a day) contain antioxidant polyphenols, which appear to prevent the oxidative damage caused by alcohol. Thus, of various alcoholic beverages consumed, red wines stand out as having low chronic toxicity. Rats given red wine do not have accelerated lipofuscin in their brains, compared to control rats while rats given equal amounts of distilled alcohol have accelerated lipofuscin accumulation[27].

Red wines, particularly Pinot Noir, Cabernet Sauvignon, Merlot, Egiodola, and Syrah varietals, are high in polyphenols such as catechins[28]. Red port wine, however, does not provide this benefit[29]. This may be a result of the early termination of fermentation in port, preventing the processing of polyphenols into bioactive, absorbable forms. Tannins are large polyphenolic molecules and are not absorbed, however, fermentation promotes decomposition into smaller, absorbable phenolic compounds.

Secondly, the higher sugar content of port is problematic. In an animal model, alcohol with a sugar content equivalent to that of port wine was significantly more damaging to the neurons than was the same amount of alcohol consumed alone[30]. These data suggest that sweet alcoholic beverages should be considered more toxic to the neurons and other cells, and suggest that red wine not be consumed with sweets. Wine consumed with a meal is absorbed more slowly, helping to mitigate peak alcohol levels, compared with the same quantity consumed on an empty stomach.

Summary for Wine

1. Alcohol is toxic. Red wine in moderation can be consumed by most adults without increased risk of chronic disease and may provide health benefits including lower risk of heart disease and obesity. Moderation means limiting intake to no more than one ounce of red wine per 30 pounds of ideal body weight day per. Other forms of alcohol cannot be justified by health benefits. Sweet wines and port should not be considered as having health benefits. The consumption of wine or other forms of alcohol with sweets or desserts may increase the toxicity of alcohol, and these combinations should be avoided.

2. Wine can increase the risk of migraines and pseudoallergic reactions: Wine contains sulfites some individuals react to (Chapter 14). Wine, depending on its fermentation, may contain biogenic amines that trigger migraines or block the enzymes that break down biogenic amines. Alcohol can inhibit these enzymes. Wines from California, for example, usually use bacteria specifically cultured to avoid production of bioamines, and thus may not provoke pseudoallergic reactions as much as wines using wild bacteria, such as traditionally used in Portugal. Foods consumed with wine, such as aged cheeses or salami, may contain biogenic amines, and alcohol can decrease the ability the body's enzymes to break these compounds down. Foods consumed with alcohol may interact and provoke migraine or other pseudoallergic reactions.

3. Alcohol is a teratogen and a carcinogen: Alcohol should not be consumed, even in moderation, during pregnancy to avoid the risk of injury to the child. Men should avoid heavy drinking for three months prior to planned conception.

Alcohol is also a carcinogen, and if health is a concern, consumption should not exceed one ounce of red wine per 30 pounds ideal body weight a day for most individuals. Some individuals may be at higher risk and should avoid alcohol completely to avoid risk of cancer (See Chapter 41). Some of the effects of alcohol are caused by an increased production of oxygen free radicals. Trimethylglycine (TMG; betaine) a vitamin-like compound found in vegetables, may attenuate this risk[31].

4. Red wine contains healthful phenol compounds: True, however, the amount per serving is less than found in chocolate, tea, coffee, plums, beans and many other foods. There is no unique health advantage to drinking wine that is not available with other foods. If red wine is enjoyed, consumption of moderate amounts is reasonable for many adults.

---

[1] National Library of Medicine Hazardous Substances Data Bank

[2] Cytochrome P450 isoform selectivity in human hepatic theobromine metabolism. Gates S, Miners JO. Br J Clin Pharmacol. 1999 Mar;47(3):299-305.PMID: 10215755

[3] Trace amines: identification of a family of mammalian G protein-coupled receptors. Borowsky B, Adham N, Jones KA, et al. Proc Natl Acad Sci U S A. 2001 Jul 31;98(16):8966-71. PMID:11459929

[4] Chocolate consumption and bone density in older women. Hodgson JM, Devine A, Burke V, Dick IM, Prince RL. Am J Clin Nutr. 2008 Jan;87(1):175-80.PMID: 18175753

[5] Does chocolate reduce blood pressure? A meta-analysis. Ried K, Sullivan T, Fakler P, Frank OR, Stocks NP. BMC Med. 2010 Jun 28;8:39.PMID: 20584271

[6] Acute effect of oral flavonoid-rich dark chocolate intake on coronary circulation, as compared with non-flavonoid white chocolate, by transthoracic Doppler echocardiography in healthy adults. Shiina Y, Funabashi N, Lee K, et al. Int J Cardiol. 2009 Jan 24;131(3):424-9..PMID: 18045712

[7] Blood pressure is reduced and insulin sensitivity increased in glucose-intolerant, hypertensive subjects after 15 days of consuming high-polyphenol dark chocolate. Grassi D, Desideri G, Necozione S, et al. J Nutr. 2008 Sep;138(9):1671-6.PMID: 18716168

[8] Continuous intake of polyphenolic compounds containing cocoa powder reduces LDL oxidative susceptibility and has beneficial effects on plasma HDL-cholesterol concentrations in humans. Baba S, Osakabe N, Kato Y, et al. Am J Clin Nutr. 2007 Mar;85(3):709-17.PMID: 17344491

[9] High cocoa polyphenol rich chocolate may reduce the burden of the symptoms in chronic fatigue syndrome. Sathyapalan T, Beckett S, Rigby AS, Mellor DD, Atkin SL. Nutr J. 2010 Nov 22;9(1):55. PMID: 21092175

[10] Regular consumption of dark chocolate is associated with low serum concentrations of C-reactive protein in a healthy Italian population. di Giuseppe R, Di Castelnuovo A, Centritto F, et al. J Nutr. 2008 Oct;138(10):1939-45.PMID: 18806104

[11] Cocoa has more phenolic phytochemicals and a higher antioxidant capacity than teas and red wine. Lee KW, Kim YJ, Lee HJ, Lee CY. J Agric Food Chem. 2003 Dec 3;51(25):7292-5.PMID: 14640573

[12] Survey of commercially available chocolate- and cocoa-containing products in the United States. 2. Comparison of flavan-3-ol content with nonfat cocoa solids, total polyphenols, and percent cacao. Miller KB, Hurst WJ, Flannigan N, et al. J Agric Food Chem. 2009 Oct 14;57(19):9169-80.PMID: 19754118

[13] The effect of polyphenol-rich dark chocolate on fasting capillary whole blood glucose, total cholesterol, blood pressure and glucocorticoids in healthy overweight and obese subjects. Almoosawi S, Fyfe L, Ho C, Al-Dujaili E. Br J Nutr. 2010 Mar;103(6):842-50. PMID: 19825207

[14] Jeanne Calment, World's Elder, Dies at 122. Whitney, CR. New York Times, August 5, 1997

[15] Formation of biogenic amines throughout the industrial manufacture of red wine. Marcobal A, Martín-Alvarez PJ, Polo MC, Muñoz R, Moreno-Arribas MV. J Food Prot. 2006 Feb;69(2):397-404. PMID:16496582

[16] Analysis of neuroactive amines in fermented beverages using a portable microchip capillary electrophoresis system. Jayarajah CN, Skelley AM, Fortner AD, Mathies RA. Anal Chem. 2007 Nov 1;79(21):8162-9. PMID:17892274

[17] Sensitization to cross-reactive carbohydrate determinants in relation to alcohol consumption. Gonzalez-Quintela A, Garrido M, Gude F, et al. Clin Exp Allergy. 2008 Jan;38(1):152-60. PMID:17979993

[18] Immunoglobulin-E reactivity to wine glycoproteins in heavy drinkers. Gonzalez-Quintela A, Gomez-Rial J, Valcarcel C, et al. Alcohol. 2011 Mar;45(2):113-22. PMID:20843643

[19] Wine-induced anaphylaxis and sensitization to hymenoptera venom. Armentia A, Pineda F, Fernández S. N Engl J Med. 2007 Aug 16;357(7):719-20. PMID:17699828

[20] The epidemiology of fetal alcohol syndrome and partial FAS in a South African community. May PA, Gossage JP, Marais AS, et al. Drug Alcohol Depend. 2007 May 11;88(2-3):259-71. PMID:17127017

[21] Maternal risk factors for fetal alcohol syndrome and partial fetal alcohol syndrome in South Africa: a third study. May PA, Gossage JP, Marais AS, et al. Alcohol Clin Exp Res. 2008 May;32(5):738-53. PMID:18336634

[22] Prenatal alcohol exposure and childhood behavior at age 6 to 7 years: I. dose-response effect. Sood B, Delaney-Black V, Covington C, Nordstrom-Klee B, Ager J, Templin T, Janisse J, Martier S, Sokol RJ. Pediatrics. 2001 Aug;108(2):E34. PMID:11483844

[23] Fetal alcohol exposure increases mammary tumor susceptibility and alters tumor phenotype in rats. Polanco TA, Crismale-Gann C, Reuhl KR, Sarkar DK, Cohick WS. Alcohol Clin Exp Res. 2010 Nov;34(11):1879-87. PMID:20662802

[24] Ethanol induces TLR4/TLR2 association, triggering an inflammatory response in microglial cells. Fernandez-Lizarbe S, Montesinos J, Guerri C. J Neurochem. 2013 Jul;126(2):261-73. PMID:23600947

[25] Effect of alcohol consumption on CpG methylation in the differentially methylated regions of H19 and IG-DMR in male gametes: implications for fetal alcohol spectrum disorders. Ouko LA, Shantikumar K, Knezovich J, Haycock P, Schnugh DJ, Ramsay M. Alcohol Clin Exp Res. 2009 Sep;33(9):1615-27. PMID:19519716

[26] Prenatal exposure to ethanol: a specific effect on the H19 gene in sperm. Stouder C, Somm E, Paoloni-Giacobino A. Reprod Toxicol. 2011 May;31(4):507-12. PMID:21382472

[27] Red wine antioxidants protect hippocampal neurons against ethanol-induced damage: a biochemical, morphological and behavioral study. Assunção M, Santos-Marques MJ, de Freitas V, et al. Neuroscience. 2007 Jun 8;146(4):1581-92. PMID:17490820

[28] Antioxidant capacities and phenolics levels of French wines from different varieties and vintages. Landrault N, Poucheret P, Ravel P, Gasc F, Cros G, Teissedre PL. J Agric Food Chem. 2001 Jul;49(7):3341-8. PMID:11453773

[29] Grape seed flavanols, but not Port wine, prevent ethanol-induced neuronal lipofuscin formation. Assunção M, de Freitas V, Paula-Barbosa M. Brain Res. 2007 Jan 19;1129(1):72-80. PMID:17156755

[30] Red Wine, but not port wine, protects rat hippocampal dentate gyrus against ethanol-induced neuronal damage--relevance of the sugar content. Carneiro A, Assunção M, De Freitas V, Paula-Barbosa MM, Andrade JP. Alcohol & Alcoholism. 2008 Jul-Aug;43(4):408-15. PMID:18445757

[31] Betaine treatment attenuates chronic ethanol-induced hepatic steatosis and alterations to the mitochondrial respiratory chain proteome. Kharbanda KK, Todero SL, King AL, Osna NA, McVicker BL, Tuma DJ, Wisecarver JL, Bailey SM. Int J Hepatol. 2012;2012:962183. PMID:22187660

18. Immune Hypersensitivity

Immune hypersensitivity refers to misdirected immune reactions. Here, the immune system recognizes something as foreign and dangerous and attacks it, sometimes furiously, although the antigen is not a threat to the body. Damage results from direct and collateral injury from the immune response.

It reminds me of experiences I had with dogs as a child. Every day as I walked home from kindergarten, my dog, Klondike, faithfully waiting for me, would see me coming up the street and run towards me to greet me. I would run too; in the opposite direction, terrified. I was scared of dogs. They were fickle creatures, much like my school teachers. I would run; Klondike would chase. When I was exhausted and could run no longer outrun him, he would nip my ankle in compliance with his instinctual imperative. We would then walk home together.

My parents had gotten that dog in an effort to help me get over my crippling cynophobia that was the result of a vicious attack by a neighbor's dog when I was three. I was sitting on the curb, a few houses up our quiet street, playing with a toy car in some sand that had washed into the gutter. The dog approached me – his face looming large above me. I pushed him away. And then he went for my face. The memories are mired with the emotion of that moment.

I had seen what big teeth he had, and I remained convinced for years that he had viciously bitten me and would have torn off my face if I had not escaped to the safety behind the screen door of my home, with him chasing after me. However, the lack of any physical injury would support my mother's contention that I had over-reacted to a playful and friendly pup. The alleged attack dog, owned by the then adolescent Dan Hicks, had apparently given me a hot lick on the face. While there was never any real danger, an overactive self-preservation mechanism initiated a reaction leading to my psycho-trauma. Once sensitized, I had a "hypersensitivity" manifest as an inordinate fear of dogs that lasted for years. I scared myself. That fear of dogs got me bitten several times, each time reinforcing my fear.

Immune hypersensitivity reactions are somewhat similar; they are inappropriate reactions to something that in itself is not a danger. The immune system reacts, usually to a substance such as food or pollen, as if it were a dangerous pathogen, by forming antibodies to it. The host can then be injured when there is an antigen - antibody binding, triggering an immune response.

Table 18-1: Hypersensitivity Reactions

Type		Onset Time	Mediators	Examples
I	Mast cell or Basophil Activation	Usually Immediate- a few minutes to two hours	IgE IgG_1, IgG_4 Other mediators	Anaphylaxis Allergic Rhinitis Asthma Mast cell activation disorders
II	Cytotoxic – Antibodies Trigger complement cascade and cell lysis.	Several hours to three days	IgG or IgM Complement	Thrombocytopenia Rheumatic Fever
IIb	Antibodies bind to cell membrane receptors and act as agonist or antagonists			Graves Disease Myasthenia Gravis Chronic Urticaria
III	Immune complexes trigger inflammation in the affected tissues	4 – 12 hours, days or weeks	IgG Complement	Glomerulonephritis Polyarteritis nodosa Reactive arthritis Systemic Lupus Serum Sickness
IV	Cell Mediated - MHC Activated CD8+ T cells kill target cells. Macrophages produce enzymes	Delayed; 2 – 3 days	T-Cells Macrophages	Poison Oak Dermatitis TB Skin tests Multiple Sclerosis Rheumatoid Arthritis Type 1 Diabetes Crohn's Disease Hashimoto's thyroiditis

The immune system uses big guns and misguided friendly fire can cause disease, organ damage, and even death. Hypersensitivity reactions, such as autoimmune diseases and allergies, were categorized in the 1960s into four classes. Although this classification is an oversimplification, it remains useful for understanding the mechanisms of hypersensitivity. Some immune hypersensitivity diseases have multiple mechanisms. The criteria have been slightly modified here to explain these conditions more clearly.

Type I Hypersensitivity

Type I Hypersensitivity reactions present as allergic reactions. Here, the immune system, using mechanisms designed to attack and destroy parasitic worms, responds to the protein it recognizes as being associated with invading pathogen. However, the protein target identified is not from a pathogen, but rather from food, pollen, insect bite, or another source that represents little threat to the body. Although Type I hypersensitivity is the most frequently recognized hypersensitivity reaction, IgE-associated Type I reactions account for only about five percent of immune hypersensitivity reactions to foods[1].

Persons with allergies have activated plasma cells that secrete IgE to specific allergens. These IgE antibodies bind to Fcε (Immunoglobulin E receptors) on the mast cells in the tissue, and to basophils in the blood. Mast cells, eosinophils, and basophils contain granules with preformed mediators that when released have both immediate and delayed effects. Thus, mast cells, eosinophils, and basophils with IgE attached are primed, loaded and ready to release these mediators if the antigen appears. When exposed to an allergen, IgE antibodies become cross-linked on the cell membrane; this opens a calcium channel. The calcium influx provokes an all or none degranulation of the mast cells and basophils, causing an immediate release of the granulocytic contents.

Mast cells and basophils release histamine, provoking vasodilation, smooth muscle spasm and increased intracellular permeability. In addition to histamine, mast cells also make and release over 200 protein and 100 non-protein inflammatory mediators[2]. Non-protein mediators include leukotrienes C4 and D4 and prostaglandins. The release of these mediators causes symptoms such as itching, hives, sneezing, coryza, and wheezing, and can include anaphylaxis. Mast cells and basophils also release heparin and chondroitin, that likely act to prevent binding of foreign bodies to cells and thus avoid endocytosis and intracellular infection. Basophils are a major source of IL-4, which stimulates differentiation of T_H0 cells to T_H2 cells, and thus, reinforcing allergic sensitivity. Eosinophilic activation triggers the release of reactive oxygen species; including peroxide, superoxide, and hypobromite; as well as several cytotoxic cationic enzymes adapted for the destruction of helminths; elastase, lipase, ribonuclease, and deoxyribonuclease. Although intended for killing worms, these agents easily cause local tissues injury.

Allergic reactions can occur within seconds of exposure, and almost always occur within a couple of hours of exposure to the antigen. Although the immediate reaction creates is most notable, there is an additional delayed inflammatory response associated with IgE-mediated degranulation. Activation of these cells promotes the generation of inflammatory eicosanoids, including leukotrienes and, prostaglandins; chemokines, cytokines and growth factors. These agents continue the inflammatory response and promote a sustained tissue reaction. Thus, treatment of severe allergic reactions requires the use of both agents to treat the immediate reaction, such as antihistamines and epinephrine, and medication to prevent injury from the delayed phase response, such as corticosteroids.

Type I reactions can also be triggered by IgG antibodies[3] or other immune mediators. In addition to immunoglobulin-induced mast cells activation, mast cell, eosinophil, and basophil degranulation can also be triggered by pharmaceutical agents, food additives, peptides, and other mediators. IgG receptors on mast cells can up-regulate or down-regulate degranulation. (See Chapter 14 on mast cell degranulation).

Type II Hypersensitivity

The immune system produces antibodies that recognize and adhere to the surface of disease-causing pathogens, such as bacteria and parasites. Some classes of antibody classes can activate the complement cascade and the activation of Membrane Attack Complex (MAC). MAC inserts itself into the target cell's membrane and forms a pore in the membrane creating a transmembrane channel. This allows cytoplasm to leak out, and calcium to flow into the cell, resulting in cell death. The complement cascade also enhances phagocytosis of antigens and promotes chemotaxis, attracting macrophages and neutrophils to the area. The complement cascade components C5a and C3a can additionally trigger mast cell degranulation. This set of reactions is used by the immune system to attack parasites and cells hijacked by viruses or hosting other intracellular pathogens.

In Type II hypersensitivity, however, the antibodies produced by the immune system bind to normal proteins on the host's own cell membranes. The antibodies can react to intrinsic antigens (proteins or glycoproteins which the cell produces) or to extrinsic antigens (a foreign molecule which has attached to the cell). When multiple IgG or IgM protein molecules bind to the cell, they can activate the classical pathway of the complement system, triggering an attack on the cell membrane, and causing the cell's destruction. In Type II hypersensitivity, the immune system creates immunoglobulins that wrongly recognize the body's own cells as foreign antigens. Hemolytic anemia, autoimmune thrombocytopenia, pemphigus, immune vasculitis, Goodpasture's syndrome and acute rheumatic fever are caused by immunoglobulin/antigen activation of the complement cascade.

In a variant of Type II hypersensitivity, sometimes referred to as Type V hypersensitivity, the antibodies bind, not to the membrane glycoproteins, but instead, to a cell surface receptor protein. The binding of the antibodies can then either inhibit or mimic the intended ligand and trigger or impair cell signaling. Grave's disease and myasthenia gravis are examples of diseases caused by antibodies acting to block or hyper-stimulate cell activity by affecting surface receptors on certain cells. About 35% of patients with chronic urticaria have IgG antibodies to IgE receptors on mast cells that trigger mast cell degranulation[4].

An outer membrane protein from the pathogen *Yersinia enterocolitica* mimics the thyroid stimulating hormone (TSH) receptor. In Grave's disease, antibodies, which form to *Yersinia*'s membrane protein, cross-react and activate the TSH receptor, causing hyperthyroidism[5]. Biofilm formation in the colon (Chapter 23) and impaired mucosal barrier increase risk for proliferation and immune response to *Yersinia*, bacteria that are normally neutralized by IgA.

Type III Hypersensitivity

Type III hypersensitivity occurs when the antigen is soluble (not attached to the cell membrane) and there are sufficient antibodies to crosslink with each other and form antibody/ antigens chains or clusters, creating immune complexes. Macrophages can usually clear large immune complexes but have difficulty binding to smaller ones. These smaller complexes may be deposited in the synovia of joints, glomeruli of the kidney, or the walls of small blood vessels, where they can induce an inflammatory response. An example is streptococcal cell wall antigen, binding with antibodies, causing post-streptococcal glomerulonephritis. These soluble immune complexes can fix complement and induce the release of chemotactic factors, thus recruiting neutrophils to the area, escalating an immune response and causing tissue damage.

Type III hypersensitivity can also occur when IgG forms to other antibodies. IgG anti-IgE antibody complexes are found in five to ten percent of patients with chronic urticaria[4].

IgG_4 usually neutralizes antigens that would otherwise bind to IgE and trigger mast cell activation. IgG_4 normally does not trigger inflammatory reactions, as it does not activate the complement system. Nevertheless, IgG_4 can participate in hypersensitivity reactions when IgG_4/antigen complexes bind to anti-IgG antibodies, usually of the IgG_1 class[6]. These IgG_1/IgG_4 immune complexes can activate the complement cascade. This may be one way in which IgG_4 reacts with food to create hypersensitivity reactions. IgG_4 may also act as a partial antagonist/agonist for mast cell activity.

Type IV Hypersensitivity

Cellular immunity protects the body from pathogens such as viruses, intracellular bacteria, and cancers by identifying non-self epitopes on the surface of cells. Cytotoxic T-cells that recognize these epitopes can induce apoptosis (self-destruction) of these cells. Apoptosis activates macrophages that phagocytize and then break down the remaining cellular debris using potent enzymes that are also used for killing and digestion of bacteria and viral particles. Cytokines from activated macrophages ramp up the immune response, recruiting T-cells and other WBCs to the area. T-cells also induce apoptosis of senile cells, which have outlived their utility.

In Type IV hypersensitivity, cytotoxic T-cells destroy host cells, mistakenly targeting them as expressing foreign epitopes or as cells that have outlived their utility. Major histocompatibility complexes (MHC) Class I and Class II are used by the body for self-recognition to prevent the immune system from attacking healthy cells. However, in Type IV hypersensitivity, CD8+ cytotoxic T cells recognize MHC Class I proteins as foreign. Macrophages act as antigen-presenting cells. They release IL-12 that stimulates CD4+ helper cells that secrete interleukin-2 and interferon-γ and mediate an inflammatory response. Activated CD8+ cells destroy the targeted cells directly while macrophages participate and sustain the inflammatory response. Other macrophages remove cellular debris. Sensitization typically develops to a specific cell membrane protein, thus attacking specific cells types in specific organs, and causing distinct disease conditions.

Type IV hypersensitivity reactions include rheumatoid arthritis, type 1 diabetes, multiple sclerosis, Hashimoto's thyroiditis, Crohn's disease, and other autoimmune diseases.

T_H17 cells, which play an important role in preventing infection by enteric bacteria, can mediate the development of Type IV hypersensitivity, including cell-mediated, autoimmune disease[7]. The role of T_H17 cell immunity in autoimmune disease is discussed in Chapter 32.

Limitations

While the four or five hypersensitivity reaction types form a helpful framework to understand diseases caused by immune reactions, immune diseases do not always fall neatly into these categories. Some diseases have multiple immune mechanisms occurring simultaneously. Other diseases may occur through additional immune mechanisms.

Hypersensitivity to Foods

Type I: Type I hypersensitivity reactions to foods are well recognized as food allergies. They are more frequently seen in children than in adults. They are discussed in chapter 11.

Type II: While only a few lectins are important as IgE allergens (peanut, wheat, and soy as examples), IgG formation to lectins is common. IgG antibodies form to both toxic and non-toxic lectins. It is not uncommon for the body to form IgG_1 to lectins, and lectins can also potentiate the formation of IgG immunoglobulins to other proteins[8]. Lectins, a type of protein common in food, are often resistant to cooking and digestion, but may be absorbed either by an abrogated mucosa or uptake by endocytosis by enterocytes.

Many lectins bind to specific glycoproteins, including those on cell membranes. Several lectins can agglutinate red blood cells, platelets or white blood cells. Some food lectins are specific to sialic acids, which are commonly the terminal sugar on membrane glycoproteins. Since many human pathogens, including malaria and cold and flu viruses depend on binding to sialic acids[9], it is not surprising that the immune system reacts to these proteins. Immunoglobulin formation to these lectins can activate complement, and damage the cells that lectins adhere to. Thus, foods can trigger Type II immune responses.

Type III: IgG reactions to food proteins, and particularly to lectins, can also induce Type III hypersensitivity reactions. IgG to circulating proteins can form immune complexes which induce an immune response. These proteins can deposit in joint spaces or in tissues where they provoke inflammation.

Type IV: Immune reaction to foods can also trigger Type IV cytotoxic hypersensitivity. Immune reactions to some food proteins can cross-react with MHC alleles in some individuals, putting them at risk for the disease. The best established of these are gluten provoking celiac disease, and cow's milk, in the pathogenesis of Type 1 diabetes in children[10].

Food-related hypersensitivity reactions may be limited to non-specific symptoms such as fatigue, myalgia, abdominal pain, constipation or diarrhea, insomnia, and irritability. They may also be specific, causing headaches, aphthous stomatitis, and joint pains, or specific autoimmune diseases.

---

[1] Food Allergy. Richard Trevino and Hamilton Dixon. Pg.7. Theime. NYAm. Acad. Otolarynglic Allergy. 1997

[2] Burning mouth syndrome and mast cell activation disorder. Afrin LB. Oral Surg Oral Med Oral Pathol Oral Radiol Endod. 2011 Apr;111(4):465-72. PMID:21420635

[3] Fc gamma receptor signaling in mast cells links microbial stimulation to mucosal immune inflammation in the intestine. Chen X, Feng BS, Zheng PY, Liao XQ, Chong J, Tang SG, Yang PC. Am J Pathol. 2008 Dec;173(6):1647-56. Epub 2008 Oct 30. PMID:18974296

[4] Pathogenesis of chronic urticaria. Kaplan AP, Greaves M. Clin Exp Allergy. 2009 Jun;39(6):777-87. Epub 2009 Apr 22. PMID:19400905

[5] Identification of outer membrane porin f protein of Yersinia enterocolitica recognized by antithyrotopin receptor antibodies in Graves' disease and determination of its epitope using mass spectrometry and bioinformatics tools. Wang Z, Zhang Q, Lu J, Jiang F, Zhang H, Gao L, Zhao J. J Clin Endocrinol Metab. 2010 Aug;95(8):4012-20. Epub 2010 May 19. PMID:20484489

[6] T cells expressing IL-2 receptor in migraine. Martelletti P. Acta Neurol (Napoli). 1991 Oct;13(5):448-56. PMID: 1776533

[7] IL-33 is a crucial amplifier of innate rather than acquired immunity. Oboki K, Ohno T, Kajiwara N, Arae K, Morita H, Ishii A, Nambu A, Abe T, Kiyonari H, Matsumoto K, Sudo K, Okumura K, Saito H, Nakae S. Proc Natl Acad Sci U S A. 2010 Oct 26;107(43):18581-6. Epub 2010 Oct 11. PMID:20937871

[8] The identification of plant lectins with mucosal adjuvant activity. Lavelle EC, Grant G, Pusztai A, Pfüller U, O'Hagan DT. Immunology. 2001 Jan;102(1):77-86. PMID:11168640

[9] Diversity in cell surface sialic acid presentations: implications for biology and disease. Varki NM, Varki A. Lab Invest. 2007 Sep;87(9):851-7. PMID:17632542

[10] Dietary intervention in infancy and later signs of beta-cell autoimmunity. Knip M, Virtanen SM, Seppä K, Ilonen J, Savilahti E, Vaarala O, Reunanen A, Teramo K, Hämäläinen AM, Paronen J, Dosch HM, Hakulinen T, Akerblom HK; Finnish TRIGR Study Group. N Engl J Med. 2010 Nov 11;363(20):1900-8. PMID:21067382

19. Immune Hypersensitivity to Foods

Why Food?

The intestines have a large exposed surface area, which unlike the skin, is adapted for absorption of water and nutrients. Thus, the intestine is the largest and most exposed surface of the body. The colon contains trillions of bacteria; it is a great place to live for anaerobic bacteria. There are plenty of nutrients, water, and a favorable, depleted-oxygen, climate-controlled environment. These bacteria function as an extra organ, helping us with digestion and nutrition. Viruses, parasites, and fungi may also see our colon as a happy place to get food, develop communities and raise their young. Sometimes, however, the bacteria upon which we depend on, behave more like miners than farmers. Some of the same bacterial species that help us can also turn on us and cause disease; and few viruses, parasites or fungi do our colons any favors. Thus, the body needs to defend itself from invaders.

The enterocyte membrane functions as a barrier that keeps bacteria and other foreign antigens inside of the lumen of the intestine and outside the body. To allow for efficient absorption of nutrients, this barrier is only one cell thick. If this barrier is breached, the gut can mobilize highly-active, immune defenses. About half of the body's entire immune cell population resides in the lamina propria of the intestines.

The immune system is adapted to recognize and destroy bacteria, viruses, fungi, ameba, worms and other pathogens. It does this by recognizing their proteins as foreign, differentiating them from the proteins of our cells. Food too comes from other living things that have proteins not so different than those of pathogens, and thus, these are foreign proteins. Foods can trigger many of the same immune reactions that the pathogens that infect our guts do.

The immune system does not usually mistake food for an aggressive pathogen; first, cooking and digestion denatures many proteins. Then, proteolytic enzymes from the stomach, pancreas and intestine sequentially cleave food proteins into peptides and single amino acids that are absorbed as nutrients. Those proteins and peptides that escape degradation are usually excluded from the lamina propria by their large size, precluding their absorption. The mucous barrier and immunoglobulins also act as barriers to entry of proteins and peptides.

Nevertheless, immune activation is not uncommon when the digestive system does not behave properly. The failure of digestion, from lack of stomach acid or enzyme activity, can increase the presence of immunogenic proteins in the lower small and the large intestine.

If the enterocyte membrane is not intact, food proteins and peptides can reach the lamina propria. This can occur if the mucosa is damaged as can happen during or after infection. Rotavirus infection, for example, damages the mucosa and activates immune cells. In doing so, it increases the risk of Type 1 diabetes[1] and celiac disease[2], by allows undigested protein from food to be presented to activated lymphocytes. Some bacteria, such as cholera, compromise the integrity of the mucosal barrier through the use of specific toxins that open the tight junctions between the enterocytes. If the normal barriers to antigens are compromised, the immune system becomes activated, making it more likely that antigen-presenting cells will gather food antigens and present them to the T cells as foreign proteins.

Additionally the M cells of the Peyer's patches in the ileum do some sampling of the chyme, as part of routine immune surveillance. Undigested food proteins and peptides may also be taken up and recognized as foreign. Lectin proteins that are not easily degraded by digestion can be taken up by M cells and presented to T cells.

Food is an ideal source of antigens to trigger the enteric immune system as it provides abundant antigens to a susceptible location, often presenting the same food proteins on a daily basis. Additionally, undigested food proteins provide fodder for dysbiosis that can stimulate hyperreactivity of the mucosal associated lymphoid tissue. Systemic infections obviously impact the immune system, but food and dysbiosis can easily act as stealth antigens.

Immunoglobulins

IgA is the most abundant immunoglobulin produced by the body. Most of the IgA produced by the body is made by cell of the lamina propria of the intestine, although it is also produced by other mucosa; IgA is present in tears and saliva, in the urinary tract, prostate, and respiratory epithelium.

IgA differs from most other antibodies, in that it does not fix complement very well and does not stimulate much of an immune response. In fact, IgA has anti-inflammatory functions. Secretory IgA (sIgA) generally triggers the release of non-inflammatory cytokines that down-regulate inflammation[3]. The principle role of sIgA is to babysit the commensal bacteria residing in the gut and keep them from causing trouble.

M cells overlay Peyer's patches in the ileum. The cells can phagocytize bacteria and other antigens and transport them to T cell lymphocytes within the Peyer's patches. The predominant T helper lymphocyte in the intestines is the T_H17 cell These cells can stimulate sIgA. T_H17 cells are common in the lamina propria of the distal small intestines and large intestines, where they help protect the body from gram-negative bacterial and fungal infections.

The T_H17 cells that have been presented antigens stimulate B-cells that then migrate from the intestine, via the lymphatic vessels to the bloodstream. The B-Cell lymphocytes then migrate back to the intestines, redistributing themselves throughout the lamina propria. Here they become plasma cells, producing sIgA to the specific antigen. Secretory IgA produced by plasma cells in the lamina propria binds to receptors on the basolateral membrane of the enterocytes. SIgA is taken up by endocytosis and transported through the cells to the microvilli where it presented on the cell's luminal surface still attached to the IgA receptor. The sIgA is then cleaved from its receptor and binds to the mucous layer where it interacts with bacteria and other antigens.

IgA acts by binding to enteric bacteria, and thus prevents the bacteria from attaching to the enterocytes; this helps preventing pathogenic growth and biofilm formation; these bacteria with sIgA, then pass harmlessly into the stool.

This process of IgA formation is rather slow; it takes about three or four weeks after exposure to an antigen for sIgA to be detected in the feces[3]. Clearly, this leisurely process is not intended as an emergency response to infection, but rather as an adaptation to the commensal bacteria taking in residence in the lumen of the colon.

When sIgA antibodies bind to food antigens, they prevent those antigens from being absorbed; however, this also diverts sIgA from its protective role in preventing bacterial biofilm formation. Large quantities of reacting food antigens can deplete sIgA and increase the risk of bacterial proliferation and intestinal dysbiosis. SIgA depletion increases the risk for adherence of the bacteria to the cells and possible infection or biofilm formation. If biofilms develop, the bacteria, such as *Clostridia*, form colonies and can produce toxins and other virulence factors which the same species does not produce as single individuals. Biofilms are discussed in Chapter 23.

IgA depletion can also occur from the disruption or loss of the mucous layer in the intestine, damage to the enterocytes, or immune dysfunction. Bacterial fermentation of amino acids can produce ammonia and sulfites which can damage the mucous layer, especially in the colon.

The mucosal immune cells of the intestine produce other classes of antibodies in addition to sIgA. IgA neutralizes bacteria and antigens, but the body also needs to protect itself from pathogens that get into the enterocytes, into the lamina propria, or beyond.

The two main classes of antibodies produced for defense against pathogens that have made their way past the mucosal barrier are IgE and IgG.

IgE and IgG are adapted to defend against different types of pathogens. IgE is adapted to fend off attacks by large invaders that are few in number, such as parasitic worms. IgE triggers degranulation mast cells, basophils, and eosinophils provoking an intense and messy, but usually localized, reaction. In contrast, IgG is adapted to the defense against very numerous, small invaders that can quickly disperse throughout the body. IgG responses are usually more direct; binding to individual bacteria or cells that have been identified as foreign. IgG can stimulate a diverse response.

IgE and IgG form not only against infectious agents, but also against food proteins that cross the enterocyte barrier. The more exposure the immune cells have to a food protein or peptide, the more likely it is to have an intense immune response. When antibodies form and react to foods in the diet, IgE and IgG immune reactions give different manifestations. In general, children are more likely to develop IgE antibodies to foods while adults are more likely to develop IgG antibodies to food.

Type I hypersensitivity reactions to foods are usually obvious. The Greeks recognized food allergies 2000 years ago. They are mediated by IgE, and there is a quick response to exposure of antigens the body is sensitized to. When a wasp sting, a rare event, is followed by wheezing, other unusual event, they are easy to associate with each other. When food is eaten and followed within an hour by itching and rash, it is not difficult to identify the association. (See IgE reactions in Chapter 11.)

In contrast, when one or more of the dozens of foods and condiments, consumed during the day, is followed by non-specific symptoms after a 24-hour delay, it is difficult to make a connection between sensitivity to a food and the response to it. IgG reactions are slow. During this delay antecedent to the adverse reaction, there is opportunity for numerous and diverse internal and external environmental factors including multiple food exposures. Thus, linking an offending agent to an adverse outcome is difficult.

The non-IgE immune response may not even give direct symptoms or signs at all. They may instead manifest much later, as a result of chronic low-level end organ damage which progresses with time and exposure, as is the case of Beta cell destruction of the pancreas, resulting in type 1 diabetes, of alterations in appetite resulting in obesity. Additionally, most patients with IgG-associated food reactions react to multiple foods; making it even more difficult to associate dietary exposure with any symptoms being experienced. Since many of the early onset symptoms associated with IgG reactions are subjective, they are often wrongly considered to be manifestations of "functional" disorders.

Table 19-1: Response to IgE and IgG to Food Antigens

Reaction	IgE	IgG
Typical time to reaction	A few minutes up to a few hours	Six to 48 hours; occasionally longer
Early Signs	Rashes, wheezing, edema, anaphylaxis	Usually none
Typical Symptoms	Itching, anxiety, bronchoconstriction, wheezing, nausea	Irritability, headache, abdominal pain, fatigue
Mode of action	Localized mast cell and basophil degranulation	Mast cell activation, immune complex formation, cytokine production, cytotoxic damage
Number of foods	Typical few	Often numerous
Skin Tests	Work well	Negative
Lab testing	Well established IgE testing	IgG or IgG$_4$ testing
Name of Reaction	Allergy	Antergy

Table 19-2: IgG Functions

Function	Description
Opsonization	The antibody binds to an antigen on the bacterial or viral surface and then binds to receptors on macrophages or other phagocytic cells that engulf and digest the particle, bacteria, or cells attached to the immunoglobulin.
Agglutination	IgG antibody can bind two antigens, and thus two bacteria, viruses, or other antigens (proteins) it recognizes. Since bacteria and other antigen-bearing particles are large, and usually have many antigen sites, with sufficient antibody clumps of bacteria, viruses or proteins can form. This limits the mobility of the pathogens and aids in localizing immune defense against them.
Complement Activation	IgG (and IgM) can activate the complement pathway by changing the conformation of the C1 complex, leading to a cascade of interactions between circulating proteins that form the Membrane Attack Complex (MAC). The MAC forms a pore in the bacteria or cell that leads to the influx of calcium, and destruction of the bacteria or cell. Complement activation can also trigger mast cell degranulation.
Antibody-Dependent Cell-Mediated Cytotoxicity	IgG (and IgE) bind to cells that are recognized as having foreign antigens, (such as virally infected cells or tumor cells) and can bind via Fc receptors to natural killer cells (NK cells) that then release cytokines and cytotoxic granules that trigger apoptosis of the cell.

Antergy

The term "food sensitivity" is often used to describe IgG-based immune reactions to foods. This term is nonspecific and inadequately conveys the harmful effects of IgG immune responses to foods, unlike the way the term allergy conveys risk of harm. The term allergy was coined in 1906 by the Austrian pediatrician, Clemens E. von Pirquet, from the Greek allos (other) and ergon (activity). Here, the term "*antergy*" is suggested to describe IgG$_1$ and IgG$_4$ induced adverse immune reactions to foods and other substances, derived from the Greek roots anti (against, opposed to, in response to) and ergon (activity).

Table 19-3: Examples of Diseases Associated with Immunoglobulin to Food

Disease	Tested Positive	Allergen Tested
Allergy, hives, asthma anaphylaxis	IgE, Skin test	Multiple
Constipation[4]	IgA, IgG	Cow's milk
Aphthous Ulcers[5]	IgA, IgG	Cow's milk
Migraine[6]	IgG	Multiple
Rheumatoid Arthritis[7]	sIgA, IgG, IgM, IgA	Multiple
Type 1 Diabetes[8]	IgA, IgG	Cow's Milk, β-lactoglobulin
Celiac Disease	sIgA, IgG, IgM	Gliadin* (Wheat)
Irritable Bowel Syndrome[9]	IgG	Multiple
Dermatitis Herpetiformis[10]	sIgA	Gliadin, Bovine β-lactoglobulin (milk)
Crohn's Disease[11]	IgG	Baker's Yeast
Atherosclerosis and Obesity[12, 13]	IgG	Multiple
Functional Dyspepsia[14]	IgG	Egg, Soybean
IgA Nephropathy[15]	IgA	Gluten (Wheat)
Inflammatory Myopathies[16]	IgA	Gliadin*
Multiple Sclerosis[17]	IgG	Gluten
Epilepsy[18]	IgA, IgG	Gliadin
Schizophrenia[19]	IgA	Gliadin, β-lactoglobulin, casein (milk)
Lymphoid Nodular Hyperplasia[20]	IgG	beta-lactoglobulin
Cerebellar Ataxia[21]	IgA, IgG	Gliadin

* Gliadin is an antigenic subfraction of gluten.

Other diseases attributed to IgG food reactions include:

- ADHD
- Fatigue
- Eczema
- Psoriasis
- Asthma
- Chronic otitis media
- Chronic rhinosinusitis
- Gallbladder disease
- Interstitial cystitis, chronic prostatitis
- Enuresis
- Insomnia
- Irritability or Rage
- Type 2 diabetes
- Tourette's syndrome
- Reynaud's phenomenon

This list is not meant to be comprehensive but rather exemplary of antergy-associated enteroimmune disease.

Food Immunogenicity

There are several lines of evidence that have demonstrated that idiosyncratic, non-allergic immune reactions to food causes disease. One line of evidence has been the use of elimination diets. Elimination diets are useful in the treatment of several disease conditions which are not IgE mediated, do not appear to be induced by pharmacologic nor toxic agents, and are not associated with food-born pathogenic organisms.

Elimination diets, however, are difficult. Not just because of compliance, but also, because most patients with antergies to food react to multiple foods; unless most, if not all reacting foods are eliminated, the disease condition may not improve. In one study, the *average patient* with migraines had elevated IgG to 24 different foods[22]. Most other studies of antergies give similar results.

Additionally, depending on the disease, recovery may not occur in just a couple of days of antigen avoidance. In chronic inflammatory diseases, such as inflammatory bowel disease or rheumatoid arthritis exacerbated by food antigens, it may take weeks for a flare-up of the disease to resolve. If a food challenge were planned, it would first require a quiescent period. If the patient has immunogenic reactions to multiple foods, avoiding one food is not helpful. Even if eliminating multiple foods, other and perhaps hidden antigens can prevent recovery. Patients cannot fast until recovery, slowly introducing one food every few days, to see if they have an exacerbation of their condition. Elimination diets provide benefits in immediate hypersensitivity reactions but are not well suited to the investigation of delayed, IgG associated, immune reactions.

In elemental diets, nutrition is given in the form of a mix of individual amino acids, sugars, and fats so that there are no antigens. Elemental diets are useful for demonstrating that a disease or condition is caused by exposure to immunogens in food. Total parenteral nutrition with elemental diets has been used to induce remission in Crohn's disease[23] but has not been found to be useful in the treatment of ulcerative colitis[24]. An oral elemental diet lasting only two weeks was found to be as effective as prednisone in achieving resolution of inflammation in patients with rheumatoid arthritis[25]. While useful in research settings, elemental diets are not practical for most patients.

Non-IgE food immunopathies may be associated with IgG as well as IgM and sIgA. In a study of rheumatoid arthritis (RA), immunoglobulins to foods were collected by aspiration of fluid from the lumen of the jejunum. IgM, sIgA, and IgG were found to be significantly associated with the presence of RA[26]. Secretory IgA was most sensitive. Jejunal aspiration with sIgA analysis, however, is not commonly available but is rather a research protocol.

Immunoglobulin G

Although IgA to foods may be more highly correlated with the presence of immune disease than IgG, testing for food immunogenicity is usually done by testing for IgG. IgA and IgM can bind to the Fcα receptors on macrophages and B cells resulting in the endocytosis of the antigen that these immunoglobulins adhered to. This allows for immune presentation and the induction of IgG antibody production to the antigen. It is likely the IgG, rather than sIgA or IgM that causes the symptomatic immune reactions. IgG reactions can explain the pathological connection between food sensitivities and clinical disease manifestations.

There are four classes of IgG; IgG_1 and IgG_4 are thoses most clearly associated with immunogenicity to foods.

Table 19-4: IgG Subtypes

Class	Binding to Lymphocyte Receptors	Complement Activation
IgG_1	CD16, CD32, CD64	Yes
IgG_2	CD32	With LPS
IgG_3	CD16, CD32, CD64	Yes
IgG_4	CD64	No

IgG antibodies, other than IgG_4, can initiate complement activation. Complement activation is a multistep cascade which leads to the formation of the membrane attack complex (MAC) that can kill a target cell or bacteria. IgG_2 appears to require a bacterial cofactor, such as LPS, to activate the complement cascade. IgG also acts by binding to receptors on white blood cells, so that the IgG antibody-antigen complex can be phagocytized.

There are three classes of IgG receptors, with several subtypes. These receptors have an array of activities, and although IgG/IgG receptor couplings induce immune cells reactivity, IgG activation of at least one receptor type reduces immune activity.

Table 19-5: IgG Receptors (FcγR)

CD16a FcγRIIIA	Expressed on macrophages, and natural killer (NK) cells. Induces cell-mediated cytotoxicity and induces cytokine release by macrophages.
CD16b FcγRIIIB	Expressed on eosinophils, macrophages, monocytes, mast cells, subsets of T cells, and dendritic cells. Induces cell activation and antimicrobial activity.
CD32 FcγRIIA	Expressed on macrophages, neutrophils, eosinophils, mast cells, platelets and Langerhans cells. Induces phagocytosis and degranulation.
CD32 FcγRIIB1	Expressed on B-cells and mast cells. Does not induce phagocytosis. Inhibits B-cell activity.
CD32 FcγRIIB2	Expressed on macrophages, neutrophils, and eosinophils. Induces phagocytosis, but inhibits cell activity.
CD64 FcγRI	A high-affinity receptor expressed on monocytes, macrophages, neutrophils, myeloid precursors, dendritic cells and mast cells. Induces phagocytosis, cell activation, and production of Reactive Oxygen Species (ROS).
FcγRIV	Expressed only by monocytes, macrophages, and neutrophils. Activated by IgG_2. Induces immune response.

FcγRIIA activation by IgG can trigger mast cell degranulation and induce airway inflammation and trigger anaphylaxis[27]. FcγRII or FcγRIII need to bind multiple antigen molecules, as do IgE receptors (FcεR), to activate cellular response. In contrast, FcγRI can be activated with a single IgG immunoglobulin-antigen complex.

IgG_1 antibodies form to foods, and it can both trigger the complement cascade and activate mast cells. IgG_1 also has other immune effects; however, it usually does not last long. Thus, its effects are limited to early antigenicity to food and may not be responsible for chronic inflammatory conditions.

IgG_4 is the IgG class of antibodies most commonly found in food immunogenicity. Similar to sIgA, the main role of IgG_4 in health is to act as a neutralizing antibody. Secretory IgA binds to pathologic, mostly gram-negative, enteric bacteria, decreasing the bacteria's adherence to enterocytes and thus prevent bacterial transport into the cell.

IgG_4 acts primarily as a neutralizing antibody, which protects the body from IgE-mediated reactions by preempting this reaction. IgG_4 binds to the antigen before it can get to the mast cell or basophil. Thus, the normal role of IgG_4 is to prevent immune reactions. IgG_4 may be required for the desensitization from IgE reactions.

The normal function of IgG_4 is to protect the organism from its immune system, with IgG_4 mitigating immune reactions. During desensitization, IgE gets downregulated with increased levels IgG_4[28]. IgG_4 neutralizes antigens by binding to them and preventing the antigen from binding to IgE on mast cells. Eventually, the plasma cells producing IgE to the antigen lack the signal to continue their work and decrease IgE production and may undergo apoptosis. It typically takes a few months to two years after an antigen exposure had been masked by IgG_4 for B cells also stand down their production of IgE antibodies.

Children with IgE food allergies will often gain IgG_4 immunity to the allergens[29] and thus prevent IgE reactions. During the first years of life, there is a transition from IgE to IgG. IgG levels, to food allergens, peak around the age of 18 months, followed by a decline. By eight years of age, levels usually come down[30]. Children who develop the highest IgG_4/IgE ratios, and have negative skin prick reactions to food allergens, are more likely to outgrow their allergies. A majority of atopic children form tolerance to IgE food allergens (wheat, milk, eggs) by the age of eight. However, many others remain hyperallergic and more than half of these children develop asthma[31].

IgG_4 does not bind complement and thus is not directly involved in cell destruction. However, IgG_4 can bind, and thus, be phagocytized by WBC-bearing CD64 receptors, including mast cells. It is only in recent years that diseases caused by IgG_4 have been recognized.

One mechanism by which IgG_4 is thought to cause food-related disease is through the formation of long-lasting, antigen-antibody complexes. These complexes are then targeted by IgG_1, forming larger immune complexes. These complexes can activate the complement cascade, which may promote malaise and fatigue, in part through direct mast cell degranulation, activated by complement factor C3a[32]. Phagocytosis of these complexes may trigger cytokine release, and the complexes may precipitate in the skin, joints or other organs causing damage. IgG_4 antibodies can also bind to mast cells through the CD64 receptors and promote activation or partial activation.

IgG_4 may induce disease processes as part of Type III hypersensitivity reactions. The IgG_4 binds to the antigens and forms circulating immune complexes in some food-induced migraines. The IgG_4 complexes then bind to anti-IgG antibodies[33]. Evidence suggests that these IgG_4/food/anti-IgG complexes induce activation of lymphocytes and the production of Interleukin-2 as a mechanism for migraine[34]. T_H17 also induces production of IL-1, which mediates Type IV hypersensitivity.

Through these mechanisms, IgG_4 activation of mast cells may contribute to a variety of inflammatory conditions including fibrosis, vasculitis, and arthritis.

Date of Birth: ▬▬▬▬ Sex: Male Age: 53

Reactive Test Results (Your blood serum reacted to these food antigens)

Almond (+1)	Coffee (+1)	Mint (+1)	Rye (+1)
Barley (+2)	Crab (+1)	Oat (+1)	Sage (+1)
Bean, Kidney (+2)	Cranberry (+2)	Orange (+1)	Sesame (+1)
Bean, Navy (+1)	Egg (+4)	Oyster (+1)	Sunflower (+1)
Blackberry (+1)	Ginger (+1)	Papaya (+1)	Tomato (+1)
Blueberry (+1)	Lentil (+1)	Peanut (+1)	Wheat (+1)
Buckwheat (+2)	Malt (+2)	Peppermint (+1)	Yeast, Baker's (+3)
Cheese (+4)	Milk, Cow's (+2)	Pineapple (+1)	Yeast, Brewer's (+2)
Chicken (+1)	Milk, Goat's (+2)	Rice (+1)	

Total number of IgG sensitivity reactions: **35**

Non-Reactive Test Results (Your blood serum did not react to these food antigens)

Alfalfa	Coco-Chocolate	Mustard	Salmon
Amaranth	Coconut	Brazil Nut	Sardine
Apple	Cod	Cashew Nut	Scallops
Apricot	Corn	Pecan	Sea Bass
Asparagus	Cumin	Nutmeg	Seed, Caraway
Avocado	Currant	Olive	Seed, Dill
Banana	Date	Onion	Rape Seed (Canola)
Basil	Duck	Oregano	Shrimp
Bay Leaf	Eggplant	Paprika	Snapper
Bean, Green	Flounder	Parsley	Sole
Bean, Lima	Garlic	Pea	Spinach
Mung Bean	Goose	Peach	Squash, Yellow
Bean, Pinto	Grape, Concord	Pear	Strawberry
Soybean	Grape, White	Pepper, B/W	Sugar, Cane
Bean, Yellow Wax	Grapefruit	Pepper, Cayenne	Tangerine
Beef	Greens, Mustard	Pepper, Green	Tapioca
Beet	Haddock	Pepper, Red	Tea
Broccoli	Halibut	Pimento	Thyme
Brussels Sprouts	Nut, Filbert	Perch	Trout
Cabbage	Horseradish	Plum	Tuna
Cantaloupe	Herring	Pork	Turkey
Carrot	Lamb	Potato, Sweet	Turnip
Catfish	Lemon	Potato, White	Vanilla
Cauliflower	Lettuce	Pumpkin	Venison
Celery	Lime	Quinoa	Walnut, Black
Cherry	Lobster	Rabbit	Walnut, English
Cucumber	Mackerel	Radish	White fish
Cinnamon	Melon, Honeydew	Raspberry	Watermelon
Clam	Millet	Rhubarb	Zucchini
Clove	Mushroom	Safflower	

Figure 19-1: Results from (total) IgG testing of foods in a 53-year-old man diagnosed with chronic prostatitis/ interstitial cystitis, causing multiple nocturia, and with chronic post nasal drip provoking dysphonia. He had reactive IgG antibodies to 35 of 154 tested food antigens. The patient reported improvement of most symptoms within a few days, and further improvement over several weeks, after eliminating reactive foods from his diet. This lab work was performed by ImmunoLabs of Fort Lauderdale, Florida.

Testing

Some labs test for total IgG while others test specifically for IgG_4 to food. An advantage of testing combined IgG is that it may catch the onset of IgG_1 reactions. IgG_1 testing gives higher sensitivity, however, advocates of IgG_4 testing voice concerns that tests including IgG_1 reactivity to food may give false positive results. This could lead to the exclusion of foods from the diet not causing problems.

IgG panels that include over 100 different foods are preferred over smaller ones as larger panels are more likely to identify the wider range of reactive foods in the diet. Foods that are highly allergenic, because of proteins that survive digestion are among those that also commonly antergenic.

Practical Pointers for Antergy Management

Most individuals with IgG antergies react to multiple foods, and these foods often comprise a sizable portion of their usual diet; this nutrition needs to be replaced. Testing a broad panel of foods not only helps identifying the foods a patient reacts to, but as importantly, provides a large number of foods the patient can eat in place of the foods eliminated from their diet.

The first step to eliminating IgG-reacting foods is to obtain an adequate supply of alternative, non-reactive foods. The patient should shop for foods and snacks from the non-reactant list and fill their pantry and refrigerator so that they have plenty of choices at home. Success requires balanced nutrition and enjoyable foods. A lack of variety, protein, palatability or convenience may lead to malnutrition, misery, and non-compliance. It may also not be practical, nor therapeutically desirable, to immediately eliminate all the IgG-reacting foods, especially when the list contains 20 or more reacting foods. It takes time for the patient to adjust to what may be an almost entirely new diet; and one which may be difficult to eat outside of the home. This adaptation takes time.

Elimination of the most highly reactive foods (3+ and 4+ foods) is recommended for the first few days, followed by the lesser reacting foods over the subsequent week. Down-regulating an overly aggressive, T_H17-dominated, immune response is a primary goal of therapy.

It has been the author's experience that the sudden withdrawal of numerous IgG-reacting foods may be associated with the development of new food antergies. This is likely a result of a continuation of the underlying immune hyper-activation and intestinal immune barrier incompetence. Along with the elimination of reacting foods, the patient should be treated for risk factors for the development of antergies, including leaky gut (Chapter 25), mast cell activation (Chapter12), and enteric dysbiosis (Chapter 23). Antioxidant and anti-inflammatory supplements should be used to calm immune hyperreactivity.

The patient should be encouraged to eat a variety foods from their "safe list" so that they can rotate the foods and avoid eating them more than twice a week. Reliance on a small number of foods increases the risk of becoming sensitized to those foods. Leftovers are best frozen or discarded to prevent eating the same foods on successive days. Four-day cycles are usually practical for items, such as nuts and fruits, but may be too long for use with grains, especially when wheat is removed from the diet. Although difficult, the patient should be encouraged to rotate grains. Also, although not as nutritious, milled white rice is less antigenic than brown rice. Milled grains are recommended until the intestinal barrier and immune regulation improves.

Complete elimination of reactive antigens should be encouraged for a period of at least several weeks to see if symptoms improve. Some patients have IgG to numerous foods, making complete elimination problematic. Although it is best to maintain complete adherence, if this is impossible, foods that are less reactive (1+) may be consumed once a week to see if they cause symptoms. Highly reactive foods should be completely avoided.

Assuming that the patient has been compliant in eliminating reactive foods and has had symptomatic improvement, the test may be repeated after several months. Foods that are no longer reactive can be added back, one at a time; to see it they provoke symptoms. Testing may also show new antergies that have developed and need to be removed from the diet. Later, an annual test is advised.

Foods, beverages, and spices which are not included on in the test panel should not be considered benign. These foods should also be eliminated for at least a couple of weeks and preferably one month until symptoms have improved. They can then be reintroduced, one food item at a time, to see if they provoke symptoms. Until symptoms have subsided, and the patient is feeling well, it is difficult to tell. When a patient is in remission, provocation of symptoms from exposure is much easier to determine.

Fortunately, most patients with food antergies respond within several days to the elimination of their reacting foods. Symptoms of irritable bowel syndrome and migraines often abate quickly with the removal of the offending antergens and recur with consumption, providing motivation for compliance with the dietary restrictions.

Wheat/Gluten: IgG immune reaction to wheat should be followed with IgA testing of anti-transglutaminase antibodies and IgG anti-gliadin antibodies to check for Gluten Disease. Testing for anti-gluten antibodies should be done while the patient is still consuming wheat, as levels will fall after eliminating it from the diet. See Chapter 22 for more on gluten disease.

Eggs and Milk: IgG reactions to eggs can be followed with separate tests for yolk and egg white so that if only one of these is positive IgG, the patient need not avoid the other. If it is only the yolk proteins that are reactive, for example, egg white can be used, allowing for preparation many baked goods. If the patient reacts to milk but not cheese, reactivity to whey, but not casein is suggested. Whey is used in some processed foods. Whey can also be tested individually from casein.

Treatment Side Effects: It is not uncommon for patients to have a period of hard stools following the change in diet. This generally lasts for no more than a couple of weeks and usually does not require treatment. The patient may, however, need to increase their intake of prebiotics (Chapter 4), especially if their usual sources of prebiotics, such as grains, have been eliminated. The patient should be encouraged to increase their consumption of fruits and vegetables that they do not have IgG to.

While IgG testing for food immunoreactions is helpful, it is imperfect. Just because an individual does not have IgG to a food does not mean that the food does not cause other problems for the patient. Moreover, new immunoreactions frequently develop in hyperreactive individuals.

Eliminating IgG-reacting foods is useful as a therapeutic trial to see if disease symptoms improve, and helps down-regulate the intestinal immune response. Although symptoms may improve, elimination of immunoreactive foods is usually insufficient therapy (with the possible exception of gluten in gluten enteropathy). If the underlying cause is not reversed, new food immunoreactivities usually develop, leading to relapse.

IgG immune response to foods is often caused by an incompetent enterocyte barrier which allows excessive contact of food proteins with dendritic presentation cells. The root causes of the disrupted barrier and incomplete digestion of proteins need to be addressed and mitigated.

Gluten, phytohemagglutinin, and other toxic lectins should be avoided as they can directly damage the enterocyte membrane. Some agents of damage, such as viral enteritis, may have come and gone; however, the reaction can be self-perpetuating. The elimination diet may help break this cycle and be curative. Inflammation, including that from the reaction to food antigens, helps maintain the T_H17 and mast cell hyperreactivity in the intestinal mucosa. The microbial biome of the large intestine can produce toxins that increase permeability and immunoreactivity. Toxoplasmosis or other infections may sustain immunoreactivity.

Healing the intestines will help diminish immune reactivity and maintenance of immune hyperreactivity. Conversely, intestinal infection may be followed by the development of new immunoreactions to foods. Foods should be rotated after intestinal infection or exposure to agents that damage the endothelial barrier, to prevent the development of new immunogenicities when the intestine is most susceptible.

Sleep and Stress: Sleep deprivation appears to stimulate the onset of new food antergies. Melatonin, released mainly during periods of rest in the intestine, helps regulate the enteric circadian rhythm and is an antioxidant for neurons in the enteric nervous system. A regular meal cycle helps maintain the enteric circadian cycle. Mast cells have receptors for melatonin, and melatonin down-regulates their response[35]. Patients should be encouraged to get sufficient sleep, and maintain regular sleeping and eating cycles. Large meals near bedtime should be avoided. Sleep is discussed in Chapter 43.

Psychological stress also stimulates adverse immune reactions. Stress increases intestinal permeability, through a corticotrophin-releasing hormone (CRH) mediated activation of mast cells in the intestinal mucosa[36], thus, increasing the risk for development of antergies. Stress has adverse effects on gastrointestinal blood flow, secretions, and motility and affects the balance GI microbiota. Melatonin protects against stress induces lesions in the GI tract[37]. Stress and its attenuation is discussed in Chapter 29.

Supplements: Supplement that help down-regulate inflammation and that help replenish the antioxidant glutathione may mitigate the development of new antergies and help resolve existing ones. One of the goals of treatment is to resolve the inflammatory process and encourage the apoptosis mast cells and down-regulation of other immune cells that sustain these immune reactions to foods.

Adequate vitamins D_3, magnesium, vitamin K_2 and a favorable dietary n3:n6 fatty acid ratio decrease the inflammatory response. Use of r-alpha lipoic acid, N-acetylcysteine and trimethylglycine may also be helpful. The diet should contain a mix of fruits and vegetables. TNF-α prevents the apoptosis of inflammatory cells; many dietary phenolic compounds decrease TNF-α production (Tables 32-1 and 32-2)

Relapse

And now we come to the saddest point of this book. Antergies can commence overnight. Foods that have provided health and nutrition one day can cause disease the next. If a patient whose condition improved through the elimination of food antergies has a sudden relapse of symptoms, a new food antergy should be suspected. If the patient reports compliance with food antergy avoidance, and especially for full-blown symptoms, new onset of antergy should be investigated. Until new test results are available, any recently introduced food, such as seasonal or rarely eaten foods that had been consumed in the 36 hours prior to the onset of symptoms should top the suspect list for elimination. This, however, does not clear more frequently eaten foods from the suspect list.

Summary

Antergies contribute to the pathogenesis and sustain many chronic inflammatory disease conditions. These include diseases such as obesity, diabetes, and schizophrenia, as well as many diseases once considered to be functional or nonorganic, such as migraine, IBS, and depression. Many disease conditions improve rapidly with the elimination of foods the patient has IgG reactivity to.

Although antergies may not be the principal cause of an inflammatory condition, antergic reactions cause the release of inflammatory cytokines that help maintain inflammatory disease activity. Abatement of antergies, thus, may provide therapeutic benefit in the treatment of any systemic inflammatory disease. Control of antergies is especially pertinent to diseases that stem from T_H17 immune activity, such as most autoimmune diseases (Chapter 32) and for neurologic diseases.

1. Antergies: IgG reactions to food: Food proteins may be absorbed and induce disease, as a result of immune hypersensitivity reactions. Comprehensive IgG testing can determine which foods cause hypersensitivity reactions, and those that do not. Elimination of reacting foods provides relief in many patients. IgG reactions may amplify mast cell activity in the intestine and support mast cell activation and prevent apoptosis. Cytokines released, largely by mast cells, can have localized or systemic adverse actions, causing disease.

2. Absorption: The immunoreactive proteins must be absorbed in order to react. In patients who are forming hypersensitivity reactions to foods, the cause of abnormal absorption should be investigated and treated. Stress and sleep deprivation can impair the intestinal mucosal barrier, increasing permeability, and thus, the formation and continued immune response to dietary proteins.

It is important to remove all reactive foods to help down regulate the over-commitment of the immune response to T_H17 lineage activation.

3. Digestion of proteins: Stomach acid, pancreatic and other enzymes are important for the digestion of proteins, and for decreasing their antigenicity. Eating at a relaxed pace, to give CCK time to respond to a meal, may help provide better digestion of proteins. Meals are eaten more slowly, it the person eats before being famished or excessively hungry.

While cooking may lower the antigenicity of some lectins, others lectins are not denatured by cooking nor digested, and some may be absorbed even when the mucosa is intact. Lectins that damage the mucosa should be eliminated from the diet. The most common offender among dietary lectins is gluten (See Chapter 22). Mucosal damage and healing are discussed in Chapter 25. Individuals who easily form antergies should avoid eating foods raw or partially cooked that are usually eaten cooked. For example, raw oysters should be avoided. Invertebrates make lectins as part of their immune defense.

4. Avoid Potatoes: There are antitrypsin proteins in certain foods that prevent adequate protein digestion, and increase the risk of an immune reaction to proteins in foods. Cooking denatures most of these; however, those in potatoes are not destroyed. Anti-trypsin enzymes can prevent enzymatic degradation of proteins and increase the antigenicity of foods. Potatoes consumption may thus increase the likelihood of developing antergies to foods consumed in the same meal with them. Potatoes and their toxins are discussed in Chapter 33.

5. Enteric dysbiosis: Bacterial overgrowth and dysbiosis may increase T_H17 activation. Intestinal biofilms can produce toxins that increase intestinal permeability. See Chapters 23 through 25. SIBO and pathogenic biofilms should be treated.

Treatment of the underlying causes is essential to long-term success. If the underlying causes are not treated, the individual will develop new antergies, and the disease will return. Dysbiosis may abate with the change in diet; however, some patients may benefit from a course of antibiotics, followed by the continued consumption of prebiotics (Chapter 4). Metronidazole, rifaximin or ciprofloxacin, may be used, but are unlikely to provide lasting benefit without the use of prebiotics to establish a healthy large intestinal biome which decreases the risk of developing new antergies. Probiotics may also provide benefit as may colonic inoculation.

6. Preventively treat the disease: Although an individual's reaction to antergies, whether IBS, migraine, thyroiditis other disease, may depend on genetic susceptibility, the disease is usually exacerbated by other factors; such as malabsorption, nutritional deficiencies, infection, stress, environmental or other factors. These factors increase immune activity, and not only maintain the disease, but often also, the patient's antergies. Removing these factors may help the patient's antergies abate.

7. Eliminate and rotate: Elimination of reactive foods can decrease immune stimulation and decrease the immune response, giving relief of the disease. Foods, which are eaten, should be rotated to decrease the risk of developing reactions to those foods.

8. Decrease inflammation: Inflammation may also be eased with the supplemental use of magnesium (Chapter 30) vitamin D (Chapter 20), and fish oil (Chapter 6). The antioxidant melatonin decreases immune hyperreactivity of the intestines, and bedtime supplementation may also be helpful (Chapter 43). The amino acid supplements N-acetylcysteine and trimethylglycine are precursors for glutathione (Chapter 40), and also appear to help with resolution of antergies. Pro-inflammatory sphingolipids help maintain the immune reactivity. R-alpha-lipoic acid, pyridoxine, and magnesium mitigate S1P levels (Chapter 10).

9. Treat mast cell activation and hyperplasia: See Chapter 12 on mast cell activation disorders and the section "Epigenetic Reset" in Chapter 30.

10. Test for and treat for pancreatic enzyme insufficiency: Inadequate proteolytic activity allows survival of antigenic proteins from food. Some patients have impared production of pancreatic enzymes. Fecal elastase and chymotrypsin tests can help assess pancreatic function and the ability to digest protein. Enzyme supplements can be used in patients with insufficient digestive enzyme activity until the underlying problem is resolved (See Chapter 8).

11. Eliminate poorly absorbed sugars: Lactose, fructose or other sugar intolerances decrease intestinal transit time and digestion of proteins; thus increase the risk of immune presentation and immune reaction.

12. Self-Monitoring: After initiating an antergen elimination diet, patients often become aware of other foods that cause symptoms. If these symptoms are consistent with allergic or antergic reactions, they should also be eliminated from the diet. Care, however, should be taken to ensure that the patient maintains a nutritionally balanced diet. New food reactions continue to form in hyperreactive individuals.

13. Maintain Healthy Behaviors: Engaging in vigorous exercise, consuming foods high in phenolic compounds, and avoiding of psychologic stress all decrease intestinal hyperpermeability, help maintain a eubiotic commensal colonic biome, and decrease levels of pro-inflammatory cytokines in the blood (Chapter 23). Maintaining adequate sleep has similar effects. These health behaviors decrease the propensity to develop new antergies to foods, and may decrease the immune sensitivity to established ones.

14: Herbs and Spices: Unfortunately, not all foods, and especially herbs and spices are often not tested even when over 100 foods are. Spices are often highly immunogenic, and thus should be avoided if not on the "safe list", until the patient has recovered enough to do a food challenge.

Additionally, as antioxidants, herbs and spices are susceptible to oxidative change. Testing of fresh herbs and spices may not reveal IgG and mast cell reactions to old, oxidized ones. Herbs and spices have the best flavors and health profiles when they are fresh and freshly ground. It is preferable to buy small packages of herbs and spices and to purchase fresh herbs and whole spices and grind them just before use so that they will be fresh and not have undergone oxidation. In general, spices should be labeled with the date the package was opened and discarded if not used within a year.

Reintroduction of IgG Positive Foods

Retesting for IgG food reactions can be done after several months to see if foods may be reintroduced. Alternatively, after a minimum of 3 months, the patient may try to reintroduce no more than one food every several days, to see if it provokes an adverse reaction. Reintroduction should begin with foods with the weakest (+1) IgG response.
In my experience, younger patients respond more quickly and often can reintroduce some foods after only a few months. Older adult patients, however, may easily require a year or two more before an antergic response abates and they are able to reintroduce the reacting food without adverse immune response. Some foods highly reactive foods, such as wheat and yeasts, may require more time than other foods. Repeat testing is appropriate serveal months to a year, depending on the age of the individual.

Patients that have developed antergies to wheat or yeast are wise to limit the consumption of these foods even after the tests become negative as they may easily become reactive again.

---

[1] Association between rotavirus infection and pancreatic islet autoimmunity in children at risk of developing type 1 diabetes. Honeyman MC, Coulson BS, Stone NL, Gellert SA, Goldwater PN, Steele CE, Couper JJ, Tait BD, Colman PG, Harrison LC. Diabetes. 2000 Aug;49(8):1319-24. PMID:10923632

[2] Rotavirus infection frequency and risk of celiac disease autoimmunity in early childhood: a longitudinal study. Stene LC, Honeyman MC, Hoffenberg EJ, Haas JE, Sokol RJ, Emery L, Taki I, Norris JM, Erlich HA, Eisenbarth GS, Rewers M. Am J Gastroenterol. 2006 Oct;101(10):2333-40. PMID:17032199

[3] The biology of intestinal immunoglobulin A responses. Cerutti A, Rescigno M. Immunity. 2008 Jun;28(6):740-50. PMID:18549797

[4] Milk protein IgG and IgA: the association with milk-induced gastrointestinal symptoms in adults. Anthoni S, Savilahti E, Rautelin H, Kolho KL. World J Gastroenterol. 2009 Oct 21;15(39):4915-8.PMID: 19842221

[5] Humoral immunity to cow's milk proteins and gliadin within the etiology of recurrent aphthous ulcers? Besu I, Jankovic L, Magdu IU, Konic-Ristic A, Raskovic S, Juranic Z. Oral Dis. 2009 Nov;15(8):560-4. Epub 2009 Jun 29.PMID: 19563417

[6] Food allergy mediated by IgG antibodies associated with migraine in adults. Arroyave Hernández CM, Echevarría Pinto M, Hernández Montiel HL. Rev Alerg Mex. 2007 Sep-Oct;54(5):162-8.PMID: 18693538

[7] The gut-joint axis: cross reactive food antibodies in rheumatoid arthritis. Hvatum M, Kanerud L, Hällgren R, Brandtzaeg P. Gut. 2006 Sep;55(9):1240-7. Epub 2006 Feb 16.PMID: 16484508

[8] Enhanced levels of cow's milk antibodies in infancy in children who develop type 1 diabetes later in childhood. Luopajärvi K, Savilahti E, Virtanen SM, Ilonen J, Knip M, Akerblom HK, Vaarala O. Pediatr Diabetes. 2008 Oct;9(5):434-41. Epub 2008 May 21. PMID:18503496

[9] Food elimination based on IgG antibodies in irritable bowel syndrome: a randomised controlled trial. Atkinson W, Sheldon TA, Shaath N, Whorwell PJ. Gut. 2004 Oct;53(10):1459-64.PMID: 15361495

[10] Comparison of the intestinal and serum antibody response in patients with dermatitis herpetiformis. Hall RP 3rd, McKenzie KD. Clin Immunol Immunopathol. 1992 Jan;62(1 Pt 1):33-41.PMID: 1728978

[11] Antibody (IgG, IgA, and IgM) to baker's yeast (Saccharomyces cerevisiae), yeast mannan, gliadin, ovalbumin and betalactoglobulin in monozygotic twins with inflammatory bowel disease. Lindberg E, Magnusson KE, Tysk C, Järnerot G. Gut. 1992 Jul;33(7):909-13.PMID: 1644330

[12] IgG antibodies against food antigens are correlated with inflammation and intima media thickness in obese juveniles. Wilders-Truschnig M, Mangge H, Lieners C, Gruber H, Mayer C, März W. Exp Clin Endocrinol Diabetes. 2008 Apr;116(4):241-5. Epub 2007 Dec 10.PMID: 18072008

[13] Eliminating Immunologically-Reactive Foods from the Diet and its Effect on Body Composition and Quality of Life in Overweight Persons. Lewis JE, Woolger JM, Melillo A, Alonso Y,

Rafatjah S, et al. J Obes Weig los Ther. (2012) 2:112. doi:10.4172/2165-7904.1000112

[14] Alterations of food antigen-specific serum immunoglobulins G and E antibodies in patients with irritable bowel syndrome and functional dyspepsia. Zuo XL, Li YQ, Li WJ, Guo YT, Lu XF, Li JM, Desmond PV. Clin Exp Allergy. 2007 Jun;37(6):823-30.PMID: 17517095

[15] Gluten sensitivity in patients with IgA nephropathy. Smerud HK, Fellström B, Hällgren R, Osagie S, Venge P, Kristjánsson G. Nephrol Dial Transplant. 2009 Aug;24(8):2476-81. Epub 2009 Mar 30.PMID: 1933286

[16] Autoantibody screen in inflammatory myopathies high prevalence of antibodies to gliadin. Orbach H, Amitai N, Barzilai O, Boaz M, Ram M, Zandman-Goddard G, Shoenfeld Y. Ann N Y Acad Sci. 2009 Sep;1173:174-9.PMID: 19758147

[17] Gluten sensitivity in multiple sclerosis: experimental myth or clinical truth? Shor DB, Barzilai O, Ram M, Izhaky D, Porat-Katz BS, Chapman J, Blank M, Anaya JM, Shoenfeld Y. Ann N Y Acad Sci. 2009 Sep;1173:343-9.PMID: 19758171

[18] Increased prevalence of silent celiac disease among Greek epileptic children. Antigoni M, Xinias I, Theodouli P, Karatza E, Maria F, Panteliadis C, Spiroglou K. Pediatr Neurol. 2007 Mar;36(3):165-9.PMID: 17352949

[19] Specific IgA antibody increases in schizophrenia. Reichelt KL, Landmark J. Biol Psychiatry. 1995 Mar 15;37(6):410-3.PMID: 7772650

[20] Colonic lymphoid nodular hyperplasia in children: relationship to food hypersensitivity. Iacono G, Ravelli A, Di Prima L, Scalici C, Bolognini S, Chiappa S, Pirrone G, Licastri G, Carroccio A. Clin Gastroenterol Hepatol. 2007 Mar;5(3):361-6.PMID: 17368236

[21] Autoantibodies in gluten ataxia recognize a novel neuronal transglutaminase. Hadjivassiliou M, Aeschlimann P, Strigun A, Sanders DS, Woodroofe N, Aeschlimann D. Ann Neurol. 2008 Sep;64(3):332-43.PMID: 18825674

[22] Diet restriction in migraine, based on IgG against foods: a clinical double-blind, randomised, cross-over trial. Alpay K, Ertas M, Orhan EK, et al Cephalalgia. 2010 Jul;30(7):829-37. PMID:20647174

[23] Enteral nutrition for maintenance of remission in Crohn's disease. Akobeng AK, Thomas AG. Cochrane Database Syst Rev. 2007 Jul 18;(3):CD005984. PMID:17636816

[24] Nutritional status and nutritional therapy in inflammatory bowel diseases. Hartman C, Eliakim R, Shamir R. World J Gastroenterol. 2009 Jun 7;15(21):2570-8. PMID:19496185

[25] Is rheumatoid arthritis a disease that starts in the intestine? A pilot study comparing an elemental diet with oral prednisolone. Podas T, Nightingale JM, Oldham R, Roy S, Sheehan NJ, Mayberry JF. Postgrad Med J. 2007 Feb;83(976):128-31. PMID:17308218

[26] The gut-joint axis: cross reactive food antibodies in rheumatoid arthritis. Hvatum M, Kanerud L, Hällgren R, Brandtzaeg P. Gut. 2006 Sep;55(9):1240-7. Epub 2006 Feb 16. PMID:16484508

[27] Human FcγRIIA induces anaphylactic and allergic reactions. Jönsson F, Mancardi DA, Zhao W, Kita Y, Iannascoli B, Khun H, van Rooijen N, Shimizu T, Schwartz LB, Daëron M, Bruhns P. Blood. 2011 Dec 2. PMID:22138510

[28] Immunologic and clinical responses to parenteral immunotherapy in peanut anaphylaxis--a study using IgE and IgG4 immunoblot monitoring. Bullock RJ, Barnett D, Howden ME. Allergol Immunopathol (Madr). 2005 Sep-Oct;33(5):250-6.PMID: 16287543

[29] High levels of IgG4 antibodies to foods during infancy are associated with tolerance to corresponding foods later in life. Tomicić S, Norrman G, Fälth-Magnusson K, Jenmalm MC, Devenney I, Böttcher MF. Pediatr Allergy Immunol. 2009 Feb;20(1):35-41. Epub 2008 Mar 12.PMID: 18346097

[30] Development of immunoglobulin G subclass antibodies to ovalbumin, birch and cat during the first eight years of life in atopic and non-atopic children. Jenmalm MC, Björkstén B. Pediatr Allergy Immunol. 1999 May;10(2):112-21.PMID: 10478613

[31] Natural history of cow's milk allergy. An eight-year follow-up study in 115 atopic children. Cantani A, Micera M. Eur Rev Med Pharmacol Sci. 2004 Jul-Aug;8(4):153-64.PMID: 15636401

[32] Activation of human mast cells by aggregated IgG through FcgammaRI: additive effects of C3a. Woolhiser MR, Brockow K, Metcalfe DD. Clin Immunol. 2004 Feb;110(2):172-80. PMID:15003814

[33] Evidence for an immune-mediated mechanism in food-induced migraine from a study on activated T-cells, IgG4 subclass, anti-IgG antibodies and circulating immune complexes. Martelletti P, Sutherland J, Anastasi E, Di Mario U, Giacovazzo M. Headache. 1989 Nov;29(10):664-70.PMID: 2613516

[34] T cells expressing IL-2 receptor in migraine. Martelletti P. Acta Neurol (Napoli). 1991 Oct;13(5):448-56. Review.PMID: 1776533

[35] Evidence of melatonin synthesis and release by mast cells. Possible modulatory role on inflammation. Maldonado MD, Mora-Santos M, Naji L, Carrascosa-Salmoral MP, Naranjo MC, Calvo JR. Pharmacol Res. 2010 Sep;62(3):282-7. PMID:19963060

[36] Psychological stress and corticotropin-releasing hormone increase intestinal permeability in humans by a mast cell-dependent mechanism. Vanuytsel T, van Wanrooy S, Vanheel H, etal. Gut. 2013 Oct 23. PMID:24153250

[37] Stress and the gut: pathophysiology, clinical consequences, diagnostic approach and treatment options. Konturek PC, Brzozowski T, Konturek SJ. J Physiol Pharmacol. 2011 Dec;62(6):591-9. PMID:22314561

20. Vitamin D₃

Vitamin D₃ (cholecalciferol) is formed when ultraviolet light, usually from sunlight, breaks the B bond in 7-dehydrocholesterol in the skin. It is transported to the liver, where it is converted into the prohormone calcifediol, and then, in the kidney or certain immune cells, it is converted to calcitriol; the active form of Vitamin D₃.

> Vitamin D₂ is made in invertebrates, such as mollusks, insects, and fungi. It is not as effective as Vitamin D₃ is in humans and is much more easily toxic. There is little reason to use it as a supplement.

Vitamin D deficiency has long been associated with rickets, a disease, once common, in children in which the bones do not calcify properly, and thus, the bones can grow bowed and deformed. Early in the 1900's, cod liver oil was used for the prevention of this disease. The taste was awful; even as an older adult, my father remembered it as a punishment. In 1923, Harry Steenbock, a professor of biochemistry at the University of Wisconsin, demonstrated that rickets in rats could be cured by exposing their feed to UV light. This process was applied to milk, and rickets became rare in the United States.

Diet is unlikely to provide sufficient vitamin D, even if a person drinks milk that has been irradiated with UV light to convert some cholesterol to vitamin D. The amount in milk may prevent rickets, but is not enough for optimal health. Sufficient vitamin D levels are essential to health, but there is a worldwide pandemic of vitamin D deficiency, even for those living under the equatorial sun.

The most common adult manifestation of severe vitamin D deficiency is osteomalacia. In this disease, there is also a failure of bone mineralization. My sister was diagnosed with fibromyalgia by a very capable rheumatologist. She had muscle aches, widespread pain and some weakness without apparent cause. However, it was osteomalacia. My sister was at risk as she is lactose intolerant and thus avoids milk, and lives in at a latitude where the UV index is too low to make vitamin D several for months of the year.

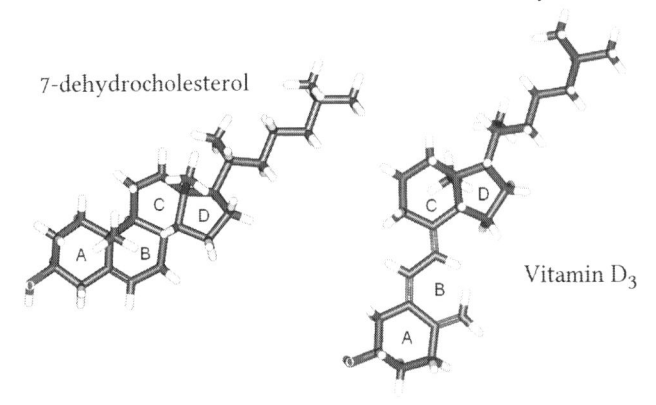

Figure 20-1: 7-dehydrocholesterol and Vitamin D₃.

To make Vitamin D₃, 7-dehydrocholesterol needs to have its "B" ring shattered by UV light. It is similar to how an opera singer can shatter a wine glass with their voice. You can wet the edge of a crystal wine glass and rub it to make it ring with a sweet vibration. Singing that same resonant frequency can make it vibrate. Sing loud enough, at the correct frequency, and the energy in the sound waves can make the glass vibrate so strongly that the glass shatters.

With 7-dehydrocholesterol, it is ultraviolet light which causes the "B" ring to vibrate, and not just any UV light, but light in a narrow section of the UVB band between 295 and 300 nm. Making the "B" ring of dehydrocholesterol vibrate is not enough; it has to shatter. In order to shatter, it takes an intensity of sunlight greater than a solar UV index of about 3. Less intense sunlight does not have sufficient energy to cause photolysis of 7-dehydrocholesterol into previtamin D₃, that can then be converted to vitamin D₃. And while a solar index of three or greater permits previtamin D formation in Caucasians, individuals with more deeply pigmented skin have built-in sunscreen, and thus, need a higher level of UV radiation to form vitamin D₃[1]. Fair skin is a rather recent adaptation that allows humans to survive in northern latitudes.

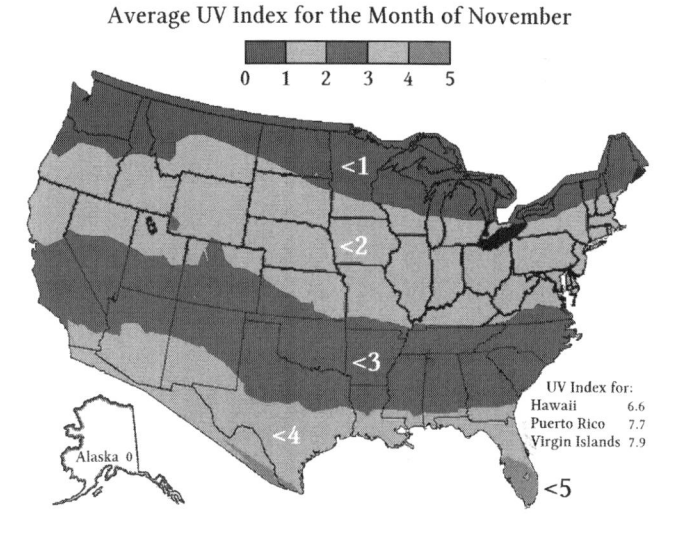

Figure 20-2: Climatologic Mean UV Index for November

Living in the north presents a problem. The map in Figure 20-2 shows the usual UV index at noon on a sunny day for the U.S.[2] during the month of November. If you live in an area that is lower than 4, you are out of luck when it comes to making Vitamin D₃ during the winter months. Individuals living Seattle make little vitamin D from October through May. Most of the population of the U.S., all of Canada, and most of Europe, New Zealand and Chile live in areas where it is impossible to get enough sunlight to make Vitamin D from sun exposure for several months of the year.

Add to this that much of the human population seems to have developed solar-phobia! Most adults and more recently most children stay indoors most hours of the day.

When people go out, it is in cars behind UV-proof glass that protects us from UV radiation. Many modern humans also are in the habit of wearing clothes, hats and sunscreen that prevents solar radiation from contacting the skin.

Unfortunately, the skin gets progressively thinner after the age of 20 and with it, the concentration of 7-dehydrocholesterol declines. An elderly person exposed to the equivalent to 15 minutes of sunshine produces about a quarter as much vitamin D as young people exposed to the same amount of sunlight[3]. Migration has increased the number of darker skinned people living in northern climates over the last few hundred years, and these people often do not produce optimal amounts of vitamin D.

For at least four months of the year, most Americans and Canadians can not form vitamin D, and many have vitamin D deficiency. Most Canadians live farther south than Paris, France, and thus Europeans also suffer from Vitamin D deficiency. New Zealand and Tasmania also have low solar indexes during their winter months.

> Vitamin D deficiency also occurs in the lower latitudes, principally among females[4].
>
> In India, it is culturally desirable to have fair skin. Girls and women avoid the sun to maintain a lighter skin color. Vitamin D deficiency is also common in Muslim countries[5] where women traditionally cover most of their skin when outside of the home, whether using a veil or not[6].

Much of the world's population does not get enough sunlight to form sufficient vitamin D during the winter months. Urbanites, even in tropical climates, may not get sufficient sun exposure to maintain optimal Vitamin D levels.

Vitamin D_3 formed in the skin, or from supplements, is converted in the liver to calcifediol, also known as 25-hydroxycholecalciferol or 25-hydroxyvitamin D ($25OHD_3$). Calcitriol ($1,25OHD_3$) is the active form of the vitamin. Vitamin D status is best reflected by the $25OHD_3$ levels in the blood as it has a long half-life.

> **Note:** This document uses the measurements:
> - International Units (IU) of Vitamin D_3 (cholecalciferol)
> - Nmol/L of $25OHD_3$
>
> For comparing with other sources:
> - 1 μg of cholecalciferol = 40 IU
> - 1 ng/mL 25OHD = 2.5 nmol/L

Vitamin D and Health

Vitamin D is a hormone with receptors present in every living cell in the body. It participates in the regulation of, at least, 200 different genes. It plays an important role in regulating inflammation[7] and fighting infection[8].

It has long been recognized that inadequate vitamin D levels are associated with bone disease. And even though these diseases seem simple enough to prevent with 400 IU of vitamin D a day, rickets continues to be seen in infants and children, especially among those with darker skin pigmentation in the United States[9] as well as in other countries[10]. Osteomalacia and osteoporosis are common in the elderly. The increased risk for low birth weight and premature births, as well as for increased risk of heart disease, and breast and prostate cancers seen among African Americans may be due to inadequate vitamin D.

Vitamin D deficiency is implicated in the pathogenesis of a large disease burden in the United States. These diseases are common because of the high susceptibility to them, at least in part, as a result of the high prevalence of vitamin D deficiency in our population. Table 20-1 provides a list of several diseases associated with inadequate vitamin D.

Table 20-1: Diseases Associated with Low Vitamin D Levels

Breast Cancer[11]	Peritonitis[17]
Colon Cancer	Asthma[18]
Prostate Cancer	Infectious diseases (Flu)
Ovarian Cancer	Respiratory Infections
Multiple Myeloma	Tuberculosis
Depression[12]	Type 1 Diabetes
Post Partum Depression	Insulin resistance[19]
Schizophrenia	Diabetic Retinopathy[20]
Bipolar Disorder	Rheumatoid Arthritis[21]
Multiple Sclerosis	Autoimmune Diseases
Cognitive Decline[13]	Loss of hearing and balance
Parkinson's Disease[14]	
	Polycystic Ovary Syndrome[22]
Atherosclerosis[15]	Obesity[23]
Endothelial Dysfunction	Obstructive Sleep Apnea in children[24]
Coronary Artery Disease	Metabolic Syndrome
Hypertension	
Rickets	Preeclampsia[25]
Osteoporosis	Premature births[26]
Osteomalacia	Fetal Growth Retardation
Myopathy[16]	Need for C-Section

Vitamin D_3 is a chemopreventive agent which arrest malignant cell differentiation. Like other steroid hormones, it is a nuclear hormone, and it regulates the expression of numerous proteins. Calcitriol suppresses the expression of genes regulated by c-MYC, a transcription factor that controls epidermal differentiation and cell proliferation[27]. Additionally, calcitriol suppresses β-catenin expression in colorectal cancer cells. β-catenin acts as a signal for cell proliferation[28]. Calcitriol also enhances activation of FoxO proteins, which are tumor suppressors and oxidative stress resistance factors[29].

In a study of US military veterans, vitamin D supplements improved chronic pain, improved sleep latency and duration, general health and social functioning[30].

Figure 2 shows the average n-3 fatty acid consumption in 31 different countries and plots them against the country's mortality rate for coronary heart disease (CHD). An inverse relationship can be seen. The lower curve shows the relationship found in most countries. There are five countries that are outliers with significantly higher CHD mortality rates for the amount of n-3 fatty acids consumed. The most extreme are the four most northern countries, Russia, Finland, Norway and Iceland. New Zealand is not as extreme an outlier, but it is as far south as these other countries are north. These data suggest that latitude has an impact on the prevalence of CHD; the mechanism for this is likely lower vitamin D levels in those populations.

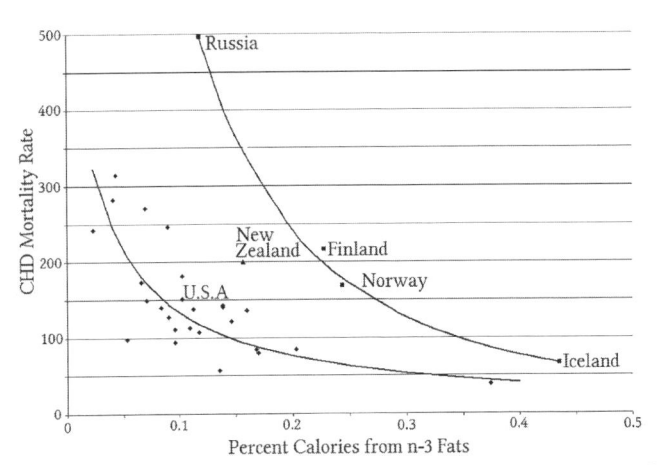

Figure 20-3: Coronary Heart Disease Mortality by percent of dietary calories from n-3 fats

Vitamin D_3 down-regulates TLR4 expression, providing an anti-inflammatory effect. As discussed in Chapter 10, TLR4 activation is required in the formation of atherosclerosis[31]. N-3 fats also down-regulate the inflammatory cascade in macrophages and other immune cells.

What Are Optimal Vitamin D Levels?

The reason that Neanderthals, Celts, and more recent Northern Europeans are fair skinned is that those with darker skin could not get enough Vitamin D, and could not survive. Women who had suffered from rickets as children often had a deformation of the pelvis that resulted in narrowing of the birth canal. Later, with pregnancy, the woman's infant could not be born, resulting in the death of both mother and child. This created a strong selective survival advantage for those with lighter skin color. But how much Vitamin D did our early ancestor's make living in the tropical savannah, enjoying the sunshine as they were being chased by lions and hunting grasshoppers? What is a normal vitamin D level for free-living humans in the natural environment in which we evolved?

In a young person, one 15-minute exposure to the summer sun can give the equivalent production of vitamin D to a dose of 10,000 IU of vitamin D_3[2]. In a study of young people from Sao Paulo, Brazil, the summertime average 25-hydroxyvitamin D_3 (25OHD) levels for medical students and indoor workers was 103 nmol/L. These were medical students and indoor workers, not outdoor laborers, or hunter-gatherers as were our ancestors, who would have spent most of every day in the sun, although some of the participants went to the beach as many as 5 days a week and spent over 30 minutes in the sun each occasion. (How can medical student get to the beach 5 times a week?!) A quarter of the participants in this study had levels above 124 nmol/liter, and the top 5 percent had levels over 165 nm/L. The highest 25OHD level in this group was 214 nmol/L[32]. Higher 25OHD levels were seen in those who frequented the beach.

People who work in the sun have higher levels: a study found that farmers in Puerto Rico had an average 25OHD level of 135 nmol/L, and lifeguards had an average of 148 nmol/L in one study and 166 nmol/L in another[33]. 25OHD levels of 100 to 200 nmol/L should be considered at normal physiologic levels for healthy young adults, and certainly not extreme or dangerous.

Another way to understand optimal Vitamin D levels is to look at what levels are required for physiologic functions, and what levels minimize disease risk.

Getting Sun

Too much sun causes aging of the skin, wrinkles and can cause skin cancer. It causes oxidative damage and lipid peroxidation. Squamous cell skin cancers and basal cell skin cancers are associated with sun exposure and are almost always curable with surgery; malignant melanoma is not. Study of the genetic mutations found in these cancers show DNA base exchanges typical of UV light – it leaves its signature in the DNA[34]. UV light can increase NK-κB and suppress AP-1; decreasing apoptosis and tissue repair[35].

Here is a strategy: Wearing a hat and sunscreen and when you go out in the sun can protect you from wrinkles and skin cancers on the head, neck and hands – the most constantly exposed areas. Make vitamin D in the skin of your arms, legs, and trunk, sparing the face of solar damage and keeping your face's youthful appearance. After 15 minutes of sun on the other parts of your body, put sunscreen on them too. Mid-day sun has a higher UVB: UVA ratio; UVB is the type that forms vitamin D[36]. Early morning and late afternoon are not good times to make vitamin D anyway.

Avoid ever getting sunburnt.

Wear sunglasses to protect your eyes. Children and especially infants' eyes are especially susceptible to UV damage, as the young lens allows much more UV light through than does the adult lens of the eye. Children need sunglasses more than adults do.

Insight to the body's optimal vitamin D requirement can be gained examining the relationship of parathyroid hormone

(PTH) with vitamin D. Vitamin D levels are inversely related to PTH levels. PTH raises calcium levels by increasing absorption of calcium from the intestine, increasing reuptake by the kidneys and by liberating calcium from the bones. When serum calcium levels are low, PTH rises to maintain the narrow physiologic range of calcium required for normal cellular function.

One action of PTH is to induce the enzyme that converts 25OHD to the active hormone 1-25OHD. 1,25OHD increases the production of the enterocyte calcium pump calbindin-D9k, which transports calcium from the intestinal lumen, into the body. The portion of calcium absorbed by the intestine increases with serum 25OHD level up to about 80 nmol/L, and then levels off[37].

In a French study of elderly women, it was found that PTH levels fell with higher 25OHD$_3$ levels, with a plateau above about 80 nmol/L of 25OHD$_3$[9]. Thus, the body scavenges bone stores of calcium to maintain serum calcium if 25OHD$_3$ levels are below 80 nmol/L (32 ng/mL); such levels are clearly deficient. Nevertheless, in a trial of vitamin D$_3$ in patients with multiple sclerosis, PTH levels continued to fall to even lower levels as 25OHD$_3$ levels increased[38], still remaining in the normal PTH range, even when 25OHD$_3$ levels averaged 385 nmol/L.

Since few urbanites have 25OHD$_3$ levels over 100 nmol/L without the use of supplements, there is limited data on the effects of higher levels. But looking at trends, most studies suggest decreasing risk of disease as 25OHD$_3$ levels rise above 75 nmol/L. There were fewer fractures and cases of colon cancer risk when vitamin D levels were at 115 nmol/L than at 90 nmol/L. In young Caucasian and Hispanic adults, bone mineral density (BMD) was highest when 25OHD3 levels were around 120 nmol/L, although (BMD) peak in African Americans at about 90 nmol/L[39]. These and other data suggest optimal levels for 25OHD$_3$ are around 90-120 nmol/l (36-48 ng/ml)[40].

Hypovitaminosis D is associated with insulin resistance. In a study of 126 Californian adults without diabetes, blood glucose levels were inversely related to 25OHD$_3$ from low levels to the upper levels present among this population, about 100 nmol/L[41]. The relationship is also seen in children and adolescents[42]. Vitamin D$_3$ levels are thus associated with improving insulin sensitivity to at least 200 nmol/liter (80 ng/ml), and perhaps higher. One pathway by which vitamin D prevents diabetes is through its activation of sphingosine kinase[43]. This enzyme lowers ceramide levels and increases S1P. Ceramide increases insulin resistance, decreases the production of insulin and induces the apoptosis of pancreatic β-cells[44]. S1P inhibits β-cells apoptosis[45].

Another measure is to look at muscular activity. Muscular contraction relies on calcium influx into the muscle cells. Several studies have found that vitamin D supplementation decreases falls among the elderly by about 20 percent[46]. In a study of over 4000 Americans over 60 years of age, time to walk 8 feet was inversely related to 25OHD levels, with a downward trend continuing with 25OHD levels between 100 and 220 nmol/L[47]. A test of the time required to stand up from a sitting position was also performed. In this test, time to stand was also inversely related to 25OHD levels, but the lowest times were associated with a 25OHD level around 125 nmol/L, after which times began to increase. The authors pointed out, however, that these higher 25OHD levels were associated with supplements given to patients with osteoporosis, and thus, the slowing in standing times may have been the result of preexisting disease rather than from higher vitamin D levels.

Vitamin D status is also related to bone density. In a study of white American men aged 30 to 79, bone density was highest in men with 25OHD$_3$ levels around 125 nmol/L (50 ng/ml)[48]; however, the decline in bone density associated with Vitamin D levels above 125 nmol/L could have been due to treatment with vitamin D in patients concerned about low bone density.

These studies suggest that optimal 25OHD$_3$ levels for health require levels of 100 to 200 nmol/L, (40 to 80 ng/ml). The current recommend range for serum 25OHD$_3$ is 75 to 185 nmol/L (30.0 to 74.0 ng/mL). The lower end of this range (less than 80 nmol/L) includes risk of osteomalacia[49].

Effect of Inflammation on 25OHD Level

Inflammation causes 25OHD levels to fall. Patients undergoing elective knee arthroplasty had a 25% decline in 25OHD levels that were observed as early as 6 hours after surgery. Levels remained below preoperative levels three months later.[50] Women with hip fractures had lower 25OHD and higher IL-6 levels a year later[51]. 25OHD levels have been found to be inversely related to obesity and insulin resistance, and to correlate with the level of inflammation. Inflammatory status may predict 25OHD level. Patients with elevated leptin and IL-6 levels had lower 25OHD levels after 30 months of follow-up[52].

The mechanism for the fall in 25OHD has not been established; however, stress and inflammation may decrease enterohepatic reuptake of fat soluble vitamins. These vitamins can be lost with malabsorption syndromes, as well. Furthermore, inflammation and stress may decrease the conversion vitamin D into 25OHD and may increase the conversion of 25OHD into 1,25OHD, the active form of this hormone, which has a short half-life.

While low levels of 25OHD3 may result from inflammation, supplementation has not been found to lower markers of inflammation. Nevertheless, vitamin D$_3$ may be helpful in some conditions associated with inflammation. In young insulin resistant patients, six months of treatment with 4000 IU of vitamin D$_3$ improved 25OHD$_3$ levels and insulin sensitivity[53].

Vitamin D₃ Toxicity

Vitamin D intake recommendations were originally set to prevent rickets. The level required for this is lower than the dose required to prevent chronic disease or optimize health. Recommended intake of vitamin D has also been kept low out of fear of toxicity. A century ago, vitamin D supplements were usually derived from natural sources, which also contained vitamin A. Vitamin D can cause toxicity, but only at levels much higher than the toxic dose for vitamin A, which can easily reach toxic levels. Some reported toxicity from vitamin D historically likely came from the use of Vitamin D₂[54] (ergosterol). Vitamin D₂ appears to *increase* inflammatory cytokine levels[55]. Additionally, very high intake levels of vitamin D can cause problems, such as hypercalcemia and kidney stones.

Vitamin D₃ can be used as rat poison. These are nocturnal creatures that avoid the sun. Rats become symptomatic with a single dose of 0.5 mg/kg of calcitriol; 1,25 OHD3, the active hormone form of vitamin D₃. This would be equivalent allometrically-adjusted dose (Chapter 40) of 5 milligrams in a 60-kg (120-pound) women. Twenty-five milligrams are equivalent to 200,000 units of calcitriol as a single dose. This is calcitriol, not the form found in over the counter vitamins.

> Vitamin D is a hormone. Cholecalciferol is a pre-prohormone that the body converts to a prohormone, which is then converted to the active hormone, calcitriol. The conversions are controlled internally; sunlight does not control vitamin D hormonal activity.
>
> Cholecalciferol is a substrate for forming the active hormone. Vitamins D, A, and K are unique in that there are no other hormones for which the body has substrate deficiencies.

In New Zealand, vitamin D (cholecalciferol,) is used to kill another nocturnal animal, the possum, which is considered to be an agricultural pest. The dose that kills 50 percent of the animals is 16.8 mg/kg[56]. That would be equivalent to 4.3 mg/kg in a human adult or 10.4 million IU of vitamin D for a 120-pound person. Large over-the-counter vitamin D capsules often contain 2000 IU. Thus, this dose would be equivalent to 5,220 capsules.

Cholecalciferol is toxic. A two-year-old boy was seen in the ER for colic and constipation and was discovered to have a serum calcium level of 14.4 mg/dL. His mother had mistakenly given him 2,400,000 IU of vitamin D₃ over four days[57]. Several cases have been studies where dilution errors caused vitamin D toxicity. This has often occurred with long time use of 100 to 1000 times the expected oral supplemental dose. In these cases, the patients become asymptomatic when 25OHD levels fall to 1000 nmol/L (400 ng/ml)[58]. As a result of a dilution error a man took about 1 million units of Vitamin D₃, (the over-the-counter, less toxic form) not just once, but once daily[59], thinking he was taking 1000 units. By the time he felt sick enough to go to the emergency room, his calcium level was 15.2 mg/dl, and his 25OHD level was 1300 nmol/L! Several patients using a supplement containing 864,000 IU of vitamin D3 daily (along with 123,500 IU of vitamin A) became symptomatic; however, 8 of the 9 patients had a disease which raised calcium levels, including squamous cell carcinoma, lymphoma, mycobacterium infection, or granulomatous disease[60]. Normally, cholecalciferol toxicity is limited by the requirement for it to be converted to the active form: calcitriol, 1-25OHD. Calcitriol is considerably more toxic than cholecalciferol or 25OHD.

High doses of Vitamin D₃ are used as a treatment for multiple sclerosis (MS). In a dosing trial, MS patients were given an accelerating dose of Vitamin D₃ beginning with the equivalent of 4000 units a day and going up to 40,000 units a day by the end of the trial. The average 25OHD level at the end of the trial was 385 nmol/L. Calcium levels were slightly *lower* by the end of the trial, remaining in the normal range. Urinary calcium remained normal, and PTH levels dropped but stayed within the normal range[61]. No toxicity was noted.

The threshold for vitamin D toxicity has been found to be around 750 nmol/L of serum 25OHD[62], with early signs including elevated calcium levels, hyperphosphatemia and increased urinary calcium. To attain a plateau level reaching of 750 nmol/L in healthy adults requires a daily dose of about 50,000 units of vitamin D a day over an extended period[63].

Ten thousand units of vitamin D₃ a day appears to be a safe dose in healthy adults, especially during winter months when vitamin D cannot be produced in the skin from sun exposure. Adults with pre-existing conditions causing hypercalcemia should use lower amounts and be monitored for 25OHD and calcium levels.

> Dietary Sources of Vitamin D
>
> Milk is treated with UV light to create some vitamin D, and this is the largest source of the vitamin D in the diet of children. This provides sufficient vitamin D that the small amount present in UV-irradiated milk has nearly eradicated rickets as a common disease in the United States and Europe.
>
> Fish that are high on the food chain can be good sources of Vitamin D. Wild salmon has nearly 1000 units of Vitamin D₃ per 3.5 oz. serving, but farmed salmon only has about 250 units per serving[2]. The higher the fish are on the food chain, the higher their vitamin D content. However, these fish are concentrated toxins, such as mercury. Thus, it is wise avoid fish from the top of the food chain as one's main source of vitamin D.
>
> Without additional supplementation, the diet is not an effective way to get sufficient vitamin D unless you are willing to eat like an Inuit. Have you had pan fried seal liver for breakfast recently?

> Can we trust the dairy? A study of 173 samples of milk from around the U.S. and British Colombia found that half of the samples had less than 80% of the amount of vitamin D listed on the label and 14% of the samples tested contained no Vitamin D at all[64]. A separate study done in New York had similar results[65].

Target Dosing

A reasonable target level for serum $25OHD_3$ is 125 nmol/L. This level could easily be expected for a young person who spent some time in the sun most days during the summer months, and is a level which seems to provide optimal bone mass and protection from multiple diseases. It is a level safe from toxicity. Additionally, it gives a large margin for variation within a healthy range. Levels below 80 nmol/L of $25OHD_3$ are associated with bone loss. Target levels should be high enough that few in the population have levels associated with risk. Taking sufficient vitamin D supplements to achieve a target level of 125 nmol/L, would place most people's 25OHD level between 100 and 150 nmol/L.

One thousand IU of vitamin D_3, taken daily, on average, raises the 25OHD3 level in healthy adults by 17.5 nmol/L (7 ng/mL) at equilibrium[66]. Thus, if an individual's $25OHD_3$ level is 60 nmol/L without supplements, 1000 IU daily would raise the level to 77.5 nmol/L at equilibrium, after about six weeks. Thus, for someone with a background level of 40 nmol/L it would take 4857 IU a day to achieve a steady state level of 125 nmol/L.

(125 nmol/L - Current level in nmol/L) / 17.5 x 1000 IU
(125 – 40) / 17.5 x 1000 = 4857 or about 5000 IU per day

1000 IU of vitamin D3 raises 25OHD3 levels by 17.5 nmol/L
1000 IU of vitamin D3 raises 25OHD3 levels by 7 ng/mL

Loading dose: To raise a low level quickly, doctors can give a large dose of Vitamin D_3. An oral dose of 300,000 units has been demonstrated to be more effective than 100,000 unit loading doses for in normalizing PTH levels[67]. A method that can be used for calculating doses for adults is to use the calculation above, and multiply it times 60 (two month's dose) to get the loading dose. For the example above, that would be 291,420 units or nearly 300,000 IU.

I suggest giving the loading dose over ten days to improve absorption, thus 30,000 units a day for ten days, followed by a daily maintenance dose. If calculations give a number over 400,000 IU, don't use that dose; do the math again. Vitamin D and other fat-soluble vitamins are best absorbed with meals, at a time when bile acids and lipase are present to help with their absorption.

25OHD3 Levels and the Intestine

Even in northern climates, although most people may not have optimal 25OHD levels, most individuals do not have levels so low as to put them risk for osteomalacia or bone loss. When 25OHD levels are low, especially in Caucasians, who make Vitamin D more easily, and for those living at lower latitudes, in malabsorption should be considered in the differential diagnosis. Malabsorption should also be considered in patients whose 25OHD levels do not rise as expected with vitamin D supplementation or injection.

Vitamin D is excreted in the bile and reabsorbed; it is easily lost in malabsorption syndrome, along with vitamins A, E and K, folate, vitamin B12, magnesium, and other minerals. Most patients with low 25OHD levels, osteomalacia, or other inflammatory conditions should be assessed for malabsorption or inflammatory disease of the intestine if the vitamin D level is low. Usually, it will not be the only deficiency present. Osteoporosis is usually the result of multiple nutrient deficiencies (Chapter 42).

Alternatively, 25OHD ($25OHD_2$ plus $25OHD_3$) may be high in some patients as a result of conversion of ergosterol, a precursor to vitamin D_2, which can be produced by overgrowth of the yeast *Candida albicans* in the intestine. In these patients, treatment for *Candida albicans* and intestinal biofilm is indicated (Chapter 23).

A Public Health Imperative

Vitamin D levels need to be raised for the entire society, in the United States and other countries. The problem has worsened with time, as the US and other temperate and northern climate countries, such as Europe and Canada, have growing populations of people with darker pigmentation, people become more urbanized stay indoors more of the time and wear sunscreen to avoid damage to the skin. Vitamin D fortification of foods is a potential way of addressing this issue.

[1] Factors that influence the cutaneous synthesis and dietary sources of vitamin D. Chen TC, Chimeh F, Lu Z, Holick MF et al. Arch Biochem Biophys. 2007 Apr 15;460(2):213-7. PMID: 17254541

[2] http://www.epa.gov/sunwise/uvimonth.htm

[3] Vitamin D and sunlight: strategies for cancer prevention and other health benefits. Holick MF. Clin J Am Soc Nephrol. 2008 Sep;3(5):1548-54. PMID: 18550652

[4] Vitamin D deficiency in rural girls and pregnant women despite abundant sunshine in northern India. Sahu M, Bhatia V, Aggarwal A, Rawat V, Saxena P, Pandey A, Das V. Clin Endocrinol (Oxf). 2009 May;70(5):680-4. PMID: 18673464

[5] 25-Hydoxyvitamin D levels among healthy Saudi Arabian women. Al-Turki HA, Sadat-Ali M, Al-Elq AH, Al-Mulhim FA, Al-Ali AK. Saudi Med J. 2008 Dec;29(12):1765-8.PMID: 19082230

[6] Hypovitaminosis D is common in both veiled and nonveiled Bangladeshi women. Islam MZ, Akhtaruzzaman M, Lamberg-Allardt C. Asia Pac J Clin Nutr. 2006;15(1):81-7. PMID:16500882

[7] Calcitriol as a chemopreventive and therapeutic agent in prostate cancer: role of anti-inflammatory activity. Krishnan AV, Moreno J, Nonn L, Swami S, Peehl DM, Feldman D. J Bone Miner Res. 2007 Dec;22 Suppl 2:V74-80. PMID: 18290727

[8] Selective inhibition of the C5a chemotactic cofactor function of the vitamin D binding protein by 1,25(OH)2 vitamin D3. Shah AB, DiMartino SJ, Trujillo G, Kew RR. Mol Immunol. 2006 Mar;43(8):1109-15. PMID: 16115686

[9] Prevention of rickets and vitamin D deficiency in infants, children, and adolescents. Wagner CL, Greer FR; American Academy of Pediatrics Section on Breastfeeding; American Academy of Pediatrics Committee on Nutrition. Pediatrics. 2008 Nov;122(5):1142-52. Erratum in: Pediatrics. 2009 Jan;123(1):197. PMID: 18977996

[10] Nutritional rickets and vitamin D deficiency in infants, children and adolescents. Unuvar T, Buyukgebiz A. Pediatr Endocrinol Rev. 2010 Mar;7(3):283-91.PMID: 20526242

[11] Scientific documentation of the relationship of vitamin D deficiency and the development of cancer. Edlich R, Mason SS, Chase ME, Fisher AL, Gubler K, Long WB 3rd, Giesy JD, Foley ML. J Environ Pathol Toxicol Oncol. 2009;28(2):133-41.PMID: 19817700

[12] The effect of vitamin D on neuropsychiatric conditions. Ashkanian M, Tehrani E, Videbech P. Ugeskr Laeger. 2010 Apr 26;172(17):1296-300. PMID: 20444398

[13] Plasma vitamin D levels and cognitive function in aging women: the nurses' health study. Bartali B, Devore E, Grodstein F, Kang JH. J Nutr Health Aging. 2014 Apr;18(4):400-6. PMID:24676321

[14] 25-hydroxyvitamin D, vitamin D receptor gene polymorphisms, and severity of Parkinson's disease. Suzuki M, Yoshioka M, Hashimoto M, et al. Mov Disord. 2012 Feb;27(2):264-71. PMID:22213340

[15] Effect of vitamin D deficiency and replacement on endothelial function in asymptomatic subjects. Tarcin O, Yavuz DG, Ozben B, et al. J Clin Endocrinol Metab. 2009 Oct;94(10):4023-30. PMID: 19584181

[16] Impact of vitamin D metabolism on clinical epigenetics. Karlic H, Varga F. Clin Epigenetics. 2011 Apr;2(1):55-61. PMID:22704269

[17] Cross-sectional study of vitamin D and calcium supplementation effects on chronic periodontitis. Miley DD, Garcia MN, Hildebolt et al. J Periodontol. 2009 Sep;80(9):1433-9.PMID: 19722793

[18] Serum vitamin D levels and severe asthma exacerbations in the Childhood Asthma Management Program study. Brehm JM, Schuemann B, Fuhlbrigge AL, et al; Childhood Asthma Management Program Research Group. J Allergy Clin Immunol. 2010 Jul;126(1):52-8.e5. 20538327

[19] Associations between concentrations of vitamin D and concentrations of insulin, glucose, and HbA1c among adolescents in the United States. Ford ES, Zhao G, Tsai J, Li C. Diabetes Care. 2011 Mar;34(3):646-8. PMID:21273498

[20] Payne J, et al "Vitamin D insufficiency in diabetic retinopathy" AAO 2010; Abstract PO223.

[21] Vitamin D and autoimmune rheumatologic disorders. Pelajo CF, Lopez-Benitez JM, Miller LC. Autoimmun Rev. 2010 May;9(7):507-10. PMID: 20146942

[22] Association of hypovitaminosis D with metabolic disturbances in polycystic ovary syndrome. Wehr E, Pilz S, Schweighofer N, et al. Eur J Endocrinol. 2009 Oct;161(4):575-82. PMID:19628650

[23] Serum 25-hydroxyvitamin D3 and body composition in an elderly cohort from Germany: a cross-sectional study. Jungert A, Roth HJ, Neuhäuser-Berthold M. Nutr Metab (Lond). 2012 May 18;9(1):42. PMID:22607088

[24] Vitamin D and tonsil disease--preliminary observations. Reid D, Morton R, Salkeld L, Bartley J. Int J Pediatr Otorhinolaryngol. 2011 Feb;75(2):261-4. PMID:21131064

[25] Vitamin D may be a link to black-white disparities in adverse birth outcomes. Bodnar LM, Simhan HN. Obstet Gynecol Surv. 2010 Apr;65(4):273-84.PMID: 20403218

[26] Wagner CL et al. "Vitamin D supplementation during Pregnancy Part 2 NICHD/CTSA Randomized Clinical Trial (RCT): Outcomes" PAS 2010; Abstract 1665.6.

[27] Vitamin D receptor as a master regulator of the c-MYC/MXD1 network. Salehi-Tabar R, Nguyen-Yamamoto L, Tavera-Mendoza LE, et al. Proc Natl Acad Sci U S A. 2012 Nov 13;109(46):18827-32. PMID:23112173

[28] Vitamin D receptor ligands, adenomatous polyposis coli, and the vitamin D receptor FokI polymorphism collectively modulate beta-catenin activity in colon cancer cells. Egan JB, Thompson PA, Vitanov MV, et al. Mol Carcinog. 2010 Apr;49(4):337-52. PMID:20043299

[29] Stimulation of Sirt1-regulated FoxO protein function by the ligand-bound vitamin D receptor. An BS, Tavera-Mendoza LE, Dimitrov V, et al. Mol Cell Biol. 2010 Oct;30(20):4890-900. PMID:20733005

[30] Improvement of pain, sleep, and quality of life in chronic pain patients with vitamin D supplementation. Huang W, Shah S, Long Q, et al. Clin J Pain. 2013 Apr;29(4):341-7. PMID:22699141

[31] The SYK side of TLR4: signalling mechanisms in response to LPS and minimally oxidized LDL. Miller YI, Choi SH, Wiesner P, Bae YS. Br J Pharmacol. 2012 Nov;167(5):990-9. PMID:22776094

[32] The effect of sun exposure on 25-hydroxyvitamin D concentrations in young healthy subjects living in the city of São Paulo, Brazil. Maeda SS, Kunii IS, Hayashi L, et al J Med Biol Res. 2007 Dec;40(12):1653-9. Epub 2007 Oct 29.PMID: 17713647

[33] Vitamin D supplementation, 25-hydroxyvitamin D concentrations, and safety. Vieth R. Am J Clin Nutr. 1999 May;69(5):842-56. PMID: 10232622

[34] Solar-UV-signature mutation prefers TCG to CCG: extrapolative consideration from UVA1-induced mutation spectra in mouse skin. Ikehata H, Kumagai J, Ono T, Morita A. Photochem Photobiol Sci. 2013 Aug;12(8):1319-27. PMID:23471200

[35] Cell fate regulated by NF-κB and AP-1-dependent signalling in human melanocytes exposed to UVA and UVB. Wäster P, Rosdahl I, Ollinger K. Br J Dermatol. 2014 Jul 21. doi: 10.1111/bjd.13278. PMID:25046326

[36] Biologically efficient solar radiation: Vitamin D production and induction of cutaneous malignant melanoma. Grigalavicius M, Juzeniene A, Baturaite Z, Dahlback A, Moan J. Dermatoendocrinol. 2013 Jan 1;5(1):150-8. PMID:24494048

[37] The Vitamin D requirement in health and disease. Heaney RP. J Steroid Biochem Mol Biol. 2005 Oct;97(1-2):13-9 PMID: 16026981

[38] Safety of vitamin D3 in adults with multiple sclerosis. Kimball SM, Ursell MR, O'Connor P, Vieth R. Am J Clin Nutr. 2007 Sep;86(3):645-51. PMID: 17823429

[39] Estimation of optimal serum concentrations of 25-hydroxyvitamin D for multiple health outcomes. Bischoff-Ferrari HA, Giovannucci E, Willett WC, Dietrich T, Dawson-Hughes B. Am J Clin Nutr. 2006 Jul;84(1):18-28. Erratum in: Am J Clin Nutr. 2006 Nov;84(5):1253. PMID:16825677

[40] Optimal serum 25-hydroxyvitamin D levels for multiple health outcomes. Bischoff-Ferrari HA. Adv Exp Med Biol. 2008;624:55-71. PMID:18348447

[41] Hypovitaminosis D is associated with insulin resistance and beta cell dysfunction. Chiu KC, Chu A, Go VL, Saad MF. Am J Clin Nutr. 2004 May;79(5):820-5. PMID:15113720

[42] Hypovitaminosis D in obese children and adolescents: relationship with adiposity, insulin sensitivity, ethnicity, and season. Alemzadeh R, Kichler J, Babar G, Calhoun M. Metabolism. 2008 Feb;57(2):183-91.PMID: 18191047

[43] 1Alpha,25-dihydroxyvitamin D3 inhibits programmed cell death in HL-60 cells by activation of sphingosine kinase. Kleuser B, Cuvillier O, Spiegel S. Cancer Res. 1998 May 1;58(9):1817-24. PMID:9581819

[44] Role of ceramide in diabetes mellitus: evidence and mechanisms. Galadari S, Rahman A, Pallichankandy S, Galadari A, Thayyullathil F. Lipids Health Dis. 2013 Jul 8;12:98. PMID:23835113

[45] Sphingosine 1-phosphate is involved in cytoprotective actions of calcitriol in human fibroblasts and enhances the intracellular Bcl-2/Bax rheostat. Sauer B, Gonska H, Manggau M, Kim DS, Schraut C, Schäfer-Korting M, Kleuser B. Pharmazie. 2005 Apr;60(4):298-304. PMID:15881612

[46] Fall prevention with supplemental and active forms of vitamin D: a meta-analysis of randomised controlled trials. Bischoff-Ferrari HA, Dawson-Hughes B, et al. BMJ. 2009 Oct 1;339:b3692. PMID: 19797342

[47] Higher 25-hydroxyvitamin D concentrations are associated with better lower-extremity function in both active and inactive persons aged > or =60 y. Bischoff-Ferrari HA, Dietrich T, Orav EJ, Hu FB, Zhang Y, Karlson EW, Dawson-Hughes B. Am J Clin Nutr. 2004 Sep;80(3):752-8. PMID:15321818

[48] Serum 25-hydroxyvitamin D and bone mineral density in a racially and ethnically diverse group of men. Hannan MT, Litman HJ, Araujo AB, TC, Holick MF, etal. J Clin Endocrinol Metab. 2008 Jan;93(1):40-6. PMID:17986641

[49] The Vitamin D requirement in health and disease. Heaney RP. J Steroid Biochem Mol Biol. 2005 Oct;97(1-2):13-9..PMID: 16026981

[50] The relation between acute changes in the systemic inflammatory response and plasma 25-hydroxyvitamin D concentrations after elective knee arthroplasty. Reid D, Toole BJ, Knox S, Talwar D, Harten J, O'Reilly DS, Blackwell S, Kinsella J, McMillan DC, Wallace AM. Am J Clin Nutr. 2011 May;93(5):1006-11. PMID:21411617

[51] Association of serum vitamin D levels with inflammatory response following hip fracture: the Baltimore Hip Studies. Miller RR, Hicks GE, Shardell MD, et al. J Gerontol A Biol Sci Med Sci. 2007 Dec;62(12):1402-6. PMID: 18166692

[52] Not a simple fat-soluble vitamin: Changes in serum 25-(OH)D levels are predicted by adiposity and adipocytokines in older adults. Ding C, Parameswaran V, Blizzard L, Burgess J, Jones G. J Intern Med. 2010 Nov;268(5):501-10. PMID:20804516

[53] Correcting vitamin D insufficiency improves insulin sensitivity in obese adolescents: a randomized controlled trial. Belenchia AM, Tosh AK, Hillman LS, Peterson CA. Am J Clin Nutr. 2013 Apr;97(4):774-81. PMID:23407306

[54] Serum levels of free 1,25-dihydroxyvitamin D in vitamin D toxicity. Pettifor JM, Bikle DD, Cavaleros M, et al. Ann Intern Med. 1995 Apr 1;122(7):511-3.PMID: 7872586

[55] The relationship between pro-resorptive inflammatory cytokines and the effect of high dose vitamin D supplementation on their circulating concentrations. Karim Y, Turner C, Dalton N, et al. Int Immunopharmacol. 2013 Nov;17(3):693-7.PMID:24007780

[56] Cholecalciferol Toxicity and Its Enhancement by Calcium Carbonate in the Common Brushtail Possum. SE Jolly, RJ Henderson, C Frampton and CT Eason. 1995 Wildlife Research 22(5) 579 – 583.

[57] Acute vitamin D intoxication in a child. Barrueto F Jr, Wang-Flores HH, Howland MA, Hoffman RS, Nelson LS. Pediatrics. 2005 Sep;116(3):e453-6. PMID:16140692

[58] Vitamin D intoxication with severe hypercalcemia due to manufacturing and labeling errors of two dietary supplements made in the United States. Araki T, Holick MF, Alfonso BD, et al. J Clin Endocrinol Metab. 2011 Dec;96(12):3603-8. PMID:21917864

[59] Vitamin D intoxication associated with an over-the-counter supplement. Koutkia P, Chen TC, Holick MF. N Engl J Med. 2001 Jul 5;345(1):66-7. PMID: 11439958

[60] Vitamin D toxicity due to a commonly available "over the counter" remedy from the Dominican Republic. Lowe H, Cusano NE, Binkley N, Blaner WS, Bilezikian JP. J Clin Endocrinol Metab. 2011 Feb;96(2):291-5. PMID:21123442

[61] Safety of vitamin D3 in adults with multiple sclerosis. Kimball SM, Ursell MR, O'Connor P, Vieth R. Am J Clin Nutr. 2007 Sep;86(3):645-51.PMID: 17823429

[62] Pharmacokinetics of vitamin D toxicity. Jones G. Am J Clin Nutr. 2008 Aug;88(2):582S-586S. Review.PMID: 18689406

[63] Vitamin D supplementation, 25-hydroxyvitamin D concentrations, and safety. Vieth R. Am J Clin Nutr. 1999 May;69(5):842-56. PMID: 10232622

[64] Vitamin D fortification in the United States and Canada: current status and data needs. Calvo MS, Whiting SJ, Barton CN. Am J Clin Nutr. 2004 Dec;80(6 Suppl):1710S-6S. PMID: 15585792

[65] Fluid milk vitamin fortification compliance in New York State. Murphy SC, Whited LJ, Rosenberry LC, Hammond BH, Bandler DK, Boor KJ. J Dairy Sci. 2001 Dec;84(12):2813-20.PMID: 11814039

[66] The Vitamin D requirement in health and disease. Heaney RP. J Steroid Biochem Mol Biol. 2005 Oct;97(1-2):13-9. PMID:16026981

[67] Superiority of a high loading dose of cholecalciferol to correct hypovitaminosis d in patients with inflammatory/autoimmune rheumatic diseases. Sainaghi PP, Bellan M, Nerviani A, et al. J Rheumatol. 2013 Feb;40(2):166-72. PMID:23242183

21. Mitochondria, Oxidation, Aging, and Disease

Different cells in the human body have different life spans. The enterocytes, which line the intestines, live about a week. Skin cells turn over quickly. Red blood cells last for about 120 days, basophils only about a week. Liver cells live until they need replacement.

Some other cells are immortal. Neurons and the retinal pigmented epithelial cells (RPE), of the eye, are "immortal," postmitotic cells that if all goes well, last a lifetime. Cardiac myocytes, of the heart, and skeletal muscle fibers are also postmitotic cells.

Of course, these cells are not immortal, but they don't have planned obsolescence and replacements, as most cells of the body do. These cells are referred to as postmitotic cells as they cannot divide and replace themselves with daughter cells. Thus, immortal cells are also dead end cells.

These postmitotic cells are not adapted for frequent replacement. Damage or death of these cells is a serious matter, as they are incapable of regeneration once we become adults. Although there are stem cells hidden some organs, such as the heart which may be coaxed into developing some new muscle cells, they cannot be relied upon to make major renovations after a disaster.

Why We Are Mortal

In the Bible, Adam and Eve ate the fruit of knowledge, relinquishing their immortality. This is why we are mortal; we traded immortality for knowledge and consciousness.

Unlike us, *Cnidaria* (jellyfish) are immortal. They do not age. When their cells are damaged, they are replaced with new ones. If a predator eats a jellyfish and spits out a couple of chunks of it, each bit can grow back into a whole identical animal.

Cnidaria do not have a brain, but they do have a neural net that allows them to react to stimuli. They can sense odors and light, and use this information to find food and avoid predators. They can coordinate their motion, and right themselves when turned over by waves. But *Cnidaria* have no adaptive response, and they cannot learn. They can be zapped with electric shocks, and will react, but never learn to avoid the stimulus, no matter how many times it is done. They do not appreciate their long lives as they have no memory of being alive. There could be a million-year-old *Cnidaria* out in the mid-Pacific, drifting in the eternal now.

Cnidaria do not have "immortal" postmitotic neurons[1]. When *Cnidaria* neurons become senescent or damaged, they are replaced. Postmitotic neurons, and the connections we form between them, in our brains are the way we learn; how we store memory; how we become who we are. Our neurons are massively interconnected. If we replaced neurons, we would lose those connections, and along with them, our memories, abilities we have learned, and ourselves. Thus, in a way, we did trade immortality for the sweet fruit of knowledge.

Telomeres and Aging

While heart and neurons are postmitotic, most other cells in our bodies can divide up to about 60 times. The number of divisions is controlled by telomeres at the ends of the chromosomes; with each cell division, the telomere shortens. When the telomere is depleted, the cell loses its ability to divide into two new cells. When the telomere wears out, the DNA unravels; the cell loses its ability to make new proteins or reproduce. Telomeric depletion is one theory of why we age.

Telomere depletion limits how many times our cells can divide into two replacement cells, but limiting this also prevents cancer growth. Mice bred with the ability to make longer telomeres do not live longer than normal mice as they are more susceptible to death from cancer.

The enzyme telomerase can add length to the telomere. Embryonic stem cells express telomerase, so, the clock restarts with conception. Immune cells and other cells that need to divide regularly also make telomerase.

Acute stress causes induction of telomerase in immune cells; however, chronic stress causes a decrease in telomerase[2]. A history of repeated major depression is also associated with shorter leukocyte telomeres[3]. Childhood adversity from abuse, neglect, or major disease causes a depletion of telomere length, which shows up in later life[4]. Women, who have been the victim of domestic-partner abuse, have shorter telomeres[5]. One year of chronic stress can cause the equivalent of six years of normal telomere depletion. Meditation and having a purpose in life are found to be associated with higher telomerase levels[6].

Emotional stress is clearly a cerebrally mediated response; this effect is mediated through neuroendocrine hormones, and thus, telomerase activity is under the direct influence of postmitotic cells. Aging of, or damage to, postmitotic cells may thus restrict telomerase expression and limit the ability to adapt to stress. Chronic inflammation associated with elevation of IL-6 and TNF-α is also associated with short leukocyte telomeres[7]. These inflammatory mediators are elevated in chronic stress reactions, inflammation, enteric bacterial dysbiosis, and in sleep deprivation.

If, from birth, the telomeres allowed 60 divisions, it would yield 2^{60} cells; enough to produce about one million trillion cells (1,152,921,504,606,850,000), while an adult only has something in the neighborhood of 50 trillion cells in their body. Thus, even one cell from a newborn could potentially produce enough cells to replace every cell in the body every week for 3695 years.

Even though telomere shortening is associated with aging, it does not affect longevity in the general population. When adults were tested and followed over time, those with shorter telomeres did not have a higher mortality; however, they did have poorer health[8]. Individuals who have shorter telomeres are more likely to be in poor health, to contract, and to die from infectious disease. Telomere depletion is likely manifested mainly as a poorer response to infection, slower healing and recovery, poor health and diminished vigor. A ten-year equivalent depletion of telomere would make a 70-year-old have the health vigor of an 80-year-old. This is a major public health and economic issue, as individuals with depleted telomeres would be expected to live just as long, but require more intensive and expensive medical care.

Although telomere depletion plays an important role in aging and the vigor of the immune response during old age, it is rather the aging and damage of the postmitotic cells which are the major contributor to the senescence and shortened survival. Prevention of premature aging needs to focus on avoidance of chronic oxidative and psychological stress, and on the promotion of health; particularly the health of the postmitotic cells.

Acute ischemia, such as heart attacks or strokes, cuts the supply of blood and oxygen, causing necrosis and massive cell death, resulting in the loss of cardiac or brain tissues. More often, however, the damage that occurs is non-necrotic tissue loss resulting from reperfusion injury, which occurs after a brief ischemic event. Although uncommon, these events can even occur in children. These injuries are devastating as recovery from them is limited. Few individuals ever return to their full, premorbid functioning.

Chronic, low-level injury also damages postmitotic tissues. The process of aging involves the slow accumulation of damage to these cells. But, what about the rest of the body; why do cells that have regenerative capacities age? The effect of aging of the postmitotic cells is not limited to the effect on the cells themselves. The neuroendocrine cells of the hypothalamus are postmitotic cells. Dysfunction of the hypothalamus has direct and indirect effects on the pituitary endocrine axis, appetite, energy, temperature control, sleep, growth hormone, sex hormones and renewal of cells throughout the body[1].

About seven percent of childhood cancer survivors who have been treated with anthracycline chemotherapeutic medications develop heart failure about 15 years after the treatment of their cancer. The younger the child, the higher the risk.

Anthracycline drugs likely act by reducing telomerase activity in many different cell types, causing senescence. This prevents the cancer cells from being able to reproduce repeatedly. Unfortunately, cardiac stem cells are one of the cell types which are affected by these medications. It is not direct damage to the cardiomyocytes, but rather damage to cardiac stem cells, caused by this toxic medication, which leads to heart failure. As the child matures, there are insufficient healthy stem cells to grow and maintain the heart. Heart failure manifests at times of increased demands: pregnancy, athletic endeavors, or with infection[9].

Mitochondria and Aging

Postmitotic cells have a high metabolic activity and use large amounts of oxygen and oxidative fuels to meet their energy demands. The energy for this activity depends on mitochondria; organelles that live in all nucleated cells. (Red blood cells and platelets are not nucleated and do not have mitochondria). The number of mitochondria in a cell ranges from a few hundred to about 100,000, depending on the metabolic demand of the cell.

The principal role of the mitochondria is to convert sugars, fats, amino acids and purines into a form of energy the cell can use for its metabolic activities. Mitochondria produce hydrogen protons and utilize their potential energy to convert ADP into ATP, a form of energy that the rest of the cell can use.

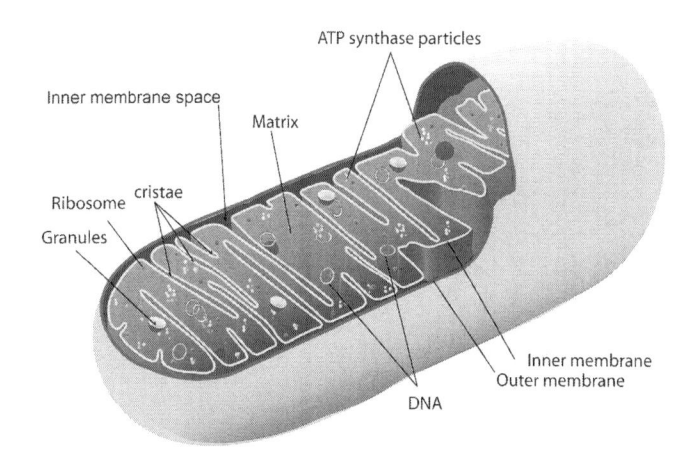

Figure 21-1: Illustration of the Membrane Structure of a Mitochondrion[10]

Electron Transport

Energy from glucose is converted within the matrix of the mitochondria by the citric acid cycle, producing reduced NAD (NADH) and succinate as energy carriers. β-oxidation of fatty acids also produces NADH and succinate within the mitochondrial matrix. These two reduced molecules are then oxidized by large inner membrane protein complexes of the electron transport chain (ETC), yielding electrons which fuel ETC proton pumps. These proton pumps transport hydrogen protons into the mitochondrial intermembrane space. The protons in the mitochondrial inner membrane space form an energy gradient compared to the matrix. They pass through ATP synthase membrane protein channels, down a concentration gradient, back into the inner membrane space, generating high-energy ATP molecules from lower energy ADP in the process.

ATP carries a high energy bond, and this energy can be transferred to other molecules. The energy from ATP drives the great majority of cellular processes which require energy, including muscular activity, ion pumps, formation of proteins, processing chemical compounds, immune response, cell division and performance of most other cell functions.

> You, my reader, are breathing and consuming oxygen. Most of consume about 400 to 500 liters of the gas each day. For each liter of O_2 consumed, 136 grams of ATP are needed and must be synthesized. That is 120 to 150 pounds of ATP. With peak exercise, O_2 consumption can increase by a factor of ten.
>
> Thus, you likely consume your weight in ATP each day. And you need to synthesize all of it. Obviously, your body does not have that much ATP. At any point in time, the body only has about 250 grams of ATP, but even on days that all we do is keep the couch warm, we use about 40 kg of ATP. During exercise, the utilization of ATP can be as high as half a kg per minute!
>
> This means that ATP needs to be recycled, over 200 times a day. Even at rest, that's about every 9 minutes. However, ATP in various organs is not used and synthesized at the same rate, During maximal exercise, the body's entire pool of ATP would need to be recycled every 30 seconds to keep up with demand[11]. Thus, in muscles such as the heart, ATP is synthesized and consumed even more quickly.

The electron transport chain is a series of four protein complexes plus Cytochrome C. These protein complexes are coded by 13 mitochondrial proteins, in addition to 74 host cell proteins. Complexes I, III and IV are proton pumps. Complex I accepts two high energy electrons from NADH, uses this energy to pump two protons into the inner membrane space, and then transfers the electrons to Coenzyme Q_{10} (CoQ_{10}), which shuttles the electrons to Complex III. Complex II accepts electrons from succinate using the intermediary $FADH_2$ to transport two electrons via CoQ_{10} to Complex III. Complex III transports two additional protons into the inner membrane space. Cytochrome C shuttles one electron at a time from Complex III to Complex IV. In the last step, Complex IV pumps out two more protons to the inner membrane space, and uses two more hydrogen protons from the matrix and combines them with oxygen (O_2) as the final electron acceptor, forming water. This requirement for oxygen is why we need to breathe. With each proton pumped, the electron gradient of the matrix gains a bit of electronegativity. H+ protons returning into the mitochondrial matrix through ATP synthase drive ATP formation.

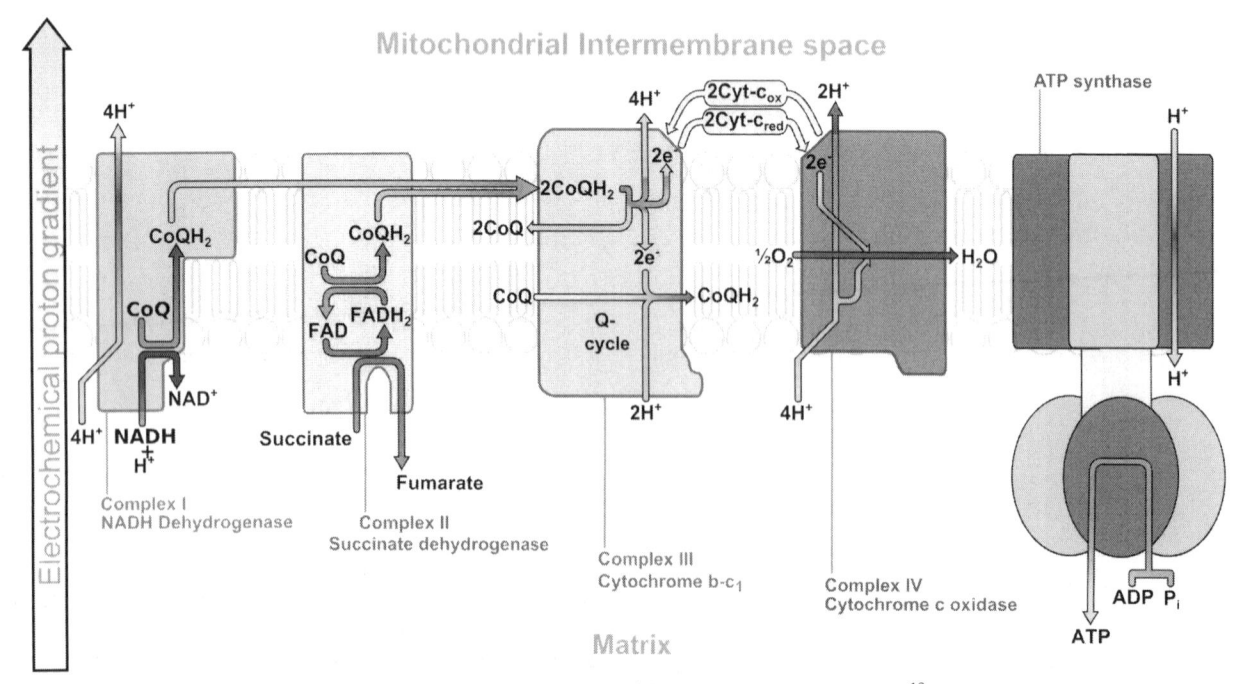

Figure 21-2: The Electron Transport of the mitochondria[12]

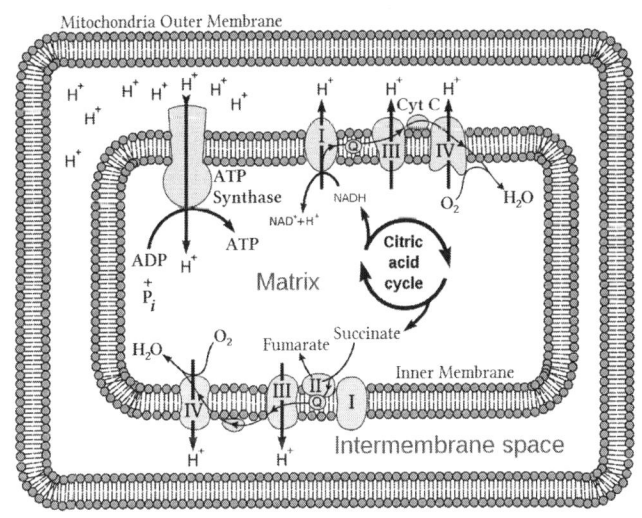

Figure 21-3: Mitochondrial Electron Transport Chain Proteins[13]

Figure 21-3 is a cartoon showing a single mitochondrion with a single ATP synthase molecule and set of electron transport chain proteins. In real life, the inner membrane of a single mitochondrion in the liver may have over 10,000 sets of these proteins. Mitochondria in the myocardium, which have profuse cristae, may have 30,000 sets of electron transport chain proteins[11].

Converting energy forms in mitochondria involves potent electrochemical processes and production of highly reactive electrons. In healthy mitochondria, a tiny amount, probably less than one-tenth of a percent of these electrons, escapes in the form of superoxide. Worn out, damaged mitochondria leak many times the amount of reactive oxygen species (ROS) than do fit mitochondria; perhaps as much as two percent of the energy can be lost into the formation of ROS in these dysfunctional mitochondria[14].

It is the NADH-dependent Complex I, which is most susceptible to the escape of electrons. These escaped electrons can then form superoxide and subsequently other ROS that can damage the cell. The reason that Complex I is most susceptible to forming superoxide radicals is not clearly established; however, it may be because it this complex manages the greatest electronegativity.

Reactive Oxygen Species

Reactive oxygen species are highly reactive molecules containing oxygen with an unpaired valence. Oxygen demands two bonds; an ROS has one, so it avidly tries to grab an electron from other molecules. This can result in significant damage to molecules exposed to ROS.

In the body, there are three major endogenous sources of reactive oxygen species: white blood cells (WBCs), 5-lipoxygenase and mitochondria. WBC in the immune system use ROS to destroy microbes and targeted cells. ROS are also used in the cell to help digest retired proteins and organelles which are being recycled, and for destroying bacteria and antigens which phagocytotic cells have engulfed. During its controlled use, ROS is vital to immune system function and to health.

ROS are like fire used to cook and heat the home; it can also burn it down. Leaky mitochondria are an important source of ROS. ROS can also be formed during the breakdown of alcohol by the enzyme CYP2E1 in the liver of habitual drinkers.

Superoxide is formed in the mitochondria when oxygen is reduced by adding and electron (with a negative charge) to an oxygen molecule. $O_2 + e^- \rightarrow O_2^{\cdot -}$. Hydrogen peroxide (HO:OH or H_2O_2) is less potent, however than hydroxyl radicals are. Hydroxyl radicals are formed when a single electron is transferred to hydrogen peroxide. In biologic systems, free intracellular iron is the supplier of this electron.

$$Fe^{2+} + H_2O_2 \longrightarrow HO^{\cdot} + OH^- + Fe^{3+}$$

Table 21-1: Some Reactive Oxygen Species

Name	Structure	Formation
Superoxide anion	$O_2^{\cdot -}$	$O_2 + e^-$
Hydrogen peroxide	H_2O_2	$O_2^{\cdot -} + H_2O$
Hydroxyl radical	$HO^{\cdot}$	HOOH + metal ion
Nitric oxide	$^{\cdot}NO$	
Peroxynitrite	$OONO^-$	$O_2^{\cdot -} + NO$
Organic peroxide	ROOH	ROOH $\rightarrow$ $RO^{\cdot}$ + $OH^{\cdot}$
Hypochlorite ion	HOCL	$H_2O_2 + Cl^-$
Ferryl radical	FeO^{2+}	Fe^2 + HOOH
Tyrosyl radical		HOCL + Tyrosine

Neutrophils and macrophages contain NADPH oxidase that forms $O_2^{\cdot -}$, and H_2O_2. These cells engulf bacteria and bathe the pathogen in H_2O_2 and $O_2^{\cdot -}$ to kill them. WBC's also contain myeloperoxidase and can form the radicals hypochlorous acid and tyrosyl, used by neutrophils to kill bacteria and other pathogens. Bacteria have antioxidant defenses, but usually, it is not enough to save them. Neutrophils can also export H_2O_2 and $O_2^{\cdot -}$ to attack cells that they cannot engulf, which can trigger apoptosis of the targeted cells.

5-lipoxygenase converts certain long chain fatty acids into leukotrienes during an immune response. The lipoxygenases (5, 12, and 15 lipoxygenases) catalyze the formation of fatty acid hydroperoxide from fatty acid and O_2. These peroxide bonds break easily and form free radicals, which act on surrounding fatty acids. Lipid peroxidation thus initiates a chain reaction providing a continuous supply of further peroxidation.

Mitochondria are the major source of non-adaptive ROS in the body, and ROS can be formed during normal cellular functioning as a result of imperfections in the capture and transfer of energy. These superoxide radicals can form hydrogen peroxide, initiate lipid peroxidation, or inactivate enzymes. Mitochondria can also trigger the formation of ROS under the influence of cytokines and during intracellular environmental events, including hypoxia.

> **Hypoxic Injury:** During ischemia, there is decreased blood flow and a decrease in oxygen delivery to the tissues. Oxidative phosphorylation (the formation of ATP using the ETC) stops as Complex IV cannot use the expended electrons to form water. Electrons get backed up, and all ETC components become fully reduced. With reperfusion, the oxygen supply returns in the presence of easily available, highly reactive electrons, and oxygen readily accepts the overabundance of electrons, forming superoxide ions. Thus, it is reperfusion that triggers the ROS induced damage.

The harmful effects of ROS include:

- Damage to the DNA
- Oxidation of amino acids in proteins
- Inactivation of enzymes (or activating and enzyme)
- Oxidation of polyunsaturated fatty acids
- Signaling apoptosis (cell death)

When ROS damage occurs, it is not a single susceptible molecule which is affected, but rather a chain reaction of stealing electrons from another molecule, and damaging the target molecule. The target, now missing an electron itself becomes a radical and can grab an electron from another molecule. During the recovery of the electron, the protein may not go back to its original conformation, so it may be crippled or dysfunctional. Thus, a free radical can set up a chain reaction wherein a single ROS radical can damage billions of molecules per second. Antioxidants act by providing a proton with a positive charge, and thus quenching the oxidation chain reaction.

ROS can easily damage DNA. Damaged to the DNA of certain genes can lead to cancer in cells that reproduce, but cancer rarely arises from postmitotic cells. DNA damage also causes errors in proteins; enzymes that are transcribed with errors or that are damaged by oxidation may not function correctly. Structural proteins with transcription errors or that are oxidized may get folded wrong, altering or defeating their function. Dysfunctional proteins that prevent the cell from undergoing apoptosis or block signals telling the cell to stop dividing can cause the cell to become cancerous. Other missense coding errors may keep proteins from functioning properly.

Between cell divisions, nuclear DNA is stored, wrapped around protein structures (histone) that stabilize and protect the DNA from damage when not in use. Most of the time only small segments of the DNA are unwound; just those that nuclear inductors stimulate so that only mRNA for proteins the cell needs at that time are made. DNA is exposed at this time and susceptible to oxidative damage.

There are multiple DNA repair mechanisms; these restore most minor manglings of the DNA; however, not all errors are repaired precisely. DNA damage can cause alterations that result in cellular dysfunction. Although the postmitotic cells do not replace themselves, they have a turnover of their organelles, membranes and membrane proteins, and in this way, they continuously refresh themselves. Although cancer rarely arises from these cells, oxidative damage and DNA errors can impair the cell's ability to make new enzymes and structural proteins.

Even though the neurons and myocytes are postmitotic, the mitochondria in these cells are not. They are replaced, on average, about every two weeks[26].

Mitochondria are unique from other organelles in our cells; they have their own DNA. It is a circular DNA like that of bacteria, and it codes for about 31 genes. Like nuclear DNA, mitochondrial DNA (mtDNA) is very susceptible to oxidative damage. In long-lived cells, damage to the mtDNA can accumulate over time. The mitochondrial circular DNA does not have histones to stabilize it, and although the mtDNA has a repair mechanism, it too, is not perfect[15]. Circular DNA does not have telomeres to limit the number of times it can undergo mitosis. Even though mitochondria usually have multiple sets of DNA, mtDNA errors may prevent the mitochondria from running efficiently.

ROS production by mitochondria provides a signal for the cell to tell which mitochondria are vigorous and productive, and which ones are geezers, leaking protons and ROS. The cell can target these weak mitochondria, tagging them through ubiquitination. This tagging allows weak mitochondria to be taken up into lysosomes for recycling. In this process worn out, polluting mitochondria are eliminated and cannibalized for their amino acids and lipids. This process selectively eliminates mitochondria with damaged DNA that makes them less efficient.

> Ubiquitin is a small molecule that can bind to proteins and acts as a label. Ubiquitination (sometimes called the kiss of death) is the process of marking proteins for the junkyard. Ubiquitination actually marks proteins for several different cells processes, including antigen processing; cell division; immune and inflammatory functions; DNA transcription and repair; and other processes. Thus, the kiss of death only refers to one aspect of this process. To mark a protein for destruction requires linking at least four ubiquitin molecules in a chain on the protein. It may be that damaged proteins are more susceptible to this labeling or just that accumulate risk with time, nevertheless, labeling targets them for removal. Proteasomes bind the proteins and cleave them into polypeptides for further processing.

> Your mitochondria came from your mother. Sperm has a contingent of them to fuel the race to the egg, but they get left out on the porch when the sperm's genetic material enters the ovum to fertilize it.
>
> The vast majority of a human female's ova are formed before her birth. They quietly wait and do almost nothing until puberty. Then, each month, a few eggs wake up and are ready to be fertilized. Thus, the ova in a 30-year-old, fertile woman only have the equivalent lifetime exposure to oxidative stress equivalent to a few months, and the mitochondria in the ova have undergone very few

divisions. This is in contrast to men who churn out a couple hundred million sperm a day well into old age. Over a thousand years, the mitochondria in the eggs have only experienced the accumulated stress and divisions that would be expected in several years.

MtDNA is often used to trace maternal lineage across multiple generations over eons. For example, mtDNA shows that Eurasians, but not Africans, interbred with Neanderthals some 37,000 years ago. Mitochondrial DNA is pretty stable, as errors in its DNA can cause problems that prevent survival. This is why mitochondrial diseases are uncommon; most mtDNA alterations severe enough to cause disease are severe enough to prevent their survival.

Mitochondria in Apoptosis

Mitochondria play a lead role in cellular apoptosis. Apoptosis is the process of programmed cell death. Apoptosis is important for the development of the embryo; it rids the tail from the pollywog as it becomes a frog, removes the web between the fingers in the developing hand, and creates the slitting of the eyelids. Not only is it essential to the development of the fetus, it also is the process by which old or unneeded cells are removed from the tissues, and by which excess immune cells are eliminated after an immune response. It has been estimated that in a healthy adult human, about 50 to 70 billion cells are removed by apoptosis each day[16]; an amount equivalent to our entire body weight each year.

Apoptosis is a different process than cellular necrosis, which occurs as a result of factors external to the cell or tissue, such as infection, toxins, or trauma. Necrosis often involves large areas of tissue, in contrast to individual cells, and in necrosis, the dead and dying cells are not generating chemokines to signal the immune system to come clear the area. Thus, an area of necrosis may require surgical intervention for the removal of the necrotic tissue. In apoptosis, the remains of the cells are removed by phagocytic cells by a process called efferocytosis without triggering inflammation.

Several diseases, including neurodegenerative conditions, such as Alzheimer's disease, Huntington's disease, and certain disease of the heart, are believed to be caused by inappropriate activation of apoptosis, leading to the loss of postmitotic cells. Other diseases, involving cells with the ability to reproduce, include cancers and autoimmune disorders. In these, there is a failure of apoptosis to eliminate harmful, senescent or unneeded cells[17].

The pathways to mitochondrial-mediated cell apoptosis rely on the balance of pro-apoptotic and anti-apoptotic proteins in the cell and on the mitochondrial membrane. The BCL-2 proteins bcl-xl, Bcl-2 and Mcl-1 are anti-apoptotic while others, such as Bad, Bax, Bak, Bnip3, and Bid, are pro-apoptotic. The sensitivity of cells to apoptotic stimuli depends on the balance between pro- and anti-apoptotic bcl-2 proteins and their activation.

One example is the activation of Procaspase-8 to Caspase-8 by stimulation of the tumor necrosis factor receptor (TNFR1) by TNF-α on the cell surface. Caspase-8 then cleaves the protein BH3 Interacting Domain Death Agonist (BID), which triggers the formation of a pore in the mitochondrial membrane, disrupting its transmembrane potential and leaking protons. This frees enzyme cytochrome C from the mitochondria. If this occurs in sufficient amounts, it triggers the activation of the cascade: Caspase-9 → Caspase-3 → Apoptosis. TNF-α is just one of many signaling molecules which can trigger apoptosis.

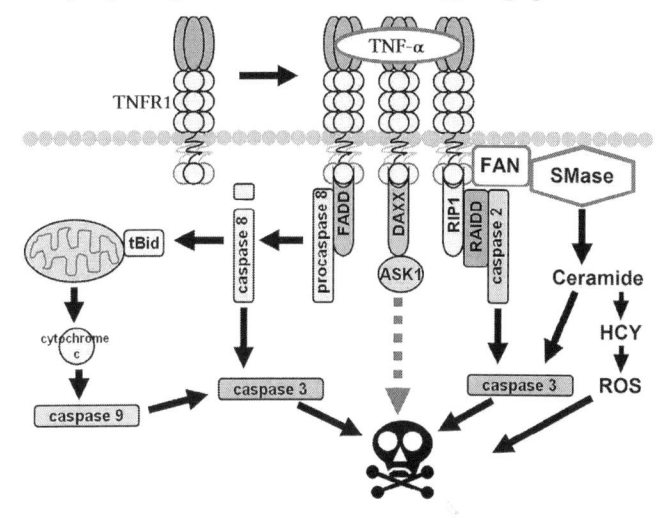

Figure 21-4: Apoptosis signaling molecules.

Tumor suppressor protein p53 helps regulate the cell cycle and prevents cancer, by arresting the cell cycle and stimulating the DNA repair, before allowing the cell cycle to restart, thus providing more time for DNA repair to occur. If the DNA damage is irreparable, p53 promotes the transcription of the pro-apoptotic proteins Bak and Bax. P53 also binds to two Bak proteins in the mitochondrial outer membrane, and if sufficient p53:Bak heterodimers form; it triggers mitochondrial apoptosis (see Figure 41-2). In unstressed cells, the amount of p53 present in a cell is balanced by continual production and removal through ubiquitination with mdm2. Expression of p53 in the cell is stimulated by oxidative stress, H_2O_2, UV-radiation, osmotic shock, DNA damage and other stressors.

Bcl-2 (B-cell lymphoma 2) is an intracellular protein that prevents apoptosis. It is so named because it was first linked to B-cell lymphoma; however, elevated expression of this protein is also associated with aggressive forms of melanoma, breast, prostate and lung cancers, which are resistant to treatment. Bcl-2 prevents activation of the protein BID, which could otherwise provoke apoptosis. Over-expression of bcl-2 prevents the elimination of aberrant cells which would otherwise undergo apoptosis, and thus, can cause cancer. Elevated bcl-2 expression has also been implicated in some autoimmune diseases, where T helper cells fail to be eliminated after the immune threat has abated.

Phagocytosis of apoptotic cells by dendritic cells may be important for the induction of T_{REG} cells that downregulate immune reactions. Thus, stymied apoptosis can maintain immune reactions after they are no longer appropriate [18].

BNIP3 is another intracellular protein which is structurally similar to Bcl-2; however, it displaces Bcl-2 and activates BID. BNIP3 is activated by certain viruses and by ischemia/reperfusion. This is a probable mechanism by which ischemia/reperfusion provokes the apoptotic loss of cardiac myocytes[26]. Ischemia/reperfusion also causes neuronal loss through apoptosis.

In oxygen deficit tissue during ischemia, xanthine and hypoxanthine accumulate. During reperfusion, the enzyme xanthine oxidase metabolizes these products, resulting in superoxide radicals[19] (pathway schematic in Figure 9-5). BNIP3 activation of BID triggers pore formation in mitochondria with addition release of free radicals and cytochrome C, leading to apoptosis of the cell.

Thus, mitochondria are essential regulators of apoptosis, for preventing the loss of needed cells and for the elimination of cancerous or superfluous immune cells. In the intestine, intraepithelial lymphocytes from the lamina propria trigger apoptosis of enterocytes when they complete their migration to the apex of the villi. Apoptosis is needed to get rid of cells that have completed their roles, as well as those which are malfunctioning. Even so, apoptosis can harm, and thus, required appropriate control.

Autophagy (self-consumption) refers to the internal destruction and recycling of organelles in the cells. This process is crucial to postmitotic cell health. Parts wear out and need replacement. Autophagy allows the cell to make new organelles and scavenge amino acids, lipids, and energy. Additionally, there are times when cells have more organelles than they require; after injury and during recovery, less work is done; muscle cells use less energy and need fewer mitochondria or other organelles. During famine and starvation, energy availability and utilization is lower; the cells scavenge proteins from surplus organelles for consumption. Autophagy also plays a role in the innate and adaptive immunity to intracellular pathogens[20].

Like other organelles, mitochondria wear out. When they do, they begin to waste energy and leak free radicals which damage the cell. Autophagy of mitochondria is called *mitophagy*. In addition to wearing out, mitochondria may be damaged during their reproduction.

When bacteria reproduce by dividing into two daughter cells, mistakes can occur, which result in mutations. Bacteria have fairly frequent mutations; although most mutations impair survival, some add survival advantage. The errors add variance. Since the reproductive rate is so high in bacteria, loss of poorly adapted individuals imparts little risk to the survival of species, compared to the advantages gained from mutations that benefit adaptation to new environments.

Mutations, however, are dangerous to postmitotic cells. When mitochondria replicate, errors can occur in the mtDNA. Over multiple generations of mitochondria, there can be populations of these organelles that are effete and inefficient. When this occurs, hydrogen ions leak out, and ROS and H_2O_2 are formed. Thus, these weak mitochondria are dangerous and need to be eliminated.

Mitochondria regularly renew themselves through a process of fusion and fission. They join together (fusion) and form larger mitochondria, and then bud off smaller mitochondria. When the components of the new, small mitochondria are weak, leaky, or have mtDNA errors, these mitochondria undergo mitophagy. Strong, healthy ones survive. These healthy mitochondria can then reproduce, forming additional, healthy mitochondria.

Table 21-2: Mitochondrial Fusion and Fission proteins[21]

Mfn1 and Mfn2	Blocking Mfn produces elongation of the mitochondria. Charcot-Marie-Tooth disease type 2A is caused by mutations in Mfn2.
OPA1	Required for inner membrane fusion. Autosomal dominant optic atrophy is caused by mutations in OPA1.
Dynamin-like protein 1 Drp1	Drp1 is a cytosolic protein recruited to mitochondria that permits mitochondrial fission. At low levels of NO, it increases fission. At high levels, Drp1 becomes nitrosylated, as occurs in Alzheimer's disease, leading to the fragmentation of mitochondria into inefficient units, and promoting neuronal cell death[22].
Fis1	Fis1 is required for mitochondrial fission

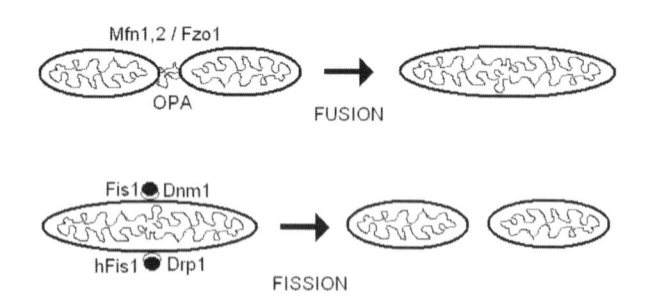

Figure 21-5: Mitochondrial Fusion and Fission

Caloric restriction activates the protein SIRT1, which activates mitophagy and mitochondrial biogenesis through the activation of PPARγ Coactivator-1α (PGC-1α). This results in the maintenance of efficient mitochondria. Exercise has the same effect on mitochondria in skeletal muscle. High-intensity interval training increases SIRT1, by activating PGC-1α and mitochondrial transcription factor A; thus, promoting skeletal muscle mitochondrial number and efficiency and improving exercise performance[26].

In health, cells maintain a balance of mitochondrial biogenesis and mitophagy to match the appropriate cellular energy demand. Excessive mitochondria are eliminated as they would both waste resources and produce damaging ROS, leading to oxidative damage. Regular turnover helps ensure efficient and vigorous mitochondria. Inactivity and excessive caloric intake, however, decrease the demand for mitochondrial efficiency and turnover. SIRT1 is down-regulated in cells that are insulin resistant. Some flavonoid phenolic compounds, including resveratrol, kaempferol, daidzein, and genistein, increase the activity of PGC-1α through activation of SIRT1[23].

During periods of nutrient restriction, the energy availability to the cells is curtailed. Most organelles in the cell may undergo autophagic degradation to scavenge nutrients. Mitochondria fuse under these conditions into long tubular mitochondria that evade degradation. These long tubular mitochondria can continue energy production while yielding some mitochondrial membrane energy conservation[24]. When the energy supply is more adequate, these long mitochondria can divide up again. In fact, mitochondria fuse and divide frequently. This mechanism allows culling of weak components.

If cells had an imbalance in favor of mitochondrial fusions, they would end up with a single, large mitochondria, but if the imbalance favored fissions they would be filled with tiny, poorly functioning mitochondria. Nevertheless, in healthy nerve cells the occurrence of mitochondrial fusions and fissions is unbalanced; there are far more fissions than would be expected[25]. This suggests that many of the fission products, along with their DNA, are eliminated.

Mitochondria thus have mechanisms for staying in shape. They not only make new DNA, proteins, and membranes, they fuse and split apart forming new mitochondria. When they split off into new mitochondria, some daughter cells will have defective DNA, and thus, have more protein defects and be less able to maintain a proper membrane potential. Some enzymes may not function. These weak mitochondria are less likely to fuse with other mitochondria and are more likely to be eliminated through phagocytosis[1].

During mitophagy, targeted mitochondria are taken up by endocytosis into autophagosomes in the cell that mature into lysosomes. Thus, effete mitochondria are harvested, broken down and eliminated along with their defective DNA. Meanwhile, higher functioning mitochondria divide and produce more healthy progeny, depending upon the needs of the cell. Exercise and starvation impel recycling the mitochondria for its component amino acids and lipids that can use as fuel; weaker mitochondria are culled first, thus selecting the strongest for survival.

With such clever mechanisms, perhaps we should never age; however, experience suggests otherwise. One problem is that excessive ROS production can cause the mitochondria to self-destruct and trigger inappropriate apoptosis in postmitotic cells. The small effete mitochondria are cleaned up pretty easily. However, large, lazy mitochondria can also form if the housekeeping is not kept up.

> I live in Florida in an area surrounded by over one million acres of state and federal forests. Each year the foresters do controlled burns of different areas of the forest. This clears out underbrush and sickly trees and provides better habitat for wildlife. Also, the pine cones need to burn to release seeds for new trees. If the foresters don't do the controlled burns, the underbrush, dead wood and vines accumulate so that, when there is a wildfire, it burns so fiercely that it results in a devastating crown fire, which can destroy large areas of mature forests. Just as fire is required for the health of some forests, regular low-level oxidative stress can help clear out the weak and poorly functioning mitochondria in the cell. Vigorous exercise or occasional inflammation can provide this stimulus. Nutrient restriction has a similar effect; nutrient restriction can promote longevity, but severe starvation can damage the muscles and heart.

If there is a large population of effete and decrepit mitochondria producing ROS, the risk of apoptosis increases. If many mitochondria are subject to oxidative stress and inflammatory cytokines, such as TNF, there may be enough damage to sufficient mitochondria to trigger apoptosis of the cell. Reperfusion injury or inflammation can trigger this.

ROS are used by white blood cells to kill bacteria. Superoxide ($O_2^{·-}$) radicals formed by mitochondria form hydroxyl radicals ($·OH$), or hydrogen peroxide (H_2O_2), which can also be converted by NOS to nitric oxide (NO).

> NO is a signaling molecule which relaxes smooth muscles in arteries, resulting in increased blood flows. Thus, when tissues are not getting sufficient oxygenation, production of NO can increase blood flow to the area. NO derived from nitroglycerin treats angina by increasing blood flow to the heart, but can also trigger migraine-like pain through vasodilatation of cephalic arteries. Viagra also acts by signaling through NO.
>
> NO is also formed in phagocytic cells as part of the immune response. NO is a potent free radical toxin to bacteria, which acts, in part, by damaging the bacteria's DNA. NO is formed by inducible nitric oxide synthase (iNOS) upon stimulation with INF-γ, but its formation is inhibited by the anti-inflammatory cytokines TGF-β and IL-10.
>
> Lipids also undergo peroxidation; this can change their metabolic activity, ant they may become toxic, or alter cellular function. NO is also a free radical which can damage host lipid membranes and produce oxidized cholesterol. In reperfusion injury, excess NO can be produced which then reacts with superoxide forming the powerful oxidant peroxynitrite.

Lipofuscin

Under inclement conditions, such as hypoxia or inflammation, as much as 10 times as much $O_2^{·-}$ is lost from mitochondria, thus forming reactive oxygen species[26] and creating dangerous amounts of ROS. Free radicals damage not only cellular proteins and DNA but also damage the cell's lipids, including those that make up the cellular membranes. These damaged lipids can impede cell function. Oxidized membrane proteins can trigger an immune response[27], for example, by activating sphingomyelinase: → ceramide → HCY → ROS injury.

Another severe consequence of protein/lipid oxidation is that while the cell does its best to break down and recycle oxidized proteins and lipid membranes, some exotic molecules created by oxidation cannot be processed by the proteasomes. The result is a plastic-like, non-biodegradable waste product called lipofuscin. Lipofuscin is the result of iron-catalyzed oxidization and polymerization of lipid and protein debris, largely of mitochondrial origin.

In renewable cells, this waste product is not as much of a problem, as it can get diluted, and the cells can be replaced. In postmitotic cells, lipofuscin collects within the cell over the body's lifetime. If lipofuscin sat quietly like old clothes in the attic, it would be bad enough. But this stuff is hazardous, more like oil-soaked rags.

Accumulation of lipofuscin is an indicator of biologic age, and the amount of lipofuscin formation among different species is inversely correlated to that species' longevity. Lipofuscin accumulation can be measured in the RPE cells of the retina, which are visible on ophthalmoscopic exam. It increases with age until about the age of 70, when it begins to disappear. Its disappearance correlates to the death of these postmitotic retinal cells[28].

Lipofuscin accumulation in cells impedes autophagocytosis of senescent organelles, including mitochondria and inhibits the degradation of proteins by proteasomes. Thus, lipofuscin promotes retention of poorly functioning mitochondria that produce more ROS. Lipofuscin also induces production of bcl-2[29], and thus prevents apoptosis and increases the risk of cancer and autoimmune disease.

Oxidative damage also inhibits the ability of mitochondria to undergo fission. This results in larger, less efficient mitochondria. These large mitochondria are less likely to undergo mitophagy, allowing for progressive enlargement and degeneration[1].

A vicious cycle of damage and lack of repairs occurs. Eventually, the cell is populated with large, poorly functioning, swollen mitochondria, which are like a dry, overgrown forest, easily set ablaze. Triggers for apoptosis at this stage can be minor events; mild ischemia and reperfusion, an inflammatory event, or even a fever, stressful exercise, or just getting excessively chilled[30]. These events can trigger pathways that activate BID, cause pore formation in the mitochondria and release of cytochrome C, triggering the caspase-9 cascade and apoptotic death of irreplaceable, postmitotic cells.

This is what old is: bloated, inefficient power plants, producing dangerous and toxic chemicals, swimming in a pool of pollution, which can self-destruct at the slightest provocation, and take the neighborhood with it.

Mitochondrial Associated Diseases

While there are some inherited mitochondrial diseases; fortunately, these are rare. Cancer is often induced as a result of oxidative damage to cellular DNA; poorly functioning mitochondria can be the source of these free radicals. Cancer survives as a result of the failure of apoptosis, which also requires the interaction of mitochondria with properly functioning and regulated proteins in the cell. Prevention of oxidative damage by maintaining the health of the mitochondria may prevent cancer. Autoimmune diseases may result from the failure of apoptosis of immune cells. Mitochondrial dysfunction is suspected as a cause of multiple diseases. Table 21-3 lists several diseases that have been suggested by at least in part caused by mitochondrial dysfunction.

Table 21-3: Some Diseases in which Mitochondrial Dysfunction is a Contributory Causes

ADHD	Amyotrophic lateral sclerosis
Alzheimer's disease	Bipolar disorder
Bulimia	Chronic fatigue syndrome
Cataplexy	Huntington's disease
Cerebellar ataxia	Irritable bowel syndrome (IBS)
Dysthymia	Leiber's congenital amaurosis
Fibromyalgia	Parkinson's syndrome
Major depression	Premenstrual dysphoric disorder
Migraine	Tinnitus
Panic disorder	Type 2 diabetes

Testing

Damage caused by oxidative and nitrosative stress cause increased levels of:

- 8-hydroxy-2-deoxyguanosine; indicating oxidative DNA damage
- Malondialdehyde (MDA); from peroxidation of polyunsaturated fatty acids
- Plasma peroxides
- Xanthine oxidase

Oxidative stress can be evaluated by testing for 8-hydroxy-2'-deoxyguanosine (8-OHdG). This is an organic acid which appears in the blood and urine. 8-OHdG can also be found in the saliva. Levels are found to be elevated after exposure to cigarette smoke. This biomarker has been used to estimate DNA damage in humans after exposure to cancer-causing agents, such as tobacco smoke, asbestos fibers, heavy metals, and polycyclic aromatic hydrocarbons[31]. Levels are increased in many disease states including type 2 diabetes, glaucoma[32], colon and other cancers, hypertension, atherosclerosis, and many other diseases[33]. 8-OHdG levels increase acutely after exercise, and these increases can be mitigated through the use of anti-oxidant vitamins and supplements[34,35]. Unfortunately, this test is not widely available and is rather expensive. Malondialdehyde (MDA) and Xanthine oxidase can also be used to indicate oxidative stress. TBAR levels are also sometimes used.

Preventive Treatment

Aging and many chronic diseases are the result of oxidative stress and its resultant damages. The best treatment is prevention; once lipofuscin has accumulated in a postmitotic cell, it is difficult to prevent aging of the cell. Prevention is far more effective in slowing aging than are any attempts to reverse it[36]. Avoid oxidative stressors, maintain healthy and vibrant mitochondria, and maintain sufficient antioxidants.

1. Avoid toxic exposures
2. Avoid chronic immune reactions
3. Participate in regular exercise to promote mitophagy
4. Avoid excessive caloric intake
5. Maintain a diet high in antioxidant nutrients and bioflavonoids.

Environmental Risks: Some oxidative damage to the cell can be prevented by avoidance of ionizing or UV radiation and potent oxidants. Radiation, tobacco smoke, air pollution and toxic chemicals should obviously be avoided.

Food Risks: Heterocyclic amines[37] (HCA), polycyclic aromatic hydrocarbons (PAH) and nitrosamines are pro-oxidants and carcinogens compounds which can form during the cooking food (especially meats and fish) at high temperatures. HCAs have been linked to prostate, pancreatic, and colon cancers and may promote obesity and type 2 diabetes[38].

The formation of HCA accelerates at cooking temperatures over 200°C (392°F). Frying foods at high temperatures increases the formation of these products. Flame grilling of foods can create temperatures of 538°C (1000°F). The temperature recommended by professional chefs for frying foods is 185°C (365°F), a temperature at which the formation of these toxins is fairly low; however, these temperatures can easily be, and often are, exceeded during cooking. The formation of HCA and other carcinogens and their prevention is discussed in Chapter 40.

Avoid Chronic Stress: Long-term stress, especially unrelenting stress with continuous sympathetic stimulus, induces inflammatory immune mediators which produce H_2O_2, a potent oxidative product. Corticosteroids inhibit autophagy. Stress and its mitigation are discussed in Chapter 29. Short bouts of stress (up to a few hours) help to induce recycling of effete mitochondria.

Avoid Chronic Inflammation: Inflammation is useful in the removal of bacteria and infected cells. Integral to the inflammatory process is the use of ROS for the killing of bacteria and cells marked for destruction. This should be a short-term process. Chronic inflammation can result from chronic exposure to toxins and stress to food immunogens, and from chronic infections.

Preventing Aging: Prevention of disease and aging requires frequent culling of effete and incompetent mitochondria. Feeble mitochondria produce ROS that form damaged proteins and lipids which become lipofuscin.

Relying on antioxidant supplements is not a viable strategy for preventing aging[39]. Antioxidants are important for quenching ROS, but by the time the ROS has been quenched, significant damage has already occurred in the mitochondria. Animal species with long life spans produce fewer superoxide radicals from complex I mitochondrial electron transport chain[40] and have fewer unsaturated phospholipid fatty acids in their cell membranes, which are susceptible to free radical damage[41]. A more viable method is to prevent the formation of free radicals.

A forty percent restriction in caloric intake can increase longevity in lab animals. This increase in longevity is accompanied by a significant decrease in the formation of ROS by Complex I proteins in the ETC. Every other day feeding of rodents has a similar effect on increasing longevity and ETC Complex I ROS production as 40% dietary restriction. It decreased mitochondrial Uncoupling Protein 2 (UCP2) and Apoptosis Inducing Factor (AIP)[42].

Neither restricting dietary carbohydrates[43] nor restricting dietary fats[44] prevent the formation of ROS by the ETC; however, a 40% restriction of dietary protein without restricting caloric intake offers a similar reduction in ROS formation to that accomplished by a 40% reduction of calories[45]. This effect can also be achieved by a 40% restriction in a single amino acid; methionine. The restriction in methionine decreases mitochondrial ROS production, without a decline in mitochondrial oxygen consumption. This dietary methionine restriction lowered mtDNA damage and decreased nuclear DNA methylation[46]. Methionine restriction likely acts by inducing selective autophagy[47] and scavenging to build new proteins Methionine restriction also increased production of SIRT1[48] and turnover of mitochondria[49]. Methionine restriction may be sufficient to reduce mitochondrial ETC Complex 1 ROS production. The methionine content in various proteinaceous foods and a methionine restricted diet are provided in Appendix H.

In contrast, methionine supplementation increases ROS production. The Western diet supplies two to three times more methionine than the adult requirement, and excess methionine can be toxic[50].

Deadly Sins and Virtues

Gluttony: Mitochondria have been compared to old cars that leak oil and are fuel-inefficient polluters. Extending this metaphor, when gas prices are low, no one seems to care about fuel economy, and the clunkers get left in service. The same is true with mitochondria. When there is plenty of fuel, there is less pressure to weed out the less efficient mitochondria. Excessive caloric intake lowers the turnover of mitochondria. High intake of methionine, found in high amounts in meat, fish and Brazil nuts, decreases turnover of mitochondria and promotes increased ROS production.

Abstinence: Low-methionine diets have been demonstrated to increase mitochondrial renewal and decrease ROS formation in multiple species, by inducing autophagy. An every-other-day methionine fast, or low methionine diet may just as efficiently reduce ROS formation. (See Appendix H.) For the non-penitent, glycine or glutamate supplementation may also function similarly to methionine restriction in preventing mitochondrial oxidative damage[51], although this may only work in yeasts[52].

Fasting, caloric restriction, and sustained exercise increase production of the ketone body, D-β-hydroxybutyrate (βOHB). βOHB increases histone acetylation and thereby, activation of FOXO3a and Mt2, two proteins that act as oxidative stress resistance factors[53].

Sloth: Exercise also stimulates the turnover of mitochondria. Exercise increases energy utilization. During vigorous exercise, the skeletal muscle cells export lactic acid for transport in the blood. Lactic acid is the principal fuel for the cardiomyocytes, and neurons during exercise when glucose levels fall. The retinal pigment epithelial cells also use lactate as fuel[54]. Lactate increases H_2O_2 production by the mitochondria and induced the expression of 673 genes, many involved in energy metabolism and several with mitochondrial reproduction[55]. Thus, exercise not only increases ROS production but also increases the creation of new proteins for mitochondria. Mitochondrial fusion and fission are influenced by the energy sources of the cell[1].

Since lactate is a fuel for the brain and is easily transported in, across the blood-brain barrier (BBB), vigorous physical exercise not only helps refresh mitochondria in the muscles, but also provides this benefit to the central nervous system. Fasting and exercise also increase the production of the ketone, 3-hydroxybutyrate (βOHB), which crosses the BBB. It is a fuel used by mitochondria[56] and may reduce oxidative stress.

Lactic acidosis is a potentially fatal adverse effect of metformin; a medication, which may be the most effective drug used in the treatment of type 2 diabetes. This drug gives a 36 percent decrease in all-cause mortality when compared to insulin and sulfonylurea medications[57]. The risk of lactic acidosis contraindicates the use of this medication in patients with kidney, liver, lung or heart insufficiencies. Metformin lowers blood sugar by inhibiting gluconeogenesis in the liver. Similarly, it can cause lactic acidosis in susceptible individuals by inhibiting lactic acid uptake in the liver for gluconeogenesis.

SPECULATION: While toxicity from lactic acidosis can be fatal, the propensity for raising lactic acid and lactic acid's effect on the mitochondria may explain some of the health benefits of this medication.

Exercise also causes an increase in cytokines, including IL-6 and TNF-α[58]. TNF-α can help to trigger apoptosis. IL-6 can either promote or impede apoptosis depending on the presence of other cytokines and cell activity. IL-6 is pro-inflammatory, and increased levels are seen in many inflammatory conditions as well as in obesity. During exercise, IL-6 can increase 100-fold[59]. Here, there is an acute, very high elevation of IL-6, versus chronic lower level exposure, in concert with the influence of other cytokines present. Exercise also increases the production of heat shock protein 72 (HSP72)[60], that blocks apoptosis[61]. These acute changes may induce mitophagy while inhibiting apoptosis.

Exercise for Mitochondrial Renewal:

Exercise which is brief and intense is much more effective for stimulating mitochondrial biogenesis, than that which is long and slow. The most efficient exercise for renewal of mitochondria may be sprints or Wingate exercises: repeated brief bouts of intense exercise lasting only 30 to 60 seconds, followed by a three- to five-minute recovery time, and then repeating the intense muscular effort. In a study using one minute, "all-out" efforts followed by 75 seconds of low-intensity recovery exercise, significant increases in SIRT1 and PGC-1α were associated with an increase in mitochondrial biogenesis[62]. This type of exercise gives the equivalent metabolic benefit of 4.5 hours of weekly endurance training in 1.5 hours of total weekly exercise time, using 30 second "all out" exercise efforts, interspaced with 4.5 minute recovery periods[63]. This requires only 9 minutes of intense exercise per week!

Exercise for efficiently increasing lactate and stimulating SIRT1 should include a warm-up period, followed by repeated bouts of intense exercise, interspaced with low-intensity, exercise recovery periods.

Longer duration exercise may also help prevent aging through the production of βOHB and induction of oxidative stress resistance factors. A small amount of caffeine, (one cup of coffee) before the exercise may increase the liberation and utilization of fat as fuel. Other than this, longer duration exercise should be performed on an empty stomach, to encourage the burning of fat as fuel, as this is the source of βOHB production. Avoiding eating for 30 minutes after the exercise may also help βOHB production.

Even with less intense exercise, there are benefits, but the exercise that gives the most health benefits is vigorous exercise that increases the heart rate and respiratory rate. Even if it is only for ten minutes, three times a week, vigorous exercise provides significant benefits.

Intemperance: Alcohol, when consumed in more than low levels, is metabolized in the liver by the cytochrome p450 enzyme CYP2E1, which creates reactive oxygen species. Alcohol can thus increase oxidative stress, and should be avoided.

Ablution and Atonement: Hot baths have some of the same beneficial metabolic effects as does exercise; using a cold clamp (cool baths during experimental conditions, or swimming in cool water) during exercise prevents most of these beneficial effects. The changes that occur with hot baths include increased levels of IL-6, epinephrine and norepinephrine release, growth hormone, cortisol, G-CSF[64] and HSP72[65], 3-hydroxybutyrate, and lactic acid[66]. Epinephrine release would be expected to promote lactate utilization[67]. The expected effects of hormones and cytokines resulting from elevated body temperature elevation from a hot bath would be to promote of mitochondrial reproduction and fission while preventing apoptosis. The net effect of exercise and hot baths, with transient elevation of body temperature, may be the increased turnover rate of mitochondria while protecting the cell from apoptosis.

Bestowing the Benefits of Exercise on the Infirm, the Incapacitated, or the Indulgent of Indolence:

Hot baths have some beneficial effects which parallel the effects of intense exercise, but without the work. The core body temperature needs to increase to about 37.5° to 38.5°C[64]. This can be done in a hot bath, hot tub, or sauna. Hot baths also help to improve glucose tolerance[68] and increase insulin sensitivity in type 2 diabetics[69]. This action is apparently mediated by normalization in the production of HSP72 in these patients. A study using a hot tub water temperature of 37.8°C to 41.0°C for 30 minutes a day found improved blood sugar levels and weight loss in insulin-dependent diabetics[70]. Hot baths have been found to be one of the most effective non-pharmacologic treatments of fibromyalgia[71]. Since lactate crosses the blood-brain barrier, hot baths should also benefit mitochondria in the brain.

Feast of Wine, Cheese, Mangoes, and Mushrooms

Active autophagy is essential for keeping cells vibrant and healthy. Several flavonoids in food have been found to induce autophagy. The bioamine spermidine also has this attribute[72]. The flavonoids that have been demonstrated to induce autophagy include resveratrol, quercetin, luteolin, and kaempferol[73].

Table 21-3: Foods high in selected flavonoids[74] and spermadine that induce autophagy

Flavonoid	Foods
Quercetin	Black elderberry, oregano, cloves, capers, red onions, shallots
Luteolin	Globe artichokes, black olives, oregano, thyme, sage
Kaempferol	Black beans, capers, caraway, cumin, cloves, red wine
Resveratrol	Cranberry, red currants, red (muscadine) wine
Spermidine	Cheddar cheese, mushrooms, mangoes, soybeans, green peas, pears, lentils, red beans, cauliflower, broccoli, corn, chicken liver, beef, potatoes, mustard seeds, and hazelnuts[75], (descending availability.)

Diets with restricted methionine, such as vegan diets, decrease mitochondrial ROS production and increase mitochondrial turnover. Lentils, beans, and most nuts other than Brazil nuts are high in protein while low in methionine. Grains are intermediate, and dairy, eggs, meats, and especially fish are high in methionine. Appendix H gives methionine content of foods.

Note: The longest lived human populations are those which consume large amounts of fish, a food very high in methionine. The effect of n-3 fats on reducing chronic inflammation or other factors in fish appears to outweigh the effect of high methionine content in this food.

Table 21-4: Antioxidants and Enzyme Cofactors

Autoxidation Enzyme Cofactors	Cofactors	Notes
Glutathione Peroxidase	Selenium, Vitamin D_3	Table 14-2 Chapter 20
Glutathione Reductase	FAD (Riboflavin) Copper Glutathione	Avoid copper as supplement unless proven deficiency. Chapter 39
Glutathione	N-acetylcysteine Zinc, SAMe	SAMe can be toxic. Chapter 39
Superoxide Dismutase SOD1 (cytoplasmic) SOD2 (Mitochondria) SOD3 (Extracellular)	Copper, Zinc Manganese Copper, Zinc	Avoid copper. Ensure adequate vitamin C to recycle copper.
Catalase	NADPH (Niacin)	
Antioxidants	Alpha lipoic acid Melatonin Taurine Vitamin C Vitamin E PQQ	
Taurine formation	Niacin, Iron, Vitamin B_6 Molybdenum	Table 14-2
Melatonin formation	Tryptophan Vitamin B_6 PQQ	Table 28-3

Nutritional Cofactors

An adequate supply of cofactors for antioxidant enzymes and ETC proteins may prevent oxidative damage and inefficient oxidative phosphorylation in the mitochondria. These cofactors are listed in Tables 21-4 and 21-5.

Vitamin C (ascorbate) is an extracellular antioxidant that acts directly on free radicals, effectively quenches ROS species including singlet oxygen, superoxide, hydroxyl, reactive nitrogen species and water-soluble peroxyl radicals. In the reaction between ascorbate and ROS species, a one-electron oxidation product is generated, an ascorbyl radical, that can be further oxidized to dehydroascorbate. Cellular reducing molecules, such as NADH, NADPH, and glutathione, can reversibly reduce one- and two-electron oxidation products, and ultimately, regenerate ascorbate. Additionally, ascorbate is utilized in the recycling of vitamin E radicals back into to vitamin E. Uric acid, bilirubin and sulfhydryl groups are other important extracellular antioxidants. Glutathione acts as an extracellular antioxidant in the alveolar fluid of the lung[76].

Carnitine is required for transport of fatty acids across the mitochondrial membrane so that the fatty acids can be used as fuel. Carnitine is produced mainly by the liver and kidneys from lysine or methionine. Carnitine also helps carry metabolic waste toxins out of the mitochondria, thus protecting them from damage. During growth, pregnancy, or other conditions of high metabolic demand, the creation of carnitine may be insufficient to supply the body's requirements for it. Supplementation may be helpful. Vitamin C is a cofactor in the synthesis of carnitine in these situations.

Table 21-5: Electron Transport Chain Cofactors

Electron Transport Chain	Cofactor	Notes
Electron Transport Chain Complex I Proteins	Niacin for NADH Riboflavin for FMN Iron, Coenzyme Q$_{10}$	CoQ$_{10}$ is made by the body but may be insufficient in old age. It is also available in the diet. Betaine, folate, and vitamin B$_{12}$ may help in the formation of adequate CoQ$_{10}$.
Cytochrome C	Iron Copper	Vitamin C helps recycle copper.
Fatty acid transport into the mitochondria	Carnitine (Acetyl-L-carnitine) Vitamin C	Non-essential amino acid, but may be insufficiently produced. Prevents lipofuscin formation and protects mitochondria. Vitamin C is required for carnitine synthesis.
Glycine amidinotransferase	Creatine	Non-essential amino acid, supplementation may help in heart failure, muscle building

Melatonin is an antioxidant formed in the pineal gland, intestines, and white blood cells from serotonin. Melatonin is lipophilic and easily crosses the blood-brain barrier and placental membranes. Melatonin is unlike most other antioxidant compounds in that it does not become a free radical when it is oxidized, but rather is converted into other antioxidant compounds. Each molecule may be able to quench up to ten reactive oxygen or reactive nitrogen species[77]. Melatonin is an important antioxidant for the mitochondrial DNA. In aged mice, melatonin increases mitochondrial function and population and decreases the production of β-amyloid protein[78].

Melatonin is an important antioxidant for neurons and has been found to be neuroprotective during induced strokes in animals, by preventing caspase-1 induced activation of IL-1β[79]. It also inhibits NF-κB activation by LPS in sepsis, preventing oxidative damage and production of inflammatory cytokines[80].

The inflammatory cytokine IL-1β can trigger programmed neuronal cell death by pyroptosis. Pyroptosis differs from apoptosis as it is a response to inflammation. In strokes, the glial cells participate in this reaction. In animal models, pyroptosis can be triggered by ischemia, rather than the ischemia/reperfusion triggered apoptosis. Medications with potential for neuronal protection during a stroke include doxycycline, minocycline, meclizine, hydroxyprogesterone, and methazolamide[81]. See TBI, Chapter 30.

> Pyrroloquinoline quinone (PQQ) (a vitamin-like compound; can increase the mass of mitochondria, and protect them as an efficient antioxidant[82]. Look for it in the fresh green vegetable aisle of your local grocery store. See Chapter 28.

Taurine is a sulfur-containing amino acid which behaves as an ROS quencher. It is formed from cysteine by enzymes that require NADH, NADPH, iron, pyridoxal phosphate[83], and perhaps molybdenum as cofactors. Treatment of mitochondrial with CoQ10 and other antioxidants takes about six months for the improvements to manifest.

Accumulation of lipofuscin can be prevented (in rats at least) with acetyl-l-carnitine supplementation, α-lipoic acid[84], and other antioxidants. Calorie restricted diets and antioxidants have also been shown to decrease the accumulation of lipofuscin.

Elimination of lipofuscin from postmitotic cells may not occur in mammals in nature. A search of the scientific literature yielded only two studies showing reversal of lipofuscin accumulation in neuronal tissue as a result of treatment; one study was performed on crustaceans[85], the other in pond snails[86] using vitamin E. Since many vitamin supplementations are associated with increased risk of cancer, if you are not a pond snail, prevention is the safer bet. See Chapters 39 and 40 on supplements and cancer prevention.

The amount of lipofuscin that accumulates in the retina increases with age, however, it varies considerably between individuals. In a study of retinal lipofuscin deposits, there was a range equivalent to 15 years more or less than that expected for the patient's calendar age. Thus, lifestyle may account for as much as 30 years variance in biologic aging[28].

Eat well: Plant foods contain hundreds of antioxidant compounds. Citrus fruits, berries, grapes (red wine), green tea, red onions, beans, and dark chocolate and coffee are among the many foods with generous supplies of phenolic compounds that are antioxidants, induce autophagy and prevent inflammation. Consuming a wide variety of fruits and vegetables provides a mix of various antioxidant compounds.

[1] Mitochondrial turnover and aging of long-lived postmitotic cells: the mitochondrial-lysosomal axis theory of aging. Terman A, Kurz T, Navratil M, Arriaga EA, Brunk UT. Antioxid Redox Signal. 2010 Apr;12(4):503-35. PMID:19650712

[2] Dynamics of telomerase activity in response to acute psychological stress. Epel ES, Lin J, Dhabhar FS, Wolkowitz OM, Puterman E, Karan L, Blackburn EH. Brain Behav Immun. 2010 May;24(4):531-9. PMID:20018236

[3] Leukocyte telomere length in major depression: correlations with chronicity, inflammation and oxidative stress--preliminary findings. Wolkowitz OM, Mellon SH, Epel ES, Lin J, et al. PLoS One. 2011 Mar 23;6(3):e17837. PMID:21448457

[4] Childhood adversities are associated with shorter telomere length at adult age both in individuals with an anxiety disorder and controls. Kananen L, Surakka I, Pirkola S, et al. PLoS One. 2010 May 25;5(5):e10826. PMID:20520834

[5] Telomere Shortening in Formerly Abused and Never Abused Women. Humphreys J, Epel ES, Cooper BA, Lin J, Blackburn EH, Lee KA. Biol Res Nurs. 2011 Mar 8. PMID:21385798

[6] Intensive meditation training, immune cell telomerase activity, and psychological mediators. Jacobs TL, Epel ES, Lin J, et al. Psychoneuroendocrinology. 2011 Jun;36(5):664-81. Epub 2010 Oct 29. PMID:21035949

[7] Cumulative Inflammatory Load Is Associated with Short Leukocyte Telomere Length in the Health, Aging and Body Composition Study. O'Donovan A, Pantell MS, Puterman E, et al. PLoS One. 2011;6(5):e19687. PMID:21602933

[8] Association between telomere length, specific causes of death, and years of healthy life in health, aging, and body composition, a population-based cohort study. Njajou OT, Hsueh WC, Blackburn EH, et al; Health ABC study. J Gerontol A Biol Sci Med Sci. 2009 Aug;64(8):860-4. PMID:19435951

[9] Juvenile exposure to anthracyclines impairs cardiac progenitor cell function and vascularization resulting in greater susceptibility to stress-induced myocardial injury in adult mice. Huang C, Zhang X, Ramil JM, et al. Circulation. 2010 Feb 9;121(5):675-83. Epub 2010 Jan 25. PMID:20100968

[10] Illustration by Mariana Ruiz Villarreal, adapted by others

[11] Principles of Biochemistry and Biophysics Chauhan, BS. University Science Press, Boston 2008, Chapter 12.

[12] Illustration by Mariana Ruiz Villarreal

[13] Illustration by Fvasconcellos, adapted by author

[14] How mitochondria produce reactive oxygen species. Murphy MP. Biochem J. 2009 Jan 1;417(1):1-13. PMID:19061483

[15] Mitochondrial DNA damage and animal longevity: insights from comparative studies. Pamplona R. J Aging Res. 2011 Mar 2;2011:807108. PMID:21423601

[16] Dysregulation of apoptosis in cancer. Reed JC. J Clin Oncol. 1999 Sep;17(9):2941-53. PMID:10561374

[17] Straw blood cell count, growth, inhibition and comparison to apoptotic bodies. Wu Y, Henry DC, Heim K, Tomkins JP, Kuan CY. BMC Cell Biol. 2008 May 20;9:26. PMID:18492269

[18] Saving death: apoptosis for intervention in transplantation and autoimmunity. Li A, Ojogho O, Escher A. Clin Dev Immunol. 2006 Jun-Dec;13(2-4):273-82. PMID:17162368

[19] Oxidative stress and autophagy in cardiac disease, neurological disorders, aging and cancer. Essick EE, Sam F. Oxid Med Cell Longev. 2010 May-Jun;3(3):168-77. PMID:20716941

[20] Autophagy-mediated antigen processing in CD4(+) T cell tolerance and immunity. Klein L, Münz C, Lünemann JD. FEBS Lett. 2010 Apr 2;584(7):1405-10. PMID:20074571

[21] Mitochondrial dynamics--fusion, fission, movement, and mitophagy--in neurodegenerative diseases. Chen H, Chan DC. Hum Mol Genet. 2009 Oct 15;18(R2):R169-76. PMID:19808793

[22] S-nitrosylation of Drp1 links excessive mitochondrial fission to neuronal injury in neurodegeneration. Nakamura T, Cieplak P, Cho DH, Godzik A, Lipton SA. Mitochondrion. 2010 Aug;10(5):573-8. PMID:20447471

[23] Isoflavones promote mitochondrial biogenesis. Rasbach KA, Schnellmann RG. J Pharmacol Exp Ther. 2008 May;325(2):536-43. PMID:18267976

[24] Tubular network formation protects mitochondria from autophagosomal degradation during nutrient starvation. Rambold AS, Kostelecky B, Elia N, Lippincott-Schwartz J. Proc Natl Acad Sci U S A. 2011 Jun 6. PMID:21646527

[25] Bcl-x L increases mitochondrial fission, fusion, and biomass in neurons. Berman SB, Chen YB, Qi B, et al. J Cell Biol. 2009 Mar 9;184(5):707-19. PMID:19255249

[26] Autophagy in health and disease. 5. Mitophagy as a way of life. Gottlieb RA, Carreira RS. Am J Physiol Cell Physiol. 2010 Aug;299(2):C203-10. Epub 2010 Mar 31. PMID:20357180

[27] A review on the oxidative and nitrosative stress (O&NS) pathways in major depression and their possible contribution to the (neuro)degenerative processes in that illness. Maes M, Galecki P, Chang YS, Berk M. Prog Neuropsychopharmacol Biol Psychiatry. 2011 Apr 29;35(3):676-92. PMID:20471444

[28] Age-related accumulation and spatial distribution of lipofuscin in RPE of normal subjects. Delori FC, Goger DG, Dorey CK. Invest Ophthalmol Vis Sci. 2001 Jul;42(8):1855-66. PMID:11431454

[29] bcl-2 protein expression in aged brain and neurodegenerative diseases. Migheli A, Cavalla P, Piva R, Giordana MT, Schiffer D. Neuroreport. 1994 Oct 3;5(15):1906-8. PMID:7841373

[30] Intracellular monocyte and serum cytokine expression is modulated by exhausting exercise and cold exposure. Rhind SG, Castellani JW, Brenner IK, et al. Am J Physiol Regul Integr Comp Physiol. 2001 Jul;281(1):R66-75. PMID:11404280

[31] 8-hydroxy-2'-deoxyguanosine (8-OHdG): A critical biomarker of oxidative stress and carcinogenesis. Valavanidis A, Vlachogianni T, Fiotakis C. J Environ Sci Health C Environ Carcinog Ecotoxicol Rev. 2009 Apr;27(2):120-39. PMID:19412858

[32] Oxidative DNA damage and total antioxidant status in glaucoma patients. Sorkhabi R, Ghorbanihaghjo A, Javadzadeh A, et al. Mol Vis. 2011 Jan 7;17:41-6. PMID:21245957

[33] Increased plasma levels of 8-hydroxydeoxyguanosine are associated with development of colorectal tumors. Sato T, Takeda H, Otake S, et al. J Clin Biochem Nutr. 2010 Jul;47(1):59-63. Epub 2010 Apr 23. PMID:20664732

[34] Vitamin E and C supplementation reduces oxidative stress, improves antioxidant enzymes and positive muscle work in chronically loaded muscles of aged rats. Ryan MJ, Dudash HJ, Docherty M, et al. Exp Gerontol. 2010 Nov;45(11):882-95. PMID:20705127

[35] Melatonin supplementation ameliorates oxidative stress and inflammatory signaling induced by strenuous exercise in adult human males. Ochoa JJ, Díaz-Castro J, Kajarabille N, et al. J Pineal Res. 2011 Apr 21. PMID:21615492

[36] Carnitine and lipoate ameliorates lipofuscin accumulation and monoamine oxidase activity in aged rat heart. Savitha S, Naveen B, Panneerselvam C. Eur J Pharmacol. 2007 Nov 21;574(1):61-5. PMID:17678889

[37] Screening for heterocyclic amines in chicken cooked in various ways. Solyakov A, Skog K. Food Chem Toxicol. 2002 Aug;40(8):1205-11.PMID: 12067585

[38] Polycyclic aromatic hydrocarbons potentiate high-fat diet effects on intestinal inflammation. Khalil A, Villard PH, Dao MA, Burcelin R, Champion S, Fouchier F, Savouret JF, Barra Y, Seree E. Toxicol Lett. 2010 Jul 15;196(3):161-7. Epub 2010 Apr 20. PMID: 20412841

[39] Is the mitochondrial free radical theory of aging intact? Sanz A, Pamplona R, Barja G. Antioxid Redox Signal. 2006 Mar-Apr;8(3-4):582-99. PMID:16677102

[40] Mitochondrial DNA damage and animal longevity: insights from comparative studies. Pamplona R. J Aging Res. 2011 Mar 2;2011:807108. PMID:21423601

[41] Correlation of fatty acid unsaturation of the major liver mitochondrial phospholipid classes in mammals to their maximum life span potential. Portero-Otín M, Bellmunt MJ, Ruiz MC, Barja G, Pamplona R. Lipids. 2001 May;36(5):491-8. PMID:11432462

[42] Effect of every other day feeding on mitochondrial free radical production and oxidative stress in mouse liver. Caro P, Gómez J, López-Torres M, Sánchez I, Naudi A, Portero-Otín M, Pamplona R, Barja G. Rejuvenation Res. 2008 Jun;11(3):621-9. PMID:18593280

[43] Carbohydrate restriction does not change mitochondrial free radical generation and oxidative DNA damage. Sanz A, Gómez J, Caro P, Barja G. J Bioenerg Biomembr. 2006 Dec;38(5-6):327-33. PMID:17136610

[44] Effect of lipid restriction on mitochondrial free radical production and oxidative DNA damage. Sanz A, Caro P, Sanchez JG, Barja G. Ann N Y Acad Sci. 2006 May;1067:200-9. PMID:16803986

[45] Protein restriction without strong caloric restriction decreases mitochondrial oxygen radical production and oxidative DNA damage in rat liver. Sanz A, Caro P, Barja G. J Bioenerg Biomembr. 2004 Dec;36(6):545-52. PMID:15692733

[46] Forty percent methionine restriction lowers DNA methylation, complex I ROS generation, and oxidative damage to mtDNA and mitochondrial proteins in rat heart. Sanchez-Roman I, Gomez A, Gomez J, Suarez H, et al. J Bioenerg Biomembr. 2011 Dec;43(6):699-708. PMID:22006472

[47] Lifespan extension by methionine restriction requires autophagy-dependent vacuolar acidification. Ruckenstuhl C, Netzberger C, Entfellner I, et al. PLoS Genet. 2014 May 1;10(5):e1004347. PMID:24785424

[48] Effect of 40% restriction of dietary amino acids (except methionine) on mitochondrial oxidative stress and biogenesis, AIF and SIRT1 in rat liver. Caro P, Gomez J, Sanchez I, et al. Biogerontology. 2009 Oct;10(5):579-92. PMID:19039676

[49] Methionine restriction decreases endogenous oxidative molecular damage and increases mitochondrial biogenesis and uncoupling protein 4 in rat brain. Naudí A, Caro P, Jové M, Gómez J, Boada J, Ayala V, Portero-Otín M, Barja G, Pamplona R. Rejuvenation Res. 2007 Dec;10(4):473-84. PMID:17716000

[50] Effect of methionine dietary supplementation on mitochondrial oxygen radical generation and oxidative DNA damage in rat liver and heart. Gomez J, Caro P, Sanchez I, Naudi A, etal J Bioenerg Biomembr. 2009 Jun;41(3):309-21. PMID:19633937

[51] Dietary glycine supplementation mimics lifespan extension by dietary methionine restriction in Fisher 344 rats. Brind J, Malloy V, Augie I, et al. FASEB Journal. 2011;25:528.2

[52] Independent and additive effects of glutamic acid and methionine on yeast longevity. Wu Z, Song L, Liu SQ, Huang D. PLoS One. 2013 Nov 7;8(11):e79319. PMID:24244480

[53] Suppression of oxidative stress by β-hydroxybutyrate, an endogenous histone deacetylase inhibitor. Shimazu T, Hirschey MD, Newman J, etal. Science. 2013 Jan 11;339(6116):211-4. PMID:23223453

[54] A metabolic switch in brain: glucose and lactate metabolism modulation by ascorbic acid. Castro MA, Beltrán FA, Brauchi S, Concha II. J Neurochem. 2009 Jul;110(2):423-40. PMID:19457103

[55] Lactate sensitive transcription factor network in L6 cells: activation of MCT1 and mitochondrial biogenesis. Hashimoto T, Hussien R, Oommen S, Gohil K, Brooks GA. FASEB J. 2007 Aug;21(10):2602-12. PMID:17395833

[56] 3-hydroxybutyrate methyl ester as a potential drug against Alzheimer's disease via mitochondria protection mechanism. Zhang J, Cao Q, Li S, Lu X, Zhao Y, Guan JS, Chen JC, Wu Q, Chen GQ. Biomaterials. 2013 Oct;34(30):7552-62. PMID:23849878

[57] Effect of intensive blood-glucose control with metformin on complications in overweight patients with type 2 diabetes (UKPDS 34). UK Prospective Diabetes Study (UKPDS) Group. Lancet. 1998 Sep 12;352(9131):854-65. PMID:9742977

[58] Heat stress, cytokines, and the immune response to exercise. Starkie RL, Hargreaves M, Rolland J, Febbraio MA. Brain Behav Immun. 2005 Sep;19(5):404-12. PMID:16061150

[59] Muscle as an endocrine organ: focus on muscle-derived interleukin-6. Pedersen BK, Febbraio MA. Physiol Rev. 2008 Oct;88(4):1379-406. PMID:18923185

[60] Effect of exercise with and without a thermal clamp on the plasma heat shock protein 72 response. Whitham M, Laing SJ, Jackson A, Maassen N, Walsh NP. J Appl Physiol. 2007 Oct;103(4):1251-6. PMID:17673560

[61] Hsp72 mediates TAp73alpha anti-apoptotic effects in small cell lung carcinoma cells. Nyman U, Muppani NR, Zhivotovsky B, Joseph B. J Cell Mol Med. 2010 Aug 27. PMID:20807285

[62] A practical model of low-volume high-intensity interval training induces mitochondrial biogenesis in human skeletal muscle: potential mechanisms. Little JP, Safdar A, Wilkin GP, Tarnopolsky MA, Gibala MJ. J Physiol. 2010 Mar 15;588(Pt 6):1011-22. PMID:20100740

[63] Sprint interval and traditional endurance training induce similar improvements in peripheral arterial stiffness and flow-mediated dilation in healthy humans. Rakobowchuk M, Tanguay S, Burgomaster KA, et al. Am J Physiol Regul Integr Comp Physiol. 2008 Jul;295(1):R236-42. PMID:18434437

[64] Human blood neutrophil responses to prolonged exercise with and without a thermal clamp. Laing SJ, Jackson AR, Walters R, Lloyd-Jones E, Whitham M, Maassen N, Walsh NP. J Appl Physiol. 2008 Jan;104(1):20-6. PMID:17901240

[65] Elevation of body temperature is an essential factor for exercise-increased extracellular heat shock protein 72 level in rat plasma. Ogura Y, Naito H, Akin S, Ichinoseki-Sekine N, etal. Am J Physiol Regul Integr Comp Physiol. 2008 May;294(5):R1600-7. PMID:18367652

[66] Metabolic and hormonal responses to exogenous hyperthermia in man. Møller N, Beckwith R, Butler PC, et al. Clin Endocrinol (Oxf). 1989 Jun;30(6):651-60. PMID:2686866

[67] Additive protective effects of the addition of lactic acid and adrenaline on excitability and force in isolated rat skeletal muscle depressed by elevated extracellular K+. de Paoli FV, Overgaard K, Pedersen TH, Nielsen OB. J Physiol. 2007 Jun 1;581(Pt 2):829-39. PMID: 17347268

[68] HSP72 protects against obesity-induced insulin resistance. Chung J, Nguyen AK, Henstridge DC, Holmes AG, Chan MH, Mesa JL, etal. Proc Natl Acad Sci U S A. 2008 Feb 5;105(5):1739-44. PMID:18223156

[69] Heat treatment improves glucose tolerance and prevents skeletal muscle insulin resistance in rats fed a high-fat diet. Gupte AA, Bomhoff GL, Swerdlow RH, Geiger PC. Diabetes. 2009 Mar;58(3):567-78. Epub 2008 Dec 10. PMID:19073766

[70] Hot-tub therapy for type 2 diabetes mellitus. Hooper PL. N Engl J Med. 1999 Sep 16;341(12):924-5. PMID:10498473

[71] Complementary and alternative medicine in the treatment of pain in fibromyalgia: a systematic review of randomized controlled trials. Terhorst L, Schneider MJ, Kim KH, et al. J Manipulative Physiol Ther. 2011 Sep;34(7):483-96. PMID:21875523

[72] Spermidine and resveratrol induce autophagy by distinct pathways converging on the acetylproteome. Morselli E, Mariño G, Bennetzen MV, etal. J Cell Biol. 2011 Feb 21;192(4):615-29. PMID:21339330

[73] Concurrent detection of autolysosome formation and lysosomal degradation by flow cytometry in a high-content screen for inducers of autophagy. Hundeshagen P, Hamacher-Brady A, Eils R, Brady NR. BMC Biol. 2011 Jun 2;9:38. PMID:21635740

74 Phenol-Explorer: http://www.phenol-explorer.eu

[75] Polyamines in foods: development of a food database. Atiya Ali M, Poortvliet E, Strömberg R, Yngve A. Food Nutr Res. 2011 Jan 14;55. PMID:21249159

[76] Birth Asphyxia and the Brain: Basic Science and Clinical Implications. Steven M. Donn, Sunil K. Sinha, Malcolm L. Chiswick. Wiley-Blackwell; 2002

[77] One molecule, many derivatives: a never-ending interaction of melatonin with reactive oxygen and nitrogen species? Tan DX, Manchester LC, Terron MP, Flores LJ, Reiter RJ. J Pineal Res. 2007 Jan;42(1):28-42. PMID:17198536

[78] Melatonin induces neural SOD2 expression independent of the NF-kappaB pathway and improves the mitochondrial population and function in old mice. García-Macia M, Vega-Naredo I, De Gonzalo-Calvo D, et al. J Pineal Res. 2011 Jan;50(1):54-63. PMID:21062349

[79] Methazolamide and melatonin inhibit mitochondrial cytochrome C release and are neuroprotective in experimental models of ischemic injury. Wang X, Figueroa BE, Stavrovskaya IG, Zhang Y, et al. Stroke. 2009 May;40(5):1877-85. PMID:19299628

[80] Antioxidants that protect mitochondria reduce interleukin-6 and oxidative stress, improve mitochondrial function, and reduce biochemical markers of organ dysfunction in a rat model of acute sepsis. Lowes DA, Webster NR, Murphy MP, Galley HF. Br J Anaesth. 2013 Mar;110(3):472-80. PMID:23381720

[81] Inhibitors of cytochrome c release with therapeutic potential for Huntington's disease. Wang X, Zhu S, Pei Z, et al. J Neurosci. 2008 Sep 17;28(38):9473-85. PMID:18799679

[82] Pyrroloquinoline quinone preserves mitochondrial function and prevents oxidative injury in adult rat cardiac myocytes. Tao R, Karliner JS, Simonis U, et al. Biochem Biophys Res Commun. 2007 Nov 16;363(2):257-62. PMID:17880922

[83] Ascorbic acid and pyridoxine in experimental anaphylaxis. Alvarez RG, Mesa MG. Agents Actions. 1981 Apr;11(1-2):89-93. PMID:6166175

[84] Neuronal mitochondrial amelioration by feeding acetyl-L-carnitine and lipoic acid to aged rats. Aliev G, Liu J, Shenk JC, Fischbach K, et al. J Cell Mol Med. 2009 Feb;13(2):320-33. PMID:18373733

[85] Reversal of a hallmark of brain ageing: lipofuscin accumulation. Fonseca DB, Sheehy MR, Blackman N, Shelton PM, Prior AE. Neurobiol Aging. 2005 Jan;26(1):69-76. PMID:15585347

[86] Lipofuscin accumulation and its prevention by vitamin E in nervous tissue: quantitative analysis using snail buccal ganglia as a simple model system. Winstanley EK, Pentreath VW. Mech Ageing Dev. 1985 Mar;29(3):299-307. PMID:3990384

22. Gluten Disease

Gluten related disease is important, not only because of its prevalence and broad effects on health, but also because it is a model for understanding many other enteroimmune disease conditions.

Grains, traditionally rice in the East, maize in the Americas, and wheat in the West, provided easily storable protein that could feed large populations year round. This freed people from the hunter-gatherer existence and allowed for specialization of trades; with this came the development of cities. Wheat has been cultivated for over 10,000 years and was key to the development of the Babylonian and Assyrian empires, followed by Egyptian, Jewish, Greek and Roman civilizations, and thus, Western civilization.

Wheat, however, is somewhat toxic. This toxicity likely gave wheat a survival advantage as a crop, as it kept grazing animals from consuming too much of it. It may prevent migrating flocks of birds or swarms of insects from destroying fields of wheat. Mammals can eat some, but cannot overgraze on wheat.

About one person in 133 in the United States has Celiac Disease[1]. In this disease, wheat makes susceptible persons seriously ill. Celiac Disease (CD) causes multiple health problems, including intestinal lymphoma that can be fatal. CD is principally a disease affecting the mucosa of the intestine; however, it can affect many organs, including the skin, brain, reproduction, and skeletal system.

Table 22-1: Frequency of Symptom in Gluten Enteropathy

Signs or Symptoms of Gluten Enteropathy[2]	Frequency Seen (% of Cases)
Abdominal Pain	80
Fatigue	80
Weight Loss	70
Diarrhea	50
Malnutrition	50
Steatorrhea	40
Bone Pain	40
Headaches	40
Peripheral Neuropathy	7
Blistering rash	5
Ataxia	3
Short Stature	2

CD is not, and should not be confused with an allergy to wheat. Wheat allergies and antergies can form to any of the many wheat protein peptides, and behave like any other food allergy or antergy. Everyone is at risk for allergies and antergies, but CD is a genetically determined disease.

Celiac Disease, also known as gluten enteropathy, is the most recognized form of gluten disease. Celiac Disease refers to a severe manifestation of gluten disease, in which several pathological conditions may present. In CD, the lining of the small intestines is severely affected, resulting in a malabsorption syndrome. A wider population can have a much milder toxic response to gluten.

CD is an autoimmune disease, and as such, requires interplay between genetic susceptibility, exposure to environmental factors, and an immune event.

1. **Genetic susceptibility**: The individual's immune system recognizes, and often misinterprets a non-pathogen as a pathogen,
2. **Exposure to an antigen**, and
3. **Presentation of the antigen** to the gastro-intestinal mucosal immune system[3].

Genetic Susceptibility

Histocompatibility Proteins: The HLA proteins are the major histocompatibility complexes (MHC) in humans for presenting cell-surface antigens. MHC Class I antigens (HLA-A, B, and C) present peptides which are produced during the normal turnover of used proteins being recycled inside of the cell. In the recycling process, proteins in the cell are broken into fragments (peptides) inside the proteasomes. A sample of these peptides is attached to MCH class I proteins that are then transported to the cell surface where they are presented on the cell surface. Proteins from intracellular pathogens, such as bacteria and viruses are also broken up, and their peptides are also presented on the cell surface. If the peptide/MCH complex is recognized as a foreign antigen, it can attract killer T-cells that can destroy the cell. Presenting a self-antigen avoids this destruction. Thus Class I antigens help protect the organism by differentiating the cell from foreign antigens and aiding in the elimination of cells harboring intracellular pathogens, such as viruses and some bacteria.

Class II MHC (HLA DO, DP, DQ, and DR antigen types) present extracellular antigens to T-cells. When antigen presenting cells (dendritic cells) phagocytize a foreign antigen, the antigen proteins are digested into peptides that are loaded into the Class II MCH. The HLA proteins grab the antigenic peptide and hold it in position presenting it to T cells. T cells can then mount an immune defense against the antigen. The T-helper cells promote the production of antibodies from B-cells to target the specific antigen. Self-antigens are suppressed by regulatory T-Cells, (T_{REG} cells), which helps to prevent autoimmune reactions.

Most HLA Class II receptors are made up of an α-protein and a β-protein, which act like a thumb and forefinger that can hold the antigen for presentation. Each person has two alleles (one from each parent) for each of these proteins, for each HLA Class II type. Thus, if an individual's mother (m) and father (f) have different HLA types they can make 4 different receptor pairs: αm-βm, αm-βf, αf-βm, and αf-βf for each Class II type.

The variation in subtype allele can provide immune adaptation to infectious disease. Thus, some individuals in a population will be able to fight a new infections disease more readily than others, depending on the subtype and disease. This variation can help some individuals in a population to survive infectious threats, depending on which disease appears and thus, helps to maintain the species. In populations that have been culled by disease, the distribution of subtypes reflects the survival advantage that helped in their environment.

Certain HLA subtypes are also associated with increased susceptibility to different autoimmune disorders, including gluten enteropathy, type 1 diabetes[4], myasthenia gravis, and Sjögren's syndrome. The genetic susceptibility for gluten enteropathy involves specific HLA DQ subtypes. A peptide fragment of gluten binds with these HLA DQ types, and is presented and recognized as a foreign antigen.

There are about 360 different antigenic pairings of the HLA-DQ in the human population. There are 84 among Caucasians in the U.S., but many of these are uncommon. Only three HLA DQ types are associated with gluten disease: DQ2.5, DQ2.2, and DQ8. Unfortunately, these are the 2nd, 3rd and 6th most common DQ alleles found in this population.

DQ8 is highly prevalent in Amerindians, from the Mississippi Valley to northern South America; as many as 90% of some Amerindian populations carry this HLA type. DQ8 is also common on the Pacific Rim and is present in about 15 percent of Scandinavians. Pre-Columbian Americans and early Scandinavians did not eat wheat, and thus there was little negative genetic selection against this allele. Now, however, these populations are exposed to and susceptible to gluten as it has become ubiquitous in the Western diet.

DQ2.5 is common in Western Europe and North and West Africa. It has its highest prevalence among populations from the Atlantic coast of Spain and of Celtic origin; two populations that also have high a prevalence of autoimmune diseases. About 13% of American Caucasians carry the DQ2.5 form. The DQ2.2 form carries some risk of gluten disease. It also is common in Asian populations.

Ninety-four percent of Europeans with gluten disease carry at least one copy of either the DQ2.5 or the DQ8 allele. Four percent have the DQ2.2 allele. Thus, at least 98% of cases of gluten disease can be explained by an HLA DQ receptor that can present gluten as an antigen to T-helper cells.

Gluten disease decreases fertility and increases the risk of death during labor for women with deformed pelvis caused by osteomalacia. Gluten disease increases the risk of death, as it increases the risk for malnutrition and susceptibility to infectious disease. Thus, gluten disease has exerted a strong negative survival pressure over the millennia. In populations that wheat was a central nutrient over the ages, few individuals carry HLA DQ types that put them at risk for this disease. In other populations where wheat has been introduced only in the last few hundred years, there is a much higher prevalence of the HLA DQ genotypes that confer susceptibility. Wheat was not a crop in the Americas, and it was too cold for it to be grown in Scandinavia. Therefore, peoples whose ancestry is from these areas have a higher likelihood of HLA susceptibility associated with CD.

Other risk factors, including environmental and other genetic factors, may additionally be required for CD. Even though 10% of the North American population has an HLA type that confers risk of gluten enteropathy, only about one percent are afflicted with the active disease. Even among identical twins, there is only 75% disease concordance[3].

Table 22-2: **HLA DQ Alleles Associated with Autoimmune Diseases:**

HLA Subtype	Prevalence among U.S. Caucasians	Percent cases of Gluten Disease	Disease Associated with HLA Type
HLA DQ-2.2	11%	4%	Celiac Disease
HLA DQ-2.5	13 %	86%	Type 1 Diabetes, Celiac Disease, Sjögren's syndrome, Lambert-Eaton syndrome, Autoimmune hepatitis, Dermatitis Herpetiformis
HLA DQ-8	10%	8%	Rheumatoid arthritis, Type 1 Diabetes, Celiac Disease

Exposure to the Antigen

Gluten is a storage protein present in wheat, barley, and rye. Gluten gives elasticity to dough, helping to hold the bubbles of gas produced by yeast, so that bread rises. This elasticity gives bread and baked goods their pleasant chewiness.

Gluten makes up about 80% of the protein in wheat. Gluten is a quaternary protein composed of two proteins subunits: prolamin and glutelin. Some of the glutelins are gliadins. There are four different gliadins in wheat (α, β, γ and ω gliadins). α, β, and γ-gliadins are associated with gluten disease. Wheat allergy can be triggered by at least 17 different wheat proteins, most frequently by α-amylase inhibitors. About 10% of baker's asthma is provoked by allergies to α- or β-gliadin[5]. Exercise-dependent wheat allergy is associated with ω-gliadin[6].

Gliadins are unusual proteins in that they are very rich in two amino acids, proline and glutamine, with about 30 to 40% of the protein mass of gliadin being composed of glutamine and 20 to 25% composed of proline. This makes gliadin difficult for mammals to digest because the digestive system's proteolytic enzymes do not cleave these bonds efficiently. It has been suggested that this was an adaptive survival mechanism for wheat and related species as it makes these grains undesirable as a staple food source. Wheat also contains α-amylase inhibitors that prevent wheat starch from being digested. Cooking denatures the enzyme α-amylase; allowing nutritive value from wheat starch.

Most dietary proteins (from milk, meat, beans or other grains) are cleaved into peptides chains no longer than ten amino acids long by proteolytic enteropeptidases. Gliadin, because of its high proline content, is more difficult to break up and is cleaved into a few dozen fragments, many of which are longer than ten amino acids in length. One 33-amino acid long fragment, the 33mer peptide (p57-89), is particularly associated with gluten disease[7]. The 33mer peptide fragment of gliadin has a high affinity to HLA-DQ2 and HLA-DQ8. This fragment, however, is not the only one that can elicit an inflammatory response. Some gliadin peptides, which are broken down by brush border exopeptidases in the glycocalyx of healthy individuals, escape digestion in individuals with damage to the enterocyte membrane[8]. (Endopeptidases and exopeptidases are described in Chapter 2).

To be susceptible to gluten disease, an individual needs to have antigen-presenting cells with an affinity for binding and presenting deaminated gliadin fragments to T-helper cells. Some gliadin fragments are taken up by endocytosis by the enterocytes lining the small intestines. The p31-43 fragment can prevent the restitution of enterocyte height and slow the activity of endosomes that are responsible for moving receptors and antibodies to the enterocyte basal cell surface membrane. This effect significantly delays endocytic activity by the enterocytes in persons with celiac disease and increases the accumulation of IgA and IL-15 and transferrin receptors on the enterocyte surface[9], and likely inhibits digestive enzyme recycling. This may in part explain the pancreatic exocrine deficiency that is common in CD. IL-15 prevents apoptosis of T-Cells and natural killer cells. In CD, IL-15 maintains hyperactivity of immune defenses and increases the number of intraepithelial lymphocytes in the intestinal mucosa. This may explain the high incidence of lymphoma associated with this disease[10].

Several gliadin protein fragments are toxic and immunogenic. The gliadin 19mer peptide appears to be toxic to all humans, regardless of HLA type; it induces numerous cytokines including TNF, INF-γ, IL23, IL27, IL12, and IL15. However, in patients with celiac disease, the increase of INF-γ is greater[11] than in other persons.

Induction of gluten disease syndrome likely results from the simultaneous actions of several gliadin fragments. Although at least two of the three fragments discussed above are toxic to individuals without genetic susceptibility to CD, the reaction to each of these three gluten fragments is more severe among those with CD.

Presentation of the Antigen

The third component required for initiating autoimmune disease is access of the antigen for presentation to the immune system. In health, under physiologic conditions, access of antigens to the gut-associated immune cells of the lamina propria is limited by competent intercellular tight junctions (TJ) that limit passage of macromolecules across the intestinal epithelial barrier.

Tight junctions bind the enterocytes together to form a continuous barrier throughout the intestine. Zonulin is a protein that participates in controlling the tight junction. In autoimmune disease, the mucosal barrier can be compromised by cholera toxin, campylobacter jejuni infection, chemotherapy, and by other agents. One of the several toxins from *Vibrio cholera* toxin acts by releasing zonulin and thus causing incompetence of the tight junctions. (Chapter 25 discusses the intestinal mucosa membrane and factors that affect it.)

In gluten disease, some gliadin protein fragments gain access to the lamina propria of the intestinal villus by passing between the enterocytes. While the zonulae adherens normally seal the space between cells, blocking the passage of molecules as large as these peptides, gluten peptides induce the enterocytes to produce zonulin, a protein that opens the channels between cells. It is not only gliadin peptides that can then enter, but also other molecules that would normally be excluded by the enterocyte barrier. This increases the changes of immune presentation of proteins from other foods and increases the risk of developing an immune response to these other proteins, as well. The breach in the epithelial barrier may also allow passage of bacterial toxins, and may increase the likelihood of bacterial translocation from the lumen of the intestine into the body.

During active gluten enteropathy (GE), there is a persistent elevation in the release of zonulin and a significant increase in intestinal permeability. Once gluten has been eliminated from the diet, zonulin levels decrease and the enterocyte barrier can return to normal. This may allow the autoimmune process to regress and allow healing of intestinal mucosal injury.

At least two, 20mer pepsin/trypsin-digested fragments of gliadin have been shown to bind to the chemokine receptor CXCR3 that triggers the release of zonulin from the tight junctions[12]. CXCR3 is expressed on the apex of the enterocytes, as well as on T_H1 and T_H17 cells[13], and it helps mediates inflammation. CXCR3 has been implicated not only in GE, but also in rheumatoid arthritis, multiple sclerosis, myasthenia gravis, Type 1 Diabetes, and other autoimmune diseases. Thus, gliadin fragments can impair the immune barrier, not only allowing passage of antigenic macromolecules, but additionally activating the T helper cells and encouraging inflammation through chemotactic activity. This effect of gluten is not restricted to individuals with genetic susceptibility to GE, and thus, gluten may be a risk factor for other autoimmune disorders.

When gliadin peptides are present and gain access to the lamina propria of the intestinal villus, certain gliadin fragments bind with tissue transglutaminase (TGM2). TGM2 is a multifunctional protein which plays a role in wound healing, apoptosis, and extracellular matrix development. One of its functions is the post-translational modification of proteins. Among other activities, TGM2 can deaminate glutamine residues in long gliadin peptides, thus, converting some glutamine molecules in proteins into glutamic acid. During this activity, some of the deaminated gliadin fragments form a covalent bond with TGM2. This TGM2-gliadin fragment complex is highly antigenic for individuals with HLA types DQ2.2, 2.5 and 8, and the immune system then easily forms antibodies to TGM2. It is these IgA and IgG anti-transglutaminase antibodies that are most useful for diagnosing *active* gluten enteropathy. TGM2 is recognized as a principal autoantigen in Celiac disease.

Another form of transglutaminase, epidermal transglutaminase (TGM3) is associated with dermatitis herpetiformis, another gliadin-related disease that is often present in patients with CD. TGM6 autoantibodies are associated with gluten ataxia[14] a disease of the cerebellum. TGM4 (prostate) or TGM7 (testes) gliadin fragment complexes may explain the decreased fertility often present in men with gluten disease.

Gluten Enteropathy: The Disease

Common morbidity in gluten enteropathy include:

- Abdominal pain, bloating, gas, or indigestion
- Constipation
- Poor appetite
- Diarrhea, either intermittent or constant
- Lactose intolerance (which resolves with elimination of gluten)
- Nausea and vomiting
- Steatorrhea (oily, foul-smelling stools that float)
- Unexplained weight loss (although people can be overweight or of normal weight)
- Growth retardation in children
- Osteoporosis

In gluten enteropathy, the villi of the intestine are damaged and flattened. This greatly decreases the absorptive surface area of the intestines. Additionally, there is a loss of pancreatic exocrine activity because of damage to enteroendocrine cells and loss of pancreatic exocrine output their activation (Chapter 8). Zymogens such as trypsin may not be activated if enteropeptidase from enterocytes is lost, and enzyme recycling is impaired[15]. Thus, malabsorption is a central feature of CD.

The mucosal damage, which characterizes gluten enteropathy, also causes a loss of intestinal brush border enzymes, such as disaccharidases (See Table 2-4). These enzymes are required for the digestion of sugars, such as lactose; thus, lactose intolerance is usually present during active GE disease. Sugar malabsorption can be associated with bloating and diarrhea, small intestinal bacterial overgrowth, and the formation of secondary bile acids; adding to GI pathology. Additionally, fats are often poorly absorbed.

In CD, the fat-soluble vitamins A, D, E, and K are lost because of fat malabsorption. Vitamin B_{12} is poorly absorbed. The loss of vitamin D and vitamin K absorption contribute to osteopenia and osteomalacia, especially in northern climates where insufficient sun exposure is available for formation of vitamin D. Vitamin A deficiency can cause night blindness. Vitamin E deficiency can cause infertility and peripheral neuropathy. Vitamin B_{12} deficiency can also cause peripheral neuropathy, and is associated with sleep disorders. Iron deficiency is also common, causing anemia. All of these are seen in CD.

Table 22-3: Nutritional Deficiencies Common in Malabsorption Syndromes, such as in Gluten Enteropathy

Malabsorption in Celiac Disease	Resulting Disease
Vitamin A	Impaired night vision.
Folate	Anemia; weakness; risk of vascular disease; cancer.
Vitamin B_{12}	Peripheral Neuropathy: tingling extremities, loss of sensation, anemia Sleep: loss of entrainment to the circadian cycle.
Vitamin D	Osteopenia: fractures Osteomalacia: bone pain Muscle weakness, impaired immunity, increased risk for cancer, diabetes.
Vitamin E	Peripheral neuropathy: tingling extremities, loss of sensation, muscle pain.
Vitamin K	Poor clotting, bruising, epistaxis, osteomalacia, osteoporosis, cancer.
Calcium	Osteopenia and osteomalacia
Iron	Anemia, growth retardation, fatigue, sleep disorders.
Fats	Weight loss, growth retardation.
Protein	Dysbiosis
Bile	Bile acid diarrhea (See Chapter 26)
Steroid Hormones	Loss and alteration of steroid hormones, altered fertility, menstrual problems, etc.

When osteopenia, osteomalacia or osteoporosis are found in men, the diagnosis of gluten enteropathy should be considered until proven otherwise[2]. The same approach should be taken with women. Lactose intolerance is common in GE secondary to the loss of brush border enzymes. This increases the risk of osteopenia, as milk, a major source of calcium and vitamin D in the Western diet, is usually avoided.

In gluten enteropathy, gliadin fragments cause proliferation and maintenance of intestinal intraepithelial leukocytes, with IL-15 preventing normal apoptosis and down-regulation of the immune response. This likely contributes to the high incidence of intestinal lymphoma in patients with CD. These intraepithelial leukocytes also may promote the early loss of enterocytes.

In CD, there is often a loss of IgA from the gut. This can impede the diagnosis of gluten disease as IgA antibodies are usually used to diagnose the disease. The lack of IgA can also impair the regulation of the mucosal immune system, and increase the risk of inflammation and bacterial overgrowth in the gut.

Gluten and Autoimmune Disease

Individuals with Gluten Disease are at high risk of autoimmune disease. Relatives without CD are also at elevated risk of autoimmune diseases. This suggests that gluten-related autoimmune disease occur without gluten enteropathy. For example, patients with multiple sclerosis[16] were found to be four times more likely, and those with Graves disease[17] to be five times as likely to have CD than others in their community.

Table 22-4: Celiac-Related Immune Diseases[2]

- Type 1 Diabetes
- Sjogren's Disease
- Rheumatoid Arthritis
- Cerebellar Ataxia
- Multiple Sclerosis[16]
- Peripheral Neuropathy
- Epilepsy
- Autoimmune Thyroid Disease
    - Hashimoto's Thyroiditis (hypothyroid)
    - Graves Disease (hyperthyroid)
- Idiopathic Dilated Cardiomyopathy
- Autoimmune Myocarditis
- Autoimmune Hepatitis
- Primary Sclerosing Cholangitis
- Primary Biliary Cirrhosis
- Alopecia
- Reproductive Disorders
- Addison's Disease
- Dermatitis Herpetiformis
- Lupus Erythematosus
- Vitiligo
- Sarcoidosis
- Infertility

Cerebellar ataxia and dermatitis herpetiformis are direct effects of antibodies to gliadin[14]. Both male and female infertility and endometriosis are more common among CD patients[18, 19, 20], with most studies indicating that infertile persons are two to three times more likely to have CD than fertile individuals.

Patients with the immune diseases listed in Table 22-4 should be evaluated for gluten disease. In a population screening of over 3000 school children only one about one-third (12 of 33) of those with biopsy-proven CD had celiac related symptoms[21], thus, lack of symptoms cannot be assumed equivalent to lack of CD and its related risks. Even if individuals do not meet the diagnostic criteria for CD, patients with a first-degree relative with CD, or HLA DQ2.5, DQ8, or DQ2.2 allele carriers may benefit from the removal of gluten from the diet. Gluten may increase the risk for autoimmune diseases due to the effects of the gluten 20mer fragment on CXCR3 and compromise of the GI epithelial tight junctions[3]. Dietary gluten may raise the risk of increased gastrointestinal intracellular permeability, increasing the risk of leaky gut syndrome (Chapter 25).

After the diagnosis of autoimmune thyroid disease, autoimmune liver disease, and type 1 diabetes associated with anti-gliadin antibodies, removal of gluten from the diet has often been found to have favorable outcomes with declines in the anti-tissue antibody levels, compared to those who continue to consume gluten[22]. The earlier the diagnosis is made, and earlier the antigens are removed, the more likely sufficient functional reserve of the affected organs will remain; thus allowing some ability for recovery.

Not all patients with these autoimmune conditions have gluten enteropathy; however, the immune reaction to gliadin peptides can trigger autoimmune disease. CD serves as a model for other autoimmune disease caused by food protein. Cow's milk protein, for example, has also been implicated in the development of type 1 diabetes (T1D) in children[23] and risk for T1D is associated with certain HLA DQ subtypes[24]. Breastfeeding followed by weaning with hydrolyzed cow's milk, where the proteins have been broken down to reduce antigenicity, has been found to decrease the risk of diabetes by about 50% in early trials among high-risk infants[4].

Removing gliadin, and other immune activators that injure the enteric mucosa, aids in healing the mucosa and normalizing enzymatic and absorptive function.

An MRI study of brain volume and intelligence in 290 Japanese school children was performed in association with data of the children's breakfast diet. Children who had a rice-based breakfast had an average I.Q. of 103.7, compared to those regularly eating wheat-based breakfasts that had an average I.Q of 99.9[25].

Dermatitis herpetiformis (DH) is a skin disease characterized by sporadic episodes of itchy, blistering dermatitis. It typically has its onset in young adulthood but may be seen in children and older persons. The rash usually affects the extensor surfaces: the elbows, knees, buttocks, and scalp. The itching usually begins about 12 hours before a new crop of blisters and lasts for about ten days, when the blisters begin to crust.

DH is caused by autoantibodies against epidermal transglutaminase (TGM3) in the skin, as a reaction to gliadin fragments. The treatment is avoiding gliadin. DH patients often have asymptomatic CD; DH is common in family members of patients with CD. Most patients with DH have antibodies to both TGM2 (tissue transglutaminase) and TGM3[26]. DH is often treated with Dapsone; however, this treatment does not prevent intestinal damage from gliadin. Patients with DH should be on a gluten-free diet.

Testing, Treatment and Secondary Prevention

Tests: IgA and IgG anti-transglutaminase antibodies are useful for diagnosing *active* gluten enteropathy; levels fall when gluten is successfully avoided. Serum citrulline is also useful to assess enterocyte mass and health (Chapter 2)[27]. Pancreatic exocrine function should also be tested.

Treatment: The essential treatment of gluten disease is a complete removal of gluten from the diet. Treatment should also include an evaluation of IgG for food antergies, (Chapter 19). If symptoms continue after gluten cessation, evaluation and treatment should be done for SIBO (Chapter 24), and for increased paracellular permeability (Chapter 25). Additionally, patients should be screened for osteoporosis and vitamin A, D, E, K and B_{12} deficiencies. Pancreatic enzyme supplements are often needed during recovery to help treat malabsorption (Chapter 8). Diarrhea may be caused by bile malabsorption, and treated as such (Chapter 26).

Gluten Avoidance: While not easy, avoiding gluten has become very much simpler in recent years. Gluten-free bread is available in health food stores as are gluten-free flour mixes, usually made of rice, tapioca, and other non-gluten sources. These are available in most large grocery stores. Pasta made from rice or beans are available at Asian food markets, and corn-based pasta is also available at larger grocery stores.

Hidden gluten needs to be eliminated, as well. Processed foods that contain hidden gluten include baked beans, dry roasted nuts, icing and frostings, licorice, salad dressings, self-basting poultry, soy sauce, thickeners, lattes, and cappuccinos. Processed foods can hide gluten, as they may be listed only as dextrin, or vinegar, which was made from wheat. Table 22-5, at the end of this chapter, gives a list of foods that may contain hidden gluten. Labels need to be read carefully to avoid gluten-containing products.

Dietary Cheating: How much cheating can a celiac patient do? None. Only tiny amounts of gliadin are needed to maintain the inflammatory state.

Even "gluten free foods" (as defined by the World Health Organization) can have up to 200 parts per million of gluten, and this can be enough to cause damage to the intestinal lining. For most patients, less than 50 mg a day should be safe[28]. This is equivalent to about one grain of wheat. This amount can easily be consumed on a wheat-free diet because of hidden wheat or contamination. Contamination can occur during food processing, transport or harvest. Wheat, barley or rye seed may grow in fields where oats are planted. Grain may be transported in a train car or stored in grain towers where other grains may have been transported or stored, and food may be processed in machinery that has been previously used for processing wheat. Oats can be contaminated with wheat, and thus should be avoided until the gluten disease becomes asymptomatic. Once asymptomatic, the small amount of contamination of oats by wheat in oatmeal or other oat products is usually insufficient to cause problems for the patient.

Lactose Intolerance: Since lactase is marginal in most adults, damage to the enterocyte membrane often manifests with lactose intolerance. Most patients with GE have lactose intolerance, which often improves with the elimination of gluten from the diet. In GE patients with lactose intolerant, lactose should be avoided until the patient has been off gluten long enough for symptoms of malabsorption to have abated. Recovery of lactose tolerance usually takes between 6 and 12 months[29]. Symptomatic patients with GE may recover more quickly if treated with pancreatic enzymes. Lactose intolerance can act as a sentinel symptom of a recurrence of intestinal damage.

Primary Prevention of Gluten Disease

About one-third of the U.S. population carries at least one copy of an HLA-DQ type that conveys a risk for CD. However, only about one percent of the population has the overt disease. Only about 40% of HLA-matched siblings of CD patients are diagnosed with the disease. This suggests that some risks for the disease may be avoided in those carrying the HLA-DQ 2.2, 2.5 and 8 subtypes. HLA type accounts for less than 50% of the risk of developing CD. Unfortunately, a considerable portion of the remaining risk may be caused by other genetic[30, 31], or epigenetic factors that are poorly amenable to intervention. This may also help explain why there are other diseases besides CD that are triggered by gliadin in the diet. CD may require exposure to gluten, genetic factors, plus environmental factors to trigger the disease. Individuals with only two of these three factors may be susceptible to various milder disease manifestations when exposed to gluten. Some known or suspected environmental risk factors may influence disease risk along with gluten include:

1. Early exposure of infants: (Epigenetic Impact) Early exposure of infants to gluten increases the risk of CD and Type 1 diabetes; delayed exposure also confers risk, albeit, lower risk. Introducing gluten (wheat, rye, and barley) and other foods, to the diet between 4 – 6 months of age imparts the least risk of CD and of other immune-mediated diseases. Children with HLA-associated risk for CD to whom wheat was introduced before four months of age were many times more likely to develop CD by the age of nine. Waiting until seven months also increased risk. Introducing oats, but not rice, before four months of age also increased the risk[32]. Chapter 11 provides recommendations for the introduction of foods to infants.

2. Breastfeeding: Breastfeeding for at least 6 months, with overlapping introduction foods including wheat, from 4 – 6 months of age decreases risk of CD. Similarly, introduction of milk at this age gives lower risk for type 1 diabetes.

3. Avoid Gluten during Gastroenteritis: Gluten should be avoided during, and for a couple of months following, diarrheal gastroenteritis, especially for children with family members with CD. Rotavirus, the most common cause of infectious gastroenteritis in children, shares antigenic recognition with the tissue transglutaminase-gliadin fragment[33]. Thus, when the body's immune system is fighting rotavirus, the T_H1 cells are activated and prone to promote immune reactivity against gliadin fragments and to promote anti-transglutaminase antibody formation. IL-15 and IL-12, which are increased in the presence of gliadin fragments, help preserve this immune memory and the inflammatory reaction. Avoidance of gluten during the aftermath of rotavirus infection may allow the immune response to normalize and avoid cross-reaction with gluten.

It is interesting to consider that of the wide array of possible HLA-DQ alleles, there are only about 360 alleles in modern man; with the number of alleles having declined over time. Peoples that did not consume wheat in pre-Columbian times have the highest incidence of HLA-DQ 2 and 8, with some populations having a 90%-prevalence. This, very likely, results from advantages conferred by these HLA subtypes. In many parts of the world, rotavirus gastroenteritis and the resulting dehydration remains a major cause of infant mortality. The HLA-DQ2 and DQ8 alleles may impart protection against this disease, and thus provide a selective advantage for survival from rotavirus gastroenteritis.

Rotavirus also affects adults. For those at risk of CD, gluten should be avoided during and for a couple of months following gastroenteritis. Even if the gastroenteritis is not rotavirus disease, small bowel mucosal damage may allow increased immune exposure to gliadin fragments that may induce an unwelcome immune response. *Toxoplasmosis gondii* infection increases immune sensitivity and anti-gluten antibodies formation, raising gluten related disease risk[34].

Recovery from Gluten Disease

Once the diagnosis of Gluten Enteropathy has been made, it is considered a lifetime diagnosis and there is a consensus that gluten needs to be excised from the diet for life.

However, if only a limited number of individuals with a genetic risk for CD develop it, why can't the inducing factors be removed? Perhaps they can.

Several studies have documented that some former CD patients can consume a diet including gluten without intestinal mucosal damage[35,36,37]. In these studies, about 15 percent of patients appear to tolerate gluten later in life. These patients are in remission; they have normal intestinal villi and normal absorption of nutrients. CD patients in remission are more likely to have been diagnosed and treated early in the course of the disease (during childhood) though genetics and other variables may also affect long-term recovery.

Most of the CD patients who become "asymptomatic" while on a diet containing gluten, however, just have milder, but ongoing disease, with a loss of bone mass (osteopenia), lactose intolerance, and flattening of the intestinal mucosa. Asymptomatic patients have elevated IgA anti-gliadin antibodies, while those in true remission do not. Thus, a person who recovers from CD on a gluten-free diet is better off strictly adhering to the diet. If, after several years, they return to consume gluten, they should be followed and tested for anti-transglutaminase and anti-gluten antibodies, even if asymptomatic. Gluten consumption should be discontinued if they have any associated symptoms or elevated antibodies or autoimmune disease. In these patients, elevated anti-gliadin or anti-transglutaminase antibodies should be seen as asymptomatic, active disease.

Lactose intolerance and other disaccharide sensitivities should be considered a symptom and a sign of active disease. GE patients often have severe lactose intolerance, which distinguishes them from the common form of lactose intolerance in adults. Most lactose intolerant adults can drink small amounts of milk, or eat small amounts of soft cheese without noticeable effect. Persons with severe lactose intolerance often report that even a small amount of milk in coffee will cause symptoms.

About half of first-degree relatives (parents, children, siblings) of CD patients exhibit features of gluten sensitivity[38]. If antibody tests are positive, indicating an immune response to gluten, it shows that these individuals are at risk for autoimmune disease and osteoporosis. This should be considered similar to "asymptomatic" gluten disease, and gluten should be eliminated from their diets.

Gluten Free Wheat Bread?

Some patients with gluten disease and some researchers have found that gliadin's immunogenicity can be mitigated by bacterial digestion during bread-making using sourdough culture. Specific lactobacilli[39] have been identified with proteolytic enzymes that degrade the 33mer peptide[40]. Trials using sourdough bread and other wheat products after treatment with these bacteria have shown good tolerance and lack of toxicity[41,42]. Sourdough fermentation can decrease the amount of intact gluten in wheat to 1/10,000 the amount present in baked goods as compared to those not processed by bacterial fermentation[43]. This digested gluten does not appear to induce toxicity or increase anti-TGM IgG in CD patients.

Gliadin is, however, not hydrolyzed by a single strain of bacterium, but rather by a pool of specific bacteria, and the process requires several hours of fermentation[44]. There is insufficient evidence to assume that all sourdough cultures, which vary according to local conditions, can render sourdough bread safe for gliadin-sensitive individuals. Even when a sourdough culture is taken from a known source to a new environment, climate, or if culture medium is fed with different flours the bacteria in the culture change. Thus, while some sourdough bread and other sourdough-processed wheat products may be safe for consumption with patients with gluten disease, other sourdough products may not be.

Although these bacteria may completely hydrolyze gliadin, other wheat proteins remain intact[45]. Thus, wheat allergy may not be diminished by the sourdough culture of the dough, depending on which protein the person reacts to. Additionally, individuals who do not tolerate bread may react to yeast, which is also highly immunogenic, and which is present in the sourdough bread.

Treatment Failure

It is not uncommon for patients with gluten enteropathy to continue to have diarrhea, bloating and abdominal pain after elimination of gluten from the diet. Bacterial dysbiosis is common in patients with celiac disease. Lactose intolerance may take several months to improve. SIBO is also common in CD patients[46], secondary to dysmotility, impaired pancreatic output, and other injury to the intestines. If abdominal symptoms continue after gluten elimination, the patient should be evaluated and treated if necessary, for SIBO, bile and sugar malabsorption (Chapters 24, 26 and 5). Pancreatic enzymes therapy is often beneficial. (Chapter 8).

Injury to the intestinal mucosa from CD exposes the enteric immune system to multiple antigens. The development of immune reaction to other foods is common in this disease. A range of symptoms may arise from immune reactions to other foods (Chapter 19); Most CD patients have multiple antergies. Testing and avoidance of reacting foods is appropriate in CD patients to speed recovery and treat secondary diseases.

Non-Celiac Gluten Disease

Gluten may increase the risk of disease even in individuals without HLA-DQ 2.2, 2.5 or 8. There are about 50 autoimmune diseases which are triggered by enteric antigens gaining access to the immune system through a compromised enteric barrier[3]. Gluten peptides can induce zonulin release and increase the risk for autoimmune disease.

Several case-control studies have shown symptomatic improvement in schizophrenic patients on gluten-free diets[47]. Patients with multi-episode schizophrenia are more than six times more likely than controls to have elevated IgG antibodies to gliadin[48]; however, in these patients, there does not appear to be an increase in HLA DQ2 or DQ8 prevalence, as there is with celiac disease. Additionally, rather than an association with α/β gliadin, in schizophrenia there appears to be an increased prevalence of antibodies to a 33 kilodalton γ-gliadin fragment[49]. An increased risk of elevated IgG tissue transglutaminase antibodies has also been found in bipolar disorder[50].

Gluten is particularly antigenic, in part because of the large post-digestive peptide fragments it creates, but also because of its effect on the enterocyte membrane and lymphoid tissue in the intestine. Gluten provokes an increase in immunogenicity; it decreases the number of T_{REG} cells[51] and increases the number of T_H17 cells in the Peyer's patches of the small intestine. Gluten also causes an increase in T_H17 cells in the pancreas that may explain its role in the causation of diabetes[52]. Gluten acts on the mucosal T-cell population, increasing the expression of proinflammatory cytokines IFN-γ, IL-17, and IL-2[53]. Thus, gluten helps potentiate enteroimmune disease. Gluten is not only a potent antigen, but also, potentiates enteroimmune reactions to other antigens.

Gluten, acting as an immune stimulator, is not required for the development of schizophrenia, bipolar disorder diabetes or other non-celiac diseases associated with gluten. Other antigens and agents, such as pathogens, which stimulate T_H17 cells in the Peyer's patches, can also increase the risk for T_H17 associated immune diseases. Gluten is not the only agent capable of this mischief. It, however, wreaks its effects efficiently and quietly, often recruiting immune response to benign dietary proteins.

Table 22-5: Food Ingredients that May Contain Gluten

Anti-caking agent (often found in spices)
Baking Powder
Binders
Caramel colorings or flavorings
Cereal fillers, protein or starch
Citric Acid
Coatings
Colorings
Corn Starch
Cyclodextrins
Dextrimaltoses
Dextrins
Dispersing Agents
Emulsifiers
Excipients (in prescription medications, for consistency)
Extracts and Flavorings (in grain alcohol)
Fillers
Flours made from wheat, barley, rye or oats
Grain alcohol (beer, ale, rye, scotch, bourbon, grain vodka)
Hydrolyzed plant protein
Hydrolyzed protein
Hydrolyzed vegetable protein
Malt, Malt Syrup or Flavoring
Maltodextrin
Modified starch, Modified food starch (made from wheat)
Mono- and di-glycerides (made using wheat starch carrier)
Natural flavorings
Oats (likely secondary to contamination with other grain)
Soy sauce (if fermented with wheat)
Starch (modified food starch, edible starch)
Starch glycolate

Textured vegetable protein
Vegetable gum
Vegetable protein or starch
Vinegars (white, or malt made from grain alcohol)
Vitamin E oil (made from Wheat Germ)
Wheat germ oil

[1] Prevalence of celiac disease in at-risk and not-at-risk groups in the United States: a large multicenter study. Fasano A, Berti I, Gerarduzzi T, et al. Arch Intern Med. 2003 Feb 10;163(3):286-92. PMID:12578508

[2] Celiac Disease. Murray, JA. PIER, American College of Physicians, June 2010.

[3] Tight junctions, intestinal permeability, and autoimmunity: celiac disease and type 1 diabetes paradigms. Visser J, Rozing J, Sapone A, Lammers K, Fasano A. Ann N Y Acad Sci. 2009 May;1165:195-205. PMID:19538307

[4] Early feeding and risk of type 1 diabetes: experiences from the Trial to Reduce Insulin-dependent diabetes mellitus in the Genetically at Risk (TRIGR). Knip M, Virtanen SM, Becker D, Dupré J, Krischer JP, Akerblom HK; for the TRIGR Study Group. Am J Clin Nutr. 2011 Jun 8. PMID:21653795

[5] Multiple wheat flour allergens and cross-reactive carbohydrate determinants bind IgE in baker's asthma. Sander I, Rozynek P, Rihs HP, et al. Allergy. 2011 May 10. PMID: 21557753

[6] Wheat dependent exercise induced anaphylaxis: is this an appropriate terminology? Wong GK, Huissoon AP, Goddard S, Collins DM, Krishna MT. J Clin Pathol. 2010 Sep;63(9):814-7. PMID:20696684

[7] Identification and analysis of multivalent proteolytically resistant peptides from gluten: implications for celiac sprue. Shan L, Qiao SW, Arentz-Hansen H, Molberg Ø, Gray GM, Sollid LM, Khosla C. J Proteome Res. 2005 Sep-Oct;4(5):1732-41.PMID: 16212427

[8] Alterations of the intestinal transport and processing of gliadin peptides in celiac disease. Matysiak-Budnik T, Candalh C, Dugave C, Namane A, Cellier C, Cerf-Bensussan N, Heyman M. Gastroenterology. 2003 Sep;125(3):696-707.PMID: 12949716

[9] Gliadin peptide P31-43 localises to endocytic vesicles and interferes with their maturation. Barone MV, Nanayakkara M, Paolella G, et al. PLoS One. 2010 Aug 18;5(8):e12246.PMID: 20805894

[10] IL-15 triggers an antiapoptotic pathway in human intraepithelial lymphocytes that is a potential new target in celiac disease-associated inflammation and lymphomagenesis. Malamut G, El Machhour R, Montcuquet N, et al. J Clin Invest. 2010 Jun 1;120(6):2131-43.. PMID: 20440074

[11] Is gliadin really safe for non-coeliac individuals? Production of interleukin 15 in biopsy culture from non-coeliac individuals challenged with gliadin peptides. Bernardo D, Garrote JA, Fernández-Salazar L, Riestra S, Arranz E. Gut. 2007 Jun;56(6):889-90. No abstract available. PMID: 17519496

[12] Gliadin induces an increase in intestinal permeability and zonulin release by binding to the chemokine receptor CXCR3. Lammers KM, Lu R, Brownley J, et al. Gastroenterology. 2008 Jul;135(1):194-204.e3. PMID:18485912

[13] CXCR3-dependent recruitment and CCR6-mediated positioning of Th-17 cells in the inflamed liver. Oo YH, Banz V, Kavanagh D, Liaskou E, Withers DR, Humphreys E, Reynolds GM, Lee-Turner L, Kalia N, Hubscher SG, Klenerman P, Eksteen B, Adams DH. J Hepatol. 2012 Nov;57(5):1044-51. PMID:22796894

[14] Gluten T cell epitope targeting by TG3 and TG6; implications for dermatitis herpetiformis and gluten ataxia. Stamnaes J, Dorum S, Fleckenstein B, Aeschlimann D, Sollid LM. Amino Acids. 2010 Nov;39(5):1183-91. PMID:20300788

[15] Conservation of digestive enzymes. Rothman S, Liebow C, Isenman L. Physiol Rev. 2002 Jan;82(1):1-18. PMID: 11773607

[16] Prevalence of celiac disease in multiple sclerosis. Rodrigo L, Hernández-Lahoz C, Fuentes D, Alvarez N, López-Vázquez A, González S. BMC Neurol. 2011 Mar 7;11:31. PMID:21385364

[17] Prospective screening for coeliac disease in patients with Graves' hyperthyroidism using anti-gliadin and tissue transglutaminase antibodies. Ch'ng CL, Biswas M, Benton A, Jones MK, Kingham JG. Clin Endocrinol (Oxf). 2005 Mar;62(3):303-6. PMID:15730411

[18] Serological testing for celiac disease in women with endometriosis. A pilot study. Aguiar FM, Melo SB, Galvão LC, Rosa-e-Silva JC, dos Reis RM, Ferriani RA. Clin Exp Obstet Gynecol. 2009;36(1):23-5. PMID:19400413

[19] Fertility disorder associated with celiac disease in males and females: fact or fiction? Khoshbaten M, Rostami Nejad M, et al. J Obstet Gynaecol Res. 2011 Oct;37(10):1308-12. PMID:21561528

[20] Primary infertility as a rare presentation of celiac disease. Rajput R, Chatterjee S. Fertil Steril. 2010 Dec;94(7):2771.e5-7. PMID:20537625

[21] Mass screening for coeliac disease using antihuman transglutaminase antibody assay. Tommasini A, Not T, Kiren V, et al. Arch Dis Child. 2004 Jun;89(6):512-5. PMID:15155392

[22] Celiac disease and autoimmune thyroid disease. Ch'ng CL, Jones MK, Kingham JG. Clin Med Res. 2007 Oct;5(3):184-92. Review.PMID: 18056028

[23] Enhanced levels of cow's milk antibodies in infancy in children who develop type 1 diabetes later in childhood. Luopajärvi K, Savilahti E, Virtanen SM, Ilonen J, Knip M, Akerblom HK, Vaarala O. Pediatr Diabetes. 2008 Oct;9(5):434-41. PMID:18503496

[24] T-cell reactivity to insulin peptide A1-12 in children with recently diagnosed type 1 diabetes or multiple beta-cell autoantibodies. Marttila J, Huttunen S, Vaarala O, et al. J Autoimmun. 2008 Sep;31(2):142-8. PMID:18565729

[25] Breakfast staple types affect brain gray matter volume and cognitive function in healthy children. Taki Y, Hashizume H, Sassa Y, Takeuchi H, Asano M, Asano K, Kawashima R. PLoS One. 2010 Dec 8;5(12):e15213. PMID:21170334

[26] Clinical, histological and immunopathological findings in 32 patients with dermatitis herpetiformis Duhring. Rose C, Bröcker EB, Zillikens D. J Dtsch Dermatol Ges. 2010 Apr;8(4):265-70, 265-71. Epub 2009 Oct 28. English, German. PMID: 19878401

[27] Citrulline as a biomarker of intestinal failure due to enterocyte mass reduction. Crenn P, Messing B, Cynober L. Clin Nutr. 2008 Jun;27(3):328-39. PMID:18440672

[28] Systematic review: tolerable amount of gluten for people with coeliac disease. Akobeng AK, Thomas AG. Aliment Pharmacol Ther. 2008 Jun 1;27(11):1044-52. Epub 2008 Feb 29. Review.PMID: 18315587

[29] Regression of lactose malabsorption in coeliac patients after receiving a gluten-free diet. Ojetti V, Gabrielli M, Migneco A, et al. Scand J Gastroenterol. 2008;43(2):174-7.PMID:17917999

[30] Evaluation of 6 candidate genes on chromosome 11q23 for coeliac disease susceptibility: a case control study. Brophy K, Ryan AW, Turner G, et al. BMC Med Genet. 2010 May 17;11:76.PMID:20478055

[31] Potential celiac patients: a model of celiac disease pathogenesis. Sperandeo MP, Tosco A, Izzo V, Tucci F, Troncone R, Auricchio R, Romanos J, Trynka G, Auricchio S, Jabri B, Greco L. PLoS One. 2011;6(7):e21281. PMID:21760890

[32] Risk of celiac disease autoimmunity and timing of gluten introduction in the diet of infants at increased risk of disease. Norris JM, Barriga K, Hoffenberg EJ, Taki I, Miao D, Haas JE, Emery LM, Sokol RJ, Erlich HA, Eisenbarth GS, Rewers M. JAMA. 2005 May 18;293(19):2343-51. PMID:15900004

[33] In celiac disease, a subset of autoantibodies against transglutaminase binds toll-like receptor 4 and induces activation of monocytes. Zanoni G, Navone R, Lunardi C, et al. PLoS Med. 2006 Sep;3(9):e358.PMID: 16984219

[34] Anti-gluten immune response following Toxoplasma gondii infection in mice. Severance EG, Kannan G, Gressitt KL, Xiao J, Alaedini A, Pletnikov MV, Yolken RH. PLoS One. 2012;7(11):e50991. PMID:23209841

[35] Long-term study of patients with coeliac disease in childhood and adolescence: latent and transient coeliac disease. Limbach A, Hoepffner W, Tannapfel A, Müller DM, Mothes T, Richter T. Klin Padiatr. 2003 Mar-Apr;215(2):76-81. German. PMID: 12677547

[36] Long-term follow-up of 61 coeliac patients diagnosed in childhood: evolution toward latency is possible on a normal diet. Matysiak-Budnik T, Malamut G, de Serre NP, et al. Gut. 2007 Oct;56(10):1379-86. PMID: 17303598

[37] Gluten tolerance in adult patients with celiac disease 20 years after diagnosis? Hopman EG, von Blomberg ME, Batstra MR, et al. Eur J Gastroenterol Hepatol. 2008 May;20(5):423-9.PMID: 18403944

[38] The natural history of gluten sensitivity: report of two new celiac disease patients resulting from a long-term follow-up of nonatrophic, first-degree relatives. Niveloni S, Pedreira S, Sugai E, et al. Am J Gastroenterol. 2000 Feb;95(2):463-8.PMID: 10685751

[39] Proteolysis by sourdough lactic acid bacteria: effects on wheat flour protein fractions and gliadin peptides involved in human cereal intolerance. Di Cagno R, De Angelis M, Lavermicocca P, De Vincenzi M, Giovannini C, Faccia M, Gobbetti M. Appl Environ Microbiol. 2002 Feb;68(2):623-33. PMID:11823200

[40] Mechanism of degradation of immunogenic gluten epitopes from Triticum turgidum L. var. durum by sourdough lactobacilli and fungal proteases. De Angelis M, Cassone A, Rizzello CG, et al. Appl Environ Microbiol. 2010 Jan;76(2):508-18. PMID:19948868

[41] Gluten-free sourdough wheat baked goods appear safe for young celiac patients: a pilot study. Di Cagno R, Barbato M, Di Camillo C, Rizzello CG, De Angelis M, Giuliani G, De Vincenzi M, Gobbetti M, Cucchiara S. J Pediatr Gastroenterol Nutr. 2010 Dec;51(6):777-83. PMID:20975578

[42] Sourdough bread made from wheat and nontoxic flours and started with selected lactobacilli is tolerated in celiac sprue patients. Di Cagno R, De Angelis M, Auricchio S, et al. Appl Environ Microbiol. 2004 Feb;70(2):1088-96. PMID:14766592

[43] Safety for patients with celiac disease of baked goods made of wheat flour hydrolyzed during food processing. Greco L, Gobbetti M, Auricchio R et al. Clin Gastroenterol Hepatol. 2011 Jan;9(1):24-9. PMID:20951830

[44] Functionality of lactic acid bacteria peptidase activities in the hydrolysis of gliadin-like fragments. Gerez CL, Font de Valdez G, Rollán GC. Lett Appl Microbiol. 2008 Nov;47(5):427-32. PMID:19146533

[45] Highly efficient gluten degradation by lactobacilli and fungal proteases during food processing: new perspectives for celiac disease. Rizzello CG, De Angelis M, Di Cagno R, et al. Appl Environ Microbiol. 2007 Jul;73(14):4499-507. PMID:17513580

[46] High prevalence of small intestinal bacterial overgrowth in celiac patients with persistence of gastrointestinal symptoms after gluten withdrawal. Tursi A, Brandimarte G, Giorgetti G. Am J Gastroenterol. 2003 Apr;98(4):839-43. PMID:12738465

[47] The gluten connection: the association between schizophrenia and celiac disease. Kalaydjian AE, Eaton W, Cascella N, Fasano A. Acta Psychiatr Scand. 2006 Feb;113(2):82-90. PMID:16423158

[48] Markers of gluten sensitivity and celiac disease in recent-onset psychosis and multi-episode schizophrenia. Dickerson F, Stallings C, Origoni A, et al. Biol Psychiatry. 2010 Jul 1;68(1):100-4. PMID:20471632

[49] Novel immune response to gluten in individuals with schizophrenia. Samaroo D, Dickerson F, Kasarda DD, Green PH, Briani C, Yolken RH, Alaedini A. Schizophr Res. 2010 May;118(1-3):248-55. PMID:19748229

[50] Markers of gluten sensitivity and celiac disease in bipolar disorder. Dickerson F, Stallings C, Origoni A, Vaughan C, Khushalani S, Alaedini A, Yolken R. Bipolar Disord. 2011 Feb;13(1):52-8. PMID:21320252

[51] Dietary gluten reduces the number of intestinal regulatory T cells in mice. Ejsing-Duun M, Josephsen J, Aasted B, Buschard K, Hansen AK. Scand J Immunol. 2008 Jun;67(6):553-9. PMID:18476878

[52] Impact of dietary gluten on regulatory T cells and Th17 cells in BALB/c mice. Antvorskov JC, Fundova P, Buschard K, Funda DP. PLoS One. 2012;7(3):e33315. PMID:22428018

[53] Dietary gluten alters the balance of proinflammatory and anti-inflammatory cytokines in T cells of BALB/c mice. Antvorskov JC, Fundova P, Buschard K, Funda DP. Immunology. 2012 Aug 22. PMID:22913724

23. Biofilms and Dysbiosis

Many bacteria are dimorphic; they can develop into two distinct phenotypic forms: a plankton form or a colony form. In the plankton form, they are drifters or swimmers. Many have flagella that act like miniscule propellers that allow them to quickly, but aimlessly, move about through fluids. If they are in a nutrient-rich environment, they wander around like children on summer vacation. They can divide into two daughter cells which swim off aimlessly. They eat, swim, multiply and get eaten.

Under the right stimulus and environmental conditions, these solitary bacteria change their form and settle down, becoming sessile (immobile), form colonies and get to work doing the adult business of bacteria: chemical processing.

Dimorphic bacteria species generate hormone-like signals for *quorum sensing* (QS), which tell other related bacteria "I'm here." When the signal strength is high enough in the bacteria's environment, it signals them to transcribe a different set of proteins, and they transition from the plankton form to the sessile, colony building form of a biofilm.

Under sufficient quorum sensing stimulus, the bacteria lose the flagella used for swimming and form pili and fimbriae. The pili are tiny hair-like appendages which allow the bacteria to link to each other and even to exchange genetic information. This is one way in which drug resistance is transferred between bacteria. The fimbriae are even smaller and shorter projections that can cover much of the surface of the bacteria, and allow them to adhere to surfaces. In the colony form, the bacteria also produce and excrete an extracellular polymeric matrix, which becomes a housing for the colony[1]. A biofilm is a bit similar to coral reefs made up of millions of individual polyps. Biofilms can form slime layers on ponds, calcify and foul pipes, and cover the bottom of ships, creating a substrate for barnacle growth.

When bacteria form biofilms as a result of QS, they not only change form and build colonies, QS also induces the formation of many other proteins. Many of these proteins are enzymes that allow the bacteria to digest a wider mix of nutrients. Biofilms are essential for waste water treatment in sewage treatment plants. They form in the sand and gravel beds used for water filtration and remove nutrients and pollutants.

Sessile bacteria in a biofilm have an array of capabilities not present in their plankton form. Although the same DNA is present, they express different proteins including enzymes that give them new capabilities, allowing some species to produce toxins or other virulence factors. There are also differences in their metabolism; how they get their nutrients, and how they spend their energy. The sessile bacteria can also influence bacteria from other species and even yeast to join the colony and add their chemical processes to the biofilm's prowess.

Once a biofilm is well established, it may produce a dispersion factor. This increases the production of planktic bacteria, and thus spread the bacteria to other areas[2].

Macrophages can easily phagocytize single bacterium but are less adept at engulfing and destroying bacteria in a biofilm. When in a biofilm, the pathogen *Pseudomonas aeruginosa* produces a protein that blocks the oxidative burst of neutrophils – preventing the WBC's ability to kill the bacteria[3]. This is a QS-dependent mechanism that planktic bacteria do not have.

Sessile bacteria in biofilms are also better at protecting themselves from antibiotics. The concentration of an antibiotic required to kill bacteria in a biofilm may be many times higher than for the same bacteria when in its planktic form[4]. There are several reasons for this:

- The high population of bacteria gives opportunity for chance mutation to evade the antibiotic.
- To get rid of toxic substances and waste products, bacteria have efficient efflux pumps. These pumps also can provide multidrug resistance[5]. Sessile bacteria dedicate much more energy to these pumps and thus are more efficient at ridding themselves of toxins including antibiotics.
- Bacteria within the colony can exchange genetic information, including plasmids for antibiotic resistance. Plasmids are an extra bit of DNA that can be transferred between bacteria, which can carry genes that provide resistance to antibiotics or for forming proteins that can act as toxins or virulence factors.
- Antibiotics are usually selected in a lab by testing their ability to inhibit growth or kill bacteria while in their planktic form, in which it is usually more susceptible.
- Antibiotics are selected on their ability to stop bacterial growth in a culture; these may not include some virulent bacteria which do not grow in culture, but which participate in the disease pathology.

When a sample is taken from an infection, the bacteria culture that grows represents only some of the bacterial species which were present in the infection, and may not include some important pathogens. Antibiotic therapy against the culturable bacteria may or may not prevent the growth of the biofilm colony.

A recent lesson from genomics is that we have often looked for and treated the wrong bacteria. *E. coli* is a predominant bacterium found in fecally contaminated water; however, it typically represents a minor bacterial population in the intestine. However, it is easy to culture. Most bacteria that reside in the colon are very difficult to culture and at presents can only be identified by their rRNA[6].

Many bacteria that thrive in mixed bacterial biofilms are not culturable. There are about 1000 species of bacteria that are common residents of the human colon, and upwards of 40,000 bacterial species that are capable of commensal habitation in the colon[7]. Most people have a minimum of about 160 different species living in their large intestine[8], many of which are difficult to culture, and some have never been grown in laboratory cultures. They have only been recently identified through bacterial RNA analysis and genomic sequencing. Biofilms causing disease are also likely to contain bacteria that are not easily cultured.

Biofilms were first to be identified as human pathogens associated with devices and implants. Urinary catheters, heart valves, IV catheters, orthopedic implants and endotracheal tubes are surfaces that support the growth and development of biofilms. These biofilm infections are very resistant to antibiotics, and removal of the device is usually required for resolution of the infections. Hospital infections thrive on these devices. The cells lining the bladder, blood vessels, and trachea are resistant to bacterial adhesion, and thus, to biofilm or colony formation.

Most of the bacteria in the mouth grow in matrix-enclosed biofilms on the surface of teeth and surrounding tissue surfaces. The common name for dental biofilm is dental plaque, which is a matrix for *Streptococcus mutans*. In this biofilm, the bacteria produce acids that dissolve the enamel of the teeth, forming dental carries. Periodontitis is another oral biofilm infection which is difficult to treat with antibiotics[9].

In recent years, chronic, non-device related infections have also proven to be biofilm infections. Pneumonia in individuals with cystic fibrosis, chronic middle-ear infections, chronic sinus infections, biliary tract infections, and osteomyelitis are usually biofilm infections[1]. It has become clear that planktic bacterial infections that require treatment by physicians are the exception and a large majority of bacterial infections that cause disease are biofilm infections. At least 80% of chronic infections are biofilm-associated infections[10].

Chronic rhinosinusitis and chronic ear infections are common diseases caused by biofilms. These infections are notoriously difficult to eradicate with antibiotics both when treating single organism or mixed flora biofilms. Antibiotics are relatively ineffective for eradicating biofilm infections, and require considerably higher antibiotic concentrations, compared to those effective for the killing planktic bacteria.

Biofilms preferentially develop on inert surfaces, such as medical devices or dead or damaged tissue; however, they can also form on living tissues[1]. Mucosal surfaces are adapted to prevent adherence by biofilm-forming bacteria. However, when the surface is damaged or disrupted, bacteria can gain a foothold, allow biofilm formation. Electron microscopy of mucosal tissue from patients with rhinosinusitis reveals biofilm formation with denudation of cilia and loss goblet cells while all control subjects had healthy-appearing cilia and goblet cells without biofilms[11,12].

Controlling inflammation and protecting mucosal cilia may impede the attachment and aggregation of bacteria that support biofilm formation[13]. Bacteria, such as entero-aggregative *Escherichia coli*, uropathogenic *E. coli*, and *Shigella flexnerie* secrete a serine protease that is a virulence factor. It degrades mucin so that the bacteria can more easily attack the cells[14].

Antigens released from sessile bacteria in biofilms stimulate the production of antibodies, but these antibodies are often not effective at targeting and assisting WBCs to kill bacteria effectively within biofilms. Instead, these antibodies may form immune complexes that damage surrounding or distant tissues. Biofilm infections are rarely resolved by the host even in individuals with intact cellular and humoral immune function[1]. Physical disruption, surfactants, and probiotics are sometimes helpful in the treatment of these infections[15]. Often, the tissue supporting the biofilm needs to be removed to clear the infection.

Dysbiosis

Dysbiosis refers to colonization of the intestine by bacteria that create a disease response. Bacteria growing in biofilms on surfaces lining the gastrointestinal mucosa differ from those living in the intestinal lumen; there is a reduction in protective mucosal organisms, such as *Bifidobacteria*, and a shift to more pathogenic species[16]. Some diseases that have been implicated in intestinal dysbiosis include:

- Irritable Bowel Syndrome[17]
- Crohn's disease and Ulcerative colitis[18]
- Obesity and Metabolic Syndrome[19]
- Allergies[20]
- Autism[21]
- Schizophrenia[22]
- Gluten enteropathy[23]
- Acne vulgaris[24]
- Chronic prostatitis[25]

Intestinal dysbiosis can cause intestinal paracellular hyper-permeability[26]; thus, this list of diseases is similar to those seen in "leaky gut syndrome" (Chapter 25).

Lipopolysaccharides

Dysbiosis and quorum sensing induces the production of bacterial toxins including lipopolysaccharides (LPS)[27]. These large lipid-polysaccharide molecules are important structural components of the outer membrane of gram-negative bacteria that helps protect bacteria from attack.

The lipid end anchors LPS into the bacterial membrane. This lipid, Lipid A, is toxic. When bacteria are killed in large numbers by immune cells, when Lipid A is released into the circulation it causes fever. At higher concentrations, it can cause diarrhea, vasodilation, capillary leaking, depletion of coagulation factors and fatal, endotoxic septic shock.

The polysaccharide in LPS, referred to as the O antigen, has considerable variation in its glycans, even among strains of the same species. The O chains are antigenic, and the target of specific antibodies.

LPS damages the mitochondrial DNA, inhibits mitochondrial reproduction and complex 1 oxidative phosphorylation[28]. It stimulates the production of quinolinic acid, which is an NMDA agonist that may provoke intestinal dysmotility and visceral pain. LPS is a Toll-Like receptor agonist (TLR4); thus, the body creates an inflammatory response to it. Lipid A invokes its inflammatory reaction via TLR4. LPS provokes CNS inflammation that participates in causing schizophrenia and other neurologic diseases. LPS stimulates the production and release of the inflammatory cytokines including TNF-α and IL1β.

Tumor Necrosis Factor-α

TNF-α is potent proinflammatory cytokine which is produced by immune cells including lymphoid lineage (monocytes and macrophages), B cells, mast cells, and dendritic cells. TNF-α can also be produced by most of the cells in the body, including neuronal support cells and endothelial cells, but usually at a lower amount than produced in inflammatory cells. LPS is a potent stimulator of TNF-α transcription. IL-1β also stimulates TNF-α production.

TNF-α acts in concert with IL-1β and IL-6 to stimulate the release of CRH, and thus, ACTH and cortisol. TNF-α induces fever and can decrease appetite. It also increases insulin and leptin resistance, and thus can be a contributory factor to type 2 diabetes and to obesity.

TNF-α is a chemoattractant and promotes the expression of adhesion molecules on endothelial cells in the blood vessels which help white blood cells migrate to areas of inflammation. TNF-α stimulates phagocytosis by macrophages and the production of PGE$_2$ and C-reactive protein.

TNF-α plays a central role in many inflammatory diseases. Prolonged low-level exposure can result in cachexia in patients with cancer, COPD, HIV, multiple sclerosis, sarcoidosis, schizophrenia and other diseases. In cachexia, there is a loss of muscle mass and weakness resulting from exposure to multiple cytokines including TNF-α. TNF-α also acts as a signaling molecule for the activation of NF-κB and MAPK, and thus can trigger apoptosis.

Table 23-1: Factors that Induce TNF-α*

Factor	Chapter
HCA, PAH (Overheated meats)	6, 40
High-fat diet	9
High fructose diet	9
Elevated uric acid levels	9
Bacterial Lipopolysaccharides (LPS)	23
Lipoteichoic acid	42
Viral, parasitic and fungal TLR-2 agonists	42
IL-1β	23
T17 Helper cells	23
Inadequate vitamin B$_{12}$ levels	30
Chronic sympathetic stimulation	31
Opiates	31
Glycoalkaloids (Potatoes)	33
Dihydrotestosterone	36
Substance P	36
Sleep deprivation	41

* Factors that mitigate TNF-α are listed in Table 31-1

LPS increases intracellular permeability[29] in the intestine and promotes the translocation of bacteria and their toxins into the body. LPS, TNF-α, and thrombin stimulate their respective receptors on endothelial cells, and this initiates signaling that increases cytosolic calcium. The increase in intracellular calcium activates myosin light chain kinase (MLCK) and RhoA, disrupting endothelial tight junctions[30]. Thus, LPS toxins from the GI tract bacteria promote increased permeability in other tissues including the blood-brain barrier and placenta.

In gluten enteropathy, there appears to be an interaction with sessile bacteria promoting the loss of goblet cells that normally produce mucin that protects the intestine from bacterial adherence, intracellular infection, and exposure to antigens[23]. Some toxic lectins can over-stimulate and exhaust the capacity of goblet cells to synthesize mucin[31]. Wheat and peanut lectins can bind to goblet cells in the human small intestinal mucosa[32].

RegIIIγ is a lectin produced by intestinal epithelial cells that binds to bacterial peptidoglycan carbohydrates, but unlike most mammalian microbe-binding C-type lectins, RegIIIγ does not recruit complement proteins and thus does not damage the bacteria[33]. Rather, this protein helps maintain commensal bacteria, by preventing them from forming biofilms. It may also prevent bacteria from adhering to each other, and exchanging information. RegIIIγ prevents gram-positive bacteria, such as *Clostridia*, from adhering to colonocytes, and helps maintain the 50 μm mucous barrier that physically separates the mucosa from bacteria[34].

Chronic exposure to alcohol downregulates the production of another endogenous lectin, Carbohydrate-Binding Protein Domain (CLEC). CLEC binds to bacteria in the intestines; By inhibiting CLEC chronic alcohol exposure promotes enteric dysbiosis[35].

Stressed lab animal have an increase in bacterial translocation across the colonic mucosa. However, if the animals are exercised for 30 minutes prior to the stress event, they have an increased in antimicrobial intestinal proteins produced by the colonocytes; including RegIIIγ and α-defensin[36]. Strenuous exercise also increases the production of sIgA in the intestine[37], which similarly, however much more specifically, binds to targeted bacteria, preventing them from forming biofilms or transmigrating across the mucosa and cause immune activation or infection. Psychological and other stress, increases the risk of adherence of bacteria to the intestinal epithelia, and thus, for forming biofilms and for bacterial transmigration. Vigorous exercise lowers this risk.

In another stress of study, 70% of lab animals that were subjected to stress had transmigration of bacteria into mesenteric lymph nodes while none of the animals pretreated with probiotics for seven days did[38]. In another study, animals were subjected to intestinal ischemia/reperfusion injury. These animals suffered disruption of the mucosa, with erosions, dysbiosis, and an increase in inflammatory cytokines in the plasma. Over 85% of the animals had translocation of bacteria to tissues outside of the intestines. Animals that were pretreated the with the probiotic bacteria, *Lactobacillus plantarum*, however, were completely protected from the bacterial translocation, had lower inflammatory cytokine levels and their intestinal epithelial recovered from the injury[39].

In a murine model of bowel inflammation, induced by *Toxoplasmosis gondii* infection, treatment with phenolic compounds reduced bacterial translocation to the kidney, liver, spleen, and blood and decreased inflammation. Treatment increased survival from zero to 20% using curcumin and to 40% for those animals receiving resveratrol. This treatment increased the proliferation and regeneration of enterocytes and T_{Reg} cells in the mucosa compared to untreated animals, and was accompanied by a shift in the microbial population of colon; favoring lactobacilli and bifidobacteria, with fewer enterobacteria and enterococci. Animals treated with resveratrol and curcumin had higher levels of the anti-inflammatory cytokine IL-10 in the lymph nodes and lower level of pro-inflammatory cytokines in the ileum[40]. These phenolic compounds are known to decrease the activation of TLR4, and decrease inflammatory activation by TNF-α.

Antibiotics play a central and life-saving role in the treatment of infections. However, their power is limited and poorly targeted. In the colon, antibiotics typically kill the most easily vulnerable planktic, commensal microbia; often leaving sessile, resistant, highly pathogenic bacteria. If the probability of bacteria developing resistance to an antibiotic is one in 10 billion bacteria, consider that the colon typically houses 100 trillion bacteria, ten thousand times more. With the high density of bacteria found in the colon, if dysfunctional, multiple QS molecules can be present in high concentration and many bacteria may be in the sessile form. The facility of biofilm to resist antibiotics also decreases the chance of antibiotic treatment success for the elimination of pathogenic bacteria from the gut. Further, many of the pathogens of concern that reside in the colon form spores which survive antibiotics and can repopulate the colon later, when the antibiotic treatment has ended[41].

Rifaximin is an antibiotic that is not systemically absorbed and is used to treat dysbiosis. Rifaximin can be very helpful in the treatment of irritable bowel syndrome with diarrhea, and has the advantage that it can work again when symptoms recur within a few weeks[42]. The problem is that dysbiosis quickly recurs. Vancomycin therapy is sometimes briefly useful in the treatment of regressive autism but only gives temporary relief[41]. Even with massive antibiotic therapy that wipes out most intestinal bacteria, the biome rebuilds itself within a few months[43]. Recall from Chapter 4 that the bacteria that thrive in the colon are those which are best adapted to the environment and the nutrient source provided for them. If the underlying habitat and nutrient mix do not change, microbial population tends to rebuild a similar community after treatment.

Defeating Biofilms
Quorum Sensing Inhibitors

It is the sessile phenotype of the microbiota that causes disease conditions. In this form, the bacteria and yeast produce toxins and virulence agents which impair the enterocyte or colonocyte barrier. For example, *Salmonella* is dependent upon other non-salmonella bacteria for quorum sensing agents that shift it to the sessile phenotype in which it become pathogenic. If the quorum sensing agents can be mitigated, bacteria behave differently.

Blocking quorum sensing is a much more desirable treatment than is killing bacteria with antibiotics. When antibiotics are used, more resistant, and perhaps more virulent, bacteria rebound. With quorum sensing inhibition, there is no Darwinian pressure to select more resistant organisms. Even when antibiotics are used, they are likely to be much more successful in the presence of quorum sensing inhibitors (QSI) as potentially pathogenic bacteria are in the planktic, non-pathogenic form.

In gram-negative bacteria, most quorum sensing systems use N-Acyl-homoserine lactones (AHL) as signal molecules. When there is sufficient signal strength, these bacteria shift from the planktic to the sessile form. Cyclic diguanylate signaling is another mechanism for stimulating biofilm formation and stimulating virulence for some bacteria including many *Clostridia* and *Vibrio* species[44].

Using a chemical structure database and virtual screening of thousands of drugs and natural compounds, 147 compounds were identified as potential QSI candidates. This subset of molecules was further modeled for three-dimensional fit to the Quorum Sensing Receptor of the *Pseudomonas aeruginosa* bacteria. The researchers sought a safe and available chemical compound that would block quorum sensing, like a key that fit perfectly into a lock, but would not turn it, but at the same time blocks the real key. They found six candidate compounds to test: three of these drugs were found to give significant inhibition of quorum sensing regulated gene expression and prevented biofilm formation in a dose-dependent manner. One of these three was salicylic acid[45]. Salicylic acid (SA) is mostly used as an anti-acne medication. SA has been assumed to act as a keratolytic agent; however, it may act as a QSI that decreases the expression of inflammatory products of sessile bacteria in the sebaceous glands.

Perhaps not coincidentally, the macrolide antibiotic erythromycin is also used for acne vulgaris. Here, its action has not been attributed to its antibiotic effect, but rather that it acted as a drying agent. A better explanation may be erythromycin's effect on decreasing the synthesis of the quorum signaling agent AHL[46]. This may explain how low-dose erythromycin, below an effective antibiotic dose, has been used for years as a chronic medication in the treatment of cystic fibrosis to prevent *Pseudomonal* lung infection[47]. Here, it is not acting as an antibiotic (to which bacteria would quickly become resistant) but rather as an anti-quorum sensing agent. Of several antibiotics tested for anti-quorum effects against *Pseudomonas aeruginosa*, the macrolide azithromycin was the most effective[48].

Mesalamine (5 – aminosalicylic acid, Rowasa), used in the treatment of inflammatory bowel disease, likely acts as a QSI after being metabolized to salicylic acid. Although mesalamine has been assumed to act as a cyclooxygenase inhibitor and to inhibit prostaglandin synthesis, 5-aminosalicylic acid may act as a quorum sensing inhibitor.

Salicylic acid is derived from willow trees. Willows usually grow in swampy or wet soils where gram-negative anaerobic bacteria flourish and form biofilms. Salicylic acid likely prevents root rot by preventing biofilm formation on the roots and bark of this tree, which lives in wet and frequently flooded areas. When the tree is injured, it increases the production of salicylic acid. This trick has worked for millions of years. It does not kill the soil bacteria, which would just be replaced by different, possibly more aggressive bacteria. Instead, it convinces the bacteria that they are in too low a density to form a biofilm. Bacteria need a critical mass to work effectively. Quorum sensing inhibitors convince the bacteria that their population is too low to get the job done, and so they remain in planktic form.

Salicylic acid is also known as 2-hydroxybenzoic acid. It is a phenolic compound. Hydroxybenzoic acids are a subclass of phenolic acid polyphenols. Although 2-hydroxybenzoic acid is not common in food, there are at least 29 other hydroxybenzoic acid phenolic compounds present in commonly consumed foods. (See Chapter 15). Polyphenols in foods are usually thought to provide benefit as antioxidants, but their primary adaptive purpose for the plant is likely to keep roots and seeds from rotting in the soil, and preventing fruit from rotting. In fruit, such as grapes, phenolic compounds are concentrated in the skin; here they act as a barrier to bacterial invasion.

Other polyphenols, especially phenolic acid polyphenols, may also affect quorum sensing. Some polyphenols have been demonstrated to reduce biofilm development using other mechanisms. Ellagic acid (EA) and tannic acid (TA) are plant polyphenols. When added to liquid culture medium, EA and TA had no effect on the growth of planktic *Escherichia coli*. However, when added in combination to a biofilm culture, these two polyphenols reduced biofilm formation of *E. coli* by about 80%. These agents impair the function of efflux pump in these bacteria[49]. Ellagic acid and salicylic acid are both hydroxybenzoic acids, both increase AMPK activity, and thereby prevent the cell (reproductive) cycle.

Tannic acid is found in oak and sumac leaves and bark but is uncommon in foods. Other tannins, (gallic acid polymers and flavone polymers) however, are present in some foods and beverages. Green and black teas and acorns are high in tannins. Chestnuts, walnuts, raspberries, blackberries and pomegranate juice are high in ellagic acid. Flavonols from cocoa and phenolics from tea have been found to increase *Lactobacillus* and *Bifidobacterium* while significantly repressing the growth of *Clostridium* species[50].

Hydroxycinnamic acids, such as caffeoylquinic and dicaffeoylquinic acids and its metabolites[51], may also be useful as QSI agents. Not only do these polyphenols impair biofilm production, they would also be expected to prevent multidrug resistance and allow for biofilm bacteria to be susceptible to treatment at a much lower concentration of antibiotics.

Prebiotic and Probiotics

Prebiotics, such as resistant carbohydrates and dietary fiber stimulate the growth of those bacteria that feed upon them. Probiotics are supplements containing the live bacteria themselves. Prebiotics usually support the growth of non-pathogenic bacteria in the colon.

In an animal model, inulin-type fructans stimulated the growth of mucosa-associated bifidobacteria and inhibited pathogenic *Salmonella enterica* biofilm[52]. Inulin-type fructans induce beneficial changes in the intestinal mucosa, including taller villi, deeper crypts, an increased number of goblet cells, and thicker mucus layer on the colonic epithelium; all which help protect the intestinal mucosa from biofilm formation[53]. Prebiotics support a beneficial microbiota by utilizing amino acids, and thus depriving pathogenic species of this fuel source, and preventing the formation of ammonia, indolamines and bioactive amines which are produced from these amino acids. A healthy commensal intestinal biome supports intestinal health and prevents injury, biofilm formation, and transmigration of bacteria across the mucosal barrier. In times of stress, prebiotics prevent the formation of inflammatory cytokines.

Carbohydrates and polyphenolic compounds that cannot be digested but are instead fermented in the colon, provide health benefits by promoting the growth of beneficial commensal organisms, and are known as prebiotics (Chapter 4). Food nutrients that are unabsorbed and promote the growth of pathogens, the development of pathogenic biofilms, and production of toxins might be dubbed "dysbiotics."

Protein Malabsorption

Clostridia, as well as some other pathogenic bacterial biofilms, thrive in a colonic environment in which there is an ample supply of proteins and amino acids. This may be due to direct utilization of the amino acids by these bacteria or as the result of production of ammonia and other metabolites of protein fermentation. Ammonia and other toxic metabolites damage the mucus layer that protects the colonocytes, thus allowing the pathogens to adhere to the epithelial membrane and form biofilms. Protein malabsorption, can thus, provide for the development of pathogenic biofilms in the colon, increase paracellular permeability, and favor translocation of bacteria across the mucosal membrane.

Supplements of pancreatic enzymes may prevent the formation of dysbiosis and biofilm formation in individuals with protein malabsorption secondary to pancreatic enzyme deficiencies. These enzymes aid in the digestion of proteins into small peptides. These peptides can then be further digested by dipeptidases on the enterocyte brush border so that the amino acids are absorbed. Pancreatic enzymes also have direct antimicrobial properties which help prevent small intestinal bacterial overgrowth (SIBO).

Damage to the enterocyte membrane from gluten, other toxins, infections, or other diseases may reduce the availability of dipeptidases and may also decrease the absorption of peptides and amino acids. Damage to the enterocytes in the small intestine can thus provoke malabsorption of proteins, peptides, and amino acids. This favors the formation of pathogenic biofilms. Treatment is approached by reversing the underlying cause.

Non-Toxic Dietary Lectins

Many nontoxic dietary lectins bind to glycoproteins on bacteria, and thus, may neutralize them in an effect similar to that of RegIIIγ and CLEC. These lectins bind to bacteria may prevent adherence of bacteria to enterocytes and help prevent biofilm formation. Table 23-2 lists some foods containing non-toxic lectins that bind bacteria. Over 500 plant lectins have been described; some of these are listed Table 7-4.

Table 23-2: Some Nontoxic Food Lectins that Bind Bacteria[54, 55]

Banana	Green Peas
Cantaloupe	Lettuce
Carrots	Sunflower Seeds
Coconut	Tomato
Cucumber	

Pathogenic vs. Commensal Microbia

Dividing microbes into pathogenic or non-pathogenic is an artificial construct. In planktic form, most anaerobic bacteria and *Candida* are innocuous and may act as commensal inhabitants of the intestine. Meanwhile, *Lactobacilli* and *bifidobacteria,* often used as probiotics, and beneficial in the gut can cause sepsis and endocarditis if present in the blood stream. Most infectious processes are polymicrobial and involve biofilm formation. The beneficial influence of *lactobacilli* and *bifidobacteria* is largely that they help modify the intestinal environment to prevent biofilm formation[56]. Most deadly hospital infections arise from commensal species from the intestine, and while often selected for bacterial resistance, these usually are no more virulent than biofilms of wild strains.

Treatment of Dysbiosis

1. Antibiotics: Specific antibiotics, such as Rifaximin or Vancomycin, have a role in the treatment of dysbiosis, but they should not be used as a sole therapy. As monotherapy, they usually only provide temporary relief. By using these agents in conjunction with other therapy for dysbiosis, there is a greater opportunity to change the make-up of the intestinal biome and to repair the underlying damage that promoted the disease state.

2. Probiotics: Probiotics, the introduction of helpful bacteria, may be helpful especially during and after the use of antibiotics, whether the antibiotics are used for treating dysbiosis or for systemic infections. Probiotics usually do not make a long-term impact on the intestinal microbiota. It is like sprinkling vegetable seeds in an abandoned lot; things may grow, but don't expect a large harvest. As explained in Chapter 4, taking a probiotic supplement with a quarter teaspoon of sodium bicarbonate as an antacid and fasting for an hour, may help increase the survival of bacteria in the supplement.

3. Prebiotics: Gut bacteria ferment sugars and proteins that arrive in the colon. The microbiota of the intestine acts like a population of weeds and wildflowers in a field. They can be plowed under, but the same species usually grow back. The weeds that thrive depend on the habitat and the nutrients available to them. The wider the diversity of plant materials in the diet, the more diverse the colonic biome will be. This lowers the risk of dominance by any species, lowering the risk of pathologic biofilm and LPS formation.

Protein, peptides, and amino acids which arrive in the cecum and colon undergo fermentation, especially in the descending colon, and are fodder for dysbiotic microbiota, often with increased *Clostridia* species and toxin production. Lactulose, a non-absorbed disaccharide prebiotic, alters the bacterial dominance and decreases the amount of ammonia and toxin produced, providing therapeutic benefit. Different fiber and other non-absorbed nutrients from the diet affect which commensal bacteria thrive.

3. Treat Protein Malabsorption: The Western diet is high in protein, and this may exceed the body's ability to digest it and absorb it as amino acids in the small intestine. Protein digestion may be impaired digestive dysfunction or lack of pancreatic or other enzymes. Damage to the small intestinal mucosa can cause the loss of dipeptides, preventing the absorption of amino acids.

Sugar malabsorption, or other conditions that decrease oral-cecal transit time, can cause dumping of unabsorbed nutrients, including proteins, into the large intestine before they have time to be absorbed. (See Chapter 24 on SIBO). Digestive problems should be addressed.

Some foods contain trypsin inhibitors that prevent protein digestion and absorption, and thus promote the growth of dysbiotic bacteria and the production of toxins[57]. Many trypsin inhibitors also inhibit chymotrypsin. Potatoes and other foods with antitrypsin/ anti-chymotrypsin activity can prevent the digestion of protein and promote biofilm formation in the colon. Protease inhibitors can be found in soy, sunflower, barley, rice[58], lima beans and potatoes, and other legumes and grains[59].

These inhibitors are proteins, many of which are denatured either by fermentation or cooking at 100°C (boiling), but are not denatured at 70°C[60], and blanching only partially inactivates these proteins[61]. Many soy-containing foods are fermented, and this usually inactivates these proteins. Potato trypsin inhibitors are heat stable and not inactivated by boiling[62]. Melons, peanuts, sunflower seeds, papaya, and tomato are often eaten raw. In fruits, the content of these anti-nutritive proteins usually declines with ripening.

Table 23-3: Plant Foods that Contain Trypsin/ Chymotrypsin Inhibitors[63]

Group	Food Plants
Squash	Squash, Pumpkins, Melons (cantaloupe), Bitter melon
Grains	Wheat, Barley
Legumes	Soy, Peanut, many others
Solanum	Potatoes, Tomato
Others	Papaya, Sunflower, Buckwheat, Sweet Potatoes, Taro, Mustard, Cabbage, Collard, Turnip Greens, Rape (canola)

Pancreatic insufficiency also prevents nutrients from being digested and absorbed. Lab test for fecal pancreatic elasetase-1 or chymotrypsin can be used to evaluate pancreatic function and to test whether adequate pancreatic enzymes are present. Fecal chymotrypsin is often low in patients with autism and Parkinson's syndrome (Chapter 35.) Individuals with pancreatic enzyme deficiency should prepare foods containing chymotrypsin inhibitors in ways that denature these proteins or avoid these foods.

Pancreatic enzyme supplements can be helpful for individuals with dysbiosis and biofilm-associated diseases, especially those with insufficient pancreatic enzyme activity. Necrotizing enterocolitis is a *Clostridia* induced biofilm disease that, at least in animals, is associated with impaired pancreatic enzyme activity[64]. Pseudomembranous colitis may also respond to pancreatic enzymes and other means to reduce protein fermentation and *Clostridia* biofilm growth in the colon.

5. Sugar Malabsorption: Simple sugars that are not absorbed in the small intestine, as a result of lactose intolerance or fructose malabsorption, as examples, reach the colon and affect the bacterial population. They can also cause a decrease intestinal transit time for the chyme that also contains other nutrients, thus also impairing protein and fat absorption. Sugars that cause symptoms due to malabsorption should be avoided. (Chapter 4),

6. Quorum Sensing Inhibitors: Certain foods contain QS inhibitors. Several studies have shown that garlic blocks QS[65, 66, 67]. Fruits, vegetables, herbs, and spices contain phenolic compounds, some of which may act as QSI agents[68] or impair bacterial efflux pumps. Certain non-toxic plant lactones may also impair biofilm formation[69]. Plant lactones are found in fruits, such as peaches and berries.

Chicken Soup: Chicken soup, traditionally used for infectious respiratory infections, inhibits neutrophil chemotaxis[70], and some of its components may act as QSI. Table 23-4 lists some foods that have shown QSI activity against at least some bacteria.

Table 23-4: Foods with QSI Activity [71 72]

Contain hydroxy benzoic acids See Table 15-5	Basil, Carrot, Oregano, Rosemary, Thyme, Blueberry, Cinnamon Strawberry
Crucifers (Iberin may be active agent)	Horseradish, Cauliflower, Cabbage, Broccoli, Garden Cress, Watercress Radish
Others	Bean Sprouts, Chamomile, Habanero, Chervil, Turmeric, Garlic, Lemongrass, Parmesan cheese, Vanilla, Water lily, Yellow Pepper

The next generation of anti-bacterial medications will likely target biofilm formation and virulence factors. These medications will be designed not to kill bacteria as this creates evolutionary pressure to evolve resistance mechanisms. Instead, these drugs will be designed to inhibit biofilm formation and the production of virulence factors[73].

These drugs may be modeled after natural biofilm-inhibiting compounds that have evolved over millions of years to protect plants from damage by biofilm infections; these include polyphenols and lactones.

A wide variety of fruits, vegetables, spices and whole grains should be eaten to ensure sufficient intake of various polyphenols. Different polyphenols may act on different anti-biofilm mechanisms and for biofilm communities housing different populations of bacteria. Refined and processed foods, which make up much of the western diet, have little available polyphenol or lactone content.

The phenolic compound chlorogenic acid (3-O-caffeoylquinic acid), which is present in large quantities in green coffee and plums, has been found to be associated with weight loss, which has been attributed to a decrease in glucose uptake from the intestines[74]. Other factors, such as QSI activity and alteration of the microbial biome of the intestine, including a reduction of inflammatory mediators which affecting appetite, offer a more compelling explanations for this weight loss.

Certain bacteria are thought to feed on QS agents, such as AHL, utilizing it as a source of nitrogen. Thus, these bacteria can lower the QS and inhibit biofilm formation. Probiotics should be selected which behave in this manner. Prebiotics may act by supporting the growth of bacteria that feed on QS agents. Low dose azithromycin may be useful as QSI for certain bacteria[75].

7. Bacterial Binding: IgA acts by binding bacteria and preventing pathogens from forming biofilms. Avoiding foods that an individual has become sensitized to will allow the gastrointestinal immune system to rededicate its IgA production to bacterial pathogens. Test for IgG (and IgE if allergic symptoms are present) to foods and avoid the reactive ones.

Lectins are carbohydrate binding proteins that adhere to specific sugars functional groups on large molecules. Lectins can bind to these sugars on bacteria, and block them from adhering to surfaces, thus preventing biofilm formation. RegIIIγ and CLELC are endogenous lectins. Several foods (Table 23-2) also contain lectins that prevent biofilm formation. Especially useful are those that are consumed raw. These lectins may also help prevent dental carries since many lectins bind to *Streptococcus mutans*, one of the bacteria responsible for dental caries[76].

Biofilms usually only form after bacteria bind to a surface, such as a foreign body or damaged mucosa or endothelium. Moreover, bacteria, bacterial toxins, and viruses bind also bind to sugar residues on cell membranes as a means for entering target cells through endocytosis.

Dietary glycosphingolipids (GSL's) also contain sugar residues that bacteria, bacterial toxins, and viruses also adhere to. These GSL's prevent the absorption of toxins such as cholera and botulism toxins, and the endocytosis of some viruses. Dietary glycosphingolipids prevent bacteria, such as *E. coli* and *Pseudomonas aeruginosa*, from adhering to colonocytes. GSL's in mother's milk may protect infants from enteric pathogens[77]. Additionally, GSL's inhibit the formation of aberrant crypts in the intestine[78] and may prevent colon cancer. There are hundreds of different GSL's in nature; however, almost all of the diversity is found outside of the animal kingdom. The food sources with the highest amounts of GSL's include dairy, eggs, soy, fish and meat, sweet potatoes, rice, millet, and spinach. Those from various plant sources provide a wider array of GSL's likely to adhere to a wide array of bacteria.

8. Exercise: RegIIIγ is an endogenous lectin that prevents biofilm formation and supports a healthy biome. Vigorous exercise increases both RegIIIγ and sIgA. Thirty minutes of vigorous exercise three times a week should increase the production of bacterial binding by RegIIIγ and sIgA.

9. Avoid Stress: Stress increases the transmigration of bacteria across the intestinal mucosa, demonstrating that it impairs immune defenses in the intestine, through multiple mechanisms; increased CRH, decreased bacterial binding by RegIIIγ and sIgA, decreased production of α and β defensins, and increased sympathetic tone, for example. Stress and its treatment are discussed in Chapter 29.

10. Control TNF-α: TNF-α is a potent proinflammatory cytokine present in many disease conditions. LPS and IL-1β both stimulate TNF-α production. LPS can be mitigated by preventing dysbiosis and biofilm production. IL-1β can be mitigated by preventing inflammation; getting sufficient sleep (see Chapter 41) and avoiding chronic stress (see Chapter 29). Diets high in fructose also increase the production of TNF-α and thus fructose consumption should be limited to less than ten percent of caloric intake (see Chapter 9).

TNF-α production can be suppressed with the phosphodiesterase-inhibiting medication pentoxifylline[79] (Trental). Phosphodiesterase inhibitors also inhibit leukotriene production and thus have anti-inflammatory effects. Like pentoxifylline, caffeine is a xanthine compound and a phosphodiesterase inhibitor[80]. Theobromine from chocolate may also inhibit phosphodiesterase activity.

Uric acid is also a xanthine compound. Both low serum uric acid levels[81,82] and high levels of serum uric acid[83] have been found to be associated with high levels of TNF-α. Caffeine acts as a nonselective, competitive inhibitor of the phosphodiesterase enzymes. If other xanthines act upon TNF-α formation as does uric acid, then additive levels of caffeine with other xanthine phosphodiesterase inhibitors may increase TNF-α production patients with elevated uric acid levels, and thus act as proinflammatory agents. Hyperuricemia should be treated. (See Chapter 9).

The phenolic compound quercetin and the vitaminer E, δ-tocotrienol, have both been found to inhibit the expression of multiple LPS-induced pro-inflammatory and pro-aging cytokines, including IL-1β, IL-6, and TNF-α and the enzyme COX2[84]. Dietary flavonoids help speed the recovery from symptoms associated with LPS and decreased levels of inflammatory cytokines, and of MDA, a marker of oxidative stress[85]. Several flavonoids from various plant foods have been found to inhibit the formation of TNF-α[86]. Table 15-4 in Chapter 15 lists several foods high in flavonoids.

11. Colonic Inoculation: A currently experimental, but effective treatment for pseudomembranous colitis, a life-threatening disease, is a fecal transplant. In this procedure, healthy person's mix of commensal colonic organisms is introduced into the colon of to a person with a pseudomembranous colitis, a disease caused by pathogenic colonic biofilm with clostridia.

Colonic inoculation, which may be accompanied by antibiotics, holds the potential for treatment of other colonic biofilm-associated diseases, including multiple sclerosis (Chapter 32) autism Chapter 35, obesity (Chapter 9), recurrent colon cancer, schizophrenia depression, OCD, and other neurologic and systemic diseases.

Summary

Patients with low fecal pancreatic elastase-1 or low fecal chymotrypsin levels should avoid protease inhibitors in foods and use pancreatic enzyme supplements to prevent excess passage of proteins into the colon. Loss of goblet cell function and production of mucin to protect the mucosa of the intestine can lead to biofilm formation.

Some phenolic compounds in foods are QSI. Polyphenols that are too large to be absorbed may provide their beneficial effects by inhibiting biofilm formation in the intestine. Lactones from fruits and berries may also inhibit biofilm formation. Non-toxic lectins that bind bacteria may decrease biofilm formation. GSL's from various sources including both plant and animal sources help prevent biofilm formation, infection and the uptake of toxins from the colon. Avoid production of LPS and TNF-α through consumption of foods high in dietary flavonoids and tocotrienol forms of vitamin E and by avoiding dysbiosis and hyperuricemia.

Pseudomembranous Colitis

Pseudomembranous colitis (PC) is an opportunistic infectious disease, caused by the spore-forming gram-positive rod, toxin-producing bacteria, *Clostridium difficile*. This is a common and difficult to treat infection. Half a million Americans get this disease each year; about 15,000 die from it. Patients often respond poorly to antibiotics and often relapse when antibiotics are withdrawn. PC is a biofilm disease that takes hold after the use of antibiotics that kill much of the commensal biome of the colon. As a spore-forming bacterium, clostridium not only recovers quickly; it also inhibits the growth of other bacteria.

It is not just caused by antibiotics. Most patients subject to this disease are elderly, inactive, and have an intestinal environment fertile and adapted for this disease. Colonic inoculation is an important treatment advance for PC, however, altering the intestinal environment can prevent this disease, and preventive methods can be used alongside other treatments to defeat it.

1. *C difficile* depend on amino acids or protein in the descending colon for nutrition. In healthy individuals, there is very little protein here. Prevent flourishing of *C difficile* by limiting the availability of the substrate that this bacteria thrives on.

- Limit protein to an appropriate level. The World Health Organization promulgates a daily intake of 0.45 grams of protein per kilogram (0.204 grams per pound) ideal body weight as the minimum daily protein intake required for maintaining nitrogen balance[87].
- Use pancreatic enzyme supplements to aid in protein digestion and absorption. The stool can be tested to see if the patient is producing inadequate enzymes by testing fecal chymotrypsin levels or fecal elastase-1 levels.
- Avoid potatoes as they contain an antitrypsin protein that impairs protein digestion. Other trypsin inhibitors should also be avoided; however, most other trypsin inhibitors found in foods are inactivated by cooking. See Table 23-3.
- Avoid lactose (milk) and limit fructose intake if there is malabsorption of these sugars: sugar malabsorption decreases oral-cecal transit time and delivers undigested nutrients, including protein, to the colon. If lactose is included in the diet lactase enzyme supplement can be used.
- Avoid proton pump inhibitors; stomach acid helps denature protein and aids in its digestion. A safer treatment for gastro-esophageal acid reflux (GERD) is provided in Chapter 40.
- Assure there is adequate fiber in the diet to support a diverse commensal bacterial population. Prebiotics may be helpful, as may be lactulose, to maintain the growth of non-toxin forming bacteria.
- Probiotics may be helpful. Fecal transplants have a high cure rate but as of this writing, in 2015, the FDA has put the brakes on this treatment.
- A diverse diet containing non-toxic lectins and glycosphingolipids helps prevent biofilm formation, by binding to bacteria and preventing biofilm formation. Exercise increases sIgA and RegIIIγ, which act similarly.
- Dietary phenolic compounds decrease the growth of *Clostridia*, likely by preventing biofilm formation in the colon as quorum sensing inhibitors, and additionally decrease TNF-α.
- Dietary polyamines (Table 10-13) and certain inulin-type fructans (table 4-4) in foods support the healthy growth of intestinal mucosa.
- Make sure that the patient has adequate levels of vitamins D_3, K_2, B_{12}, and folate. These are typically low in malabsorption syndromes.

The bland, mechanically soft diet, often found in hospitals and nursing homes is unlikely to these dietary elements, or to provide them with sufficient diversity to help form a balanced, healthy, commensal colonic biome. Even worse is parenteral nutrition. Just fasting allows an increase in bacterial transmigration from the gut into the bloodstream. Many of the most deadly hospital infections, including *Klebsiella* and *Pseudomonas* are caused by commensal bacteria transmigration from the intestine into the bloodstream. Total parenteral nutrition, fasting or diets that fail to impede biofilm formation can thus cause disease and death in debilitated patients.

> Enteroimmunopathy and Infectious Disease:
>
> Chronic opportunistic infectious diseases can take hold in individuals with impaired T_H1 immunity secondary to enteroimmune disease dominated by TH17 immune activation. Several of these are listed in Table 10-4 in Chapter 10. For example, *Mycobacterium avium* complex (MAC) is an infection more likely to occur and progress in individuals with HIV, with chronic lung disease and patients with enteroimmunopathies that redeploy the immune system.
>
> MAC is an intracellular pathogen; the body depends on T_H1 cells for immune response. In enteroimmunopathies, inflammatory cytokines promote and sustain the dominance of T_H17 T cell lineages at the expense of T_H1 and T_H2 activity. Rheumatoid arthritis[88] and Crohn's disease are risk factors for MAC. Crohn's disease is also a risk factor for chronic Ebstein Barr and *Stenotrophomonas maltophilia* infections[89]. Treatment of MAC should include treatment of the underlying immune imbalance as these patients are at increased risk for disease progression[90] and development of drug resistance.
>
> MAC infection is in part protected against by non-specific immunity. Mannose-binding lectin (MBL), a protein produced by the liver, can activate the complement system and destroy certain pathogens including *Mycobacterium*.
>
> A treatment approach for opportunistic infection in patients with enteroimmunopathy includes the following steps along with appropriate an antibiotic regimen:
>
> 1. The inclusion of a Quorum Sensing Inhibitor: For MAC this would usually be azithromycin. Natural QSI, such as phenolic compounds, especially those that are small enough to be systemically absorbed, should be included in the diet.
>
> 2. Testing for and elimination of IgG food antergens, as described in Chapter 19. Food and environmental allergens should also be eliminated where possible.
>
> 3. Treat intestinal dysbiosis; including the use of prebiotics and pancreatic enzymes if fecal chymotrypsin or pancreatic elastase-1 levels are found to be low.
>
> 4. Enhancement of MBL production. Growth hormone and thyroid hormone (T_3) increase production of MBL in the liver. These are circadian hormones released during the first part of sleep. Thus, maintenance of normal circadian sleep and meal cycles should be encouraged. Slow-release melatonin, 3 to 5 mg, should be given just before bedtime. Sleep and circadian cycles are discussed in Chapter 43. If the patient requires thyroid supplementation, liothyronine sodium (Cytomel; T3) should be given, using physiologic doses only, at bedtime so that its peaks follows the normal circadian cycle peaking around midnight. Thyroxine (T_4) is best taken in the morning, and should be taken on an empty stomach, and not with supplements, as these can alter its absorption.
>
> 5. Vitamins A and D inhibit MAC growth[91]. Zinc (10 mg a day) can be used to help convert β-carotene into active forms of vitamin A with less risk of toxicity than from using retinol. (See Chapter 37 and 40). Vitamin D should be supplemented to maintain a serum level of 125 nmol/L of 25OHD3.

[1] Biofilms: microbes and disease. Aparna MS, Yadav S. Braz J Infect Dis. 2008 Dec;12(6):526-30. PMID:19287843

[2] A fatty acid messenger is responsible for inducing dispersion in microbial biofilms. Davies DG, Marques CN. J Bacteriol. 2009 Mar;191(5):1393-403. Epub 2008 Dec 12. PMID:19074399

[3] Identity and effects of quorum-sensing inhibitors produced by Penicillium species. Rasmussen TB, Skindersoe ME, Bjarnsholt T, et al. Microbiology. 2005 May;151(Pt 5):1325-40. PMID:15870443

[4] Type IV pili and the CcpA protein are needed for maximal biofilm formation by the gram-positive anaerobic pathogen Clostridium perfringens. Varga JJ, Therit B, Melville SB. Infect Immun. 2008 Nov;76(11):4944-51. PMID:18765726

[5] Clinically relevant chromosomally encoded multidrug resistance efflux pumps in bacteria. Piddock LJ. Clin Microbiol Rev. 2006 Apr;19(2):382-402. PMID:16614254

[6] Molecular monitoring of the intestinal flora by denaturing high performance liquid chromatography. Goldenberg O, Herrmann S, Marjoram G, Noyer-Weidner M, Hong G, Bereswill S, Göbel UB. J Microbiol Methods. 2007 Jan;68(1):94-105. PMID:16904779

[7] Gastrointestinal microbiology enters the metagenomics era. Frank DN, Pace NR. Curr Opin Gastroenterol. 2008 Jan;24(1):4-10. PMID:18043225

[8] A human gut microbial gene catalogue established by metagenomic sequencing. Qin J, Li R, Raes J, et al; MetaHIT Consortium, Bork P, Ehrlich SD, Wang J. Nature. 2010 Mar 4;464(7285):59-65. PMID: 20203603

[9] Periodontitis: an archetypical biofilm disease. Schaudinn C, Gorur A, Keller D, Sedghizadeh PP, Costerton JW. J Am Dent Assoc. 2009 Aug;140(8):978-86. PMID:19654249

[10] Pneumococcal biofilms. Moscoso M, García E, López R. Int Microbiol. 2009 Jun;12(2):77-85. PMID:19784927

[11] Bacterial biofilms in surgical specimens of patients with chronic rhinosinusitis. Sanclement JA, Webster P, Thomas J, Ramadan HH. Laryngoscope. 2005 Apr;115(4):578-82. PMID:15805862

[12] Chronic rhinosinusitis and biofilms. Ramadan HH, Sanclement JA, Thomas JG. Otolaryngol Head Neck Surg. 2005 Mar;132(3):414-7. PMID:15746854

[13] Biofilms in chronic rhinosinusitis. Suh JD, Cohen NA, Palmer JN. Curr Opin Otolaryngol Head Neck Surg. 2010 Feb;18(1):27-31. PMID:19940770

[14] The serine protease motif of Pic mediates a dose-dependent mucolytic activity after binding to sugar constituents of the mucin substrate. Gutiérrez-Jiménez J, Arciniega I, Navarro-García F. Microb Pathog. 2008 Aug;45(2):115-23. PMID:18538533

[15] Eradicating chronic ear, nose, and throat infections: a systematically conducted literature review of advances in biofilm treatment. Smith A, Buchinsky FJ, Post JC. Otolaryngol Head Neck Surg. 2011 Mar;144(3):338-47. PMID:21493193

[16] Mucosal biofilm communities in the human intestinal tract. Macfarlane S, Bahrami B, Macfarlane GT. Adv Appl Microbiol. 2011;75:111-43. PMID:21807247

[17] Gastrointestinal microbiota in irritable bowel syndrome: present state and perspectives. Salonen A, de Vos WM, Palva A. Microbiology. 2010 Nov;156(Pt 11):3205-15. PMID:20705664

[18] The bowel microbiota and inflammatory bowel diseases. Tannock GW. Int J Inflam. 2010 Aug 5;2010:954051. PMID:21188223

[19] Role of gut microflora in the development of obesity and insulin resistance following high-fat diet feeding. Cani PD, Delzenne NM, Amar J, Burcelin R. Pathol Biol (Paris). 2008 Jul;56(5):305-9. Epub 2008 Jan 30. PMID:18178333

[20] Probiotics: use in allergic disorders: a Nutrition, Allergy, Mucosal Immunology, and Intestinal Microbiota (NAMI) Research Group Report. Isolauri E, Salminen S; Nutrition, Allergy, Mucosal Immunology, and Intestinal Microbiota (NAMI) Research Group Report. J Clin Gastroenterol. 2008 Jul;42 Suppl 2:S91-6. PMID:18542035

[21] Differences between the gut microflora of children with autistic spectrum disorders and that of healthy children. Parracho HM, Bingham MO, Gibson GR, McCartney AL. J Med Microbiol. 2005 Oct;54(Pt 10):987-91. PMID:16157555

[22] Increased urinary excretion of a 3-(3-hydroxyphenyl)-3-hydroxypropionic acid (HPHPA), an abnormal phenylalanine metabolite of Clostridia spp. in the gastrointestinal tract, in urine samples from patients with autism and schizophrenia. Shaw W. Nutr Neurosci. 2010 Jun;13(3):135-43. PMID:20423563

[23] Role of intestinal bacteria in gliadin-induced changes in intestinal mucosa: study in germ-free rats. Cinova J, De Palma G, Stepankova R, Kofronova O, Kverka M, Sanz Y, Tuckova L. PLoS One. 2011 Jan 13;6(1):e16169. PMID:21249146

[24] Acne vulgaris, probiotics and the gut-brain-skin axis - back to the future? Bowe WP, Logan AC. Gut Pathog. 2011 Jan 31;3(1):1. PMID:21281494

[25] Chronic prostatitis and small intestinal bacterial overgrowth: effect of rifaximin. Weinstock LB, Geng B, Brandes SB. Can J Urol. 2011 Aug;18(4):5826-30. PMID:21854715

[26] Changes in gut microbiota control inflammation in obese mice through a mechanism involving GLP-2-driven improvement of gut permeability. Cani PD, Possemiers S, Van de Wiele T, et al. Gut. 2009 Aug;58(8):1091-103. PMID:19240062

[27] Quorum sensing affects biofilm formation through lipopolysaccharide synthesis in Klebsiella pneumoniae. De Araujo C, Balestrino D, Roth L, Charbonnel N, Forestier C. Res Microbiol. 2010 Sep;161(7):595-603. PMID:20600864

[28] Lipopolysaccharide-induced mitochondrial DNA depletion. Choumar A, Tarhuni A, Lettéron P, et al. Antioxid Redox Signal. 2011 Dec 1;15(11):2837-54. PMID:21767162

[29] Paracellular permeability is increased by basal lipopolysaccharide in a primary culture of colonic epithelial cells; an effect prevented by an activator of Toll-like receptor-2. Hanson PJ, Moran AP, Butler K. Innate Immun. 2011;17(3):269-82. PMID:20472611

[30] Regulation of endothelial junctional permeability. Vandenbroucke E, Mehta D, Minshall R, Malik AB. Ann N Y Acad Sci. 2008 Mar;1123:134-45. PMID:18375586

[31] Biological Effects of Plant Lectins on the Gastrointestinal Tract:Metabolic Consequences and Applications. Pusztai, A., Bardocz, S. Trends. Glycosci. Glycotechnol. 8:149-165

[32] Characterization of glycoconjugates of human gastrointestinal mucosa by lectins. I. Histochemical distribution of lectin binding sites in normal alimentary tract as well as in benign and

malignant gastric neoplasms. Fischer J, Klein PJ, Vierbuchen M, Skutta B, Uhlenbruck G, Fischer R. J Histochem Cytochem. 1984 Jul;32(7):681-9. PMID:6330198

[33] Symbiotic bacteria direct expression of an intestinal bactericidal lectin. Cash HL, Whitham CV, Behrendt CL, Hooper LV. Science. 2006 Aug 25;313(5790):1126-30. PMID:16931762

[34] The antibacterial lectin RegIIIgamma promotes the spatial segregation of microbiota and host in the intestine. Vaishnava S, Yamamoto M, Severson KM, Ruhn KA, Yu X, Koren O, Ley R, Wakeland EK, Hooper LV. Science. 2011 Oct 14;334(6053):255-8. PMID:21998396

[35] Enteric dysbiosis associated with a mouse model of alcoholic liver disease. Yan AW, Fouts DE, Brandl J, et al. Hepatology. 2011 Jan;53(1):96-105. PMID:21254165

[36] The effects of moderate exercise on chronic stress-induced intestinal barrier dysfunction and antimicrobial defense. Luo B, Xiang D, Nieman DC, Chen P. Brain Behav Immun. 2013 Nov 27. pii: S0889-1591(13)00544-8. PMID:24291325

[37] Effects on secretory IgA levels in small intestine of mice that underwent moderate exercise training followed by a bout of strenuous swimming exercise. Godínez-Victoria M, Drago-Serrano ME, Reyna-Garfias H, et al. Brain Behav Immun. 2012 Nov;26(8):1300-9. PMID:22884415

[38] Probiotics prevent bacterial translocation and improve intestinal barrier function in rats following chronic psychological stress. Zareie M, Johnson-Henry K, Jury J, et al. Gut. 2006 Nov;55(11):1553-60. PMID:16638791

[39] Lactobacillus plantarum prevents bacterial translocation in rats following ischemia and reperfusion injury. Wang B, Huang Q, Zhang W, Li N, Li J. Dig Dis Sci. 2011 Nov;56(11):3187-94. PMID:21590333

[40] Anti-inflammatory effects of resveratrol, curcumin and simvastatin in acute small intestinal inflammation. Bereswill S, Muñoz M, Fischer A, et al. PLoS One. 2010 Dec 3;5(12):e15099. PMID:21151942

[41] Therapy and epidemiology of autism--clostridial spores as key elements. Finegold SM. Med Hypotheses. 2008;70(3):508-11. PMID:17904761

[42] Effects of rifaximin treatment and retreatment in nonconstipated IBS subjects. Pimentel M, Morales W, Chua K, et al. Dig Dis Sci. 2011 Jul;56(7):2067-72. PMID:21559740

[43] Molecular monitoring of the intestinal flora by denaturing high performance liquid chromatography. Goldenberg O, Herrmann S, Marjoram G, Noyer-Weidner M, Hong G, Bereswill S, Göbel UB. J Microbiol Methods. 2007 Jan;68(1):94-105. PMID:16904779

[44] c-di-GMP turn-over in Clostridium difficile is controlled by a plethora of diguanylate cyclases and phosphodiesterases. Bordeleau E, Fortier LC, Malouin F, Burrus V. PLoS Genet. 2011 Mar;7(3):e1002039. PMID:21483756

[45] Computer-aided identification of recognized drugs as Pseudomonas aeruginosa quorum-sensing inhibitors. Yang L, Rybtke MT, Jakobsen TH, et al. Antimicrob Agents Chemother. 2009 Jun;53(6):2432-43. PMID:19364871

[46] A low concentration of azithromycin inhibits the mRNA expression of N-acyl homoserine lactone synthesis enzymes, upstream of lasI or rhlI, in Pseudomonas aeruginosa. Kai T, Tateda K, Kimura S, Ishii Y, Ito H, Yoshida H, Kimura T, Yamaguchi K. Pulm Pharmacol Ther. 2009 Dec;22(6):483-6. PMID:19393329

[47] Regulatory effects of macrolides on bacterial virulence: potential role as quorum-sensing inhibitors. Tateda K, Standiford TJ, Pechere JC, Yamaguchi K. Curr Pharm Des. 2004;10(25):3055-65. PMID:15544497

[48] Effects of antibiotics on quorum sensing in Pseudomonas aeruginosa. Skindersoe ME, Alhede M, Phipps R, et al. Antimicrob Agents Chemother. 2008 Oct;52(10):3648-63. PMID:18644954

[49] Dietary plant components ellagic acid and tannic acid inhibit Escherichia coli biofilm formation. Hancock V, Dahl M, Vejborg RM, Klemm P. J Med Microbiol. 2010 Apr;59(Pt 4):496-8. PMID:19959627

[50] Prebiotic evaluation of cocoa-derived flavanols in healthy humans by using a randomized, controlled, double-blind, crossover intervention study. Tzounis X, Rodriguez-Mateos A, Vulevic J, et al. Am J Clin Nutr. 2011 Jan;93(1):62-72. PMID:21068351

[51] Chlorogenic acids from green coffee extract are highly bioavailable in humans. Farah A, Monteiro M, Donangelo CM, Lafay S. J Nutr. 2008 Dec;138(12):2309-15. PMID:19022950

[52] Modulation of gut mucosal biofilms. Kleessen B, Blaut M. Br J Nutr. 2005 Apr;93 Suppl 1:S35-40. PMID:15877893

[53] Studies with inulin-type fructans on intestinal infections, permeability, and inflammation. Guarner F. J Nutr. 2007 Nov;137(11 Suppl):2568S-2571S. PMID:17951504

[54] Lectin-like constituents of foods which react with components of serum, saliva, and Streptococcus mutans. Gibbons RJ, Dankers I. Appl Environ Microbiol. 1981 Apr;41(4):880-8. PMID:6786220

[55] Lectins in the United States diet: a survey of lectins in commonly consumed foods and a review of the literature. Nachbar MS, Oppenheim JD. Am J Clin Nutr. 1980 Nov;33(11):2338-45. PMID:7001881

[56] Study of human microecology by mass spectrometry of microbial markers. Osipov GA, Verkhovtseva NV. Benef Microbes. 2011 Mar 1;2(1):63-78. PMID:21831791

[57] Effect of diets containing potato protein or soya bean meal on the incidence of spontaneously-occurring subclinical necrotic enteritis and the physiological response in broiler chickens. Fernando PS, Rose SP, Mackenzie AM, Silva SS. Br Poult Sci. 2011 Feb;52(1):106-14. PMID:21337205

[58] Evolutionary families of peptidase inhibitors. Rawlings ND, Tolle DP, Barrett AJ. Biochem J. 2004 Mar 15;378(Pt 3):705-16. PMID:14705960

[59] MEROPS The Peptidase Database Rawlings, N.D., Barrett, A.J. & Bateman, A. (2010) MEROPS: the peptidase database. Nucleic Acids Res 38, D227-D233.

[60] Inactivation of trypsin inhibitors in sweet potato and taro tubers during processing. Kiran KS, Padmaja G. Plant Foods Hum Nutr. 2003 Spring;58(2):153-63. PMID:12906353

[61] Nutritive value and effect of blanching on the trypsin and chymotrypsin inhibitor activities of selected leafy vegetables. Mosha TC, Gaga HE. Plant Foods Hum Nutr. 1999;54(3):271-83. PMID:10716408

[62] Purification and characterization of a heat-stable serine protease inhibitor from the tubers of new potato variety "Golden Valley". Kim MH, Park SC, Kim JY, et al. Biochem Biophys Res Commun. 2006 Aug 4;346(3):681-6. PMID:16777063

[63] http://merops.sanger.ac.uk/cgi-bin/inhibitors.pl?id=S01.151

[64] Effect of diets containing potato protein or soya bean meal on the incidence of spontaneously-occurring subclinical necrotic enteritis and the physiological response in broiler chickens. Fernando PS, Rose SP, Mackenzie AM, Silva SS. Br Poult Sci. 2011 Feb;52(1):106-14. PMID:21337205

[65] Garlic blocks quorum sensing and promotes rapid clearing of pulmonary Pseudomonas aeruginosa infections. Bjarnsholt T, Jensen PØ, Rasmussen TB, et al. Microbiology. 2005 Dec;151(Pt 12):3873-80. PMID:16339933

[66] Garlic blocks quorum sensing and attenuates the virulence of Pseudomonas aeruginosa. Harjai K, Kumar R, Singh S. FEMS Immunol Med Microbiol. 2010 Mar;58(2):161-8. PMID:19878318

[67] Garlic as an inhibitor of Pseudomonas aeruginosa quorum sensing in cystic fibrosis--a pilot randomized controlled trial. Smyth AR, Cifelli PM, Ortori CA, et al. Pediatr Pulmonol. 2010 Apr;45(4):356-62. PMID:20306535

[68] Influence of polyphenols on bacterial biofilm formation and quorum-sensing. Huber B, Eberl L, Feucht W, Polster J. Z Naturforsch C. 2003 Nov-Dec;58(11-12):879-84. PMID:14713169

[69] Effects of plant lactones on the production of biofilm of Pseudomonas aeruginosa. Cartagena E, Colom OA, Neske A, Valdez JC, Bardón A. Chem Pharm Bull (Tokyo). 2007 Jan;55(1):22-5. PMID:17202695

[70] Chicken soup inhibits neutrophil chemotaxis in vitro. Rennard BO, Ertl RF, Gossman GL, Robbins RA, Rennard SI. Chest. 2000 Oct;118(4):1150-7. PMID:11035691

[71] Screening for quorum-sensing inhibitors (QSI) by use of a novel genetic system, the QSI selector. Rasmussen TB, Bjarnsholt T, Skindersoe ME, et al. J Bacteriol. 2005 Mar;187(5):1799-814. PMID:15716452

[72] Food as a source for quorum sensing inhibitors: iberin from horseradish revealed as a quorum sensing inhibitor of Pseudomonas aeruginosa. Jakobsen TH, Bragason SK, Phipps RK, et al. Appl Environ Microbiol. 2012 Apr;78(7):2410-21. PMID:22286987

[73] Paradigm shift in discovering next-generation anti-infective agents: targeting quorum sensing, c-di-GMP signaling and biofilm formation in bacteria with small molecules. Sintim HO, Smith JA, Wang J, Nakayama S, Yan L. Future Med Chem. 2010 Jun;2(6):1005-35. PMID:21426116

[74] The use of green coffee extract as a weight loss supplement: a systematic review and meta-analysis of randomised clinical trials. Onakpoya I, Terry R, Ernst E. Gastroenterol Res Pract. 2011;2011. pii: 382852. PMID:20871849

[75] Once-weekly azithromycin in cystic fibrosis with chronic Pseudomonas aeruginosa infection. Steinkamp G, Schmitt-Grohe S, Döring G, et al. Respir Med. 2008 Nov;102(11):1643-53. PMID:18701270

[76] Inhibition of bacterial adherence to saliva-coated through plant lectins. Oliveira MR, Napimoga MH, Cogo K, et al. J Oral Sci. 2007 Jun;49(2):141-5. PMID:17634727

[77] Sphingolipids in food and the emerging importance of sphingolipids to nutrition. Vesper H, Schmelz EM, Nikolova-Karakashian MN, Dillehay DL, Lynch DV, Merrill AH Jr. J Nutr. 1999 Jul;129(7):1239-50. PMID:10395583

[78] Colonic cell proliferation and aberrant crypt foci formation are inhibited by dairy glycosphingolipids in 1, 2-dimethylhydrazine-treated CF1 mice. Schmelz EM, Sullards MC, Dillehay DL, Merrill AH Jr. J Nutr. 2000 Mar;130(3):522-7. PMID:10702579

[79] Inhibition of cytokine release from alveolar macrophages in pulmonary sarcoidosis by pentoxifylline: comparison with dexamethasone. Tong Z, Dai H, Chen B, Abdoh Z, Guzman J, Costabel U. Chest. 2003 Oct;124(4):1526-32. PMID:14555589

[80] Caffeine's Vascular Mechanisms of Action. Echeverri D, Montes FR, Cabrera M, Galán A, Prieto A. Int J Vasc Med. 2010;2010:834060. PMID:21188209

[81] Hyponatremia, hypophosphatemia, and hypouricemia in a girl with macrophage activation syndrome. Yamazawa K, Kodo K, Maeda J, Omori S, Hida M, Mori T, Awazu M. Pediatrics. 2006 Dec;118(6):2557-60. PMID:17142545

[82] Uric acid is associated with features of insulin resistance syndrome in obese children at prepubertal stage. Gil-Campos M, Aguilera CM, Cañete R, Gil A. Nutr Hosp. 2009 Sep-Oct;24(5):607-13. PMID:19893872

[83] Increased reactive oxygen species and tumor necrosis factor-alpha production by monocytes are associated with elevated levels of uric acid in pre-eclamptic women. Peraçoli MT, Bannwart CF, Cristofalo R, et al. Am J Reprod Immunol. 2011 Dec;66(6):460-7. doi: 10.1111/j.1600-0897.2011.01016.x. PMID:21623992

[84] Inhibition of nitric oxide in LPS-stimulated macrophages of young and senescent mice by δ-tocotrienol and quercetin. Qureshi AA, Tan X, Reis JC, Badr MZ, Papasian CJ, Morrison DC, Qureshi N. Lipids Health Dis. 2011 Dec 20;10:239. PMID:22185406

[85] Effect of quercetin on lipopolysaccharide induced-sickness behavior and oxidative stress in rats. Sah SP, Tirkey N, Kuhad A, Chopra K. Indian J Pharmacol. 2011 Apr;43(2):192-6. PMID:21572657

[86] Effects of antioxidant polyphenols on TNF-alpha-related diseases. Kawaguchi K, Matsumoto T, Kumazawa Y. Curr Top Med Chem. 2011;11(14):1767-79. PMID:21506932

[87] Protein and Amino Acid Requirements in Human Nutrition: Report of a Joint WHO/FAO/UNU Expert Consultation. World Health Organization ISBN-13: 9789241209359 December 2007

[88] Clinical significance and antibiotic susceptibilities of nontuberculous mycobacteria from patients in Crete, Greece. Gitti Z, Mantadakis E, Maraki S, Samonis G. Future Microbiol. 2011 Sep;6(9):1099-109. PMID:21958147

[89] Prevalence of infectious pathogens in Crohn's disease. Knösel T, Schewe C, Petersen N, Dietel M, Petersen I. Pathol Res Pract. 2009;205(4):223-30. PMID:19186006

[90] Three sisters of pulmonary Mycobacterium avium complex disease. Inoue T, Tanaka E, Sakuramoto M, et al. Kansenshogaku Zasshi. 2005 May;79(5):341-7. PMID:15977574

[91] Vitamins A & D inhibit the growth of mycobacteria in radiometric culture. Greenstein RJ, Su L, Brown ST. PLoS One. 2012;7(1):e29631. PMID:22235314

24. Small Intestinal Bacterial Overgrowth

In contrast to the colon, the small intestine, especially the upper portion of the small intestine, is nearly devoid of bacteria. The body invests considerable effort into destroying bacteria in the upper intestine, through several mechanisms. Gastric acid and enzymes kill most of the bacteria ingested with food. Several pancreatic enzymes destroy bacteria and viruses and bile acids also have antibacterial activity. Salivary glands and the intestinal mucosa produce lysozyme that kills bacteria by attacking their cell walls. The glycocalyx over the brush border denies most bacteria access to adhere to the enterocytes. Mucin, produced by goblet cells, and IgA, formed by plasma cells in the intestinal villi bind to bacteria and keep them from adhering to the intestinal mucosa or to other bacteria, so that those that survive are flushed through the small intestine and not able to reproduce or form biofilms (Chapter 23.)

Table 24-1: Concentration of viable bacteria per gram of contents

	Stomach	Jejunum	Ileum	Colon
Bacteria per gram	0 to 10^3	$0 - 10^4$	$10^5 - 10^8$	$10^{10} - 10^{12}$

Some bacteria may evade destruction, survive, and grow in the small intestine, especially when there are problems with digestion, such as lack of stomach acidity[1]. This can occur in old age, from medication use, or lack of enzyme activity as seen in chronic pancreatitis. However, when colonization of the upper portion of the small intestine occurs, it usually is not by aerobic bacteria from the mouth, but by anaerobic bacteria which have entered the small intestine retrograde from the colon, through the ileal cecal valve. Colonization of the small intestine by these enteric bacteria is referred to as small intestinal bacterial overgrowth (SIBO).

When SIBO occurs, the bacteria ferment food in the small intestine, and thus, may cause production of gas, bloating, nausea, vomiting and diarrhea; the same set of symptoms observed in sugar malabsorption syndromes where fermentation of these sugars occurs in the colon. In SIBO, however, the glucose, as well as other sugars and other nutrients, are fermented in the small intestine, an area not adapted to house bacteria or their byproducts.

The signs and symptoms of SIBO are similar to those for lactose, fructose and other sugar malabsorption syndromes, and the same as for irritable bowel syndrome: abdominal bloating, cramping pain, flatulence, nausea, and diarrhea.

Table 24-2: Disease Effects of SIBO

Effect	Secondary Effects[12]
Fermentation of sugars	Production of hydrogen or methane gasses Abdominal bloating with distension, abdominal cramping pain, flatulence, nausea, and diarrhea. (Bloating is a symptom; distension is a sign. Acidification of chyme: decreases the efficiency of pancreatic enzymes in food digestion.
Bacterial deconjugation of bile acids in the upper intestine	Bile acids are reabsorbed without forming micelles, thus leading to fat malabsorption: loss of vitamins A, E, D, and K, and steatorrhea Secondary bile acid lithocholic acid forms, which is toxic to enterocytes
Enterocyte injury	Loss of brush border enzymes: ➢ Disaccharides – less digestion and more fermentation of the sugars. ➢ Peptidases – loss of amino acid uptake, fermentation of amino acids; ammonia and biogenic amine production.
Fermentation of vitamin B_{12} by anaerobic bacteria	Increased risk of vitamin B_{12} deficiency, anemia, and elevated homocysteine with associated disease risks. Levels of vitamin K and folate may be normal or high as a result of bacterial synthesis of these vitamins.
Immune activation by bacteria	Increased levels of IL-6, IgM, and IgA_2. Increased intraepithelial lymphocytes in the small intestine. May increase risk of an immune response to foods as well as to bacteria. May cause depression.
Bacterial Translocation	Bacteria may be able to move across the epithelial membrane into lymph nodes, the bloodstream, and other organs. They induce inflammatory cytokines and inflammation. May cause infections in the lymph nodes, lungs, and other organs in immune-compromised individuals.
Loss of nutrient absorption	Weight loss Steatorrhea: bulky fatty stools Iron deficiency Hypoproteinemia

Diagnosis

The diagnosis of SIBO is made by finding a bacterial population in the small intestine exceeding 10^5–10^6 organisms/mL. This can be done using endoscopy; an endoscope is passed down the esophagus, through the stomach and duodenum where it meets the jejunum and aspirating fluid found at that point. A less costly and invasive test is the hydrogen breath test (HBT), which also is used for testing sugar malabsorption syndromes. This test measures hydrogen production resulting from the fermentation of carbohydrates by intestinal bacterial

The Hydrogen Breath Test (HBT):

In the HBT, after fasting, an individual breathes into a gas analyzer that measures hydrogen gas in the exhaled breath. The patient then takes a test load of the suspect sugar and is retested, usually over a two hour or longer period. In normal patients, hydrogen levels start and stay low, below ten parts per million until fermentation of the test sugar takes place. Several sugars are commonly used:

Carbohydrate	Diagnostic Use	Rise Over Baseline[2]
Lactose	Lactose Intolerance	20 ppm
Fructose	Fructose Malabsorption	20 ppm
Lactulose	Intestinal transit time (Inaccurate)	20 ppm
Inulin	Intestinal transit time	20 ppm
Glucose	Small Intestine Bacterial Overgrowth	12 ppm

In both lactose intolerance and fructose malabsorption, sugars, which are normally absorbed in the small intestine, pass into the cecum and colon unabsorbed. Here, they ferment, resulting in gas formation. Some of the gasses are absorbed into the bloodstream and exhaled the breath where it can be measured. When sugars are not absorbed in the small intestine, it typically takes about one and a half hours for gas levels fermentation to rise. A rise in H_2 levels of over 20 ppm above baseline is considered a positive test for malabsorption.

Some patients have shorter or longer oral-cecal transit times (OCTT). OCTT is influenced by diet, the test meal, subsequent meals, and ability to digest sugars. Non-digested sugars decrease the OCTT[3]. The presence of these sugars and their fermentation products affect the mechanisms that regulate intestinal motility[4].

Lactulose is an artificial disaccharide. The body lacks enzymes necessary to cleave it into monosaccharides; therefore, it is not absorbed. It too is fermented by colonic bacteria. It has been often used to test how long it takes for a test meal to pass from the mouth into the colon, as it will show a peak of gas after colonic fermentation begins. The time required for the H_2 to rise from fasting baseline by 20 ppm is used as the oral-cecal transit time. Lactulose has been used to test for SIBO; however, it has a very low sensitivity (31%)[5]. Lactulose greatly reduces OCTT; in one study the OCTT for a test meal was 85 minutes for liquid lactulose, 162 minutes with solid lactulose, and 292 minutes for inulin[3]. Lactulose HBT may have diagnostic utility, but it does not give an accurate diagnosis of SIBO or OCTT.

Inulin is not a sugar, but rather non-digestible fructan found in the diet, that is fermented by intestinal bacteria. It is useful for HBT of OCTT and gives accurate results comparable to other methods that do not affect OCTT[6], such as inert beads that can be seen on X-ray. Typical OCTT using inulin is about 300[7] to 400[6] minutes, which is consistent with the duration of a normal migrating motor complex (see below). A rise in bacterially generated gas during an inulin HBT in less than 60 minutes would be consistent with SIBO.

Most microbes use glucose, and thus in SIBO glucose is easily fermented, and gas produced. In SIBO, the gas peak occurs earlier after the test meal than for colonic fermentation, as fermentation occurs in the small intestine. A rise of H_2 by 12 ppm above baseline is considered a positive test for SIBO. While more sensitive than lactulose, the glucose HBT, still, only has a sensitivity of 44%, compared with the culture of endoscopic aspirate from the upper small intestine[5]. The rise in gas production usually occurs in SIBO in less than one hour.

Hydrogen breath test is best performed as a Hydrogen-Methane Breath Test, as *Methanobrevibacter* populations in the intestine of many patients convert hydrogen, created during fermentation, into methane. About 30 percent of patients with SIBO only have an elevation of methane gas[8]. *Methanobrevibacter* metabolize two hydrogen gas (H_2) molecules into one molecule of methane (CH_4). In patients colonized with these bacteria, the H_2 level may not rise, and if CH_4 is not tested for, a false negative result can occur. This is more often found in patients with constipation.

HBT can also give false negative results in patients with slower intestinal transit times. The duration of the test is usually two to three hours while normal OCTT is about five hours, and a positive test relies on the rapid transit, often associated with impaired absorption of sugars.

False-negative results can occur for glucose HBT in SIBO if the bacterial overgrowth is further along the ileum as the glucose may be absorbed by the small intestine before it arrives at the affected area[2].

The reported prevalence of SIBO greatly depends on the diagnostic method used. About five percent of healthy young adults and fifteen percent of healthy older adults have a positive glucose HBT, but it is rare for these asymptomatic adults to have positive duodenal aspirates.

SIBO has very similar symptoms to irritable bowel syndrome (IBS) and is commonly diagnosed in both IBS and fibromyalgia (FM). In a study in which lactulose breath test was used, 84 percent of IBS patients and 100 percent of FM patients had positive lactulose HBT. The H_2 peak occurred at about 135 to 150 minutes after the test meal was consumed[9]. These results, however, are more consistent with a rapid OCTT than SIBO. When duodenal aspirates were tested only four percent of IBS patients had positive tests; nevertheless, intestinal dysmotility is common among IBS patients[10]. The glucose-HBT is also commonly positive in IBS patients, with near half of IBS patients having a positive glucose breath test, with about 30 percent of these patients producing only methane[11].

There are several possible explanations for the disparity in testing between duodenal aspirations and HBT in IBS and FM. One explanation is that a positive HBT with a negative test for bacteria on duodenal aspirates in IBS and FM patients represents a true case of SIBO where bacterial growth lays distal to the duodenum and beyond the reach of endoscopic. At present, there is no clinical test that directly assesses the pathological growth of bacteria in the small intestine beyond the first several inches of the jejunum. Alternatively, a positive HBT in IBS and FM may not reflect SIBO, but rather rapid OCTT that may be associated with bacterial dysbiosis of the large intestine.

Which of these or other possible explanations for the disparity in test results is most accurate, may not be as salient as the diagnostic information that HBT provides. A positive HBT may represent proximal or distal SIBO or rapid OCTT with colonic fermentation; nevertheless, it represents dysbiosis in any of these situations. A positive HBT that guides treatment that symptomatic relief has value even when it does not clearly define the causal mechanism.

Causation

SIBO is usually caused by impaired or disorganized enteric motility and found in constipation, inflammatory bowel disease, diabetic autonomic neuropathy, IBS[12], or other condition in which orderly peristalsis is disrupted. SIBO is common in patients with gastroparesis[13], a condition in which the stomach does not empty well as a result of lack of muscular contractions of the stomach walls. Blind loop syndrome, where a pouch or section of the intestine does not have normal motility, also causes a form of SIBO.

Gastrointestinal Motility 101

The clothes washer in my home has two basic motions: wash, where the clothes get agitated back and forth in the wash water, and the spin cycle that gets rid of most of the water in the clothes before taking them out to dry. The gastrointestinal tract has similar activity, with two basic motions: segmentation (wash) and peristalsis (spin dry).

Peristaltic motion in the esophagus, under vagal nerve control, squeezes food forward; delivering the food bolus to the stomach. The contraction moves forward in a traveling wave contraction, with the muscles ahead relaxing so that the bolus is propelled forward.

When a meal begins, the stomach muscles relax so that the stomach can expand and hold more food. The pyloric sphincter closes, and the stomach makes about 3 or 4 gentle mixing waves per minute to mix the food with acid and enzymes. As digestion proceeds, the mixing motion gets more intense and changes to a peristaltic-like motion. During this activity, the pyloric sphincter allows 10 to 15 milliliters of chyme to pass into the duodenum with each contraction. The muscular motion of the stomach is under parasympathetic control through the vagal nerve.

Segmentation and tonic contractions are ring-like contractions of the muscular layers surrounding the intestines, which are stimulated by the presence of food in the small intestine. Segmentation isolates the food into an area and then slowly sloshes it back and forth about 12 to 16 times a minute like toothpaste in a tube. This agitation mixes the chyme with enzymes and enhances mixing so that nutrients are better exposed to the mucosa for absorption. Tonic contractions isolate one area of the intestine from another and prolong the intestinal transit time so that more nutrients can be absorbed.

Peristalsis is a segmental contraction of the muscular walls of the intestine that propels the chyme forward, distally, towards the exit. This usually occurs at the end of digestion, to prepare for the next meal, but will also occur in the presence of irritation, so that the intestine can rid itself of potentially toxic agents.

The intestines are innervated by both sympathetic and parasympathetic innervations. The sympathetic activity decreases blood flow to the intestines and tightens sphincters. The general effect is to decrease parasympathetic, vegetative activities and divert blood flow to the muscles and brain (for fight or flight activities). Parasympathetic activity, through the vagal nerve, stimulates digestive activities and increases blood flow to the GI tract.

Both segmentation and peristalsis are under the influence of the vagal nerves but are largely mediated by serotonin release from the enterochromaffin cells of the intestine. The presence of food causes the release of serotonin into the lamina propria which stimulates segmental contraction of the musculature of the intestine. Serotonin also acts as a vasodilator in the intestines, increasing blood flow, and thus absorption of nutrients.

Higher amounts of serotonin can be released in the presence of irritants. When higher levels of serotonin are released, it stimulates peristalsis. This helps spread irritants out over a wider area, so they are less concentrated. However, with sufficient stimulation and serotonin release, a generalized peristalsis occurs, resulting in diarrhea. Serotonin is also absorbed into the bloodstream and carried to the brain where high levels stimulate nausea and vomiting as a result of stimulation of $5HT_3$ receptors[14]. Thus, serotonin not only stimulates digestion; it provides a defense mechanism for ridding the body of toxins.

Serotonin is only one of several hormonal agents which act on gastrointestinal motility.

Table 24-3: Some Gastrointestinal Motility Hormones

Hormone	Effect on Gastrointestinal Motility
Serotonin	Activates cholinergic excitatory motor neurons and NO inhibitory motor neurons; it leads to contraction of smooth muscle and coordinated relaxation; generating pressure waves.
Melatonin	Reinforces migrating motor complex (MMC)[15]. Melatonin increases blood flow and acts as an antioxidant[16] that protects the autonomic nervous system.
VIP	Induces relaxation of smooth muscle (the lower esophageal sphincter, sphincter of Oddi) and intestinal wall muscles in front of a peristaltic wave.
Nitric Oxide (NO)	Induces relaxation of smooth muscle in front of a peristaltic wave.
Substance P	Causes contraction of smooth muscle in the intestinal wall behind the peristaltic wave.
Galanin	Causes contraction of smooth muscle in the intestinal wall.
CCK	Inhibits gastric emptying, stimulates gall-bladder contraction. Helps prepare for the migrating motor complex peristalsis.
Somatostatin	Inhibits intestinal motility.
Neurotensin	Causes relaxation of circular smooth muscles in the intestinal wall.
Enkephalins	Increase pyloric sphincter contractions, relaxation of smooth muscles of the intestinal wall.
Motilin	Mediates migrating motor complex peristalsis between meals.
GLP-1[17]	Delays gastric emptying and inhibits the migrating motor complex.
Xenin	Increases propagation of aboral contractions during phase III MMC.

The motor activity of the intestines depends on electrical pacemaker cells located in the outer muscular layer of the stomach and intestine. These cells are not unlike pacemaker cells in the heart. Acetylcholine from vagal nerve fibers increases the electrical activity and spike potentials while epinephrine from sympathetic nerves decreases this activity. This activity helps to coordinate the muscular activity of the intestine.

During the fasting state, the motor activity of the GI tract becomes modified, and there are cycles of migrating motor activity stimulated by a migrating electrical wave; the Migrating Motor Complex (MMC), which begins either in the antrum of the stomach (the portion nearest the jejunum) or in the jejunum. The MMC electrical wave travels from the stomach or jejunum to the distal ileum at a rate of about 5 cm per minute. A new MMC begins about every 90 minutes during fasting.

The MMC has three phases: in phase I, there is myoelectric quiescence, in phase II, there is irregular myoelectrical spiking, and in phase III, there are bursts of regular, intense myoelectric activity that migrate arboreally and trigger peristaltic activity. Phase III activity is followed by another cycle of phase I quiescence.

Because the wall of the small intestine is about 700 cm long, it takes longer than 90 minutes for the MMC to travel from the stomach to the terminal ileum; (700 / 5 = 140). Thus, a new wave begins while the previous wave is still traveling. A meal will interrupt the MMC, but 90 to 120 minutes later the MMC waves will begin again, starting from the positions along the intestine where they left off. The interruption of the MMC is mediated by cholecystokinin[18].

The MMC promotes a long, continuous peristaltic cleaning wave which clears the stomach and small intestine of its contents. The MMC is mediated in part by the hormone motilin under vagal stimulus. The MMC and the long peristaltic wave are responsible for the growling of the belly often associated with hunger.

The length of time it takes for non-absorbed food constituents to go from the mouth to the end of the ileum is referred to as the oral-cecal transit time (OCTT). Considering that the delay from the onset of a meal to the initiation of the next MMC at the antrum of the stomach is about 120 minutes; that it requires about 40 minutes for the MMC contraction wave to develop; and that at a rate of 5 cm/minute it would be expected to take the MMC 140 minutes to travel from the stomach to the end of the ileum; a normal OCTT should take around 300 minutes if the MMC is not interrupted by a meal. This is the amount of time required for inulin to produce H_2 in normal patients.

An OCTT less than 140 minutes in an adult is not consistent with a normal MMC peristaltic wave, but rather represents peristaltic activity associated with stimuli such as irritants or pathology that promote clearing of the intestinal contents.

Circadian Influences

GI motility is additionally mediated by CLOCK (Circadian Locomotor Output Cycles Kaput) genes expressed in intestinal epithelial cells and in the enteric neurons which help control circadian rhythms[19]. Gastric emptying times are longer for solid foods in the evening than in the morning. MMC propagation velocity in the small intestine is slower at night; only about 2.9 cm/minute, as compared to 6.4 cm/minute during the day[20]. Colonic motility is low at night but increases in the morning.

Disruption of the circadian cycle by alterations in sleep time and meal times can provoke changes in GI motility. Disruption of circadian rhythms, such as occurs with shift work or time zone traveling, can lead to gastrointestinal symptoms including bloating, abdominal pain, diarrhea, or constipation[19].

MMC begin in either the stomach or the jejunum. The hormone motilin increases the output of serotonin. 5HT$_4$ antagonists can block both gastric and duodenal initiated MMC while 5HT$_3$ inhibitors only block gastric MMC[21]. Somatostatin and motilin appear to interact to support MMC[22]. Tegaserod, a medication used for IBS with constipation, is a 5HT$_4$ agonist.

Glucagon-like peptide-1 (GLP-1) is released after food intake and increases insulin excretion from the pancreas. GLP-1 inhibits gastric emptying, increases satiety and inhibits small bowel motility in the antrum and duodenum. GLP-1 inhibits the MMC both in healthy individuals and individuals with IBS[23]. A GLP-1 analog has been found to inhibit small intestine motility, and relieve IBS pain during an acute attack[24].

Motilin is released by the presence of bile acids in the blood stream, and thus an intact enterohepatic circulation of bile acids appears to trigger MMC[25]. Bile acid sequestrants often cause constipation, by removing bile acids from the enterohepatic circulation.

Causation of SIBO
Myenteric Motility Disorders

The most prevalent cause of SIBO is gastrointestinal dysmotility. Normally, the GI track moves its contents forward during the fasting state with migrating motor complexes. There are several disease states where the MMC is abnormal, and retrograde pressure waves can occur, preventing normal clearing of the intestinal contents.

Gastroparesis is commonly associated with SIBO. Gastroparesis, a disorder of abnormal emptying of the stomach, is most often associated with long-standing diabetes as a result of autonomic neuropathy. It can also occur as the result of viral infections or ischemia.

Small intestinal dysmotility is common among patients with SIBO[26]. As in gastroparesis, intestinal dysmotility can result from long-standing diabetes, chronic renal failure or other dysautonomias, secondary to neuropathy. Intestinal dysmotility, common among patients with IBS or FM, is likely neuropathic in nature, secondary to inflammatory injury to the enteric nervous system.

Morphine has been demonstrated to provoke SIBO in lab animals as it impairs the MMC[35]. Casomorphin, a peptide formed during the digestion of the protein casein from milk, acts as an opiate receptor agonist and slows the MMC[27]. Wheat, spinach, and digested blood also contain peptides similar to casomorphin[28], which may slow MMC activity.

Connective tissue diseases may also interfere with bowel motility as in the case of scleroderma, polymyositis, and other diseases. Here, the muscles of the intestine are damaged, and this can cause pseudo-obstruction. Portal hypertension and liver cirrhosis are also associated with high risk for SIBO as a result of intestinal dysmotility.

Table 24-4: Risk factors for SIBO

Class	Condition[29]
Motility Disorders	Gastroparesis Gastroesophageal reflux disease (GERD)[30] Small bowel dysmotility Celiac disease Chronic intestinal pseudo-obstruction Irritable Bowel Syndrome Dysautonomia Liver cirrhosis, Portal hypertension Chronic renal failure Scleroderma[31]
Hypochlorhydria	Autoimmune atrophic gastritis Atrophic gastritis secondary to chronic *Helicobacter pylori* infection Gastric bypass surgery Hypothyroidism Use of antacids Use of H$_2$ Inhibitors (e.g.; Zantac, Tagamet) Proton pump inhibitor medications (PPI; e.g.: Nexium, Prilosec)
Pancreatic Enzyme Insufficiency (PEI)	Multiple Causes See PEI in Chapter 8
Structural/Anatomic disorder; in which chyme is diverted from moving into the colon.	Small intestine diverticula Small intestine strictures (from radiation, medications, Crohn's disease) Surgically created blind loops Resection of ileocecal valve Fistulas between proximal and distal bowel Gastric resection
Medications: Antibiotics Acid suppressants Morphine	Recurrent use of antibiotics can select resistant organisms Medications that block stomach acid production can allow survival of ingested bacteria Opiates suppress GI motility
Organ System Dysfunction	Chronic pancreatitis Cystic Fibrosis Immunodeficiency states Crohn's disease Celiac disease Malnutrition Alcohol Abuse

Inflammatory activity in the lamina propria of the small intestine may also trigger myometrium activity, which may be uncoordinated and lead to dysmotility. Bacterial activity in the small intestine may provoke an inflammatory reaction and worsen dysmotility; thus, SIBO may be self-promoting.

Bacterial fermentation of carbohydrates in the small intestine causes acidification of the chyme. Lowering the pH of the chyme decreases the activity of many digestive enzymes and can impair the digestion of proteins. The undigested proteins and large protein fragments raise the risk that these proteins and peptides will be presented to the immune system and become recognized as antigens. Immune reactions to food can cause dysmotility.

Fermented amino acids form biogenic amines that can affect both the enteric and central nervous systems. Ammonia produced by fermentation of amino acids is associated with hepatic encephalopathy in patients with liver cirrhosis[32]. Loss of digestive enzyme activity and undigested proteins also lead to fermentation of the proteins by bacteria, promoting biofilm and toxin formation (Chapter 23).

In SIBO, bile is deconjugated by bacteria in the small intestine. These bile acids may be reabsorbed early, thus preventing absorption of fats and fat-soluble vitamins. Some bacteria convert bile acids into secondary bile acids that act as irritants, promoting dysmotility. Loss of bile acids can diminish the MMC during the fasting state.

Morphine can at high dose inhibit, or at low dose stimulate MMC[33]. The dependence that develops can cause symptoms during withdrawal[34]. Opiates can promote SIBO and bacterial translocation[35]. Bacterial translocation occurs in SIBO, with bacteria crossing the enterocyte membrane, and then making their way to mesenteric lymph nodes, liver, and the spleen. In lab animals, induced acute pancreatitis disturbs the MMC and is associated with the development of SIBO and bacterial translocation[36].

Structural Motility Disorders

Similar to problems with nerve or motor propulsion, portions of the GI tract that are not able to flush material through, are at high risk for bacterial overgrowth. The simplest example is diverticula which can form along the small intestine, but which do not participate in motor contractions. Surgically created blind loops, such as the Billroth procedure, also provide an environment for SIBO. Intestinal strictures as may occur in some disease condition, such as Crohn's disease, and can prevent normal propulsion of the chyme, increasing the risk for SIBO.

Loss of Antimicrobial Action

Loss of the antimicrobial action of the GI tract increases the ability of bacteria to survive in what is otherwise a hostile environment for microbes.

Patients who do not produce stomach acid (achlorhydria or due to use of proton pump inhibitors, such as omeprazole), may have as many as $10^4 - 10^8$ microorganisms per milliliter of stomach contents; while normal stomach acid kills most ingested bacteria. Most of the bacteria ingested are not from food, but rather from the mouth, teeth, and the upper airway. These are usually aerobic bacteria; however, the bacteria associated with symptoms in SIBO are mainly anaerobic bacteria that colonize the colon. These anaerobes are common in our environment and exposure to intact skin or ingestion of them in small amounts does not normally cause disease.

The most common causes for loss of stomach acidity are medication: antacids, H_2 blockers and proton pump inhibitors (PPI) used for symptoms of heartburn and ulcers. Other causes of achlorhydria include chronic infection with *Helicobacter pylori*, hypothyroidism, and autoimmune atrophic gastritis.

SIBO is common in patients with gastroesophageal reflux disease (GERD) and in IBS, two conditions in which patients are commonly prescribed PPI medications that decrease stomach acid. As many as half of GERD patients[30] and IBS patients treated with PPI have SIBO. However, the risk of SIBO appears not to be influenced by the use of PPI medications[37]. Both GERD and IBS are diseases in which there is gastrointestinal dysmotility. Patients using PPI for non-dysmotility conditions are not at increased risk for SIBO[30].

Bile has antimicrobial activity as do pancreatic enzymes. Pancreatic deficiency and loss of bile acids due to medications (bile acid sequestrants) or to ileostomy surgery are risk factors for SIBO. Pancreatic deficiency is highly associated with SIBO, and while this may be related to the antimicrobial actions of pancreatic enzymes, it is almost certainly related to the actions of pancreatic enzymes on motor activity of the gallbladder and intestines.

The small intestine also produces lysozyme, IgA, and mucin which protect the intestine from bacterial overgrowth. This can be disrupted in disease conditions, such as Celiac disease, where there is damage to the intestinal mucosa. Immunodeficient patients are at increased risk of SIBO. Immune sensitization to foods can divert antibacterial-IgA production to IgA, which binds to foods. Lack of IgA for binding bacteria allows bacterial survival and biofilm formation.

Other Risk Factors for SIBO

In addition to supplying lysozyme, IgA, and mucin, the mucosa of the small intestine produces enzymes for cleaving carbohydrates into monosaccharides that are easily absorbed. The non-absorbed saccharides not only provide food for growth of bacteria in the intestine, but also increase peristaltic activity. When there is damage to the mucosa, as in gluten enteropathy, the brush border enzymes are lost. When the MMC is not properly coordinated, it supports SIBO by increasing the retrograde motion of the chyme.

Chronic alcoholics are at increased risk of SIBO. This may occur as a result of neuropathy as well as loss of bactericidal proteins made by the mucosa[38]. Overuse of antibiotics may be a risk factor for SIBO as it promotes the growth of resistant organisms over susceptible organisms. This results in loss of a balanced commensal community and allows overgrowth and biofilm formation of potentially harmful organisms.

The Kynurenine Pathway

The amino acid tryptophan is the precursor of the monoamine neurotransmitter serotonin and melatonin. Tryptophan can be diverted from the production of serotonin and metabolized through the kynurenine pathway, in which tryptophan is converted to 3-hydroxy-L-kynurenine (3HKA) and quinolinic acid (QA). The kynurenine pathway is stimulated by bacterial lipopolysaccharides (LPS) from enteric bacteria, and by the cytokines interferon-gamma (INF-γ), tumor necrosis factor (TNF) and interleukins 1 and 6 (IL-1, IL-6). Thus, the kynurenine pathway is stimulated by pathologic anaerobic biofilm growth and inflammation.

3HKA is cytotoxic and generates oxygen radicals that can kill bacteria and infected cells. QA is an NMDA receptor agonist and a neuro-excitotoxin. Although the kynurenine pathway has been associated with neurologic disease, there is little research available on its impact on the GI system, that area where this pathway almost certainly evolved. Figure 31-2 illustrates the kynurenine pathway.

Glutamate receptors, including NMDA receptors, promote tonic contractions of the GI musculature[39]. Additionally, the NMDA receptor incites visceral pain[40]. Histamine, released as a result of mast cell activation, also acts on NMDA receptors[41]. NMDA receptor antagonists have been suggested for use in treatment of IBS[42] and fibromyalgia[43].

The production of QA, resulting from bacterial LPS production and inflammation, likely mediates cramping and other visceral pain, and may provoke intestinal dysmotility. QA may provoke pain in SIBO, IBS, and fibromyalgia, and contribute to the pathology other malabsorption syndromes.

QA is neurotoxic and may cause long-term damage to the motor neurons of the intestine that regulate intestinal motility; to secretory neurons that regulate endocrine and exocrine secretions; and to sensory neurons that respond to stretch, tonicity, glucose and amino acids. QA and 3HKA may be responsible for the gastrointestinal nervous system neuropathy seen in fibromyalgia and IBS.

SIBO Prevalence and Disease Association

SIBO is unusual in healthy young adults but is more common in older adults; with about 15% of older adults having positive hydrogen breath tests indicating SIBO. This is not part of normal aging, but rather the result of disease.

Table 24-5 lists common diseases associated with SIBO. Patients having these conditions should be asked about symptoms of SIBO, and tested if the typical symptoms are present: bloating, abdominal cramping pain, abdominal distension, flatulence, nausea, and diarrhea.

Patients with gluten enteropathy should be tested for SIBO if their symptoms fail to resolve after elimination of gluten from the diet. Patients with hepatic encephalopathy, chronic pancreatitis or cystic fibrosis should be tested even if they do not report symptoms. In diseases that cause abdominal pain and diarrhea, such as Crohn's disease, symptoms caused by SIBO can be attributed to the underlying condition even when the underlying condition is not active. Thus, testing these patients for SIBO can be helpful. SIBO is a common cause of chronic diarrhea, and it should be included in its differential diagnosis.

Table 24-5: Some Diseases in which SIBO is Common

Chronic Diarrhea
Diabetes
Irritable Bowel Syndrome
Rosacea[44]
Scleroderma
Gastroesophageal Reflux Disease
Gastroparesis
Hepatic Encephalopathy
Chronic Pancreatitis
Cystic Fibrosis
Gluten Enteropathy
Crohn's Disease
Irritable Bowel Syndrome
Fibromyalgia
Post Billroth surgery

SIBO and Sleep

Disruption of the circadian cycle can cause intestinal dysmotility, which is the major risk factor for SIBO. IBS and GERD are common among shift workers and associated with sleep disorders. Nurses on rotating shifts are twice as likely to have a functional bowel disorder as those working day shifts[45]. Missing meals during the day or feeding at night may also disrupt gastrointestinal circadian cycles[46,47].

Glucose, insulin, ghrelin, leptin, and GLP-1 follow meal patterns[48]. Nighttime eating can offset the intestinal circadian rhythm, and nighttime meals result in increase blood sugar and triglyceride levels, compared to the same meal consumed during the day[49]. Shift workers are at increased risk of obesity, cardiometabolic disease[50], and breast cancer[51]. They have increased triglyceride levels, BMI, waist circumference and obesity. Shift workers also have blunted response to insulin, ghrelin, and xenin[52].

In night eating syndrome (NES), the sleep cycle remains typical, but patients wake to eat at night. There is an attenuated nocturnal rise in the plasma concentrations of melatonin and leptin and a greater increase in the concentrations of cortisol. Ghrelin, a hunger hormone, has its cycle delayed by about 5 hours in these patients[53]. NES may respond to bright light therapy. It may also respond to morning[54] or evening meals[55] high in tryptophan, the precursor of serotonin and melatonin. Ensuring adequate vitamin B_6 for conversion of tryptophan to serotonin, and daytime exposure to bright light may enhance entrainment to a normal circadian cycle[56] for sleep and for the MMC.

Treatment of SIBO

1. Antibiotics: A first line of treatment of SIBO is antibiotic treatment. Rifaximin (400 mg three times a day for ten days) has shown favorable results in several studies and is also effective in treating many patients with IBS[57]. Rifaximin may require the presence of bile acids to be effective, thus limiting its effectiveness in the small intestine[58]. Several other antibiotic regimens (ciprofloxacin, metronidazole, and others) have been found to be of similar efficacy and are less costly.

Although SIBO, as diagnosed by HBT, is common in children with IBS symptoms[59], rifaximin treatment was found not to be of benefit in children with chronic abdominal pain with positive HBT[60].

Antibiotic treatment usually provides only temporary benefits, as the treatment does not address the underlying problem, and the small intestine will likely re-colonize and have new biofilm formation if the root causes remain. Repeated treatment with rifaximin is effective but increases the risk of developing resistant organisms.

Use of quorum sensing (QS) inhibitors may help prevent biofilm formation and the production of LPS by enteric bacteria. Azithromycin and erythromycin have some QS inhibiting activity. Some phenolic compounds and lactones in foods also inhibit QS. (See Chapter 23.)

2. If possible, reverse the underlying cause: Celiac, Crohn's disease, and hypothyroidism should be treated. Gluten enteropathy needs strict avoidance of gluten as well as treatment of SIBO. Diabetics require good blood sugar and blood pressure control to prevent neuropathy. Alcohol excesses should be avoided. Treating the underlying causes of gastrointestinal dysmotility is often difficult. It is often not possible to reverse existing organ damage. Diverticula do not disappear, and surgically created blind pouches are not easily corrected.

Medications that inhibit normal peristalsis may need to be eliminated. This includes some antidepressants. Intestinal dysmotility may be worsened by some medications, including medications used to treat the symptoms of SIBO, such as antidiarrheal medications. Opiates notably inhibit the MMC and decrease gastrointestinal movement.

3. Intestinal Motility: Even when antibiotics are effective, the effect is usually temporary. After antibiotic treatment with rifaximin for SIBO in patients with IBS, symptoms reoccurred, on average, in 40 days[61].

If, after antibiotic treatment, patients are treated with low dose bedtime erythromycin (50 mg), used not as an antibiotic but as a motilin analog, the average reoccurrence is delayed for 138 days. Low-dose erythromycin stimulates MMC phase III activity[62]. The drug tegaserod, a 5HT$_4$ agonist, at a dose of 2 to 6 mg, taken at bedtime delayed occurrence for 195 days[61].

4. Malabsorption: Non-absorbed sugars not only ferment in the large intestine; they have a direct effect on peristalsis and OCTT. Lactose and fructose should be avoided in individuals who do not absorb them well. Sorbitol should be avoided until the individual is well enough to test to see if it is tolerated. Beans and other gas-producing foods should be avoided until the individual is well and added back slowly or taken with *Beano* to avoid bloating (see Chapter 5). Lactose and fructose breath testing may be appropriate in individuals suspected with non-absorption, after antibiotic treatment of SIBO.

Protein malabsorption can also cause dysbiosis and symptoms. Malabsorption of proteins increases production of ammonia and *Clostridial* and other bacterial toxins. A stool test for chymotrypsin or elastase may be helpful to determine if pancreatic enzyme production is sufficient. Protein malabsorption is discussed in Chapter 7.

Malabsorption may cause vitamin and mineral deficiencies that require treatment. Vitamins A, D, E, K, B$_{12}$, folate, and magnesium are easily lost in malabsorption syndromes including SIBO. See Chapter 39 for the use of supplements.

5. GERD: Gastroesophageal reflux disease (GERD), a risk factor for SIBO may be successfully treated with 3 mg of melatonin[63] and 5 to 10 mg of zinc[64]. This treatment avoids the used of acid inhibitors that promote SIBO.

6. Melatonin: Although melatonin is thought of as a hormone of the pineal gland, about 90 percent of the body's melatonin is made by enterochromaffin cells in the mucosa of the intestine. Melatonin reinforces the MMC[65]. Sublingual melatonin, which is rapidly absorbed, may cause brief abdominal cramping as a result of this. Melatonin also slows the speed of MMC propagation. Melatonin at bedtime can increase MMC organization during the nighttime sleep cycle, and help prevent SIBO. Melatonin is also an antioxidant and has anti-inflammatory actions.

Maintaining a regular circadian eating and sleeping cycle may help prevent SIBO. Disruption of the circadian sleep cycle decreases melatonin production and increases risk gastroesophageal reflux disease and IBS. Serotonin production during the day can be enhanced by a breakfast high in tryptophan and adequate vitamin B$_6$, along with exposure to sunshine. Melatonin production can be enhanced by a similar diet, and avoiding bright light in the evening and with the use of melatonin supplements. Melatonin at bedtime is helpful in the treatment of IBS and protects the gastrointestinal mucosa[66].

Eating anything more than a light snack should be avoided during the hour before bedtime so that both the endogenous and supplemental melatonin can help form orderly MMC waves. Maintaining a regular sleep and meal cycle should be included in the treatment of SIBO and other diseases associated with intestinal dysmotility. Shift work, especially rotating shift work, should be avoided in affected patients.

7. Prebiotics and probiotics: Probiotics, a mix of commensal bacteria (*Lactobacillus casei, Lactobacillus plantarum, Streptococcus faecalis* and *Bifidobacterium brevis*) as a supplement, was found to be more effective in the treatment of SIBO than was metronidazole[67]. The prebiotic fiber, hydrolyzed guar gum, was found to be more effective than rifaximin in successfully treating SIBO with positive HBT[68]. Fructose oligosaccharides (FOS) (Chapter 4) support beneficial commensal bacteria, decreasing the production of LPS and thus, would be expected to decrease kynurenine products.

8. Pancreatic Exocrine Function: Pancreatic enzymes supplements may help in the treatment of SIBO. Try to resolve any other underlying causes of postcibal asynchrony. This is discussed in the section on pancreatic exocrine function in Chapter 8.

9. Avoid inflammation from food immunogens: Inflammation in the intestinal lamina propria, resulting from reactions to food immunogens, can cause the release of histamine and other inflammatory mediators which can impair normal GI motility and increase risk for SIBO. Testing for food immunogens is covered in Chapter 19.

10. Spicy Foods: Hot foods, such as chili peppers, can increase the symptoms in patients with gastric motility disorders including GERD and IBS. Chronic use of spicy foods may down-regulate this sensitivity. Thus, small amounts of hot peppery spices used on a regular basis may improve motility by making the intestine less sensitive to irritants[69].

11. Bile Acid Sequestrants: Even though bile acids are needed in for normal MMC function and have anti-bacterial actions, bile acid sequestrants may be helpful in treating it. In patients with SIBO or rapid OCTT, bile that has been fermented into secondary bile acids is reabsorbed and recycled into the hepato-enteric circulation. The secondary bile acids, lithocholic acid and deoxycholic acid, are irritants and may disrupt the MMC. Bile acid sequestrants can slow OCTT[70] and may be helpful in the treatment of IBS with diarrhea. Bile acid sequestrants may also absorb and help eliminate bacterial toxins. Fiber from grain binds to bile salts in the colon, and helps in its elimination[71]. See the section on Bile Acid Malabsorption in Chapter 26.

12. DHA: The n-3 fatty acid, docosahexaenoic acid, helps normalize electrical conduction of the heart and nerves. DHA has the potential benefit of normalizing migrating motor complexes in those with SIBO.

Infantile Colic

Infantile colic is a disease with a very similar presentation to SIBO and sugar malabsorption syndromes; there is bloating, abdominal distension, abdominal pain, vomiting and foul-smelling diarrhea. It is not uncommon for an infant with colic to spent 3 hours a day crying. Colic usually occurs about the time that artificial formulas are introduced.

In a small study, glucose hydrogen breath tests were found to be positive in about half of infants with colic; suggesting SIBO. As in other pediatric trials, antibiotic treatment was not helpful[72]. Infantile colic may be triggered by fruit juices with sorbitol or foods with high fructose-to-glucose ratios[73]. Removal of lactose from the diet is also helpful in most infants with colic; the lactose-free formula is associated with decreased production of hydrogen gas[74].

Studies have also shown that colicky infants have a different distribution of intestinal bacteria than infants without colic[75]. The microbiota is more likely to have gas-forming strains of enteric bacteria[76], and coliform bacteria; *Escherichia coli* were found to be more abundant in colicky infants[77]. Certain strains of the commensal enteric lactobacilli (*L. delbrueckii*, and *L. plantarum MB 456*) have been found to inhibit the growth of gas forming *E. coli*[78].

Infantile colic occurs in infants as their intestines become colonized by bacteria from the environment. Colic is most commonly caused by dysbiosis. Infant formula with probiotics can be helpful for introducing beneficial bacteria. Mother's milk contains galactose oligosaccharides, which act as a prebiotic and promote the colonization of the colon with beneficial commensal bacteria.

Some infants respond to lactose-free formula, suggesting lactase deficiency; however, this deficiency is most likely secondary to damage to the brush border and loss of brush border enzymes.

SIBO may be present in infants due to dysmotility of the intestine. Feeding infants as soon as they are hungry allows hunger to guide the feeding patterns. Development of regular feeding and sleeping patterns helps develop normal enteric motility and decrease the risk of SIBO-induced colic.

Fruit juice is inappropriate for infants less than 4 months of age. Fruits, such as apples, have higher amounts of fructose than glucose and thus may be associated with malabsorption. Many fruits and their juices contain sorbitol, which is very poorly absorbed and thus subject to fermentation. Rice cereal usually does not cause gas production while other cereals contain fructans which ferment and produce gas.

[1] Increased incidence of small intestinal bacterial overgrowth during proton pump inhibitor therapy. Lombardo L, Foti M, Ruggia O, Chiecchio A. Clin Gastroenterol Hepatol. 2010 Jun;8(6):504-8. PMID: 20060064

[2] How to interpret hydrogen breath tests. Ghoshal UC. J Neurogastroenterol Motil. 2011 Jul;17(3):312-7. PMID:21860825

[3] Gastric emptying and orocaecal transit time of meals containing lactulose or inulin in men. Clegg M, Shafat A. Br J Nutr. 2010 Aug;104(4):554-9. PMID:20370945

[4] Effect of lactose on oro-cecal transit in lactose digesters and maldigesters. He T, Priebe MG, Welling GW, Vonk RJ. Eur J Clin Invest. 2006 Oct;36(10):737-42. PMID:16968470

[5] Utility of hydrogen breath tests in diagnosis of small intestinal bacterial overgrowth in malabsorption syndrome and its relationship with oro-cecal transit time. Ghoshal UC, Ghoshal U, Das K, Misra A. Indian J Gastroenterol. 2006 Jan-Feb;25(1):6-10. PMID:16567886

[6] In vivo evaluation of a colonic delivery system using isotope techniques. Verbeke K, de Preter V, Geboes K, Daems T, van den Mooter G, Evenepoel P, Rutgeerts P. Aliment Pharmacol Ther. 2005 Jan 15;21(2):187-94. PMID:15679769

[7] Inulin is an ideal substrate for a hydrogen breath test to measure the orocaecal transit time. Geboes KP, Luypaerts A, Rutgeerts P, Verbeke K. Aliment Pharmacol Ther. 2003 Oct 1;18(7):721-9. PMID:14510746

[8] Results of small intestinal bacterial overgrowth testing in irritable bowel syndrome patients: clinical profiles and effects of antibiotic trial. Majewski M, McCallum RW. Adv Med Sci. 2007;52:139-42. PMID:18217406

[9] A link between irritable bowel syndrome and fibromyalgia may be related to findings on lactulose breath testing. Pimentel M, Wallace D, Hallegua D, Chow E, Kong Y, Park S, Lin HC. Ann Rheum Dis. 2004 Apr;63(4):450-2.PMID:15020342

[10] Small intestinal bacterial overgrowth in patients with irritable bowel syndrome. Posserud I, Stotzer PO, Björnsson ES, Abrahamsson H, Simrén M. Gut. 2007 Jun;56(6):802-8. PMID:17148502

[11] Results of small intestinal bacterial overgrowth testing in irritable bowel syndrome patients: clinical profiles and effects of antibiotic trial. Majewski M, McCallum RW. Adv Med Sci. 2007;52:139-42. PMID:18217406

[12] Small intestinal bacterial overgrowth: roles of antibiotics, prebiotics, and probiotics. Quigley EM, Quera R. Gastroenterology. 2006 Feb;130(2 Suppl 1):S78-90. PMID:16473077

[13] Small intestinal bacterial overgrowth in gastroparesis: are there any predictors? Reddymasu SC, McCallum RW. J Clin Gastroenterol. 2010 Jan;44(1):e8-13. PMID:20027008

[14] Serotonin and its role in colonic function and in gastrointestinal disorders. Costedio MM, Hyman N, Mawe GM. Dis Colon Rectum. 2007 Mar;50(3):376-88. PMID:17195902

[15] Melatonin and serotonin effects on gastrointestinal motility. Thor PJ, Krolczyk G, Gil K, Zurowski D, Nowak L. J Physiol Pharmacol. 2007 Dec;58 Suppl 6:97-103. PMID:18212403

[16] Melatonin and serotonin effects on gastrointestinal motility. Thor PJ, Krolczyk G, Gil K, Zurowski D, Nowak L. J Physiol Pharmacol. 2007 Dec;58 Suppl 6:97-103. PMID:18212403

[17] Endogenous glucagon-like peptide 1 controls endocrine pancreatic secretion and antro-pyloro-duodenal motility in humans. Schirra J, Nicolaus M, Roggel R, Katschinski M, Storr M, Woerle HJ, Göke B. Gut. 2006 Feb;55(2):243-51. PMID:15985560

[18] Endogenous CCK disrupts the MMC pattern via capsaicin-sensitive vagal afferent fibers in the rat. Rodríguez-Membrilla A, Vergara P. Am J Physiol. 1997 Jan;272(1 Pt 1):G100-5. PMID:9038882

[19] Role of clock genes in gastrointestinal motility. Hoogerwerf WA. Am J Physiol Gastrointest Liver Physiol. 2010 Sep;299(3):G549-55. PMID:20558764

[20] Circadian variation in the propagation velocity of the migrating motor complex. Kumar D, Wingate D, Ruckebusch Y. Gastroenterology. 1986 Oct;91(4):926-30. PMID:3743969

[21] Mechanism of interdigestive migrating motor complex in conscious dogs. Nakajima H, Mochiki E, Zietlow A, Ludwig K, Takahashi T. J Gastroenterol. 2010 May;45(5):506-14. PMID:20033824

[22] Relationship between interdigestive migrating motor complex and gut hormones in human. Tomita R. Hepatogastroenterology. 2009 May-Jun;56(91-92):714-7. PMID:19621688

[23] GLP-1 suppresses gastrointestinal motility and inhibits the migrating motor complex in healthy subjects and patients with irritable bowel syndrome. Hellström PM, Näslund E, Edholm T, Schmidt PT, Kristensen J, Theodorsson E, Holst JJ, Efendic S. Neurogastroenterol Motil. 2008 Jun;20(6):649-59. PMID:18298441

[24] GLP-1: broadening the incretin concept to involve gut motility. Hellström PM. Regul Pept. 2009 Aug 7;156(1-3):9-12. PMID:19362109

[25] Role of bile acids in duodenal migrating motor complexes in dogs. Kajiyama Y, Irie M, Enjoji A, Ozeki K, Ura K, Kanematsu T. Dig Dis Sci. 1998 Oct;43(10):2278-83. PMID:9790466

[26] Interdigestive and postprandial motility in small-intestinal bacterial overgrowth. Stotzer PO, Björnsson ES, Abrahamsson H. Scand J Gastroenterol. 1996 Sep;31(9):875-80. PMID:8888434

[27] Effect of casein and beta-casomorphins on gastrointestinal motility in rats. Daniel H, Vohwinkel M, Rehner G. J Nutr. 1990 Mar;120(3):252-7. PMID:2319342

[28] Opioid receptor ligands derived from food proteins. Teschemacher H. Curr Pharm Des. 2003;9(16):1331-44. PMID:12769741

[29] Small intestinal bacterial overgrowth: a comprehensive review. Dukowicz AC, Lacy BE, Levine GM. Gastroenterol Hepatol (N Y). 2007 Feb;3(2):112-22. PMID:21960820

[30] Increased incidence of small intestinal bacterial overgrowth during proton pump inhibitor therapy. Lombardo L, Foti M, Ruggia O, Chiecchio A. Clin Gastroenterol Hepatol. 2010 Jun;8(6):504-8. PMID:20060064

[31] Small intestinal bacterial overgrowth in patients suffering from scleroderma: clinical effectiveness of its eradication. Parodi A, Sessarego M, Greco A, Bazzica M, Filaci G, Setti M, Savarino E, Indiveri F, Savarino V, Ghio M. Am J Gastroenterol. 2008 May;103(5):1257-62. PMID:18422815

[32] Role of small intestinal bacterial overgrowth and delayed gastrointestinal transit time in cirrhotic patients with minimal hepatic encephalopathy. Gupta A, Dhiman RK, Kumari S, Rana S, Agarwal R, Duseja A, Chawla Y. J Hepatol. 2010 Nov;53(5):849-55. PMID:20675008

[33] Dose- and time-dependent biphasic response to morphine on intestinal migrating myoelectric complex. Sarna SK, Lang IM. J Pharmacol Exp Ther. 1985 Sep;234(3):814-20. PMID:2993596

[34] Myoelectric activity of the small intestine during morphine dependence and withdrawal in rats. Kuperman DA, Sninsky CA, Lynch DF. Am J Physiol. 1987 Apr;252(4 Pt 1):G562-7. PMID:3565571

[35] The role of interdigestive small bowel motility in the regulation of gut microflora, bacterial overgrowth, and bacterial translocation in rats. Nieuwenhuijs VB, Verheem A, van Duijvenbode-Beumer H, Visser MR, Verhoef J, Gooszen HG, Akkermans LM. Ann Surg. 1998 Aug;228(2):188-93. PMID:9712563

[36] Interdigestive small bowel motility and duodenal bacterial overgrowth in experimental acute pancreatitis. Van Felius ID, Akkermans LM, Bosscha K, Verheem A, Harmsen W, Visser MR, Gooszen HG. Neurogastroenterol Motil. 2003 Jun;15(3):267-76. PMID:12787336

[37] Proton pump inhibitor therapy does not affect hydrogen production on lactulose breath test in subjects with IBS. Law D, Pimentel M. Dig Dis Sci. 2010 Aug;55(8):2302-8. PMID:19834807

[38] Enteric dysbiosis associated with a mouse model of alcoholic liver disease. Yan AW, Fouts DE, Brandl J, Stärkel P, Torralba M, Schott E, Tsukamoto H, Nelson KE, Brenner DA, Schnabl B. Hepatology. 2011 Jan;53(1):96-105. PMID:21254165

[39] The effects of excitatory amino acids on isolated gut segments of the rat. Janković SM, Milovanović D, Matović M, Irić-Cupić V. Pharmacol Res. 1999 Feb;39(2):143-8. PMID:10072705

[40] Role of peripheral N-methyl-D-aspartate (NMDA) receptors in visceral nociception in rats. McRoberts JA, Coutinho SV, Marvizón JC, Grady EF, Tognetto M, Sengupta JN, Ennes HS, Chaban VV, Amadesi S, Creminon C, Lanthorn T, Geppetti P, Bunnett NW, Mayer EA. Gastroenterology. 2001 Jun;120(7):1737-48. PMID: 11375955

[41] Histamine in the nervous system. Haas HL, Sergeeva OA, Selbach O. Physiol Rev. 2008 Jul;88(3):1183-241. PMID:18626069

[42] Effects of the N-methyl-D-aspartate receptor on temporal summation of second pain (wind-up) in irritable bowel syndrome. Zhou Q, Price DD, Callam CS, Woodruff MA, Verne GN. J Pain. 2011 Feb;12(2):297-303. PMID:21146468

[43] Effects of the N-methyl-D-aspartate receptor antagonist dextromethorphan on temporal summation of pain are similar in fibromyalgia patients and normal control subjects. Staud R, Vierck CJ, Robinson ME, Price DD. J Pain. 2005 May;6(5):323-32. PMID:15890634

[44] Small intestinal bacterial overgrowth in rosacea: clinical effectiveness of its eradication. Parodi A, Paolino S, Greco A, Drago F, Mansi C, Rebora A, Parodi A, Savarino V. Clin Gastroenterol Hepatol. 2008 Jul;6(7):759-64. PMID:18456568

[45] Functional bowel disorders in rotating shift nurses may be related to sleep disturbances. Zhen Lu W, Ann Gwee K, Yu Ho K. Eur J Gastroenterol Hepatol. 2006 Jun;18(6):623-7. PMID:16702851

[46] Feeding cues alter clock gene oscillations and photic responses in the suprachiasmatic nuclei of mice exposed to a light/dark cycle. Mendoza J, Graff C, Dardente H, Pevet P, Challet E. J Neurosci. 2005 Feb 9;25(6):1514-22. PMID:15703405

[47] Restricted feeding uncouples circadian oscillators in peripheral tissues from the central pacemaker in the suprachiasmatic nucleus. Damiola F, Le Minh N, Preitner N, Kornmann B, Fleury-Olela F, Schibler U. Genes Dev. 2000 Dec 1;14(23):2950-61. PMID:11114885

[48] Effect of a phase advance and phase delay of the 24-h cycle on energy metabolism, appetite, and related hormones. Gonnissen HK, Rutters F, Mazuy C, Martens EA, Adam TC, Westerterp-Plantenga MS. Am J Clin Nutr. 2012 Oct;96(4):689-97. PMID:22914550

[49] Circadian aspects of postprandial metabolism. Morgan L, Hampton S, Gibbs M, Arendt J. Chronobiol Int. 2003 Sep;20(5):795-808. PMID:14535354

[50] The impact of the circadian timing system on cardiovascular and metabolic function. Morris CJ, Yang JN, Scheer FA. Prog Brain Res. 2012;199:337-58. PMID:22877674

[51] A meta-analysis on dose-response relationship between night shift work and the risk of breast cancer. Wang F, Yeung KL, Chan WC, Kwok CC, Leung SL, Wu C, Chan EY, Yu IT, Yang XR, Tse LA. Ann Oncol. 2013 Nov;24(11):2724-32. PMID:23975662

[52] Appetite-regulating hormones from the upper gut: disrupted control of xenin and ghrelin in night workers. Schiavo-Cardozo D, Lima MM, Pareja JC, Geloneze B. Clin Endocrinol (Oxf). 2012 Dec 1. PMID:23199168

[53] Circadian rhythm profiles in women with night eating syndrome. Goel N, Stunkard AJ, Rogers NL, Van Dongen HP, Allison KC, O'Reardon JP, Ahima RS, Cummings DE, Heo M, Dinges DF. J Biol Rhythms. 2009 Feb;24(1):85-94. PMID:19150931

[54] A tryptophan-rich breakfast and exposure to light with low color temperature at night improve sleep and salivary melatonin level in Japanese students. Wada K, Yata S, Akimitsu O, Krejci M, Noji T, Nakade M, Takeuchi H, Harada T. J Circadian Rhythms. 2013 May 25;11(1):4. PMID:23705838

[55] Evening intake of alpha-lactalbumin increases plasma tryptophan availability and improves morning alertness and brain measures of attention. Markus CR, Jonkman LM, Lammers JH, Deutz NE, Messer MH, Rigtering N. Am J Clin Nutr. 2005 May;81(5):1026-33. PMID:15883425

[56] Can breakfast tryptophan and vitamin B6 intake and morning exposure to sunlight promote morning-typology in young children aged 2 to 6 years? Nakade M, Akimitsu O, Wada K, Krejci M, Noji T, Taniwaki N, Takeuchi H, Harada T. J Physiol Anthropol. 2012 PMID:22738346

[57] Review of rifaximin as treatment for SIBO and IBS. Pimentel M. Expert Opin Investig Drugs. 2009 Mar;18(3):349-58. PMID: 19243285

[58] Bile acids improve the antimicrobial effect of rifaximin. Darkoh C, Lichtenberger LM, Ajami N, Dial EJ, Jiang ZD, DuPont HL. Antimicrob Agents Chemother. 2010 Sep;54(9):3618-24. PMID:20547807

[59] Prevalence of small intestinal bacterial overgrowth in children with irritable bowel syndrome: a case-control study. Scarpellini E, Giorgio V, Gabrielli M, Lauritano EC, Pantanella A, Fundarò C, Gasbarrini A. J Pediatr. 2009 Sep;155(3):416-20. PMID:19535093

[60] Double-blind, placebo-controlled antibiotic treatment study of small intestinal bacterial overgrowth in children with chronic abdominal pain. Collins BS, Lin HC. J Pediatr Gastroenterol Nutr. 2011 Apr;52(4):382-6. PMID:21240023

[61] Low-dose nocturnal tegaserod or erythromycin delays symptom recurrence after treatment of irritable bowel syndrome based on presumed bacterial overgrowth. Pimentel M, Morales W, Lezcano S, Sun-Chuan D, Low K, Yang J. Gastroenterol Hepatol (N Y). 2009 Jun;5(6):435-42. PMID:20574504

[62] Comparison between physiologic and erythromycin-induced interdigestive motility. Björnsson ES, Abrahamsson H. Scand J Gastroenterol. 1995 Feb;30(2):139-45. PMID:7732336

[63] The potential therapeutic effect of melatonin in Gastro-Esophageal Reflux Disease. Kandil TS, Mousa AA, El-Gendy AA, Abbas AM. BMC Gastroenterol. 2010 Jan 18;10:7. PMID:20082715

[64] Zinc salts provide a novel, prolonged and rapid inhibition of gastric acid secretion. Kirchhoff P, Socrates T, Sidani S, et al. Am J Gastroenterol. 2011 Jan;106(1):62-70. PMID:20736941

[65] Melatonin and serotonin effects on gastrointestinal motility. Thor PJ, Krolczyk G, Gil K, Zurowski D, Nowak L. J Physiol Pharmacol. 2007 Dec;58 Suppl 6:97-103. PMID:18212403

[66] Gut clock: implication of circadian rhythms in the gastrointestinal tract. Konturek PC, Brzozowski T, Konturek SJ. J Physiol Pharmacol. 2011 Apr;62(2):139-50. PMID:21673361

[67] Comparative clinical efficacy of a probiotic vs. an antibiotic in the treatment of patients with intestinal bacterial overgrowth and chronic abdominal functional distension: a pilot study. Soifer LO, Peralta D, Dima G, Besasso H. Acta Gastroenterol Latinoam. 2010 Dec;40(4):323-7. PMID:21381407

[68] Clinical trial: the combination of rifaximin with partially hydrolysed guar gum is more effective than rifaximin alone in eradicating small intestinal bacterial overgrowth. Furnari M, Parodi A, Gemignani L, Giannini EG, Marenco S, Savarino E, Assandri L, Fazio V, Bonfanti D, Inferrera S, Savarino V. Aliment Pharmacol Ther. 2010 Oct;32(8):1000-6. PMID:20937045

[69] Are rice and spicy diet good for functional gastrointestinal disorders? Gonlachanvit S. J Neurogastroenterol Motil. 2010 Apr;16(2):131-8. PMID:20535343

[70] Effects of chenodeoxycholate and a bile acid sequestrant, colesevelam, on intestinal transit and bowel function. Odunsi-Shiyanbade ST, Camilleri M, McKinzie S, Burton D, Carlson P, Busciglio IA, Lamsam J, Singh R, Zinsmeister AR. Clin Gastroenterol Hepatol. 2010 Feb;8(2):159-65. PMID:19879973

[71] Randomized, double-blinded, placebo-controlled study of effect of wheat bran fiber and calcium on fecal bile acids in patients with resected adenomatous colon polyps. Alberts DS, Ritenbaugh C, Story JA, Aickin M, Rees-McGee S, Buller MK, Atwood J, Phelps J, Ramanujam PS, Bellapravalu S, Patel J, Bextinger L, Clark L. J Natl Cancer Inst. 1996 Jan 17;88(2):81-92. PMID:8537982

[72] The role of small bowel bacterial overgrowth in infantile colic. Hochman JA, Simms C. J Pediatr. 2005 Sep;147(3):410-1. PMID:16182688

[73] Association between infantile colic and carbohydrate malabsorption from fruit juices in infancy. Duro D, Rising R, Cedillo M, Lifshitz F. Pediatrics. 2002 May;109(5):797-805. PMID:11986439

[74] Dietary treatment of colic caused by excess gas in infants: biochemical evidence. Infante D, Segarra O, Luyer BL. World J Gastroenterol. 2011 Apr 28;17(16):2104-8. PMID:21547129

[75] Intestinal microflora in breastfed colicky and non-colicky infants. Savino F, Cresi F, Pautasso S, Palumeri E, Tullio V, Roana J, Silvestro L, Oggero R. Acta Paediatr. 2004 Jun;93(6):825-9. PMID:15244234

[76] Bacterial counts of intestinal Lactobacillus species in infants with colic. Savino F, Bailo E, Oggero R, Tullio V, Roana J, Carlone N, Cuffini AM, Silvestro L. Pediatr Allergy Immunol. 2005 Feb;16(1):72-5. PMID:15693915

[77] Molecular identification of coliform bacteria from colicky breastfed infants. Savino F, Cordisco L, Tarasco V, Calabrese R, Palumeri E, Matteuzzi D. Acta Paediatr. 2009 Oct;98(10):1582-8. Epub 2009 Jul 9. PMID:19604166

[78] Antagonistic effect of Lactobacillus strains against gas-producing coliforms isolated from colicky infants. Savino F, Cordisco L, Tarasco V, Locatelli E, Di Gioia D, Oggero R, Matteuzzi D. BMC Microbiol. 2011 Jun 30;11:157. PMID:21718486

25. Leaky Gut Syndrome

Leaky gut syndrome is the common, and colorful, name for symptoms associated with an increased passage of large molecules between the enterocytes lining the intestine.

Typically, it refers to paracellular hyperpermeability of the small intestine. In this state, the tight junctions between the enterocytes fail to exclude large molecules that are normally kept out of the lamina propria of the small intestine.

The continuous layer of enterocytes lining the gastrointestinal tract forms a barrier between the external environment (the lumen of the intestine) and the organism. The enterocytes are bound together by tight junctions near the cells apices that limit passage of the intestinal contents within the intestinal lumen, through this barrier, to water and other small molecules.

The integrity of the enterocyte barrier is essential for health. If the barrier is incompetent, the immune cells of the gut can be inundated with non-pathogenic antigens, such as food proteins and form reactions to them. This can result in allergies and antergies to foods, the development of autoimmune disease, and the induction of mast cells activation disorders. Loss of the epithelial border competence can also allow exposure to viruses, bacteria, and bacterial toxins, food, contaminants and other molecules into the blood and lymphatics, which would normally be excluded or degraded by the enterocytes.

When the tight junctions open, due to physiologic stimulus, disease or toxins, larger molecules can pass between the cells. Incompetence of the paracellular tight junctions can allow passage of large molecule between the enterocytes. Disruption of the mucous layer overlaying the enterocytes can give bacteria abnormal access to the enterocytes, which may affect the tight junctions. For example, *Vibrio cholerae* secretes toxins including Zonula Occludens Toxin, which activates an intracellular pathway, in the enterocytes, that results in actinomycin contraction and production of a protein (zonulin). Zonulin opens the tight junctions and increases paracellular permeability.

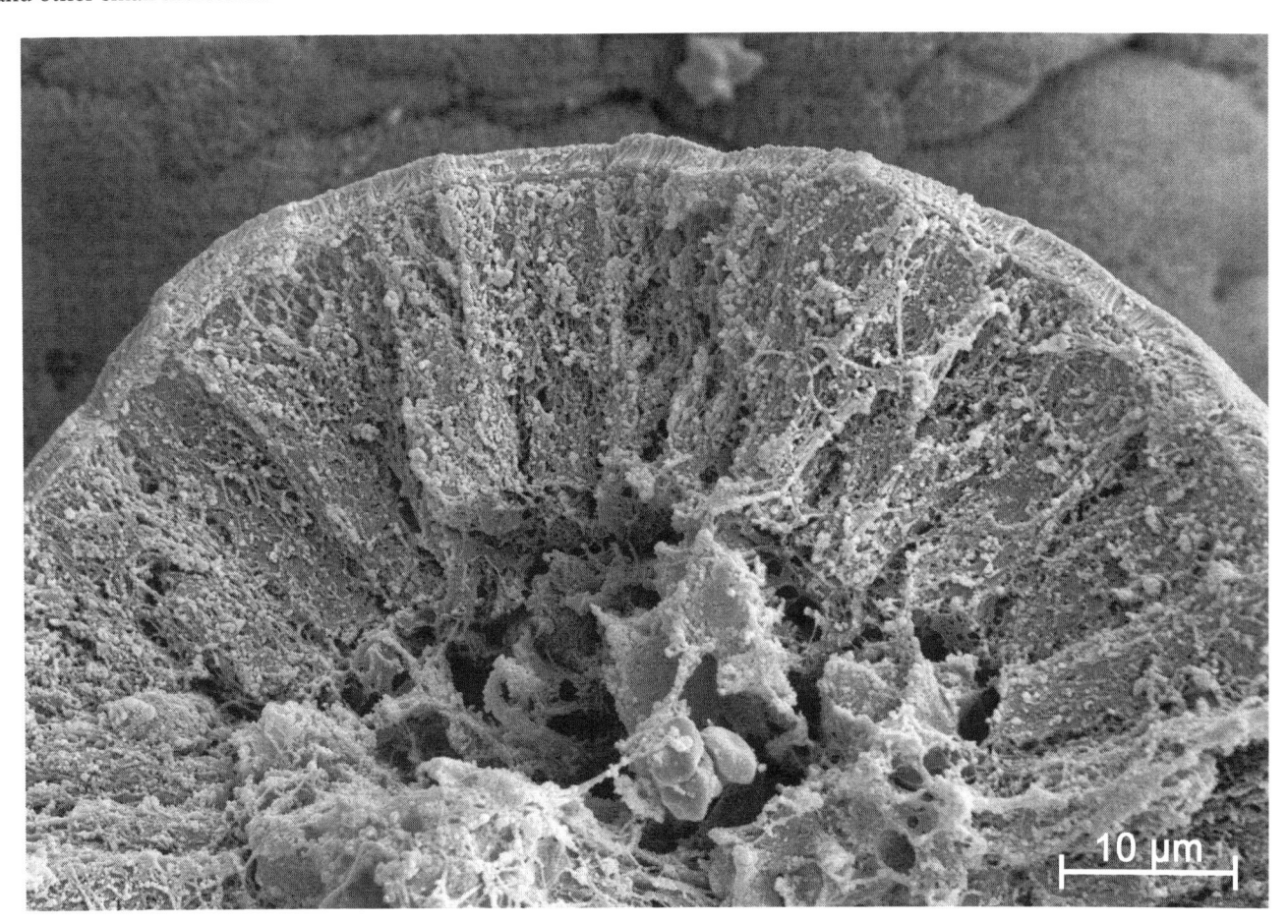

Figure 25-1: Electron Micrograph of the tip of an intestinal villus. The micrograph shows cross-sections of about a dozen enterocytes covered with microvilli. Tight junctions closely bind the apices of the cells together. Micrograph provided by courtesy of Tomsz Skrzypek, Ph.D., John Paul II Catholic University of Lublin.

The tight junctions surround the apex of the entire cell. These junctions are made up of at least 19 different proteins including zonulin, occludin, and claudins. These proteins link the cells like zip-locks so that only very tiny molecules can seep through. Humans have 24 different claudin genes. Claudin-15 is the one most highly expressed in the small intestine; claudin-4 and claudin-7 are highly expressed in the colon[1]. The presence of different claudin proteins, expressed by cells in various areas of the intestines and other tissues, allows various tissues to allow passage or blockage of various compounds.

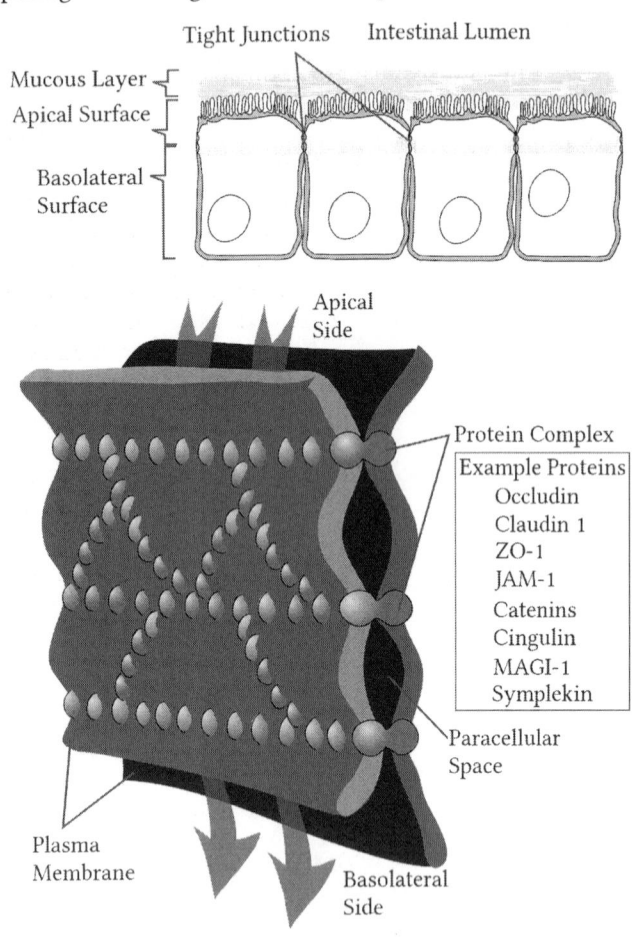

Figure 25-2: Tight Junctions[2]

These junctions are not static seals but rather dynamic; opening and closing according to regulation by cellular signaling. For nutrients to enter the body, they must pass through the enterocytes (transcellular absorption) or between the cells (paracellular absorption). Tight junctions can act as channels for absorption of molecules that are not soluble or don't have carriers to cross the enterocyte membrane, and open under certain conditions, allowing molecules to slip in. For example, after a meal where glucose is present the junctions will open some, under the influence of sodium-dependent glucose transport protein 1 (SGLT1). Actin fibrils in the enterocytes can pull the junctions open when stimulated. This permits an increased influx of water and other small molecules to enter the lamina propria during a time when sodium and glucose pumps have created a positive osmotic gradient. Thus, the space between cells is a regulated channel for absorption of nutrition. Milk proteins have been found to help close tight junctions, and this may have a beneficial effect on infants. Estrogen (estradiol) also decreases enterocyte paracellular permeability[3].

These channels are subject to pathological processes. Cholera toxins can hijack control over the tight junctions, adding to its virulence. Increased intestinal permeability, resulting from malfunction of the intra-enterocyte junctions, can result from dietary state, toxins, inflammatory mediators, mast cell products, neuronal or humoral signals, and viral or microbial pathogens. Genetic alterations of the occludin or claudin proteins can also affect their functions. Mast cell activation can also increase paracellular permeability. During anaphylaxis, large amounts of water leak into the bowel, causing cramping, diarrhea, and dehydration, and can contribute to shock.

Table 25-1: Examples of Factors that can Increase Intestinal Permeability

Nutrients (Functional)	Glucose, amino acids, mid-chain free fatty acids, oligosaccharides (benefits uptake of nutrients)
Bacterial toxins:	Cholera zonula occludens toxin (Zot) Toxins from *Bacteroides*, *Clostridium*[63] Lipopolysaccharides (LPS)[4]
Infections:	Bacteria (e.g.; *Campylobacter*) Viruses (e.g.; *Rotavirus*) Protozoa (e.g.; *Giardia*)
Stress Hormones	Corticotropin-releasing hormone (CRH)[5,6]
Cytokines	Tumor Necrosis Factor-alpha (TNF-α), Interferon-γ, IL-4
Medications:	Aspirin, non-steroidal anti-inflammatory medications (NSAIDs)[7], Cytotoxic drugs, Chemotherapeutics
Irritants and toxins:	Alcohol, Secondary Bile Acids, Carrageen, Dextrin sulfate[8]
Food Toxins:	Saponin, Pore Forming Protein (oyster mushrooms)[9] Lectins: Phytohemagglutinin and other toxic lectins[10] Glycoalkaloids: Poorly stored potatoes[11], eggplants Gliadin fragments
Injury	Burns to the skin[12] Heart failure (ischemia) Fracture[13]
Nutritional Deficiencies	Vitamin A[37] and zinc deficiencies[14]
Young Age	Infants, especially premature infants
Mast cell degranulation	Mast cell tryptase[15] Immune modulators and cytokines, histamine, other compounds
Disrupted Sleep Cycle	Increases CRH. Alters GI motility leading to SIBO
Oxidative Stress	Damages mucosa

> ### Bacterial Translocation
>
> Within a few hours of injury, bacteria from the gut can migrate from the bowel into the lamina propria of the intestine, into the lymphatic system[16], and into diverse organs[13]. Perhaps this is an adaptive process; an injured animal licks its wounds and swallows the bacteria from the contaminated wound. These bacteria can then be quickly presented to the immune system to help fight infection.
>
> A much more dangerous process is usually seen. Injury may induce bowel ischemia and inflammation, favoring pathogenic bacteria and production of LPS. In infants[17], immune-compromised patients, and hospitalized patients; for example, burn patients, bacterial translocation from the gut is the source of bacteria for bloodstream and blood-disseminated infections. Antibiotics used in these patients can kill beneficial bacteria that usually keep biofilm formation in check. Sessile bacteria may become more invasive as a result of toxin production.
>
> Upon entry to the lamina propria, most bacteria are phagocytized by macrophages. Most of those which escape are taken up by the mesenteric lymph nodes; however, bacteria can also pass into the peritoneum and into the bloodstream where they can cause and spread infection[18]. Hospitalized patients on parenteral nutrition (IV feeding) are also at increased risk for bacterial translocation and sepsis as dietary fiber, non-toxic food lectins and other nutrients, which help prevent biofilm formation and maintain the commensal *bifidobacteria* and *lactobacilli* in the gut, are not provided. Furthermore, glycine, a major fuel for distal small intestinal enterocytes, and short chain fatty acids, fuel for the colonocytes, are not available to the intestinal mucosa during parenteral nutrition, leaving these cells at increased susceptibility.

Mucosal injury and inflammatory reactions result when bacterial proteins gain access to the lamina propria of the intestinal mucosa, causing systemic inflammatory processes. The bacterial translocation from the lumen into the lamina propria is not required; inflammatory molecules from the bacteria are sufficient to cause systemic inflammation and mast cell activation (See Table 12-3).

Increased inter-enterocyte permeability has been found in patients, and family members of patients, with type 1 diabetes, Crohn's disease, autism, and gluten enteropathy[19]. One of the peptide fragments of gluten causes the release of zonulin, and thus, increases permeability not just for those with a genetic propensity for celiac disease, but for most animals[20]. Normally, only peptides smaller than about ten amino acids long can slip through the paracellular absorption pathway. The 33mer gluten peptide is a 33 amino acid chain that has must be presented as an antigen for development of anti-glutaminase antibodies.

Certain bacterial infections, notably *Campylobacter* infections, often precede the development of irritable bowel syndrome. Infection with this bacterium can increase paracellular permeability between enterocytes for up to a year after infection. *Helicobacter pylori*, the bacteria responsible for most peptic ulcer disease, increases permeability between the cells lining the stomach.

Increased intestinal permeability can allow the passage of incompletely digested dietary protein and peptide fragments, pieces of bacterial glycoproteins, and other molecules to enter the interior of the body where they are presented to the immune system. This can set up immune reactions.

Some toxins that open tight junctions on the enterocytes may have similar effects on tight junctions in other organs if the toxin gains access to the blood. This may include tight junctions of the blood-brain barrier, kidneys, and placenta, and thus allow compounds access to privileged areas they are usually excluded from. Different cell types have different claudins and may react specifically with various molecular compounds. The tight junctions of the enterocytes protect the body from the contents of the gut; the blood-brain barrier protects the brain from molecules that would affect its function. The placental barrier separates the mother's blood from that of the fetus. Antigens, toxins and other peptides and molecules can promote chemotaxis of mast cells into the intestinal endothelium, where they take up residence in the lamina propria of the villi. These mast cells are part of the immune system and can produce cytokines and other chemical mediators that affect health. The long-term stimulation of mast cell production increases the risk for development of mast cell activation disorders. (Chapter 12).

Most dietary protein is enzymatically degraded into oligopeptides or amino acids that are then absorbed. The peptides and some proteins are absorbed by endocytosis into the enterocytes, where they are degraded into amino acids by lysosomes within these cells. In this way, the proteins are degraded into non-immunogenic amino acids. A small percentage of proteins and peptides are transported intact through the M-cells that overlay the Peyer patches in the small intestine. These proteins are presented to the immune cells in the Peyer patches, which promote the development of T helper cells, usually either T_H17 or T_{REG} cells. Thus, this process acts in the development of sIgA, which neutralizes antigens and acts in the development of antigenic tolerance.

In normal conditions, the enterocytes form a well-regulated barrier which limits exposure of macromolecules and antigenic materials in the lumen of the gut to the immune cells of the intestine. Many other molecules which are absorbed by the enterocytes are broken down by intracellular enzymes; for example, histamine is absorbed and broken down by monoamine oxidase in the enterocytes.

PPAR-γ agonists can mitigate colonic inflammation and barrier dysfunction induced by stress, and mitigates the stress-induced decrease in IgA production[21]. PPAR-γ agonists are discussed in Chapter 31.

Abnormal function of the enterocyte barrier, with increased intestinal permeability has been found in many disease conditions. Table 25-2 lists several diseases that are associated with increased intestinal paracellular permeability (IIPP). The first group includes those in which IIPP is likely causal of the disease. The second group of conditions causes IIPP. Patients with autism and their family members have been found to be more likely to have IIPP; thus, this is likely part of the causal web for this disease. Vitamin A and Zinc deficiencies cause IIPP, as does H. pylori and some other infections, burns and head trauma.

Table 25-2: Diseases Associated with Increased Intestinal Paracellular Permeability (IIPP)

Conditions caused by IIPP	Diabetes[32,22] Obesity[23] Crohn's disease[24] Irritable bowel syndrome[25] Multiple sclerosis[26] Autism[27]
Conditions causing IIPP	Gluten enteropathy[28] Bacterial enteritis[29] Traumatic brain injury[30] Neonatal maternal deprivation[25*] Congestive heart failure[31] Portal hypertension (liver disease)[32] Rotavirus infection[33] Paracytic infections[34] Aspirin and NSAIDS[35] Alcohol abuse[32] Cancer chemotherapy[36] Vitamin A deficiency[37] Zinc deficiency[38] Oxidative stress[39] Helicobacter pylori infection[40] Severe burns[41]

IIPP can also be caused by losses or damage to the enterocytes. Some agents will denude the villi of enterocytes. More commonly, problems are caused by agents that increase paracellular permeability through their action on the tight junctions. Increased paracellular permeability can also permit bacterial translocation across the epithelial barrier, which can lead to systemic infection[42].

IIPP also acts in the pathogenesis of many other diseases. Impaired enterocyte and colonocytes membranes allow food and microbial antigens increased exposure to the immune cells of the lamina propria. This allows absorption of toxins, bioamines and other substances from the gut that are not absorbed by normal mucosa. IIPP is a contributing cause in the initiation and maintenance of mast cell, enteroimmune (Table 19-3) and autoimmune diseases (Table 33-1). These diseases include multiple sclerosis, type 1 diabetes, migraine, Parkinson's disease, schizophrenia and many other conditions.

Pathogenesis

Bacterial Toxins: The claudins are a class of proteins in the tight junction. During inflammation and in response to certain pathogens, claudin can be internalized by the cell; resulting in an increase in paracellular permeability. Several toxins have been found to induce claudin internalization; including H. Pylori associated factors, E. coli cytotoxic necrotizing factor-1 and *Clostridium perfringens* enterotoxin[43]. In small intestinal bacterial overgrowth (SIBO), there is a change from in bacterial populations, the numbers of *bifidobacteria* and *lactobacilli* falls and the number of pathogenic, toxin-producing bacteria that increase paracellular permeability rises. Biofilm formation is associated with IIPP[44]. LPS has been shown to increase paracellular permeability[22].

Cytokines: Cytokines induce production of claudins and impair the tight junction. IL-6 increases tight junction permeability by stimulating the expression of channel-forming claudin-2[45]. Interleukin-1β also increases intestinal paracellular permeability. Yet another inflammatory cytokine, TNF-α, promotes a significant increase in claudin-1 expression and tight junction dysfunction. Inflammation is also associated with a decrease production of the tight junction (TJ) proteins ZO-1 and occludin[46]. Thus, inflammatory processes that increase production of these cytokines cause IIPP.

Oxidative Stress: Oxidative stress can also increase paracellular permeability, not only between enterocytes but also in many other tissues, including the brain, lung, kidneys and bladder, as a result of its effects on the tight junction protein claudin[47]. Oxidative stress induces increased gastric paracellular permeability by its action on claudin-3[48]. Aspirin increases gastric paracellular permeability by inhibiting the production of claudin-7[49]. Oxidative damage diminishes claudin-2 in the lung[50].

Zinc Deficiency: Zinc increases the expression of the tight junction proteins occludin and ZO-1[51]. Zinc supplements reduce the incidence and severity of diarrheal disease in children. In one study, zinc supplements (20 for 10 – 14 days), lowered the risk of diarrhea in children for three months[52]. Oxidative stress from alcohol depletes free zinc availability, resulting in zinc deprivation and epithelial barrier disruption[53].

Alcohol: Not only does alcohol induce IIPP, this increase in permeability allows entry of endotoxins that promote alcoholic liver disease[54]. Exposure to alcohol may affect which claudins are expressed by the cells, and this affects

---

* Neonatal Maternal Deprivation is an epigenetic condition which is produced in rats by separating from their mothers for a few hours daily in the first 2 weeks of life. These animals have an accentuated reaction to stress throughout their lives.

their function and epithelial permeability[55]. Alcohol can increase permeability six-fold. Interestingly, this increased permeability is mediated by proteins that help control the circadian rhythm. This provides direct evidence that the circadian genes participate in the regulation of intestinal permeability[56].

In the respiratory system, an increase in paracellular permeability between alveolar cells can increase exposure to allergens and may increase the risk of asthma. Alcohol increases this permeability in the lung. Claudins may also be induced by injury[57] as a protective mechanism.

Airborne Hazard

The epithelial cells lining the airways have tight junctions between cells, very similar to those in the intestines. Dust mite turds are sufficiently small to become easily airborne and small enough to get deep into the lungs. These fecal pellets contain a proteolytic enzyme that breaks down the protein occludin. Occludin holds the tight junctions of the respiratory mucosa together, allowing the fecal pellet antigens (Der p 1) to pass between the cells. Sensitization occurs after dendritic cells in the lungs that pick up these antigens move to the lymph nodes and present the mite enzyme to T_H2 cells. The T_H2 cells activate B cells to make specific IgE antibodies to Der p 1 antigen. These IgE antibodies attach to mast cells in the lungs and other areas of the body. When more Der p 1 gets into the airway and gets past the tight junction, preformed-IgE on mast cells bind to the proteolytic enzyme in the dust mite turds, triggering degranulation that can result in an asthmatic reaction.

Another agent that can cause increased IIPP is zonula occludens toxin (Zot), one of the several toxins produced by the pathogen *Vibrio cholera*. It is not the toxin that causes the profuse watery diarrhea, but rather another toxin that provides increased virulence. Zot toxin was instrumental in understanding how the tight junctions act; as it causes the temporary opening of the tight junctions in certain areas of the small intestine.

Gliadin: Gliadin, one of the subunits of the protein gluten from wheat (as well as in barley and rye), is an example of a protein that can affect the enterocyte tight junctions. Specific peptides resulting from digestive enzymatic cleavage of gliadin (amino acid peptides 31-43 and 57-89) trigger the release of the peptide zonulin from the apical surface of the enterocyte[58]. These peptides act as agonists on the CXCR3 chemokine receptor that is present on the surface of the enterocyte and also on lymphocytes. This activation promotes the release of the protein zonulin from the enterocyte luminal surface. Zonulin shares an N-terminal, eight amino acid sequence with Cholera Zonula Occludens toxin which triggers the disassembly of the tight junctions between the surrounding cells. This allows the entry of other peptides into the lamina propria, where they are taken up by dendritic cells and presented as antigens to the lymphocytic immune cells of the gut[59]. Here they induce cytokine release and the development of antibody production[58].

Other peptide fragments from gliadin can also cause CXCR3 activation on immune cells, and these also promote the production of multiple inflammatory cytokines, including IL-6, TNF-α, and INF-γ. The immune reaction by gliadin peptide fragments is enhanced in individuals with celiac disease, and production of the cytokine IL-8 is especially elevated in this population[58]. The 33mer gliadin peptide, aa57–89, is associated with anti-transglutaminase antibody production.

Gliadin fragment-induced release of zonulin does not just cause gluten enteropathy; it participates in the pathology of Type 1 Diabetes (T1D) and other autoimmune diseases[60]. The gluten fragment opens the tight junction and allows passage of other antigens that induce other diseases. Immune reactions to milk proteins, for example, are thought to induce the autoimmune destruction of pancreatic β-cells T1D. The specific susceptibility of the individual to different antigens involves their HLA type and other genetic traits.

Phytohemagglutinin: Under-cooked kidney beans contain the toxic lectin, phytohemagglutinin, which causes rapid growth cycling of the enterocytes, and early loss of these cells before they reach the tip of the villi. There is not only a loss of cell coverage, but the immature cells also produce less brush border digestive enzymes. Goblet cells are also affected and may "burnout" and fail to produce protective mucin, allowing bacterial adherence to the enterocytes, overgrowth, biofilm formation, and translocation. Other toxic lectins may have similar effects (See Chapter 7 on proteins).

CRH: Corticotropin-Releasing Hormone (CRH) is a peptide hormone secreted by the paraventricular nucleus of the hypothalamus in response to stress. CRH modulates the stress response. It triggers the formation of proopiomelanocortin; that is cleaved into ACTH, as well as β-endorphin, α-MSH, and β-MSH in the pineal gland. ACTH stimulates the adrenal cortex to produce cortisone and other steroid hormones. CRH is also produced by T-lymphocytes, the placenta, and mucosal crypt cells of the colon. Both CRH receptors; CRHR1 and CRHR2, are expressed in the GI tract.

Both physical and psychological stresses promote enterocyte paracellular permeability via CRH. CRH induces the release of Nerve Growth Factor (NGF), and likely other mediators, from colonic mast cells that increase enterocyte paracellular permeability[25].

Maternal deprivation, or stress at an early age in animals, can induce a significant increase of CRF, CRHR1, and CRHR2 mRNA expression in the adrenal cortex, a decrease in CRHR1 and CRHR2 mRNA expression in the amygdala, and an increase in the number of mast cells in the hypothalamus. This effect makes the animal more sensitive to stress hormones into adulthood[25], and thus, increase the risk of IIPP resulting from various stressors.

Mast Cells: The hormone neurotensin (NT) is released from neuroendocrine cells of the gut by ingestion of fat. NT helps in the early absorption of fat by facilitating the uptake of the bile acid taurocholate through the mucosa of the proximal small intestine. This early absorption of fat may be used as a signal affecting satiety or preparing the body for a fat load that will soon be absorbed by the ileum.

NT acts by stimulating mast cells degranulation. Mast cell products mediate the uptake of the bile acid taurocholate in the jejunum by opening tight junctions and increasing paracellular permeability in the jejunum. These effects appear to be mediated by the release of histamine and the leukotriene, LTC_4. NT induced uptake of taurocholate can be impeded by the use of the anti-leukotriene medication zileuton and by the H_1 blocker diphenhydramine[61].

Mast Cell Activation Disorders: Mast cell activation increases paracellular permeability in pathological conditions including food allergy, IgG_4, stress, enteritis, and ischemia. Nitric oxide (NO) at the levels normally produced by the intestinal epithelium help to maintain the epithelial barrier, whereas the excessive NO released by inflammatory cells can damage the epithelial barrier. Normal levels of NO stabilize the mucosal mast cells, inhibiting mast cell activation[61].

The substrate for NO synthase is L-arginine. Nitric oxide synthase is unusual in that it requires six cofactors. These include tetrahydrobiopterin (BH4), NADPH, FAD, FMN, heme, and calmodulin. The dietary factors which support nitric oxide synthase are the B vitamins, niacin, riboflavin and folate, and the minerals iron, magnesium, zinc, and calcium. Folate (especially 5-methyltetrahydrofolate; 5-MTHF) helps to recycle BH4. Magnesium is a cofactor for several enzymes involving NADPH recycling. Vitamin C protects the endothelial barrier as a cofactor in NO protection of the endothelium[62]. Elevated uric acid levels impair the production of NO; thus a high fructose diet and alcohol impair NO production. (See Chapter 9: Metabolic Syndrome.)

Table 25-3: Cofactors for Nitric Oxide Synthase

NO Synthase Substrate and Cofactors	Nutrient Cofactor
Substrate:	L-Arginine
Tetrahydrobiopterin (BH4)	Folate (5-MTHF), Zinc, Iron, Niacin
NADPH	Niacin, Magnesium
FAD, FMN	Riboflavin, Magnesium, Zinc
Heme	Iron
Calmodulin	Calcium
Required for NO action on epithelial barrier	Vitamin C

SIBO and inflammation can increase the number of mast cells in the lamina propria of the intestine, causing mast cell hypertrophy. This may increase the risk for mast cell activation disorders (See Chapter 12).

More than 50 different autoimmune diseases are associated with HLA class I and class II histocompatibility antigens. Individuals with who carry certain HLA types are at greatly increased risk for these diseases. HLA antigens are important in immune recognition to prevent the immune system from recognizing self-epitopes on cells as foreign antigens, and thus prevent autoimmunity. When the enterocyte barrier is compromised, food proteins and peptides are presented as antigens that may cross-react with self-antigens. This can result in autoimmune disease where the immune system attacks host cells. Thus, susceptibility to the disease depends on the individual's HLA type and exposure to an antigen that cross-reacts with it. Several autoimmune diseases follow intestinal exposure to antigens through a compromised enterocyte barrier[63].

Usual Requirements for Autoimmune Disease:

1. Genetic Susceptibility (HLA type)

2. Antigen that cross-reacts with self-antigen (often dietary protein but may be ingested pollen, bacteria, yeast, or another antigen)

3. Presentation of the antigen to gut immune cells; often as a result of a compromised epithelial barrier and paracellular exposure. Some proteins may be presented through endocytosis.

NSAIDs: Aspirin and NSAID medications increase enterocyte paracellular permeability, perhaps by inhibiting the production of PGE_2, which promotes increased mucous production. A second mechanism may be the diversion of the eicosanoid pathway away from prostaglandin formation by COX1 inhibition, and towards increased production of leukotrienes (see Chapter 15).

Summary

When the enterocyte barrier is compromised, it allows larger molecules to gain access to the lamina propria of the intestine, thus gaining direct access to immune cells or absorption into the blood stream. Damage to the enterocyte monolayer can also be accompanied by loss of enterocyte surface enzymes, including disaccharidases, dipeptidases, and diamine oxidase. Intracellular proteolytic enzymes are also lost with the loss of the enterocytes. Loss of proteolytic enzymes and peptidases increases the risk for immunogenic peptides to be available for immune presentation

A compromised intestinal mucosa can allow access of multiple antigens to the enteric immune system and thus allow the passage of food toxins, such as bioamines and bioactive peptides, and bacterial toxins, such as LPS, into the blood stream. Low levels of bioactive amines, which are normally broken down with an intact mucosal barrier, may cause symptoms when the barrier is compromised. Food allergies and antergies are much more likely to develop when the enteric immune system is inundated with food proteins. IgA normally binds to enteric bacteria and neutralizes them, thus preventing an inflammatory response. Loss of IgA, resulting from the loss of the mucus layer to which it normally binds, disrupted enterocyte function, or decreased production, can increase the inflammatory response to bacteria and other antigens in the gut.

Testing for Increased Intestinal Permeability

Lactulose-mannitol test: The lactulose-mannitol test can be used to test for small intestinal hyperpermeability. In this test, a fasting patient is given a drink containing equal amounts of lactulose and mannitol, and their urine is collected over the following six hours. These sugars are not metabolized. The amount that is absorbed should appear in the urine within 6 hours. Mannitol, a monosaccharide, passively diffuses between intact enterocytes, but lactulose is a larger molecule, and little is absorbed if the mucosa is intact. About 14 percent of the mannitol is absorbed by healthy mucosa; however, less than half of one percent of lactulose should be absorbed. Less than three percent as much lactulose as mannitol should appear in the urine if the mucosal barrier is intact.

If less mannitol is absorbed, it may indicate carbohydrate malabsorption.

Sucrose absorption test: The sucrose absorption test can be used to test for abnormal permeability of the stomach and duodenum. Sucrose is not normally absorbed intact. Sucrose, table sugar, is broken down by disaccharidases (oligo-1,6-glucosidase and sucrose alpha-glucosidase) present in the small intestine; if these enzymes are active, there should be very little sucrose absorbed below the duodenum, even if there is increased paracellular permeability. If sucrose is absorbed, it indicates absorption above the jejunum. Sucrose found in a five-hour urine collection following a test dose of sucrose indicates increased permeability in the stomach and or duodenum.

Treating Paracellular Hyperpermeability

Treatment for prevention or recovery from food associated pathologies should provide assurance that the enterocyte membrane is functioning normally. The first step in the treatment of paracellular hyperpermeability is to reverse the underlying causes: eliminate irritants, toxins, and deficiencies, and treat any infections.

1. Gliadin: Eliminate gliadin from the diet: worldwide, wheat is mankind's most highly consumed plant protein; this, however, does not make it safe. Rather, it makes diseases caused by it common.

2. Treat Dysbiosis: Lipopolysaccharides produced by pathogenic bacterial biofilms strongly increase paracellular permeability. Certain other bacterial toxins additionally impair the patency of the enterocyte membrane. Preventing dysbiosis and biofilm formation are essential to the maintenance of a healthy enterocyte membrane. Treat infections and bacterial overgrowth. Antibiotics may be used for a rapid response, but prebiotics and probiotics help restore eubiosis. Prebiotics were found, in an animal model, to alter gut microbiota, decrease inflammatory stress, and improve tight junction function through a GLP-2 mediated mechanism[64]. Prebiotic foods are needed for sustained integrity of the mucosal barrier (Chapter 4.) Testing for fecal chymotrypsin or elastase levels and treating with pancreatic enzymes when low is often helpful in treating dysbiosis and preventing toxin formation. See Chapter 23 on Biofilms and Dysbiosis.

3. Avoid producing TNF-α: TNF-α greatly increases paracellular permeability. TNF-α formation can be prevented by avoiding dysbiosis, as well as by many dietary bioflavonoids (Table 15-4), certain medications, and other compounds. Mitigation of TNF-α is discussed in treatment item 10 in Chapter 23.

4. Avoid Malabsorption: Avoid poorly absorbed foods that promote small intestinal bacterial overgrowth, such as milk in lactose intolerant individuals, and high-fructose diets in individuals with fructose malabsorption.

5. Secondary Bile Acids: Prevent secondary bile acid formation by preventing malabsorption syndromes and bacterial overgrowth. Secondary bile acid accumulation can be treated with bile acid sequestrants which will eliminate them. See Item 5 Chapter 26.

6. Immune Reactants: Avoid foods to which there are allergies or antergies. Not only IgE, but other antibodies, including IgG_4, can also trigger mast cell degranulation. See Chapters 11 and 19.

7. Avoid Mast Cell Degranulation. See Chapter 14.

8. Treat Mast Cell Activation Disorders: Antihistamines, for example, Zyrtec and Pepcid (cetirizine and famotidine) help to avoid some of the effects of histamine release from mast cells and basophils. It is sometimes more effective to use both an H_1 and an H_2 blocker. Famotidine is preferred H_2 blocker as it does not inhibit the enzyme ALDH. Anti-leukotriene medications and mast cell stabilizers are also sometimes helpful. See Chapter 12.

9. Avoid aspirin and nonsteroidal anti-inflammatory medications: If an anti-inflammatory is required, a cyclooxygenase 2 inhibitor, such as celecoxib, which also inhibits ALOX-5 and leukotriene formation, is preferable. Table 15-4 in Chapter 15 lists some foods, high in flavonoids, which also inhibit ALOX-5 and leukotriene production.

10. Avoid alcohol: If alcohol is to be used, it should be limited to red wine in small amounts. See Chapter 17.

11. Treat Nutritional Deficiencies: The fat-soluble vitamins (A, D, E, and K) can be depleted in malabsorption conditions and with chronic diarrhea where there is a rapid small intestinal transit time. Magnesium, folate and zinc and vitamin B_{12} may also be wasted. Treat nutritional deficiencies, especially vitamin A using β-carotene (see Chapter 39) and zinc, which are essential for tight junction function.

Zinc supplementation may improve enterocyte barrier. A reasonable supplement for adults with malabsorption or compromised enterocyte barrier is 25 mg of zinc, daily for two weeks, followed by 10 mg a day, taken with meals.

NO production is dependent on several cofactors and sufficient supply of L-arginine. The diet should supply sufficient folate and vitamin C, 5-methyltetrahydrofolate, tetrahydrobiopterin (THB). Supplements may be helpful in some cases[65]. Endogenous production of THB requires the cofactors folate, zinc, iron and niacin. Supplements of N-acetyl cysteine may help speed recovery of mucous production in patients with a compromised enterocyte barrier or damage to goblet cells.

12. Avoid Oxidative Stress: Many foods with phenolic compounds have antioxidant activates. These compounds may not need to be absorbed by the body to provide benefit. First, they protect the food from forming toxic peroxides. Additionally, they may protect the enterocytes from oxidative compounds formed in the lumen of the intestine. Fermentation of polyphenolic compounds frees phenolics for absorption, whether the fermentation occurs in the wine vat or in the colon.

Isothiocyanates in garlic and broccoli, for example, increase the transcription of antioxidant enzymes – this is the major antioxidant effect by which food decreases the risk of cancer and other diseases.

Old, worn-out mitochondria increase the production of ROS. Mitochondria can be renewed with exercise and diet (Chapter 21). Chronic inflammation and alcohol create oxidative stress.

Melatonin is an important endogenous antioxidant for the GI system which helps to protect the mucosa[66]. A dose of 3 mg of melatonin at bedtime has been found to have a therapeutic effect on the GI system, helping to heal mucosa.

13. Breastfeed Infants: Infants are born with high intestinal permeability. Breast milk helps develop the mucosal barrier and a commensal intestinal microbiota. Breast milk contains polyamines, spermidine, spermine, and putrescine, present in human and other mammalian milks, aid in growth and maturation factors for the GI system[67] and help with the development of the mucosal barrier. This may decrease the risk for development of food allergies[68]. It is preferable to breastfeed infants exclusively for at least four months and to continue breastfeeding at least into the 9th month of life. Avoid the introduction of gliadin (wheat, barley, and rye) and cow's milk until the infant is four to six months old, and then give small amounts, skipping days (See Chapter 11.)

14. Avoid Emotional Stress: Emotional stress can impair the intestinal barrier through the effects of CRH. Be especially nice to babies and pregnant women. Maternal stress and stress on infants can increase the reaction to stress for the child's entire lifetime. See stress and epigenetics in Chapter 29.

15. Dietary Polyamines: Dietary polyamines may be helpful for the maintenance and restoration of the enterocyte barrier in adults, especially spermadine. Diets rich in vegetables, fruits, and legumes should supply plenty of polyamines (Table 13-10.)

16. PPAR-γ agonists: Agents that activate PPAR-γ may help normalized the enteric barrier, as well as those of the CNS. Natural PPAR-γ agonists include the n-3 fatty acid DHA. PPAR-γ agonists are discussed in Chapter 31.

17. Treat Hyperuricemia if Present: Hyperuricemia is a risk factor for diabetes, but also for IIPP by impairing NO production. Avoid hyperuricemia by limiting the intake of alcohol and fructose in the diet. See Chapter 9.

18. Consume a Varied Diet: The flavonoid polyphenol quercetin has been shown to upregulate the protein claudin-4 within the epithelial tight junction[69]. Flavonoids have been found to mitigate the induction of inflammatory cytokines by of LPS. Foods especially rich in quercetin include dark chocolate, capers, oregano, red onions, shallots and orange juice.

Polyphenols and lectins in fruits and vegetables can help control the formation of biofilms and the production of virulence factors that increase IPP. A mix of foods high in polyphenols is essential to a healthy diet. See Chapter 23 on Biofilms.

19. Potatoes: Potatoes should be avoided in individuals with increased intracellular permeability and especially in patients with Inflammatory Bowel Disease; (see Box: "Potatoes and IBD," Chapter 33.) Potatoes contain glycoalkaloids that can increase intracellular permeability. The glycoalkaloid content of potatoes can be minimized by using freshly harvested potatoes, peeling the potatoes and discarding the skins, by boiling rather frying the potatoes, and discarding damaged tubers or tubers with a greenish tint to the skin or area below the skin. Eggplants also contain toxic glycoalkaloids, especially in the skin, and should also be avoided. Lectins in potatoes may increase mast cell degranulation which increases intestinal intracellular permeability in atrophic individuals or individuals with MACD. See Chapter 14 for mast cell degranulation agents.

Some toxic lectins, such as those in beans, cause a rapid turnover of enterocytes, and loss of coverage of the villi. Cooking beans in boiling temperatures degrades the lectins, while lower temperatures do not. Cooking beans in a pressure cooker completely degrades phytohemagglutinin.

20. Sleep In sleep deprivation, there is an increase in inflammatory cytokine production which would favor tight junction dysfunction. Cytokine production in sleep deprivation is discussed in detail in Chapter 41.

21. Other Organs may be Affected: Keep in mind that agents which increase enterocyte paracellular permeability may also increase intracellular permeability in the brain, bladder, placenta, kidneys, lungs and other organs.

[1] BioGPS at biogps.gnf.org

[2] Illustration by Mariana Ruiz Villarreal

[3] Oestradiol decreases colonic permeability through oestrogen receptor beta-mediated up-regulation of occludin and junctional adhesion molecule-A in epithelial cells. Braniste V, Leveque M, Buisson-Brenac C, Bueno L, Fioramonti J, Houdeau E. J Physiol. 2009 Jul 1;587(Pt 13):3317-28. PMID:19433574

[4] Paracellular permeability is increased by basal lipopolysaccharide in a primary culture of colonic epithelial cells; an effect prevented by an activator of Toll-like receptor-2. Hanson PJ, Moran AP, Butler K. Innate Immun. 2011;17(3):269-82. PMID:20472611

[5] Pathways involved in gut mucosal barrier dysfunction induced in adult rats by maternal deprivation: corticotrophin-releasing factor and nerve growth factor interplay. Barreau F, Cartier C, Leveque M, et al. J Physiol. 2007 Apr 1;580(Pt 1):347-56. PMID:17234701

[6] Corticotropin releasing factor signaling in colon and ileum: regulation by stress and pathophysiological implications. Larauche M, Kiank C, Tache Y. J Physiol Pharmacol. 2009 Dec;60 Suppl 7:33-46. PMID: 20388944

[7] Correlation between cyclical epithelial barrier dysfunction and bacterial translocation in the relapses of intestinal inflammation. Porras M, Martín MT, Yang PC, Jury J, Perdue MH, Vergara P. Inflamm Bowel Dis. 2006 Sep;12(9):843-52.PMID: 16954803

[8] Bacteria penetrate the inner mucus layer before inflammation in the dextran sulfate colitis model. Johansson ME, Gustafsson JK, Sjöberg KE, Petersson J, Holm L, Sjövall H, Hansson GC. PLoS One. 2010 Aug 18;5(8):e12238.PMID: 20805871

[9] Interaction between food substances and the intestinal epithelium. Shimizu M. Biosci Biotechnol Biochem. 2010;74(2):232-41. Epub 2010 Feb 7. Review.PMID: 20139625

[10] Modulation of immune function by dietary lectins in rheumatoid arthritis. Cordain L, Toohey L, Smith MJ, Hickey MS. Br J Nutr. 2000 Mar;83(3):207-17. PMID:10884708

[11] Potato glycoalkaloids adversely affect intestinal permeability and aggravate inflammatory bowel disease. Patel B, Schutte R, Sporns P, Doyle J, Jewel L, Fedorak RN. Inflamm Bowel Dis. 2002 Sep;8(5):340-6. PMID:12479649

[12] Commensal microflora induce host defense and decrease bacterial translocation in burn mice through toll-like receptor 4. Chen LW, Chang WJ, Chen PH, Hsu CM. J Biomed Sci. 2010 Jun 12;17:48. PMID:20540783

[13] Bacterial translocation from the gastrointestinal tract in healthy and injured rats. Nikitenko VI, Stadnikov AA, Kopylov VA. J Wound Care. 2011 Mar;20(3):114-22. PMID:21537294

[14] Zinc deficiency induces membrane barrier damage and increases neutrophil transmigration in Caco-2 cells. Finamore A, Massimi M, Conti Devirgiliis L, Mengheri E. J Nutr. 2008 Sep;138(9):1664-70.PMID: 18716167

[15] Mast cell tryptase controls paracellular permeability of the intestine. Role of protease-activated receptor 2 and beta-arrestins. Jacob C, Yang PC, Darmoul D, et al. J Biol Chem. 2005 Sep 9;280(36):31936-48. PMID:16027150

[16] Role of lymphatics in bacterial translocation from intestine in burn rats. Feng YQ, Wang DC, Wang K, Leng XF, Xiao H, Guo DF. Zhonghua Shao Shang Za Zhi. 2011 Feb;27(1):49-53. PMID:21591343

[17] Procession to pediatric bacteremia and sepsis: covert operations and failures in diplomacy. Bateman SL, Seed PC. Pediatrics. 2010 Jul;126(1):137-50. PMID:20566606

[18] Review article: bacterial translocation in the critically ill--evidence and methods of prevention. Gatt M, Reddy BS, MacFie J. Aliment Pharmacol Ther. 2007 Apr 1;25(7):741-57. PMID:17373913

[19] Alterations in intestinal permeability. Arrieta MC, Bistritz L, Meddings JB.Gut. 2006 Oct;55(10):1512-20. PMID: 16966705

[20] Gliadin induces an increase in intestinal permeability and zonulin release by binding to the chemokine receptor CXCR3. Lammers KM, Lu R, Brownley J, et al. Gastroenterology. 2008 Jul;135(1):194-204.e3. PMID:18485912

[21] The role of PPARgamma on restoration of colonic homeostasis after experimental stress-induced inflammation and dysfunction. Ponferrada A, Caso JR, Alou L, et al. Gastroenterology. 2007 May;132(5):1791-803. PMID:17484875

[22] De novo lipogenesis maintains vascular homeostasis through endothelial nitric-oxide synthase (eNOS) palmitoylation. Wei X, Schneider JG, Shenouda SM, Lee A, Towler DA, Chakravarthy MV, Vita JA, Semenkovich CF. J Biol Chem. 2011 Jan 28;286(4):2933-45. PMID:21098489

[23] Changes in gut microbiota control metabolic endotoxemia-induced inflammation in high-fat diet-induced obesity and diabetes in mice. Cani PD, Bibiloni R, Knauf C, Waget A, Neyrinck AM, Delzenne NM, Burcelin R. Diabetes. 2008 Jun;57(6):1470-81. PMID:18305141

[24] Gut permeability to lactulose and mannitol differs in treated Crohn's disease and celiac disease patients and healthy subjects. Vilela EG, Torres HO, Ferrari ML, Lima AS, Cunha AS. Braz J Med Biol Res. 2008 Dec;41(12):1105-9. PMID:19148373

[25] Pathways involved in gut mucosal barrier dysfunction induced in adult rats by maternal deprivation: corticotrophin-releasing factor and nerve growth factor interplay. Barreau F, Cartier C, Leveque M, Ferrier L, Moriez R, Laroute V, Rosztoczy A, Fioramonti J, Bueno L. J Physiol. 2007 Apr 1;580(Pt 1):347-56. PMID:17234701

[26] Multiple sclerosis patients have peripheral blood CD45RO+ B cells and increased intestinal permeability. Yacyshyn B, Meddings J, Sadowski D, Bowen-Yacyshyn MB. Dig Dis Sci. 1996 Dec;41(12):2493-8. PMID:9011463

[27] Alterations of the intestinal barrier in patients with autism spectrum disorders and in their first-degree relatives. de Magistris L, Familiari V, Pascotto A, et al. J Pediatr Gastroenterol Nutr. 2010 Oct;51(4):418-24. PMID:20683204

[28] A comparison of antibody testing, permeability testing, and zonulin levels with small-bowel biopsy in celiac disease patients on a gluten-free diet. Duerksen DR, Wilhelm-Boyles C, Veitch R, Kryszak D, Parry DM. Dig Dis Sci. 2010 Apr;55(4):1026-31. PMID:19399613

[29] Increased rectal mucosal enteroendocrine cells, T lymphocytes, and increased gut permeability following acute Campylobacter enteritis and in post-dysenteric irritable bowel syndrome. Spiller RC, Jenkins D, Thornley JP, Hebden JM, Wright T, Skinner M, Neal KR. Gut. 2000 Dec;47(6):804-11. PMID:11076879

[30] Splanchnic ischemia and gut permeability after acute brain injury secondary to intracranial hemorrhage. Hernández G, Hasbun P, Velasco N, Wainstein C, Bugedo G, Bruhn A, Klaassen J, Castillo L. Neurocrit Care. 2007;7(1):40-4. PMID:17603761

[31] Altered intestinal function in patients with chronic heart failure. Sandek A, Bauditz J, Swidsinski A, et al. J Am Coll Cardiol. 2007 Oct 16;50(16):1561-9. PMID:17936155

[32] Intestinal permeability in patients with chronic liver diseases: Its relationship with the aetiology and the entity of liver damage. Cariello R, Federico A, Sapone A, et al. Dig Liver Dis. 2010 Mar;42(3):200-4. PMID:19502117

[33] Lactulose-mannitol intestinal permeability test in children with diarrhea caused by rotavirus and cryptosporidium. Diarrhea Working Group, Peru. Zhang Y, Lee B, Thompson M, et al. J Pediatr Gastroenterol Nutr. 2000 Jul;31(1):16-21. Erratum in: J Pediatr Gastroenterol Nutr 2000 Nov;31(5):578. PMID:10896065

[34] Impact of anti-Giardia and anthelminthic treatment on infant growth and intestinal permeability in rural Bangladesh: a randomised double-blind controlled study. Goto R, Mascie-Taylor CG, Lunn PG. Trans R Soc Trop Med Hyg. 2009 May;103(5):520-9. PMID:18789466

[35] Susceptibility to gut leakiness: a possible mechanism for endotoxaemia in non-alcoholic steatohepatitis. Farhadi A, Gundlapalli S, Shaikh M, Frantzides C, Harrell L, Kwasny MM, Keshavarzian A. Liver Int. 2008 Aug;28(7):1026-33. PMID:18397235

[36] Gastrointestinal permeability in ovarian cancer and breast cancer patients treated with paclitaxel and platinum. Melichar B, Hyspler R, Dragounová E, Dvorák J, Kalábová H, Tichá A. BMC Cancer. 2007 Aug 9;7:155. PMID:17688683

[37] Association of vitamin A and zinc status with altered intestinal permeability: analyses of cohort data from northeastern Brazil. Chen P, Soares AM, Lima AA, Gamble MV, Schorling JB, Conway M, Barrett LJ, Blaner WS, Guerrant RL. J Health Popul Nutr. 2003 Dec;21(4):309-15. PMID:15038585

[38] Perturbed zinc homeostasis in rural 3-5-y-old Malawian children is associated with abnormalities in intestinal permeability attributed to tropical enteropathy. Manary MJ, Abrams SA, Griffin IJ, et al. Pediatr Res. 2010 Jun;67(6):671-5. PMID:20496476

[39] Dietary Grape-Seed Procyanidins Decreased Postweaning Diarrhea by Modulating Intestinal Permeability and Suppressing Oxidative Stress in Rats. Song P, Zhang R, Wang X, He P, Tan L, Ma X. J Agric Food Chem. 2011 May 6. PMID:21534629

[40] Effect of Helicobacter pylori and eradication therapy on gastrointestinal permeability. Implications for patients with seronegative spondyloarthritis. Di Leo V, D'Inca R, Bettini MB, Podswiadek M, Punzi L, Mastropaolo G, Sturniolo GC. J Rheumatol. 2005 Feb;32(2):295-300. PMID:15693091

[41] Effects of enteral supplementation with glutamine granules on intestinal mucosal barrier function in severe burned patients. Peng X, Yan H, You Z, Wang P, Wang S. Burns. 2004 Mar;30(2):135-9. PMID:15019120

[42] Perioperative symbiotic treatment to prevent postoperative infectious complications in biliary cancer surgery: a randomized controlled trial. Sugawara G, Nagino M, Nishio H, Ebata T, Takagi K, Asahara T, Nomoto K, Nimura Y. Ann Surg. 2006 Nov;244(5):706-14. PMID:17060763

[43] Regulation and roles for claudin-family tight junction proteins. Findley MK, Koval M. IUBMB Life. 2009 Apr;61(4):431-7. PMID:19319969

[44] Changes in gut microbiota control inflammation in obese mice through a mechanism involving GLP-2-driven improvement of gut permeability. Cani PD, Possemiers S, Van de Wiele T, et al. Gut. 2009 Aug;58(8):1091-103. PMID:19240062

[45] Interleukin-6 (IL-6) regulates claudin-2 expression and tight junction permeability in intestinal epithelium. Suzuki T, Yoshinaga N, Tanabe S. J Biol Chem. 2011 Sep 9;286(36):31263-71. PMID:21771795

[46] Increase in the Tight Junction Protein Claudin-1 in Intestinal Inflammation. Poritz LS, Harris LR 3rd, Kelly AA, Koltun WA. Dig Dis Sci. 2011 Jul 12. PMID:21748286

[47] Claudins: Control of Barrier Function and Regulation in Response to Oxidant Stress. Overgaard CE, Daugherty BL, Mitchell LA, Koval M. Antioxid Redox Signal. 2011 May 9. PMID:21275791

[48] Oxidative stress induces gastric epithelial permeability through claudin-3. Hashimoto K, Oshima T, Tomita T, Kim Y, Matsumoto T, Joh T, Miwa H. Biochem Biophys Res Commun. 2008 Nov 7;376(1):154-7. Epub 2008 Sep 5. PMID:18774778

[49] Aspirin induces gastric epithelial barrier dysfunction by activating p38 MAPK via claudin-7. Oshima T, Miwa H, Joh T. Am J Physiol Cell Physiol. 2008 Sep;295(3):C800-6. PMID:18667601

[50] Role of Claudins in Oxidant-Induced Alveolar Epithelial Barrier Dysfunction. Sun Y, Minshall RD, Hu G. Methods Mol Biol. 2011;762:291-301. PMID:21717365

[51] Supplemental zinc reduced intestinal permeability by enhancing occludin and zonula occludens protein-1 (ZO-1) expression in weaning piglets. Zhang B, Guo Y. Br J Nutr. 2009 Sep;102(5):687-93. PMID:19267955

[52] Role of zinc in pediatric diarrhea. Bajait C, Thawani V. Indian J Pharmacol. 2011 May;43(3):232-5. PMID:21713083

[53] The role of zinc deficiency in alcohol-induced intestinal barrier dysfunction. Zhong W, McClain CJ, Cave M, Kang YJ, Zhou Z. Am J Physiol Gastrointest Liver Physiol. 2010 May;298(5):G625-33. Epub 2010 Feb 18. PMID:20167873

[54] Evidence that chronic alcohol exposure promotes intestinal oxidative stress, intestinal hyperpermeability and endotoxemia prior to development of alcoholic steatohepatitis in rats. Keshavarzian A, Farhadi A, Forsyth CB, et al. J Hepatol. 2009 Mar;50(3):538-47. PMID:19155080

[55] Chronic alcohol ingestion alters claudin expression in the alveolar epithelium of rats. Fernandez AL, Koval M, Fan X, Guidot DM. Alcohol. 2007 Aug;41(5):371-9. PMID:17889313

[56] Role of intestinal circadian genes in alcohol-induced gut leakiness. Swanson G, Forsyth CB, Tang Y, Shaikh M, Zhang L, Turek FW, Keshavarzian A. Alcohol Clin Exp Res. 2011 Jul;35(7):1305-14. PMID:21463335

[57] Claudin-4 augments alveolar epithelial barrier function and is induced in acute lung injury. Wray C, Mao Y, Pan J, Chandrasena A, Piasta F, Frank JA. Am J Physiol Lung Cell Mol Physiol. 2009 Aug;297(2):L219-27. PMID:19447895

[58] Identification of a novel immunomodulatory gliadin peptide that causes interleukin-8 release in a chemokine receptor CXCR3-dependent manner only in patients with coeliac disease.Lammers KM, Khandelwal S, Chaudhry F, Kryszak D, Puppa EL, Casolaro V, Fasano A.Immunology. 2011 Mar;132(3):432-40. PMID:21091908

[59] Gliadin induces an increase in intestinal permeability and zonulin release by binding to the chemokine receptor CXCR3. Lammers KM, Lu R, Brownley J, et al. Gastroenterology. 2008 Jul;135(1):194-204.e3. PMID:18485912

[60] Tight junctions, intestinal permeability, and autoimmunity: celiac disease and type 1 diabetes paradigms. Visser J, Rozing J, Sapone A, Lammers K, Fasano A. Ann N Y Acad Sci. 2009 May;1165:195-205. PMID:19538307

[61] Involvement of mast cells in basal and neurotensin-induced intestinal absorption of taurocholate in rats. Gui X, Carraway RE. Am J Physiol Gastrointest Liver Physiol. 2004 Aug;287(2):G408-16. PMID:14693504

[62] Nitric oxide mediates tightening of the endothelial barrier by ascorbic acid. May JM, Qu ZC. Biochem Biophys Res Commun. 2011 Jan 14;404(2):701-5. PMID:21156160

[63] Pathological and therapeutic implications of macromolecule passage through the tight junction; p. 697-722. Fasano, A. Tight Junctions. Marcelino Cereijido, ed. CRC Press, Inc.; Boca Raton, FL: 2001.

[64] Changes in gut microbiota control inflammation in obese mice through a mechanism involving GLP-2-driven improvement of gut permeability. Cani PD, Possemiers S, Van de Wiele T, Guiot Y, Everard A, Rottier O, Geurts L, Naslain D, Neyrinck A, Lambert DM, Muccioli GG, Delzenne NM. Gut. 2009 Aug;58(8):1091-103. PMID:19240062

[65] Nitric oxide mediates tightening of the endothelial barrier by ascorbic acid. May JM, Qu ZC. Biochem Biophys Res Commun. 2011 Jan 14;404(2):701-5. Epub 2010 Dec 13. PMID:21156160

[66] Evaluation of urinary 6-hydroxymelatonin sulphate excretion in women at different age with irritable bowel syndrome. Wisniewska-Jarosinska M, Chojnacki J, Konturek S, et al. J Physiol Pharmacol. 2010 Jun;61(3):295-300. PMID:20610859

[67] Estimation of 24-hour polyamine intake from mature human milk. Dorhout B, van Beusekom CM, Huisman M, Kingma AW, de Hoog E, Boersma ER, Muskiet FA. J Pediatr Gastroenterol Nutr. 1996 Oct;23(3):298-302. PMID: 8890081

[68] Are milk polyamines preventive agents against food allergy? Dandrifosse G, Peulen O, El Khefif N, Deloyer P, Dandrifosse AC, Grandfils C. Proc Nutr Soc. 2000 Feb;59(1):81-6. PMID:10828177

[69] Quercetin enhances intestinal barrier function through the assembly of zonula [corrected] occludens-2, occludin, and claudin-1 and the expression of claudin-4 in Caco-2 cells. Suzuki T, Hara H.J Nutr. 2009 May;139(5):965-74. PMID:19297429

26. Irritable Bowel Syndrome

Irritable Bowel Syndrome (IBS) is a condition characterized by recurrent episodes of abdominal pain that is relieved by defecation. Additionally there is a change in the form and frequency of stools and commonly, abdominal bloating. IBS is usually associated with either loose stools (IBS with diarrhea: IBS-D) or hard difficult to pass stools (IBS with constipation: IBS-C). IBS-D patients tend to be on the lookout for bathrooms where ever they go as they may suddenly require the use of one at nearly any moment. In contrast, IBS-C patients may only have a bowel movement once or twice a week. Another set of IBS patients alternate between constipation and diarrhea; this is designated as IBS-A.

A diagnosis of IBS is made three times more commonly among women than men, and the prevalence increases at menopause. IBS is the most common diagnosis made by gastroenterologists; it affects somewhere between 12 and 22% of the population[1]; about one in 6 persons.

IBS had been considered to be a "functional disease" without physical lesions. The 40 million Americans affected by IBS often do not appreciate the lack of diagnostic test, lack of understanding of the disease, or of targeted treatment. Until recently IBS had neither lab test nor physical finding even on colonoscopy and microscopy; it remains a diagnosis of exclusion, after ruling out other, usually more dangerous, disease entities. IBS is not a single pathological condition, but rather caused by multiple, often overlapping, pathologies. A single patient may have several processes contributing to the causation of IBS. The causation of these processes is diverse; thus, treatment, without knowing the causes in a specific patient is likely to yield poor results. The good news is that we can now find causation for most of those suffering from IBS, and thus provide more targeted treatment.

The Pathology

There are two common processes in IBS: increased or disorganized peristalsis and increased intestinal paracellular permeability.

The predominant neuroendocrine cells of the intestines are the enterochromaffin cells (EC cells) which produce and release the neurotransmitter serotonin. EC cells have an essential role in GI homeostasis; they help regulate secretion of stomach acid, stimulate peristalsis and trigger visceral pain. Somatostatin inhibits the release of serotonin by limiting calcium influx through the L-type calcium channels that modulate serotonin release.

EC cells are affected by the central nervous system, the enteric nervous system, and by the contents of the intestinal lumen. Serotonin controls both gut motility and secretion and is implicated in pathologic conditions, such as vomiting, diarrhea, and irritable bowel syndrome. Serotonin secretion stimulates 5-HT$_3$ receptors on vagal afferent nerve fibers to the central nervous system. Stimulus can trigger nausea, and sufficient stimulus can cause vomiting.

The EC cells have microvilli that face the intestinal lumen. This surface membrane contains receptors that can activate the release of serotonin from secretory granules located at the basolateral pole of these cells. Here, serotonin (5-HT) can activate other enterocytes, goblet cells, neurons and smooth muscle cells; resulting in an increase in secretions, motility, and pain. An increase in motility, caused by irritants, promotes redistribution and dilution of the irritant from an area where it may be overly concentrated. If this stimulation involves a large area, it can result in cramping pain and diarrhea. This mechanism likely contributes to the pain and diarrhea experienced in IBS-D and IBD [2].

The population of EC cells can increase within a few days of the onset of intestinal inflammation, along with an increase in N and D enteroendocrine cells. N cells produce neurotensin, which is proinflammatory in the colon and stimulates mast cell activity. D cells produce and release somatostatin, which suppresses the release of motilin, VIP, and some other GI hormones. In inflammatory bowel disease (IBD) and some other chronic inflammatory disorders, however, D cells numbers are decreased.

Inflammation slows the reuptake of serotonin by EC cells, permitting sustained response to it[3]. Thus, in chronic inflammation, somatostatin, which normally down-regulates motilin and 5-HT release, is diminished, and more EC cells may be present. Furthermore, downregulation of 5-HT reuptake by these cells can increase the secretory, peristaltic and pain response to EC cell stimulation. With chronic stimulation, however, excessive amounts of somatostatin or 5-HT may lead to tachyphylaxis, causing receptor desensitization or loss of intestinal neurons. Alternations in response may impair or disorganize peristalsis, resulting in constipation or diarrhea.

Tryptophan, the substrate for production of serotonin and melatonin, can be diverted in the presence of bacterial lipopolysaccharides (LPS), IL-1β, IL-6, TNF-α, and INF-γ, into the kynurenine pathway. SIBO and enteric biofilms produce LPS that can induce the neurotoxin quinolinic acid and the oxidant 3H-kynurenine. These agents may promote IBS by damaging enteric neurons. LPS also causes oxidative stress. Oxidative stress may increase the risk of mast cell mutations and the development of aberrantly-behaved clones. The tryptophan/kynurenine pathway is further discussed in Chapter 31.

IBS patients have higher levels of motilin and serotonin, and very elevated levels of somatostatin in their blood, compared to healthy controls. IBS-D patients have a shorter resting period between migrating motor complex (MMC) cycles, short phase II duration, and longer phase III MMC, with greater electrical amplitude and faster propagation of the MMC wave. Patients with IBS-C have a longer phase I and II and a shorter phase III MMC activity. "Gastrointestinal Motility 101" in Chapter 24 provides further explanation of the MMC.

Table 26-1: IBS-C vs. IBS-D GI Motility Differences

Alterations in IBS[4, 5]	IBS – C Constipation	IBS – D Diarrhea
Plasma somatostatin	Very High	Very High
Plasma serotonin (5-HT)	High	High
Phase III plasma motilin	Low	High
MMC phase I and II duration	Long	Short
MMC phase III duration	Short	Long
MMC total cycle duration	Long	Short
MMC amplitude	Low	High
MMC propagation velocity	Fast	Fast

EC cell luminal surfaces have G protein-coupled receptors for glutamine, tyrosine and glucose; bile salt transporter proteins; and certain taste and olfactory receptors. Activation of these receptors occurs when they are exposed to the substances the receptors transports or reacts to, and this can trigger the release of serotonin[39].

The action of the receptors and transporters on the surfaces of EC cells explains some reactions to food ingestion. For example, for many people, coffee in the morning acts a purgative, inducing a bowel movement. Other individuals are highly sensitive to trace amines in foods. Trace amines may result from bacterial fermentation of food. Tyramine, for example, can be found at significant levels in some foods, such as wines, cheeses, and chocolate. In patients with carcinoid tumors, these foods can cause diarrhea by triggering the release of serotonin. Consumption of the agents listed in Table 26-3 may promote the release of serotonin into the lamina propria of the intestine, which stimulates intestinal motility. In patients with IBS, this stimulation may provoke symptoms. Bile acids stimulate the release of serotonin from EC cells via the hormone motilin.

Bile acid malabsorption (BAM) diarrhea: BAM is one of the most common causes of chronic diarrhea; it is present in about 28 percent of IBS-D patients[6], and a common cause of chronic diarrhea in other diseases. BAM causes bile acid diarrhea (BAD) when excessive amounts of bile acid (BA) enter the colon and enhance mucosal permeability and reactivity. This allows an increase in water and electrolyte secretion into the colon. Additionally BA's accelerates colonic transit by stimulating propulsive colonic contractions, causing diarrhea. It is predominantly the secondary bile acids that cause these effects.

BA's are recycled several times a day. After being excreted by the liver and concentrated in the gallbladder, they are released with meals, to aid in the absorption of fats. In health, BA's are almost completely reabsorbed by Ileal Bile Acid Transporter (IBAT) proteins in the brush border membrane of enterocytes in the terminal ileum. Uptake of BA into the enterocytes stimulates production of the hormone, Fibroblast Growth Factor-19 (FGF19). The BA's are then transported into the portal venous bloodstream bound to albumin and returned to the liver for reuse. FGF19 provides hormonal feedback that informs the liver that sufficient BA's available; thus, FGF19 down-regulates the synthesis of new bile acids by the liver.

It is normal for a small portion of the BA's to enter the colon; some BA binds to dietary fiber and is thus lost, and a very small amount evades ileal uptake and recycling. Once in the colon, BA's are conjugated into secondary bile acids by colonic bacteria, and some are reabsorbed. About 20% of the bile acid pool is comprised of these secondary BA's. With each meal, about three percent of the bile pool enters the colon, and about half is reabsorbed. About five percent of the BA pool is lost each day and replaced by the liver.

Bile acids in the colon alter and are altered by the colonic biome. Bile acids are metabolized by bacteria in the colon to secondary bile acids that increase the risk of irritable bowel syndrome, inflammatory bowel disease, and colonic cancer. The biome also changes; there is an increase in *E. coli* and a decrease in *Bifidobacterium* with increased colonic BA.

Bile acid malabsorption often occurs in Crohn's disease, celiac disease and after ileal resection, due to the loss of bile acid absorptive surface area in the terminal ileum. In inflammatory conditions, injury or loss of ileal enterocytes, FGF19 production is also diminished. Deficient FGF19 feedback causes the liver to increases bile acid synthesis and output, and further increases the amount of BA's that enter the colon[7]. Thus, more BA's are produced in a situation where the ileal capacity for BA uptake is already compromised. The increased flow of BA into the colon causes an increased conjugation into secondary BA and further increases irritation, permeability, and diarrhea.

BAM diarrhea is common in cancer patients, particularly those treated with radiation to the abdomen or pelvis that injures the quickly growing enterocytes. Pancreatic resection and chemotherapy also cause BAM[8]. BAM may also occur with malabsorption, due to rapid ileal transit that decreases the contact time of bile laden chyme with the absorptive surface, such as with lactose intolerance. The rapid transit increases the formation of secondary BA's. SIBO is also associated with BAM, likely because of bacterial conversion of primary BA's to secondary BA's. Pancreatic insufficiency and cholecystectomy are associated with BAD, perhaps due to inadequate micelle function. Without sufficient bile, pancreatic lipase and colipase, fat absorption is inefficient, and little fat or fat-soluble vitamins are absorbed, causing fat malabsorption, steatorrhea, and fat-soluble vitamin deficiencies. An increase in secondary BA's may be to blame.

Most patients with BAM and BAD benefit from treatment with bile acid sequestrants. Newly synthesized bile acids are primary BA's and less likely to provoke BAD. Thus, even with a higher amount of new BA's synthesized by the liver, there is a lower proportion of secondary BA's that are motilin stimulants. The sequestrants preferentially remove secondary bile acids by diluting them with new primary BA's.

In Europe, BAM is tested for using the SeHCAT test using a radioactive bile acid tracer. After administration, levels tested after a few hours and then again after seven days. If there is a normal 95% daily recycling of bile acids, seventy percent should remain after seven days ($0.95^7 = 0.70$). In a positive (abnormal) test, less than 15% of the tracer remains; about a 77% percent daily recycling efficiency. Low SeHCAT retention correlates highly with bile acid sequestrant treatment success[9]. C4 estimates hepatic bile acid synthesis (see Table 26-1). Serum FGF19 estimates bile acid uptake from the ileum.

BAM causes altered enteroendocrine activity and intracellular permeability; features common in all IBS. BAM explains the mechanism of disease in many patients but does not explain the underlying pathology of IBS. or even the cause of BAM.

Some of the conditions causing IBS include parasitic infestations, pancreatic insufficiency, and acute and chronic infection. SIBO, food allergies, gluten intolerance, food antergies and mast cell activation disorder are also associated with IBS. Additionally, many patients have subclinical inflammatory bowel disease, rather than IBS, that should be treated for what it is.

Dysbiosis: The lab test that is most frequently abnormal in IBS is dysbiosis; with poor growth of commensal organisms *Lactobacillus* and *Bifidobacterium*. The question remains whether this dysbiosis is the primary cause of IBS or if occurs as in reaction to other processes. The loss of these commensal organisms may occur from the use of antibiotic medications, lack of prebiotics in the diet, (which are often avoided by IBS patients as they increase bloating and gas) or because of overgrowth of competing organisms. About two percent of IBS patients have occult blood in their stools, and one percent has *C. difficile*[45]. Hemoglobin in the stool increases the growth of *Candida* and encourages biofilm formation.

Foods high in lactose, fructose, or sorbitol can cause meteorism. IBS patients are hypersensitive to stretching of the intestines, and maldigestion of sugars exacerbates symptoms. Non-absorbed sugars also promote rapid oral cecal transit time (OCTT). As a result, these sugars ferment in the cecum and colon, causing gas and bloating. Patients with IBS-D typically have short OCTT. Heavy growth of microbiota that produces methane is associated with IBS-C; meanwhile, bacterial fermentation that yields hydrogen is detected more frequently in patients with IBS-D[10]. Malabsorption also promotes SIBO and the formation of secondary bile acids, which act as mucosal irritants. Short OCTT also delivers unabsorbed proteins and fats to the colon that support toxin-producing bacterial species and biofilm development.

Post-infectious IBS (PI-IBS): About ten percent of IBS patients have an acute onset of the condition that coincides with an infectious, often food-borne, gastroenteritis. Among the pathogens associated with acute-onset PI-IBS are the gram-negative *Campylobacter, Escherichia coli, Salmonella,* and *Shigella*. PI-IBS presents more commonly as IBS-D (70%) while sixty percent of non-PI-IBS is IBS-C[11]. In PI-IBS, there is hyperplasia of lamina propria intraepithelial lymphocytes, T cells, serotonin-containing enteroendocrine cells and mast cells, and increased mucosal permeability. IBS patients with PI-IBS have a better prognosis, as the disease often resolves after five to six years.

Campylobacter jejuni causes IBS in both children and adults[12]. Intestinal *Campylobacter* infection can disrupt the enterocyte tight-junctions, and increase paracellular permeability for months following the infection[13,14]. This breach of enterocyte tight-junctions impairs the mucosal barrier and allows food proteins and peptides and bacterial toxins and debris into contact with dendritic and other immune cells in the lamina propria. The immune response can recruit mast cells into the mucosa. Mast cell activity releases histamine, which acts as a chemotactic agent for more mast cells.

Campylobacter jejuni is ubiquitously found in farm animals; it is often present in the feces of dairy cows, cattle, and poultry[15]. About 40% of poultry shed *Campylobacter* in their feces. Between five and 15% of pet dogs and cats carry *Campylobacter jejuni* in their intestines[16,17]. Most human cases of *C. jejuni* infection appear to arise from food-borne exposure, although exposure can also come from pets and other animals.

Campylobacter infection may initiate gluten enteropathy in susceptible individuals[18]. Initiation occurs after exposure of the enteric immune system to gluten resulting from the increased paracellular permeability effected by this disease. Gluten peptides then further contribute to paracellular permeability in IBS. Gluten often causes GI symptoms in patients with IBS that do not have celiac disease[19], but IBS patients are four times more likely to have celiac disease-related antibodies than are healthy controls[20]. *Campylobacter* enteritis can also trigger the onset of chronic small intestinal bacterial overgrowth (SIBO)[21] that promotes increased intestinal permeability[22].

SIBO is commonly found in patients with IBS; it is two to nine times more prevalent in IBS patients than in healthy, asymptomatic individuals[23,24]. Increased intestinal permeability is also found in IBS; however, it does not necessarily correlate to the presence of SIBO[25]. Some of the diagnoses of SIBO in IBS, however, may be false positives, resulting from the abnormally short oral-cecal transit times in IBS (see Chapter 24). The presence of SIBO indicates that there is aberrant intestinal motility; this contributes to conditions favorable to increased intracellular permeability; decreased OCTT favors bile passage to the colon.

The augmented intestinal permeability in IBS may result from specific bacteria in the intestinal biome and the toxins they produce. Some bacterial species increase intestinal permeability in SIBO[26] while others do not[27]. Spore forming bacteria enhance the synthesis of serotonin from enterochromaffin cells[28], as do those that produce short-chain fatty acids[29]. Serotonin slows colonic activity; excess can cause IBS-C constipation. Biofilm formation promotes LPS production and increased kynurenine production. In a study of patients with severe IBS, 89% (compared to 11% of controls) had LPS antibodies to the obligate intracellular bacteria, *Chlamydia trachomatis* in enteroendocrine cells and macrophages of the small bowel mucosa[30].

Mast Cell Activation: In PI-IBS due to *Shigella* enteritis, the mast cell population in the lamina propria doubled among cases, as compared to controls, three years later. Certain other immune and enterochromaffin cells numbers also increase[31]. The increase of mast cells in PI-IBS has been confirmed in other studies[32]. Increased intestinal permeability, allowing access of antigens from the lumen of the intestine to the enteric immune system, facilitates the development of mast cell hyperplasia lamina propria in the and the development of antibodies that can trigger mast cell activity in IBS. IBS is common in mast cell activation disorders, and mast cell hyperplasia is usual in the mucosa of the small intestines in IBS[33]. Mast cell hyperplasia is also found in "functional" dyspepsia[34].

The release of mast cells products in areas lying close to nerve terminals in the GI mucosa may explain the pain experienced in IBS[35]. IBS-D patients have an increase in serine protease in the stool. This mast cell mediator nearly doubles colonic mucosal paracellular permeability[36]. Hyperplasia of colonic mast cells in IBS is associated with fatigue, depression[37], and abdominal bloating[38]. Recently introduced corticotropin-releasing hormone antagonists, for the treatment of IBS, likely help by preventing mast cell activation and decreasing paracellular permeability.

Although there is hyperplasia other immune cell populations in the intestinal lamina propria in patients with IBS[38], symptoms of this disease can largely be explained by mast cell activity. Like other mast cell disorders, mast cell behavior, rather than mast cell number, in IBS explains the activity and symptoms of the disease. Understanding IBS as a mast cell activation disorder helps direct attention to mechanisms for, and intervention in the disease.

IgG Antibodies in IBS: IgG to foods are commonly elevated in IBS[39]. In a Chinese study, after testing for and eliminating common foods to which the patients had IgG reactivity, 65% of patients had either remarkable or complete remission of IBS symptoms after elimination of IgG reacting foods[40]. Another study, which looked specifically at IgG$_4$ levels in 16 common foods, found great improvement after three and six months of dietary elimination of these foods[41]. Yet another study that looked at IgG levels for 29 foods found improvement among those adhering to the elimination diet, with continued improvement in symptoms over the 12-week trial. The improvement resulting from a diet where IgG reactive foods were avoided gave better results in this study than did the medication treatment arm, using tegaserod[42].

In these studies, testing was limited to the commonly eaten foods, often panels of only a dozen foods. Complete resolution of IBS symptoms should not be expected unless nearly all IgG food antergens have been eliminated from the diet. In studies that included testing for IgG to yeast[1, 42], it was the most common IgG reactant found, affecting about 85% of patients with IBS. However, IgG to yeast was not tested for in several of these studies. The natural food colorant, annatto, has been reported by patients to be a common trigger for IBS. However, a test for it is not commonly available. Molds may be another trigger, which are not usually tested for. Molds are commonly, but mostly unintentionally, consumed in foods. Blue cheese is an example where is mold intentionally eaten.

The list of foods that are most commonly reactive on IgG testing includes those that cause IgE food allergies. Skin prick sensitivity testing and IgE titers for foods, however, are not useful in identifying foods, that when avoided, provide relief of IBS symptoms[43]. IgG$_4$ may be formed in response to repeated exposure to foods for which there are IgE antibodies. In its functional role in health, IgG$_4$ neutralizes antigens, thus preventing IgE allergic reactions. IgG$_4$, however, can directly and indirectly trigger mast cell degranulation. IgG$_1$ antigens can also cause immune activation. IgG$_1$ is commonly formed to lectins in foods.

If exposure to a food antigen is eliminated, IgG production for that antigen diminishes over time; in contrast, continued exposure supports sustained or increased antibody production. IgG$_4$ can form immune complexes with the antigen and IgG$_1$, and thus, can cause disease. IgE pollinosis and environmental allergens may also stimulate IgG$_4$ antibody formation as suggested by the common immunoreactions to molds in IBS. Thus, environmental allergens may support antergies to foods. Appendix A provides a brief list of common environmental antigens and their cross-reacting foods.

The beneficial response of IBS to the elimination of IgG reacting foods likely results from the prevention of mast cell activation. The elimination of antergens may also allow the downregulation of intestinal mucosal immunity, and reduce reactive paracellular permeability.

For IgG testing and elimination to be most effective in IBS or other conditions, as wide a range of foods as is practical should be tested. Then, only those foods found to be non-reactive should be included in the patient's diet. After the person improves, additional foods that were not tested may be added, one every couple of days to see it they react.

Pancreatic Exocrine Insufficiency: Pancreatic exocrine insufficiency is common in IBS, secondary to loss of digestive enteroendocrine cells[44]. This decreases digestion of proteins that both act as antigens and encourage intestinal dysbiosis, with decreased growth of commensal organisms and supports overgrowth biofilms forming LPS.

Table 26-2: Pathology and Tests in IBS Patients[45]

Condition (Prevalence)	Test
Bile acid malabsorption (BAM) (28%)	Serum FGF19 (elevated) Serum 7 α-hydroxy-4-cholesten-3-one (C4) (low) Fecal Bile acids (48-hour sample)
Colonic dysbiosis (73%)	Low growth of commensals: *Lactobacillus, Bifidobacterium*
Infectious Disease	Stool culture, EIA tests
SIBO	Chapter 24
Mast Cell Activation	Fecal tryptase or other tests for MCAS. See Chapter 12 Fecal serine protease (IBS-D)
Celiac disease or gliadin intolerance	IgA and IgG Antigliadin antibodies, See below, And Chapters 22 and 24
Antergies	IgG to foods. See Chapter 19
Parasite infestations (7.5%)	Stool test for ova and parasites (e.g.: *Giardia, Blastocystis*, etc.)
Pancreatic exocrine insufficiency	Fecal Elastase-1, Chymotrypsin, ^{13}C mixed-triglyceride breath test
Subclinical Inflammatory Bowel Disease (IBD) (15%)	Fecal Calprotectin, Eosinophil Protein X, Eosinophil Cationic Protein. If elevated, the diagnosis is likely IBD rather than IBS. See Chapter 34

See Appendix C for lab tests

Other Diseases diagnosed as IBS: About 14% of IBS patients have elevated levels of fecal eosinophil protein X, (EPX) and 12% have elevated fecal calprotectin and other have elevated fecal eosinophil cationic protein (ECP). These individuals should be considered as having inflammatory bowel disease, rather than IBS, even if the disease is not identified on colonoscopy. IBD is covered in Chapter 34. About 7 percent of IBS patients have intestinal parasites[45]. These may cause IBS-like symptoms (not IBS), or increase the risk of IBS by altering intestinal mucosal permeability and activity.

Non-immune Food Triggers for IBS

Several foods have been found to be common triggers for IBS symptoms. Most of these, such as citrus, chocolate and banana and tomato are common allergens and most likely act through immune mechanisms. Others, however, may have a more pharmacologic response.

Caffeine: Caffeine is a stimulant for the large intestine, and causes an increase in motor activity and pressure in the transverse and descending colon within four minutes of drinking a caffeinated beverage[46], and thus, can increase pain, as a result of abnormal sensitivity to stretch receptors in the intestine in patients with IBS. Caffeine also relaxes the internal anal sphincter muscles, and thus, can provoke fecal incontinence in patients with IBS-D. Chocolate and tea also contain theobromine, a molecule closely related to caffeine. Thus, caffeine is likely to worsen the symptoms of IBS.

Additionally, caffeine consumption can disturb sleep. Quality sleep is important for normalization of the migrating motor complex (MMC) and recovery from IBS. (See Chapters 24 and 42.) Stress and sleep deprivation may increase the production of CRH, a mast cell degranulator.

Nightshades: Potatoes and tomatoes have been identified as causing adverse reactions in IBS[32]. Eggplant is another member of the nightshade group (*Solanum* genus) that may provoke IBS. These nightshades contain glycoalkaloids, including solanine, which in toxic amounts, causes abdominal cramping, nausea, vomiting, and diarrhea. The toxin damages mitochondria and can cause apoptosis. Individuals with IBS, as well as those with Inflammatory Bowel Disease (IBD), may be uniquely sensitive to the alkaloid toxins in potatoes[47],[48]. The amount of alkaloids in potatoes varies greatly, depending on the potato cultivar, the climate and season grown, and on harvest and storage techniques. These alkaloids are not destroyed by cooking but are concentrated by frying in oil.

A more probable cause for GI sensitivity to potatoes and eggplant among IBS and IBD patients is reaction to lectins that survive cooking and digestion, and which, directly elicit mast cell degranulation[49] (See Chapter 14.) Eggplants, also contain toxic alkaloids and lectins which may induce degranulation. Nightshades also contain trypsin inhibitors that inactivate some pancreatic enzymes (Table 23-3). Tomatoes alkaloids and lectins are considered to be nontoxic. If tomatoes provoke adverse reactions in IBS, the cause is most likely immunogenic. Potatoes' role in IBD is further discussed in Chapter 33.

Table 26-3: Agents that Release Serotonin from EC cells[39]

Agent Class	Agents
Trace Amines	Tyramine, Octopamine
Amino Acid	Glutamine, Tyrosine
Secondary Bile Salt	Sodium deoxycholate
Tastes	Caffeine (bitter), Umami (protein)
Other	Sucralose
Olfactants	Thymol (thyme), Eugenol (cloves)

Foods high in trace amines, certain flavors and aromas that are detected by receptors in the gut, and sucralose may also stimulate the release of serotonin from EC cells and trigger IBS symptoms.

Treatment of IBS

IBS is a multifactorial disease; an approach eliminating these multiple factors helps with healing. Antergies, mast cell activation, intestinal paracellular permeability (IPP) and SIBO if present, should be treated.

1. TEST!: Test to find the underlying cause of IBS so that treatment can be directed at the underlying causes of the disease. Tables 26-2 and 34-1 show some of the most productive tests for understanding pathology in IBS.

2. Secondary Bile Acids: Malabsorption can cause dumping of chyme into the cecum, where BA's and nutrients ferment. Bile also increases the release of motilin. Secondary BA's stimulate intestinal propulsion and increase paracellular permeability, provoking IBS symptoms. Glycine or trimethylglycine (betaine) (500 mg B.I.D. or T.I.D.) may improve ileal mucosal health and absorption including that of BA's; thus increasing FGF19 and prevent the formation of primary and secondary BA's.

BA sequestrants bind BA's, preventing their reabsorption and promote the generation of primary BA's. The bile acid sequestrant colesevelam (Welchol) is the preferred agent, with a dose of one or two 625mg tablets before meals for patients with IBS-D. Cholestyramine or colestipol may be used but are not as potent bile acid sequestrants. A side effect of these medications can be constipation, but this may be avoided by using low doses. Patients with IBS-C may respond to a single bedtime tablet of colesevelam. This low, bedtime-dose avoids interference with the absorption of nutrients. Bile acid sequestrant side-effects including the loss of lipid soluble vitamins; thus, they should not be used be used as a primary, chronic therapy, but rather, for short periods to get a patient feeling better, while addressing the underlying causes of the IBS. Supplementation of vitamins A, D, E, and K should accompany the use of these medications. Dietary fiber, especially from grains, also binds to bile acids and helps to increase BA turnover.

3. Prebiotics and Probiotics: Probiotics in unison with prebiotics is often helpful for commensal depletion in IBS. Dietary inulins increase the proliferation of *Lactobacillus,* and *Bifidobacterium* and fructose-oligosaccharides decrease *C. difficile* growth. Prebiotics and probiotics are discussed in Chapter 4. Probiotics may be helpful, especially following the use of wide-spectrum antibiotics; however, dietary fiber that act as prebiotics maintain the effect.

4. Treat Infection: Active infections causing bacterial gastroenteritis, or parasites, such as *Giardia*, should also be treated with appropriate antibiotics. Parasitosis causes an imbalanced enteric ecology.

The antibiotic rifaximin (1200 mg/day for ten days) reduces gastrointestinal symptoms in patients with IBS-D with SIBO. Some patients require a double dose to achieve resolution of symptoms[50]. The benefit of treatment with this antibiotic is usually temporary, as it is not treating the underlying condition, and thus fermentation and IBS symptoms usually reoccur. Treatment with rifaximin can be repeated with renewed, although temporary, benefit[51]. The benefits are also limited to IBS without constipation. Ciprofloxacin and metronidazole may be as effective, and available at lower costs. Use of these antibiotics can put the patient at risk for pseudomembranous colitis, and further disruption of the commensal bacteria biome in the colon.
A diet that contains adequate prebiotic fiber, phenolic compounds, and glycosphingolipids for the support of eubiosis (as compared to dysbiosis) is needed for long-term improvement. Antibiotic treatment should be considered, at best, a jump-start towards health.

Treatment of SIBO is covered in Chapter 24. When lactulose breath tests are used to test for SIBO in the diagnosis of IBS, tests are positive in about half the patients. Nevertheless, when bacterial aspirates from the jejunum are performed, SIBO is rare[52]. About half of patients with IBS have a positive glucose hydrogen/methane breath-test, and most of these patients respond to antibiotic treatment[53]. While the fermentation is not occurring in the proximal small intestine, it is occurring. Avoidance of poorly absorbed sugars, especially fructose, lactose, and sorbitol, may especially help those patients with IBS-D and rapid OCTT. Use of lactase and Beano may provide relief for those consuming dairy or legumes

5. Treat for Mast Cell Activation: IBS is a mast cell enterocolitis[54]. Preventing mast cell activation can not only help eliminate symptoms, but with time, may allow the number of mast cells in the intestinal mucosa to return to normal.

Use of histamine blockers and leukotriene inhibitors may help attenuate the results of mast cell activity and help to prevent the increased paracellular permeability that maintains disease activity. Eighty percent of the H_1 blocker fexofenadine is excreted unchanged into the bile[55]. It is thus, recycled, and can act locally on immune cells of the intestinal mucosa.

Mast cell stabilizers (cromolyn sodium) and COX2 inhibitors may also be helpful in some patients. Pyridoxine (vitamin B_6) may help stabilize mast cells[56], aids in the formation of serotonin and melatonin, and may limit kynurenine pathway toxicity. Vitamin B_6 should be supplemented if levels are low and R-lipoic acid may be helpful. (See Chapter 39.)

Chapter 12 provides further detail on mast cell activation disorders and their treatment. Mast cell degranulation may be avoided by eliminating foods, medications, and other factors which trigger mast cell degranulation. (Chapter 14)

6. Eliminate IgG Reacting Foods from the Diet: Eliminating antergens from the diet often provides excellent results for many months; however, symptoms often reappear as new immunogenicities form. If the underlying propensity to forming IgG immunogenicity to foods remains, new food sensitivities are likely to develop, and the disease response can reoccur. Test for food antergies using a broad array of IgG tests for food; the goal is not only to remove reacting foods, but also to provide a list of "safe foods" which do not trigger reactions. Even with a panel of over 100 foods, there will be foods that are not tested, and thus, which the patient may be reacting to. Reacting foods should be eliminated for at least six months, and then retesting may be done. After 2 months per decade of age, foods items can be reintroduced, to see if they trigger symptoms. One or two foods can be introduced to the diet about each week as it may take one or more days to provoke symptoms from eating a reacting food. Further details on treating antergies are given in Chapter 19.

7. Treat Intestinal Hyperpermeability. IBS patients should be tested for gliadin and transglutaminase antibodies to diagnose if gluten enteropathy is present. Wheat should be avoided even if no antibodies to wheat or gluten are found, at least until the patient is asymptomatic.

Zinc supplementation may improve enterocyte barrier by in increasing the expression of the tight junction proteins occludin and ZO-1[57]. Oxidative stress from alcohol depletes free zinc availability, resulting in zinc deprivation and epithelial barrier disruption[58]. Zinc supplements reduced the incidence and severity of diarrheal disease in children; 20 mg of zinc for 10 – 14 days gave some protection from diarrhea for up to three months[59]. A reasonable dose for a zinc supplement for adults with IBS is 10 to 15 mg a day.

The flavonoid quercetin may help improve the enterocyte barrier as it has been shown to upregulate claudin-4 within the epithelial tight junction[60]. Other flavonoids may also provide this benefit. The treatment of intestinal hyperpermeability is discussed in Chapter 25.

8. Digestive Enzymes: Pancreatic enzyme insufficiency is common in IBS due to loss of enteroendocrine cells in the intestinal mucosa (See pancreatic exocrine insufficiency (PEI), Chapter 8). Digestive enzyme supplements help patients with PEI. Enzyme deficiencies cause steatorrhea, malabsorption, SIBO, and dysbiosis. Patients with low enzyme activity should avoid trypsin inhibitors: Table 23-3. Enzyme supplements can be helpful during recovery.

9. Melatonin: Melatonin is an important endogenous antioxidant which scavenges both reactive oxygen and reactive nitrogen species. Melatonin is produced in the pineal gland, however, less well recognized is the role of melatonin in the gut and the gonads. The GI tract produces considerably more melatonin than does the pineal gland.

Melatonin is a non-recyclable antioxidant; once it accepts an ROS or radical, it cannot be used again, as can many other antioxidants. Thus, in oxidative stress melatonin can be depleted. Melatonin helps protect the gastrointestinal mucosa from oxidative damage. It has an anti-inflammatory effect, acts as a smooth muscle relaxant in the gut, and slows intestinal transit time. In women with IBS, levels of the melatonin metabolite, 6-hydroxymelatonin sulfate (6-HMS) are higher than those of control subjects[61]. This suggests a higher rate of depletion and a higher level of oxidative stress. Melatonin levels are significantly lower in IBS patients than in age and gender- matched controls[62].

Serotonin and melatonin metabolism are altered in IBS[63]. Melatonin also plays an important role in the regulation of pancreatic enzyme release via afferent vagal stimulation[64]. Melatonin supplements have been found to decrease abdominal and rectal pain and urgency in the treatment of IBS[65, 66]. The dose used in these studies was 3 mg at bedtime. Melatonin may also help treat mast cell hyperplasia (Chapter 29; Epigenetics).

A diet with adequate tryptophan, vitamin B_6, and Pyrroloquinoline quinone help ensure serotonin and melatonin production. Additionally, regular meal times and exposure to bright sunlight during the day, avoidance of meals and bright light at night, and regular sleep times help entrain a normal intestinal MMC cycle. Dietary flavonoids increase the endogenous production of antioxidant enzymes.

Avoidance of alcohol is suggested. The most relevant other oxidants are those arising from bacterial production of LPS and the production of toxic kynurenine products. Avoid intestinal biofilm formation, as described in Chapter 23.

10. Fighting Fear of Flatus: Patients with IBS often limit their diet to palatable, low fiber, easy to digest foods that help avoid symptoms, and thus avoid foods that provide nutrients needed for sustaining a eubiotic colonic bacterial biome. Such a diet, however, supports maintenance and progression of the disease. Patients need to understand that they won't attain health if they are afraid of foods that make them fart, and that mild, dry flatus is a sign of a healthy cecal biome, while large amounts of wet nasty farts often indicate malabsorption of sugars or protein. Symptomatic relief may be required before a patient is willing to modify their diet sufficiently to improve GI function. For example, the best sources of fructose oligosaccharide fiber are onions and garlic; foods that the patient may associate with an increase in symptoms. See Chapter 4 for details.

11. Initiating Treatment: Therapy can be initiated providing symptomatic relief: a trial of digestive enzymes, probiotics, melatonin, and low dose zinc may be used even before any test results are available; these treatments bear very little risk and very often provide benefit at low costs. A therapeutic trial using these makes sense for most patients. Follow with a gradual introduction of a mix of dietary fibers; fruits grains and vegetables, so that the intestinal microbiota gradually adapts to the new foods over a few weeks. Onion and garlic may be introduced well cooked: for example, in soup or stew, to improve their digestibility. In some patients, elimination of caffeine can be helpful. Bile acid sequestrants often give rapid relief.

Testing for, and elimination of, immune reacting foods should be done in patients with suspected mast cell involvement. If the patient is compliant and does not improve, make sure that gluten intolerance, leaky gut, SIBO, and mast cell activation disorder, parasitosis and IBD have been ruled out or adequately treated. As with any disease, understanding and eliminating the underlying causes is required for long-term recovery.

Inform the patient that it will take time for the intestines to normalize. Even if IBS patients achieve rapid symptomatic improvement, it is important that they understand that it will likely take time to restore normal GI motility and to normalize mast cell activity and population. It should be emphasized that a return to old habits will most likely set the stage for a return of the disease.

[1] Treating irritable bowel syndrome with a food elimination diet followed by food challenge and probiotics. Drisko J, Bischoff B, et al. J Am Coll Nutr. 2006 Dec;25(6):514-22. PMID:17229899

[2] Luminal regulation of normal and neoplastic human EC cell serotonin release is mediated by bile salts, amines, tastants, and olfactants. Kidd M, Modlin IM, et al. Am J Physiol Gastrointest Liver Physiol. 2008 Aug;295(2):G260-72. PMID: 18556422

[3] Enteroendocrine cells and 5-HT availability are altered in mucosa of guinea pigs with TNBS ileitis. O'Hara JR, Ho W, Linden DR, Mawe GM, Sharkey KA. Am J Physiol Gastrointest Liver Physiol. 2004 Nov;287(5):G998-1007. PMID: 15231483

[4] High interdigestive and postprandial motilin levels in patients with the irritable bowel syndrome. Simrén M, Björnsson ES, et al. Neurogastroenterol Motil. 2005 Feb;17(1):51-7. PMID:15670264

[5] Small intestine motility and gastrointestinal hormone levels in irritable bowel syndrome. Zhao JH, Dong L, Hao XQ. Nan Fang Yi Ke Da Xue Xue Bao. 2007 Oct;27(10):1492-5. PMID:17959521

[6] Systematic review with meta-analysis: the prevalence of bile acid malabsorption in the irritable bowel syndrome with diarrhoea. Slattery SA, Niaz O, Aziz Q, Ford AC, Farmer AD. Aliment Pharmacol Ther. 2015 Apr 27. PMID:25913530

[7] Bile Acid diarrhea: prevalence, pathogenesis, and therapy. Camilleri M. Gut Liver. 2015 May 23;9(3):332-9. PMID:25918262

[8] Are bile acid malabsorption and bile acid diarrhoea an important cause of diarrhoea complicating cancer therapy? Phillips F, Muls AC, Lalji A, et al. Colorectal Dis. 2015 Feb 28. PMID:25728737

[9] Systematic review: the prevalence of idiopathic bile acid malabsorption as diagnosed by SeHCAT scanning in patients with diarrhoea-predominant irritable bowel syndrome. Wedlake L, A'Hern R, Russell D, et al. Aliment Pharmacol Ther. 2009 Oct;30(7):707-17. PMID:19570102

[10] Small intestinal bacterial overgrowth in irritable bowel syndrome: are there any predictors? Reddymasu SC, Sostarich S, et al. BMC Gastroenterol. 2010 Feb 22;10:23. PMID: 20175924

[11] Histopathological alterations in post-infectious irritable bowel syndrome in Bangladeshi population. Bhuiyan MR, Majumder TK, Raihan AA, Roy PK, Farha N, Kamal M. Mymensingh Med J. 2010 Apr;19(2):275-81. PMID:20395926

[12] An outbreak of acute bacterial gastroenteritis is associated with an increased incidence of irritable bowel syndrome in children. Thabane M, Simunovic M, Akhtar-Danesh N, et al. Am J Gastroenterol. 2010 Apr;105(4):933-9. PMID:20179687

[13] Disruption of tight junctions and induction of proinflammatory cytokine responses in colonic epithelial cells by Campylobacter jejuni. Chen ML, Ge Z, Fox JG, Schauer DB. Infect Immun. 2006 Dec;74(12):6581-9. PMID:17015453

[14] Campylobacter and IFNgamma interact to cause a rapid loss of epithelial barrier integrity. Rees LE, Cogan TA, Dodson AL, et al. Inflamm Bowel Dis. 2008 Mar;14(3):303-9. PMID:18050297

[15] Dynamics of endemic infectious diseases of animal and human importance on three dairy herds in the northeastern United States. Pradhan AK, Van Kessel JS, Karns JS, et al. J Dairy Sci. 2009 Apr;92(4):1811-25. PMID:19307664

[16] Campylobacter excreted into the environment by animal sources: prevalence, concentration shed, and host association. Ogden ID, Dallas JF, MacRae M, et al. Foodborne Pathog Dis. 2009 Dec;6(10):1161-70. PMID:19839759

[17] Prevalence and shedding patterns of Campylobacter spp. in longitudinal studies of kenneled dogs. Parsons BN, Williams NJ, Pinchbeck GL, et al. Vet J. 2010 Nov 18. PMID:21094061

[18] Clinical onset of celiac disease after an episode of Campylobacter jejuni enteritis. Verdu EF, Mauro M, Bourgeois J, Armstrong D. Can J Gastroenterol. 2007 Jul;21(7):453-5. PMID:17637949

[19] Gluten causes gastrointestinal symptoms in subjects without celiac disease: a double-blind randomized placebo-controlled trial. Biesiekierski JR, Newnham ED, Irving PM, et al. Am J Gastroenterol. 2011 Mar;106(3):508-14. PMID:2122483

[20] Yield of diagnostic tests for celiac disease in individuals with symptoms suggestive of irritable bowel syndrome: systematic review and meta-analysis. Ford AC, Chey WD, Talley NJ, et al. Arch Intern Med. 2009 Apr 13;169(7):651-8. PMID:19364994

[21] ICC density predicts bacterial overgrowth in a rat model of post-infectious IBS. Jee SR, Morales W, Low K, et al. World J Gastroenterol. 2010 Aug 7;16(29):3680-6. PMID:20677340

[22] Intestinal permeability and function in dogs with small intestinal bacterial overgrowth. Rutgers HC, Batt RM, Proud FJ, et al. J Small Anim Pract. 1996 Sep;37(9):428-34. PMID:8887203

[23] Small intestinal bacterial overgrowth in irritable bowel syndrome: systematic review and meta-analysis. Ford AC, Spiegel BM, Talley NJ, Moayyedi P. Clin Gastroenterol Hepatol. 2009 Dec;7(12):1279-86. PMID:19602448

[24] Prevalence of small intestinal bacterial overgrowth in children with irritable bowel syndrome: a case-control study. Scarpellini E, Giorgio V, Gabrielli M et al. J Pediatr. 2009 Sep;155(3):416-20. PMID:19535093

[25] The Relationship between Small-Intestinal Bacterial Overgrowth and Intestinal Permeability in Patients with Irritable Bowel Syndrome. Park JH, Park DI, Kim HJ, et al. Gut Liver. 2009 Sep;3(3):174-9. PMID:20431742

[26] Clostridium perfringens epsilon toxin increases the small intestinal permeability in mice and rats. Goldstein J, Morris WE, Loidl CF, et al. PLoS One. 2009 Sep 18;4(9):e7065. PMID:19763257

[27] Luminal bacteria and small-intestinal permeability. Riordan SM, McIver CJ, Thomas DH, Duncombe VM, Bolin TD, Thomas MC. Scand J Gastroenterol. 1997 Jun;32(6):556-63. PMID:9200287

[28] Indigenous bacteria from the gut microbiota regulate host serotonin biosynthesis. Yano JM, Yu K, Donaldson GP, et al. Cell. 2015 Apr 9;161(2):264-76. PMID:25860609

[29] Gut microbes promote colonic serotonin production through an effect of short-chain fatty acids on enterochromaffin cells. Reigstad CS, Salmonson CE, Rainey JF 3rd, et al. FASEB J. 2015 Apr;29(4):1395-403. PMID:25550456

[30] Chlamydia trachomatis antigens in enteroendocrine cells and macrophages of the small bowel in patients with severe irritable bowel syndrome. Dlugosz A, Törnblom H, Mohammadian G, et al. BMC Gastroenterol. 2010 Feb 16;10:19. PMID:20158890

[31] Increased immunoendocrine cells in intestinal mucosa of postinfectious irritable bowel syndrome patients 3 years after acute Shigella infection--an observation in a small case control study. Kim HS, Lim JH, Park H, Lee SI. Yonsei Med J. 2010 Jan 31;51(1):45-51. PMID:20046513

[32] Histopathological alterations in post-infectious irritable bowel syndrome in Bangladeshi population. Bhuiyan MR, Majumder TK, Raihan AA, Roy PK, Farha N, Kamal M. Mymensingh Med J. 2010 Apr;19(2):275-81.PMID:20395926

[33] Decreased expression of serotonin in the jejunum and increased numbers of mast cells in the terminal ileum in patients with irritable bowel syndrome. Wang SH, Dong L, Luo JY, et al. World J Gastroenterol. 2007 Dec 7;13(45):6041-7. PMID:18023097

34 Duodenal mastocytosis, eosinophilia and intraepithelial lymphocytosis as possible disease markers in the irritable bowel syndrome and functional dyspepsia. Walker MM, Talley NJ, Prabhakar M, et al. Aliment Pharmacol Ther. 2009 Apr 1;29(7):765-73. PMID:19183150

35 Activated mast cells in proximity to colonic nerves correlate with abdominal pain in irritable bowel syndrome. Barbara G, Stanghellini V, De Giorgio R, et al. Gastroenterology. 2004 Mar;126(3):693-702.PMID:14988823

36 Increased faecal serine protease activity in diarrhoeic IBS patients: a colonic lumenal factor impairing colonic permeability and sensitivity. Gecse K, Róka R, Ferrier L, et al. Gut. 2008 May;57(5):591-9. PMID:18194983.

37 Mast cells and cellularity of the colonic mucosa correlated with fatigue and depression in irritable bowel syndrome. Piche T, Saint-Paul MC, Dainese R, et al. Gut. 2008 Apr;57(4):468-73. PMID:18194987

38 Mucosal immune activation in irritable bowel syndrome: gender-dependence and association with digestive symptoms. Cremon C, Gargano L, Morselli-Labate AM, Santini D, et al. Am J Gastroenterol. 2009 Feb;104(2):392-400. PMID:19174797

39 Food-specific serum IgG4 and IgE titers to common food antigens in irritable bowel syndrome. Zar S, Benson MJ, Kumar D. Am J Gastroenterol. 2005 Jul;100(7):1550-7.PMID: 15984980

40 The therapeutic effects of eliminating allergic foods according to food-specific IgG antibodies in irritable bowel syndrome. Yang CM, Li YQ. Zhonghua Nei Ke Za Zhi. 2007 Aug;46(8):641-3. PMID: 17967233

41 Food-specific IgG4 antibody-guided exclusion diet improves symptoms and rectal compliance in irritable bowel syndrome. Zar S, Mincher L, Benson MJ, Kumar D. Scand J Gastroenterol. 2005 Jul;40(7):800-7.PMID: 16109655

42 Food elimination based on IgG antibodies in irritable bowel syndrome: a randomized controlled trial. Atkinson W, Sheldon TA, Shaath N, Whorwell PJ. Gut. 2004 Oct;53(10):1459-64. PMID:15361495

43 Alterations of food antigen-specific serum immunoglobulins G and E antibodies in patients with irritable bowel syndrome and functional dyspepsia. Zuo XL, Li YQ, Li WJ, et al. Clin Exp Allergy. 2007 Jun;37(6):823-30.PMID: 17517095

44 Is irritable bowel syndrome an organic disorder? El-Salhy M, Gundersen D, Gilja OH, et al. World J Gastroenterol. 2014 Jan 14;20(2):384-400. PMID:24574708

45 Frequency of abnormal fecal biomarkers in irritable bowel syndrome. Goepp J, Fowler E, McBride T, Landis D. Glob Adv Health Med. 2014 May;3(3):9-15. PMID:24891989

46 Is coffee a colonic stimulant? Rao SS, Welcher K, Zimmerman B, Eur J Gastroenterol Hepatol. 1998 Feb;10(2):113-8. PMID: 9581985

47 Naturally occurring glycoalkaloids in potatoes aggravate intestinal inflammation in two mouse models of inflammatory bowel disease. Iablokov V, Sydora BC, Foshaug R, et al. Dig Dis Sci. 2010 Nov;55(11):3078-85. PMID: 20198430

48 Potato glycoalkaloids adversely affect intestinal permeability and aggravate inflammatory bowel disease. Patel B, Schutte R, Sporns P. Inflamm Bowel Dis. 2002 Sep;8(5):340-6.PMID: 12479649

49 Potato lectin activates basophils and mast cells of atopic subjects by its interaction with core chitobiose of cell-bound non-specific immunoglobulin E. Pramod SN, Venkatesh YP, Mahesh PA. Clin Exp Immunol. 2007 Jun;148(3):391-401. PMID:17362264

50 High-dose rifaximin treatment alleviates global symptoms of irritable bowel syndrome. Jolley J. Clin Exp Gastroenterol. 2011;4:43-8. PMID:21694871

51 Effects of Rifaximin Treatment and Retreatment in Nonconstipated IBS Subjects. Pimentel M, Morales W, Chua K, et al. Dig Dis Sci. 2011 Jul;56(7):2067-72. PMID:21559740

52 Small intestine bacterial overgrowth in patients with irritable bowel syndrome. Carrara M, Desideri S, Azzurro M, et al. Eur Rev Med Pharmacol Sci. 2008 May-Jun;12(3):197-202. PMID:18700692

53 Results of small intestinal bacterial overgrowth testing in irritable bowel syndrome patients: clinical profiles and effects of antibiotic trial. Majewski M, McCallum RW. Adv Med Sci. 2007;52:139-42. PMID:18217406

54 A clinicopathologic study... systemic mastocytosis ... and ... mucosal mast cell density in IBS.... Doyle LA, et al . Am J Surg Pathol. 2014 Jun;38(6):832-43. PMID:24618605

55 Comparative pharmacology of the H1 antihistamines. del Cuvillo A, Mullol J, Bartra J, Dávila I, Jáuregui I, Montoro J, Sastre J, Valero AL. J Investig Allergol Clin Immunol. 2006;16 Suppl 1:3-12. PMID:17357372

56 Ascorbic acid and pyridoxine in experimental anaphylaxis. Alvarez RG, Mesa MG. Agents Actions. 1981 Apr;11(1-2):89-93. PMID:6166175

57 Supplemental zinc reduced intestinal permeability by enhancing occludin and zonula occludens protein-1 (ZO-1) expression in weaning piglets. Zhang B, Guo Y. Br J Nutr. 2009 Sep;102(5):687-93. PMID:19267955

58 The role of zinc deficiency in alcohol-induced intestinal barrier dysfunction. Zhong W, McClain CJ, Cave M, Kang YJ, Zhou Z. Am J Physiol Gastrointest Liver Physiol. 2010 May;298(5):G625-33. PMID:20167873

59 Role of zinc in pediatric diarrhea. Bajait C, Thawani V. Indian J Pharmacol. 2011 May;43(3):232-5. PMID:21713083

60 Quercetin enhances intestinal barrier function through the assembly of zonula [corrected] occludens-2, occludin, and claudin-1 and the expression of claudin-4 in Caco-2 cells. Suzuki T, Hara H.J Nutr. 2009 May;139(5):965-74. PMID:19297429

61 Evaluation of urinary 6-hydroxymelatonin sulphate excretion in women at different age with irritable bowel syndrome. Wisniewska-Jarosinska M, Chojnacki J, Konturek S, et al. J Physiol Pharmacol. 2010 Jun;61(3):295-300. PMID:20610859

62 Melatonin improves bowel symptoms in female patients with irritable bowel syndrome: a double-blind placebo-controlled study. Lu WZ, Gwee KA, Moochhalla S, Ho KY. Aliment Pharmacol Ther. 2005 Nov 15;22(10):927-34. PMID:16268966

63 Serum serotonin concentration and urine 5-hydroxyindole acetic acid excretion in patients with irritable bowel syndrome. Moskwa A, Chojnacki J, Wiśiewska-Jarosińska M, et al. Pol Merkur Lekarski. 2007 May;22(131):366-8. PMID: 17679369

64 Brain-gut axis in the modulation of pancreatic enzyme secretion. Jaworek J, Nawrot-Porabka K, Leja-Szpak A, Konturek SJ. J Physiol Pharmacol. 2010 Oct;61(5):523-31.PMID: 21081795

65 A preliminary study of melatonin in irritable bowel syndrome. Saha L, Malhotra S, Rana S, Bhasin D, Pandhi P. J Clin Gastroenterol. 2007 Jan;41(1):29-32. PMID:17198061

66 Melatonin improves abdominal pain in irritable bowel syndrome patients who have sleep disturbances: a randomised, double blind, placebo controlled study. Song GH, Leng PH, Gwee KA, et al. Gut. 2005 Oct;54(10):1402-7. PMID:15914575

27. Interstitial Cystitis, Bladder Pain Syndrome and Chronic Prostatitis

Interstitial Cystitis/ Bladder Pain Syndrome is a chronic condition affecting the urinary bladder. This disease causes discomfort or pain in the pelvic area that can be severe, but relieved by urination. It can be accompanied by urinary frequency, with micturition as frequently as every ten minutes needed to gain relief. The names Interstitial Cystitis (IC), Bladder Pain Syndrome (BPS), and IC/BPS are used for this condition.

There are no diagnostic physical signs or urologic findings that confirm the diagnosis of IC/BPS. There are no standard laboratory tests for it. Its diagnosis is determined by symptoms and the exclusion of mimicking disorders; IC/BPS is a diagnosis of exclusion.

The diagnostic criteria for IC/BPS are:

- Pain, pressure, or discomfort in the pelvic area
- Daytime urinary frequency greater than ten times, or urgency due to pain, pressure, or discomfort
- Pain that worsens as the bladder fills, and
- Ruling out other causes.

The *Pelvic Pain and Urgency/Frequency Patient Symptom Scale* is given in Appendix F. This scale is useful for the diagnosis and for monitoring response to IC/BPS therapy.

IC/BPS is not a rare condition. Between 2.7 and 6.5 percent of women over the age of 18 meet the diagnostic criteria for IC/BPS; between 3 and 8 million American women have this disease[1]. Although not rare, it is less common in men. IC/BPS is often misdiagnosed as overactive bladder, prostatitis, urethritis, trigonitis, or other non-specific conditions.

IC/BPS has considerable comorbidity. Over a third of patients with BPS have depressive symptoms and half report a history of panic attacks[2]. Nearly ninety percent of women with BPS report sexual dysfunction[3]. IC/BPS can be a debilitating condition which can prevent the individual from working or participating in social activities.

Chronic Prostatitis

Male chronic pelvic pain syndrome, also know as chronic prostatitis (CP) or nonbacterial prostatitis, shares many similarities with IC/BPS[4]. It is a common condition accounting for 1.5 million physician visits annually in the United States. Although bacteria cause less than one in ten cases of prostatitis, antibiotics are usually prescribed for this disease. CP can cause chronic pelvic pain[5], difficulty with urination, painful urination, and sexual dysfunction[6], including ejaculatory pain and decreased libido[7]. Similar to IC/BPS, chronic prostatitis is a disease of exclusion.

If bladder pain and urinary frequency, with pain relief upon urination in IC/BPS, seems reminiscent to the abdominal pain with relief by defecation in IBS-D, it is not by chance. Although both were once considered functional diseases and remain diagnoses of exclusion, these conditions share common pathologies.

Not only does IC/BPS share pathology with IBS, these diseases share patients; thirty percent of patients with IC/BPS have IBS. About twenty percent of IC/BPS patients suffer from migraines or fibromyalgia[8], and half have known allergies[9]. Also, like IBS, a high percentage of men with chronic prostatitis have positive lactulose hydrogen breath tests, suggesting SIBO[10]. Similar to IBS, IC/BPS is a mast cell activation disorder[11].

Mast cells lead the immune response to bladder infections. Mast cells are activated by antigens present on fimbriated *E. coli,* for example. Mast cell activation, initiated by bacteria or other antigens, releases histamine and bradykinin, which induce pain, and prostaglandins that act on local nerve endings, lowering the threshold of pain. Histamine also provokes detrusor irritability and bladder contraction; this stimulates the emptying the bladder of infected urine and causes the sensation of urgency. The release of TNF-α and leukotriene B_4 from mast cells initiates chemotaxis of inflammatory cells, to help fight the infection, causing pyuria[12].

In the short term, as with an infrequent urinary tract infection, mast cell activation is responsible for many of the symptoms of cystitis but helps clear the infection. With prolonged or chronic bladder wall mast cell activation, as with chronic infection or antergies, however, mast cell activation not only causes the chronic cystitis but can lead to fibrosis of the bladder, which causes it to be less distensible. This can cause chronic urinary frequency, nocturia, bladder pain with filling, and micturition; even when mast cell activation is no longer present.

Electron microscopy has revealed two[13] to four-fold[9] increases in the mast cell population of the bladder mucosa in IC/BPS and shown that as many as ninety percent of these mast cells are in an activated state. Pain, in an animal model of IC/BPS, has been shown to be mediated by histamine[14], and blocked by H_1 blockers and by neurokinin antagonists that prevent mast cell degranulation[15].

Methylhistamine; the major metabolite of histamine, and tryptase; a marker of mast cell population, are elevated in the urine of patients with IC[13]. There is also evidence that chronic prostatitis may also be a mast cell activation disorder[16, 17]. In experimental models, mast cell infiltration of the prostate occurs as an early change[18].

The hypothalamic stress hormone, Corticotropin-releasing hormone (CRH), is a mast cell activator that increases paracellular permeability of the bladder. CRH also induces production of vascular endothelial growth factor (VEGF)[19] that may be involved in the pathology of IC/BPS. Hypersecretion of CRH occurs during chronic stress. Alcohol also increases CRH release.

Food and IC/BPS

The triad of pain that worsens with certain foods and beverages, worsens with bladder filling, and improves with urination is found in 97% of IC/BPS cases. The role of food in triggering BPS is so pronounced that it has been suggested to be part of the diagnostic criteria for the disease. The foods that are most frequently reported to exacerbate IC/BPS are coffee, tea, soda, alcoholic beverages, citrus fruits and juices, artificial sweeteners and hot peppers[20].

Testing and treatment for IC/BPS is similar to that for IBS. This testing and treatment regimen may also be helpful in chronic prostatitis.

Treatment

As with other mast cell activation disorders (MACD), the treatment is multifactorial. These treatments are briefly stated here and given in more detail in previous chapters.

1. Treat MCAD: H_1 and H_2 antagonists are often helpful in patients with IC/BPS and chronic prostatitis[21, 22]. These agents do not prevent mast cell degranulation but rather prevent the action of histamine released from the mast cells. H_2 antagonists appear to be more effective in IC/BPS than are H_1 antagonists, although both can be most used in combination to increase efficacy.

Cimetidine, ranitidine, and famotidine have been found to be effective H_2 antagonists for the treatment of mast cell-associated bladder pain in an animal model, with ranitidine being the most effective[21]; Famotidine was nearly as effective. Famotidine has the added advantage that it does not impair the breakdown of histamine; as do many other H_2 blockers. These agents have short half-lives and may be best used as twice-daily medications.

The H_1 blocker hydroxyzine was only mildly helpful in a human trial[23] and not was effective in animal models[21] of IC/BPS; nevertheless, diphenhydramine and cetirizine both reduced pain. Cetirizine is an active metabolite of hydroxyzine, which is largely excreted unchanged in the urine[24]. Ebastine, acrivastine, and levocetirizine are also largely excreted unchanged in the urine, which may aid in efficacy; however, it has not been demonstrated that having a histamine antagonist active in the urine is helpful. It would only be helpful if the medication acted locally on the mucosa. Cetirizine can be used as a once-daily medication. Cetirizine can cause drowsiness; thus, it may be best used at bedtime.

H_2 antagonist: Famotidine (Pepcid) is preferred. Ranitidine (Zantac), or Nizatidine (Axid) may be used as alternatives.

H_1 antagonist: Cetirizine (Zyrtec) is preferred. Loratadine (Claritin) and fexofenadine may be used as alternatives.

Side effects may be mitigated by using these medications at bedtime. However, they may provide less daytime relief.

Other medications that may be helpful are mast cell stabilizers (cromolyn, ketotifen) and leukotriene antagonist medications, such as zileuton. (See Chapter 12 for more on treatment of MCAD).
The COX2 inhibitor celecoxib may be helpful. Inflammatory eicosanoid production may also be lowered with n-3 fatty acid supplements (fish oil), vitamin D, and tocotrienols (See cancer prevention Chapter 40).

2. Avoid Mast Cell Degranulation: Allergens that bind to IgE cause mast cell degranulation, as can IgG complexes. Potatoes and sulfites in foods and medications can also provoke degranulation in some individuals, especially when the body is under oxidative stress. Opiates and some other medications can trigger mast cells degranulation. (Chapter 14 has further discussion on prevention and treatment of mast cell degranulation.

3. IgG Food Antergy Testing and Treatment: IgG reactions may support the formation of mast cell hypertrophy. Test for IgG antibodies to food and eliminate these from the diet. (See Chapter 19). If more than a few percent of food items are positive on IgG testing, it is indicative of increased paracellular permeability. Intracellular permeability for the bladder (and prostate) may not be identical to that of the intestine, but there is certainly overlap in agents that impair the tight junctions and agents which improve it.

If multiple food immunogenicities are found, or the diagnosis of IBS co-exist in the patient, treatment for IBS should be initiated as described in Chapter 26. Removal of reacting antergens can give rapid remission of symptoms.

In addition to antergens, patients should avoid foods that commonly exacerbate IC/BPS: coffee, tea, soda, alcoholic beverages, citrus fruits and juices, artificial sweeteners and hot peppers

4. Endothelial Barrier Normalization: CRH increases paracellular permeability, likely through its action on mast cells. Chronic stress should be mitigated (Chapter 29), and alcohol should be avoided.

Oxidative stress can cause an increase in paracellular permeability (PP) not only between enterocytes but in many other tissues, including the brain, lung, kidneys and bladder mucosa, resulting from its effects on the tight-junction protein, claudin[25]. Thus, antioxidants may be used, especially if oxidative stress is evident.

Oxidative stress can be tested using 8-Hydroxy-2'-deoxyguanosine (8-OHdG), which is a marker of oxidative damage to DNA or MDA. Alcohol increases oxidative stress and depletes zinc availability at the tight junctions. Betaine, from a diet with green leafy vegetables, may help prevent oxidative injury from alcohol.

Oxidative stress can be treated by mitochondrial renewal, by avoiding exposure to pro-oxidants (Table 40-5 in Chapter 40) and a diet high in phenolic compounds and isothiocyanates. Melatonin may be used as an antioxidant at 3 mg at bedtime.

Zinc has long been used in prostate health. Here, it may induce expression of proteins for the epithelial tight junctions. Twenty-five milligrams of zinc oxide or sulfate may be used as a daily starting dose that can be decreased to 10 mg daily after a couple of weeks.

Supplements that increase nitric oxide (NO) production may be helpful. The body uses L-arginine to make NO. L-arginine, given at a dose of 1500 mg a day, has been tested in clinical trials of IC/BPS, and found to help reduce symptoms in some patients[26]. Nitric oxide synthase is unusual in that it requires multiple cofactors. The dietary factors which are required for NO production and function are shown in Table 25-3 in Chapter 25.

The flavonoid quercetin has been shown to upregulate the protein claudin-4 within the epithelial tight junction[27]. In a trial of this agent for IC/BPS, there were significant improvements in symptoms when quercetin was used (500 mg twice a day).

A layer of glycosaminoglycans protects the bladder mucosa. Loss or damage of this protective layer exposes the mucosal epithelium to direct exposure to urine. Intravesical instillation of the non-sulfated glycosaminoglycan hyaluronic acid has been found to give symptomatic relief in IC/BPS. Oral supplementation with chondroitin sulfate, a sulfated glycosaminoglycan, also gave symptomatic relief[28]. N-acetyl cysteine and L-Taurine may help promote a normal glycosaminoglycan layer in the bladder. N-acetyl cysteine is also an anti-oxidant.

5. Test for SIBO and Treat if Present: Small intestinal bacterial overgrowth, or biofilm formation in the large intestine, can promote the production of quinolinic acid that acts as an NMDA agonist and promotes visceral type pain. Testing and treatment of SIBO is appropriate, especially if symptoms consistent with SIBO or IBS are present. Treatment of SIBO is covered in Chapter 24.

6. Gluten Free Diet: Gliadin peptides from wheat disrupt the tight junction in the intestines by the release of zonulin. Gliadin peptides also trigger immune reactions by binding to transglutaminase. In Celiac disease, antibodies to tissue transglutaminase contribute to damage of the small intestine. In dermatitis herpetiformis, epidermal transglutaminase is the predominant autoantigen. Gliadin peptides and prostate transglutaminase may be a causal factor in chronic prostatitis and the loss of fertility common in celiac disease. Patients with IC/BPS and CP may benefit from a gluten-free diet.

7. Antiinflammatory Agents: Minocycline, which readily enters the prostate, has been used in the treatment of chronic prostatitis for 40 years[29], however, it had been assumed to provide benefit as an antibiotic agent. More recent understanding reveals that minocycline acts as an anti-inflammatory agent by blocking Toll-like receptor-2 (TLR-2) stimulated activation of inflammatory transcription factors. Minocycline helps in chronic prostatitis by inhibiting the expression of inflammatory cytokines IL-6, IL-8, IL-13, and G-CSF[30].

Other agents which down-regulate TLR-2, such as vitamin D_3, zinc, or which stimulate PPAR-γ, such as DHA from fish oil, and may be useful in treating IC/BPS and chronic prostatitis. See Figure 42-2 and Table 42-3.

Supplement Summary: Supplements should be considered a secondary treatment to aid in recovery when initiating primary treatments to remove the underlying causes of the disease.

Supplement List: May be helpful in the initial treatment of IC/PBS and chronic prostatitis.

- Zinc — 10 - 15 mg daily
- Vitamin D_3 — 5000 IU daily
- Magnesium citrate — 300 mg daily
- Vitamin K_2 — Menatetrenone: MK_4; 5 mg daily
- R-α-lipoic acid — 50 – 100 mg daily
- Vitamin C — 50 mg 2 – 3 times daily
- Melatonin — 3 mg at bedtime
- Quercetin — 500 mg twice daily
  or
  Curcumin — 800 mg daily
- N-acetyl cysteine — 1000 mg daily
- DHA (Fish Oil) — 500 mg twice daily

Foods especially rich in quercetin include dark chocolate, black elderberries, capers, oregano, red onions, and shallots (See Table 31-2.)

[1] Prevalence of Symptoms of Bladder Pain Syndrome / Interstitial Cystitis Among Adult Females in the United States. Berry SH, Elliott MN, Suttorp M, et al. J Urol. 2011 Jun 15. PMID:21683389

[2] Depressive disorders and panic attacks in women with bladder pain syndrome / interstitial cystitis: a population-based sample. Watkins KE, Eberhart N, Hilton L, et al. Gen Hosp Psychiatry. 2011 Mar-Apr;33(2):143-9. PMID:21596207

[3] Prevalence and correlates of sexual dysfunction among women with bladder pain syndrome/interstitial cystitis. Bogart LM, Suttorp MJ, Elliott MN, Clemens JQ, Berry SH. Urology. 2011 Mar;77(3):576-80. PMID:21215432

[4] Similarities between interstitial cystitis and male chronic pelvic pain syndrome. Moldwin RM. Curr Urol Rep. 2002 Aug;3(4):313-8. PMID:12149163

[5] Chronic pelvic pains represent the most prominent urogenital symptoms of "chronic prostatitis". Krieger JN, Egan KJ, Ross SO, Jacobs R, Berger RE. Urology. 1996 Nov;48(5):715-21; discussion 721-2. PMID:8911515

[6] Distinguishing chronic prostatitis and benign prostatic hyperplasia symptoms: results of a national survey of physician visits. Collins MM, Stafford RS, O'Leary MP, Barry MJ. Urology. 1999 May;53(5):921-5. PMID:10223484

[7] Sexual dysfunction in men with chronic prostatitis/chronic pelvic pain syndrome: improvement after trigger point release and paradoxical relaxation training. Anderson RU, Wise D, Sawyer T, Chan CA. J Urol. 2006 Oct;176(4 Pt 1):1534-8; discussion 1538-9. PMID:16952676

[8] Interstitial cystitis/painful bladder syndrome and associated medical conditions with an emphasis on irritable bowel syndrome, fibromyalgia and chronic fatigue syndrome. Nickel JC, Tripp DA, Pontari M, Moldwin R, et al. Urol. 2010 Oct;184(4):1358-63. PMID:20719340

[9] Activation of bladder mast cells in interstitial cystitis: a light and electron microscopic study. Theoharides TC, Sant GR, el-Mansoury M, et al Urol. 1995 Mar;153(3 Pt 1):629-36. PMID:7861501

[10] Chronic prostatitis and small intestinal bacterial overgrowth: effect of rifaximin. Weinstock LB, Geng B, Brandes SB.Can J Urol. 2011 Aug;18(4):5826-30. PMID:21854715

[11] Histamine and mucosal mast cells in interstitial cystitis. Enerbäck L, Fall M, Aldenborg F. Agents Actions. 1989 Apr;27(1-2):113-6. PMID:2750582

[12] Type 1 fimbriated Escherichia coli-mast cell interactions in cystitis. Abraham S, Shin J, Malaviya R. J Infect Dis. 2001 Mar 1;183 Suppl 1:S51-5. PMID:11171015

[13] Activation of bladder mast cells in interstitial cystitis. Letourneau R, Sant GR, el-Mansoury M, Theoharides TC. Int J Tissue React. 1992;14(6):307-12. PMID:1306530

[14] Mast cell-derived histamine mediates cystitis pain. Rudick CN, Bryce PJ, Guichelaar LA, Berry RE, Klumpp DJ. PLoS One. 2008 May 7;3(5):e2096. PMID:18461160

[15] Pharmacologic attenuation of pelvic pain in a murine model of interstitial cystitis. Rudick CN, Schaeffer AJ, Klumpp DJ. BMC Urol. 2009 Nov 12;9:16. PMID:19909543

[16] Cell relationship in a Wistar rat model of spontaneous prostatitis. Keith IM, Jin J, Neal D Jr, Teunissen BD, Moon TD. J Urol. 2001 Jul;166(1):323-8. PMID:11435894

[17] Age-related alterations in inflammatory response during experimental autoimmune prostatitis. Morón G, Maletto B, Orsilles M, Depiante-Depaoli M, Pistoresi-Palencia MC. Mech Ageing Dev. 2000 Sep 1;118(1-2):71-85. PMID:10989126

[18] Increased endogenous estrogen synthesis leads to the sequential induction of prostatic inflammation (prostatitis) and prostatic pre-malignancy. Ellem SJ, Wang H, Poutanen M, Risbridger GP. Am J Pathol. 2009 Sep;175(3):1187-99. PMID:19700748

[19] Corticotropin-releasing hormone-receptor 2 is required for acute stress-induced bladder vascular permeability and release of vascular endothelial growth factor. Boucher W, Kempuraj D, Michaelian M, Theoharides TC.BJU Int. 2010 Nov;106(9):1394-9. PMID:20201838

[20] Effect of comestibles on symptoms of interstitial cystitis.Shorter B, Lesser M, Moldwin RM, Kushner L. J Urol. 2007 Jul;178(1):145-52. PMID:17499305

[21] Pharmacologic attenuation of pelvic pain in a murine model of interstitial cystitis. Rudick CN, Schaeffer AJ, Klumpp DJ. BMC Urol. 2009 Nov 12;9:16. PMID:19909543

[22] Oral cimetidine gives effective symptom relief in painful bladder disease: a prospective, randomized, double-blind placebo-controlled trial. Thilagarajah R, Witherow RO, Walker MM. BJU Int. 2001 Feb;87(3):207-12. PMID:11167643

[23] A pilot clinical trial of oral pentosan polysulfate and oral hydroxyzine in patients with interstitial cystitis. Sant GR, Propert KJ, Hanno PM, Burks D, et al; Interstitial Cystitis Clinical Trials Group. J Urol. 2003 Sep;170(3):810-5. PMID:12913705

[24] Comparative pharmacology of the H1 antihistamines. del Cuvillo A, Mullol J, Bartra J, et al. J Investig Allergol Clin Immunol. 2006;16 Suppl 1:3-12. PMID:17357372

[25] Claudins: Control of Barrier Function and Regulation in Response to Oxidant Stress. Overgaard CE, Daugherty BL, Mitchell LA, Koval M. Antioxid Redox Signal. 2011 May 9. PMID:21275791

[26] A randomized double-blind placebo-controlled crossover trial of the efficacy of L-arginine in the treatment of interstitial cystitis. Cartledge JJ, Davies AM, Eardley I. BJU Int. 2000 Mar;85(4):421-6. PMID:10691818

[27] Quercetin enhances intestinal barrier function through the assembly of zonula [corrected] occludens-2, occludin, and claudin-1 and the expression of claudin-4 in Caco-2 cells. Suzuki T, Hara H.J Nutr. 2009 May;139(5):965-74. PMID:19297429

[28] Complementary and alternative therapies as treatment approaches for interstitial cystitis. Whitmore KE. Rev Urol. 2002;4 Suppl 1:S28-35. PMID:16986031

[29] Treatment of chronic prostatitis. Comparison of Minocycline and Doxycycline. Brannan W. Urology. 1975 May;5(5):626-31. PMID:1093309

[30] Toll-Like Receptor-2 Plays a Fundamental Role in Periodontal Bacteria-Accelerated Abdominal Aortic Aneurysms. Aoyama N, Suzuki JI, Ogawa M, et al. Circ J. 2013 Feb 13. PMID:23412709

28. Headaches

Comorbidity of Migraine

Migraine is more than a painful inconvenience and a day of lost wages. Migraine with aura is associated with an elevated risk of vascular disease, stroke, and heart attack. Since comorbidity often indicates co-existing causation, these associations can give clues to the underlying causes of the headaches and suggest a direction for preventive treatment. Successful preventive therapy of migraine can also be expected to decrease the risk of its associated comorbid conditions.

Table 28-1: Common Comorbidities of Migraine

Migraine Type	Comorbidities[1]	Risk Ratio
Migraine with Aura	Transient Ischemic Attacks	4.3
	Strokes	2.8
	Cerebellar Infarcts	
	Patent foramen ovale[2,3]	2.0 – 3.0
	Angina	3.0
	Myocardial Infarction	2.9
	Suicidal Ideation	1.8 – 2.4
	Suicidal Attempt	4.3
Migraine (without aura)	Myocardial Infarction	1.9
Migraine (Not differentiated)	Major Depression	2.2 – 3.1
	Bipolar Disorders	2.9 – 7.3
	General Anxiety Disorder	3.9 – 5.3
	Panic Disorder	3.0 – 5.1
	Agoraphobia	2.4
	Social Phobia	3.4
	Restless Leg Syndrome	2.5
	Fibromyalgia	
	Irritable Bowel Syndrome	
	Celiac Disease	
	Chronic Fatigue Syndrome	
	Reynaud's Phenomenon	
	Systemic Lupus (SLE)	
	Narcolepsy	
	Obesity[17]	
	Epilepsy[4]	
	Enuresis[5]	

How Headaches Happen

It may be helpful to begin by explaining the causation of the most popular headache on the planet. More people have experienced these than any other type; it is the headache most clearly associated with dietary intake: hypothermic sphenopalatine cephalgia.

RED FLAG HEADACHE WARNINGS

Some headaches are caused by dangerous conditions that require urgent medical attention. People with migraines or other headaches are not immune to headaches from by strokes, tumors, infections, or vascular disease. Any of the following signs may be an indication of a dangerous condition which requires urgent medical evaluation:

- Increasing headache frequency and severity.
- New headache onset below the age of 5 or after the age of 50.
- Worst headache ever.
- New onset of seizures.
- Headache accompanied by systemic symptoms, (fever, chills, weight loss).
- New headaches in a person with immunodeficiency or a history of cancer.
- Neurologic signs or symptoms such as loss of movement or sensation.
- Thunderclap Headache; severe headache with an onset to peak in pain within seconds or minutes.
- Headache brought on by exertion, strain or positional changes.

Hypothermic Sphenopalatine Cephalgia

This headache feels like a vice-grip clamping down inside one's face. It is excruciating, yet at times, comical as the victim realizes that the intense lancing pain is the self-induced result of a foolish and lustful rush to consume a sweet, frozen treat. Hypothermic sphenopalatine cephalgia is best known as an ice-cream headache, or brain freeze. Boys are more susceptible to get ice cream headaches than are girls[2], perhaps resulting from the males' greater endowment of lust for consumption and paucity of poise.

Fortunately, brain freeze usually lasts less than 30 seconds, unless you are one of the unfortunate few in whom it can last as long as 10 minutes[6]. Similar headaches can be caused by plunging into cold water[7] or exposure to cold weather.

Hypothermic sphenopalatine cephalgia usually occurs on warm days about 30 seconds after eating something very cold, provoking cooling of the palate and pharynx. One of the main jobs of the sphenopalatine ganglion is to control blood flow to the nasal mucosa so that air is warm and humidified before going into the lungs. When the area is cooled very quickly by eating ice cream, the stimulus triggers a reflex action in the sphenopalatine ganglion that quickly relaxes the nasopalatine artery walls, in an attempt to increase blood flow to the area to warm air passing by. But, since the tissue is cold, and the air is warm, actual blood flow to the area may remain the same or may even decrease. It is like a river reaching a wide area; flow slows by 25 to 35%[8]. The engorgement and stretching of the walls of the arteries cause pain via stretch receptors. These pain receptors are of the same type as those activated with broken bones, where the periosteum is stretched, or with intestinal pain with colic where the gut wall is stretched.

Individuals, who are subject to migraines, are more susceptible to ice cream headaches[1], as similar mechanisms are responsible for headache pain. Migraines, however, not only can last for hours or days, they include other symptoms and risks beyond those of a mere brain freeze.

Engorgement of intracranial arteries is also the mechanism by which nitroglycerin[9], used for angina to increase blood flow to the heart, can provoke headaches. Nitroglycerin headaches are also common in factory workers where explosives are made. Nitroglycerine is metabolized into nitrate in the mitochondria. Nitrate is then metabolized to NO (nitric oxide), a potent vasodilator, especially during ischemic conditions.

Nitroglycerin headaches, however, are not true migraines. They can give the pain of the migraines but lack the prodrome, nausea, and photophobia. Nitroglycerin headaches in normal subjects are usually short lasting; however, they can last hours and be severe in those prone to headaches. Nitroglycerin can reproduce the usual migraine pain in migraineurs, provoke tension headaches in those susceptible to tension headaches and cause cluster headaches in those susceptible to them. This suggests that NO is involved in these headaches as well[10]. Histamine receptors (H_1R) in the large intracranial arteries release NO upon stimulation with histamine[11]; NO is also part of the mechanism for histamine-associated headaches.

The oxidative S-nitrosylation of NO can also promote delayed migraine[10]. In this reaction, NO is attacked by oxygen radicals resulting in the formation of peroxynitrite radicals. Migraine headaches may be the result of endothelial dysfunction, a process mediated by oxidative stress[12]. In endothelial dysfunction, there is impaired vascular reactivity, inflammation, and increased coagulability. Nitric oxide is not only a potent vasodilator but is also a mediator of inflammation. During both migraine and migraine-free periods, migraineurs suffer sustained nitrosative stress[13,14]. NO only lasts for a few seconds and is rapidly oxidized to nitrite and nitrate. Migraineurs, especially those with migraine with aura, have elevated nitrite and nitrate levels, especially during migraine attacks. NO and its products can be measured and used as markers of inflammatory response. Additionally, the inflammatory marker hsCRP is elevated in migraine[15].

Although the brain itself does not have innervation for pain, the intracranial vessels, meninges, and dura mater do. The dura is innervated by the ophthalmic ramus of the first branch of the trigeminal nerve, which arises in the trigeminal ganglion. These nerves then project by secondary neurons to the trigeminal nucleus caudalis in the brain stem and from there to brain areas where pain is experienced[16].

The trigeminal nerve is the largest cranial nerve. It has multiple functions, including sensory; including pain and pressure innervation, to the face. It has three branches, which helps explain the distribution of headache pain.

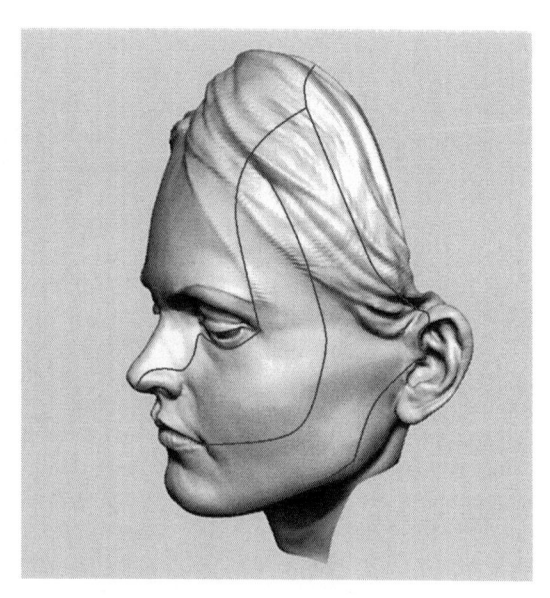

Figure 28-1: Surface sensory divisions of the three branches of the Trigeminal nerve and distribution to the face: Ophthalmic nerve (frontal area), Maxillary nerve (zygomatic arch area), and Mandibular nerve (jaw and sideburn area). The cervical plexus innervates the anterior neck, and the back of the head is innervated by the dorsal rami of cervical nerves (Image by Selwy).

CGRP

The trigemino-cerebrovascular system provides a feedback mechanism to ensure a steady supply of blood to the brain. If blood flow to the brain is reduced, the trigeminal nerve rapidly reacts in a reflex action to normalize the blood flow. This action is mediated by the release of CGRP (Calcitonin Gene-Related Peptide), the most potent peptide vasodilator known.

CGRP is formed in motor nerves and ganglion in response to nerve injury and is also involved in the transmission of neurogenic inflammatory pain. CGRP is present in especially high concentrations in the trigeminal ganglion. Cytokines, including TNF-α, IL-1β, and IL-6, increase the production of CGRP through the MAPK signaling pathway. TNF-α and IL-6 have been found to be elevated at the onset of migraines[17]. Thus, inflammation, immune reactions, stress, and sleep deficits increase the production of inflammatory cytokines and increase the risk of migraines.

Nitroglycerin increases the release of CGRP, with an exaggerated release in individuals subject to headaches[10]. Kynurenic acid can mitigate the trigeminal nociception induced by nitroglycerin or NO by decreasing CGRP release[18] and by inhibiting the activation of glutamate receptors[19]. Kynurenic acid, a product of tryptophan metabolism, is discussed in more depth in Chapter 31.

The neuroexcitatory amino acid glutamate is also released from the trigeminal neurons, along with CGRP, in response to the activation of calcium channels. Glutamate may play a role in cortical spreading depression, which is associated with aura in migraine[20].

Serotonin 5HT$_{1B}$ receptor agonist medications known as triptans that are used for migraines decrease CGRP release from the trigeminal neurons and also act as potent vasoconstrictors. The toxin ergotamine, for this reason, was used for migraine and to treat post-partum hemorrhage.

Elevated CGRP levels have been reported, in several conditions where inflammation is implicated, including migraine, sepsis, acute exacerbation of asthma and psoriasis[17]. CGRP causes delayed type migraine in part by triggering mast cell degranulation. The cranial dura tissue which covers the brain is invested with a large number of mast cells which are found close to nerve endings of the meningeal nociceptors. Degranulation of these nociceptors can cause meningeal inflammation. It is not only histamine release, but also other mediators, such as prostanoids, leukotrienes, cytokines (TNF-alpha and IL-6 and endothelin-1), chemokines, and tryptase which promote headache pain[21].

Notably, an injection of CGRP will trigger a migraine in migraineurs, but only promote a sense of mild head fullness in non-migrainuers[17]. This suggests that migraine is a mast cell activation disorder, where mast cell hyperplasia and/or hyperactivity promote a migrainous reaction to CGRP.

CGRP has anti-inflammatory actions that should limit the vasodilatory effect triggered by inflammatory mediators, and thus, limit the headache. However, glutamate[22], mast cell mediators, and NO may directly or indirectly stimulate CGRP production or release, and thus, setup a positive feedback loop which maintains the headache, sometimes as a delayed cyclic headache, which can cycle for days.

Immediate Vs. Delayed Migraine

Nitroglycerin and ice cream can trigger headaches within a minute. CGRP can also give an immediate headache, but can also be involved in extended or delayed headaches which may require 24 hours or more to manifest. This delay between the exposure and onset of a migraine can make it difficult to determine the association between the causative exposure and the headache.

Migraines provoked by IgG food immunogenicities are often delayed by 12 to 36 hours following the consumption of a reacting immunogen. CGRP can help explain how NO triggers delayed onset migraine headaches[23]. The inflammatory cytokine IL-1β can also induce CGRP through a mechanism in which IL-1β promotes expression of COX2 that stimulates the production of PGE$_2$. When this occurs in the trigeminal nerve, inflammatory prostaglandins activate neurons to release GCRP about 24 hours after the exposure to IL-1β[24]. Most food-related headaches involve an inflammatory process and act through a delayed mechanism. NO nitrosylation also gives a delayed migraine. GCRP then promotes various symptoms, depending on the patient.

$$IL\text{-}1\beta \rightarrow COX2 \rightarrow PGE2 \rightarrow CGRP$$

Generalized schema for migraines:

CGRP → Mast cell degranulation → Histamine → NO production → Vasodilation → Pain

CGRP → Mast cell degranulation → Other mast cell mediators → Nausea, irritability, etc.

Glutamate → Neuroexcitation → Aura

This schema provides opportunities for intervention at various points in the development of headaches.

Table 28-2: Effectors of Migraine and Potential Control Points

Effector	Causes	Therapy
CGRP (and glutamate)	Inflammatory cytokines increase release. Low tryptophan levels increase CGRP release. NO increases release.	Avoid inflammatory cytokines: Treat infections, avoid antergens. Get adequate sleep and avoid chronic stress. Dietary tryptophan.
Mast cell degranulation	Mast cell activation disorder (MCAD) – excessive mast cells deposition in tissue, mast cell degranulation.	Treat MCAD: See Chapter 12.
Histamine	Mast cell degranulation. Impaired histamine catabolism.	Supply nutrients, and avoid enzyme inhibitors: See Table 13-6
Nitric Oxide production	Histamine release from mast cells. Oxidative stress increases nitrosylation of NO. Increased CGRP release.	Avoid immunogens. Avoid and treat oxidative stress: See Chapter 21.
Glutamate	Inflammatory cytokines increase release. Increased release of NO. Low serotonin levels. Increased glutamate release. Decreased conversion to GABA. Decreases kynurenic acid	As above. Oxidative stress; Chapter 21. See Table 28-3. See Table 28-4. Magnesium and vitamin B$_6$
IL-1β	Increase CGRP release.	Table 40-2, Chapter 40
TNF-α	Increase CGRP release.	Item 8, Page 206

Serotonin agonists ("triptan" medications) can both prevent and abort migraine attacks by preventing the release of CGRP and glutamate[20]. 5-hydroxytryptophan, the precursor of serotonin, has also been used prophylactically against migraine. L-tryptophan is an essential amino acid utilized in the formation of proteins, as well as for the formation of the neurotransmitter serotonin, the vitamin niacin, melatonin and other molecules. It is the least abundant of the eight major essential amino acids in the diet, and as a result of this, serotonin depletion can occur.

Tryptophan depletion, promoted by feeding a multi-amino acid supplement deficient in tryptophan, was found to induce nausea, photophobia and migraines in migraineurs and cause nausea in control individuals after 8 hours[25]. The body converts tryptophan into 5-hydroxy- tryptophan (5-HTP). In a trial using 600 mg of 5-HTP daily, 71 percent of migraineurs experienced a decrease in the intensity of headache pain[26]. In another study, 5-HTP reduced the frequency of migraines[27]. Tryptophan depletion can induce motion sickness, which migraineurs are especially susceptible to[28]. Tryptophan depletion may also provoke the depletion of kynurenic acid.

Probably more common than dietary tryptophan deficiency, however, is failure L-tryptophan conversion into serotonin because of the diversion of tryptophan to other products. Tryptophan can be diverted into the kynurenine pathway by bacterial LPS and certain inflammatory cytokines; thus depleting serotonin (see Chapter 31.) Phenotypic variations in genetic alleles may affect the conversion of tryptophan to serotonin. A significant portion of the tryptophan available for conversion to serotonin can also be converted to niacin (vitamin B_3). Thus, niacin supplements may spare tryptophan so that it is more available for conversion to serotonin.

Table 28-3: Enzymes and Cofactors for Serotonin and Melatonin Production

Enzyme	Reaction	Cofactor
Tryptophan 5-monooxygenase	Tryptophan to 5-hydroxytryptophan (5-HTP) *(Rate-limiting step)*	Iron, Tetrahydro-biopterin [requires Folate (5-MTHF), Zinc, Iron, Niacin]
Aromatic L-amino acid decarboxylase	5-HTP to Serotonin	Pyridoxal-5-phosphate (vitamin B_6) Pyrroloquinoline quinone (PQQ)
Aralkylamine N-acetyl-transferase	Serotonin to N-acetylserotonin	Acetyl-CoA (Carnitine required)
Acetyl-serotonin N-methyl-transferase	N-acetylserotonin to Melatonin	S-adenosyl-L-methionine (SAMe) See below

Tetrahydrobiopterin is a required cofactor for the enzyme tryptophan hydroxylase, which converts tryptophan into 5-HTP. This is the rate-limiting step in the production of serotonin. 5-HTP is then converted to serotonin by aromatic L-amino acid decarboxylase, an enzyme requiring vitamin B6 and PQQ. See Figure 31-2.

The Star Dust Vitamin

Pyrroloquinoline quinone (PQQ) is an essential nutrient that is found in a healthful diet[29], and which meets the definition of a vitamin. Foods rich in PQQ include legumes, leafy vegetables, and some fruits. In a NASA space probe, an organic molecule was found in the tail of a comet, which was identified as PQQ. PQQ is thought to be a component of interstellar dust, which was deposited on earth along with water from comets, and which may have helped in the early formation of life on the planet[30].

PQQ is an antioxidant, but can act as a pro-oxidant depending on the redox state of the environment; for example, the availability of reduced glutathione[31]. PQQ can induce the production of new mitochondria in aging cells[32] and appears to be required for the induction of lymphocytes in the Peyer's patches in the ileum[33]. PQQ was found, in an animal model, to protect the heart from ischemia/reperfusion injury as effectively as the beta blocker metoprolol[34]. PQQ has been found to be protective against glutamate-induced neurotoxicity[35], to prevent neuropathic pain and muscular atrophy after nerve injury[36] and prevent apoptosis of neurons in the hippocampus[37].

The estimated minimum daily dietary intake of PQQ for health is about 150 mcg. PQQ supplements, however, usually are sold containing about 10 mg (10,000 mcg.)

Melatonin and Migraine

Melatonin, a hormone formed from serotonin, can be helpful in preventing and treating migraine. Urinary 6-sulphatoxymelatonin, a metabolic end product of melatonin, is lower in migraine patients during migraines[38], as well as when they are not having a migraine[39]. Melatonin receptors in the trigeminal nucleus indirectly activate opioid receptors, potentiate GABA, and inhibit lipoxygenase and cyclooxygenase 2; thus, inhibiting the formation of inflammatory eicosanoids[40]. Melatonin is an antioxidant that lowers the formation of nitrosyl products.

In one clinical trial of migraineurs, 2 mg of melatonin an hour before bedtime over eight weeks did not reduce migraine attack frequency[41]. In another, 3-month trial, 3 mg of melatonin 30 minutes before bedtime was associated with a 50%, or greater, reduction of migraines in 75% of the patients, and eliminated migraines completely in 25% of the patients[42]. In another study of children aged 6 to 16, 3 mg of melatonin at bedtime was effective in reducing or eliminating headaches in 90% of the children[43].

Sleep disorders can increase the incidence of migraines, perhaps through an increase in inflammation and IL-6 associated with sleep deprivation. Melatonin may reduce migraine as a result of improved sleep. For initiating sleep, melatonin may be most effective using a low dose (0.3 to 1.0 mg sublingually) when getting into bed to sleep (lights off). To sustain sleep, 3 to 5 mg of slow-release melatonin is often effective. Migraineurs have increased sensitivity to suppression of melatonin by light[44]. Bright and fluorescent light (which contains more light in the blue end of the spectrum) should be avoided in the evenings before sleep.

Glutamate

Glutamate is an excitatory neurotransmitter. Excessive release of glutamate or activation of glutaminergic neurons may cause migraine, particularly in migraine with aura.

The enzyme glutamine synthetase in the astrocyte converts glutamate (and ammonia) into the amino acid glutamine that is used as an energy source by neurons. Glutamate, the by-product of the energy use, is exported back into the extracellular space by neurons, and astrocytes recycle it into fuel again, and exported into the extracellular space so that it is available for the neurons. Glutamate is also an excitatory neurotransmitter that increases alertness and decreases reaction time. Excessive or unbalanced glutamate, however, can act as an excitotoxin.

Ammonia, which can be produced in the colon from the fermentation of unabsorbed amino acids, is also neuroexcitotoxin. Ammonia is also taken up by astrocytes, and, and if not metabolized efficiently to glutamine can cause swelling of the astrocytes and vasoconstriction. Ammonia can activate the NMDA receptor, induce NO synthesis[45] and release glutamate from astrocytes[46].

Glutamate can also be converted in the astrocyte to GABA; an inhibitory neurotransmitter. The herbal calmative agents *Centella asiatica* (gotu kola) and *Valeriana officinalis* (valerian) stimulate glutamate decarboxylase activity by over 40% while *Melissa officinalis* (lemon balm) inhibits 4-aminobutyrate aminotransferase activity[47]. Thus, these herbs increase GABA and decrease glutamate. The anticonvulsant medication pregabalin stimulates glutamate decarboxylase and GABA production while valproic acid inhibits its removal by 4-aminobutyrate aminotransferase. The benzodiazepines, which are used as anti-anxiety, anticonvulsive and sedative agents, also act by enhancing GABA availability.

Excessive glutamate activity induces neurotoxicity and apoptosis, especially in the presence of hypoglycemia or hypoxia. Neuroprotectins prevent neuronal cell death otherwise induced by glutamate[48]. Neuroprotectin D1 (NDP1) is an eicosanoid formed from the n-3 fatty acid docosahexaenoic acid (DHA). Both DHA and NPD1 limit hippocampal electrically induced hyperexcitability. NPD1 has been found to protect retinal pigmented epithelium (RPE) cells from oxidative stress and apoptosis[49]. Thus, DHA may help protect the brain from glutamate-induced hyperexcitability, from migrainous aura, and may also protect the retina from macular degeneration.

Table 28-4: Glutamate, Glutamine, GABA Metabolism[50]

Enzyme	Substrate	Product	Cofactors and Effectors
Glutamate decarboxylase	Glutamate	γ-amino-butyrate (GABA)	Pyridoxal-5-Phosphate Valerian ↑ Gotu kola ↑
Glutamate-ammonia ligase	Glutamate Ammonia	Glutamine	Magnesium
Phosphate-activated Glutaminase	Glutamine	Glutamate	
4-aminobutyrate aminotransferase	γ-amino-butyrate	Glutamate	*Melissa officinalis* ↓

Mast Cell Degranulation

CGRP is a mast cell degranulator, as discussed above. Immune reactions to food can trigger migraines, likely through mast cell activation and degranulation. Dietary sulfites and potato lectin are known to provoke mast cell degranulation but have not been associated with migraine.

Migraine and Food Antergies

Mast cells have IgG receptors that can trigger mast cell activity. This is not restricted to degranulation, but can include more limited response, including the release of IL-1β. After the release of IL-1β, it takes about 3 hours for cells in the ganglia to produce COX2, and then, at least another hour for peak production of PGE2. From the time of release of IL-1β to peak output of CGRP is at least 24 hours[24].

Many migraineurs associate certain foods as triggers for migraines. In studies using an oligoantigenic or elemental diet, most patients get relief of migraine and reintroduction of the foods causes a reoccurrence of symptoms[51]. In a study of children with epilepsy, over half of those with migraine and/or hyperactivity had relief from migraines and seizures during an oligoantigenic diet. The seizures reoccurred when the diet was reintroduced. Children with seizures but no migraine or hyperactivity did not respond to this diet. This suggests that seizures due to traumatic or ischemic brain injury do not respond to diet but those due to enteroimmune mechanism do[4]. In a study of children with migraine and enuresis, the bed wetting stopped in more than half the children on the oligoantigenic diet and, for the most part, reoccurred when the previous diet was reintroduced[5].

In a blinded study protocol, migraineurs were tested for IgG antibodies to 266 different foods. Patients were then randomized to either a diet that included the reacting food or one eliminating those foods for six weeks, before crossing over to the other diet. Patients in the active treatment arm that eliminated IgG reactive foods had fewer migraine attacks, decreasing in number by more than 30%[52].

A similar study tested for IgG antergens to 108 foods. The patients were placed on diets eliminating the foods that they had elevated IgG antibodies to. After one month, two-thirds of the patients that eliminated the IgG-reacting foods from their diets had complete remission of their migraines. In the study, 100% of migraineurs had IgG antibodies to foods while only 26% of control individuals had IgG antibodies at least one of the 108 foods tested[53].

Food antergies are a common cause of migraines. The presence of these antibodies suggests that the enterocyte barrier is compromised. In most individuals, elimination of IgG-reacting foods from the diet, will downregulate immune reaction to the food antigens. After some time, usually six months to a year, the food can often be reintroduced. Food antergies may continue to develop if there is continued stimulation from cross-reacting antigens, an inflammatory milieu, or compromised enterocyte membrane. If the underlying stimulus for antergen formation is not eliminated, patients will develop new immune reactions to foods, and the migraines will reoccur.

Patients with multiple IgG immunoreactivities to foods would be expected to have T_H17 dominated immune defenses, a state maintained by intestinal dysbiosis and intestinal paracellular hyperpermeability. These patients have an altered immune reactivity, and an intestinal environment which supports quorum sensing and biofilm formation in the gut. For the long-term resolution of headaches, associated with immune reactivity from the intestines, dysbiosis, and paracellular hyperpermeability need to be resolved. Stress, sleep deprivation, intestinal biofilm, poor nutrition, toxic lectins and other stimuli can promote antergies.

Infectious Agents

Migraine frequency has also been associated with non-food antibodies. In a study of migraineurs, 59% had antibodies to *Chlamydia pneumoniae* while only 21% of controls did[54]. In another study, 44% of migraineurs had antibodies to *Toxoplasmosis gondii* while only 25% of controls did[55]. These highly prevalent infections may contribute to migraine, or may reflect host immunity impairment. *Chlamydia* antibodies have been found in many neurological conditions including schizophrenia[56], but proving ongoing infection or improvement with treatment has been elusive[57]. While *Toxoplasmosis* can infect the brain, cause headaches, and remain a chronic infection, it also causes inflammatory changes in the gut and increases sensitivity to gluten. An association between *Toxoplasmosis* antibodies and risk for neurologic disease has also been found in numerous studies[58] and is discussed in Chapter 31.

Pets are frequent carriers of *Campylobacter jejuni*. *C. jejuni* infection often precedes the onset of IBS, migraine, and the neurological disease, Guillain-Barre syndrome[59]. This infection damages the enterocyte barrier and increases intestinal paracellular permeability for up to a year after infection. *C. jejuni* may increase the systemic absorption of bacterial LPS, which may affect the CNS, through inducing 5-HTP diversion into the kynurenine pathway. *C. jejuni* produces endotoxins and GM1 ganglioside, which may cause acute inflammatory polyneuropathy. The association of infections with migraine may reflect the immune response to the organism, toxins produced by the organism, or in the case of intracellular parasites such as *Toxoplasmosis* and *Chlamydia*, may reflect their effects on cell metabolism.

Migraine and Trace Amines

The bioamine, tyramine, can provoke migraines. Trace Amine (TA) receptors are a class of cell surface protein receptors that bind to certain amines that are normally found in the blood only at very low levels. These bioamines include tyramine, tryptamine, octopamine, synephrine and β-phenylethylamine. Four human TA receptors have been identified (1, 3, 4, and 5); all map to chromosome 6q23.2[60]. The TA_1 receptor binds tyramine and β-phenylethylamine. Both these trace amines can trigger migraine headaches.

At low levels, tyramine acts on arterial tissue as a vasoconstrictor; however, when higher levels are present, it is a vasodilator[61]. Vasodilatation explains headache pain as seen in migraine, but it does not account for the auras, photophobia, or some other migraine symptoms. Ice cream and nitrates do not give auras, but tyramine does. The ability of tyramine to cause migraine with aura is explained by the presence of TA_1 receptors, which are found in multiple areas of the brain[6,62].

A meta-analysis of published studies between 1966 and 2001 concluded that oral challenges with biogenic amines had failed to show any significant relationships between tyramine or phenylethylamine and headache[63]. However, in other studies, where triggering foods were removed, the number of migraine attacks declined significantly. Tyramine and other biogenic amines targeting the TA receptors may act in concert with other risk factors to yield their effects. Two likely factors that affect the entry of trace amines into the blood stream are intestinal paracellular permeability and catabolic enzymes. Normally, these amines should not bypass the enterocyte tight junctions. Alcohol, often cited as a cofactor in trace amine-related migraines, can increase paracellular permeability. Other factors that increase paracellular permeability, such as gliadin, are discussed in Chapter 25. Enzymes at the brush border of the enterocytes include AOC1, which breaks down histamine and trace amines. There is competitive inhibition of this enzyme by the trace amines. Additionally, alcohol inhibits the catabolism of the amines by AOC1, by inhibiting the downstream catabolism of AOC1 products. The enterocytes absorb some of the trace amines. MAO is an important intracellular enzyme for bioactive amine catabolism. It too is under competitive inhibition by other trace amines and is inhibited by alcohol. In the presence of alcohol or other factors that increase intestinal permeability or decrease the enzymatic break-down of bioactive amines, trace amines may have more pronounced effects than they would under normal circumstances.

Food Nitrites and Migraine

Nitrites are commonly used to preserve color in lunch-, smoked-, and cured meats. Nitrites have been suggested as the cause of "hot-dog headaches"[64], but there are no trials confirming this, only anecdotal reports. If hot dogs do cause migraine, the migraine may be triggered by biogenic amines produced by bacterial fermentation of the meat, rather than from the nitrite preservatives in the meat.

While the nitrite content of hotdogs may not trigger migraine, there are additional reasons to avoid cured meats containing nitrite; they are carcinogenic. Children were found to have an increased risk of brain cancer if their mothers ate hotdogs or sausage during pregnancy[65]. They are also a likely carcinogen for leukemia in children[66] and for colon cancer[67]. The N-nitroso compounds formed while cooking these meats may be the causative compound. Alternatively, HCAs formed during cooking of meat are known carcinogens (See Chapter 40).

Additive Effects

Multiple food and non-food stimuli can trigger migraines, and thus, it is a difficult endeavor to sort out which stimulus triggered a specific headache. Often, there are plenty of factors to point to, and the accumulative effects of food and other stimuli can act in concert. Although migraineurs may identify provocative stimuli, the effects may not be reliably reproduced when the stimuli are isolated.

When trace amines act as a trigger, there is likely a threshold to the response. Consumption of red wine one day, or a brownie, banana, orange juice, aged cheese, and wheat on different days may achieve the threshold for migraine, however, a combination these foods, or foods and stress, or lack of sleep may easily exceed the threshold for migraine.

Trace amine associated migraines may be prevented by avoiding foods high in tyramine, phenylethanolamine, and other bioactive amines. For long-term prevention, it is desirable to treat the multiple underlying issues that may include an impaired intestinal mucosal barrier, antergies, oxidative stress and other factors.

Migraine Prophylaxis

The basis for preventive treatment of migraine is to mitigate the inflammatory state. Inflammation supports the formation of inflammatory cytokines, which stimulate CGRP release, and immune reactions that support mast cell hyperplasia and degranulation. Elimination of IgG reacting foods often gives resolution of intractable migraines within days. Many patients, however, will relapse (forming new immune reactions to foods) in the following months if the underlying inflammatory condition is not treated.

Table 28-5: Migraine Prophylaxis

1. Eliminate IgG food antergens from the diet.	See Chapter 19
2. Treat intestinal hyperpermeability, dysbiosis, and biofilm formation.	See Chapters 23 and 25
3. Prevent mast cell activation.	See Chapter 12
4. Avoid dietary trace amines.	See Chapter 13
5. Use N-3 fatty acid DHA as a neuroprotectant.	See Chapter 6
6. Decrease inflammation from TLR activation.	See Chapters 20, 30, and 31
7. Treat oxidative stress.	See Chapter 21
8. Avoid emotional and social stress.	See Chapter 29
9. Get sufficient sleep.	See Chapter 41
10. Prevent PGE2 production.	Below
11. Use supplements to improve coenzyme activity.	Below

Prevent PGE$_2$ Production

Avoiding inflammation and immune activation which induces activation and release of IL-1β can prevent the induction of PGE2 and the release of CGRP.

IL-1β induces production of the enzyme PTGS2 (COX2), which converts arachidonic acid into PGE$_2$. This process can be inhibited by the use of medications that inhibit the COX2 enzyme, including aspirin and non-steroidal anti-inflammatory medications, even after the initiation of the immune event.

The production of PGE2 can also be mitigated by a diet low in n-6 fatty acids, or less efficiently by a diet high in n-3 fatty acids. (See Chapter 6.) Adequate vitamin D and tocotrienol forms of vitamin E also inhibit the enzyme PTGS2 (COX2) as illustrated in Figure 41-2.

IL-1β formation may be mitigated by avoiding chronic stress, sleep deprivation, and intestinal dysbiosis. Mitigation of TNF-α production is discussed in Chapters 23 and 31.

Use of Supplements for Migraine Prevention

The best source of vitamins and mineral is a balanced diet, containing limited amounts of refined foods that have been stripped of nutrients to increase shelf life. Supplements may be helpful, however, especially during the time prior to attaining control of the headaches.

Enzyme cofactor supplements are often helpful for the prophylaxis of migraines. The cofactors most often cited as helpful are riboflavin[68] and magnesium[69]. This may suggest a bottleneck in the catabolism of N-methylhistamine by MAO or AOC1. Both these enzymes require the cofactor FAD, which use riboflavin. The coenzymes utilized in the metabolism of histamine are shown in Table 13-6. Riboflavin is also a cofactor for the formation of NO from NOS, for mitochondrial Complex I and II proteins and in many other reactions. See Table 25-3 in Chapter 25 for NO cofactors.

Table 28-6: Enzyme Cofactor Supplements Often Helpful for Migraine Prevention

Magnesium (organic salt)	200 – 350 mg daily
Riboflavin	5 mg twice daily
Pyridoxine (vitamin B$_6$)	25 mg daily
Folate (5-MTHF preferred for supplement)	400 mcg to 600 mcg daily
Zinc	10 to 20 mg daily
Vitamin D$_3$ (if needed)	See Chapter 12
Tocotrienols	10 mg daily
Melatonin	3 to 6 mg slow release at bedtime
Niacin	See below
PQQ and TMG	From Diet

5-Hydroxytryptophan (5-HTP): is a substrate for the production of serotonin and melatonin. It can also be converted back to tryptophan and enter the kynurenine pathway. 5-HTP 100 to 200 mg three times daily is helpful in migraine prevention in some individuals. Serotonin is a calming neurotransmitter. Melatonin can be helpful especially in patients with sleep delay disorders and migraine, or light-induced migraine[70]. Kynurenic acid is an NMDA antagonist, is neuroprotective, and blocks CGRP release. The kynurenine pathway has both neuroprotective and neurotoxic products. (See Chapter 31.)

Magnesium: Magnesium blocks the ion channel on the NMDA receptor and acts as an antagonist, blocking excessive glutaminergic activation[71] and excitotoxicity[72]. Magnesium is also useful in treating post-operative pain[73]. Migraineurs have been found to have lower Mg levels than matched controls[74].

Magnesium is not effective for the acute treatment of migraine, in part, because it is only slowly absorbed from the intestine and has side effects when given IV[75]. Nevertheless, magnesium has been found to be helpful in decreasing the frequency and severity of migraines when used as a prophylactic agent[76].

Pyridoxine-5-phosphate (PLP, aka P5P) is required for the production of kynurenic acid. With insufficient PLP, this pathway produces the neurotoxic compound 3-hydroxy-kynurenine. PLP is also a coenzyme for the conversion of 5-HTP to serotonin. Treatment of migraine using 5-HTP should include treatment with pyridoxine, but may use pyridoxine alone. PLP is also required for conversion of glutamate to GABA. Magnesium is also a cofactor for converting the kynurenine pathway toxin, quinolinic acid into niacin. PLP and magnesium are needed for the catabolism of ceramide and sphingosine-1-phosphate.

PQQ and TMG: PQQ is needed for the formation of serotonin and melatonin. TMG (Trimethylglycine; Betaine) helps recycle SAMe, which is also needed for the formation of melatonin and in many other reactions including the catabolism of histamine. Folate, vitamin B$_{12}$, and PLP also help recycle SAMe using a different pathway. PQQ, TMG, and folate are found in fresh vegetables and whole grains.

Niacin: Several studies have shown niacin can terminate migraine headaches; however, most of these studies used IV niacin. Large oral doses (500 mg) were also successfully used, but niacin causes unpleasant side effects (including severe flushing, tingling, and nausea), and many patients refuse this treatment after one experience with it. These large doses of niacin are thought to induce the production of PGD$_2$ that increases cerebral blood flow, thereby ending the migraine[77]. The increased efferent flow might relieve tension on blood vessels.

Niacin has also been used to prevent migraine, tension, and other headaches. These trials for headache prophylaxis used large doses of niacin (over 300 mg daily). The super-physiological doses required, along with side effects and possible toxicity of chronic high dose (slow release niacin) relegate niacin to a secondary tier treatment for migraine headaches, which is better avoided unless other preventive treatments options have failed.

Caution: Niacin may act as a feedback mechanism which inhibits the conversion of the kynurenine pathway neurotoxic end product quinolinic acid into nicotinamide. High dose niacin should not be given without pyridoxine-5-phosphate to decrease the risk of excess quinolinic acid formation.

Other Antimigraine Agents

Ginger: 500 to 600 mg of dry powdered ginger at the onset of an aura is helpful in some patients. It can be repeated every 4 hours as needed.

Feverfew: Feverfew is sometimes used for the prevention of migraine. Although feverfew is often recommended for migraine, results vary, as do the formulations of various preparations. Feverfew is sometimes associated with rebound headaches when discontinued. Although several mechanisms of action have been proposed, it is not clear how this agent works. It typically takes several weeks before it becomes effective. Feverfew can cause an immune reaction in some individuals. Feverfew should not be used during pregnancy,

Histame: Histame is a proprietary dietary supplement containing the enzyme amine oxidase, copper containing 1 (AOC1), used to neutralize histamine and other bioamines in the intestines. This product may be helpful to some patients with migraine.

Avoid Enzyme Inhibitors

Pyridoxal-5-phosphate (vitamin B$_6$) can be inhibited by isoniazid, hydrazine, oral contraceptives, and yellow dye 5; these agents may increase the risk of migraine. Vitamin B$_6$ (PLP) is a coenzyme in the conversion of tryptophan to serotonin and in the kynurenine pathway as discussed above.

Aldehyde dehydrogenases (ALDH) are enzymes involved in the catabolism of histamine. They are inhibited through competitive inhibition by alcohol, disulfiram, and some medications, including certain H_2 blockers (cimetidine, ranitidine, and nizatidine, but not famotidine) and by some mushrooms.

Alcohol can compete for an enzymatic catabolism of aldehyde, and thus, may slow the catabolism of histamine; this may contribute to its action on migraine. Alcohol also depletes zinc availability and increases endothelial permeability[78]. This allows increased exposure to immunogens, exogenous biogenic amines, and agents cuasing mast cells degranulation to otherwise protected tissues. Alcohol creates oxidative stress. Alcohol should be avoided in patients with frequent migraines and by those in whom it is a known contributor to migraines.

| Table 28-7: Botox Injection Utility for Migraines |||
Headache Type	Prevalence Type	Botox Helps[79]
Exploding Migraine	45%	11% Response
Imploding Migraine	36%	70 % Response
Ocular Migraine	19%	70 % Response

Patients, who described headache pain as crushing or clamping, as if an external force was being applied, are described as have imploding migraines. Patients who describe the headache pain as a pressure building up inside the head are as described as having an exploding migraine. Other patients describe an eye popping or ocular migraine. Only those with imploding headaches or ocular migraines are likely to get relief from Botox treatment of external muscles. This suggests that the exploding migraine involves intracranial arteries, while the imploding and ocular migraines involve extracranial arteries which are in reach of the Botox injection.

[1] Comorbidities of migraine. Wang SJ, Chen PK, Fuh JL. Front Neurol. 2010 Aug 23;1:16. PMID:21188255

[2] Patent Foramen Ovale in Children with Migraine Headaches. McCandless RT, Arrington CB, Nielsen DC, Bale JF Jr, Minich LL. J Pediatr. 2011 Mar 22. PMID:21450305

[3] Prevalence of patent foramen ovale in patients with migraine. Tatlidede AD, Oflazoğlu B, Celik SE, Anadol U, Forta H. Agri. 2007 Oct;19(4):39-42. PMID:18159578

[4] Oligoantigenic diet treatment of children with epilepsy and migraine. Egger J, Carter CM, Soothill JF, Wilson J. J Pediatr. 1989 Jan;114(1):51-8. PMID:2909707

[5] Effect of diet treatment on enuresis in children with migraine or hyperkinetic behavior. Egger J, Carter CH, Soothill JF, Wilson J. Clin Pediatr (Phila). 1992 May;31(5):302-7. PMID:1582098

[6] Ice-cream headache--a large survey of 8359 adolescents. Fuh JL, Wang SJ, Lu SR, Juang KD. Cephalalgia. 2003 Dec;23(10):977-81. PMID: 14984231

[7] Ice cream headache. Ice cream headache occurred during surfing in winter. Harries M. BMJ. 1997 Sep 6;315(7108):609. PMID: 9302987

[8] Ice cream headache. Cerebral vasoconstriction causing decrease in arterial flow may have role. Sleigh JW. BMJ. 1997 Sep 6;315(7108):609. PMID: 9302986

[9] Effect of nitroglycerin on cerebral circulation measured by transcranial Doppler and SPECT. Dahl A, Russell D, Nyberg-Hansen R, Rootwelt K. Stroke. 1989 Dec;20(12):1733-6. PMID:2512693

[10] Headache-type adverse effects of NO donors: vasodilation and beyond. Bagdy G, Riba P, Kecskeméti V, Chase D, Juhász G. Br J Pharmacol. 2010 May;160(1):20-35. PMID:20331608

[11] Histamine and histamine intolerance. Maintz L, Novak N. Am J Clin Nutr. 2007 May;85(5):1185-96. PMID:17490952

[12] Migraine and biomarkers of endothelial activation in young women. Tietjen GE, Herial NA, White L, Utley C, Kosmyna JM, Khuder SA. Stroke. 2009 Sep;40(9):2977-82. PMID:19608996

[13] Increased nitric oxide stress is associated with migraine. Gruber HJ, Bernecker C, Lechner et al. Cephalalgia. 2010 Apr;30(4):486-92. PMID:19673897

[14] Increased nitrosative and oxidative stress in platelets of migraine patients. Yilmaz G, Sürer H, Inan LE, Coskun O, Yücel D. Tohoku J Exp Med. 2007 Jan;211(1):23-30. PMID:17202769

[15] Migraine and biomarkers of endothelial activation in young women. Tietjen GE, Herial NA, White L, Utley C, Kosmyna JM, Khuder SA. Stroke. 2009 Sep;40(9):2977-82. PMID:19608996

[16] Treatment of migraine attacks based on the interaction with the trigemino-cerebrovascular system. Link AS, Kuris A, Edvinsson L. J Headache Pain. 2008 Feb;9(1):5-12. PMID:18217201

[17] Calcitonin gene-related peptide: A molecular link between obesity and migraine? Recober A, Goadsby PJ. Drug News Perspect. 2010 Mar;23(2):112-7. PMID:20369076

[18] Kynurenate derivative attenuates the nitroglycerin-induced CamKIIα and CGRP expression changes. Vámos E, Fejes A, Koch J, Tajti J, Fülöp F, Toldi J, Párdutz A, Vécsei L. Headache. 2010 May;50(5):834-43. PMID:19925620

[19] Kynurenine metabolites and migraine: experimental studies and therapeutic perspectives. Fejes A, Párdutz A, Toldi J, Vécsei L. Curr Neuropharmacol. 2011 Jun;9(2):376-87. PMID:22131946

[20] Release of glutamate and CGRP from trigeminal ganglion neurons: Role of calcium channels and 5-HT1 receptor signaling. Xiao Y, Richter JA, Hurley JH. Mol Pain. 2008 Apr 16;4:12. PMID:18416824

[21] Mast cell degranulation activates a pain pathway underlying migraine headache. Levy D, Burstein R, Kainz. PMID:17459586

[22] Pathogenesis of migraine: from neurotransmitters to neuromodulators and beyond. G. D'Andrea G. Leon, A Neurological Sciences, Vol 31, Supp 1, 1-7, DOI: 10.1007/s10072-010-0267-8

[23] Headache-type adverse effects of NO donors: vasodilation and beyond. Bagdy G, Riba P, Kecskeméti V, Chase D, Juhász G. Br J Pharmacol. 2010 May;160(1):20-35. PMID:20331608

[24] IL-1β stimulates COX-2 dependent PGE2 synthesis and CGRP release in rat trigeminal ganglia cells. Neeb L, Hellen P, Boehnke C, Hoffmann J, Schuh-Hofer S, Dirnagl U, Reuter U. PLoS One. 2011 Mar 4;6(3):e17360. PMID:21394197

[25] Tryptophan depletion increases nausea, headache and photophobia in migraine sufferers. Drummond PD. Cephalalgia. 2006 Oct;26(10):1225-33. PMID:16961791

[26] 5-Hydroxytryptophan versus methysergide in the prophylaxis of migraine. Randomized clinical trial. Titus F, Dávalos A, Alom J, Codina A. Eur Neurol. 1986;25(5):327-9. PMID:3536521

[27] Comparison of the effect of 5-hydroxytryptophan and propranolol in the interval treatment of migraine. Maissen CP, Ludin HP. Schweiz Med Wochenschr. 1991 Oct 26;121(43):1585-90. PMID:1947955

[28] Effect of tryptophan depletion on symptoms of motion sickness in migraineurs. Drummond PD. Neurology. 2005 Aug 23;65(4):620-2. PMID:16116130

[29] Levels of pyrroloquinoline quinone in various foods. Kumazawa T, Sato K, Seno H, Ishii A, Suzuki O. Biochem J. 1995 Apr 15;307 (Pt 2):331-3. PMID:7733865

[30] Interstellar and Cometary Dust in Relation to the Origin of Life. F.R. Krueger and J. Kissel. Advances in Astrobiology and Biogeophysics, 2006, 2006, 325-339, DOI: 10.1007/3-540-33088-7_12

[31] Role of glutathione in augmenting the anticancer activity of pyrroloquinoline quinone (PQQ). Shankar BS, Pandey R, Amin P, Misra HS, Sainis KB. Redox Rep. 010;15(4):146-54. PMID:20663290

[32] Pyrroloquinoline quinone stimulates mitochondrial biogenesis through cAMP response element-binding protein phosphorylation and increased PGC-1alpha expression. Chowanadisai W, Bauerly KA, Tchaparian E, Wong A, Cortopassi GA, Rucker RB. J Biol Chem. 2010 Jan 1;285(1):142-52. PMID:19861415

[33] Influence of adding pyrroloquinoline quinone to parenteral nutrition on gut-associated lymphoid tissue. Omata J, Fukatsu K, Murakoshi S, Moriya T, Ueno C, Maeshima Y, Okamoto K, Saitoh D, Yamamoto J, Hase K. JPEN J Parenter Enteral Nutr. 2011 Sep-Oct;35(5):616-25. PMID:21508181

[34] Comparison of pyrroloquinoline quinone and/or metoprolol on myocardial infarct size and mitochondrial damage in a rat model of ischemia/reperfusion injury. Zhu BQ, Simonis U, Cecchini G, Zhou HZ, Li L, Teerlink JR, Karliner JS. J Cardiovasc Pharmacol Ther. 2006 Jun;11(2):119-28. PMID:16891289

[35] The neuroprotective action of pyrroloquinoline quinone against glutamate-induced apoptosis in hippocampal neurons is mediated through the activation of PI3K/Akt pathway. Zhang Q, Shen M, Ding M, Shen D, Ding F. Toxicol Appl Pharmacol. 2011 Apr 1;252(1):62-72. PMID:21320517

[36] Effect of pyrroloquinoline quinone on neuropathic pain following chronic constriction injury of the sciatic nerve in rats.Gong D, Geng C, Jiang L, Aoki Y, Nakano M, Zhong L. Eur J Pharmacol. 2012 Dec 15;697(1-3):53-8. PMID:23063836

[37] Pyrroloquinoline quinone rescues hippocampal neurons from glutamate-induced cell death through activation of Nrf2 and up-regulation of antioxidant genes. Zhang Q, Ding M, Gao XR, Ding F. Genet Mol Res. 2012 Aug 16;11(3):2652-64. PMID:22843070

[38] Low urinary 6-sulphatoxymelatonin concentrations in acute migraine. Masruha MR, de Souza Vieira DS, Minett TS, Cipolla-Neto J, Zukerman E, Vilanova LC, Peres MF. J Headache Pain. 2008 Aug;9(4):221-4. PMID:18594760

[39] Urinary 6-sulphatoxymelatonin levels are depressed in chronic migraine and several comorbidities. Masruha MR, Lin J, de Souza Vieira DS, et al. Headache. 2010 Mar;50(3):413-9. PMID:19817880

[40] Melatonin: a hormone that modulates pain. Ambriz-Tututi M, Rocha-González HI, Cruz SL, Granados-Soto V. Life Sci. 2009 Apr 10;84(15-16):489-98. PMID:19223003

[41] Prophylaxis of migraine with melatonin: a randomized controlled trial. Alstadhaug KB, Odeh F, Salvesen R, Bekkelund SI. Neurology. 2010 Oct 26;75(17):1527-32. PMID:20975054

[42] Melatonin, 3 mg, is effective for migraine prevention. Peres MF, Zukerman E, da Cunha Tanuri F, Moreira FR, Cipolla-Neto J. Neurology. 2004 Aug 24;63(4):757. PMID:15326268

[43] Melatonin to prevent migraine or tension-type headache in children. Miano S, Parisi P, Pelliccia A, Luchetti A, Paolino MC, Villa MP. Neurol Sci. 2008 Sep;29(4):285-7. PMID:18810607

[44] Melatonin secretion is supersensitive to light in migraine. Claustrat B, Brun J, Chiquet C, Chazot G, Borson-Chazot F. Cephalalgia. 2004 Feb;24(2):128-33. PMID:14728708

[45] Glutamine as a mediator of ammonia neurotoxicity: A critical appraisal. Albrecht J, Zielińska M, Norenberg MD. Biochem Pharmacol. 2010 Nov 1;80(9):1303-8. PMID:20654582

[46] Ammonia triggers exocytotic release of L-glutamate from cultured rat astrocytes. Görg B, Morwinsky A, Keitel V, et al. Glia. 2010 Apr 15;58(6):691-705. PMID:20014275

[47] Effects of traditionally used anxiolytic botanicals on enzymes of the gamma-aminobutyric acid (GABA) system. Awad R, Levac D, Cybulska P, Merali Z, Trudeau VL, Arnason JT. Can J Physiol Pharmacol. 2007 Sep;85(9):933-42. PMID:18066140

[48] Neuroprotectins A and B, bicyclohexapeptides protecting chick telencephalic neuronal cells from excitotoxicity. I. Fermentation, isolation, physico-chemical properties and biological activity. Kobayashi H, Shin-Ya K, Nagai K, et al. J Antibiot (Tokyo). 2001 Dec;54(12):1013-8. PMID:11858654

[49] Neurotrophins induce neuroprotective signaling in the retinal pigment epithelial cell by activating the synthesis of the anti-inflammatory and anti-apoptotic neuroprotectin D1. Bazan NG. Adv Exp Med Biol. 2008;613:39-44. PMID:18188926

[50] Effects of traditionally used anxiolytic botanicals on enzymes of the gamma-aminobutyric acid (GABA) system. Awad R, Levac D, Cybulska P, et al. Can J Physiol Pharmacol. 2007 Sep;85(9):933-42. PMID:18066140

[51] Is migraine food allergy? A double-blind controlled trial of oligoantigenic diet treatment. Egger J, Carter CM, Wilson J, et al. Lancet. 1983 Oct 15;2(8355):865-9.PMID: 6137694

[52] Diet restriction in migraine, based on IgG against foods: a clinical double-blind, randomised, cross-over trial. Alpay K, Ertas M, Orhan EK, Ustay DK, Lieners C, Baykan B. Cephalalgia. 2010 Jul;30(7):829-37. PMID:20647174

[53] Food allergy mediated by IgG antibodies associated with migraine in adults. Arroyave Hernández CM, Echavarría Pinto M, Hernández Montiel HL. Rev Alerg Mex. 2007 Sep-Oct;54(5):162-8.. PMID: 18693538

[54] Association between Chlamydia pneumoniae IgG antibodies and migraine. Lu Q, Xu J, Liu H. J Headache Pain. 2009 Apr;10(2):121-4. PMID:19238508

[55] Is Toxoplasma gondii a causal agent in migraine? Koseoglu E, Yazar S, Koc I. Am J Med Sci. 2009 Aug;338(2):120-2. PMID:19564786

[56] The association of infectious agents and schizophrenia. Krause D, Matz J, Weidinger E, Wagner J, Wildenauer A, Obermeier M, Riedel M, Müller N. World J Biol Psychiatry. 2010 Aug;11(5):739-43. PMID:20602604

[57] Chlamydophila pneumoniae Infection and Its Role in Neurological Disorders. Contini C, Seraceni S, Cultrera R, Castellazzi M, Granieri E, Fainardi E. Interdiscip Perspect Infect Dis. 2010;2010:273573. PMID:20182626

[58] Toxoplasma gondii and other risk factors for schizophrenia: an update. Torrey EF, Bartko JJ, Yolken RH. Schizophr Bull. 2012 May;38(3):642-7. PMID:22446566

[59] Guillain-Barré syndrome: an update. Vucic S, Kiernan MC, Cornblath DR. J Clin Neurosci. 2009 Jun;16(6):733-41. PMID:19356935

[60] Trace amines: Identification of a family of mammalian G protein-coupled receptors. Beth Borowsky, Nika Adham, Kenneth A. Jones, et al. Proc Natl Acad Sci U S A. 2001 Jul 31;98(16):8966-71. PMID: 11459929

[61] Characterization of the vasorelaxant activity of tyramine and other phenylethylamines in rat aorta. Varma DR, Deng XF, Chemtob S, Nantel F, Bouvier M. Can J Physiol Pharmacol. 1995 Jun;73(6):742-6.PMID: 7585347

[62] Biochemistry of neuromodulation in primary headaches: focus on anomalies of tyrosine metabolism. D'Andrea G, Nordera GP, Perini F, et al. Neurol Sci. 2007 May;28 Suppl 2:S94-6. PMID: 17508188

[63] Intolerance to dietary biogenic amines: a review. Jansen SC, van Dusseldorp M, Bottema KC, Dubois AE. Ann Allergy Asthma Immunol. 2003 Sep;91(3):233-40; PMID: 14533654

[64] A possible role for nitric oxide in glutamate (MSG)-induced Chinese restaurant syndrome, glutamate-induced asthma, 'hot-dog headache', pugilistic Alzheimer's disease, and other disorders. Scher W, Scher BM. Med Hypotheses. 1992 Jul;38(3):185-8. PMID:1381038

[65] A meta-analysis of maternal cured meat consumption during pregnancy and the risk of childhood brain tumors. Huncharek M, Kupelnick B. Neuroepidemiology. 2004 Jan-Apr;23(1-2):78-84. PMID:14739572

[66] Cured and broiled meat consumption in relation to childhood cancer: Denver, Colorado (United States) Sarasua S, Savitz DA. Cancer Causes Control. 1994 Mar;5(2):141-8. PMID: 8167261

[67] Total N-nitroso compounds and their precursors in hot dogs and in the gastrointestinal tract and feces of rats and mice: possible etiologic agents for colon cancer. Mirvish SS, Haorah J, Zhou L, Clapper ML, Harrison KL, Povey AC. J Nutr. 2002 Nov;132(11 Suppl):3526S-3529S. PMID:12421882

[68] Riboflavin. Monograph. Altern Med Rev. 2008 Dec;13(4):334-40. PMID:19152481

[69] Therapeutic uses of magnesium. Guerrera MP, Volpe SL, Mao JJ. Am Fam Physician. 2009 Jul 15;80(2):157-62. PMID:19621856

[70] Headache due to photosensitive magnesium depletion. Durlach J, Pagès N, Bac P, Bara M, Guiet-Bara A. Magnes Res. 2005 Jun;18(2):109-22. PMID:16100849

[71] Antidepressant-like activity of magnesium in the chronic mild stress model in rats: alterations in the NMDA receptor subunits. Pochwat B, Szewczyk B, Sowa-Kucma M, et al. Int J Neuropsychopharmacol. 2014 Mar;17(3):393-405. PMID:24067405

[72] Magnesium sulfate protects against the bioenergetic consequences of chronic glutamate receptor stimulation. Clerc P, Young CA, Bordt EA, et al. PLoS One. 2013 Nov 13;8(11):e79982. PMID:24236167

[73] Effect of intravenous magnesium sulphate on postoperative pain following spinal anesthesia. A randomized double blind controlled study. Kumar M, Dayal N, Rautela RS, Sethi AK. Middle East J Anesthesiol. 2013 Oct;22(3):251-6. PMID:24649780

[74] Blood Magnesium levels in migraineurs within and between the headache attacks: a case control study. Samaie A, Asghari N, Ghorbani R, Arda J. Pan Afr Med J. 2012;11:46. PMID:22593782

[75] The use of intravenous magnesium sulphate for acute migraine: meta-analysis of randomized controlled trials. Choi H, Parmar N. Eur J Emerg Med. 2014 Feb;21(1):2-9. PMID: 23921817

[76] The effects of magnesium, L-carnitine, and concurrent magnesium-L-carnitine supplementation in migraine rophylaxis. Tarighat Esfanjani A, Mahdavi R, Ebrahimi Mameghani M, et al. Biol Trace Elem Res. 2012 Dec;150(1-3):42-8. PMID:22895810

[77] The treatment of migraines and tension-type headaches with intravenous and oral niacin (nicotinic acid): systematic review of the literature. Prousky J, Seely D. Nutr J. 2005 Jan 26;4:3. PMID:15673472

[78] Evidence that chronic alcohol exposure promotes intestinal oxidative stress, intestinal hyperpermeability and endotoxemia prior to development of alcoholic steatohepatitis in rats. Keshavarzian A, Farhadi A, Forsyth CB, et al. J Hepatol. 2009 Mar;50(3):538-47. PMID:19155080

[79] Migraine prophylaxis with botulinum toxin A is associated with perception of headache. Burstein R, Dodick D, Silberstein S. Toxicon. 2009 Oct;54(5):624-7. PMID:19344670

29. Stress and the Hypothalamic Pituitary Axes

A couple gazelles are grazing when one spots a cheetah. They take off running. One says to the other, "What's the use? There's no way we can outrun a cheetah moving at over 100 kilometers per hour!" The other replies, "I don't need too outrun her; I just need to outrun you."

The body is designed for rapid response to danger. In the event of imminent danger, we can quickly respond to a rush of adrenalin (epinephrine), with an increase in heart rate, and then shunting of blood away from the intestines and kidneys to the muscles, brain and eyes; so that we can fight or flee. This reaction is designed to give us *a few minutes* of intense activity, during which time we can either evade or rebuff an attack. Another adaptive response system helps to accommodate acute injury; cortisol decreases the immune response and inflammation at a time when immobilization (by inflamed muscles, for example,) would hamper escape and survival.

These are functional short-term adaptive responses that increase survival advantage when confronted by predators, and increase success when acting as a predator. These acute stress responses are adapted for short-term deployment to respond to intense survival situations. During these events, the autonomic nervous system shifts dominance to the sympathetic branch; with adrenergic response, and to the hypothalamic/pituitary/adrenal (HPA) axis mediated release of corticosteroids.

Stress and the Sympathetic Immune System

The sympathetic nervous system releases norepinephrine (NE) and Neuropeptide Y (NPY) from peripheral nerve terminals. NE is also released into the bloodstream from the adrenal gland along with epinephrine. Peripherally, NE participates in the flight or fight response. Its job is to cause vasoconstriction of vegetative areas, such as the gut, to shunt blood to the muscles and brain. NE also helps to release glucose to support increased muscular activity, and to make lactate available as a fuel for the brain during the fight or flight reaction. Neuropeptide Y enhances the vasoconstrictive effect of NE.

NE is also a neurotransmitter that acts on the CNS, increasing alertness. NE enhances the anti-inflammatory effect of cortisol. In acute stress, estrogen inhibits IL-6 and the breakdown of catecholamines. This helps down-regulate HPA axis activation after the event. In chronic stress, however, this negative feedback loop fails; in this situation sympathetic nerve endings release NE and Neuropeptide Y, which along serotonin, increase the production of inflammatory cytokines by immune cells.

The sympathetic nervous system provides the primary pathway for neural regulation of immune function. NE, which is delivered by nerve endings in the various immune tissues, is the main mediator for this, and β_2-adrenergic receptors are the principal sympathetic receptors in the immune tissues. CD8+ and CD4+ T cells have β-adrenergic receptors. The parasympathetic branch of the autonomic system, in contrast, does not innervate any immune organ[1].

In chronic stress, such as social stress, sympathetic innervation to the lymph nodes develops via nerve growth factor (NGF). This increase in growth of nerve endings is very specific and limited to the paracortex area of the lymph nodes, the area populated by T cells.

This chronic β-adrenergic response down-regulates T_H1 immunity and up-regulates TGF-β, IL-6, and IL-8 production[2]. The presence of TGF-β and IL-6 together promotes the transformation of naïve T helper 4+ cells into T_H17 cells[3]. These stress-induced changes increase the production of INF-γ and decrease the production of INF-β by more than 80%, thus altering the balance of the immune system in its capacity to respond to various disease threats.

Chronic stress increases arborization of sympathetic nerve fibers in the skin, resulting in an increase in substance P and an increase in degranulated mast cells in the skin[4]. Mast cell activation can cause atopic dermatitis or urticaria, and can cause hair follicles to go into telogen, the resting phase; thus causing temporary hair loss[5].

Macaque troops are large and have dominant, aggressive, alpha males. The alpha males spend much of their daily routine harassing and intimidating the less dominant members of the troop. There are high social stress and frequent bite wounds to non-dominant males and females. The chronic stress-induced immune changes may provide a survival advantage for response to contaminated wounds, such as bites; where enteric anaerobes would cause infections and in which the T_H17 response is protective. This shift in immunity, however, decreases the body's ability to fight viral or other intracellular infections. Social stress in the lower primates has been shown to increase the proliferation of SIV, a virus similar to HIV, in primates[6]. The chronic stress in these animals is associated with smaller body size, poorer health, and shorter life span.

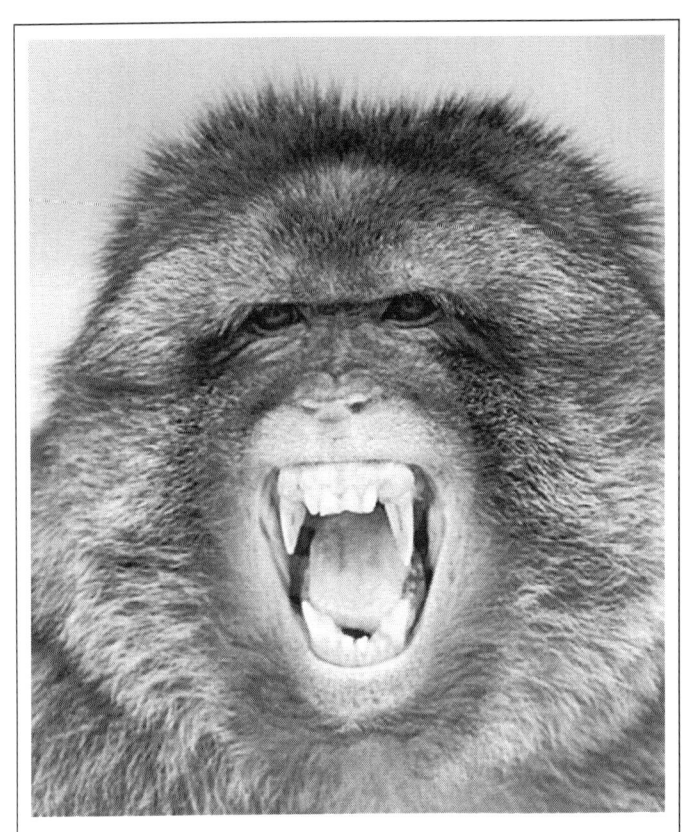

Figure 29-1: Big Macaque Attack

Baboon troops in natural settings have a hierarchal social structure, with aggressive, dominant males enjoying the perks of frequent grooming and mating opportunities. There is plenty of free time for the dominant males to harass lower-ranked troop members. Low-ranking male baboons in the wild show physiological stress, with elevated basal levels of glucocorticoids, elevated cholesterol and hypertension. They are also more susceptible to anxiety behaviors[7] and can suffer from depressive-like behavior.

Low-ranking baboons have some coping mechanisms that lower glucocorticoid levels. Subordinate males with high rates of covert "stolen copulations" do not show elevated basal glucocorticoid concentrations. Other subordinate males initiate fights with weaker baboons to displace aggression after losing a fight. These behaviors are associated with normal, rather than low, glucocorticoid levels[8].

In one wild baboon troop, which lost its most aggressive and dominant males, a new culture developed, in which the rewards of grooming and sexual access were distributed based on cooperative engagement, rather than aggressive dominance. The males in this troop had lower levels of stress hormones[7].

In males, sexual activity, or at least confidence in having access to sexual activity, appears to reduce stress.

Since about half the body's immune cells reside in the intestine, this population this area is greatly affected by chronic stress. Noradrenergic fibers are highly branched in the lamina propria of the intestinal mucosa in association with lymphoid tissue. As in lymph nodes, sympathetic nerves predominate in zones where T cells aggregate in Peyer's patches, and mast cells immediately under the epithelium are selectively associated with enteric sympathetic nerves. Sympathetic stimulus favors IgE, IgG$_1$ and IgG$_4$ production[2]. Thus, social stress, as well as other chronic stressors, can upregulate immune sensitivity in the gut, through the action of the sympathetic immune system and thereby, stress promotes immune activity that can result in food allergies and anteries.

Chronic Stress and the HPA Axis

The hypothalamus is an area of the brain that controls numerous homeostatic functions including hunger/satiation, thirst, sleep/wakefulness, circadian cycles, and body temperature. Most of these systems are regulated by hormone feedback loops. There are at least nine hypothalamic hormones, and most of these hormones mediate the production and release of pituitary hormones.

There are four hypothalamic-pituitary end organ loops, one for each of the four hypothalamic releasing hormones:

1. The hypothalamic-pituitary-adrenal axis (HPA):
   CRH → ACTH → Cortisol
2. The hypothalamic-pituitary-thyroid axis (HPT):
   TRH → TSH → T_3, T_{r3}, T_4
3. The hypothalamic-pituitary-gonadal axis (HPG):
   GnRH → LH → Sex hormones
4. The hypothalamic-pituitary-hepatic axis (HPH):
   GHRH → GH → IGF-1

Feedback from end-organ hormones, as well as other molecules, provide signals to hypothalamic receptors. This feedback creates a loop, in which the hypothalamus senses the activity of endocrine organs by sensing the end-organ hormones, and along with other signals, the body uses this information to regulate the pituitary hormone output. This allows the hypothalamus to regulate the hormonal balance of the body, maintain homeostasis in the face of a changing environment and allows the body to respond to a variety of stressors. This provides the body greater ability to adapt to injury, infection, famine, and other challenges.

Famine, for example, is a risky environment for pregnancy. Mammals have a limited number of pregnancies during their reproductive life, and each is a major depletion of her reproductive capacity. During famine, both the mother and fetus are at risk of malnourishment, which can compromise the survival of the mother, child, and other children the mother may already have. Bearing a child into a famine or hostile environment where the child is unlikely to survive is a poor reproductive strategy. Thus, during famine or other chronic stress conditions, sex drive and fertility diminish as the hypothalamus lowers GnRH output.

Table 29-1: HPA Axis Hormones

Hypothalamic Hormone	Pituitary Action	Site and Hormones
Corticotropin Releasing Hormone (CRH)	ACTH release	Adrenal Cortex: Cortisol Aldosterone
Thyrotropin Releasing Hormone (TRH)	TSH (Thyroid Stimulating Hormone	Thyroid Gland: Thyroxine (T4), Triiodothyronine (T3), and reverse T3 (Tr3)
Gonadotropin Releasing Hormone (GnRH)	LH (Luteinizing hormone) FSH (Follicle stimulating hormone)	Gonads: Testosterone, Progesterone, Estrogen
Gonadotropin Inhibiting Hormone (RFRP-3)	Prevents the onset of puberty	Hypothalamus: Inhibits GnRH production
Growth Hormone Releasing Hormone (GHRH)	GH (Growth hormone)	Liver: IGF-1
Somatostatin	Inhibits GH and TSH release	Pituitary
Dopamine	Inhibits prolactin release	Pituitary
Oxytocin		Breast: Milk let-down reflex Emotional bonding Uterine contraction
Vasopressin		Kidneys: Increases reabsorption of water
Hypocretin		Brain: Wakefulness (See Chapter 41 on sleep)

The HPA axis mediates the response to injury and infection through its control of steroid hormones, especially glucocorticoids. Cortisol is the principal glucocorticoid in humans

Glucocorticoids have three main actions. They prepare the body for fight of flight by:

- Simulating the release of adrenaline from chromaffin cells in the adrenal gland
- Raise blood glucose levels through gluconeogenesis
- Suppressing inflammation and the immune response.

Corticosteroids help terminate the immune response to acute infection. This prevents immune activity from over-utilizing resources and creating excessive damage to the tissues around an infection. At the outset of an infection, inflammatory cytokines are produced that recruit more immune cells and upregulate the immune response. Later, when the battle against the microbes has been won, it is time to clean up, and go back to "peacetime" immune activity. Cortisol helps with this. The HPA axis is stimulated by inflammatory cytokines. In contrast, these cytokines suppress the HP-Gonadal axis; lowering hypothalamic secretion of Gonadotropin Releasing Hormone (GnRH), and thereby decreasing luteinizing hormone and sex hormones production. Inflammatory cytokines similarly suppress the growth hormone axis. The hypothalamic pituitary hormonal axes respond to cytokines and focus the body's resources on adapting to the situation at hand.

Glucocorticoids, such as cortisol, suppress the induction of inflammatory responses in immune cells including lymphocytes, macrophages, and dendritic cells. They inhibit the production of inflammatory cytokines including IL-1β and TNF and promote induction of anti-inflammatory cytokines, such as IL-10 by dendritic cells and macrophages. Glucocorticoids also induce apoptosis of T lymphocytes, macrophages, and dendritic cells and decreased the production of antibodies by B lymphocytes, leading to down-regulation of the immune response.

In health, ACTH is released from the pituitary during the sleep cycle so that there is a clear peak in the release of cortisol at about eight o'clock in the morning. After injuries or physical or emotional trauma, dysfunctional, chronic stress reaction can occur. In this event, the HPA axis feedback mechanism cycle is disrupted; the A.M. peak is lost, and cortisol levels are elevated much of the day. Disruption of the HPA homeostasis can impair the immune system and can cause increased appetite, excess adipose accumulation especially in the abdomen, fatigue, and other problems.

> Chronic stress is associated with shorter stature in children. Children who enter day care before 18 months of age were significantly shorter six months later than those who were kept home[9]. Children raised in hostile environments have growth delays that may never be completely recovered[10,11]. Increases in glucocorticoids are associated with decreased output of GH and IGF-1.

Persistent, unrelenting stress can cause chronic stress. This occurs if living in a condition where there are constant or frequent threats or intimidation; where assaults, or threats of assault, may even occur multiple times daily. This may happen in dysfunctional families, where there is sibling rivalry, where there is verbal or emotional abuse or intimidation. Working in a dangerous environment, where there is continuous adjusting to changing risk or peril, or dealing with menace can cause chronic stress. It often occurs in caretakers of disabled children and with intimate partner abuse.

A more pernicious form of chronic stress occurs in some individuals where stress becomes the usual response to their environment, even when the stressor no longer is present. In this situation, there may be an unusually low threshold for stress response and reinforcement.

In some individuals, the threshold for triggering a stress response is set so low that non-threat events in a safe environment trigger the stress response. These individuals have adaptive hyper-vigilance. This can result from a home environment that is a continuous threat, in which the individual has learned to be constantly prepared to respond danger. Individuals exposed to an environment of adversity during childhood have low thresholds for stress response and are susceptible to the development of chronic stress response. In utero stress can increase this susceptibility.

Epigenetics of Stress

Stressful events during the third trimester of pregnancy, as well as those in early life, can influence future stress reactions for the child's entire life. Stress during this time can even set up a multi-generational stress reaction. Mice pups whose mothers spend more time grooming (licking) them are less likely to have chronic stress responses throughout their lives[12]. Conversely, female offspring of low-grooming mothers, do little grooming of their pups, resulting in subsequent generations of low-grooming, easily-stressed mice. When pups from low-grooming dams are raised by average dams, they retain the low-grooming/high-stress phenotype. However, if these pups are raised by a high-grooming dam, they become low-stress/high-groomers. Similarly, if female pups from low-stress/high-grooming females are raised by average dams, they retain the high-grooming phenotype, but if raised in stressful environments by low-grooming dams, they become low-grooming/high-stress mothers. Maternal bonding style is passed generation to generation in humans as well[13].

Epigenetic imprinting, which when adaptive, can provide a survival advantage in hostile environments. In humans and other primates, epigenetics influences culture. When raised in stressful, hostile environments, males are more aggressive, and females are less social and less nurturing.

Nutritional deprivation during critical periods of development can result in stable adaptations which promote "aggressive" storage of fat, obesity and risk for type 2 diabetes; dehydration during pregnancy can increase sodium retention and risk of hypertension in the offspring[14]. Epigenetic programming may assist survival into a harsh environment but is dysfunctional if the environmental conditions no longer suit that adaptation.

Epigenetic effects may be more deeply ingrained into the DNA than just maternally imbuing stress-prone reactivity or preference for obesogenic diets being programmed into the child[15]. Epigenetic modifications of the sperm or ova can influence transgenerational changes, independent of the offspring's environment[16].

Epigenetic influences do not change the DNA sequence, but rather, affect the transcription of various genes. DNA in the nucleus is wound around histones that help stabilize it, and prevent it from being damaged. For gene expression to take place, the section of DNA to be transcribed needs to be detached from the histone so that mRNA can be made, and new proteins can be produced. The DNA is held in place on the histone by acetylation, and when stimulated, deacetylase enzymes specifically free up the appropriate section of DNA so that mRNA for the right proteins can be transcribed.

Epigenetic imprinting allows for environmental adaptation. This imprinting occurs through several mechanisms. The first is methylation of the DNA. In methylation, some cytosine molecules in the DNA are converted to 5-methylcytosine, which like cytosine, pairs with guanine. 5-methylcytosine, however, binds more tightly to the histones, which impedes acetylation of the DNA; thus lowering the expression of methylated areas of DNA and that control how easily genes are expressed by the cell. Methylation of DNA is a stable modification that is usually transcribed by DNA methyltransferases to daughter cells.

Another potential process for epigenetic modifications can be the effect of the histone selection. There are several different histone proteins, and these have differing amounts and placement of the amino acid lysine in their protein structure. The enzyme histone acetyltransferase (HAT) induces acetylation of these lysine molecules. Histones that are more highly acetylated have a more open chromatin structure, allowing for more active transcription. The enzyme histone deacetylase (HDAC) removes the acetyl group, thus giving a tighter winding of chromatin and thus quieting or silencing transcription.

During meiosis and mitosis, the DNA remains mostly connected to the histone, and DNA replication usually inserts the same histone to a given area of DNA. If, however, the DNA is in use during cell replication, the DNA may be disassociated from the histone, and a different histone, or differently modified histone, may be substituted. RNA present in the cell during cell division also contributes the activity of the new cells. Thus, cellular activity and environmental conditions during replication can influence the ease of DNA transcription in the daughter cells and subsequent generations of the cell.

Thus, if a mother is stressed in the final trimester of pregnancy, if raised in a stressed environment from their time of birth, or subjected to stress as young children, the offspring may become more adept at responding adversity, and have a lower threshold for activating a stress response throughout their life. This is not fun but does provide survival advantages for the species.

Infants that are raised in a low-stress caring environment, being held and stroked, are less reactive to stress. Lack of touch (grooming) in pups increases methylation, and thus decreased expression of glucocorticoid receptors in the brain[17], changing the sensitivity of CRH feedback.

Aggressiveness is influenced by events and the environment in early life. (See box "Nurture, Nature, Rage and Violence" in Chapter 37.) Infants born to women pregnant during the terrorist attacks on September 11, 2001, had lower cortisol levels; the genome can carry maternal transmission of anxiety disorders and susceptibility for PTSD across generations[18]. How we adapt to our environment, our personalities, our cultures as a society, and the diseases we are susceptible to may be highly impacted by influences during our early life.

Either hypermethylation, with decreased gene expression; or hypomethylation, with increased gene expression, can cause pathologic adaptations. Schizophrenia and bipolar disorder have both been linked to hypomethylation of the gene for membrane-bound catechol-O-methyltransferase, which increases dopamine degradation in the frontal lobe[19].

Dietary excess in one generation can alter energy utilization in subsequent generations[20]. Much of the disease burdens we identify as familial, such as metabolic syndrome associated with obesity, hypertension, diabetes, and heart disease is likely epigenetic, rather than genetic[21] modifications. This may also be the case for depression, anxiety, PTSD[22], and irritable bowel syndrome[23]. Susceptibility to cancer is more often due to epigenetic influences than genetic aberrations in the DNA sequence. Intelligence is more likely epigenetic than a genetic trait[24].

Epigenetic Reset

Although epigenetic modifications are usually stable and are preserved when cells divide, cells can re-adapt to a changing environment. During embryogenesis, most epigenetic imprinting is reset. When cells divide, epigenetic influences from the past may be overwritten and be impacted by the current environment if the influences are sufficiently strong.

Starting a new life gives the opportunity to reset the degree of methylation for the environment the offspring is born into. The fetal environment, however, is not pristine; it is its mother's womb, and that environment is shaped by the mother's epigenetic imprinting, her health and nutritional status and behavior. If she is diabetic or obese, it will affect the epigenetic imprinting of the fetus developing in her. As growing infants and children, epigenetic imprinting continues to be affected by the environment the dividing cells are exposed to, both internal and external.

The most salient epigenetic imprinting of sperm occurs during spermatogenesis in early adolescence and the 90 days leading up to sperm production[25]. In females, the most critical times are during oocytogenesis, which occurs before or shortly after birth, and the period of oogenesis and development, thus including the weeks before and the months of pregnancy. These are times when the health and environment of the parents most affect the lifetime health of the offspring. Toxins, such as alcohol, should be avoided by prospective parents especially during these times.

Epigenetic imprinting may be amenable to modification and thus treatment during adult life[17]. Resetting can occur during cell division. Thus, fetal development, and growth during infancy and youth are times epigenetic changes occur most readily. Effecting epigenetic changes during adulthood is less responsive, perhaps requiring years of exposure, habits and an environment which favors the new settings, during the time that cells are replaced in the organ. These changes can be beneficial when they improve health and well-being, or destructive when they promote disease and misery.

Diet, especially maternal diet and diet during youth, can affect epigenetically induced susceptibility to obesity, diabetes, cardiovascular disease, cancer, and congenital disease[26]. The stress response can also be affected.

Appropriate levels of DNA methylation, with neither hypo- nor hypermethylation, is most likely when there is an adequate, but not excess level of folate, vitamins B_{12} and B_6, docosahexaenoic acid (DHA), and betaine[27]. The n-3 fatty acids DHA and EPA found in fish oil may reverse hypermethylation[28, 32].

Genistein, from soybeans; epigallocatechin-3-gallate (EGCG), present in green tea; and sulforaphane, present in cruciferous vegetables, inhibit DNA methyltransferases and HDAC, and lower the risk of cancer. Maternal ingestion of up to two cups of green tea a day during pregnancy and lactation is safe and likely decreases the risk of cancer in the offspring. Butyrate, present in cheese also inhibits HDAC[26]. Curcumin is an inhibitor of HAT, and it may erase epigenetic imprinting in sperm. However, excess curcumin could potentially inhibit spermatogenesis[29].

Exposure to maternal undernutrition, obesity, stress, and gestational diabetes increase the risk for chronic disease in the offspring through epigenetic mechanisms. Melatonin decreases this risk, in part as an antioxidant, and likely as an epigenetic modifier[30]. Melatonin is an essential antioxidant that easily crosses the placenta and which rises to high levels during pregnancy. Melatonin may also act by inhibiting DNA methyltransferase[31], and thus, inhibit the transference of epigenetic imprinting onto the offspring. Ensuring sufficient sleep, darkness, tryptophan, and cofactors for melatonin production may help reset epigenetic encoding that promotes health.

Table 29-2 list several nutritional factors that affect epigenetic imprinting. Even though they may act in opposite directions, they may provide a benefit by preventing previous epigenetic settings, and allowing new, more adaptive response to the current, hopefully benign, environment.

Table 29-2: Epigenetic Reset Factors[26, 30]

Folate Vitamin B$_{12}$ Vitamin B$_6$ Betaine (TMG)	Methyl donation – provide for SAMe synthesis and homocysteine recycling Ensure availability of methyl groups thus, preventing hypomethylation
N-3 fatty acids EPA and DHA	Promote reversal of hypermethylation[28, 32]
ECGC (green tea) Sulforaphane (cruciferous vegetables)	HDAC and DNA methyltransferase inhibitors. Also inhibit NF-κB activation. Dietary intake is associated with decreased risk of cancer;
Genistein (soy)	Maternal intake associated with decreased risk of cancer and chronic disease in later life.
Butyrate (cheese) Diallyl sulfide (from garlic)	Histone deacetylase inhibitor.
Indole-3-carbinol (cruciferous vegetables)	Regulates microRNA expression. Provides transplacental protection from lung cancer carcinogens.
Melatonin	Inhibits DNA methyltransferase, antioxidant.
Curcumin	Inhibits histone acetyltransferase.

Stressful experiences can reinforce the stress response. When a chronically stressed individual knows that they have a maladaptive reaction to stress, it often adds to their stress, as they are anxious that they will not be able to control their response or react appropriately to situations. For example, individuals with panic attacks may have considerable anxiety about having a panic attack while in public.

Situations are especially stressful when they are novel, unpredictable and out of the individual's control. Acute glucocorticoids exposure stimulates a stronger emotional memory to adverse events, for example, but chronic exposure causes memory deficits for declarative (facts) memory retrieval[33]. Very high, acute corticosteroids levels may also decrease adverse memory creation.

In post-traumatic stress disorder (PTSD), there is chronic vigilance and a low threshold for a stress reaction. The stress response is no longer dependent on real threats in the environment, but rather on perceived threats, which may be seen almost everywhere.

Chronic stress stimulates the HP-Adrenal axis and leads to prolonged suppression of HP Gonadal axis[34], which can be manifest as amenorrhea, for example. In chronic stress or chronic illness, the homeostasis of the hypothalamic-pituitary-end organ axes can become dysfunctional.

Chronic stress and activation of the HP-Adrenal axis leads to increased cortisol output inducing a loss of lean body mass (muscle and bone mass) due to decreased IGF-1 and lowered anabolic steroid production. Chronically elevated cortisol stimulates proliferation of adipocytes leading to visceral obesity. Adipocytes are metabolically and hormonally active, and secrete IL-6 and TNF-α. IL-6 and TNF-α, overproduced by the expanded visceral adipose tissue, further stimulate the HP-Adrenal axis, forming a pathologic positive feedback loop.

IL-6 and TNF-α act on the liver to produce C-reactive protein (CRP) and fibrinogen. These proteins increase the risk of stroke and atherosclerosis. IL-6 can promote the formation of the inflammatory mediator PGE$_2$ in the brain; one effect of which is to induce INF-γ, which stimulates the shunting of tryptophan into the kynurenine pathway, with potential for neurotoxin production (see Chapter 31).

In chronic stress, cortisol increases the proliferation of fat cells. Leptin released from the fat cells should quell hunger and help stop further weight gain by antagonizing the effect of Neuropeptide Y (NPY) in the hypothalamus; however, TNF-α blocks sensitivity to leptin. This mechanism is helpful during an acute injury or infection to rebuild energy stores, but dysfunctional when it occurs as a chronic condition. TNF-α has been implicated in both insulin and leptin resistance in the hypothalamus[35]. Additionally, agouti-related protein (AGRP), which can be elevated by stress[36], has a long-term effect on increasing appetite and can do so in chronic stress.

Leptin also has an immunostimulatory effect on naïve T helper cells and T$_H$1 cells; inducing the production of INF-γ, TNF-α, and more leptin. Leptin also activates macrophages and monocytes to produce TNF-α, IL-1, and IL-6, which can lead to autoimmunity and tissue damage[37].

Stress can also affect the HP-Thyroid axis. Both IL-1β and IL-6 decrease basal TSH release and IL-1β also decreases TRH transcription[38]. IFN-γ can decrease serum T$_4$ and T$_3$ in a dose-dependent manner, and elevated TNF-α can cause low T$_3$ syndrome. Additionally, vasopressin (AVP) and NPY, which can be elevated by norepinephrine during stress, also decrease TSH output[39]. These cytokines contribute to the low T$_3$ syndromes, which often occur in long-term critical illness. While TSH, T$_4$, and T$_3$ release are diminished during chronic stress, rT$_3$ appears to be less affected[40].

Chronic stress, resulting in excess cortisol production, thus can lead to the development of the Metabolic Syndrome with:

- Stimulation of appetite and adipocyte proliferation,
- Accumulation of excess adipose tissue around the heart and in the abdominal cavity that presents as abdominal obesity,
- Suppression of GH and IGF-1, causing loss of lean body mass (muscle and bone) and decreased growth in children and adolescents,
- Suppression of sex hormones, causing loss of fertility and reproductive drive and sexual dysfunction.
- Suppression of thyroid hormonal activity.

STRESS!!!
↓
HYPOTHALAMUS

CRH → Increases Paracellular Permeability
         Promotes Anxiety and Fear
         Induces Mast Cell Degranulation
↓
PITUITARY
↓
ACTH
↓
ADRENAL CORTEX
↓
CORTISOL → ↓GROWTH HORMONE
              ↓IGF-1
              Loss of Lean Body Mass
              (Muscle and Bone)
↓
ADIPOCYTES → Proliferation → Visceral Obesity
↓
Apoptosis and ← IL-6, TNF-α → | Insulin Resistance
Inflammation | Dyslipidemia
↓ | Atherosclerosis
LIVER | Hypertension
↓ | Hypercoagulability
C-REACTIVE PROTEIN
FIBRINOGEN →

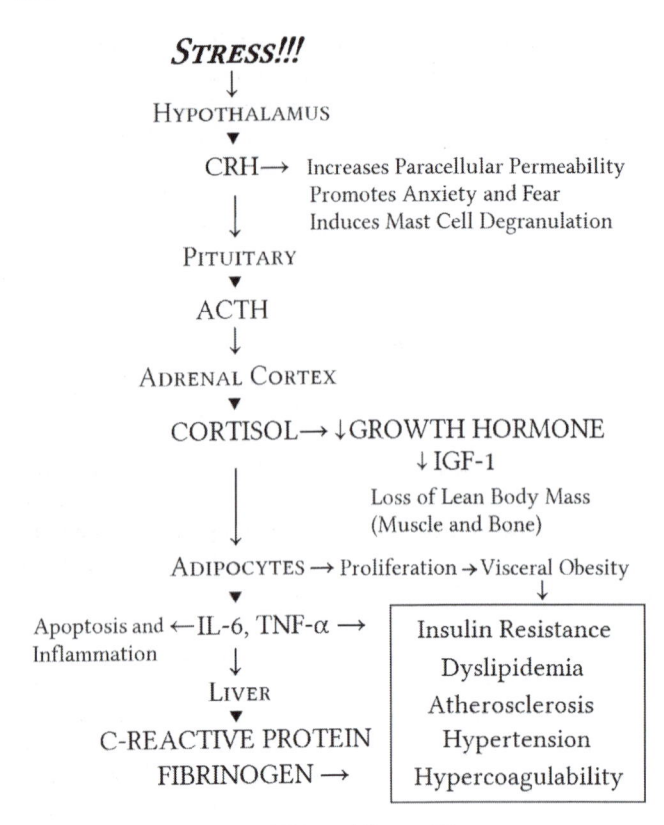

Figure 29-2: HPA and Stress Hormones

Recall from Chapter 9 on metabolic syndrome, that elevated serum uric acid levels are associated with elevated TNF-α, IL-6, and CRP[41]. These same factors are elevated and contribute to metabolic syndrome in chronic stress. In both cases, they act on the HPA axis. The deleterious effects of stress are not limited to metabolic syndrome. IL-6 is associated with a low threshold for pain, fatigue and depression. The effect of IL-6 is seen in fibromyalgia, depression, chronic fatigue syndrome and other disorders.

While acute distress does not appear to have an immediate effect on the hypothalamic-pituitary-gonadal (HPG) axis[42], it is suppressed by chronic stress. This effect is principally mediated by CRH, but also by noradrenergic and gamma-amino-butyric acid (GABA) neurons[43]. Stress-induced elevations in adrenal glucocorticoids cause an increase in Gonadotropin Inhibiting Hormone (RFRP-3) that contributes to hypothalamic suppression of reproductive function[44]. Chronic stress appears to have different effects on the HPG axis of women and men; this may explain the increased prevalence of major depression and other stress-related diseases in women[45]. When women have insufficient fat mass, they may become amenorrheic. This effect appears to be mediated through decreased production of leptin, by "hungry" adipocytes; low leptin levels inhibit the production of kisspeptin. Kisspeptin, a small protein hormone, stimulates GnRH release that induces LH and FSH, which stimulate sex hormone production. Kisspeptin also effects CRH, vasopressin, and oxytocin gene expressions[46]. TNF-α blocks sensitivity to leptin, and thus kisspeptin production, thereby abrogating the GnRH axis during chronic stress and inflammatory disease.

Corticosteroids also inhibit the release of GHRH, and thus, of GH and IGF-1. These hormones are essential for growth and healing but are inhibited during chronic stress.

Corticotropin Releasing Hormone

CRH levels are elevated in chronic stress and with alcohol use. CRH acts on the amygdala; increasing the sense of fear and anxiety[47]. Elevated CRH may contribute to impulsive and violent behaviors.

Individuals with depression have hypersecretion of CRH and hypercortisolemia. CRH has been found to be elevated in veterans with PTSD[48], however, contrary to the situation observed in depression; those with PTSD have CRH hypersecretion but have low ACTH and cortisol levels[49]. Severe maternal stress, or exposure to alcohol during the second and third semesters of pregnancy exposes the fetus to excessive levels of CRH and cortisol, resulting in susceptibility to Major Depressive Disorder[50]. Transient gastric irritation in neonatal animals can cause increased CRH release later in life, accompanied by anxious and depressive-like behaviors[51].

Elevated CRH levels increase paracellular permeability and mast cell activation. The increase in permeability is mediated through CRH receptors, $CRHR_1$ and $CRHR_2$. This increased permeability can promote immune reactivity to foods, and increase the absorption of LPS and other toxins. CRH may be a factor in the etiology of irritable bowel syndrome[52] and other inflammatory disorders of the intestine. CRH induces mast cell degranulation and release of histamine, which in concert with elevated IL-8, caused by chronic sympathetic stress, are chemotactic for mast cell recruitment to the affected area. CRH can also increase paracellular permeability of the bladder and increase production of vascular endothelial growth factor (VEGF)[53], and thereby promote interstitial cystitis.

CRH increases the permeability of the blood-brain barrier and increases degranulation of mast cells in the dura matter. This degranulation selectively releases IL-6, IL-8, and vascular VEGF. This may increase the risk for migraines. An inducible mouse model of multiple sclerosis, experimental allergic encephalomyelitis (EAE), fails to develop in mice bred to be deficient in CRH[54].

The increase in CRH release provoked by alcohol is mediated by acetaldehyde, a breakdown product of alcohol[55]. Aldehydes are also created by the breakdown of histamine. Thus, it may be possible to at least partially mitigate the acetaldehyde-associated increase in CRH by assuring sufficient aldehyde dehydrogenase (ALDH) enzyme cofactors (magnesium and niacin), and by avoiding agents that inhibit ALDH (disulfiram, H_2 blockers other than famotidine).

Prostaglandin E_2 and $PGF_{2\alpha}$ increase CRH RNA expression. Low plasma docosahexaenoic acid (DHA) levels are associated with greater cerebrospinal fluid CRH levels[56];

thus, DHA likely lowers CRH expression. Higher rates of violent behavior are found in populations with high n-6 dietary fats and lower rates found in populations with higher intake of the n-3 fatty acid DHA[57]. DHA lowers PGE_2 production. DHA may also act on depression by increasing the number of serotonin $5-HT_{1A}$ receptors in the hippocampus[58].

Since CRH can trigger mast cell activation, and mast cell products (inflammatory eicosanoids and histamine catabolism) may increase CRH production, a positive feedback cycle of CRH activity can occur, maintaining high CRH output, supporting chronic stress reactions. CRH affects the intestinal mucosa, causing increased paracellular permeability, mast cell activation, and risk of immune reaction to foods; thus promoting mast cell hypertrophy. CRH can thus promote a long-term, positive feedback loop for chronic immune-related stress, and emotional events, triggering high CRH, can initiate chronic immune-mediated stress.

A shift to a lower n-6: n-3 ratio in the diet, and the addition of DHA through supplementation of fish oil or consumption of cold water fish, such as salmon, may help break this cycle. This can shift the eicosanoid balance towards anti-inflammatory products, which do not induce CRH production. Immune-mediated stress should be treated along with emotional stress if present.

Summary: Restitution of the Hypothalamic Pituitary Axes

Restoration of the HPA begins with the elimination of its causation. Stress should be considered a disease in itself and treatment provided. In chronic stress, the original stressor may have come and gone; nevertheless, the HPA cycle can continue to be dysfunctional. Restoration of the circadian sleep cycle is important to the restoration of the HPA axis.

Treatment of depression is given in Chapter 31. Treatment for chronic sympathetic hyperactivity and PTSD and anxiety are discussed in Chapter 32.

1. Sleep: A regular circadian cycle is essential to normalizing the hypothalamic-pituitary axes. There are over 600 different genes transcribed in the pituitary that have two-fold or greater difference in transcription between day and night[59]. ACTH and CRH feedback is under pineal circadian control, as is thyroid stimulating hormone (TSH). Sleep deprivation decreases TSH output[60]. Sleep deprivation or disruption of the circadian cycle shifts T_H0 immune cell development towards the T_H17 lineage, increasing the risk of autoimmune disease and immune reactions to foods[61].

Nighttime sleep should be regular and adequate. Although napping can supplement nighttime sleep, the circadian cycle cannot be patched by daytime naps. The genes and hormones that guide the circadian cycle are entrained by light[62]. Sleep at night should take place in a dark room, which preferably gives a natural increase in lighting at dawn. In urban areas with street lights, this can be difficult, however "alarm" clocks are available which slowly increase light in the morning for a more natural wakening. Melatonin at bedtime may be useful to help reset the circadian cycle (0.3 to 3 mg) and also acts as an antioxidant.

Regular meals and regular nighttime sleep also help maintain the circadian cycle of the GI tract and help avoid SIBO (Chapter 24). Avoid caffeine and excess chocolate after 2 P.M. Sleep is discussed in detail in Chapter 43.

2. Normalize thyroid function if abnormal: Thyroid function should be checked in patients with enteroimmunopathies and those having stress reactions. Hashimoto's thyroiditis is an autoimmune disorder common in patients with food anergies.

Although T_4 has a long half-life, it is normally released by the thyroid in the morning. Thyroxine (T_4) replacement should be preferably taken in the morning without food, as calcium (and other minerals) in food prevent its absorption. Taking T_4 without food, and getting good absorption is more important than timing. The thyroid gland normally releases T_3 during the first hours of sleep[63]. Thus, if Cytomel (liothyronine), a synthetic T_3 is used, it is best taken at bedtime.

When oral corticosteroids are prescribed, they should be given in the morning, to mimic the natural peak output that occurs around 8 a.m.

3. Repair membrane function: Stress, on its own, contributes to the disruption of membrane function through the actions of CRH. The enterocyte membrane is not isolated in this respect, and other membrane barriers are at risk, including the blood-brain barrier, the placenta barrier, the kidney glomeruli and the lung membranes. All are affected by CRH and stress. In the intestine, CRH increases mast cell activation and the likelihood of forming immune reactions to foods, which further cause membrane dysfunction and other problems. Adrenergic activation from stress also increases immunoreactivity of T_H17 lymphocytes and promotes immune sensitivity to food and autoimmune disorders. Dispelling stress reactions is essential for successful, long-term remission of mast cell activation associated diseases, autoimmune diseases, and other enteroimmunopathies.

Avoiding immune reaction to foods is essential to breaking the CRH enteroimmune cycle, where CRH induces increased mast cell development, increased permeability and increased T_H17 response to foods, and thus increased stress and HP adrenal axis activity. Riboflavin (vitamin B_2) and zinc may help improve tight junction function affected by CRH. Treatment of food sensitivities is discussed in Chapter 19. Treatment of mast cell activation disorder is given in Chapter 12.

Alcohol has a negative effect on membrane function and should be avoided. Magnesium citrate (200 to 350 mg daily) and niacin or niacinamide (10 mg daily) may help ALDH activity and help clear acetaldehyde, a toxin that increases CRH output. Chapters 17 and 41 provide more information about alcohol. Chapter 25 further discusses the repair of enterocyte membrane function.

4. Promote a healthy n-6:n-3 fatty acid balance: Minimize dietary n-6 fats, and consume or supplement n-3 fats especially DHA and EPA. One gram of DHA twice daily as an adult supplemental dose. N-3 and n-6 fats are discussed in Chapter 6. Vitamin D levels should be checked to make sure that they are adequate. (Discussed in Chapter 20).

6. Friends and family: We are social creatures. Friendships and open communication reduce stress. Family is also the source of much of the stress in our lives. Lack of kindness and responsibility are the root of much family discord and stress.

Family stress and history of abuse need to be part of the evaluation and management of immune-related diseases. Family counseling or crisis intervention may be required. Patients should be evaluated not only as victims, but also as perpetrators of abuse, and treatment offered. Perpetration of abuse is often a maladaptive response to chronic stress. Many perpetrators are themselves the victim of abuse, and they may welcome treatment. An intimate partner violence screening assessment based on the validated HITS assessment is given in Appendix D on page 414.

Gentle touch has been shown helpful for stress reduction[64] and MLD, a form of gentle massage, has also been found to be helpful in the treatment of fibromyalgia[65]. In this therapy, light, lingering pressure is applied. This may be similar to the sensory stimulation which was reported as helpful for anorexia[66]. Just being held or hugged in a non-sexual manner can be therapeutic. Being groomed reduces stress in primates, including humans. Having the hair gently brushed appears to reduce the stress response.

Avoid alcohol; see the note on alcohol and intimacy in Chapter 17. Particularly in men, sexual frustration is stressful. Intimacy, which provides a sexual outlet, helps mitigate stress for men. Just having that confidence that the outlet is available is often helpful.

Emotional Distress

Psychological distress occurs when there is an imperative to alter a situation when we lack the ability to do so. It stems from largely from a lack of control. When a problem is lodged in our consciousness, resisting resolution, it sits there, eating at us. Imagine that you have bills to pay, and no funds to pay then, and to miss payment deadlines would cause severe consequences. This would cause constant worry as you are forced to keep the bill in mind because it needs resolution. You remain under stress until the payment is made. If you could pay the bill, the stress would be eliminated.

In the workplace environment, supervisors suffer less from stress, as they have more control than those subservient to them. When individuals are placed in a position where they are made accountable for a situation but lack the ability to alter it, it causes stress. In situations where a person is overwhelmed by the future and feels that they cannot resolve the problem, there is stress.

Women have suffered more stress in their traditional role in the family, as they have been more responsible for caregiving but had little control over external factors that caused the problems. Women are often caretakers, and may face challenging situations that defy remedy. It is not uncommon for women to sacrifice their financial well-being to care for an aging parent; this sacrifice is less common among men.

Chronic stress is a learned behavior, which becomes the body's normal state. The brain often needs to be retrained, and the positive feedback cycle broken. Vigorous exercise, hot baths, movies, and emotional retraining can be helpful.

Addressing Stress

1. Acknowledge the stress.

2. Identify the things causing the stress.

3. Sort out what you have control over and what you do not control. Figure out what you can fix, what you cannot fix, and where you can gain control over.

4. Take control of the things that you can control. If you can fix the problem, act on it.

5. If you cannot remedy the situation, then acknowledge that it is out of you hands, and thus, it is not your responsibility. Give it to the person or entity where responsibility lies. Faith in a high power is helpful, as you can cede your lack of control and outcome to the will of God. Sometimes you just need to let go.

Mother Goose voiced the sentiment:

> For every ailment under the sun
> There is a remedy, or there is none;
> If there be one, try to find it;
> If there be none, never mind it.

This is concept is also expressed in the serenity prayer:

> Great Spirit, give me the courage to do what needs be done,
> Serenity to accept what cannot be remedied,
> And the insight to know the one from the other."

I have a friend who graduated 2nd in his class in medical school. He was rewarded with a prestigious position at a university hospital. One night at the hospital he had a patient whose condition was rapidly deteriorating. He had complete responsibility for the situation, and no backup that night. His attempts to stabilize the patient's condition where failing. He was terrified, almost paralyzed by fear as the patient condition worsened. The stress became so intense that he panicked and actually hid under a bed. My friend had assumed the patient's demise was a result of his lack of medical expertise. More likely, he lacked the depth of experience to understand that no one would have been able to save the patient.

My friend had not been a doctor long enough to have "insight to know one from another." This brilliant and caring young doctor abandoned his career in medicine – it had become far too stressful for him. Sometimes we need help to figure out what can be done and what cannot. Ask for help.

6. Make a plan of action with a schedule or calendar. This can help take control of stress situations. Missing from the prayer of serenity is a request for serenity during the unfolding of time; having too little time to accomplish what needs to be done, as well as having to wait for things to happen, is stressful. Having a plan can help organize time, and give some relief from it. When everything is arranged on a schedule, the problems may become more manageable. In the plan, try to deal with each stressor as an independent issue. The plan may include accepting loss and contingency plans.

7. Choose battles wisely. Choose battles you are sure to win, and avoid those that are not winnable. Only take on those in between after considering the risk and benefits of the struggle. Decline opportunities for stress by saying, "No, thank you" to people who treat you as if you were a source of cheap or free therapy or labor, or as an emotional dumping ground.

8. Avoid unneeded stressors that come into your like through electrical wires. These include:

- Telephone calls from relatives or others who drain you like vampires do;
- Media filled demagoguery that spew fear and loathing;
- Media that show graphic ugliness and violence;
- Internet time killers like social media and video games that keep you indoors sitting;
- Being a couch potato;
- Avoid rumination and focusing on the negative.

9. Focus on the present. You only have control over the present. Talk to a friend or counselor about how you feel to acknowledge and describe the stressors and your feelings. Be in the moment. Watch your body and relax when you notice defensive posturing. Remember to breathe. Yoga may be helpful.

10. Take care of yourself. Exercise: walk, swim, jog, play, get some sun. Get a massage. Take a hot bath. Regular, vigorous exercise helps reduce stress; walking or running 3 miles, at least three times a week is helpful. See Chapter 21 for exercise recommendations and reasoning.

11. Forgive and ask for forgiveness. Forgive yourself while you are at it.

> "Resentment is like drinking poison and waiting for it to kill your enemy."
> ~Nelson Mandela
>
> "Malice drinks one-half of its own poison."
> ~Seneca

12. Don't sweat the little stuff. Remember, it is almost all little stuff.

13. Approach a crisis as an opportunity for change.

14. Remember, a masterpiece can be painted on any canvas.

What Not to Do

Medications, such as benzodiazepines may be helpful for getting through a short-term crisis; however, they are not appropriate as a chronic fix, rather they are like buying on credit; you pay more later. Short-term fixes do not resolve chronic problems. For chronic problems, the payment just builds up. Use of tobacco, alcohol, and medications, such as benzodiazepines for relief from stress is like spending more than you earn and relying on credit cards to make payments. Drugs will not resolve social or financial problems and will likely worsen it. Most medications or herbs that relieve anxiety should only be used as short-term bridges over storm swollen rivers.

Haste is the enemy of accuracy and wisdom. Avoid making decisions while upset or during emotionally charged circumstances. Better decisions are made when we are calm and thinking clearly, not under the influence of norepinephrine. In a study of patients that had attempted suicide, 24% had deliberated their decision less than 5 minutes, and 71% had spent less than an hour contemplating it[67]. If you feel your heart pounding against your chest wall, you might want to wait on any life altering decisions.

A short-term break in activities, vacation, or taking the time to adjust to a new situation can be helpful to recover from stress or a traumatic event. Taking a break to recover from illness, injury or trauma makes sense. However, avoiding friends and family; withdrawing from the world and procrastination is unlikely to help in the long run. It makes sense to catch your breath and take the time to review important decisions, but just delaying unpleasant situations that will not go away, can just add stress.

Anxiety often results from resisting the experience of anxiety. It is like trying not to think about the monkey – the harder you try, the more he is in your consciousness. Every time you check to see if you are thinking about the monkey – there he is again.

Acceptance Based Therapy teaches that rather than trying to control negative thoughts and emotions, it helps to observe them dispassionately; let them come and go. The goal is to change one's relationship with their thoughts and feelings, rather than the impossible task of changing emotions created in response to a situation.

As a young man, I got caught in a strong rip current swimming at a beach on the Pacific coast of Mexico, that I later learned was notorious for frequent drownings. I tried to swim back to the beach, but it was becoming surprisingly smaller in the distance. I was becoming exhausted and realized there was no way I was going overcome the force of the current. I must have actually listened to my father at least once as I remembered his advice on rip currents: to relax and to take a new and leisurely, diagonal tact towards shore. The goal was not to get back to where I started, but rather to get to a piece of safe, dry ground. I swam a diagonally towards the shore, and I ended up about nearly a kilometer down from where I had left my gear. If I had fought the current with all my might, I likely would have joined other victims of the tide. When I just went for a ride, all I had to do was relax and keep moving with my goal in sight.

Try to view emotions only as information that is being presented to you. Anxiety and fear are temporary feelings that will pass. Try to understand that those emotions may be more related to events that occurred long in the past than to the present situation. Every time the smoke detector goes off, it does not mean your house is on fire. Take a look and see what is causing the alarm to activate before you go screaming and running from the building. That is what these emotions are for – they are an alarm to let you know there may be in danger. Look to see what actions, if any, are appropriate, and make a decision to act or not. If you do not get upset about the alarm going off, it will usually turn itself off within a couple of minutes.

Be receptive and look for humor in every scene you play in life. Sometimes life presents dark humor, but if you cast it as a comedy, it is much more likely to have a happy ending.

The Sweet Spot for Playing, Learning, and Working

When we are using skills that we have acquired in a challenging situation and meeting the demands of the challenge, it is fun. Whether the challenge is playing tennis, skateboarding, caring for a patient, solving equations, preparing a feast, or playing a computer game; when we are actively using skills or competency and successfully meeting a challenge, it is fun. "Flow" is the psychological term described by Mihaly Csikszentmihalyi for this state of energized focus with full involvement[68]. It is also described as being "in the zone" or "in the groove." It is a state where the mind is focused on the activity, is relaxed, and aroused at the same time.

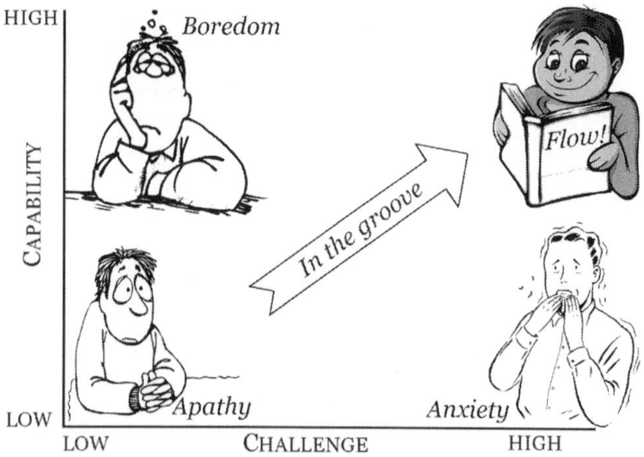

Figure 29-3: Flow Diagram

If the challenge is too low for our set of skills, we become bored, when we face difficult challenges for which we are unprepared or unable to accomplish, stress can result.

One strategy for avoiding stress is to remove the challenge. Sometimes referred to as in-school dropouts, students may quit trying if the challenge is excessive. Adults also avoid challenges that create stress. This can create apathy: a situation where there is no challenge and no skill development. Apathy may be a reasonable response to excessive challenge in the face of inadequate skill as it can be less destructive than stress. If we do not have the capabilities required to meet the challenge, and we cannot just walk away or zone out, it can be very stressful, especially if the challenge is accompanied by real or perceived threat of harm.

An imperative in computer game design is the progressive escalation of the challenge as the player builds skill. If the game starts off too difficult, the player will become frustrated and quit. If the game does not provide a progressive challenge, it becomes boring[69]. It is the job of game makers, teachers, managers and parents to match the challenge to the skill level of a gamer, student, and employee while training them and helping them increase their skills. One of the major complaints of students and employees is boredom; they feel that their skills are not being utilized, and then school and work are not fun.

Good leaders (including parents, teachers, and managers, or doctors trying to effect behavioral changes in patients) make sure that challenge is appropriate for those they work with and that it does not cause distress. Keeping people in the flow, where they are interested and challenged, produces the best results; learning is more effective; employees are more productive; people enjoy and take pride in their accomplishments. Great teachers and leaders set demand levels sufficiently high to keep those they are responsible for engaged and active, and avoid intimidation or hostility as a means of keeping them on task.

> A stress reduction prayer:
>
> *Lord, make me a channel of your peace;*
> *where there is hatred, let me bring love;*
> *Where there is injury, help me bring healing,*
> *where there is wrong, let me sow forgiveness;*
> *where there is discord, let me create harmony;*
> *where there is error, help me bring truth;*
> *where there is doubt, let me create faith;*
> *where there is despair, let me bring hope,*
> *where there are shadows, let me bring light;*
> *where there is sadness, let me bring joy.*
>
> *Lord, grant that I may seek rather to*
> *comfort than to be comforted;*
> *to understand, than to be understood;*
> *to love, than to be loved.*
>
> *It is by self-forgetting that one finds.*
> *It is by forgiving that one is forgiven.*
> *It is by surrendering our fatigued bodies to sleep*
> *that we can awaken to your glory.*
>
> Adapted from Francis of Assisi

[1] Autonomic innervation and regulation of the immune system (1987-2007). Nance DM, Sanders VM. Brain Behav Immun. 2007 Aug;21(6):736-45 PMID:17467231

[2] The sympathetic nerve--an integrative interface between two supersystems: the brain and the immune system. Elenkov IJ, Wilder RL, Chrousos GP, Vizi ES. Pharmacol Rev. 2000 Dec;52(4):595-638. PMID:11121511

[3] Th17 cells: from precursors to players in inflammation and infection. Awasthi A, Kuchroo VK. Int Immunol. 2009 May;21(5):489-98. PMID:19261692

[4] Further exploring the brain-skin connection: stress worsens dermatitis via substance P-dependent neurogenic inflammation in mice. Pavlovic S, Daniltchenko M, Tobin DJ, Hagen E, Hunt SP, Klapp BF, Arck PC, Peters EM. J Invest Dermatol. 2008 Feb;128(2):434-46. PMID:17914449

[5] Stress exposure modulates peptidergic innervation and degranulates mast cells in murine skin. Peters EM, Kuhlmei A, Tobin DJ, Müller-Röver S, Klapp BF, Arck PC. Brain Behav Immun. 2005 May;19(3):252-62. PMID:15797314

[6] Personality and serotonin transporter genotype interact with social context to affect immunity and viral set-point in simian immunodeficiency virus disease. Capitanio JP, Abel K, Mendoza SP, Blozis SA, McChesney MB, Cole SW, Mason WA. Brain Behav Immun. 2008 Jul;22(5):676-89. PMID:17719201

[7] A pacific culture among wild baboons: its emergence and transmission. Sapolsky RM, Share LJ. PLoS Biol. 2004 Apr;2(4):E106. PMID:15094808

[8] Styles of male social behavior and their endocrine correlates among low-ranking baboons. Virgin CE Jr, Sapolsky RM. Am J Primatol. 1997;42(1):25-39. PMID:9108969

[9] The effect of day care attendance on infant and toddler's growth. Zmiri P, Rubin L, Akons H, Zion N, Shaoul R. Acta Paediatr. 2011 Feb;100(2):266-70. PMID:20825606

[10] Final height in psychosocial short stature: is there complete catch-up? Gohlke BC, Stanhope R. Acta Paediatr. 2002;91(9):961-5. PMID:12412873

[11] Growth delay as an index of allostatic load in young children: predictions to disinhibited social approach and diurnal cortisol activity. Johnson AE, Bruce J, Tarullo AR, Gunnar MR. Dev Psychopathol. 2011 Aug;23(3):859-71. PMID:21756437

[12] Nongenomic transmission across generations of maternal behavior and stress responses in the rat. Francis D, Diorio J, Liu D, Meaney MJ. Science. 1999 Nov 5;286(5442):1155-8. PMID:10550053

[13] Intergenerational transmission of parental bonding among women. Miller L, Kramer R, Warner V, Wickramaratne P, Weissman M. J Am Acad Child Adolesc Psychiatry. 1997 Aug;36(8):1134-9. PMID:9256594

[14] Gestational programming: population survival effects of drought and famine during pregnancy. Ross MG, Desai M. Am J Physiol Regul Integr Comp Physiol. 2005 Jan;288(1):R25-33. PMID:15590994

[15] Maternal Methyl Donors Supplementation during Lactation Prevents the Hyperhomocysteinemia Induced by a High-Fat-

Sucrose Intake by Dams. Cordero P, Milagro FI, Campion J, Martinez JA. Int J Mol Sci. 2013 Dec 16;14(12):24422-37. PMID:24351826

[16] Plastics derived endocrine disruptors (BPA, DEHP and DBP) induce epigenetic transgenerational inheritance of obesity, reproductive disease and sperm epimutations. Manikkam M, Tracey R, Guerrero-Bosagna C, Skinner MK. PLoS One. 2013;8(1):e55387. PMID:23359474

[17] Epigenetic effects of glucocorticoids. Weaver IC. Semin Fetal Neonatal Med. 2009 Jun;14(3):143-50. PMID:19217839

[18] Maternal, not paternal, PTSD is related to increased risk for PTSD in offspring of Holocaust survivors. Yehuda R, Bell A, Bierer LM, Schmeidler J. J Psychiatr Res. 2008 Oct;42(13):1104-11. PMID:18281061

[19] Hypomethylation of MB-COMT promoter is a major risk factor for schizophrenia and bipolar disorder. Abdolmaleky HM, Cheng KH, Faraone SV, et al. Hum Mol Genet. 2006 Nov 1;15(21):3132-45. PMID:16984965

[20] Progressive, transgenerational changes in offspring phenotype and epigenotype following nutritional transition. Burdge GC, Hoile SP, Uller T, Thomas NA, Gluckman PD, Hanson MA, Lillycrop KA. PLoS One. 2011;6(11):e28282 PMID:22140567

[21] Genetic and epigenetic control of metabolic health. Schwenk RW, Vogel H, Schürmann A. Mol Metab. 2013 Sep 25;2(4):337-347. PMID:24327950

[22] A review on the evidence of transgenerational transmission of posttraumatic stress disorder vulnerability. Yahyavi ST, Zarghami M, Marwah U. Rev Bras Psiquiatr. 2013 Dec 23;0:0. PMID:24402183

[23] Susceptibility to stress induced visceral hypersensitivity in maternally separated rats is transferred across generations. van den Wijngaard RM, Stanisor OI, van Diest SA, et al. Neurogastroenterol Motil. 2013 Dec;25(12):e780-90. PMID:23965154

[24] Maternal intake of methyl-donor nutrients and child cognition at 3 years of age. Villamor E, Rifas-Shiman SL, Gillman MW, Oken E. Paediatr Perinat Epidemiol. 2012 Jul;26(4):328-35. PMID:22686384

[25] Immunohistochemical Analysis of Histone H3 Modifications in Germ Cells during Mouse Spermatogenesis. Song N, Liu J, An S, Nishino T, Hishikawa Y, Koji T. Acta Histochem Cytochem. 2011 Aug 27;44(4):183-90. PMID:21927517

[26] Impact of epigenetic dietary compounds on transgenerational prevention of human diseases. Li Y, Saldanha SN, Tollefsbol TO. AAPS J. 2014 Jan;16(1):27-36. PMID:24114450

[27] Effects of altered maternal folic acid, vitamin B12 and docosahexaenoic acid on placental global DNA methylation patterns in Wistar rats. Kulkarni A, Dangat K, Kale A, Sable P, Chavan-Gautam P, Joshi S. PLoS One. 2011 Mar 10;6(3):e17706. PMID:21423696

[28] Altered maternal micronutrients (folic acid, vitamin B(12)) and omega 3 fatty acids through oxidative stress may reduce neurotrophic factors in preterm pregnancy. Dhobale M, Joshi S. J Matern Fetal Neonatal Med. 2012 Apr;25(4):317-23. PMID:21609203

[29] Histone acetylase inhibitor curcumin impairs mouse spermiogenesis-an in vitro study. Xia X, Cai H, Qin S, Xu C. PLoS One. 2012;7(11):e48673. PMID:23144926

[30] Roles of melatonin in fetal programming in compromised pregnancies. Chen YC, Sheen JM, Tiao MM, Tain YL, Huang LT. Int J Mol Sci. 2013 Mar 6;14(3):5380-401. PMID:23466884

[31] Epigenetic regulation: a new research area for melatonin? Korkmaz A, Reiter RJ. J Pineal Res. 2008 Jan;44(1):41-4. PMID:18078446

[32] Fatty acids and epigenetics. Burdge GC, Lillycrop KA. Curr Opin Clin Nutr Metab Care. 2013 Dec 7. PMID:24322369

[33] Glucocorticoid therapy-induced memory deficits: acute versus chronic effects. Coluccia D, Wolf OT, Kollias S, Roozendaal B, Forster A, de Quervain DJ. J Neurosci. 2008 Mar 26;28(13):3474-8. PMID: 18367613

[34] Chronic stress, visceral obesity and gonadal dysfunction. Kyrou I, Tsigos C. Hormones (Athens). 2008 Oct-Dec;7(4):287-93. Review.PMID: 19121989

[35] Modulation of hypothalamic PTP1B in the TNF-alpha-induced insulin and leptin resistance. Picardi PK, Caricilli AM, de Abreu LL, Carvalheira JB, Velloso LA, Saad MJ. FEBS Lett. 2010 Jul 16;584(14):3179-84. Epub 2010 Jun 2.PMID: 20576518

[36] Relation between the hypothalamic-pituitary-thyroid (HPT) axis and the hypothalamic-pituitary-adrenal (HPA) axis during repeated stress. Helmreich DL, Parfitt DB, Lu XY, Akil H, Watson SJ. Neuroendocrinology. 2005;81(3):183-92. PMID:16020927

[37] Neural regulation of innate immunity: a coordinated nonspecific host response to pathogens. Sternberg EM. Nat Rev Immunol. 2006 Apr;6(4):318-28. PMID: 16557263

[38] Two novel mutations of the TSH-beta subunit gene underlying congenital central hypothyroidism undetectable in neonatal TSH screening. Baquedano MS, Ciaccio M, Dujovne N, Herzovich V, Longueira Y, Warman DM, Rivarola MA, Belgorosky A. J Clin Endocrinol Metab. 2010 Sep;95(9):E98-103. PMID:20534762

[39] The hypothalamus-pituitary-thyroid axis in critical illness. Mebis L, van den Berghe G. Neth J Med. 2009 Nov;67(10):332-40. PMID:19915227

[40] Thyroid hormone regulation by stress and behavioral differences in adult male rats. Helmreich DL, Tylee D. Horm Behav. 2011 Aug;60(3):284-91. PMID:21689656

[41] Elevated serum uric Acid is associated with high circulating inflammatory cytokines in the population-based colaus study. Lyngdoh T, Marques-Vidal P, Paccaud F, Preisig M, Waeber G, Bochud M, Vollenweider P. PLoS One. 2011;6(5):e19901. Epub 2011 May 20. PMID:21625475

[42] Are salivary gonadal steroid concentrations influenced by acute psychosocial stress? A study using the Trier Social Stress Test (TSST). Schoofs D, Wolf OT. Int J Psychophysiol. 2011 Apr;80(1):36-43. PMID:21256897

[43] Corticotrophin-releasing factor and stress-induced inhibition of the gonadotrophin-releasing hormone pulse generator in the female. Li XF, Knox AM, O'Byrne KT. Brain Res. 2010 Dec 10;1364:153-63. PMID:20727865

[44] Stress increases putative gonadotropin inhibitory hormone and decreases luteinizing hormone in male rats. Kirby ED, Geraghty AC, Ubuka T, Bentley GE, Kaufer D. Proc Natl Acad Sci U S A. 2009 Jul 7;106(27):11324-9. PMID:19541621

[45] Stress response circuitry hypoactivation related to hormonal dysfunction in women with major depression. Holsen LM, Spaeth SB, Lee JH, Ogden LA, Klibanski A, Whitfield-Gabrieli S, Goldstein JM. J Affect Disord. 2011 Jun;131(1-3):379-87. PMID:21183223

[46] Effects of kisspeptin on parameters of the HPA axis. Rao YS, Mott NN, Pak TR. Endocrine. 2011 Jun;39(3):220-8. PMID:21387128

[47] Omega-3 status and cerebrospinal fluid corticotrophin releasing hormone in perpetrators of domestic violence. Hibbeln JR, Bissette G, Umhau JC, George DT. Biol Psychiatry. 2004 Dec 1;56(11):895-7. PMID:15576068

[48] Elevated plasma corticotrophin-releasing hormone levels in veterans with posttraumatic stress disorder. de Kloet CS, Vermetten E, Geuze E, Lentjes EG, Heijnen CJ, Stalla GK, Westenberg HG. Prog Brain Res. 2008;167:287-91. PMID:18037027

[49] Returning from war with invisible wounds. PRIME Education, Inc. 2010. www.primeinc.org

[50] Intrauterine factors as determinants of depressive disorder. Weinstock M. Isr J Psychiatry Relat Sci. 2010;47(1):36-45. PMID:20686198

[51] Transient gastric irritation in the neonatal rats leads to changes in hypothalamic CRF expression, depression- and anxiety-like behavior as adults. Liu L, Li Q, Sapolsky R, Liao M, Mehta K, Bhargava A, Pasricha PJ. PLoS One. 2011 May 12;6(5):e19498. PMID:21589865

[52] Role of corticotropin-releasing hormone in irritable bowel syndrome and intestinal inflammation. Fukudo S. J Gastroenterol. 2007 Jan;42 Suppl 17:48-51. PMID:17238026

[53] Corticotropin-releasing hormone-receptor 2 is required for acute stress-induced bladder vascular permeability and release of vascular endothelial growth factor. Boucher W, Kempuraj D, Michaelian M, Theoharides TC. BJU Int. 2010 Nov;106(9):1394-9. PMID:20201838

[54] Corticotropin-releasing hormone and the blood-brain-barrier. Theoharides TC, Konstantinidou AD. Front Biosci. 2007 Jan 1;12:1615-28. PMID:17127408

[55] Ethanol modulates corticotropin releasing hormone release from the rat hypothalamus: does acetaldehyde play a role? Cannizzaro C, La Barbera M, Plescia F, Cacace S, Tringali G. Alcohol Clin Exp Res. 2010 Apr;34(4):588-93. PMID:20102575

[56] Omega-3 status and cerebrospinal fluid corticotrophin releasing hormone in perpetrators of domestic violence. Hibbeln JR, Bissette G, Umhau JC, George DT. Biol Psychiatry. 2004 Dec 1;56(11):895-7. PMID:15576068

[57] Essential fatty acids and their role in conditions characterised by impulsivity. Garland MR, Hallahan B. Int Rev Psychiatry. 2006 Apr;18(2):99-105. PMID:16777664

[58] The role of 5-HT(1A) receptors in fish oil-mediated increased BDNF expression in the rat hippocampus and cortex: A possible antidepressant mechanism. Vines A, Delattre AM, Lima MM, Rodrigues LS, Suchecki D, Machado RB, Tufik S, Pereira SI, Zanata SM, Ferraz AC. Neuropharmacology. 2011 Jun 29. PMID:21740919

[59] Pineal function: impact of microarray analysis. Klein DC, Bailey MJ, Carter DA, Kim JS, Shi Q, Ho AK, Chik CL, Gaildrat P, Morin F, Ganguly S, Rath MF, Møller M, Sugden D, Rangel ZG, Munson PJ, Weller JL, Coon SL. Mol Cell Endocrinol. 2010 Jan 27;314(2):170-83. PMID:1962238

[60] Changes in serum TSH and free T4 during human sleep restriction. Kessler L, Nedeltcheva A, Imperial J, Penev PD. Sleep. 2010 Aug;33(8):1115-8. PMID: 20815195

[61] Retinoid-related orphan receptors (RORs): critical roles in development, immunity, circadian rhythm, and cellular metabolism. Jetten AM. Nucl Recept Signal. 2009;7:e003. PMID:19381306

[62] Cones are required for normal temporal responses to light of phase shifts and clock gene expression. Dollet A, Albrecht U, Cooper HM, Dkhissi-Benyahya O. Chronobiol Int. 2010 Jun;27(4):768-81. PMID:20560710

[63] Free triiodothyronine has a distinct circadian rhythm that is delayed but parallels thyrotropin levels. Russell W, Harrison RF, Smith N, Darzy K, Shalet S, Weetman AP, Ross RJ. J Clin Endocrinol Metab. 2008 Jun;93(6):2300-6. Epub 2008 Mar 25. PMID:18364382

[64] Healing by Gentle Touch Ameliorates Stress and Other Symptoms in People Suffering with Mental Health Disorders or Psychological Stress. Weze C, Leathard HL, Grange J, Tiplady P, Stevens G. eCAM 2007;4(1)115–123.

[65] Comparison of manual lymph drainage therapy and connective tissue massage in women with fibromyalgia: a randomized controlled trial. Ekici G, Bakar Y, Akbayrak T, Yuksel I. J Manipulative Physiol Ther. 2009 Feb;32(2):127-33. PMID:19243724

[66] Inducing sensory stimulation in treatment of anorexia nervosa. Grunwald M, Weiss T. QJM. 2005 May;98(5):379-80. PMID:15833769

[67] Characteristics of impulsive suicide attempts and attempters. Simon OR, Swann AC, Powell KE, et al. Suicide Life Threat Behav. 2001;32(1 Suppl):49-59. PMID:11924695

[68] Flow: The Psychology of Optimal Experience. Mihaly Csikszentmihalyi, Harper Collins 2008

[69] The Game Maker's Apprentice. Jacob Habgood and Mark Overmars. Technology in Action. 2006

30. IMMUNOEXCITOTOXIC CNS INJURY

Traumatic Brain Injury and Immunocytotoxicity

The immune mechanisms through which traumatic brain injury (TBI) and stroke incur damage, and the agents that can mitigate this damage, offer valuable insight into understanding and treating enteroimmune inflammatory disorders affecting the central nervous system. Additionally, understanding TBI allows secondary preventive treatment of these conditions that can limit damage to the non-recoverable, post-mitotic neurons, which occurs in the hours following injury.

For most injuries, if the patient lives through the acute trauma and blood loss, the chances of surviving increase every hour, over the next several days. During the Vietnam War, for example, only three percent of casualties, among U.S. soldiers who made it to the hospital, died. Forty percent of those fatalities, however, were head injuries[1]. Patients with TBI, rather than improving in the days after the injury, often deteriorate. This is because TBI creates an immunocytotoxic cascade in the brain in the hours and days following the injury. In TBI, especially closed head injury, it is not the original trauma to the CNS, but rather the immunoexcitotoxic reaction to the injury that worsens the patient's condition. Furthermore, patients who survive the acute phase of TBI often suffer from chronic neuroexcitotoxic inflammatory disease that persists and progresses with time.

Over five million Americans have long-term disability from TBI[2]. These injuries occur in motor vehicle accidents, falls, sporting injuries. They are common sequelae from blast injuries among military veterans of Iraq and Afghanistan. Even relatively minor head injuries that do not involve loss of consciousness can result in TBI. Although not well recognized, traumatic spinal cord injury may be even more common. It can result in non-impingement radicular symptoms, including paresthesias and weakness, and results in chronic neuropathic pain.

The most common initial event in TBI is a concussion. This injury occurs, as a result of acceleration-deceleration and rotational forces upon the CNS. Rotational acceleration, as may occur in boxing or vehicle collisions from the side, requires less force to cause a concussion[3]. A concussion usually involves motion of the brain in opposing force to that of the skull.

A concussion may result in the loss of consciousness; however, in a study of high school and college athletes, only nine percent of concussions resulted in the loss of consciousness[4]. At the time of the initial injury, there is typically an immediate onset of a short-term neurologic impairment, with spontaneous recovery. The injured may merely feel dazed, be momentarily disoriented, or have difficulty thinking.

In the first seconds, the concussion provokes a mass regional depolarization of the neurologic tissue. There are potassium efflux and calcium influx into the neurons. This triggers the widespread release of the excitatory neurotransmitter glutamate, which triggers further depolarization and electrolyte flux through potassium channels, allowing further entry of calcium into, and potassium out of the neurons. Neuronal activity is suppressed by this widespread depolarization. Sodium-potassium pump activity is accelerated to restore function.

In the first few hours after the injury, more serious events follow. The large influx of intracellular calcium activates second-messenger systems in the cells. Meanwhile, the increased workload to restore polarization can exhaust ATP stores and trigger anaerobic metabolism of energy stores. The large release of glutamate, especially during hypoxia, is neuroexcitotoxic. These events result in the formation of reactive oxygen and nitrogen species. Dysfunction of aquaporin water channels can cause brain swelling. Vasospasm, which occurs as an intrinsic immune reaction, decreases decrease blood flow to areas of the injury. In severe injuries, there is often brain swelling and increased intracranial pressure, thus, further limiting blood flow and oxygenation. Hypoxia, followed by reperfusion, creates free radicals that can trigger neuronal cell death through apoptosis.

Additionally, in TBI, there is often bleeding within the CNS. This may be focal intracranial hemorrhage, but more commonly is petechial hemorrhage, with numerous tiny capillary bleeds. Along with debris from to the neurons and other tissues of the CNS, blood extravasated into CNS tissues needs to be cleared. Microglia, the principal immune cells of the CNS, become activated by heme from red blood cells and cellular debris from neurons and other brain tissue detritus. Once activated they produce inflammatory cytokines that further damages the CNS, killing more neurons and reinforcing the inflammatory response. This process may last weeks, or become a chronic inflammatory process.

> Children and teenagers are at increased risk of severe cerebral edema with TBI. Second Impact Syndrome, a rare but catastrophic injury, can occur when a second concussion occurs before the resolution of the first injury.
>
> Women appear to be more susceptible to TBI than are men. Men may be at less risk due to their increased neck musculature or cranial mass that may afford greater protection from injury.

Postconcussion Syndrome: After a concussion, patients often remain symptomatic for several days to weeks. Headache and difficulty with memory are two of the most common post-concussive symptoms. A tool for assessing Postconcussion Syndrome is given in Appendix K.

Posttraumatic Headaches

Post-concussive headaches may have various or multiple overlapping causes. Some are migrainous; intracranial and vascular. TBI exacerbates migraines in migraineurs. These patients often report increased frequency or even daily migraine during the post-concussive period. Commonly, cervicogenic cephalgia, arises from injury to the cervical spine; herniated disks, spinal stenosis, or injury to facet joints can occur from the same injuries causing TBI. These headaches may be caused by injury to, or compression of, cervical nerves C1 to C3. More commonly, injury to the lower cervical and high thoracic nerves promote trigger point spasm and myalgia in the muscles of the neck and upper back that cause headaches. TBI patients often have sleep disturbances, exacerbating headaches and may have tension or rebound headaches, worsened by analgesic use. Other patients may have pain or tenderness directly from the injury to the soft tissues or bone of the head and face. Migraine is discussed in Chapter 28. Trigger point treatment is discussed in Appendix J.

The hippocampus is crucial for the formation of new declarative memory. Atrophy of the hippocampus often occurs in moderate to severe TBI. After mild TBI, postconcussion symptoms usually abate over the first three months.

Table 31-1: Postconcussion Symptoms

Type	Postconcussion Symptoms[5]
Somatic	Fatigue; sleep disturbance, headache, blurred or double vision, sensitivity to light, dizziness, nausea, and/or vomiting, noise sensitivity, tinnitus, nocturia.
Emotional	Irritability, depressed affect, restlessness, feeling frustrated.
Cognitive	Forgetfulness, poor concentration, taking longer to think.

About 13 percent of U.S. Army soldiers who incurred mild TBI serving in Afghanistan or Iraq have long-term residual TBI symptoms; these individuals are about four times more likely to suffer from PTSD. They suffer from poorer visual memory and slower reaction times[6]. Five years after "moderated" TBI as many as 60% of these soldiers had vestibular dysfunction, and 72% had hearing loss[7].

Chronic Traumatic Encephalopathy: TBI, even from relatively minor injury, especially when repeated, can result in chronic traumatic encephalopathy (CTE). CTE is a progressive disease that begins with emotional and cognitive disorders and progresses to deterioration of motor functions. As many as 80% of patients have irritability, poor insight or judgment, depression and paranoia, and about 60% suffer from inappropriate outbursts of anger, aggression, and apathy. Several studies have shown increased rate of crime and conduct disorders following TBI[8]. In one study, patients hospitalized for TBI during childhood and adolescence had a 5.7 times higher prevalence of conduct disorders and a 6.8 times higher rate of criminality, most of which was violent crime[9].

Stage I CTE has similar symptoms to those of post-concussive syndrome; however, the symptoms fail to abate after three months. Instead, they progress to stage II CTE, in which there are the additional symptoms of irritability, outburst of anger, or aggression and depression. Drug and alcohol abuse is common in stage II CTE.

Microglia are specialized monocytes that reside in the brain and act as macrophages for the CNS. They comprise about one-fifth of the cells in the brain, but most exist in a resting state. During an infection or after injury microglia quickly activate. They can divide and create new microglia.

Activated microglia act as antigen presenting cells and are phagocytic and cytotoxic, destroying infectious agents and foreign antigens. They also remove dead cells in the brain. Additionally, microglia secrete neurotrophic factors key to neuronal survival. Thus, normal levels of activation are important for brain health. However, when over-activated, these cells produce proinflammatory neurotoxins and free radicals[10]. This overactivity can damage the brain.

Glial cell-derived neurotrophic factor, (GDNF), is produced by glial cells and promotes the growth of neurons during development. In the adult brain, however, while still produced by astrocytes, GDNF is mostly produced by neurons, especially in the striatum. From here, it is transported to the midbrain, via dopaminergic neurons. GDNF is essential for dopaminergic and motor neuronal survival and re-growth of neurons after injury.

The rate-limiting enzyme, tyrosine hydroxylase, (TH) converts tyrosine into L-DOPA; the precursor of dopamine, epinephrine and norepinephrine. Cofactors for TH include O_2 and Fe^{2+}. TH activity is a source of H_2O_2 and other reactive oxygen species. GDNF not only modulates TH and excitatory activity, it also prevents ROS associated injury from TH activity[11]. Loss of GDNP and increased TH activity impair the survival of dopaminergic cells; this can lead to Parkinson's disease and amyotrophic lateral sclerosis (ALS).

Loss of GDNF may also cause the drug and alcohol abuse seen in CTE. The ventral tegmental area (VTA) of the midbrain functions in the reward system, affecting motivation, cognition, and addiction. GDNF applied to the VTA suppresses alcohol consumption. GDNF decreases voluntary alcohol consumption and craving by its actions on the VTA, decreases the potential for drug abuse, and may help prevent addiction to psycho-stimulants[11,12,13].

Dopamine activates the reward system; dopamine promotes alcohol and drug craving and addiction. Neuronal injury often increases the production of heat shock protein 90 (HSP90). HSP90 acts as a chaperone for TH protecting it from degradation, and thus, HSP90 increases TH level and activity. Alcohol consumption also increases TH binding to HSP90. GDNF appears to diminish the binding of TH to HSP90, thereby subjecting it to normal degradation, thus, reducing TH activity, along with the reward stimulus from alcohol or drug use[11].

> In the VTA, GDNF has a positive autoregulatory feedback loop: GDNF upregulates and maintains its own expression. GDNF acts through specific tyrosine kinase receptors, and the activation of MEK/ERK1/2 and Akt/PI3K, which increase the transcription of GDNF and proteins it regulates. Disruption of GDNF's autoregulatory feedback cycle, from reductions in levels of endogenously produced GDNF, prevents the subsequent activation of the loop; even a short disruption may prevent GDNF production[14]. During the inflammatory response, GDNF production is suppressed by PGE2 through its activation of the prostaglandin receptor, EP1. PGF2 and thromboxane, however, increase GDNF production, through activation of EP4[15]. Addiction treatment is discussed below.

In stage II CTE, social and cognitive difficulties often lead to financial difficulties, bankruptcy, job loss, perpetration of physical abuse. Relationships, obviously, become difficult as social and cognitive functioning decline, and divorce often occurs.

Stage III CTE is often cut short by suicide, overdose, or death from unintentional injury, thus precluding progression to stage IV CTE. In stage IV CTE, there is a greater loss of motor function; some patients develop the mask-like facies, tremor, wide propulsive gait, and the bradykinesia of Parkinson's disease. There may be dysarthric speech, balance disorders, ocular muscle abnormalities, and deafness. Some patients develop dementia.

Table 30-2: Chronic Traumatic Encephalopathy Stages

Stage I CTE: Headache, loss of concentration and attention, dizziness.
Stage II CTE: Depression, mood swings, explosivity, short-term memory loss, difficulties with attention and concentration, headache. Drug or alcohol abuse is common.
Stage III CTE: Executive dysfunction and cognitive impairment. Cerebral atrophy, cognitive impairment with memory loss, executive dysfunction, loss of attention and concentration, depression, explosivity and visuospatial abnormalities. Mood disorders, irritability, outbursts of violent or aggressive behavior, confusion, and speech abnormalities. A high rate of substance abuse, suicide, and overdose deaths.
Stage IV CTE: Dementia, profound short-term memory loss, executive dysfunction, attention and concentration loss, explosivity and aggression, paranoia, depression, impulsivity and visuospatial abnormalities. Word finding difficulty. Parkinson's disease-like motor dysfunction[16].

CTE symptoms progress with cognitive and emotional decline followed by eventual motor deterioration. Even in early CTE, perivascular neurofibrillary tangles can be found in the sulci of the frontal cortex. Remarkably, neurofibrillary tangles are present in about a third of CTE patients after TBI within hours of the injury[17].

CTE has two pathophysiologic forms; in one, there is abundant hyperphosphorylated Tau protein and amyloid plaques, similar, or identical to those in Alzheimer's disease (AD); in the other form there is heavy production of tau, without the formation of plaque. Individuals with the APOE4 genotype are at elevated risk for AD and for the AD form of CTE[18].

TBI is common among professional football players. In football, the injuries may be mild but repeatedly occur over years of play, and many players develop CTE. Professional football players are four times more likely to develop Alzheimer's disease (AD) or amyotrophic lateral sclerosis (ALS) than the general population[19].

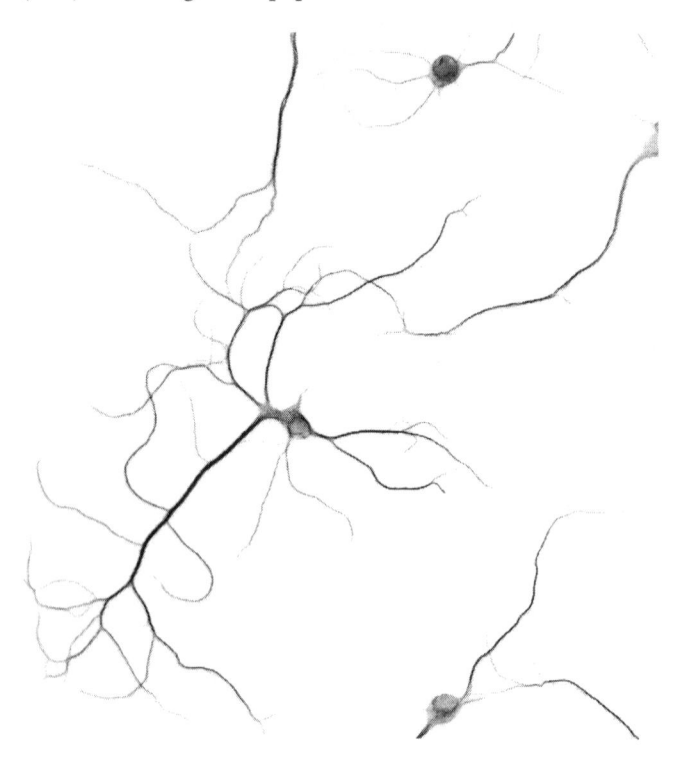

Figure 30-1: Neurons; tubular protein content revealed by fluorescent stain[20]. Only tubular protein is visualized.

> **Microtubule-Associated Protein Tau:**
>
> Microtubules (MT) are part of the cell's cytoskeleton. MT are assemblies of α and β tubulin proteins, which rapidly assemble into helical spirals that form long, thin, stiff tubes, which provide structure, allow cells to move and form projections. MT are dynamic, with typical half-lives of 5 to 10 minutes. Length can be added to one end of the MT while the other end is disassembled. MT are required for the formation of axons and dendrites that project from the soma of a neuron, and they participate in cell migration.
>
> Tau is a microtubule-associated protein that helps stabilize MT α and β tubulin assembly structures in neurons. Tau protein must be dephosphorylated by serine/threonine protein phosphatases before it adheres to, and properly stabilizes the MT. Quinolinic acid (QA) inhibits the expression of serine/threonine protein phosphatases, and thereby, causes hyperphosphorylation of Tau and a reactive upregulation of Tau transcription.

> Hyperphosphorylated Tau causes irregular, dysfunctional microtubules and promotes MT disruption. This impairs neurons from forming new axons and dendrites, resulting in memory loss and neurodegeneration. Glutamate and NMDA also increase phosphorylation of Tau. This association suggests that QA acts as an excitotoxin via NMDA receptors and that it promotes inflammatory activation of microglia[16]
>
> Neuroexcitotoxic damage impairs neuronal growth and repair; the attempts at repair promote Tau formation. This excess, hyperphosphorylated Tau easily aggregates into insoluble neurofibrillary tangles, which are typical in AD, CTE, and several other neurologic diseases. The quinolinic acid formation pathway is illustrated in Figure 31-2.

Injury Timeline

In the first hours after a concussion, there is swelling in the brain. The swelling is made more severe by hypoxia and metabolic acidosis, which results from hypoxia. The swelling contributes to ischemic damage and disruption of the blood-brain barrier (BBB). In the first 12 hours after the injury there is impairment of the BBB, may be bleeding, leakage of plasma and fluids into the intracellular spaces, and alterations of the normal osmotic gradient.

After 24 hours, secondary processes are being caused by inflammation. In an animal model of TBI, there were two peaks in brain edema and ischemia; the first peaking at around six hours, and the second, induced by inflammation, triggered by the release of heme from RBC's, at about 72 hours after the injury[21].

CT scans are often used in emergency medicine in the first hours following head injury to evaluate the patient for intracranial hemorrhage or skull fracture. Conventional neuroimaging tools, however, such as CT and MRI, do not reveal concussive injury.

Table 30-3: Phases of Traumatic Brain Injury

Time Frame	Events
First seconds: Immediate	Concussion, regional depolarization, brief neurologic impairment.
First hours: Acute reaction	Excitotoxic reaction, ischemia/reperfusion, oxidative injury; massive death of neurons.
First days: Acute-delayed reaction	Microglial activation and immune response further damage neurons adjacent to the injury locus. Second wave of injury from heme and iron.
First weeks: Post-acute phase	Activated microglia either continue inflammation or begin repair.
Months to years: Chronic phase	Chronic inflammatory response with slow, and often, widespread neuronal loss.

Immunocytotoxicity

Most injuries involve physical trauma; so it might be expected that TBI causes shearing of axons. However, this is not what usually occurs[22]. The damage to axons does not occur at the time of injury but rather occurs later, as a result of inflammatory activity. One of the first events in TBI is the release of glutamate. Glutamate, an excitatory neurotransmitter, is the most abundant neurotransmitter in the brain; 90% of synapses in the cerebral cortex have glutamate receptors. Glutamate is stored in vesicles in nerve endings, and released when the nerve fires; upon depolarization. Glutamate stimulation enhances attention, learning, memory, and alertness. Excessive glutamate stimulus, however, is excitotoxic. When over-activated, there is the generation of reactive oxygen and nitrogen species (ROS and RNS) production of lipid oxidation products, nitric oxide (NO) and prostaglandins.

Glutamate receptors, like other neuroreceptors, are either metabotropic or ionotropic receptors. The metabotropic glutamate receptors are surface G proteins which act through signal cascades within the cell. The ionotropic glutamate receptors; NMDA, AMPA and kainate receptors, in contrast, are ion channel receptors. When activated, these ion channels allow the flux of ions; such as the influx of Na^+ and Ca^{++} and efflux of K^+ from the cell. NMDA receptor activation allows an influx of calcium, which is excitatory. The excess calcium causes oxidative stress in the cell's mitochondria, activating caspase-3, which can trigger the apoptotic cascade and neuronal cell death[23]. TNF-α potentiates this pathway.

In TBI, glutamate-induced excitotoxic injury is responsible for immediate, delayed, and chronic neuronal injury and death. A fluid concussive model for TBI found that the calcium content of hippocampal neurons remained elevated for more than 30 days after the injury[24], suggesting a long-term increase susceptibility to excitotoxic activity.

One mechanism thought to be responsible for the increased long-term susceptibility to excitotoxicity is changes within the glutamate AMPA receptor. In normal conditions, all AMPA receptors undergo translational RNA editing that makes the AMPA (GluR2) receptor channel impermeable to calcium. However, after hypoxia/ischemia, TBI[25], excitotoxic levels of glutamate[26], or in neurodegenerative diseases, this editing is impaired. Lack of editing makes AMPA channels in affected neurons permeable to calcium. Stretching of axons, from injury or swelling, may also cause alterations that impair AMPA editing. Sporadic amyotrophic lateral sclerosis (ALS) has been attributed to neuro-excitotoxicity caused by excessive calcium influx secondary to impaired editing of AMPA receptors[27]. This damage becomes especially evident as motor neuron disease. Several antidepressant medications; including tricyclics, such as amitriptyline; and SSRI's, such as sertraline, have been found to bind to[28], and increase RNA editing of AMPA receptors[29], and thus, may help restore neuronal resilience to excitotoxicity.

Ischemia/Reperfusion Injury

TBI results from ischemic reactions followed by reperfusion. Brain edema, generalized depolarization, with its increased energy demand, and other TBI mechanisms induce ischemia, followed by reperfusion.

Ischemia/reperfusion (I/R) injury is a generalized mechanism which occurs in during and after stroke[30] concussion, myocardial infarction[31], ischemic lung injury[32], intestinal ischemia[33], and in the liver, kidney, and other organ transplants[34]. I/R trauma results in the activation of toll-like receptors, notably TLR4 and TLR2[35] and perhaps other TLR's. Most of the tissue damage that results from ischemia occurs, as a result of the innate immune response which occurs after reperfusion; as a result of oxidative damage through the creation of ROS and RNS, and the activation of the nuclear transcription factor NF-κB.

Toll-like receptors respond to infectious agents; TLR4 is activated by LPS from microbial cell walls of gram-negative bacteria and TLR2 by lipoteichoic acid from cell walls of gram-positive bacteria. TLR's are also activated by certain endogenous compounds which are produced during injury. TLR's may be activated by heat-shock proteins, β-amyloid, stathmin; a regulator of microtubule disassembly, α-synuclein; from presynaptic terminals, and from other molecules released by degenerating cells, including heme. Oxidized lipoproteins and hyaluronan can also activate certain TLR's.

In mice, TLR4 blocking antibodies were found to mitigate I/R damage to the CNS induced by occluding the common carotid arteries[36]. Mice genetically missing functional TLR4 have decreased microglial activation and pro-inflammatory cytokine production, and preserved spinal cord function after thoracic artery occlusion/reperfusion[37].

I/R activates the MyD88 pathway via TLR4 and TLR2, thus, activating nuclear transcription factor NF-κB. NF-κB then moves into the nucleus, where it transcribes segments of the DNA for several proinflammatory proteins, raising the level of inflammatory cytokines including TNF-α, IL-1β, IL-6, IL-8, and IFN-γ. NF-κB increases transcription for COX2[38], increasing PGE2 synthesis, and iNOS, which in an inflammatory environment, produces high levels of NO. NO reacts with superoxide, forming toxic peroxynitrite. Cellular stress products such as H_2O_2, TNF-α, and arachidonic acid activate sphingomyelinase; peroxynitrite specifically activates the acidic sphingomyelinase isomers[39]. Even transient focal cerebral ischemia induces large increases in acidic sphingomyelinase activity that induces excitotoxicity, proinflammatory cytokine production, and neuronal apoptosis[40].

NF-κB activation not only promotes the generation of intracellular free radicals, but it is also is activated by them. Hydrogen peroxide, for example, can trigger nuclear translocation of NF-κB into the nucleus. This suggests a positive feedback loop, wherein NF-κB activation induces generation of free radicals that in turn further activate NF-κB. This process can reach a tipping point at which apoptosis occurs. Evidence suggests that ROS activates or potentiates NF-κB through a TLR4-dependent mechanism. Thus, extracellular ROS can promote the generation of intracellular ROS. A wide array of antioxidants prevent the NF-κB nuclear translocation and activation; targeting TLR4-mediated NF-κB pathway with antioxidants or other TLR4 interdiction may limit ROS-induced cellular damage.

The TLR-mediated immune reaction after an ischemic event in the CNS promotes microglial activation that can continue for at least several months. The pro-inflammatory response is not restricted to the site of ischemic injury; it can spread to other areas of the CNS[41].

TLR2-deficient mice do not have significantly different production of the inflammatory cytokines, IL1β, IL-6, or TNF-α; however, they have significantly reduced activation of microglia in the days following an ischemic event. Three days after I/R injury, TLR2-deficient mice had a 47% smaller volume of stroke damage. However, at seven days, the TLR2-deficient mice had a 32% greater volume of indirect ischemic damage. This indirect damage results from the microglial immune response. TLR2 promotes microglial activation, but it also promotes the transition of microglial activity from inflammation to repair functions[42]. Thus, TLR2 activation is important after an injury, to down-regulate the inflammatory processes and initiate repair and regrowth.

Heme

A secondary event in TBI or intracerebral hemorrhage or spinal cord injury is the enzymatic lysis of hemoglobin, from red blood cells, into heme an iron. In head injuries, there is often bleeding from small capillaries in multiple areas of the brain. It takes some time to for the RBC's to be broken down and for hemoglobin to be lysed. Iron and heme levels usually peak about 72 hours after head injury or cerebral hemorrhage[43].

Iron released into the CNS increases the production of the excitotoxin quinolinic acid (QA)[44] and may activate microglia and increases the production of free radicals[45]. Heme is an agonist for TLR4 activity and activates microglia via the MyD88/TRIF signaling pathway. The breakdown of hemoglobin is associated with a second wave or brain edema and neurologic damage, peaking three days after the injury[46].

Microglial Activation

The microglia are immune cells, originally derived from the bone marrow during fetal life. New microglia are supplied by reproduction in the CNS. They behave, principally, as an innate immune system, without the benefit of antibodies, which are too large to pass through the blood-brain barrier (BBB). When activated, microglia produce immune defense factors, including pro-inflammatory cytokines, chemokines, prostaglandins, proteases, free radicals, NO, and the excitotoxic neurotransmitters; glutamate, aspartate, and QA. Microglia have cytokine receptors, and thus, their activation recruits other microglia to the area of injury.

Microglia also participate in phagocytosis of bacteria, and exogenous and endogenous cellular debris. After injury or infection, microglia in the brain phagocytize irreversibly damaged neurons and cellular debris; recycling, and clearing space for the recovery of new and recovering cells. Compounds in the neuronal debris further stimulate and maintains these activities and the production of cytokines, chemokines, and other inflammatory factors, which recruit more microglia to the area. This can provoke wider neuronal damage in which viable and healthy neurons may be killed.

Microglia can produce BDNF, basic fibroblast growth factor, and other growth factors. Activated astrocytes produce GDNF, release trophic compounds, and support the regrowth of neuronal connections. The normally quiescent NG-2 oligodendrocyte precursor cells become active; multiplying and differentiating into to mature myelin-producing oligodendrocytes. These cells are responsible for myelination of nerve fibers and construction of new neuronal circuits. ND-2 cells can migrate from undamaged areas of the brain[47], and at least in the hypothalamus, act as stem cells, capable of forming new neurons[48]. The brain, thus, can repair and generation of some new neurons.

Sphingomyelinase, induced by I/R, causes the formation of ceramide and other sphingolipids within stressed cells. This can activate apoptosis and destruction of injured neurons. S1P is created and exported as a distress signal from less severely damaged cells. Microglia are derived from the same lineage as macrophages, and similarly, S1P can promote migration, phagocytosis, and microglial proliferation and survival. Activation of S1P receptors on neurons increases excitation and nociception, the perception of pain. The population distribution of the various S1P receptors on target cells depends on the internal and external environment of these cells. The response to S1P is mediated by cytokines and other signaling factors; S1P can induce production of proinflammatory cytokines in astrocytes and prevent astrocyte proliferation. It can maintain the destruction or promote repair and regrowth. In a less stressful milieu, S1P inhibits axonal demyelination and induces myelination of axons by microglia and promote proliferation and survival of neural progenitor cells[49].

The inflammatory process inhibits the repair and recovery processes, and oligodendrocytes needed for repair, become susceptible to apoptosis[50]. After spinal cord and brain injury that results in the death of GPR17+ neurons and oligodendrocytes, there is a proliferation and migration of GPR17+ microglia/macrophages into the area of the lesion[51,52]. GPR17 is a surface receptor for leukotrienes, LTD$_4$ and LTE$_4$, and uracil nucleotides, including those that are precursors for glycosphingolipids. When microglia are activated, they can behave as phagocytotic macrophages, capable of causing progressive neuronal cell loss. GPR17 also induces activation of astrocytes and NG-2 cells, however, after injury; these repair cells are repressed, and the activated microglia continue the inflammatory reaction, further impairing neurologic functioning and repair, and at times promoting neural loss.

A component of the injury pathway occurs at a result of mitogen-activated protein kinase (MAPK) p38α. P38α helps induce phagocytosis of axonal debris and β-amyloid. It also induces production of IL-8, chemokines, and may induce IL-1β, IL-6, IL-12, and TNF-α in microglia. In a murine model of multiple sclerosis, p38α in dendritic cells was necessary for the disease progression and maintenance of the TH$_{17}$ response. Both, in the early aftermath of TBI and during a chronic lower level inflammation, microglial activation is dependent on MAPK p38α[53]. Other factors also contribute to the chronic inflammatory response. In TBI, proinflammatory cytokines, including GM-CSF, IFN-γ and TNF are amplified by hypoxia[54]. GM-CSF enhances TLR4 and CD14 expressions in microglia and increases inflammatory reactivity, inducing NF-κB nuclear translocation and thus, the production of IL-1β, IL-6, TNF-α, COX2 and NO by microglia. Induction of TLR4 and CD14 by GM-CSF also up-regulates production of ERK1/2 and p38[55]. Depending on the concentrations of various cytokines in the cell's environment, the inflammatory signals can promote inflammatory cell proliferation, which may also trigger the killing of other cells, or may trigger apoptosis of the inflammatory cells and the down-regulation of inflammation. TNF-α can also trigger the TRAF6→RIP→P13K pathway, for example. The combination of IL-1β and TNF-α can activate CASP8 and the apoptotic cascade.

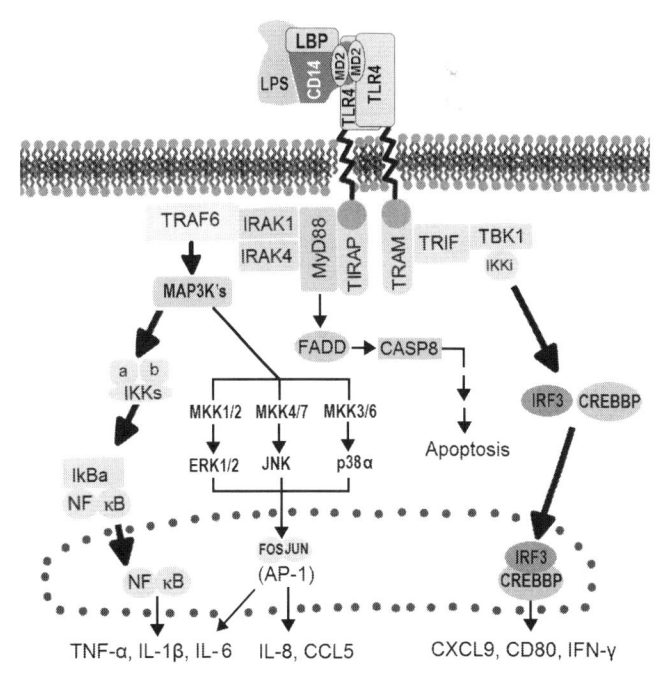

Figure 30-2: TLR4 Cascade

Cerebral edema after TBI is mediated through microglial release of IL-6 in a TLR4 dependent mechanism[56]. Microglia appear to be both necessary, and sufficient, to cause vasospasm through TLR4-MyD88-dependent activity[57]. TNF-α promotes brain edema and axonal swelling and apoptosis of neurons and oligodendrocytes[58]. TNF-α activity can be potentiated by the presence of bacterial LPS. Vasospasm and edema can cause ischemia, followed by reperfusion, which provokes oxidative damage to neurons. Hypoxia increases production of ROS by mitochondria. P38α is activated by reactive oxygen species[59].

The presence of inflammatory cytokines prevents microglia from switching from an inflammatory mode to their repair mode. In health, there are only very small amounts of pro-inflammatory cytokines in the brain. After injury or during disease states, TNF-α, IL-1β, and IL-6 act as neurotrophic factors that maintain microglia in an inflammatory reactive state. Low levels of cytokines or even high level of a single pro-inflammatory cytokine will not trigger axonal destruction. The combination of high levels of the cytokines TNF-α and IL-1β in concert will, however, trigger axonal loss and neurodegeneration. TNF-α, alone, does not activate the kynurenine pathway where tryptophan is converted to QA; it requires the presence of IL-1β or IL-6. IL-1β increases the sensitivity of the NMDA receptors. The neuronal damage effected by pro-inflammatory cytokines is dependent upon microglia and the excitotoxins they produce. IL-1β is the principal activator of microglial inflammation. TNF-α up-regulates astrocyte glutaminase, which converts glutamine into the excitatory neurotransmitter glutamate. (Figure 32-3). Neurons can tolerate fairly high levels of glutamate or LPS if exposed to one of these compounds at a time, but in combination, much lower levels can be neurotoxic.

The Imperfect Blood-brain Barrier

Another mechanism in TBI is the temporary disruption of the blood-brain barrier, at least in certain areas. This allows, at least temporary, exposure of the CNS to circulating cytokines and toxins, which are normally excluded from the CNS. Even brief exposure to these agents may induce long-acting effects.

The BBB isolates the CNS, including the spinal cord, from many compounds in the bloodstream and helps protects it from most blood-born microbes. Nevertheless, the brain contains several circumventricular organs (CVO's) which lack a BBB; these organs sample substances in the blood to sense what is going on in the body. The CVO's include the posterior pituitary, pineal gland, subfornical organ and other CVO's that participate in electrolyte and fluid homeostasis, hormonal control, cardiovascular regulation and energy homeostasis.

There are four choroid plexuses (CP's), one for each ventricle. The CP's produce enough cerebral spinal fluid (CSF) to flush the ventricles about every 6 hours. The CP's, also, actively transport substances out of the CSF, helping to remove excess neurotransmitters, metabolites, wastes, toxins and foreign substances from the CSF. The CP's may allow entry of inflammatory cytokines, and even allow inflammatory WBC's across the BBB, especially after TBI, ischemia, infection, or other injuries. Oxidative stress[60], infection, proinflammatory cytokines[61], zinc deficiency, bacterial toxins, such as LPS[62], and other agents which increase intestinal paracellular permeability, (Chapter 25) may also increase BBB permeability, especially at the CP's. Some tumor cells produce substance P, which induces TNF-α production; TNF-α impairs the tight junctions of the BBB, thus allowing metastasis of cancer cells to the brain[63]. Ingress of proinflammatory cytokines and migration of immune cells into the CNS can activate microglia.

Somatic inflammation, present at the time of TBI or stroke can worsen neuronal damage; passage of inflammatory cytokines from peripheral sources that increase microglial activation and inflammatory activity. Patients with inflammatory somatic conditions, thus, more susceptible to TBI and CTE.

Even after a neurologic injury event which is followed by repair, the microglia may remain primed for activity and be hypersensitive to inflammatory signals. Microglia may be primed even by minor injury. They can also be primed or reactivated by exposure to cytokines, both of neuronal or somatic origin. With sustained inflammatory stimuli, microglia remain chronically activated, and rather than switching to repair mode, they remain inflammatory. Systemic immune activation, outside of the CNS increases and maintains microglia activation within the CNS[18]. Thus once primed, the microglia may stay primed for extended periods, sustained by even low levels of systemic inflammation. This may explain why older adults are more susceptible to TBI from relatively minor trauma, and why diabetic patients and those with other inflammatory conditions are more susceptible to severe sequelae from cerebral vascular events.

TBI is not the only process that primes microglia – it is an immune mechanism common to multiple conditions, including ischemia, antergic or allergic reactions, heavy metal toxicities, and infections. Most chronic CTE patients do not have a single activator, but rather have several exposures that activate and help maintain microglial activation and immuno-cytotoxicity. Psychological stress after stroke also potentiates neuroinflammation through a TLR4→NF-κB mediated pathway and increases the ischemic area from stroke[64] or TBI.

The proinflammatory cytokines from central and systemic sources also cause cognitive impairment. IL-1β and TNF-α are associated with poorer cognitive performance and lower levels of BDNF[65]. These cytokines likely explain many of the behavior effects which occur in TBI and other CNS diseases[66,67], as well as those seen with systemic infections. Improvements in cognition, mood, memory, and attention deficits imparted by inflammatory cytokines, even in long-standing disease, can occur within minutes of anti-TNF-α treatment[68]. A trial in which paraspinal etanercept was given improved stroke-related neurologic dysfunction present one to three years after the stroke within minutes of administering the medication[69]. Thus stroke, like TBI, can be understood as a chronic inflammatory condition.

Factors that promote inflammatory cytokines support the continued neuro-immunocytotoxic damage seen in CTE and other central neuropathies. These same mechanisms of injury also underlie neuropathology causing AD, ALS, MS, schizophrenia, and other diseases of the CNS.

Table 30-4: Exemplary factors that activate microglia[18]

Neurologic Trauma	Alcohol
Ischemia or hypoxia	Aluminum, Mercury, Copper
Infectious agents:	Environmental toxins
Herpes encephalopathy	Systemic immune stimulation
Toxoplasmosis gondii[70]	Brain aging

Neuro-immunoexcitotoxic Prevention

While only limited restoration of postmitotic neurons after extensive CNS damage is likely to be achieved, neurologic function can be improved, and the sustained loss of viable neurons abated. If neuroglial activity is shifted from an inflammatory state to one that supports repair and regrowth of axons and dendrites, memory, behavior and function can improve. In health, the brain is dynamic and able to repurpose intact areas to improve function.

Primary, secondary, and tertiary prevention of CTE and other neuro-immune encephalopathies needs to focus on limiting microglial activation and oxidative injury. Treatment can modify inappropriate microglial activation and excitotoxic inflammation from defensive and destructive behavior to repair, regrowth, and maintenance. This requires normalization of cytokines; both those from outside of the microglia and those produced by these cells.

Minocycline: Minocycline, a tetracycline antibiotic, which can cross the blood-brain barrier, has been found to have neuroprotective benefits in various experimental inflammatory CNS disease models, including TBI, ischemia, ALS, Parkinson's disease, Huntington's disease, Alzheimer's disease, and multiple sclerosis (MS). Minocycline inhibits microglial activation. It decreases prostaglandin-endoperoxide synthase 2 (PTGS2 aka COX2) activity, through the repression of poly (ADP - ribose) polymerase-1 activity, caspase-1 and caspase-3 expression, and the subsequent release of cytochrome C from the mitochondria. Minocycline also chelates excess calcium after injury[71].

The point at which minocycline intervenes in the inflammatory cascade has not been established. Its wide range of anti-inflammatory activities suggests that it acts early in the inflammatory pathway, activity, perhaps affecting TIRAP/MYD88. Table 30-5 lists and compares the activities of minocycline with those of quercetin.

Minocycline may be useful in the treatment of neurological disease and injury. Women, however, often discontinue its use as it promotes *Candida* vaginosis. Flavonoid supplements, such as quercetin, and other phenolic compounds, such as resveratrol[72], curcumin[73], and luteolin[74] provide similar benefits and merit study. Quercetin has been shown to cross the blood-brain barrier readily[75].

Minocycline, as a single agent, however, has limited efficacy in the treatment of TBI. If treated before the injury, minocycline reduces the IL-1β rise that occurs within the first hours after the injury, but does it does not prevent it if given subsequent to the injury. Even after the injury, however, minocycline prevents neuronal damage by suppressing inflammation and apoptosis. Minocycline has a synergistic effect in preventing nerve damage and in restoring the ability to learning subsequent to TBI when administered in conjunction with n-acetylcysteine (NAC)[76].

Table 30-5: Antiinflammatory Actions of Minocycline

Anti-inflammatory Effect	Minocycline[77]	Quercetin[78]
Inhibits phospholipase A2 and prostaglandin production	✓	✓
Inhibits AP-1 Pathway	✓	✓
Inhibits IKK-β release of NF-κB	✓	✓
Inhibits ROS production	✓	✓
Inhibits apoptosis	✓	✓
Inhibits excitotoxicity	✓	✓*
Binds intracellular Ca++	✓	

* Inhibits IDO activity and QA production by inhibiting the production of IL-1β, IL-6, and TNF-α.

NAC: The nutritional supplement N-acetyl cysteine crosses the BBB and replenishes glutathione, (GSH) the principle antioxidant of the brain. This prevents mitochondrial damage, apoptosis, and the oxidative stress that promotes inflammatory signaling. NAC decreases the production of IL-1 β, IL-6 and TNF-α. GSH is a strong inhibitor of sphingomyelinase[39]. GSH also modulates NMDA receptors by activating glutamate-cystine anti-porters; removing glutamate from the synaptic cleft, thus preventing excitotoxicity. GSH allows for conversion of PGE2 to PGF2α, and thus for the production of GDNF. The combined effects of lowering oxidative stress, dampening inflammation, and avoiding excitotoxicity act to increase Bcl-2; thus, preventing neuronal apoptosis, and increasing BDNF; resulting in increase neurite growth. NAC also increases the release of dopamine. NAC is helpful for schizophrenia and bipolar disorder, especially in reducing negative symptoms[79].

O₂: Hyperbaric oxygen therapy can significantly reduce TBI-induced microglial activation, TNF-α expression, and neuronal apoptosis, even several days after an injury[80].

Betaine: Betaine, also known as trimethylglycine, may also decrease neuroimmune cytotoxicity. Betaine is an osmolyte that maintains cellular hydration and protects protein conformation and aids in the proper folding of new proteins[81]. Betaine decreases the risk of excitotoxicity. Like vitamin D3 and zinc, betaine, inhibits TLR4 expression[82], and likely helps dampen microglia activation. Betaine-GABA Transporter (BGT-1) is upregulated in astrocytes after excitotoxic injury. Intracellular betaine protects cells against injury by preventing osmotic stress[83] and by recycling homocysteine into SAMe; it prevents oxidative stress incurred by acid SMase. Betaine protects the mitochondria by increasing the endogenous production of SAMe[84]. SAMe increases glutathione activity and has been shown to provide some benefit in early AD[85] and schizophrenia[86]. Betaine prevents Tau hyper-phosphorylation[87], inhibits LPS induced NO production in activated microglia[88]. Betaine is used in doses as high as 6 grams a day to treat hyperhomocysteinemia.

Zinc: Zinc supplementation may increase resilience to TBI. In an animal model of TBI to the frontal cortex, which causes depressive-like behavior, zinc supplementation with oral and injected zinc decreased anhedonia, and oral zinc supplement improved post-traumatic cognition[89]. In another study, post-TBI anxiety behaviors were more severe in injured rodents with inadequate dietary zinc, and milder in those receiving a zinc supplemented diet[90]. Zinc may provide neuroprotection by decreasing expression of TLR4, decreasing glutamate activity in NMDA synapses, by aiding in the transformation of beta-carotene to 9-cis RA, as a cofactor for SOD, or through other mechanism, such as supporting the BBB. Zinc is further discussed in Chapter 37. Excessive zinc should be avoided, as zinc release in the hippocampus can increase protein ubiquitination and cause neuronal death[91], and can induce ceramide activity.

Pyrroloquinoline quinone (PQQ): Pyrroloquinoline quinone is a water-soluble, vitamin-like compound, present in green vegetables. PQQ prevents neuroinflammation and neuronal loss, at least in part by preventing glutamate-induced neuron excitotoxicity[92]. PQQ protects neurons by activating the phosphorylation of Akt and suppressing glutamate-induced phosphorylation of c-Jun N-terminal protein kinase (JNK)[93]. PQQ may function through activation of PPAR-γ co-activator 1-alpha (PGC-1α).

PQQ may inhibit NMDA excitotoxicity and inhibits iNOS activity and oxidative damage after spinal cord injury[94]. PQQ prevents neuropathic pain after nerve injury[95]. In animal disease models, PQQ has been found to decrease the formation of neurofibrillary tangles, prevent Parkinson's disease, ischemic damage, and help in the recovery of TBI. Administration of 10 mg/kg PQQ in rats was very effective in regenerating nerves and normalizing behavior after severe traumatic brain injury[96]. In another study, 1mg/kg of PQQ was ineffective but 3 mg/kg and 10 mg/kg reduced cerebral ischemic infarct area[97]. If adjusted for body surface area, 10mg/kg would be about 1.5 mg/kg for a human adult, more than has been used in any human study to date.

Amitriptyline (AMI): AMI, a tricyclic medication, is a very effective inhibitor of TLR2 and TLR4. It most likely acts by preventing TLR2 or TLR4 from forming dimmers on the cell's surface membranes, perhaps by blocking MD2[98]. Like several other antidepressants, AMI is also an effective, functional inhibitor of acid sphingomyelinase (FIASMA). FIASMA's cause acid SMase enzymes to detach from the inner lysosomal membrane, exposing them to proteolysis[99], rather than blocking enzymatic activity. (See Appendix M). AMI also increases the production of BDNF, GDNF, VEGF and other neuronal growth factors[100] and increases AMPA RNA editing (See above). Thus, this medication is a good candidate for post-injury prevention and treatment of TBI.

Low dose AMI, 10 mg[101], has been shown to be effective in the treatment of spinal stenosis. While it is often used for the treatment of neuropathic pain, AMI is not especially effective as a treatment for pain[102], but rather, is helpful for neuroinflammation. High-dose AMI, commonly used for depression, causes considerable cholinergic side-effects. Bedtime dosing helps promote sleep through its antihistaminic action. This is helpful in injured patients, who commonly suffer from insomnia. AMI, thus, may provide secondary benefits by lowering levels of proinflammatory cytokines associated with sleep deprivation. (Chapter 42).

PPAR-γ: PPAR-γ agonists may help decrease neuroinflammation and mitigate damage to the CNS and spinal cord after injury. PPAR-γ is highly expressed in adipocytes; in the immune cells, including monocytes, B, T and dendritic cells and microglia; colonic and other epithelial cells; and retinal cells. PPAR-γ agonists are used in the treatment of diabetes; in adipocytes, they increase insulin sensitivity, lipid storage, and proliferation of pancreatic β cells. PPAR-γ activity is anti-inflammatory and increases cell differentiation, which may inhibit the proliferation of a variety of cancers[103]. Several PPAR-γ activators, which cross the BBB, have been studied for their effect on neuroinflammatory disease.

PPAR-γ is an intracellular protein that forms a heterodimer with retinoid X receptor (RXR) protein. Beta-carotene and vitamin A compounds modulate the RXR activity, with the vitamin A compound, 9-cis retinoic acid, activation RXR most specifically, while β-apo-13-carotenone, antagonizes it[104]. The heterodimer complex enters the cell's nucleus, where it binds to peroxisome proliferator response elements (PPRE) in the DNA sequence. A PPRE is a specific DNA sequence; AGGTCA is separated by a single or double nucleotide, and then repeated. PPAR thus binds to and promote the transcription of dozens of specifically "labeled" genes.

PPAR-γ induces the transcription of segments of DNA that include genes for the antioxidant enzymes catalase and superoxide dismutases, for anti-proliferative response and decreased IL-6 production. PPAR-γ induces IκB-α, which impedes NF-κB activity. The PPAR-γ/RXRs heterodimer increases transcription of the catechol-O-methyltransferase,

(COMT) enzyme that degrades catecholamines, DRD3 (dopamine receptor 3), and HTR2A (5-HT$_{2A}$, serotonin) receptor. PPAR-γ agonists inhibit pro-inflammatory cytokine signaling pathways by inhibiting STAT→ Janus kinase signaling and increase the production of SOCS (suppressor of cytokine signaling) proteins. PPAR-γ agonists are generally anti-inflammatory. However, since they induce so many receptors, enzymes, and other proteins, their effects are complex, and their activity is mediated by the cells and the environments in which they appear. They induce TNF-α, and dependent upon the milieu, can induce apoptosis of pro-inflammatory cells, thus reducing inflammation.

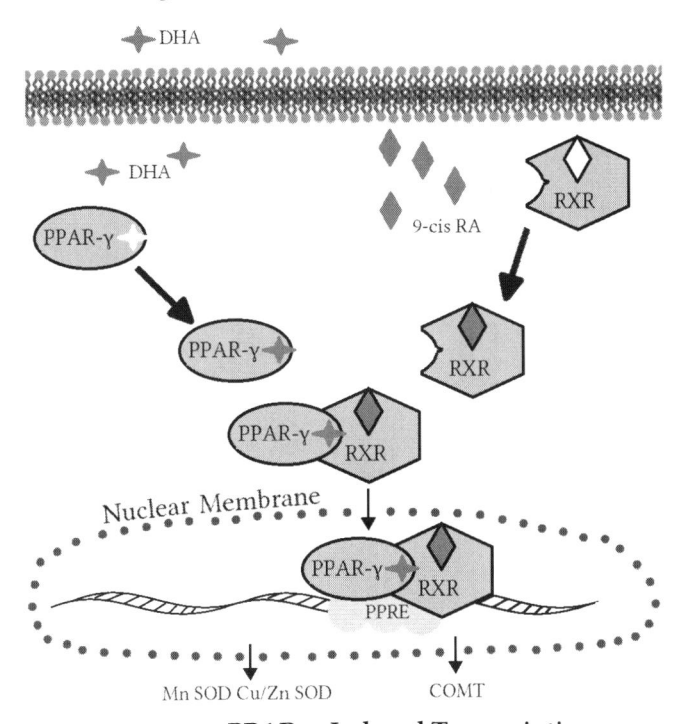

Figure 30-3: **PPAR-γ Induced Transcription**

Animals pretreated with PPAR-γ agonists are protected from ROS-induced damage after ischemia/reperfusion. PPAR-γ agonists reduce microglial activation, lesion size, motor dysfunction and neuropathic pain after spinal cord injury[105]. They have been found to improve the cognition of AD patients and reduce symptoms in Parkinson's disease[106].

Table 30-6: PPAR-γ Activators

Class	PPAR-γ Activators
Certain HMG-CoA reductase inhibitors	**Simvastatin, Atorvastatin**
Certain NSAIDS	Indomethacin, ibuprofen, diclofenac flufenamic acid, fenoprofen
Certain fatty acids	**DHA, EPA, LA**
Certain cannabinoid agonists	**Cannabidiol**
Thiazolidinediones	**Pioglitazone, Rosiglitazone**
Angiotensin II receptor antagonists	Telmisartan, irbesartan, candesartan

Bold: Best demonstrated to prevent neuronal loss

Cannabinoids: There are at least 60 cannabinoids present in marijuana[107]. While some of these have potential benefits in TBI, marijuana has obvious problems in ambulatory patients, has persistent negative effects on reward behaviors[108], and may impede brain development, which is not complete in humans until about the age of 27 to 28. Frequent adolescent marijuana-users have lower IQ's as adults, with an apparent loss of as much as 10 IQ points. Those who use marijuana only as adults do not appear to suffer from this loss[109]. Marijuana use causes dependence, and THC may be neurotoxic.

Killer Weed

Rats deficient in magnesium can have behavioral disturbances associated with neuro-excitotoxicity. One of these is aggressive behavior in which they kill mice. Correcting the deficiency inhibits this behavior[110]. Some rats are dirty rotten, "natural killer rats", while most are not. However, about 60% of the rats that do not exhibit muricidal behavior will do so when treated with delta-9-tetrahydrocannabinol (THC). When mild magnesium deficiency was induced in non-muricidal rats, 100 percent of them became killer rats when given THC, even at low doses of THC. TCH induces neurotoxicity in these animals, even at low doses in the presence of mild magnesium deficiency[111]. Magnesium deficiency is common in humans.

This does not rule out the use of CB agonists. CB$_1$ receptors are mainly expressed in the CNS and are responsible for the psychoactive effects of marijuana. CB$_2$ receptors are mainly present on immune cells, and thus, provide the immune modulation, and provide pain relief. Other CB receptors have been implicated in microglial migration[112].

Most of the medicinal effects of cannabis likely result from cannabidiol, not from THC, the compound most responsible for marijuana's psycho-activity. In a porcine model, cannabidiol modulated excitotoxicity, oxidative stress, and inflammation through its effect on CB$_2$ and 5-HT$_{1A}$ receptors. Cannabidiol appears to be a weak antagonist for CB$_1$ and exerts its activity through formation of CB$_2$/5-HT$_{1A}$ dimers on the microglia membrane[113]. Cannabidiol inhibits microglial activity in the spinal cord and has protective effects in a mouse model of multiple sclerosis[114]. Cannabidiol also has potent anti-cancer effects. It activates PPAR-γ and induces COX2, inducing apoptosis of cancer cells[115]. It may similarly act in the elimination of excess activated microglia and other immune cells.

NSAIDs and aspirin: Aspirin and NSAIDs decrease inflammation, and some NSAIDs, such as indomethacin, ibuprofen, and diclofenac, are also agonists for PPAR-γ, and thus decrease activation of NF-κB. While helpful in animal models of Alzheimer's disease (AD), there have been numerous observational studies and trials using these medications to prevent neuro-inflammatory disease, mostly in studies of AD. A review of the trials showed they were ineffective and increased mortality[116]. Some studies suggest that if given prior to the onset of dementia, COX1 inhibitors may slow disease progression, but increase it if given after disease onset[117]. These medications do not appear especially effective and have considerable toxicity. The NSAIDs, indomethacin, and naproxen decrease cerebral blood flow[118] and might increase ischemic damage after neurologic injury or stroke.

NSAIDs, as COX inhibitors, block the production of PGE2. PGE2, through its activation of EP1, increases the production of the inflammatory cytokines IL-6 and TNF-α and inhibits the production of GDNF. NSAIDS also block the production of PGF2 and thromboxane which increase the production of GDNF. NSAIDs may fail to provide benefit in brain injury, as a result of their effects on GDNF and upon other nerve growth factors[15].

Conversion of PGE2 to PGF2α requires NADPH and is inhibited by oxidized glutathione (GSSG). Thus, adequate energy (ATP) and antioxidant availability are required to reduce products of oxidation in the cell to enzymatically process PGE2 to PGF2α.

ARB's: While these medications used in the treatment of hypertension activate PPAR-γ and showed promise in laboratory models[119], angiotensin-receptor blockers are not effective in preventing cerebral damage. ARB's have been well studied in multiple, large trials including tens of thousands of patients at high-risk cardiovascular events. These trials failed to reach a statistically significant reduction in stroke[120]. These studies perhaps looked at the wrong endpoint; a PPAR-γ agonist would not be expected to prevent stroke, but rather decrease the damage it caused. Nevertheless, ARB's also failed to decrease total mortality. These medications are unlikely to be effective for secondary prevention of TBI.

Statin Medications: Several of the "statin" drugs, used to lower cholesterol, increase PPAR-γ. Several have been used in experimental models of TBI. Simvastatin, atorvastatin, and lovastatin show benefit; pravastatin was found to be ineffective. Of these, simvastatin has been found to be the most effective[121,122]. These medications increase cerebral blood flow after injury[123] and increase BDNF and neurogenesis[124]. Simvastatin promotes neurogenesis after stroke in an animal model[125]. In an animal model of subarachnoid hemorrhage, simvastatin helped with recovery, however; performance deteriorated if the medication was discontinued after two weeks; a period characterized by vasoconstriction[126]. When simvastatin was administered orally beginning one day after TBI, it reduced IL-1β, but not IL-6 or TNF-α, and the benefits to neurologic function, while statistically significant were rather small[127]. When administered immediately after ischemic injury, atorvastatin dramatically reduced infarct size and brain water content and attenuated the expression of HMGB1, RAGE, TLR4, and NF-κB[128]. (HMGB1 is secreted by immune cells, is a nuclear transcription factor for inflammatory proteins and an activating ligand for TLR2). Atorvastatin suppresses HMGB1 induced TLR4 up-regulation[129]. After TBI, statins increase vascularization and neurogenesis[130].

Among patients using any statin medication, there is a 29% decrease in risk for AD[131]. Trails using statins to treat patients with AD, however, have failed to provide benefit[132,133,134]. Thus, simvastatin may help prevent neuroinflammatory disease but is not helpful after AD is diagnosed.

Niaspan, a slow-release form of niacin, reduces HMGB1, RAGE, TLR4 and MMP-9 (which induces abrogation of the BBB after CNS injury) in rats after stroke[135]. Similar to the statin medications, Niaspan increases neuronal and vascular remodeling after stroke in animal models[136].

A study that compared minocycline and simvastatin found that minocycline decrease CNS lesion size in animals after TBI, while simvastatin did not, and that inflammatory markers were lowered within 24 hours with minocycline, but that it took 72 hours for simvastatin to do so, with further effect after 7 days[137].

Docosahexaenoic acid: DHA activates PPAR-γ in the CNS, and thus, it prevents neuroinflammation. Animals consuming 10 mg/kg/day of DHA had nearly six times fewer β-amyloid positive axons than unsupplemented animals subjected to TBI[138]. Animals receiving a high-DHA diet for 12 days prior to concussive injury had normal levels of brain-derived neurotrophic factor (BDNF) and CREB, and nearly normal levels of superoxide dismutase (SOD) and Sir2, while those on a normal diet had 25 - 35 percent declines in these proteins[139]. In animals with spinal cord injury, a combination of injected and oral DHA improved motor recovery[140] and decreased damage to myelin and to serotonergic fibers[141]. DHA, in the treatment of neurologic trauma, is effective when an injection (500 nmol/kg of DHA) is given acutely at the time of injury, but provides little benefit from oral post injury treatment alone[142]. Pretreatment is also effective[143]. Thus, DHA supplements, used by individuals such as soldiers and athletes who are at high risk of injury, may prevent neurologic injury.

DHA increased BDNF levels after TBI in animals and counteracted learning impairments[144]. Oral fish oil restored dopamine release in the CNS after TBI, while olive oil did not[145]. Dietary n-6 and saturated fats worsened outcomes after TBI[146,147]. There is only very limited experience treating acute head injury in humans with n-3 fatty acids; however, early results are promising[148].

Dietary DHA appears to prevent chronic disease when it is consumed over much of the lifetime[149] and has been found to improve functioning in elderly humans with mild cognitive impairment[150]. Neuroprotectins, formed from DHA, prevent neurons from glutaminergic excitotoxic damage[151]. Dietary DHA supplied prior to ischemic injury, reduces ischemic lesion area, prevents microglial activation, decreases COX2 and IL-1β levels and increases levels of the anti-apoptotic molecule Bcl-2 in the brain,[152]. N-3 fatty acids may also reduce pain in patients with chronic neuropathic pain[153,154].

Thiazolidinediones: Thiazolidinediones (TZD's) are PPAR-γ agonist used in the treatment of diabetes. There are two thiazolidinediones approved for use in the United States; rosiglitazone and pioglitazone. Between these, rosiglitazone has a higher binding affinity for PPAR-γ while pioglitazone crosses the BBB more readily than rosiglitazone. A meta-analysis of 22 animal studies found both TZD's have similar efficacy in limiting infarct volume and maintaining functional outcome (recovery) after brain injury[155].

In a murine model of TBI, pioglitazone given 15 minutes after a controlled head injury decreased lesion size was by 55%, and microglial activation was averted[156]. In a different study rosiglitazone diminished TBI lesion size when the medication was injected 5 minutes after the injury and repeated 6 and 24 hours after the injury[157]. Rosiglitazone has also been found to be neuroprotective after spinal cord injury[158]. In another study, comparing rosiglitazone and pioglitazone, only pioglitazone was found to prevent inflammatory brain injury[159]. Both medications prevent vascular dementia in disease models where the vascular disease is caused by homocysteine or diabetes[160],[161].

In a very elucidating study, TZD's were administered three hours after middle cerebral artery occlusion. In animals in which the occlusion was relieved 2 hours into the experiment, before the medication was delivered, infarct volume was similar to animals that did not receive the medication. In animals in which the occlusion was removed three hours and 15 minutes into the experiment, *15 minutes after* the medication was delivered, brain injury volume was significantly reduced.

This experiment demonstrates that TZD's, like most agents, prevents the oxidative damage that occurs with reperfusion. It highlights that preventive treatment is most effective when given prior to reperfusion. This study also found that the most effective doses of these medications was quite small; 1 mg/kg for rosiglitazone and 0.1 mg/kg for pioglitazone[162]. Even when given 24 hours after an ischemic event, rosiglitazone has been demonstrated to reduce the eventual injury volume and improve neurological outcome[163].

Magnesium

Magnesium (Mg) is a cofactor for over 300 metabolic functions. These include protein synthesis, cellular energy production and storage, phosphate transfer reactions, reproduction, stabilization of mitochondrial membranes, glucose transport, insulin secretion, DNA and RNA synthesis, DNA repair, carbohydrate oxidation, and neurotransmitter synthesis. It helps convert the neurotoxic metabolite quinolinic acid into niacin and a cofactor for enzymes in the sphingolipid metabolism and helps signal inflammatory cells to switch from the warpath to one of repair and healing. Mg is an NMDA antagonist, as it blocks the NMDA ion channel[164] and thereby protects against glutamate neuro-excitotoxicity[165].

Pain: Magnesium deficiency increases nociception in patients with suboptimal Mg, increasing perception and reaction to pain[166]. Having adequate Mg levels may prevent central sensitization otherwise induced by nociceptive peripheral stimuli; Mg competes with calcium entry into the cell and blocks NMDA glutamate receptors. Mg was found to reduce postoperative throat pain from intubation during surgery in patients given a 610 mg dose of Mg Citrate, containing about 140 mg of elemental Mg, as a lozenge 30 minutes prior to surgery[167]. NMDA receptors are located centrally, in the spinal cord, and peripherally, as well as in the intestine. In the intestine, NMDA activity induced by inflammation increases visceral sensitivity[168]. Treatment with Mg decreases post-operative ileus after abdominal surgery from 4.2 days among controls to 2.3 days in those receiving IV magnesium. Those receiving magnesium also requested less morphine for pain[169].

Marginal Mg status promotes chronic inflammation and contributes to the causation of migraine headaches, Alzheimer's disease, ADHD, hypertension, cardiovascular and cerebrovascular disease, sudden cardiac death, cancer, diabetes, obesity, and poorer quality sleep[170,171,172,173,174]. Mg deficiency also lowers the threshold for seizures[175] and depressive-like behavior in rats[176] and increases the risk for eclampsia, and suicide[177] in humans. Mg was found to improve insomnia in a trial among elderly patients. Here, they used 500 mg of the poorly absorbed magnesium oxide daily[178]. Low Mg and Zn levels have been found to be highly correlated with depression and mania scores in adults with mood disorders[179]. For example, in a 20 year follow-up study of 4500 young adults, those with the highest dietary Mg intake at baseline had only 53% the prevalence of type 2 diabetes as those in the lowest quartile of Mg intake upon follow-up. In this population, Mg intake was also inversely associated with the inflammatory marker, hs-CRP, fibrinogen, and IL-6[180].

Magnesium is the most common dietary insufficiency in the Western diet, and second only to vitamin D as a nutritional deficiency. About half of Americans consume less Mg in their diet than the estimated average amount required for health[181]. Dietary calcium levels have increased in recent years, and calcium may compete with Mg for absorption. Malabsorption syndromes, including Crohn's disease, gluten enteropathy, regional enteritis, and chronic diarrhea can cause hypomagnesemia. Hypomagnesemia is often associated with low vitamin D levels[182]. This may often be secondary to malabsorption. Low Mg levels can result from alcoholism or diuretic use, and are common in older adults[183]. Proton pump inhibitors decrease Mg absorption by about five percent[184]. This can be significant in populations where intake and absorption of Mg is already marginal or deficient.

In animal models, magnesium protects against I/R damage of the small intestine. This protection occurs through activation of the PI3K/Akt signal pathway, which inhibits the generation of ROS and apoptotic signaling. PI3K promotes the phosphorylation of Akt, which inhibits the production of BAD and caspase-9 and promotes the transcription of anti-apoptotic proteins, including eNOS[185]. (See Figure 41-2.) Activation of the PI3K/Akt pathway has been demonstrated to protect the brain from I/R damage[186,187,188]. Mg (MgSO$_4$) attenuates endotoxin-induced upregulation of NF-κB and other inflammatory mediators and enhances PI3K/Akt activity[189].

Additionally, Mg dampens glutamate activation of NMDA excitotoxic activity[190]. Extracellular Mg inhibits the NMDA channel[191], decreasing its activity and preventing the release of glutamate. It competes with calcium, decreasing the calcium influx. This may directly prevent excitotoxic damage at the time of TBI or ischemia. Magnesium also protects neuronal mitochondria. By preventing calcium influx, Mg also competes with calcium channels on smooth muscles, and may inhibit reactive cerebral vasoconstriction which causes ischemia. Mg is a cofactor in sphingosine phosphorylation, decreasing inflammation.

Magnesium is an effective agent in preventing ischemic damage in animal models of stroke. When Mg was administered within two hours of ligation of the middle cerebral artery, it decreased infarct size and increased survival. Other studies have shown decreased infarct size when Mg was administered prior to ischemia[192]. Mg given at the time of a concussion also attenuates TBI associated depression and anxiety[193].

In humans, Mg used in the treatment of stroke has shown only minimal benefit. Its use has been more successful in the treatment of subarachnoid hemorrhage (SAH), a disease in which reactive vasoconstriction, beyond the ischemic threshold, provokes injury. In SAH, Mg mitigates the delayed cerebral ischemia and provides better long-term outcomes. The best data for use of Mg in human studies is in the prevention of neonatal cerebral ischemia and the prevention of cerebral palsy[192], especially in preterm infants[194].

Treatment of TBI with magnesium, however, is difficult. Intestinal absorption of Mg absorption is restricted. All studies of magnesium for the prevention of ischemic injury have used injected Mg. Parenteral Mg administration allows attainment of levels higher than those that can be achieved through the diet, thus making it difficult to predict the impact of oral treatment. Secondly, for Mg to be effective in preventing ischemic damage, it needs to be administered prior to the glutamate release and calcium influx of the excitotoxic event. This likely explains the failure of Mg treatment in human trials of Mg for stroke, where near immediate treatment would be required for efficacy. Parenteral Mg would need to be administered within the first hours after a concussion to prevent TBI.

Nevertheless, as Mg deficiency is prevalent among those eating the Western diet, with a paucity of green vegetables, legumes, fruits and whole grains. Mg supplementation may curtail damage in TBI. Thus, especially for athletes and soldiers who are at high risk of TBI, and pregnant women, whose children are at risk, should be encouraged to use magnesium supplementation to optimize blood levels.

Athletes may be enticed to use magnesium supplements regularly if made aware of its performance enhancing effect[195,196]. Mg increases glucose availability and utilization by muscle during exercise[197].

As supplements, magnesium hydroxide, oxide or oxalate may be helpful for constipation. They have very low intestinal absorption; about four to five percent bioavailability[198]. It is a poor choice as a Mg supplement. Organic salts of Mg have higher intestinal absorption than inorganic salts. Magnesium lactate and Mg gluconate appear to have the most favorable absorption[199]. Mg citrate has nearly as high an absorption and is readily available. Mg supplements also vary in the percent of elemental Mg they contain. Sixty-one percent of the elemental mass of magnesium oxide is Mg while only five percent of magnesium gluconate is. This makes for very large pills. Mg citrate, at 16% magnesium, has smaller, easier to swallow pills.

The daily estimated average dietary requirement for Mg is 440 mg for men and 320 mg for women. The 2003-2006 NHANES study found that without supplements, most Americans do not get enough in their diets. A 100 mg daily supplement of Mg should be sufficient for most adults to maintain optimal Mg levels; however, higher doses can be recommended for the acute treatment of TBI or spinal cord injury. Supplementation with 200 to 400 mg of elemental Mg a day may be used in adults and children over the age of eight[200]. Vitamin D increases the absorption of Mg[201], and thus, vitamin D insufficiency worsens Mg depletion.

Mg supplements may provide benefit to patients with traumatic CNS injury as it decreases neuropathic pain[202,203]. In a double-blinded study, a six-week program of Mg supplementation diminished neuropathic pain and increased spinal range of motion at a six-month follow-up assessment[204]. It may also reduce anxiety[205].

Mg is mostly eliminated through the kidneys. Patients with renal insufficiency can be at risk of hypermagnesemia. Caution and testing should be used if Mg supplements are administered to patients with renal insufficiency; however this is mainly a concern in parenteral Mg treatment.

Folate: A 10-fold improvement in axon regrowth and functional recovery after CNS injury occurred when mice received 80 μg/kg of folic acid[206]. Using surface area ratio conversion, this is equivalent to about 6.5 μg/kg for adult humans, similar to the recommended 400 μg daily intake.

Vitamin B$_{12}$: At levels not much below those considered normal, vitamin B$_{12}$ deficiency can cause poor memory, depression, fatigue, mania, and psychosis[207,208]. Vitamin B$_{12}$ deficiency has long been known to cause irreversible neuropathies.

Methylcobalamin is a cofactor for the enzyme methyltransferase, which helps recycle homocysteine into methionine, as shown in figure 30-4. Methionine is required for the formation of S-adenosylmethionine (SAMe), which is necessary for methylation of myelin sheath phospholipids. Additionally, vitamin B_{12}, along with folate and betaine, prevents the accumulation of homocysteine, which is toxic to cerebral endothelial cells via its activation of acid sphingomyelinase, which promotes intracellular ceramide accumulation[209].

Another form of vitamin B_{12}, adenosylcobalamin, is a required cofactor for the enzyme, methyl malonyl coenzyme A mutase (MCM). MCM resides in the mitochondria. Here, several amino acids and odd-chain fatty acids are broken down into methyl malonic acid (MMA). MMA is converted into methyl malonyl-CoA and then isomerized by MCM, into succinyl-CoA. Succinyl-CoA a key element of the TCA cycle, which provides a source of energy for the cell. This may explain the relief from fatigue associated with vitamin B_{12} injections. Patients with inborn errors of metabolism, which cause methyl malonic acidemia, had an average full-scale IQ around 79 if the MDM dysfunction results in hyperammonemia but have normal IQ levels if hyperammonemia is prevented[210]. (See Chapter 35 for more on the effects of ammonia on the brain.)

Cobalamin, perhaps specifically hydroxocobalamin, is not anti-inflammatory, but rather an inflammatory regulator. It appears to decrease ROS but increase reactive nitrogen species; lowers TNF-α and IL-1β, COX2, and HMGB1, but raises IL-6. Cobalamin also protects against endotoxin damage[211].

Vitamin B_{12} is also neurotrophic. While vitamin B_{12} deficiency increases TNF-α, it decreases epidermal growth factor (EGF) levels in the brain and spinal cord. A lack of EGF causes neuropathy and contributes to neurodegeneration[212], likely through a decreased activity by astrocytes. IL-6 is a myelinotrophic cytokine. Vitamin B_{12} deficiency, as a result of high TNF-α and low EGF and IL-6, induces myelin damage[213] and increases the number of cells positive for glial fibrillary acidic protein (GFAP)[214]. As many as 40% of older adults have impaired absorption of vitamin B_{12}. Vitamin B_{12} is excreted into the bile and reabsorbed into the enterohepatic circulation. Thus, it is easily lost in malabsorption syndromes.

Vitamin K: While vitamin K is not an antioxidant and does not quench free radicals, it appears to prevent oxidative damage. Glutamate induces oxidative damage resulting in neurotoxicity when glutathione is depleted. Vitamin K_1 (phylloquinone) and K_2 (MK-4, menatetrenone) protect against cystine or glutathione depletion-induced oxidative death of oligodendrocytes and immature neurons. This protection is afforded with vitamin K levels easily within upper normal physiologic levels. In vitro, Vitamin K_1 and K_2 both protect oligodendrocytes when supplied prior to, or at the time of cysteine depletion, however, vitamin K_1 is only marginally effective in preventing cell death three hours later, while vitamin K_2 is protective at higher, but physiologic concentrations for about 6 hours. Vitamin K_3 (menadione) is toxic to oligodendrocytes[215].

Vitamin K does not prevent glutathione depletion directly, but rather prevents the generation of ROS. Vitamin K_2 suppresses inflammation and the effect of TNF-α, by increasing the production of IκB, the protein that binds NF-κB, inactivating it[216].

Vitamin K also plays an essential role in the growth, development, and repair of the brain, as it participates in the biosynthesis of sphingolipids required for neuronal proliferation, differentiation, and axonal myelinization. The main form of vitamin K found in the brain is MK-4[217].

Vitamin K is easily and quickly depleted by a deficient diet. In a study of both young and older adults, where vitamin K was limited in the diet, serum vitamin K_1 levels fell to from about 1.2 nM/L to 0.3 nM/L within one week[218]. Vitamin K depletion easily occurs in malabsorption and enteroimmunopathy. Vitamin E (α-tocopherol) interferes with vitamin K activity[219] and lowers vitamin K (MK-4) levels in the brain[220]. Long-term low vitamin K_1 intake is associated with age-related cognitive decline[221].

Vitamin D: Acute kidney injury, caused by I/R, is common in critically ill patients. Low vitamin D levels are associated with a 60 percent increase in mortality among surgical ICU patients and a 73% increased risk of acute kidney injury[222]. D protects the kidney by reducing upregulation of TLR4 and translocation of NF-κB into the nucleus[223]. Vitamin D may also activate PPAR-γ[224].

Melatonin: Melatonin attenuates I/R injury by suppressing the interaction between TLR4/TRIF and TLR4/MyD88, and thus, NF-κB activation[225]. Melatonin inhibits the expression of MyD88 and TLR4-mediated production of TNF-α, IL-1β, IL-6, IL-8, and IL-10 in LPS-stimulated macrophages and attenuates LPS-induced upregulation of COX2 and iNOS in macrophages[226]. Melatonin is an antioxidant for the brain.

The antioxidant vitamin E also helps mitigate mild traumatic brain injury and associated learning disabilities[227].

Exercise: Aerobic fitness and exercise prevent age-related decline in cognitive function. Exercise increases BDNF and improves mood and neuroplasticity[228]. A meta-analysis of 29 randomized controlled trials of exercise in adults, including three trials with patients with mild cognitive impairments, found significant improvements in memory, attention, processing speed and executive function over a one-year period[229]. A follow-up study of adults shows that the distance walked correlates well with cortical volume nine years later. Neurogenesis in the hippocampal dentate gyrus, one of the few areas that give rise to new neurons, is increased by exercise. BDNF has been found to correlate with the degree of lactate elevation during exercise[230].

Rats subjected to TBI were randomized to running exercise or not. Those randomized to running for three weeks had increased levels of the nerve growth factor, neurotropin-3 (NT-3), and these animals had smaller infarct volume and better functional recovery than sedentary animals[231]. In another murine model of TBI, animals subjected to percussive brain injury, most inflammatory markers were diminished in animal supplemented with the PPAR-γ agonist DHA with voluntary exercise as compared to those with given DHA alone[232]. Rats forced to run on a treadmill for 30 minutes once daily for ten days, two days following TBI had lower levels of Bax and increased levels of Bcl-2, indicating a decrease in neuronal apoptosis. Exercise alleviated short-term memory impairment and limited DNA fragmentation and caspase-3 expression in the hippocampus of these animals[233].

Short bouts of low-level exposure to these cytokines, such as those occurring during exercise, may down-regulate the inflammatory response.

PPAR-γ Coactivator-1α (PGC-1α) helps integrate environmental signals, not only as a coactivator of PPAR-γ, but also through CREBB, thyroid hormone receptor-β, and NRF1. NRF1 is a transcription factor for mitochondrial proteins. Many of the cognitive benefits of exercise appear to be mediated through PGC-1α[234]. Exercise increases PGC-1α, and this effect may be mediated by lactate that is produced during vigorous exercise[235].

TBI Prevention

Athletes are frequently exposed to head trauma. Football, hockey, and soccer players, pugilists and other have repeated blows to the head. For these individuals, a cocktail of nutritional supplements including DHA, zinc, NAC, r-alpha-lipoic acid, betaine, and bioflavonoid compounds may prevent microglial activation from an injury sustained during practice and play. These and other nutritional supplements could be used on a regular basis. The near-immediate loss of neurons following head or spinal cord trauma needs to be prevented by giving the medication prior to reperfusion. These supplements would also suppress chronic microglial inflammatory activity.

Brain injury preventive supplements and medications might also be given episodically. A cocktail of supplements could be given to athletes prior to a game; for example, or to pregnant women at the onset of labor. Under other circumstances, medications or supplements could be given immediately after an incident when TBI or other brain or spinal cord injury may occur. For example, after a rear-end collision, most patients deny significant injury at the scene of the accident, and they are correct, as the injury occurs during the following hours. These individuals often have increasing pain and disability related to spinal cord trauma in the hours and days following the accident. Treatment administered immediately after an accident to prevent TBI, traumatic spinal cord injury, or in stroke or suspect stroke patients has the potential to greatly reduce injury.

A nutritional supplement/medication cocktail to prevent CNS injury could be used immediately after an accident, stroke or injury. A medication cocktail or a combination of pharmaceuticals and nutraceuticals of higher potency is warranted in high-risk situations. Risk of toxic side effects, which might occur with long-term use or these medications, is of less concern when the medication is used as a single dose prior to a full evaluation of the patent's injury by a physician. For example, rosiglitazone, which appears to be more effective than pioglitazone if given after the injury[155], may cause myocardial injury when used as a chronic medication. A single dose immediately following an injury or the onset of stroke symptoms could mitigate brain damage, and allow time for medical evaluation of the patient. Thus, coaches, emergency medical technicians, medics, and soldiers subjected to percussive injury may be able to prevent severe injury with the use of a single dose administered at the scene of the event, while the need for continued treatment can be considered later.

Opiates: Most opiate analgesics potentiate neuro-inflammation as they bind to MD2/TLR4 and act as agonists[236]. Through this mechanism, they may also increase extracellular dopamine levels and increase the potential for addiction. Opiates are inappropriate for chronic pain, especially neuropathic pain, as they increase sensitization to pain[237]. The κ-opioid receptor, however, may inhibit TLR4/NF-κB signaling[238]. The opioid antagonist naloxone has sometimes been employed, in an off-label use, in the treatment of multiple sclerosis[239]. Naloxone has potential for providing treatment benefits by impairing TLR4 activity. Other opiates should be avoided.

Polypharmacy

In TBI, as in other neurologic diseases, it is not a single enzyme or protein, but rather multiple proteins cascades which are involved in the disease pathology. Many therapeutic agents provide benefit; however, further benefits are often available using the synergistic effects of compounds that affect different components of the pathological process. A therapeutic approach which addresses multiple pathways using several compounds can be more effective, and may be able to use smaller doses, associated with fewer and less severe side effects. For example, minocycline provides more effect when given with NAC. (Minocycline should not be dosed at the same time as Mg, as they bind to one another, preventing absorption).

Especially when using nutritional supplements, combining compounds often provides benefit, and unrecognized nutritional inadequacies can be compensated for. Various supplements may have differing effects on different cell types of different parts of inflammatory pathways. A cocktail approach, with several neuroprotective compounds acting on various pathways, is more likely to provide benefit than a single agent, affecting a single pathway.

In a study of aged dogs with Alzheimer's-like dementia, a combination of bioflavonoids and antioxidants increased executive function, visual discrimination, and memory[240]. In a study of rodents, a combination of melatonin, zinc, EPA, DHA, curcumin, piperine from black pepper, uridine, and choline reduced hippocampal atrophy and prevented neurodegeneration and depression[241].

In a study of retired football players diagnosed as having TBI and cognitive impairment, a poly-nutrient supplement was given, which included antioxidants, ginkgo, and vinpocetine to enhance blood flow, fish oil and multivitamins for six months. There were improvements in attention, memory, reasoning, information processing speed and accuracy. SPECT scans of the brain demonstrated increased brain perfusion[242]. In a similar, randomized study, these nutrients or placebos were provided to healthy adults. The supplements increased executive function, information processing efficiency, improved mood, and decreased hostility[243].

In acute brain or spinal cord injury, from trauma or stroke, the window for preventing loss of postmitotic neurons is extremely limited, and the consequences of this loss are severe. A shotgun approach, using optimal doses of several neuroprotective compounds with low toxicity offers the possibility of preventing damage to the CNS.

A combination of minocycline, a TZD, and NAC at the time of injury may prevent severe CNS damage. Other compounds, such as 9-cis-RA to enhance PPAR-γ activity. Zinc and manganese, to help assure SOD function, and magnesium might be used if minocycline is not part of the mixture. (Caution needs to be used to avoid compounds that might bind to minocycline (Mg^{++} and Zn^{++}) and decrease its bioavailability. In a hospital setting, IV or IM magnesium sulfate may be used, and other injected medications would provide the advantage of immediate and predictable bioavailability. Quercetin, which does not bind metal ions could be used in place of minocycline.) Most of these pharmaceuticals are, however, only available by prescription, and thus, currently unavailable to accident victims during the limited time window critical for effective injury prevention.

Amitriptyline (AMI) is a potent TLR4/TLR2 inhibitor with strong sedation effects. The sedation makes it undesirable for use as an immediate treatment in TBI, as cognitive slowing, drowsiness and difficulty in awakening are symptoms of severe TBI. This side-effect is especially pronounced in naïve patients. Its use could mask a deterioration of the patient's condition. AMI is appropriate during the post-acute phase of TBI and traumatic spinal cord injury to limit microglial hyper-activation. This medication is likely best used from the second day after the injury for about one month. Low dose AMI Here, its bedtime sedation is helpful, as it helps with neuropathic pain and sleep disturbances which are common in post-concussive syndromes. After the first month, post-acute phase, AMI's suppressive effect on TLR2 activation may limit the generation of new neurons and neurites, and thus, recovery. Co-administration of Mg may be overcome this through its activation of PI3K.

Melatonin, which also improves sleep, is appropriate for the long-term recovery phase of treatment of TBI, as it inhibits the TLR4 pathway without impacting the PI3K pathway that signals microglia to work in repair. Melatonin can be used in conjunction with low dose (10mg) AMI.

A mix of available nutritional supplements, although perhaps with less effective, would be available without a prescription and thus more readily accessible to patients at the time of injury or onset of symptoms of suspected stroke. Such a combination could include quercetin and curcumin to impede activation of the TLR4 cascade, DHA as a PPAR-γ agonist, NAC, melatonin and r-α-lipoic acid as antioxidants, and PPQ as an additional neuroprotective agent. Magnesium, manganese, zinc, betaine, vitamins D_3, K_2, and B_{12} should also be helpful.

Shiva the Destroyer: HMGB1

The protein, high-mobility group box1 (HMGB1), amplifies neuroinflammation and can promote cell death. HMGB1 has various functions. As a nuclear protein, it binds to the DNA, facilitates transcription and is involved in the regulation of gene expression and the stabilization of nucleosomes. In the cytosol, it promotes autophagy. When released from cells, either after cell death or when actively secreted by immune cells, HMGB1 activates the TLR2 inflammatory cascade[244,245]. HMGB1 release is thought to disrupt the BBB, and facilitate the transmigration of inflammatory cells and cytokines into the CNS. HMGB1 interacts with RAGE (receptor for advanced glycation end-products), to increase the increasing recruitment of leukocytes across endothelial barriers[246]. In rats subjected to TBI, RAGE expression increased six hours after TBI and peaked after one day. Levels then began to fall slowly, remaining higher than the sham-injury animals for six days after TBI[247]. The presence of AGE products in diabetics may explain the potentiated ischemic and traumatic injury these patients suffer.

HMGB1 levels begin to rise in the hours following TBI. Nevertheless, HMGB1 also promotes remodeling and recovery after stroke. HMGB1 induces neuron outgrowth, plasticity and enhances stem and progenitor cell recruitment, proliferation and differentiation after brain injury. Low IL-1β levels potently up-regulate HMGB1 in astrocytes, which is exported to the cell's cytoplasm[247]. This is thought to promote neurovascular repair and aid in functional recovery after an ischemic event[247].

Akt (protein kinase B) can activate NF-κB, and increase the production of inflammatory cytokines. Akt also binds to Bax and inactivate it. This prevents Bax from making pores in the outer mitochondrial membrane and thus, mitochondrial apoptosis through the caspase cascade. Akt also activates the cascade, Akt→Rheb→mTOR→S6K. S6K activates ribosomal translation of mRNA into protein. Akt, additionally, activates the ubiquitination, and thereby, proteolysis of the tumor suppressor protein, FOXO. Thus, Akt promotes growth and proliferation, including tumors.

PI3K is one of the several activators of Akt. TLR2 activation stimulates PI3K while TLR4 activation appears not to. Thus, stimulation of TLR2 promotes both the destruction of cells and repair and growth. The endogenous agonist for TLR2 after injury may be HMGB1. At the onset of injury, in the presence of high levels of proinflammatory cytokines, HMGB1 promotes cell death. When levels of the cytokines have fallen, the HMGB1 →TLR2→PI3K →Akt pathway may be essential for signaling and promoting repair of injured tissues.

Interdiction of HMGB1, TLR2, and Akt activation during the first minutes and hours after TBI of ischemic injury may be able to prevent microglial activation and attenuate neuronal loss; however, excessive suppression in the following days may impede recovery. During the acute phase, in the presence of the proinflammatory cytokines, IL-1β, IL-6, TNF-α, and reactive oxygen and nitrogen species, and other inflammatory mediators, HMGB1, Akt and other mediators facilitate the destruction of compromised cells and tissue, but can also damage uncompromised tissue. Later, when the inflammatory cytokines are at lower levels, these same mediators activate repair and re-growth. HMGB1 can be thought of as an accelerant that potentiates both injury and repair. It likely has similar effects in the growing and developing brain, helping to remodel it and facilitate development and learning.

Some medications with potential for attenuation of the destruction of viable post-mitotic neurons after TBI or stroke only have a narrow window for use; they should be given in the minutes following an injury. HMGB1 inhibitors may provide benefit even when delayed for a few hours after injury[248]. However, caution must be used not excessively to dampen the repair functions endowed to HMGB1 and Akt via TLR2 activity. Patients with stroke or severe TBI should have their inflammatory status monitored, and be weaned off anti-HMGB1 and anti-TLR2 medications when pertinent inflammatory markers normalize, in the days or weeks following the injury.

Angiotensin receptor antagonists, including telmisartan, irbesartan, and candesartan may have utility in the acute treatment of TBI[249] and stroke as they inhibit RAGE/HMGB1 and mildly activate PPAR-γ. However, they have shown little benefit in clinical trials, where they were applied several hours to days after the injury[250]. These medications must be administered within four hours of the injury to provide efficacy, buy likely should only be continued for the first several days[248]. Amitriptyline also inhibits TLR2 function. Magnesium, in contrast, helps activate PI3K and thus, is essential for neurological growth and repair.

The mechanisms active in microglial activation, neuroexcitation, and neuroinflammation are not in themselves pathological. They are essential to not only to protect the brain from infection, but are integral to learning and development. The brain prunes old connections and develops new ones, in order for us to learn and adapt. Caution should be applied to the chronic use of medications that greatly impede the inflammatory response in the CNS; they may prevent inflammation, but may also limit growth, repair, development and learning, as may be the case with chronic marijuana use.

Drug and Alcohol Abuse in CTE: Especially for CTE patients with alcohol abuse, therapy that increasing GDNF production provides benefit. Drug seeking, however, while prevented by adequate GDNF levels in the brain, may be enhanced by higher levels of GDNF[251], unless other measures are used to prevent it. The GDNF causes long-term increases in ERK that induced TH expression in the ventral tegmental area. This is dependent on NMDA glutamate activity[252]. Calming NMDA activity can decrease drug craving. Thus, both excess NMDA and low GDNF (and BDNF) activities should be treated together.

Calcitriol, the active form of vitamin D_3, has been found to increase levels of GDNF mRNA, in vitro, by over 18 times. The addition of the vitamin A compound, retinoic acid, had additive effects[253]. In animals, calcitriol has been found to increase GDNF[254], and within days, help restore TH function in the striatum of animals with a chemically-induced form of Parkinson's disease[255].

The tricyclic antidepressant, amitriptyline, also increases expression of GDNF, as well as BDNF, fibroblast growth factor-2 (FGF-2), and VGEF mRNA's in astrocyte cultures[256]. Amitriptyline acts by enhancing the phosphorylation of CREB[257]. Caberoline, used in the treatment of prolactinomas, and rasagiline, used in the treatment of Parkinson's disease also increase GDNF[11].

Excitotoxic, NMDA-induced glutaminergic activity can be mitigated by reducing by avoiding the formation of quinolinic acid through the kynurenine pathway by LPS and TNF-α, and by adequate supply of pyridoxal-5-phosphate (PLP), so that the NMDA antagonist, kynurenic acid is formed. PLP is also a required cofactor for glutamate decarboxylase (GAD) which converts glutamate to GABA.

Magnesium also inhibits glutamate activity, as a competitor for calcium channel flux, and is a cofactor for the enzyme glutamate-ammonia ligase, which converts glutamate to glutamine. This enzyme is inhibited by quinolinic acid; QA levels in the neuroglia can become elevated during inflammation and activation. The herbs *Centella asiatica* (gotu kola) and *Valeriana officinalis* (valerian) stimulate GAD, while *Melissa officinalis* (lemon balm) inhibits the formation of glutamate[258], and may be helpful (Table 28-4). Although valproate inhibits the conversion of GABA to glutamate, it inhibits cell growth[259] and repair and should be avoided in TBI.

Alcohol seeking behavior is additionally mediated by acetaldehyde (ACD) in the brain. In the brain, alcohol is oxidized to ACD by the enzyme catalase, using H_2O_2 as a co-substrate. Alpha-lipoic acid, an H_2O_2 scavenger, reduces voluntary alcohol intake in animals[260],[261].

Lipid rafts are also important in neuron for growth factor signaling, cell adhesion and guidance of axon elongation and for some synaptic transmissions. The GDNF receptor Ret is located in lipid rafts[11]. Lipid rafts are important in neuroinflammation as the TLR's occupy these rafts and as a result of the high concentration of sphingolipids in them. Alpha-lipoic acid prevents H_2O_2 induced ASMase activation and may help stabilize the lipid rafts.

TBI Secondary Prevention Summary

The brain has limited capacity for generating new neurons. Preventing neuronal loss is much less steep a challenge than attempting to restore neurons in AD, PD, TBI, or other neurologic diseases.

Immediate treatment at the time of injury helps limit CNS damage, especially in the case of reperfusion injury. Even late treatment can prevent the ongoing damage and may help with functional recovery.

Attempting to decrease neuroinflammation without treating systemic inflammation is likely to limit success.

The selection of nutraceuticals and pharmaceuticals for the prevention and treatment of CNS injury depends on the timing of when they are employed and the severity of the injury:

- Before trauma
- At the moment of trauma or within the first hour
- Within the first several hours
- After the first several hours, within the first days
- Treatment for post conclusive injury
- Treatment for CTE

Obviously, primary prevention of injuries by avoiding risk and engineering safety into our lives is critical. Appendix L gives instructions for adjusting the front seats of vehicles to reduce injury from accidents. Helmets prevent some of the injuries to bicyclists, workers, and athletes. Tragically, TBI, especially in children, is often the result of intentional injury. Prevention of domestic violence requires non-judgmental screening and provision of treatment for the perpetrator. Perpetration of domestic violence should be considered a disease condition until proven otherwise, and treatment provided. A screening tool is provided in Appendix D. TBI is a common cause of domestic abuse, and thus, a cause of TBI. Perpetrators should be screened for PTSD, rage, depression, TBI, and history of being abused.

Before an Injury: Prior to injury nutraceuticals can be used to prevent immunocytotoxic reaction in the event of CNS trauma. This is recommended for individuals at high risk, such as athletes, soldiers, and near-term pregnant women. Like all of us, these individuals should maintain a healthy diet, with a high n-3: n-6 ratio, diverse phenolic compounds, sufficient magnesium, and vitamin D_3 and B_{12}, and get sufficient sleep.

Pre-game TBI Prevention: In addition to a healthy diet, when risk will be high over the ensuing hours, supplements may be given before a game, or during labor, to lower risk of neuro-immunocytotoxic damage. These might be given by a coach or midwife to ensure that the subject has the nutrients onboard during the high-risk period, given as a single dose.

- DHA – 500 to 1000 mg
- Magnesium citrate or another organic Mg salt– 600 mg
- Vitamin K_2 – 5 mg
- Phenolic compounds
- Vitamin D_3 – 6000 IU
- Zinc – 10 mg
- N-Acetyl cysteine – 500 mg
- Betaine – 500 mg
- R-α-lipoic acid – 100 mg
- PQQ – 10 mg
- Folate 400 μg

Immediately post-injury: Even for minor head or back injury, nutraceutical supplements are recommended to prevent immunocytotoxic activation. The supplements recommended for pregame treatment would be appropriate for minor injury, other than adding 10 mg of vitamin K_2.

If the trauma is more than mild, a combination of supplements and medications should be used. The loss of consciousness is not required for significant injury. It the injured appears shaken, dazed or confused, the injury can cause TBI. Patients often deny any problem because of embarrassment, confusion, or because it is the easiest answer. Asking the injured if they are OK and getting an affirmation is non-informative.

Disorientation, taking time to gather their wits, wanting to be still, or having an "adrenaline rush" all suggest a significant injury. The feeling of an "adrenaline-rush" is often the result of a massive excitotoxic glutamic discharge. The head does not need to be hit to cause a concussion. Side-impacts during motor vehicle accidents often cause concussion without the injured hitting their head.

Asking a person that has been in an accident about symptoms that suggest a concussion is more helpful in determining the need for follow-up care:

- Did you feel disoriented, even for a few seconds?
- Did it take some time to gather your wits?
- Did you lose a moment?
- Did it take some time to figure out what happened?
- Did you feel an adrenaline rush or very excited?

The goal of immediate treatment is to minimize excitotoxic and oxidative injury which occurs as a result of reperfusion injury. Similar supplements to those used for pregame prevention can be used until pharmaceuticals can be given. Most pharmaceuticals that would be helpful require a prescription and are not available over the counter.

- DHA – 2000 mg
- Magnesium citrate – 600 mg
- Vitamin K_2 – 45 mg
- Phenolic compounds 1000 mg
- Vitamin D_3 – 10,000 IU
- N-Acetyl cysteine – 1000 mg
- Betaine – 1000 mg
- R-α-lipoic acid – 100 mg
- PQQ – 0.5 mg/kg
- Folate – 400 µg

These represent fairly large doses but with extremely low risk. This is not meant as a substitute for medical treatment, but only an immediate preventive to acute prevent oxidative and excitotoxic injury in the first hours after injury. Even when a patient is immediately transported to an emergency medical facility, it is likely that damage, which could have been prevented, will occur by the time a patient is seen by a physician. These supplements could easily be kept on hand and given to the injured person without the requirement of a prescription.

Prescription medications that could be made available to for immediate treatment are:

- Rosiglitazone: 1 mg/kg (or 0.1 mg/kg for pioglitazone)
- Minocycline 100 mg
- Sertraline 25 mg

For example, soldiers could carry single-dose packs of these medications, along with nutraceuticals, to use if exposed to a blast or other CNS trauma. They could be prescribed for this use by team doctors for football players, or for other sports for use in case of injury. These would not be used in the place of medical evaluation and further treatment, but rather as immediate preventive treatment, until the evaluation could be done, where a decision could be made whether further treatment was indicated. These medications may be continued if the injury warrants it.

First days after trauma: In the days after the trauma, CNS injury usually worsens. These same nutraceuticals and medications can continue to be used. Low-dose amitriptyline and melatonin may be added and continued over the following weeks.

Immediately after the injury: The TLR response is part of the non-specific immune system for response to injury. This includes mounting an attack against microbes and destruction of tumor cells, eliminating non-viable cells, cleaning up the debris from the destruction of pathogens or killed endogenous materials. TLRs are also signals for rebuilding and supporting growth.

Thus, the goal is not to suppress TLR activity, but rather, after a traumatic brain injury, to help move the microglia from the cleanup phase into the repair and regrowth phase.

Post-concussive injury, CTE, long-term TBI: The highest number of individuals requiring treatment for TBI is the large population with established pot-concussive TBI, CTE, or spinal cord traumatic injury. The same supplements used in primary prevention can be used for secondary prevention. Getting activated neuroglia to repair and support regrowth, myelinization, and neurogenesis requires normal, low levels of TNF-α and LPS, ceramide and avoidance of opiates. Magnesium, vitamin D_3, and PPARγ ligands help move activated microglia and astrocytes into a repair mode. During any phase of treatment, the same supplements will be helpful.

Antioxidants: Glutathione (GSH) is the principal antioxidant of the CNS. Under excitotoxic stress, GSH becomes oxidized to GS:SG. Excess glutamate stimulates acid SMase and prevents the absorption of cysteine by the neuron, which is required for the formation of GSH; thus contributing to GSH depletion[262]. Oxidative damage to the CNS, associated with low GSH, has been found in patients with major depressive disorder, bipolar disorder, and schizophrenia[263]. Several nutrients help form and recycle glutathione to its reduced state. These include:

Cysteine: available from N-acetyl cysteine
Alpha-lipoic acid
Betaine
FAD: from vitamin B2 (riboflavin)
NAD: from niacin or tryptophan
Dietary glycine and serine and choline

Additionally, melatonin is an important antioxidant for the central, peripheral and enteric nervous systems.

Vitamin B12: Adequate vitamin B12 levels are important throughout primary and secondary prevention. B12 tablets are, however, poorly absorbed, and B12 needs to be mixed with saliva or injected to be well absorbed. For this reason, it is not listed to be taken in combination with the other nutraceuticals. It needs be administered as a separate oral compound or injected.

Sphingolipids: Magnesium, alpha-lipoic acid, vitamin B12, and vitamin D_3 all act to decrease the inflammatory aspects of this pathway. Amitriptyline, sertraline, fluoxetine, are all antidepressants that are FIASMA's and lower aSMase activity, amlodipine inhibits aSMase activity, and diltiazem increases it. Tomatidine, from green tomatoes, is one of few natural compounds that have been found to inhibit aSMase. Appendix M gives FIAMSA activity of common medications.

Other medications: Patients suffering from TBI, neuro-inflammatory disease, or recent stroke with hyperlipidemia, who are using statin medications, may benefit from the use of atorvastatin or simvastatin. Likewise, such patients may benefit from the choice of pioglitazone if they are diabetic.

Although a very useful medication, amitriptyline is easily toxic and has a prolonged half-life (up to 27 hours) in some patients. Children appear to be especially susceptible to its toxicity[264]. To decrease the risk of toxic exposure, use a low dose and dispense no more than a 30-day supply at a time.

Drug and Alcohol Abuse Prevention in CTE

1. Enhance GDNF production: Vitamin D3 should be given at therapeutic levels (6,000 to 10,000 IU daily). Monitor 25-hydroxy D3 levels to keep them between 90 and 150 nmol/L (36-60 ng/ml). A loading dose of vitamins D and B_{12} should be considered for patients with low levels. Beta-carotene and low dose zinc (10 mg/day) can be used to increase retinoic acid availability.

Akt/PI3K activity increases GDNF transcription. Supplement magnesium at around 600 mg daily with an organic salt such as Mg citrate or Mg ascorbate.

PGF_2 induces GDNF transcription. NADPH is required for conversion of PGE2 to PGF2, and NADPH required niacin and reduced glutathione. Reduced glutathione levels can be enhanced as outlined above, under "Antioxidants".

Amitriptyline and other tricyclic medications raise GDNF. Low-dose bedtime amitriptyline (10 mg) can be added to, using no more than 25 mg. Amitriptyline doses of 10 mg have been shown to be effective in spinal stenosis[265]. Doses as low as 5 mg have been shown to be sufficient to provide benefit when used in combination with other agents[266]. Low-dose therapy avoids most side effects and toxicity. Amitriptyline is useful to help restore sleep after injury, and this alone provides benefit. Ten to 20 mg is usually sufficient to help with sleep. Low dose amitriptyline may be used in combination with melatonin to improve sleep in patients with insomnia.

2. Control Glutamate excitotoxicity: Magnesium should be supplied at about 400 mg daily using an organic magnesium salt. Vitamin B_6 at a dose of 10 mg daily is easily sufficient for most individuals. Valerian, gotu kola, and lemon balm may be used to reduce glutamate activity.

Avoid induction of quinolinic acid production from LPS and TNF-α. LPS production can be avoided by preventing and treating dysbiosis (Chapters 23 – 25). TNF-α levels can be lowered by treating inflammation and through a diet rich in bioflavonoids.

Some antidepressant medications, including amitriptyline and sertraline, increase AMPA RNA editing, and help restore the ability of this membrane protein to exclude Ca^{++} and thus, Ca^{++} induced excitotoxicity. It is probably not coincidental that these medications are also FIASMA's.

3. Reduce H_2O_2: Alpha-lipoic acid is generally well tolerated at a dose of 500 to 600 mg daily; however, doses over 1000 mg can cause nausea. R-α-lipoic acid is the biologically active isomer while the S-α-lipoic acid isomer is not. R-α-lipoic acid sodium is recommended at a dose of 50 to 100 mg a day.

Betaine is a particularly good choice as it decreases the risk of excitotoxicity, protects the cell from HCY induced activation of acid SMase and TLR4 induced inflammatory cascade. Betaine also protects the liver from alcohol toxicity and protects the mitochondria.

The treatment suggested here for drug and alcohol craving may also be useful for treating aggressive and antisocial behavior or the lack of judgment seen in patients with CTE.

> **Addendum:** Since most post-concussion syndrome resolves on its own, many neurologists take a wait and see approach, occasionally giving analgesics for headaches during this three-month period. In my experience, most concussive injury severe enough and lasting long enough to elicit a neurology referral, responds poorly to tincture of time. Yesterday was a banner day for me; I had first visits with four stage 1 CTE patients; none had been treated for it, one was a medical doctor. Each of them could have been treated from the day of their accident with miniscule risk.
>
> Here is my general Rx for my post-concussion and CTE patients, in otherwise good health. This combination is not too hard to find nor expensive and helps prevent migraine and other pain. I ask the patients to purchase at least enough for two months of treatment.
>
> - Vitamin D_3 – 10,000 IU daily for one week, Followed by 6000 IU Daily
> - Magnesium citrate – 200 mg daily
> - Riboflavin 10 - 25 mg
> - Betaine – 500 mg
> - R-α-lipoic acid (sodium)– 100 mg
> - N-Acetyl cysteine – 500 mg
> - Melatonin 3 mg at bedtime
> - Cinnamon (Chinese cassia) 1000 mg (one rounded ¼ teaspoon of ground cinnamon)

[1] Clinical trials in head injury. Narayan RK, Michel ME, Ansell B, J Neurotrauma. 2002 May;19(5):503-57. PMID:12042091

[2] Traumatic Brain Injury in the United States: Emergency Department Visits, Hospitalizations, and Deaths 2002–2006. Faul M., Xu L., Wald M. M., Coronado V. G. Centers for Disease Control and Prevention, National Center for Injury Prevention and Control. Atlanta, GA. 2010.

[3] Concussion and mild head injury. Anderson T, Heitger M, Macleod AD. Practical Neurology. 2006;6;342-357. http://pn.bmj.com/cgi/content/full/6/6/342

[4] Epidemiology of concussion in collegiate and high school football players. Guskiewicz KM, Weaver NL, Padua DA, et al. Am J Sports Med. 2000 Sep-Oct;28(5):643-50. PMID:11032218

[5] Patient Characterization Protocols for Psychophysiological Studies of Traumatic Brain Injury and Post-TBI Psychiatric Disorders. Rapp PE, Rosenberg BM, Keyser DO, et al. Front Neurol. 2013; 4: 91. PMID:23885250

[6] Residual effects of combat-related mild traumatic brain injury. Kontos AP, Kotwal RS, Elbin RJ, et al. J Neurotrauma. 2013 Apr 15;30(8):680-6. PMID:23031200

[7] Vertigo after head injury--a five year follow-up. Berman JM, Fredrickson JM. J Otolaryngol. 1978 Jun;7(3):237-45. PMID:151151

[8] Prevalence of traumatic brain injury in juvenile offenders: a meta-analysis. Farrer TJ, Frost RB, Hedges DW. Child Neuropsychol. 2013;19(3):225-34. PMID:22372420

[9] Association of traumatic brain injury with criminality in adolescent psychiatric inpatients from Northern Finland. Luukkainen S, Riala K, Laukkanen M, Hakko H, Räsänen P. Psychiatry Res. 2012 Dec 30;200(2-3):767-72. PMID:22560660

[10] Role of cytokine p40 family in multiple sclerosis. Brahmachari S, Pahan K. Minerva Med. 2008 Apr;99(2):105-18. PMID:18431321

[11] GDNF--a potential target to treat addiction. Carnicella S, Ron D. Pharmacol Ther. 2009 Apr;122(1):9-18. PMID:19136027

[12] Excessive alcohol consumption is blocked by glial cell line-derived neurotrophic factor. Carnicella S, Amamoto R, Ron D. Alcohol. 2009 Feb;43(1):35-43. PMID:19185208

[13] Positive autoregulation of GDNF levels in the ventral tegmental area mediates long-lasting inhibition of excessive alcohol consumption. Barak S, Ahmadiantehrani S, Kharazia V, Ron D. Transl Psychiatry. 2011;1. pii: e60. PMID:22238721

[14] Positive autoregulation of GDNF levels in the ventral tegmental area mediates long-lasting inhibition of excessive alcohol consumption. Barak S, Ahmadiantehrani S, Kharazia V, Ron D. Transl Psychiatry. 2011;1. pii: e60. PMID:22238721

[15] Eicosanoid receptor subtype-mediated opposing regulation of TLR-stimulated expression of astrocyte glial-derived neurotrophic factor. Li X, Cudaback E, Breyer RM, et al. FASEB J. 2012 Jul;26(7):3075-83. PMID:22499581

[16] The spectrum of disease in chronic traumatic encephalopathy. McKee AC, Stern RA, Nowinski CJ, et al. Brain. 2013 Jan;136(Pt 1):43-64. PMID:23208308

[17] Chronic traumatic encephalopathy in athletes: progressive tauopathy after repetitive head injury. McKee AC, Cantu RC, Nowinski CJ, et al. J Neuropathol Exp Neurol. 2009 Jul;68(7):709-35. PMID:19535999

[18] Immunoexcitotoxicity as a central mechanism in chronic traumatic encephalopathy-A unifying hypothesis. Blaylock RL, Maroon J. Surg Neurol Int. 2011;2:107. PMID:21886880

[19] Neurodegenerative causes of death among retired National Football League players. Lehman EJ, Hein MJ, Baron SL, Gersic CM. Neurology. 2012 Nov 6;79(19):1970-4. PMID:22955124

[20] Image from Dieter Brandner and Ginger Withers of Whitman College.

[21] Aquaporin 9 in rat brain after severe traumatic brain injury. Liu H, Yang M, Qiu GP, Zhuo F, Yu WH, Sun SQ, Xiu Y. Arq Neuropsiquiatr. 2012 Mar;70(3):214-20. PMID:22392116

[22] All roads lead to disconnection?--Traumatic axonal injury revisited. Büki A, Povlishock JT. Acta Neurochir (Wien). 2006 Feb;148(2):181-93; PMID:16362181

[23] Molecular mechanisms of cognitive dysfunction following traumatic brain injury. Walker KR, Tesco G. Front Aging Neurosci. 2013 Jul 9;5:29. PMID:23847533

[24] Traumatic brain injury causes a long-lasting calcium (Ca2+)-plateau of elevated intracellular Ca levels and altered Ca2+ homeostatic mechanisms in hippocampal neurons surviving brain injury. Sun DA, Deshpande LS, Sombati S, et al. Eur J Neurosci. 2008 Apr;27(7):1659-72. PMID:18371074

[25] Mild in vitro trauma induces rapid Glur2 endocytosis, robustly augments calcium permeability and enhances susceptibility to secondary excitotoxic insult in cultured Purkinje cells. Bell JD, Ai J, Chen Y, Baker AJ. Brain. 2007 PMID:17664176

[26] Exposure of neurons to excitotoxic levels of glutamate induces cleavage of the RNA editing enzyme, adenosine deaminase acting on RNA 2, and loss of GLUR2 editing. Mahajan SS, Thai KH, Chen K, Ziff E. Neuroscience. 2011 Aug 25;189:305-15. PMID:21620933

[27] Profound downregulation of the RNA editing enzyme ADAR2 in ALS spinal motor neurons. Hideyama T, Yamashita T, Aizawa H, et al. Neurobiol Dis. 2012 Mar;45(3):1121-8. PMID:22226999

[28] Antidepressant interactions with the NMDA NR1-1b subunit. Raabe R, Gentile L. J Biophys. 2008;2008:474205. PMID:20107576

[29] Effects of antidepressants on GluR2 Q/R site-RNA editing in modified HeLa cell line. Sawada J, Yamashita T, Aizawa H, et al. Neurosci Res. 2009 Jul;64(3):251-8. PMID:19447293

[30] Reduced cerebral ischemia-reperfusion injury in Toll-like receptor 4 deficient mice. Cao CX, Yang QW, Lv FL, et al. Biochem Biophys Res Commun. 2007 Feb 9;353(2):509-14. PMID:17188246

[31] Toll-like receptors: new players in myocardial ischemia/reperfusion injury. Ha T, Liu L, Kelley J, Kao R, Williams D, Li C. Antioxid Redox Signal. 2011 Oct 1;15(7):1875-93. PMID:21091074

[32] Local and remote tissue injury upon intestinal ischemia and reperfusion depends on the TLR/MyD88 signaling pathway.

Victoni T, Coelho FR, Soares AL, et al. Med Microbiol Immunol. 2010 Feb;199(1):35-42. PMID:19941004

[33] Activation of the MyD88 signaling pathway inhibits ischemia-reperfusion injury in the small intestine. Watanabe T, Kobata A, Tanigawa T, et al. Am J Physiol Gastrointest Liver Physiol. 2012 Aug 1;303(3):G324-34. PMID:22628037

[34] Roles of toll-like receptors signaling in organ transplantation. Li T, Chen G, Zhang Z. Zhong Nan Da Xue Xue Bao Yi Xue Ban. 2011 Dec;36(12):1125-33. PMID:22246357

[35] Dynamic expression of toll like receptor 2 and 4 in a rat model of myocardial ischemia/reperfusion injury. Liu QP, Pan KY, Zhou X, et al. Zhongguo Ying Yong Sheng Li Xue Za Zhi. 2013 Jul;29(4):326-30. PMID:24175554

[36] TLR4-mediated MyD88-dependent signaling pathway is activated by cerebral ischemia-reperfusion in cortex in mice. Gao Y, Fang X, Tong Y, Liu Y, Zhang B. Biomed Pharmacother. 2009 Jul;63(6):442-50. PMID:18804339

[37] Toll-like receptor 4-dependent microglial activation mediates spinal cord ischemia-reperfusion injury. Bell MT, Puskas F, Agoston VA, et al. Circulation. 2013 Sep 10;128(11 Suppl 1):S152-6. PMID:24030400

[38] TLR2 and TLR4 in the brain injury caused by cerebral ischemia and reperfusion. Wang Y, Ge P, Zhu Y. Mediators Inflamm. 2013;2013:124614. PMID:23864765

[39] BRENDA, accessed April 2014. http://www.brenda-enzymes.org/php/result_flat.php4?ecno=3.1.4.12

[40] Pivotal role for acidic sphingomyelinase in cerebral ischemia-induced ceramide and cytokine production, and neuronal apoptosis. Yu ZF, Nikolova-Karakashian M, Zhou D, Cheng G, Schuchman EH, Mattson MP. J Mol Neurosci. 2000 Oct;15(2):85-97. PMID: 11220788

[41] Live imaging of Toll-like receptor 2 response in cerebral ischaemia reveals a role of olfactory bulb microglia as modulators of inflammation. Lalancette-Hébert M, Phaneuf D, Soucy G, Weng YC, Kriz J. Brain. 2009 Apr;132(Pt 4):940-54. PMID:19153151

[42] Toll-like receptor 2 deficiency leads to delayed exacerbation of ischemic injury. Bohacek I, Cordeau P, Lalancette-Hébert M, Gorup D, Weng YC, Gajovic S, Kriz J. J Neuroinflammation. 2012 Aug 8;9:191. PMID:22873409

[43] Accelerated hemolysis and neurotoxicity in neuron-glia-blood clot co-cultures. Jaremko KM, Chen-Roetling J, Chen L, Regan RF. J Neurochem. 2010 Aug;114(4):1063-73. PMID:20497302

[44] Regulation of quinolinic acid neosynthesis in mouse, rat and human brain by iron and iron chelators in vitro. Stachowski EK, Schwarcz R. J Neural Transm. 2012 Feb;119(2):123-31. PMID:21833493

[45] Pathogenic implications of iron accumulation in multiple sclerosis. Williams R, Buchheit CL, Berman NE, LeVine SM. J Neurochem. 2012 Jan;120(1):7-25. PMID:22004421

[46] Heme activates TLR4-mediated inflammatory injury via MyD88/TRIF signaling pathway in intracerebral hemorrhage. Lin S, Yin Q, Zhong Q, et al. J Neuroinflammation. 2012 Mar 6;9:46. PMID:22394415

[47] Extensive regenerative plasticity among adult NG2-glia populations is exclusively based on self-renewal. Robins SC, Villemain A, Liu X, Djogo T, Kryzskaya D, Storch KF, Kokoeva MV. Glia. 2013 Oct;61(10):1735-47. PMID:23918524

[48] Evidence for NG2-glia derived, adult-born functional neurons in the hypothalamus. Robins SC, Trudel E, Rotondi O, Liu X, Djogo T, Kryzskaya D, Bourque CW, Kokoeva MV. PLoS One. 2013 Oct 29;8(10):e78236. PMID:24205170

[49] An update on the biology of sphingosine 1-phosphate receptors. Blaho VA, Hla T. J Lipid Res. 2014 Jan 23. PMID:24459205

[50] Myelin loss and oligodendrocyte pathology in white matter tracts following traumatic brain injury in the rat. Flygt J, Djupsjö A, Lenne F, Marklund N. Eur J Neurosci. 2013 Jul;38(1):2153-65. PMID:23458840

[51] The P2Y-like receptor GPR17 as a sensor of damage and a new potential target in spinal cord injury. Ceruti S, Villa G, Genovese T, Mazzon E, Longhi R, Rosa P, Bramanti P, Cuzzocrea S, Abbracchio MP. Brain. 2009 Aug;132(Pt 8):2206-18. PMID:19528093

[52] Changes of the GPR17 receptor, a new target for neurorepair, in neurons and glial cells in patients with traumatic brain injury. Franke H, Parravicini C, Lecca D, Zanier ER, Heine C, Bremicker K, Fumagalli M, Rosa P, Longhi L, Stocchetti N, De Simoni MG, Weber M, Abbracchio MP. Purinergic Signal. 2013 Sep;9(3):451-62. PMID:23801362

[53] The p38α MAPK regulates microglial responsiveness to diffuse traumatic brain injury. Bachstetter AD, Rowe RK, Kaneko M, Goulding D, Lifshitz J, Van Eldik LJ. J Neurosci. 2013 Apr 3;33(14):6143-53. PMID:23554495

[54] Post-Traumatic Hypoxia Is Associated with Prolonged Cerebral Cytokine Production, Higher Serum Biomarker Levels, and Poor Outcome in Patients with Severe Traumatic Brain Injury. Yan EB, Satgunaseelan L, Paul E, Bye N, et al. J Neurotrauma. 2014 Jan 9. PMID:24279428

[55] GM-CSF increases LPS-induced production of proinflammatory mediators via upregulation of TLR4 and CD14 in murine microglia. Parajuli B, Sonobe Y, Kawanokuchi J, et al. J Neuroinflammation. 2012 Dec 13;9:268. PMID:23234315

[56] High mobility group box protein-1 promotes cerebral edema after traumatic brain injury via activation of toll-like receptor 4. Laird MD, Shields JS, Sukumari-Ramesh S, et al. Glia. 2014 Jan;62(1):26-38. PMID:24166800

[57] The role of microglia and the TLR4 pathway in neuronal apoptosis and vasospasm after subarachnoid hemorrhage. Hanafy KA. J Neuroinflammation. 2013 Jul 13;10:83. PMID:23849248

[58] Tumor necrosis factor-α antagonist reduces apoptosis of neurons and oligodendroglia in rat spinal cord injury. Chen KB, Uchida K, Nakajima H, Yayama T, Hirai T, Watanabe S, Guerrero AR, Kobayashi S, Ma WY, Liu SY, Baba H. Spine (Phila Pa 1976). 2011 Aug 1;36(17):1350-8. PMID:21224756

[59] The p53 Transcription Factor Modulates Microglia Behavior through MicroRNA-Dependent Regulation of c-Maf. Su W, Hopkins S, Nesser NK, et al. J Immunol. 2014 Jan 1;192(1):358-66. PMID:24319262

[60] Specific role of tight junction proteins claudin-5, occludin, and ZO-1 of the blood-brain barrier in a focal cerebral ischemic insult. Jiao H, Wang Z, Liu Y, Wang P, Xue Y. J Mol Neurosci. 2011 Jun;44(2):130-9. PMID:21318404

[61] Enhancement of Blood-brain Barrier Permeability and Reduction of Tight Junction Protein Expression Are Modulated by Chemokines/Cytokines induced by Rabies Virus Infection. Chai Q, He WQ, Zhou M, Lu H, Fu ZF. J Virol. 2014 Feb 12. PMID:24522913

[62] Lipopolysaccharide precipitates hepatic encephalopathy and increases blood-brain barrier permeability in mice with acute liver failure. Chastre A, Bélanger M, Nguyen BN, Butterworth RF. Liver Int. 2013 Jun 19. PMID:23910048

[63] The proinflammatory peptide substance P promotes blood-brain barrier breaching by breast cancer cells through changes in microvascular endothelial cell tight junctions. Rodriguez PL, Jiang S, Fu Y, Avraham S, Avraham HK. Int J Cancer. 2014 Mar 1;134(5):1034-44. PMID:23934616

[64] Toll-like receptor 4 is involved in subacute stress-induced neuroinflammation and in the worsening of experimental stroke. Caso JR, Pradillo JM, Hurtado O, Leza JC, Moro MA, Lizasoain I. Stroke. 2008 Apr;39(4):1314-20. PMID:18309167

[65] Correlation of acute phase inflammatory and oxidative markers with long-term cognitive impairment in sepsis survivors rats. Biff D, Petronilho F, Constantino L, et al. Shock. 2013 Jul;40(1):45-8. PMID:23603768

[66] Klebsiella pneumoniae meningitis induces memory impairment and increases pro-inflammatory host response in the central nervous system of Wistar rats. Barichello T, Simões LR, Valvassori SS, et al. J Med Microbiol. 2014 Jan;63(Pt 1):111-7. PMID:24105840

[67] Depressive-like-behavior and proinflammatory interleukin levels in the brain of rats submitted to pneumococcal meningitis. Barichello T, Dos Santos I, Savi GD, et al. Brain Res Bull. 2010 Jul 30;82(5-6):243-6. PMID:20450961

[68] Rapid improvement of chronic stroke deficits after perispinal etanercept: three consecutive cases. Tobinick E. CNS Drugs. 2011 Feb;25(2):145-55. PMID:21254790

[69] Selective TNF inhibition for chronic stroke and traumatic brain injury: an observational study involving 629 consecutive patients treated with perispinal etanercept. Tobinick E, Kim NM, Reyzin G, et al CNS Drugs. 2012 Dec;26(12):1051-70. PMID:23100196

[70] Migratory activation of primary cortical microglia upon infection with Toxoplasma gondii. Dellacasa-Lindberg I, Fuks JM, Arrighi RB, Lambert H, Wallin RP, Chambers BJ, Barragan A. Infect Immun. 2011 Aug;79(8):3046-52. PMID:21628522

[71] Acute minocycline treatment mitigates the symptoms of mild blast-induced traumatic brain injury. Kovesdi E, Kamnaksh A, Wingo D, Ahmed F, Grunberg NE, Long JB, Kasper CE, Agoston DV. Front Neurol. 2012 Jul 16;3:111. PMID:22811676

[72] Resveratrol decreases inflammation in the brain of mice with mild traumatic brain injury. Gatson JW, Liu MM, Abdelfattah K, et al. J Trauma Acute Care Surg. 2013 Feb;74(2):470-4; discussion 474-5. PMID:23354240

[73] Brain and spinal cord interaction: a dietary curcumin derivative counteracts locomotor and cognitive deficits after brain trauma. Wu A, Ying Z, Schubert D, Gomez-Pinilla F. Neurorehabil Neural Repair. 2011 May;25(4):332-42. PMID:21343524

[74] Luteolin downregulates TLR4, TLR5, NF-κB and p-p38MAPK expression, upregulates the p-ERK expression, and protects rat brains against focal ischemia. Qiao H, Zhang X, Zhu C, Dong L, Wang L, Zhang X, Xing Y, Wang C, Ji Y, Cao X. Brain Res. 2012 Apr 11;1448:71-81. PMID:22377454

[75] Quercetin permeability across blood-brain barrier and its effect on the viability of U251 cells. Ren SC, Suo QF, Du WT, et al. Sichuan Da Xue Xue Bao Yi Xue Ban. 2010 Sep;41(5):751-4, 759. PMID:21302433

[76] Minocycline plus N-acetylcysteine synergize to modulate inflammation and prevent cognitive and memory deficits in a rat model of mild traumatic brain injury. Haber M, Abdel Baki SG, Grin'kina NM, Irizarry R, Ershova A, Orsi S, Grill RJ, Dash P, Bergold PJ. Exp Neurol. 2013 Nov;249:169-77. PMID:24036416

[77] Novel therapeutic targets in depression: minocycline as a candidate treatment. Soczynska JK, Mansur RB, Brietzke E, et al. Behav Brain Res. 2012 Dec 1;235(2):302-17. PMID:22963995

[78] Quercetin and Nf-kB/ AP-1 induced cell apoptosis (Homo sapiens). Pico A, Boye C, Nuno. wikipathways.org/index.php/Pathway:WP2435 Accessed 2-20-2014

[79] N-acetylcysteine in psychiatry: current therapeutic evidence and potential mechanisms of action. Dean O, Giorlando F, Berk M. J Psychiatry Neurosci. 2011 Mar;36(2):78-86. PMID:21118657

[80] Microglial activation induced by traumatic brain injury is suppressed by postinjury treatment with hyperbaric oxygen therapy. Lim SW, Wang CC, Wang YH, Chio CC, Niu KC, Kuo JR. J Surg Res. 2013 Oct;184(2):1076-84. PMID:23726237

[81] Expression of organic osmolyte transporters in cultured rat astrocytes and rat and human cerebral cortex. Oenarto J, Görg B, Moos M, Bidmon HJ, Häussinger D. Arch Biochem Biophys. 2014 Oct 15;560:59-72. PMID:25004465

[82] Betaine protects against high-fat-diet-induced liver injury by inhibition of high-mobility group box 1 and Toll-like receptor 4 expression in rats. Zhang W, Wang LW, Wang et al. Dig Dis Sci. 2013 Nov;58(11):3198-206. PMID:23861108

[83] Changes in GABA transporters in the rat hippocampus after kainate-induced neuronal injury: decrease in GAT-1 and GAT-3 but upregulation of betaine/GABA transporter BGT-1. Zhu XM, Ong WY. J Neurosci Res. 2004 Aug 1;77(3):402-9. PMID:15248296

[84] Betaine treatment attenuates chronic ethanol-induced hepatic steatosis and alterations to the mitochondrial respiratory chain proteome. Kharbanda KK, Todero SL, King AL, et al. Int J Hepatol. 2012;2012:962183. PMID:22187660

[85] Possible role of S-adenosylmethionine, S-adenosyl-homocysteine, and polyunsaturated fatty acids in predementia syndromes and Alzheimer's disease. Panza F, Frisardi V, Capurso C, et al. J Alzheimers Dis. 2009;16(3):467-70. PMID:19276539

[86] Improvement of aggressive behavior and quality of life impairment following S-adenosyl-methionine (SAM-e) augmentation in schizophrenia. Strous RD, Ritsner MS, Adler S, et

al. Eur Neuropsychopharmacol. 2009 Jan;19(1):14-22. PMID:18824331

[87] Betaine Alleviates Hypertriglycemia and Tau Hyperphosphorylation in db/db Mice. Jung GY, Won SB, Kim J, Jeon S, Han A, Kwon YH. Toxicol Res. 2013 Mar;29(1):7-14. PMID:24278623

[88] Recognition of betaine as an inhibitor of lipopolysaccharide-induced nitric oxide production in activated microglial cells. Amiraslani B, Sabouni F, Abbasi S, Nazem H, Sabet M. Iran Biomed J. 2012;16(2):84-9. PMID:22801281

[89] Use of zinc as a treatment for traumatic brain injury in the rat: effects on cognitive and behavioral outcomes. Cope EC, Morris DR, Scrimgeour AG, Levenson CW. Neurorehabil Neural Repair. 2012 Sep;26(7):907-13. PMID:22331212

[90] Zinc supplementation provides behavioral resiliency in a rat model of traumatic brain injury. Cope EC, Morris DR, Scrimgeour AG, et al. Physiol Behav. 2011 Oct 24;104(5):942-7. PMID:21699908

[91] Zinc in traumatic brain injury: from neuroprotection to neurotoxicity. Morris DR, Levenson CW. Curr Opin Clin Nutr Metab Care. 2013 Nov;16(6):708-11. PMID:23945221

[92] Pyrroloquinoline quinine protects rat brain cortex against acute glutamate-induced neurotoxicity. Zhang Q, Ding M, Cao Z, Zhang J, Ding F, Ke K. Neurochem Res. 2013 Aug;38(8):1661-71. PMID:23686346

[93] The neuroprotective action of pyrroloquinoline quinone against glutamate-induced apoptosis in hippocampal neurons is mediated through the activation of PI3K/Akt pathway. Zhang Q, Shen M, Ding M, Shen D, Ding F. Toxicol Appl Pharmacol. 2011 Apr 1;252(1):62-72. PMID:21320517

[94] Pyrroloquinoline quinone attenuates iNOS gene expression in the injured spinal cord. Hirakawa A, Shimizu K, Fukumitsu H, Furukawa S. Biochem Biophys Res Commun. 2009 Jan 9;378(2):308-12. PMID:19026989

[95] Effect of pyrroloquinoline quinone on neuropathic pain following chronic constriction injury of the sciatic nerve in rats. Gong D, Geng C, Jiang L, et al.Eur J Pharmacol. 2012 Dec 15;697(1-3):53-8. PMID:23063836

[96] The neuroprotective effect of pyrroloquinoline quinone on traumatic brain injury. Zhang L, Liu J, Cheng C, Yuan Y, Yu B, Shen A, Yan M. J Neurotrauma. 2012 Mar 20;29(5):851-64. PMID:22040225

[97] Neuroprotection by pyrroloquinoline quinone (PQQ) in reversible middle cerebral artery occlusion in the adult rat. Zhang Y, Feustel PJ, Kimelberg HK. Brain Res. 2006 Jun 13;1094(1):200-6. PMID:16709402

[98] Evidence that tricyclic small molecules may possess toll-like receptor and myeloid differentiation protein 2 activity. Hutchinson MR, Loram LC, Zhang Y, et al. Neuroscience. 2010 Jun 30;168(2):551-63. PMID:20381591

[99] Functional Inhibitors of Acid Sphingomyelinase (FIASMAs): a novel pharmacological group of drugs with broad clinical applications. Kornhuber J, Tripal P, Reichel M, Mühle C, et al. Cell Physiol Biochem. 2010;26(1):9-20. PMID:20502000

[100] Tricyclic antidepressant amitriptyline indirectly increases the proliferation of adult dentate gyrus-derived neural precursors: an involvement of astrocytes. Boku S, Hisaoka-Nakashima K, Nakagawa S, et al. PLoS One. 2013 Nov 18;8(11):e79371. PMID:24260208

[101] The effectiveness of tricyclic antidepressants on lumbar spinal stenosis. Orbai AM, Meyerhoff JO. Bull NYU Hosp Jt Dis. 2010;68(1):22-4. PMID:20345358

[102] Amitriptyline for neuropathic pain and fibromyalgia in adults. Moore RA, Derry S, Aldington D, Cole P, Wiffen PJ. Cochrane Database Syst Rev. 2012 Dec 12;12:CD008242. PMID: 23235657

[103] Therapeutic implications of targeting energy metabolism in breast cancer. Sakharkar MK, Shashni B, Sharma K, et al. PPAR Res. 2013;2013:109285. PMID:23431283

[104] The formation, occurrence, and function of β-apocarotenoids: β-carotene metabolites that may modulate nuclear receptor signaling. Harrison EH, dela Sena C, Eroglu A, Fleshman MK. Am J Clin Nutr. 2012 Nov;96(5):1189S-92S. PMID:23053561

[105] Mechanisms of anti-inflammatory and neuroprotective actions of PPAR-gamma agonists. Kapadia R, Yi JH, Vemuganti R. Front Biosci. 2008 Jan 1;13:1813-26. PMID:17981670

[106] Pharmacological manipulation of peroxisome proliferator-activated receptor γ (PPARγ) reveals a role for anti-oxidant protection in a model of Parkinson's disease. Martin HL, Mounsey RB, Mustafa S, Sathe K, Teismann P. Exp Neurol. 2012 Jun;235(2):528-38. PMID:22417924

[107] The pharmacologic and clinical effects of medical cannabis. Borgelt LM, Franson KL, Nussbaum AM, Wang GS. Pharmacotherapy. 2013 Feb;33(2):195-209. PMID:23386598

[108] Tentative evidence for striatal hyperactivity in adolescent cannabis-using boys: a cross-sectional multicenter fMRI study. Jager G, Block RI, Luijten M, Ramsey NF. J Psychoactive Drugs. 2013 Apr-Jun;45(2):156-67. PMID:23909003

[109] Persistent cannabis users show neuropsychological decline from childhood to midlife. Meier MH, Caspi A, Ambler A, et al. Proc Natl Acad Sci U S A. 2012 Oct 2;109(40):E2657-64. PMID:22927402

[110] Inhibition of mouse-killing behaviour in magnesium-deficient rats: effect of pharmacological doses of magnesium pidolate, magnesium aspartate, magnesium lactate, magnesium gluconate and magnesium chloride. Bac P, Pages N, Herrenknecht C, Teste JF. Magnes Res. 1995 Mar;8(1):37-45. PMID:7669506

[111] Magnesium deficiency reveals the neurotoxicity of delta-9-tetrahydrocannabinol (THC) low doses in rats. Bac P, Pages N, Herrenknecht C, Maurois P, Durlach J. Magnes Res. 2003 Mar;16(1):21-8. PMID:12735479

[112] N-arachidonoyl glycine, an abundant endogenous lipid, potently drives directed cellular migration through GPR18, the putative abnormal cannabidiol receptor. McHugh D, Hu SS, Rimmerman N, et al. BMC Neurosci. 2010 Mar 26;11:44. PMID:20346144

[113] Mechanisms of cannabidiol neuroprotection in hypoxic-ischemic newborn pigs: role of 5HT(1A) and CB2 receptors. Pazos

MR, Mohammed N, Lafuente H, et al. Neuropharmacology. 2013 Aug;71:282-91. PMID:23587650

[114] Cannabidiol inhibits pathogenic T cells, decreases spinal microglial activation and ameliorates multiple sclerosis-like disease in C57BL/6 mice. Kozela E, Lev N, Kaushansky N, et al. Br J Pharmacol. 2011 Aug;163(7):1507-19. PMID:21449980

[115] COX-2 and PPAR-γ confer cannabidiol-induced apoptosis of human lung cancer cells. Ramer R, Heinemann K, Merkord J, et al. Mol Cancer Ther. 2013 Jan;12(1):69-82. PMID:23220503

[116] Aspirin, steroidal and non-steroidal anti-inflammatory drugs for the treatment of Alzheimer's disease. Jaturapatporn D, Isaac MG, McCleery J, Tabet N. Cochrane Database Syst Rev. 2012 Feb 15;2:CD006378. PMID:22336816

[117] Non-steroidal anti-inflammatory drugs and cognitive function: are prostaglandins at the heart of cognitive impairment in dementia and delirium? Cunningham C, Skelly DT. J Neuroimmune Pharmacol. 2012 Mar;7(1):60-73. PMID:21932048

[118] Effect of non-steroid anti-inflammatory drugs on neurovascular coupling in humans. Szabo K, Rosengarten B, Juhasz T, Lako E, Csiba L, Olah L. J Neurol Sci. 2014 Jan 15;336(1-2):227-31. PMID:24262992

[119] Attenuation of focal brain ischemia by telmisartan, an angiotensin II type 1 receptor blocker, in atherosclerotic apolipoprotein E-deficient mice. Iwai M, Inaba S, Tomono Y, , et al. Hypertens Res. 2008 Jan;31(1):161-8. PMID: 18360031

[120] Potential of the angiotensin receptor blockers (ARBs) telmisartan, irbesartan, and candesartan for inhibiting the HMGB1/RAGE axis in prevention and acute treatment of stroke. Kikuchi K, Tancharoen S, Ito T, et al. Int J Mol Sci. 2013 Sep 13;14(9):18899-924. PMID:24065095

[121] Restoration of cognitive deficits after statin feeding in TBI. Chauhan NB, Gatto R. Restor Neurol Neurosci. 2011;29(1):23-34. PMID:21335666

[122] Statins increase neurogenesis in the dentate gyrus, reduce delayed neuronal death in the hippocampal CA3 region, and improve spatial learning in rat after traumatic brain injury. Lu D, Qu C, Goussev A, Jiang H, et al. J Neurotrauma. 2007 Jul;24(7):1132-46. PMID:17610353

[123] Simvastatin and atorvastatin improve behavioral outcome, reduce hippocampal degeneration, and improve cerebral blood flow after experimental traumatic brain injury.Wang H, Lynch JR, Song P, et al. Exp Neurol. 2007 Jul;206(1):59-69. PMID:17521631

[124] Simvastatin-mediated upregulation of VEGF and BDNF, activation of the PI3K/Akt pathway, and increase of neurogenesis are associated with therapeutic improvement after traumatic brain injury. Wu H, Lu D, Jiang H, Xiong Y, et al. J Neurotrauma. 2008 Feb;25(2):130-9. PMID:18260796

[125] Therapeutic benefit of treatment of stroke with simvastatin and human umbilical cord blood cells: neurogenesis, synaptic plasticity, and axon growth. Cui X, Chopp M, Shehadah A, Zacharek A, et al. Cell Transplant. 2012;21(5):845-56. PMID:22405262

[126] Simvastatin treatment duration and cognitive preservation in experimental subarachnoid hemorrhage. Takata K, Sheng H, Borel CO, Laskowitz DT, Warner DS, Lombard FW. J Neurosurg Anesthesiol. 2009 Oct;21(4):326-33. PMID:19955895

[127] Simvastatin attenuates microglial cells and astrocyte activation and decreases interleukin-1beta level after traumatic brain injury. Li B, Mahmood A, Lu D, Wu H, Xiong Y, Qu C, Chopp M. Neurosurgery. 2009 Jul;65(1):179-85; discussion 185-6. PMID:19574840

[128] Atorvastatin protects rat brains against permanent focal ischemia and downregulates HMGB1, HMGB1 receptors (RAGE and TLR4), NF-kappaB expression. Wang L, Zhang X, Liu L, et al. Neurosci Lett. 2010 Mar 8;471(3):152-6. PMID:20100543

[129] Statins attenuate high mobility group box-1 protein induced vascular endothelial activation : a key role for TLR4/NF-κB signaling pathway. Yang J, Huang C, Yang J, Jiang H, Ding J. Mol Cell Biochem. 2010 Dec;345(1-2):189-95. PMID:20714791

[130] Simvastatin-mediated upregulation of VEGF and BDNF, activation of the PI3K/Akt pathway, and increase of neurogenesis are associated with therapeutic improvement after traumatic brain injury. Wu H, Lu D, Jiang H, et al. J Neurotrauma. 2008 Feb;25(2):130-9. PMID:18260796

[131] Statins and cognition: a systematic review and meta-analysis of short- and long-term cognitive effects. Swiger KJ, Manalac RJ, Blumenthal RS, Blaha MJ, Martin SS. Mayo Clin Proc. 2013 Nov;88(11):1213-21. PMID:24095248

[132] A randomized, double-blind, placebo-controlled trial of simvastatin to treat Alzheimer disease. Sano M, Bell KL, Galasko D, et al. Neurology. 2011 Aug 9;77(6):556-63. PMID:21795660

[133] Atorvastatin therapy lowers circulating cholesterol but not free radical activity in advance of identifiable clinical benefit in the treatment of mild-to-moderate AD. Sparks DL, Sabbagh MN, Connor DJ, et al. Curr Alzheimer Res. 2005 Jul;2(3):343-53. PMID:15974900

[134] Cochrane review on 'Statins for the treatment of dementia'. McGuinness B, O'Hare J, Craig D, Bullock R, Malouf R, Passmore P. Int J Geriatr Psychiatry. 2013 Feb;28(2):119-26. PMID:22473869

[135] Niaspan reduces high-mobility group box 1/receptor for advanced glycation endproducts after stroke in type-1 diabetic rats. Ye X, Chopp M, Liu X, Zacharek A, Cui X, Yan T, Roberts C, Chen J. Neuroscience. 2011 Sep 8;190:339-45. PMID:21683770

[136] Niaspan increases axonal remodeling after stroke in type 1 diabetes rats. Yan T, Chopp M, Ye X, Liu Z, Zacharek A, Cui Y, Roberts C, Buller B, Chen J. Neurobiol Dis. 2012 Apr;46(1):157-64. PMID:22266016

[137] Comparison of the Effect of Minocycline and Simvastatin on Functional Recovery and Gene Expression in a Rat Traumatic Brain Injury Model. Haar CV, Anderson GD, Elmore BE, et al. J Neurotrauma. 2014 Jan 20. PMID:24308531

[138] Docosahexaenoic acid reduces traumatic axonal injury in a rodent head injury model. Bailes JE, Mills JD. J Neurotrauma. 2010 Sep;27(9):1617-24. PMID:20597639

[139] The salutary effects of DHA dietary supplementation on cognition, neuroplasticity, and membrane homeostasis after brain trauma. Wu A, Ying Z, Gomez-Pinilla F. J Neurotrauma. 2011 Oct;28(10):2113-22. PMID:21851229

[140] A combination of intravenous and dietary docosahexaenoic acid significantly improves outcome after spinal cord injury. Huang WL, King VR, Curran OE, et al. Brain. 2007 Nov;130(Pt 11):3004-19. PMID:17901087

[141] Docosahexaenoic acid prevents white matter damage after spinal cord injury. Ward RE, Huang W, Curran OE, et al. J Neurotrauma. 2010 Oct;27(10):1769-80. PMID:20698757

[142] Improved outcome after spinal cord compression injury in mice treated with docosahexaenoic acid. Lim SN, Huang W, Hall JC, et al. Exp Neurol. 2013 Jan;239:13-27. PMID:23026410

[143] Docosahexaenoic acid pretreatment confers protection and functional improvements after acute spinal cord injury in adult rats. Figueroa JD, Cordero K, Baldeosingh K, et al. J Neurotrauma. 2012 Feb 10;29(3):551-66. PMID:21970623

[144] Dietary omega-3 fatty acids normalize BDNF levels, reduce oxidative damage, and counteract learning disability after traumatic brain injury in rats. Wu A, Ying Z, Gomez-Pinilla F. J Neurotrauma. 2004 Oct;21(10):1457-67. PMID:15672635

[145] Oral fish oil restores striatal dopamine release after traumatic brain injury. Shin SS, Dixon CE. Neurosci Lett. 2011 Jun 8;496(3):168-71. PMID:21514362

[146] Omega-3 fatty acids improve recovery, whereas omega-6 fatty acids worsen outcome, after spinal cord injury in the adult rat. King VR, Huang WL, Dyall SC, et al. J Neurosci. 2006 Apr 26;26(17):4672-80. PMID:16641248

[147] A saturated-fat diet aggravates the outcome of traumatic brain injury on hippocampal plasticity and cognitive function by reducing brain-derived neurotrophic factor. Wu A, Molteni R, Ying Z, Gomez-Pinilla F. Neuroscience. 2003;119(2):365-75. PMID:12770552

[148] Therapeutic use of omega-3 fatty acids in severe head trauma. Lewis M, Ghassemi P, Hibbeln J. Am J Emerg Med. 2013 Jan;31(1):273.e5-8. PMID:22867826

[149] ω-3 fatty acids in the prevention of cognitive decline in humans. Cederholm T, Salem N Jr, Palmblad J. Adv Nutr. 2013 Nov 6;4(6):672-6. PMID:24228198

[150] Docosahexaenoic acid-concentrated fish oil supplementation in subjects with mild cognitive impairment (MCI): a 12-month randomised, double-blind, placebo-controlled trial. Lee LK, Shahar S, Chin AV, Yusoff NA. Psychopharmacology (Berl). 2013 Feb;225(3):605-12. PMID:22932777

[151] Neuroprotectins A and B, bicyclohexapeptides protecting chick telencephalic neuronal cells from excitotoxicity. I. Fermentation, isolation, physico-chemical properties and biological activity. Kobayashi H, Shin-Ya K, Nagai K, et al. J Antibiot (Tokyo). 2001 Dec;54(12):1013-8. PMID:11858654

[152] Accumulation of dietary docosahexaenoic acid in the brain attenuates acute immune response and development of postischemic neuronal damage. Lalancette-Hébert M, Julien C, Cordeau P, Bohacek I, et al. Stroke. 2011 Oct;42(10):2903-9. PMID:21852616

[153] Omega-3 fatty acids for neuropathic pain: case series. Ko GD, Nowacki NB, Arseneau L, Eitel M, Hum A. Clin J Pain. 2010 Feb;26(2):168-72. PMID:20090445

[154] Metabolomics uncovers dietary omega-3 fatty acid-derived metabolites implicated in anti-nociceptive responses after experimental spinal cord injury. Figueroa JD, Cordero K, Serrano-Illan M, et al. Neuroscience. 2013 Dec 26;255:1-18. PMID:24042033

[155] Administration of thiazolidinediones for neuroprotection in ischemic stroke: a pre-clinical systematic review. White AT, Murphy AN. J Neurochem. 2010 Nov;115(4):845-53. PMID: 20964688

[156] Pioglitazone attenuates mitochondrial dysfunction, cognitive impairment, cortical tissue loss, and inflammation following traumatic brain injury. Sauerbeck A, Gao J, Readnower R, et al. Exp Neurol. 2011 Jan;227(1):128-35. PMID:20965168

[157] PPARgamma agonist rosiglitazone is neuroprotective after traumatic brain injury via anti-inflammatory and anti-oxidative mechanisms. Yi JH, Park SW, Brooks N, Lang BT, Vemuganti R. Brain Res. 2008 Dec 9;1244:164-72. PMID:18948087

[158] PPARγ agonist rosiglitazone is neuroprotective after traumatic spinal cord injury via anti-inflammatory in adult rats. Zhang Q, Hu W, Meng B, Tang T. Neurol Res. 2010 Oct;32(8):852-9. PMID:20350367

[159] Pioglitazone reduces secondary brain damage after experimental brain trauma by PPAR-γ-independent mechanisms. Thal SC, Heinemann M, Luh C, Pieter D, Werner C, Engelhard K. J Neurotrauma. 2011 Jun;28(6):983-93. PMID:21501066

[160] Pharmacological investigations on potential of peroxisome proliferator-activated receptor-gamma agonists in hyperhomocysteinemia-induced vascular dementia in rats. Sain H, Sharma B, Jaggi AS, Singh N. Neuroscience. 2011 Sep 29;192:322-33. PMID:21777659

[161] Behavioral and biochemical investigations to explore pharmacological potential of PPAR-gamma agonists in vascular dementia of diabetic rats. Sharma B, Singh N. Pharmacol Biochem Behav. 2011 Dec;100(2):320-9. PMID:21893084

[162] Extension of the neuroprotective time window for thiazolidinediones in ischemic stroke is dependent on time of reperfusion. Gamboa J, Blankenship DA, Niemi JP, et al. euroscience. 2010 Oct 27;170(3):846-57. PMID:20691766

[163] Delayed post ischemic treatment with Rosiglitazone attenuates infarct volume, neurological deficits and neutrophilia after embolic stroke in rat. Allahtavakoli M, Moloudi R, Arababadi MK, Shamsizadeh A, Javanmardi K. Brain Res. 2009 May 19;1271:121-7. PMID:19332033

[164] Antidepressant-like activity of magnesium in the chronic mild stress model in rats: alterations in the NMDA receptor subunits. Pochwat B, Szewczyk B, Sowa-Kucma M, et al. Int J Neuropsychopharmacol. 2014 Mar;17(3):393-405. PMID:24067405

[165] Magnesium sulfate protects against the bioenergetic consequences of chronic glutamate receptor stimulation. Clerc P, Young CA, Bordt EA, Grigore AM, Fiskum G, Polster BM. PLoS One. 2013 Nov 13;8(11):e79982. PMID:24236167

[166] Role of NMDA receptors in the trigeminal pathway, and the modulatory effect of magnesium in a model of rat temporomandibular joint arthritis. Cavalcante AL, Siqueira RM, Araujo JC, et al. Eur J Oral Sci. 2013 Dec;121(6):573-83. PMID:24206074

[167] Oral magnesium lozenge reduces postoperative sore throat: a randomized, prospective, placebo-controlled study. Borazan H, Kececioglu A, Okesli S, Otelcioglu S. Anesthesiology. 2012 Sep;117(3):512-8. PMID:22797283

[168] N-methyl-D-aspartate receptor antagonist therapy suppresses colon motility and inflammatory activation six days after the onset of experimental colitis in rats. Érces D, Varga G, Fazekas B, et al. Eur J Pharmacol. 2012 Sep 15;691(1-3):225-34. PMID:22796676

[169] Magnesium Can Decrease Postoperative Physiological Ileus and Postoperative Pain in Major non Laparoscopic Gastrointestinal Surgeries: A Randomized Controlled Trial. Shariat Moharari R, Motalebi M, et al. Anesth Pain Med. 2013 Dec 6;4(1):e12750. PMID:24660146

[170] Magnesium in disease prevention and overall health. Volpe SL. Adv Nutr. 2013 May 1;4(3):378S-83S. PMID:23674807

[171] Implications of magnesium deficiency in type 2 diabetes: a review. Chaudhary DP, Sharma R, Bansal DD. Biol Trace Elem Res. 2010 May;134(2):119-29. PMID:19629403

[172] Suboptimal magnesium status in the United States: are the health consequences underestimated? Rosanoff A, Weaver CM, Rude RK. Nutr Rev. 2012 Mar;70(3):153-64. PMID: 22364157

[173] Magnesium supplementation improves indicators of low magnesium status and inflammatory stress in adults older than 51 years with poor quality sleep. Nielsen FH, Johnson LK, Zeng H. Magnes Res. 2010 Dec;23(4):158-68. PMID:21199787

[174] Magnesium: its role in nutrition and carcinogenesis. Blaszczyk U, Duda-Chodak A. Rocz Panstw Zakl Hig. 2013;64(3):165-71. PMID:24325082

[175] Effect of magnesium chloride and magnesium L-aspartate on seizure threshold in rats under conditions of dietary magnesium deficiency. Spasov AA, Iezhitsa IN, Kharitonova MV, Kravchenko MS. Bull Exp Biol Med. 2007 Aug;144(2):214-6. PMID:18399283

[176] Dietary magnesium restriction reduces amygdala-hypothalamic GluN1 receptor complex levels in mice. Ghafari M, Whittle N, Miklósi AG, et al. Brain Struct Funct. 2014 May 8. PMID:24807818

[177] Zinc, magnesium and NMDA receptor alterations in the hippocampus of suicide victims. Sowa-Kućma M, Szewczyk B, Sadlik K, Piekoszewski W, Trela F, Opoka W, Poleszak E, Pilc A, Nowak G. J Affect Disord. 2013 Dec;151(3):924-31. PMID:24055117

[178] The effect of magnesium supplementation on primary insomnia in elderly: A double-blind placebo-controlled clinical trial. Abbasi B, Kimiagar M, Sadeghniiat K, et al. J Res Med Sci. 2012 Dec;17(12):1161-9. PMID:23853635

[179] Nutrient intakes are correlated with overall psychiatric functioning in adults with mood disorders. Davison KM, Kaplan BJ. Can J Psychiatry. 2012 Feb;57(2):85-92. PMID:22340148

[180] Magnesium intake in relation to systemic inflammation, insulin resistance, and the incidence of diabetes. Kim DJ, Xun P, Liu K, Loria C, Yokota K, Jacobs DR Jr, He K. Diabetes Care. 2010 Dec;33(12):2604-10. PMID:20807870

[181] Magnesium, inflammation, and obesity in chronic disease. Nielsen FH. Nutr Rev. 2010 Jun;68(6):333-40. PMID:20536778

[182] Relationship of Serum Magnesium and Vitamin D Levels in a Nationally-Representative Sample of Iranian Adolescents: The CASPIAN-III Study. Kelishadi R, Ataei E, Ardalan G, et al. Int J Prev Med. 2014 Jan;5(1):99-103. PMID: 24554998

[183] http://ods.od.nih.gov/factsheets/Magnesium-HealthProfessional/. Accessed 3/20.2014

[184] Modeling and simulation of the effect of proton pump inhibitors on magnesium homeostasis. 1. Oral absorption of magnesium. Bai JP, Hausman E, Lionberger R, Zhang X. Mol Pharm. 2012 Dec 3;9(12):3495-505. PMID:23051182

[185] The role of phosphoinositide-3-kinase/Akt pathway in propofol-induced postconditioning against focal cerebral ischemia-reperfusion injury in rats. Wang HY, Wang GL, Yu YH, Wang Y. Brain Res. 2009 Nov 10;1297:177-84. PMID:19703434

[186] Neuroprotective effect of humanin on cerebral ischemia/reperfusion injury is mediated by a PI3K/Akt pathway. Xu X, Chua CC, Gao J, Chua KW, Wang H, Hamdy RC, Chua BH. Brain Res. 2008 Aug 28;1227:12-8. PMID:18590709

[187] The phosphatidylinositol-3 kinase/Akt pathway mediates geranylgeranylacetone-induced neuroprotection against cerebral infarction in rats. Abe E, Fujiki M, Nagai Y, et al. Brain Res. 2010 May 12;1330:151-7. PMID:20206146

[188] Simvastatin acutely reduces ischemic brain damage in the immature rat via Akt and CREB activation. Carloni S, Girelli S, Buonocore G, Longini M, Balduini W. Exp Neurol. 2009 Nov;220(1):82-9. PMID:19664625

[189] Phosphoinositide 3-kinase/Akt pathway is involved in mediating the anti-inflammation effects of magnesium sulfate. Su NY, Peng TC, Tsai PS, Huang CJ. J Surg Res. 2013 Dec;185(2):726-32. PMID:23859135

[190] Permeant ion effects on external Mg2+ block of NR1/2D NMDA receptors. Qian A, Johnson JW. J Neurosci. 2006 Oct 18;26(42):10899-910. PMID:17050728

[191] NR2 subunit-dependence of NMDA receptor channel block by external Mg2+. Qian A, Buller AL, Johnson JW. J Physiol. 2005 Jan 15;562(Pt 2):319-31. PMID:15513936

[192] Magnesium treatment for neuroprotection in ischemic diseases of the brain. Westermaier T, Stetter C, Kunze E, et al. Exp Transl Stroke Med. 2013 Apr 25;5(1):6. PMID:23618347

[193] Magnesium attenuates post-traumatic depression/anxiety following diffuse traumatic brain injury in rats. Fromm L, Heath DL, Vink R, Nimmo AJ. J Am Coll Nutr. 2004 Oct;23(5):529S-533S. PMID:15466958

[194] Perinatal neuroprotection. Salmeen KE, Jelin AC, Thiet MP. F1000Prime Rep. 2014 Jan 2;6:6. eCollection 2014. PMID:24592318

[195] Magnesium enhances exercise performance via increasing glucose availability in the blood, muscle, and brain during exercise. Chen HY, Cheng FC, Pan HC, et al. PLoS One. 2014 Jan 20;9(1):e85486. PMID:24465574

[196] On the significance of magnesium in extreme physical stress. Golf SW, Bender S, Grüttner J. Cardiovasc Drugs Ther. 1998 Sep;12 Suppl 2:197-202. PMID:9794094

[197] Effects of magnesium on exercise performance and plasma glucose and lactate concentrations in rats using a novel blood-sampling technique. Chen YJ, Chen HY, Wang MF, Hsu MH, Liang WM, Cheng FC. Appl Physiol Nutr Metab. 2009 Dec;34(6):1040-7. PMID:20029512

[198] Bioavailability of US commercial magnesium preparations. Firoz M, Graber M. Magnes Res. 2001 Dec;14(4):257-62. PMID:11794633

[199] Study of magnesium bioavailability from ten organic and inorganic Mg salts in Mg-depleted rats using a stable isotope approach. Coudray C, Rambeau M, Feillet-Coudray C, et al. Magnes Res. 2005 Dec;18(4):215-23. PMID:16548135

[200] Therapeutic uses of magnesium. Guerrera MP, Volpe SL, Mao JJ. Am Fam Physician. 2009 Jul 15;80(2):157-62. PMID:19621856

[201] Magnesium absorption: mechanisms and the influence of vitamin D, calcium and phosphate. Hardwick LL, Jones MR, Brautbar N, Lee DB. J Nutr. 1991 Jan;121(1):13-23. PMID:1992050

[202] Efficacy of intravenous magnesium in neuropathic pain. Brill S, Sedgwick PM, Hamann W, Di Vadi PP. Br J Anaesth. 2002 Nov;89(5):711-4. PMID:12393768

[203] Relief of neuropathic pain with intravenous magnesium. Tanaka M, Shimizu S, Nishimura W, et al. Masui. 1998 Sep;47(9):1109-13. PMID:9785788

[204] A double-blinded randomised controlled study of the value of sequential intravenous and oral magnesium therapy in patients with chronic low back pain with a neuropathic component. Yousef AA, Al-deeb AE. Anaesthesia. 2013 Mar;68(3):260-6. PMID:23384256

[205] Effects of elevation of brain magnesium on fear conditioning, fear extinction, and synaptic plasticity in the infralimbic prefrontal cortex and lateral amygdala. Abumaria N, Yin B, Zhang L, et al. J Neurosci. 2011 Oct 19;31(42):14871-81. PMID:22016520

[206] Folate regulation of axonal regeneration in the rodent central nervous system through DNA methylation. Iskandar BJ, Rizk E, Meier B, Hariharan N, Bottiglieri T, Finnell RH, Jarrard DF, Banerjee RV, Skene JH, Nelson A, Patel N, Gherasim C, Simon K, Cook TD, Hogan KJ. J Clin Invest. 2010 May;120(5):1603-16. PMID:20424322

[207] The neuropsychiatry of vitamin B12 deficiency in elderly patients. Lachner C, Steinle NI, Regenold WT. J Neuropsychiatry Clin Neurosci. 2012 Winter;24(1):5-15. PMID:22450609

[208] Psychotic disorder and extrapyramidal symptoms associated with vitamin B12 and folate deficiency. Dogan M, Ozdemir O, Sal EA, et al. J Trop Pediatr. 2009 Jun;55(3):205-7. PMID:19095695

[209] Homocysteine induces cerebral endothelial cell death by activating the acid sphingomyelinase ceramide pathway. Lee JT, Peng GS, Chen SY, Hsu CH, Lin CC, Cheng CA, Hsu YD, Lin JC. Prog Neuropsychopharmacol Biol Psychiatry. 2013 Aug 1;45:21-7. PMID:23665108

[210] Neurocognitive phenotype of isolated methylmalonic acidemia. O'Shea CJ, Sloan JL, Wiggs EA, et al. Pediatrics. 2012 Jun;129(6):e1541-51. PMID:22614770

[211] Biphasic modulation of NOS expression, protein and nitrite products by hydroxocobalamin underlies its protective effect in endotoxemic shock: downstream regulation of COX-2, IL-1β, TNF-α, IL-6, and HMGB1 expression. Sampaio AL, Dalli J, Brancaleone V, et al. Mediators Inflamm. 2013;2013:741804. PMID:23781123

[212] Further evidence for the involvement of epidermal growth factor in the signaling pathway of vitamin B12 (cobalamin) in the rat central nervous system. Scalabrino G, Tredici G, Buccellato FR, Manfridi A. J Neuropathol Exp Neurol. 2000 Sep;59(9):808-14. PMID:11005261

[213] Cobalamin and normal prions: a new horizon for cobalamin neurotrophism. Scalabrino G, Veber D. Biochimie. 2013 May;95(5):1041-6. PMID:23328344

[214] The multi-faceted basis of vitamin B12 (cobalamin) neurotrophism in adult central nervous system: Lessons learned from its deficiency. Scalabrino G. Prog Neurobiol. 2009 Jul;88(3):203-20. PMID:19394404

[215] Novel role of vitamin k in preventing oxidative injury to developing oligodendrocytes and neurons. Li J, Lin JC, Wang H, Peterson JW, et al. J Neurosci. 2003 Jul 2;23(13):5816-26. PMID:12843286

[216] Vitamin K2 stimulates osteoblastogenesis and suppresses osteoclastogenesis by suppressing NF-κB activation. Yamaguchi M, Weitzmann MN. Int J Mol Med. 2011 Jan;27(1):3-14. PMID:21072493

[217] Menaquinone-4 concentration is correlated with sphingolipid concentrations in rat brain. Carrié I, Portoukalian J, Vicaretti R, Rochford J, Potvin S, Ferland G. J Nutr. 2004 Jan;134(1):167-72. PMID:14704312

[218] Dietary induced subclinical vitamin K deficiency in normal human subjects. Ferland G, Sadowski JA, O'Brien ME. J Clin Invest. 1993 Apr;91(4):1761-8. PMID:8473516

[219] Vitamin E and K interactions--a 50-year-old problem. Traber MG. Nutr Rev. 2008 Nov;66(11):624-9. PMID:19019024

[220] Vitamin E decreases extra-hepatic menaquinone-4 concentrations in rats fed menadione or phylloquinone. Farley SM, Leonard SW, Labut EM, et al. Mol Nutr Food Res. 2012 Jun;56(6):912-22. PMID: 22707266

[221] Lifelong low-phylloquinone intake is associated with cognitive impairments in old rats. Carrié I, Bélanger E, Portoukalian J, Rochford J, Ferland G. J Nutr. 2011 Aug;141(8):1495-501. PMID:21653572

[222] Association of low serum 25-hydroxyvitamin D levels and acute kidney injury in the critically ill. Braun AB, Litonjua AA, Moromizato T, et al. Crit Care Med. 2012 Dec;40(12):3170-9. PMID:22975885

[223] Renoprotective effect of paricalcitol via a modulation of the TLR4-NF-κB pathway in ischemia/reperfusion-induced acute kidney injury. Lee JW, Kim SC, Ko YS, et al. Biochem Biophys Res Commun. 2014 Feb 7;444(2):121-7. PMID:24434153

[224] Involvement of peroxisome proliferator-activated receptor gamma in vitamin D-mediated protection against acute kidney injury in rats. Kapil A, Singh JP, Kaur T, Singh B, Singh AP. J Surg Res. 2013 Dec;185(2):774-83. PMID:24011919

[225] Melatonin inhibits type 1 interferon signaling of toll-like receptor 4 via heme oxygenase-1 induction in hepatic ischemia/reperfusion. Kang JW, Lee SM. J Pineal Res. 2012 Aug;53(1):67-76. PMID: 22288937

[226] Melatonin modulates TLR4-mediated inflammatory genes through MyD88- and TRIF-dependent signaling pathways in lipopolysaccharide-stimulated RAW264.7 cells. Xia MZ, Liang YL, Wang H, Chen X, Huang YY, Zhang ZH, Chen YH, Zhang C, Zhao M, Xu DX, Song LH. J Pineal Res. 2012 Nov;53(4):325-34. PMID:22537289

[227] Vitamin E protects against oxidative damage and learning disability after mild traumatic brain injury in rats. Aiguo Wu, Zhe Ying, Gomez-Pinilla F. Neurorehabil Neural Repair. 2010 Mar-Apr;24(3):290-8. PMID:19841436

[228] The influence of exercise on cognitive abilities. Gomez-Pinilla F, Hillman C. Compr Physiol. 2013 Jan;3(1):403-28. PMID:23720292

[229] Aerobic exercise and neurocognitive performance: a meta-analytic review of randomized controlled trials. Smith PJ, Blumenthal JA, Hoffman BM, et al. Psychosom Med. 2010 Apr;72(3):239-52. PMID:20223924

[230] Physical exercise as a preventive or disease-modifying treatment of dementia and brain aging. Ahlskog JE, Geda YE, Graff-Radford NR, Petersen RC. Mayo Clin Proc. 2011 Sep;86(9):876-84. PMID:21878600

[231] Spontaneous Wheel Running Exercise Induces Brain Recovery via Neurotrophin-3 Expression Following Experimental Traumatic Brain Injury in Rats. Koo HM, Lee SM, Kim MH. J Phys Ther Sci. 2013 Sep;25(9):1103-7. PMID:24259924

[232] Exercise facilitates the action of dietary DHA on functional recovery after brain trauma. Wu A, Ying Z, Gomez-Pinilla F. Neuroscience. 2013 Sep 17;248:655-63. PMID:23811071

[233] Treadmill exercise inhibits traumatic brain injury-induced hippocampal apoptosis. Kim DH, Ko IG, Kim BK, et al. Physiol Behav. 2010 Dec 2;101(5):660-5. PMID:20888848

[234] Effect of exercise on mouse liver and brain bioenergetic infrastructures. E L, Lu J, Burns JM, Swerdlow RH. Exp Physiol. 2013 Jan;98(1):207-19. PMID:22613742

[235] Lactate administration reproduces specific brain and liver exercise-related changes. E L, Lu J, Selfridge JE, Burns JM, Swerdlow RH. J Neurochem. 2013 Oct;127(1):91-100. PMID:23927032

[236] Evidence that opioids may have toll-like receptor 4 and MD-2 effects. Hutchinson MR, Zhang Y, Shridhar M, et al. Brain Behav Immun. 2010 Jan;24(1):83-95. PMID:19679181

[237] Opioid activation of toll-like receptor 4 contributes to drug reinforcement. Hutchinson MR, Northcutt AL, Hiranita T, et al. J Neurosci. 2012 Aug 15;32(33):11187-200. PMID:22895704

[238] κ-Opioid receptor stimulation modulates TLR4/NF-κB signaling in the rat heart subjected to ischemia-reperfusion. Lin J, Wang H, Li J, Wang Q, Zhang S, Feng N, Fan R, Pei J. Cytokine. 2013 Mar;61(3):842-8. PMID:23402995

[239] Pilot trial of low-dose naltrexone and quality of life in multiple sclerosis. Cree BA, Kornyeyeva E, Goodin DS. Ann Neurol. 2010 Aug;68(2):145-50. PMID:20695007

[240] A combination cocktail improves spatial attention in a canine model of human aging and Alzheimer's disease. Head E, Murphey HL, Dowling AL, et al. J Alzheimers Dis. 2012;32(4):1029-42. PMID:22886019

[241] Neuroprotective and cognitive enhancing effects of a multi-targeted food intervention in an animal model of neurodegeneration and depression. Borre YE, Panagaki T, Koelink PJ, et al. Neuropharmacology. 2013 Nov 25;79C:738-749. PMID:24286859

[242] Reversing brain damage in former NFL players: implications for traumatic brain injury and substance abuse rehabilitation. Amen DG, Wu JC, Taylor D, Willeumier K. J Psychoactive Drugs. 2011 Jan-Mar;43(1):1-5. PMID:21615001

[243] Effects of brain-directed nutrients on cerebral blood flow and neuropsychological testing: a randomized, double-blind, placebo-controlled, crossover trial. Amen DG, Taylor DV, Ojala K, Kaur J, Willeumier K. Adv Mind Body Med. 2013 Spring;27(2):24-33. PMID:23709409

[244] Attenuation of myocardial injury by HMGB1 blockade during ischemia/reperfusion is toll-like receptor 2-dependent. Mersmann J, Iskandar F, Latsch K, et al. Mediators Inflamm. 2013;2013:174168. PMID:24371373

[245] ASC/caspase-1/IL-1β signaling triggers inflammatory responses by promoting HMGB1 induction in liver ischemia/reperfusion injury. Kamo N, Ke B, Ghaffari AA, et al. Hepatology. 2013 Jul;58(1):351-62. PMID:23408710

[246] Biphasic actions of HMGB1 signaling in inflammation and recovery after stroke. Hayakawa K, Qiu J, Lo EH. Ann N Y Acad Sci. 2010 Oct;1207:50-7. PMID:20955426

[247] Expression of HMGB1 and RAGE in rat and human brains after traumatic brain injury. Gao TL, Yuan XT, Yang D, et al. J Trauma Acute Care Surg. 2012 Mar;72(3):643-9. PMID:22491548

[248] Delayed inhibition of angiotensin II receptor type 1 reduces secondary brain damage and improves functional recovery after experimental brain trauma. Timaru-Kast R, Wyschkon S, Luh C, et al. Crit Care Med. 2012 Mar;40(3):935-44. PMID:21926585

[249] Candesartan, an angiotensin II AT₁-receptor blocker and PPAR-γ agonist, reduces lesion volume and improves motor and memory function after traumatic brain injury in mice. Villapol S, Yaszemski AK, Logan TT, et al. Neuropsychopharmacology. 2012 Dec;37(13):2817-29. PMID:22892395

[250] Potential of the angiotensin receptor blockers (ARBs) telmisartan, irbesartan, and candesartan for inhibiting the HMGB1/RAGE axis in prevention and acute treatment of stroke. Kikuchi K, Tancharoen S, Ito T, et al. Int J Mol Sci. 2013 Sep 13;14(9):18899-924. PMID:24065095

[251] Role of ventral tegmental area glial cell line-derived neurotrophic factor in incubation of cocaine craving. Lu L, Wang

X, Wu P, et al. Biol Psychiatry. 2009 Jul 15;66(2):137-45. PMID:19345340

[252] Regulation of ERK (extracellular signal regulated kinase), part of the neurotrophin signal transduction cascade, in the rat mesolimbic dopamine system by chronic exposure to morphine or cocaine. Berhow MT, Hiroi N, Nestler EJ. J Neurosci. 1996 Aug 1;16(15):4707-15. PMID:8764658

[253] 1,25-Dihydroxyvitamin D3, an inducer of glial cell line-derived neurotrophic factor. Naveilhan P, Neveu I, Wion D, Brachet P. Neuroreport. 1996 Sep 2;7(13):2171-5. PMID:893098

[254] 1,25-Dihydroxyvitamin D(3) increases striatal GDNF mRNA and protein expression in adult rats. Sanchez B, Lopez-Martin E, Segura C, et al. Brain Res Mol Brain Res. 2002 Dec;108(1-2):143-6. PMID:12480187

[255] 1,25-Dihydroxyvitamin D3 administration to 6-hydroxydopamine-lesioned rats increases glial cell line-derived neurotrophic factor and partially restores tyrosine hydroxylase expression in substantia nigra and striatum. Sanchez B, Relova JL, Gallego R, et al. J Neurosci Res. 2009 Feb 15;87(3):723-32.PMID:18816795

[256] Tricyclic antidepressant amitriptyline indirectly increases the proliferation of adult dentate gyrus-derived neural precursors: an involvement of astrocytes. Boku S, Hisaoka-Nakashima K, Nakagawa S, et al. PLoS One. 2013 Nov 18;8(11):e79371. PMID:2426020

[257] Antidepressants induce acute CREB phosphorylation and CRE-mediated gene expression in glial cells: a possible contribution to GDNF production. Hisaoka K, Maeda N, Tsuchioka M, Takebayashi M. Brain Res. 2008 Feb 27;1196:53-8. PMID:18234163

[258] Effects of traditionally used anxiolytic botanicals on enzymes of the gamma-aminobutyric acid (GABA) system. Awad R, Levac D, Cybulska P, Merali Z, Trudeau VL, Arnason JT. Can J Physiol Pharmacol. 2007 Sep;85(9):933-42. PMID:18066140

[259] Valproic acid, a molecular lead to multiple regulatory pathways. Kostrouchová M, Kostrouch Z, Kostrouchová M. Folia Biol (Praha). 2007;53(2):37-49. PMID:17448293

[260] Reduction in central H(2)O(2) levels prevents voluntary ethanol intake in mice: a role for the brain catalase-H(2)O(2) system in alcohol binge drinking. Ledesma JC, Baliño P, Aragon CM. Alcohol Clin Exp Res. 2014 Jan;38(1):60-7. PMID:24033657

[261] Alpha-lipoic acid reduces ethanol self-administration in rats. Peana AT, Muggironi G, Fois G, Diana M. Alcohol Clin Exp Res. 2013 Nov;37(11):1816-22. PMID:23802909

[262] Oxidative glutamate toxicity involves mitochondrial dysfunction and perturbation of intracellular Ca2+ homeostasis. Pereira CF, Oliveira CR. Neurosci Res. 2000 Jul;37(3):227-36. PMID: 10940457

[263] Decreased levels of glutathione, the major brain antioxidant, in post-mortem prefrontal cortex from patients with psychiatric disorders. Gawryluk JW, Wang JF, Andreazza AC, Shao L. Int J Neuropsychopharmacol. 2011 Feb;14(1):123-30. PMID:20633320

[264] Significant toxicity in a young female after low-dose tricyclic antidepressant ingestion. Grover CA, Flaherty B, Lung D, Pageler NM. Pediatr Emerg Care. 2012 Oct;28(10):1066-9. PMID:23034495

[265] The effectiveness of tricyclic antidepressants on lumbar spinal stenosis. Orbai AM, Meyerhoff JO. Bull NYU Hosp Jt Dis. 2010;68(1):22-4. PMID:20345358

[266] Effect of low-dose triple therapy using gabapentin, amitriptyline, and a nonsteroidal anti-inflammatory drug for overactive bladder symptoms in patients with bladder pain syndrome. Kwon WA, Ahn SH, Oh TH, Lee JW, Han DY, Jeong HJ. Int Neurourol J. 2013 Jun;17(2):78-82. PMID:23869272

31. Mood and Thought Disorders

We're a bunch of sick puppies! During the course of any one year, over one-quarter of Americans adults suffer from at least one mental disorder[1]. Mostly, we are anxious and depressed. How did life get so hard?

Table 31-1: Prevalence of Common Mental Disorders in the United States

Mental Disorder	Prevalence
Anxiety Disorders	18.1%
Mood Disorders	9.5%
Impulse-Control Disorders	8.9%
Substance Abuse Disorders	3.8%

Depression has its benefits

It may be easier to understand depression if considering it as a set of functional adaption behaviors then enhance survival. It may not enhance it as a pleasurable experience, however, over the last several dozen, millions of years; depression has helped mammals and perhaps of other animals to survive hard times. Depression represents a cluster of behaviors, which while being devoid of fun, allow creatures to endure environmental perturbations.

In times of danger and famine, anxiety gives animals an edge, keeping them safer and less likely to be a victim of predation. Typically, males become more aggressive during famine while females become timid and anxious. Females respond by being less sexually responsive and less fertile; this saves reproduction to more propitious times when the survival of offspring has a greater assurance.

Depression is also functional during disease and after severe injury. It provides a quiescent time for healing. Rats that survive sepsis from perforation of the large intestine show depression-like symptoms[2]. Depressive behaviors help animals conserve and store energy. Long, cold winters can be dangerous times to be out foraging; not only do animals need to look for food; they need to avoid being food. There are times when it is safer to curl up in a den and conserve energy; to sleep and stay warm and dry. Even a short winter storm with gloomy, wet days and dark skies may be enough to trigger the hibernation imperative; melancholy is a safer bet than getting wet, stranded and hypothermia.

Additionally, bereavement is a natural response to loss. We are social animals, and we form strong emotional bonds. Loss or breaking of those bonds hurts. We are saddened by the suffering of those around us, and a reversal of fortune can cause disappointment or despair.

Thus, it may seem a reasonable intuitive that depression is the psychological result of experiencing a loss or hard times, resulting in a prolonged reactive sadness. Having a chronic disease might easily be understood to cause loss of social interaction and standing, loss of financial security, anxiety, and pain, leading to psychological stress. Most folks who are depressed attribute their depression to an event or events the broke their happiness.

Depression, while sometimes triggered by a stressful event, is an inflammatory condition. We may be saddened to hear of a tragedy, or cry watching a movie; these are short-term responses. Most long-term depressive behaviors, in contrast, are mediated through inflammatory mechanisms.

Depression is much more commonly a disease behavior than an adaptive psychological response. Even when psychological stress or trauma initiates the inflammatory response, depression enduring after an adaptive period indicates an inflammatory problem. A major depressive episode is not a psychological event but rather, is a physiologic disease process.

Fibromyalgia, irritable bowel syndrome, acne, migraine, and traumatic brain injury are inflammatory diseases in which depression is a common comorbidity. Depression is intertwined with many other chronic diseases. Chronic lung diseases, heart diseases, diabetes, and cancers are also associated with high prevalence of depression. Chronic disease may lead to sedentary behavior, problems with sleep, boredom and isolation, and drug or alcohol abuse. Figure 30-1 diagrams some of the interactions between somatic disease and depression.

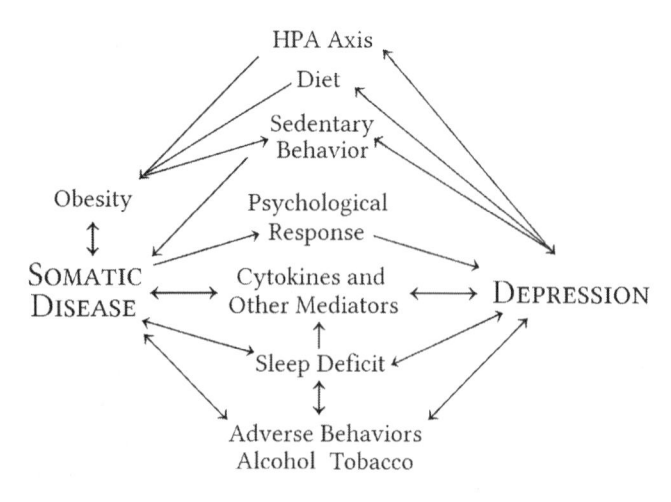

Figure 31-1: Causal web: chronic disease and depression.

Chronically ill individuals often use tobacco, alcohol or drugs to self-regulate, self-medicate and assuage their pain, boredom, and inability to adapt to their reconfigured life; often they see themselves as having gone from vital and capable to infirm and dependent overnight.

It is also not uncommon for depression to lead the way to chronic disease. In follow-up studies, depression is a risk factor for subsequent development of obesity[3]. Depression is associated with sedentary behavior and sleep disturbances. Sedentary behavior promotes survival of inefficient mitochondria that produce reactive oxygen species (ROS) and nitrosative radicals. Alcohol use promotes ROS. ROS lead to an inflammatory milieu that promotes depression. Individuals suffering from depression may eat poorly, binge eat, or select sweet, palatable foods that increase the risk of obesity, diabetes, and other diseases. Thus, depression may act as a risk factor for somatic disease.

Many diseases, which have depression as a comorbidity, share etiologic causation with it. For example, lower levels of n-3 fatty acids are a risk factor for congestive heart failure[4], ventricular fibrillation, cardiac arrest[5], asthma[6], and inflammatory diseases, such as Crohn's disease [7], and acne[8], as well as for depression[9]. In these conditions, there may be a positive feedback loop, wherein the diseases build upon each other.

Considering the comorbidities between anxiety, depression, bipolar disorder and schizophrenia with heart disease, metabolic syndrome[10], and chronic lung disease, the role of inflammation as an underlying cause should not come as a surprise. Many of the somatic disorders associated with enteroimmune diseases have depression as a co-morbidity; depression is not a separate disease, but rather, another manifestation of same inflammatory condition in many patients with fibromyalgia, irritable bowel syndrome, inflammatory bowel disease.

Mood and thought disorders and many degenerative diseases of the CNS share similar pathologic etiologies; understanding one disease gives greater insight to other related diseases. The differences between the diseases may depend on inflammatory pathway or pathways involved, genetic or epigenetic dispositions, developmental age at which the disease develops, "dose" of various contributing component factors or other influences. Since causation is not uniform among all patients, neither is treatment; not all patients respond to a single silver bullet,

The causal web between somatic disease and depression is often too intertwined to distinguish cause and consequence. Fortunately, untangling the web is not required for successful secondary prevention; the goal is to excise the causal links. Treatment involves removing the underlying causes of depression and any associated disease conditions. Treating sleep deprivation, getting physical activity, eating a healthful diet, and avoiding causal agents can help resolve depression and other diseases.

Biology of Mood Disorders

Important inflammatory mechanisms that contribute to depression and other mood disorders include:

- **The Tryptophan/Kynurenine pathway**
- **Neurotrophic Factors**
- **Sphingolipids**

The tryptophan pathway can be thought of as a homeostatic mechanism for controlling alertness and excitability versus rest, relaxation, and time for growth and repair. Neurotrophic factors, such as BDNF, act on growth, maintenance and repair of nerves. Sphingolipids help direct the propagation of the inflammatory response.

For many years, the monoamine hypothesis was the dominant explanation for depression; low serotonin, norepinephrine, or dopamine activity in the brain explained depressive behavior, and medications that increased the availability of these neurotransmitters relieved depression. While this model has some validity, it fails to explain most of what is going on in depression. The deficits in this model can explain why antidepressant medications that only affect the monoamine pathways are not especially effective. In mild to moderate depression, these medications are little if any more effective than placebos; nevertheless, they have significant, although limited, efficacy in treating severe depression[11]. And when these antidepressants do work, it is largely through mechanisms beyond their effects on monoamines.

The Tryptophan Pathway

The essential amino acid tryptophan is a precursor of the neurotransmitter serotonin and the neurohormone melatonin. Serotonin acts as a calming influence. Melatonin helps in sleep and acts as an anti-oxidant for central nervous system (CNS), as well as for the autonomic and gastrointestinal nervous systems. Tryptophan is also the precursor for the *kynurenine pathway*. The kynurenine pathway affects the NMDA receptors, which act in alertness, memory, and learning. The tryptophan pathway is illustrated in Figure 31-2.

Over 95% of the tryptophan absorbed by the body that is not used to build proteins goes to the kynurenine pathway. Less than 1% goes to form serotonin in the CNS. Thus, even small deficits in the tryptophan supply or shifts into the kynurenine pathway make less available for serotonin and melatonin. This occurs during inflammatory conditions or dietary protein deficits. In the kynurenine pathway, tryptophan is metabolized by the rate-limiting enzyme, indoleamine 2, 3-dioxygenase (IDO), into N-formyl-kynurenine, which is then converted into kynurenine and its metabolites. IDO is expressed at high levels in the gut, especially when induced by inflammation and biofilm produced LPS[12]. Thus, gastrointestinal inflammation can lead to a depletion of tryptophan availability, and limit of serotonin and melatonin for the enteric, autonomic, and central nervous systems.

Experimental diets low in tryptophan can be used to induce serotonin depletion. This diet provides sufficient amounts of other essential amino acids but insufficient tryptophan. As protein is formed free tryptophan is depleted, which causes serotonin insufficiency.

Short-term diet-induced tryptophan depletion studies confirm that serotonin can play a role in depression, but limits that role considerably. In some studies, about half of the patients treated with SSRI medications for depression had a relapse of depressive ideation within seven hours of beginning a tryptophan depletion diet[13]. However, neither change in mood[14,15,16] nor anxiety[17] was seen in most studies of these studies. More consistently, tryptophan depletion decreased personal and positive memory, increased attention to neutral information[18], and increased recognition of negative facial expressions[19].

These findings indicate that tryptophan and serotonin depletion have little, if any, direct effect on mood. They do, however, promote a negative bias on memory and attention. This change in memory and perception can promote depression-congruent biases, which especially affect females[20]. Serotonin depletion alone does not explain depression; medications that solely augment serotonin do not resolve depression. Serotonin appears to influence perception, rather than mood.

Serotonin is a major neurotransmitter for the gut, where it mediates GI motility. Melatonin also modulates GI motility and acts as a neuroprotective antioxidant. The total amount of melatonin made in the gastrointestinal tract is well over 100 times that made in the pineal gland, the site of melatonin production in the brain[21]. In general, the effect of serotonin in the gut is to increase peristaltic tone; while melatonin decreases peristaltic tone, increases blood flow and acts as an antioxidant[22], especially at night. Tryptophan depletion may have more impact on depression as a result of its effect on the gut than its effect on the CNS. Tryptophan has been found to be low in individuals with sugar malabsorption[23] (e.g., lactose intolerance, fructose malabsorption: see Chapter 3) and in irritable bowel syndrome[24]. Melatonin is helpful in the treatment of IBS. (See Chapter 26)

Tryptophan and Napping

Thanksgiving and Christmas feasts are special days for midday over-eating, which often include turkey. Many people notice drowsiness and the urge to nap after these feasts. This drowsiness has been attributed to tryptophan.

It's not that simple. Turkey is a low-fat meat and high in protein but is only an average source of tryptophan. The drowsiness, however, has more to do with the rest of the meal – particularly the carbohydrates. A Thanksgiving feast can easily exceed 3500 calories, with many of those calories in the form of carbohydrates. Carbohydrates promote the release of insulin, which increases the uptake of branched-chain amino acids and glucose into the muscles, but leaves tryptophan behind, available for conversion to serotonin[25]. Serotonin can cross the blood-brain barrier, and some is converted to melatonin, which makes us drowsy[26]. Other neural-hormonal effects of a large meal also likely play a role.

Milk is high in tryptophan, calcium, and sugars. This may explain why milk-based desserts, high in protein and carbohydrates, help us relax and are comfort foods. Pie with ice cream, a bowl of cereal with milk, or cookies and milk, or just a glass of warm milk an hour before bedtime, provide some extra tryptophan which can be converted into serotonin. In the pineal gland, serotonin can be utilized to form melatonin, which helps with sleep. Milk has one of the highest percentages of tryptophan per gram of protein of any food. Calcium, also available in milk, helps in the conversion of serotonin to melatonin.

If you want to stay awake after lunch and your job does not accommodate siestas, have a meal high in protein, but avoid meals heavy in carbohydrates.

The metabolic steps for conversion of tryptophan to serotonin and melatonin, as well as required the coenzymes, which may be used as supplements to ensure normal processing, are listed in Table 28-3.

The Kynurenine Pathway

The kynurenine pathway has several metabolites that affect behavior through effects on the central nervous system. The various compounds formed can cause calming, sickness behavior or agitation.

The first and rate-limiting step in the kynurenine pathway is the conversion of tryptophan into N-formyl-L-kynurenine by the enzymes tryptophan 2, 3-dioxygenase (TDO) or by indoleamine 2, 3- dioxygenase (IDO). TDO prefers L-tryptophan as a substrate while IDO has a much greater affinity for D-tryptophan[27]. TDO is found exclusively in the liver of mammals[28] and regulates serum tryptophan concentrations, whereas IDO is found ubiquitously in all tissues and is involved in activating the immune response. Iron in heme, as a cofactor, forms reactive epoxides with oxygen that generate N-formyl kynurenine from tryptophan[29]. IDO and TDO are present in many bacteria, including species that inhabit the colon, and process proteins fermentation products.

Table 31-2: Induction of IDO

Mediator	Typical Immune Mechanism
Interferon-γ (INF-γ)	T_H1 immune activation – Viral disease or intracellular bacteria
Bacterial Lipopolysaccharides	LPS; usually from anaerobic bacteria. Suggests biofilm formation, increased intestinal paracellular permeability, or bacterial translocation. May occur in contaminated wounds.
TNF plus IL-1 or TNF plus IL-6	Inflammatory cytokines. Multiple sources, often from intestinal (T_H17) immune function.

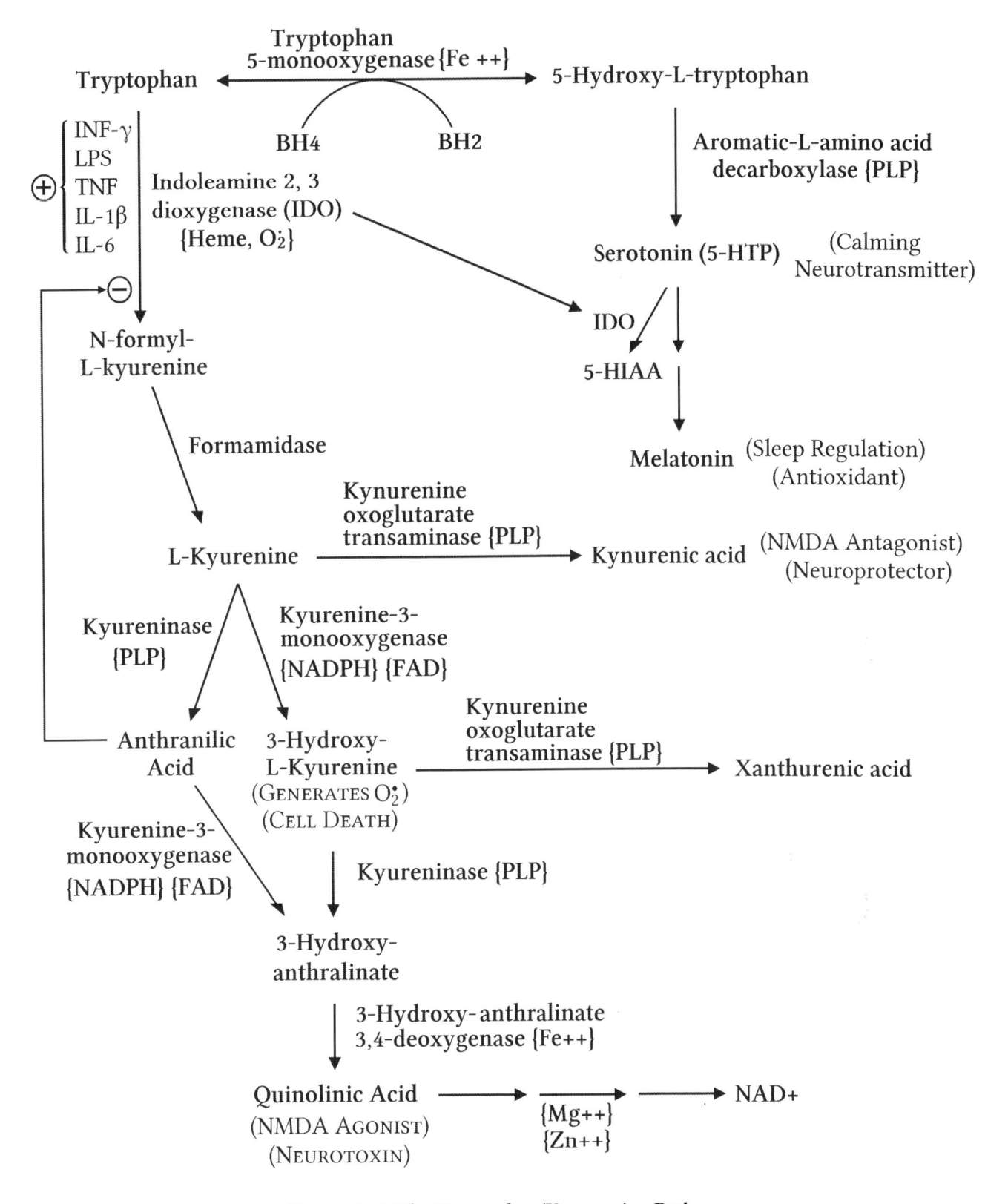

Figure 31-2: The Tryptophan/Kynurenine Pathway

Enzyme cofactors are shown in { } Brackets.
Fe^{++} = Iron, Mg^{++} = Magnesium, PLP = Pyridoxal-5-Phosphate (vitamin B6), FAD = Riboflavin (vitamin B2). $O_2^{\cdot}$ = superoxide anion, BH4 = Tetrahydrobiopterin, BH2 = Dihydrobiopterin, INF-γ = Gamma interferon, LPS = lipopolysaccharides. ⊖ = Inhibits, ⊕ = Enhances. TDO = Tryptophan 5-monooxygenase. Zn^{++} = Zinc.

At the beginning of this chapter, survival advantages were attributed to depression. For example, injured animals will often crawl into a hole or up a tree, and not move, sometimes for several days, giving them time to recover. This behavior may be in part a result of the kynurenine pathway. Kynurenine is increased in septic animals[30]. Stimulation of the kynurenine pathway is induced by LPS, INF-γ, or a combination of TNF-α and either IL-1β or IL-6.

In addition to infection, the kynurenine pathway may be activated in immune reactions to cancer, and limit cancer cell growth. It also acts in protecting the female reproductive organs from infection[31]. Kynurenine and its metabolites regulate blood flow to the placenta and downregulate immune rejection of the fetus[32].

Kynurenine can be metabolized to kynurenic acid by an enzyme requiring the vitamin B6 compound, pyridoxal-5-phosphate (PLP). Kynurenic acid is the only known endogenous *antagonist* for the N-methyl-D-aspartate (NMDA) receptor, although PQQ may also act in this function. It is also an antagonist for nicotinic receptors in the brain. Kynurenic acid (KA) acts as an important neuroprotective agent, as it can prevent excitotoxicity. TDO, present in the liver, is induced by Vitamin D[33]. Here is may help quell the immune response and increase KA. Additionally, the kynurenine pathway produces nicotinamide for production of NAD; a coenzyme used for energy conversion in the Complex I proteins in mitochondria, as well as for many enzymatic reactions, including recycling of antioxidants including glutathione.

Thus, kynurenine does very good things. But like any system, if it gets thrown out of balance, there can be a very dark side to its power. Excess kynurenic acid can decrease cognition[34], and if too far out of balance, excess it may even cause confusion and psychotic symptoms.

The kynurenine pathway compound 3-hydroxy-L-kynurenine (3HKA) has cytotoxic effects, as a result of its ability to generate free radicals. 3HKA also has the effect of down-regulating T_H17 cells and up-regulating T_{REG} cells, thus, lowering the immune response to enteric pathogens[35]. Kynurenic acid may also promote a shift in CD4+ T cell response which increases production of T_{REG} cells and down-regulates immune response[36].

The kynurenine pathway evolved to promote survival. Kynurenic acid as an NMDA antagonist is calming and neuroprotective. Together 3HKA and KA may help fight infection, get the animal to stay quiet and rest, and set the stage to down-regulate the immune system, and later, have quinolinic acid kick in as an NMDA agonist and get the animal moving again. Macrophages and monocytes peripherally, and dendritic cells and microglia in the CNS are immune cells that produce IDO. The enzyme IDO is induced in these cells by the stimulus of interferon-γ (INF-γ), bacterial LPS, or TNF plus IL-1 or IL-6[37]. IDO helps depletes tryptophan which prevents the microbes from forming proteins; impeding microbial growth.

The kynurenine pathway has been implicated in several neurologic disorders including AIDS-dementia complex, Huntington's disease, schizophrenia, Alzheimer's disease, seizure disorders, multiple sclerosis and bipolar disorder[38]. It may play a role in the pathology of autism. Activation of the kynurenine pathway may also trigger post-partum depression and anxiety[39], somatization syndromes[40], and premenstrual syndrome.

Quinolinic acid (QA) is a potent NMDA receptor agonist that increases excitotoxicity and increases rage reactions. It decreases glutamate removal from the synapse and inhibits glutamine synthase (AKA glutamate-ammonia ligase); thus, QA limits removal of both the excitatory neural transmitter glutamate and the neurotoxin ammonia. QA increases phosphorylation of tau; thus, it impedes neurite growth by impairing the formation of microtubules and increases the formation of β-amyloid neurofibrillary tangles, promoting Alzheimer's and some other neurodegenerative diseases. QA also induces the formation of the cytokine IL-1β[41].

The kynurenine metabolite, 3-HKA, generates free radicals, which are useful in killing bacteria and cancer cells, but in the brain can kill neurons[42].

Diseases or conditions in which INF-γ is elevated increase IDO, as well. These include rheumatoid arthritis, malaria, and cancers. IDO not only metabolize tryptophan into N-formyl-L-kynurenine; thus lowering its availability for conversion to serotonin, but converts of serotonin to 5-HIAA, a compound that facilitates the transmission of pain. This helps to decrease activity in injured animals, which helps with healing; however, depression is also associated with increased pain. The conversion of serotonin to 5-HIAA also lowers its conversion to melatonin, which may additionally impair sleep. Tryptophan depletion on its own can cause a milieu of negative perception. Thus, inflammatory conditions leading to IDO activation can lead to depletion of tryptophan, serotonin, and melatonin, and promote neurologic dysfunction, neurotoxicity, increased perception of pain and sleep dysfunction.

Lipopolysaccharides, from biofilm formation in the intestine, also induce IDO and increase transit of tryptophan into the kynurenine pathway. Patients with major depression have been found to have an increase in IgM and IgA antibodies to LPS from the cell walls of gram-negative enterobacteria. These LPS antibodies are also associated with an increase in fatigue, autonomic and gastrointestinal symptoms, and subjective feeling of infection[43]. The presence of LPS antibodies results from intestinal dysbiosis and overgrowth of gram-negative enterobacteria, often accompanied by hyperpermeability of the intestinal mucosa. The production of INF-γ by natural killer cells and T-killer cells triggers the kynurenine cascade and the depletion of tryptophan, serotonin, and melatonin.

Kynurenine produced by the intestine and other organs can easily pass the blood-brain barrier, where astrocytes can form kynurenic acid, or glial cells can metabolize it into toxic compounds. While kynurenine crosses the blood-brain barrier, neither kynurenic acid nor quinolinic acid can. Thus, the activity of the kynurenine pathway in the CNS, whether calming or neurotoxic depends on the milieu within the CNS, and how this compound is metabolized there.

Astrocytes cannot produce the enzyme kynurenine-3-monooxygenase (KMO) whereas microglia can; while microglia produce IDO but astrocytes, apparently, cannot. In schizophrenia, there is a loss of microglia, thus a decline in the quinolinic acid path and an accumulation of kynurenic acid[44]. The loss of microglia may be the result 3-hydroxy-kynurenine toxicity. Different dynamics in the kynurenine pathway may result in various neuro-immune responses associated with differences in the activation of the enzyme IDO[45].

Immune reactions to foods can also induce IDO production. Normally, IDO and the products of the kynurenine pathway help fight infection. In immune reaction to food, there is no infection to battle and no resolution. There is a positive feedback cycle of IDO induction of kynurenine by inflammatory cytokine products, and a reactive down-regulation of T_H17 cells which fight enteric infections, thus allowing more LPS producing bacteria to grow. This may support the growth of fungi[46] and promote intestinal dysbiosis that can trigger a new wave of inflammation. Serotonin is a major neurotransmitter in the enteric nervous system, and of melatonin, an antioxidant. Both participate in the regulation of peristalsis. Depletion of these compounds and the production of 3HK, QA, and 5-HIAA may increase abdominal pain and peristaltic dysfunction resulting in dysbiosis and symptomatic disease.

Pyridoxal-5-phosphate (PLP), the biologically active form of vitamin B_6, is a cofactor for over 160 enzymatic reactions, including in the formation of neuroprotective kynurenic acid and serotonin. Studies of the U.S. population indicate that between 19 and 27% have levels of PLP low enough to be associated with elevated markers of inflammation[47]. PLP levels have been found to be inversely associated with 3-HK levels, with a steep rising slope in 3-HK when PLP levels are below about 20 nmol/L. PLP levels are also inversely associated with C-reactive protein, WBC, and neopterin levels[48].

Neopterin is a biomarker of cellular immune activity, as it is produced by macrophages upon stimulation by INF-γ. Neopterin levels are elevated in many inflammatory conditions, including chronic fatigue syndrome, depression, fatigue, and so-called "somatization" disorders[49,50].

In patients with inflammatory conditions, PLP becomes sequestered or depleted, and thus, even with normal intake PLP levels fall and 3-HK levels rise. Adding a daily dose of 40 mg of pyridoxine greatly raise PLP and normalizes 3-HK levels in these patients, within several weeks[48]. Magnesium and zinc may also help normalize kynurenine metabolite levels and lower inflammation. Magnesium is discussed in more detail in Chapter 30; zinc herein below.

Neurotrophic Factors

Depressive behaviors may be induced during famine when there is insufficient food and under chronic stress. During these times, the body utilizes muscle as s protein source and growth is inhibited. One of the neurohormones involved is brain-derived neurotrophic factor (BDNF). Patients with severe illnesses or major depressive disorder (MDD) have low BDNF levels. When BDNF is administered to obese, sedentary, lab animals, it causes a spontaneous increase in exercise and decrease in appetite, accompanied by weight loss. The site of this action is the paraventricular nucleus, an area that controls appetite and energy utilization[51].

In the hippocampus, BDNF supports neuronal survival and the development of new neurons. BDNF plays a role in the consolidation of declarative and spatial memory. This is the memory for facts and places. When an animal goes foraging for food, it is helpful to remember how to get home, and how to later to go back and find the place that the food was available. If it is a seasonal fruit, for example, it helps to relate the food to the time of year the fruit is ready, how to get there, the dangers to be avoided, landmarks, how much fruit was available, waterholes along the way, etc. BDNF helps create these memories.

Social defeat stress, an animal model of depression, induces long-term down-regulation of BDNF. Social defeat moves the animal down in status, in a hierarchical group. The change in BDNF is long-term and is the result of repressive histone methylation in the hippocampus[52]. Methylation of the BDNF gene in lymphocytes occurs in humans with depression. It distinguishes cases from controls so well that lymphocyte BDNF gene methylation has been advocated as a biomarker for diagnosis of depression[53].

Histones are proteins that act like a spool that DNA is coiled around, providing stability. Segments of DNA get un-wrapped by nuclear transcription factors when a protein is needed. Methylation is one of several covalent bonding processes that can bind DNA to the histone, thus making that particular section of DNA resistant to access for transcription. DNA methylation can thus limit specific sets of proteins and shape metabolism and behavior for long periods, indeed, sometimes for the life of the animal.

This type transcription modulation is the basis of epigenetics; wherein prenatal, perinatal, or chronic influences can induce long-term changes in the animal's metabolism. Maternally deprived rats have lower levels of the neurotrophins BDNF, NT-3 and NFG than control animals, manifest depressive behaviors and have increased production of ACTH when stressed[54]. Chronic treatment with the tricyclic antidepressant, imipramine, reverses this DNA methylation, allowing an increase in the transcription of BDNF[55,56]. The n-3 fatty acids EPA and DHA may also reverse this hypermethylation[57]. Administration of these fatty acids promotes higher levels of BDNF[58]. The low serum BDNF levels found in depressed human subjects normalizes with successful treatment of depression[59].

Chronic stress and chronic exposure stimulation of glucocorticoid receptors cause downregulation of BDNF in the hippocampus and in animals decreases motivation to find food and to engage in goal-directed activity[60].

Hyponeophagia is the avoidance or anxiety-induction in animals subjected to novel feeding environments. It is an animal model of depression, used to assess the efficacy of anti-depressants. Successful treatment of hyponeophagia is dependent upon hippocampal neurogenesis. If the development of new neurons in blocked, treatment is ineffective. BDFN is essential for this neuro-neogenesis[61].

In patients with major depression, recovery correlates well with normalization of BDNF levels[62]. When several antidepressant medications were compared in human cell cultures, the tricyclic medication amitriptyline raised BDNF levels, while paroxetine, mirtazapine, and venlafaxine did not[63]. Nevertheless, successful treatment with SSRI medications normalizes BDNF levels. Mice genetically selected with reduced ability to make BDNF do not respond to SSRI treatment.

While SSRI medications block serotonin transporters (SERT) with the first dose, several weeks of treatment are required for clinical benefit. SSRI's provide benefit by upregulation of BDNF in hippocampal astrocytes. Serotonin stimulus increases the expression of BDNF[64]. Ironically, it appears that chronic extracellular serotonin exposure caused by SSRI medications induces the downregulation of $5HT_{1A}$ serotonin receptors in the dorsal raphe, and this stimulates BDNF production. Depression is not relieved by increasing serotonin levels, but rather the indirect downregulation of serotonin receptors, which induces BDNF production[61].

BDNF not only acts in the hippocampus, but also has effects on the amygdala; a neural hub of mood regulation that is affected in major depressive disorder (MDD). Low BDNF is associated with a down-regulated transcription of γ-aminobutyric acid (GABA), somatostatin (SST), tachykinin, neuropeptide Y (NPY) and cortistatin in the amygdala[65]. These neurohormones help explain some symptoms of depression.

Table 31-3: Effects of Neurohormonal Downregulation of in Depression

Neurohormone	Expected Effect of Down-Regulation
γ-aminobutyric acid	Increases anxiety
Somatostatin	Increased nociception and hyperalgesia (increased pain)[66]
Neuropeptide Y	Decreases appetite, memory, and learning; increases nociception and hyperalgesia.
Tachykinin	Increases anxiety, psychosis, and nausea.
Cortistatin	Impairs deep (slow-wave) sleep[67]

Although BDNF is the most well-studied neurotrophin, it is only one of several neurotrophic factors, and it only explains some of the behavioral and cognitive patterns seen in depression and other mood disorders. In depression, there is a loss of motivation, sadness, self-recrimination, sleep disturbances, and rumination. Depression is often accompanied by anxiety, worry, and outbursts of defensive rage. Some of these patterns, such as anxiety, rage, and early morning wakening can be easily understood to be adaptive to dangerous environmental conditions; they help keep the animal alert and on guard. A high neuronal to astrocyte BDNF level may induce anxiety.

Other cognitive and behavioral patterns, such as guilt, low self-esteem, and sadness require another explanation. Other neurotrophic factors may mediate depression and other mood disorders. Earlier in this chapter, changes in perception and memory were attributed to serotonin depletion. The kynurenine pathway likely explains other alterations in behavior and mood.

Neurotrophins support the growth and maintenance of neurons and their axons and dendrites. They include NGF (Nerve Growth Factor), BDNF (Brain-Derived Neurotrophic Factor), (NT-3) Neurotropin-3 and (NT-4) Neurotropin-4. There are also glial cell-derived neurotrophic factors, although neurons may also make them. These nerve growth factors are active in repairing nerves or replacing nerve cells after injury, and also have activity in peripheral tissues. Although the brain is made up mostly of postmitotic neurons, it has some capacity for new neuronal development, especially at the hippocampus.

The glial cell-derived neurotrophic factor (GDNF) family promotes the growth of dopaminergic neurons. Thus, deficient availability of GDNF neurotrophic factors may play a role in the causation of Parkinson's syndrome and schizophrenia. As cited in the section on the kynurenine pathway, there is a loss of glial cells in schizophrenia.

The neurotrophins (NGF, BDNF, NT-3, and NT-4) act via TrkB membrane receptors (neurotrophic tyrosine kinase receptor, type 2). Activation of TrkB receptors appears to be essential for an antidepressant effect. Mice do not respond to antidepressants if TrkB signaling is inhibited. While SSRI's and some other antidepressants increase BDNF, every antidepressant medication tested for its effect on TrkB, increased TrkB signaling, by inducing autophosphorylation of TrkB. BDNF is not needed if TrkB is directly stimulated. The antidepressant response to TrkB activation occurs even when monoamine activation is inhibited[68].

BDNF also regulates and stabilizes the excitatory glutamate receptors on neurons. Agents that potentiate the AMPA receptor activity have been shown to have antidepressant-like effects. Several antidepressants bind to and potentiate AMPA activity[69]. Amitriptyline and sertraline have been shown to promote AMPA RNA editing, which prevents neuro-excitotoxicity[70].

Table 31-4: Neurotrophic Factors

Neurotrophin Family	Function
NGF Nerve growth factor	NGF is critical for the maintenance and survival of sensory and sympathetic neurons.
BDNF Brain-derived Neurotrophic Factor	A neurotrophic factor present in several areas of the brain, including in the hippocampus. Low levels are associated with major depressive disorder (MDD) and bipolar disorder. BDNF is associated with the development of declarative memory.
NT-3 Neurotrophin-3	NT-3 is a neurotrophic protein in the NGF family of neurotrophins. It supports the survival of neurons and promotes growth and differentiation of new neurons and synapses. Its levels are low during MDD[71].
NT-4 Neurotrophin-4	NT-4 is a neurotrophic protein in the NGF family of neurotrophins.
GDNF Family	**Function**
GDNF Glial cell-derived neurotrophic factor	Promotes survival and differentiation of dopaminergic neurons. It prevents apoptosis of motor neurons. Deficits may play a role in depression and Parkinson's disease. Levels are low during MDD.
Artemin	Artemin is a glial cell line-derived neurotrophic factor. Artemin supports the survival of peripheral neuron populations and at least one population of dopaminergic CNS neurons. Levels are low during MDD.
Persephin and Neurturin	These proteins are glial cell line-derived neurotrophic factors.

The SLC6A4 gene (SERT), codes for the serotonin membrane transporter protein. Genetic alterations or decreased expression of the SERT protein have been implicated in Major Depressive Disorder, antisocial personality disorder, alcohol abuse, and obsessive-compulsive disorder as well as in other mental conditions. Similar to the BDNF gene, it has been demonstrated that the SERT gene is more highly methylated in adults who suffered physical or sexual abuse as children[72,73].

Genetic polymorphisms of genes, such as BDNF and SERT may explain heightened susceptibility to MDD and other mental disorders. Environmental influences, such as physical or emotional abuse, trauma, and stress, especially during early life can also increase susceptibility to these diseases through methylation or other covalent bonding of the DNA to histones, which then decrease gene expression.

In multiple sclerosis, there is an increased activity of neurotrophic factors[74,75]. These neurotrophic factors are important for regrowth and repair of nerves, but when under the influence of inflammatory cytokines or oxidative stress, the neuroglia respond with inflammatory activity.

Sphingolipids

Patients suffering from depression have been found to have elevated ceramide levels; particularly short-chain, saturated ceramides 18:0, 20:0, and 16:0[76,77]. Palmitic acid (16:0) ceramide is endogenously produced; 18:0 and 20:0 ceramides are derived from dietary saturated animal fats. Animals genetically or pharmaceutically treated to increase brain ceramide show depression-like behavior even in the absence of stress[78]. Elevated 16:0 ceramide prevents neuronal growth, proliferation, maturation and survival by intracellular nutrient deprivation[79]; starvation behavior.

Sphingolipids are immune modulators. Sphingosine-1-phosphate (S1P) activates of microglia. In an inflammatory milieu, S1P promotes microglial proliferation, migration, and phagocytotic activity. Activation of S1P receptors on neurons increases excitation, which can manifest as irritability, and nociception, the perception of pain. The enzyme acid sphingomyelinase (acid SMase), frees sphingomyelin from the cell membrane, and converts it to ceramide. Ceramide-1-phosphate (C1P) prevents apoptosis and promotes survival of inflammatory cells. Acid SMase is induced by cellular and oxidative stress. Acid SMase levels have been also found to be elevated in patients with major depressive disorder[80]. Several of the most effective antidepressant medications; sertraline, amitriptyline, and fluoxetine, are potent functional inhibitors of acid SMase (See Chapter 30).

Elevated homocysteine (HCY) is associated with not only with MMD but also with rage (anger attacks)[81], and with white matter and vascular lesions in the brain[82], as HCY is toxic to cerebral endothelial cells. HCY exerts its effect via its activation of acid sphingomyelinase, which promotes intracellular ceramide accumulation[83] and production of S1P.

Sphingolipid associated neuroinflammation and depression may be prevented by preventing the development of pro-inflammatory sphingolipids. Avoiding a diet high in saturated fats acids and fructose may provide a balance of membrane sphingolipids that are less inflammatory. Lower HCY levels can be maintained by a diet with sufficient vitamins to maintain sufficient SAMe to recycle it to methionine; folate, vitamin B_{12}, and betaine. Vitamin B_6 also helps remove HCY, and additionally is a cofactor for S1P lyase, which metabolizes S1P. HCY and methionine recycling are discussed below.

Perhaps most importantly, prevention of sphingolipid induced depression and neuroinflammation should be approached by avoiding oxidative and other cellular stressors that activate acid SMase. Magnesium, alpha-lipoic acid, and vitamin D_3 decrease acid SMase activity. N-acetyl cysteine, which helps generate the CNS antioxidant glutathione and melatonin may also help prevent acid SMase activity. Sphingolipids are also discussed in chapters 9, 10, and 30. TNF-α and IL-1β, which induce the kynurenine pathway, also induce sphingosine kinase, and production of the immune cell activator, S1P[84].

Emotional Stress

Neurogenesis, the generation of new neurons via mitotic cell division in adults, is limited in the human brain. One area where neurogenesis does occur is the hippocampus; however stress impairs neurogenesis in this area. Neurogenesis is very sensitive to glucocorticoids and is inhibited by elevated levels[85]. Short-term stress; a single episode of one to three hours of stress, increases memory and learning, and this is mediated by an increase in BDNF. Chronic or repeated stress, however, decreases the expression of BDNF in the hippocampus[86]. Stress also decreases BDNF in the prefrontal cortex[87].

During stress, cortisol is released. A single dose of short-acting corticosteroid, given within six hours of a traumatic experience, increases BDNF levels and decreases the risk of development of Post Traumatic Stress Disorder (PTSD)[88].
The high density of cortisol receptors in the hippocampus makes it more susceptible to chronic stress than most areas of the brain. Long-term or severe stress or high-dose corticosteroid therapy causes atrophy of the hippocampus. This atrophy can usually be reversed with relief of the stress; however, stress in young children, especially in the prenatal and neonatal period, can result in persistent, life-long epigenetic changes in BDNF expression. Please be nice to babies and pregnant women.

Atrophy of the hippocampus is one of the first anatomical changes seen in Alzheimer's disease. Decreases in hippocampus volume are also seen in schizophrenia, bipolar disorder, MDD, PTSD and chronic stress. This volume loss is associated with learning and memory deficits and mood dysregulation. In PTSD and MDD, there is a decrease in the survival of mature neurons in the hippocampus[89]. A particular polymorphism of the BDNF gene (val66met) is a risk factor for both PTSD and bipolar disorder. Trauma-induced epigenetic changes and contemporaneous stress are also important contributors to the onset of these illnesses in individuals with the altered allele[90].

Elevation in TNF-α and IL-6 levels are associated with loss of hippocampal volume and decreased BDNF production[91]. Chronic physical or emotional stress increases levels of the pro-inflammatory cytokines IL-1β, TNF-α, and IL-6 and lowers the expression of anti-inflammatory cytokines TGF-β and IL-10[92]. Individuals with a history of stress during childhood or recent stress, have higher levels of inflammatory cytokines, lower BDNF expression, and smaller hippocampal volumes than control individuals do[93]. Proinflammatory cytokines decrease BDNF levels and are the likely mechanism by which interferon therapy provokes depressive symptoms[94].

IL-1β impairs the release of the neurotransmitter acetylcholine and the production of NGF. This is thought to be how IL-1β causes memory impairment. The n-3 fatty acid EPA treatment has been found to prevent IL-1β induced memory impairment[95]. NFG also required for the survival of sensory and sympathetic neurons.

Chronic stress increases several proinflammatory mediators. Four weeks of mild, chronic stress raises the expression of IL-1β, TNF-α, and IL-6 and lowers expression of anti-inflammatory cytokines TGF-β and IL-10 in the brains of lab animals[96]. Thus, chronic stress raises the activity IDO and shifts tryptophan away from serotonin and melatonin production and towards kynurenine. Sleep deprivation also causes an increase in serum levels of the inflammatory cytokines IL-1β, TNF, IL-6 and lowers levels of anti-inflammatory cytokines.

The phenolic compound curcumin reverses the corticosteroid-induced depression of BDNF[97], and associated depressive-like behaviors in animals, increases hippocampal BDNF[98], and increases hippocampal neurogenesis[99]. Although the phenolic compound curcumin is not itself an antioxidant, it induces enzymes with antioxidant activity[100].

Chronic stress decreases phosphorylation of the nuclear transcription factor CREB, preventing its activity. Curcumin blocks the stressed induced decline in CREB phosphorylation in the hippocampus[101]. The effect of curcumin is most likely shared by a diverse array of flavonoid compounds from grape, citrus, cocoa, and other sources, which reverse the stress-induced suppression of neurogenesis[102,103,104,105].

Effects of Dietary Fats

A high-fat diet can induce oxidative stress and production of inflammatory cytokines. After several weeks on a high-fat diet, rats were found to have a decrease in BDNF in the hippocampus, a decreased numbers of newly generated cells in the dentate gyrus of the hippocampus, and an increased level of malondialdehyde (MDA), a marker of oxidative stress. MDA, resulting from lipid peroxidation, reduces the growth of neural progenitor cells, but treatment with BDNF can restore growth[106]. A high cholesterol diet can also elevate IL-1β in the hippocampus[107]. Diets high in fat decrease BDNF expression[108,109], likely as a result of oxidative stress and impaired production of DHA.

In general, dietary n-6 fatty acids promote the formation of inflammatory eicosanoids, such as PGE$_2$ while n-3 fatty acids promote the formation of anti-inflammatory eicosanoids. Prostaglandin E$_2$ is associated with loss of impulse behavior control in the periaqueductal gray area (PAG) of the brain, facilitating rage. (See Chapter 37) PGE$_2$ is also associated with neurotoxicity and cell death after ischemia[110]. COX2, an enzyme that produces PGE$_2$, is induced by stimulation of NMDA receptors. COX2 inhibitors have been shown to have beneficial effects in the early treatment of schizophrenia and depression. PGE$_2$ induces the production of cytokines, including INF-γ, which increase the activity of IDO and the conversion of tryptophan to kynurenine[26]. Phospholipase A$_2$ and COX2, sequential enzymes required for PGE$_2$ production, have been shown to participate in the induction of depression in patients who are treated with interferon-α[111]. Vitamin D$_3$

and tocotrienol forms of vitamin E inhibit COX2 and thus limit PGE$_2$ formation. See Figure 40-2, Chapter 40.

Arachidonic acid (AA), a 20-carbon n-6 fatty acid, is the precursor for the formation of PGE$_2$. Eicosapentaenoic acid (EPA) is the 20-carbon chain n-3 fatty acid which parallels AA. EPA has been shown to be useful in the treatment of depression[112], schizophrenia[113], and other mood disorders. The n-3 fatty acid docosahexaenoic acid (DHA) also inhibits the formation of COX2 and other inflammatory mediators (see Chapter 31).

Depression has been found to respond better to fish oil supplements with a higher eicosapentaenoic acid (EPA) to docosahexaenoic acid (DHA) ratio, than to one with a high DHA to EPA ratio. This suggests that somatic inflammation has a large impact on depression. Excessive formation of arachidonic acid-based eicosanoids elicits an inflammatory response. It would be expected that a large dose of EPA would be required to treat somatic inflammation. In a review of fish oil trials for depression, the trials using larger doses of EPA rather than DHA had stronger therapeutic effects against depression[114]. The effect of EPA on depression likely results from a shift from proinflammatory to anti-inflammatory cytokines and prostaglandins.

DHA mainly affects the electrical conduction in the heart (helping to avoid death by arrhythmias) and the nervous system. DHA affects bipolar disorder in part, by increasing the expression of the neurotrophin BDNF. BDNF levels are reduced in several neurologic diseases including Alzheimer's disease, depression, obsessive-compulsive disorder, schizophrenia, and bipolar disorder. DHA released from phospholipids of the neuronal cell membrane increase BDNF synthesis by activating MAPK signaling that phosphorylates CREB (cAMP response element-binding protein), a transcription factor for BDNF[115]. DHA also induces production of PPARγ and thereby reduces inflammation and neurotoxicity. (See Chapter 31.)

High intakes of fish may be protective from bipolar disorder. In countries where the annual per capita of fish is over about 75 pounds a year, there are low rates for this disease[116]. In lab animals, DHA deficiencies cause alterations in the dopaminergic systems. Post-mortem examinations of the orbitofrontal cortex of patients with bipolar disorder (BPD) have found the tissues in this area to have low DHA content[117]. BPD patients also have been found to have lower DHA levels in their red blood cell membranes compared to control subjects[118].

In an experiment, mice were fed either a diet with safflower oil (high in n-6 but lacking n-3 fatty acids) or perilla oil (high in n-3 fatty acids) for four weeks. The hippocampus and striatum, but not the cortex of the brains, were found to be low in DHA in the animals on the high n-6 diet. NGF was unchanged between the diets, but BDNF levels were significantly lower in the safflower oil diet[119]. The addition of EPA to an n-3 deficient diet was able to restore DHA levels but did not fully restore NGF levels in the hippocampus, even though NGF levels were elevated in the piriform cortex[120].

EPA supplements in patients with BPD have had limited success; they help with depressive symptoms, but not with mania. DHA, however, appears to provide benefit. In a study of adolescents using 1.5 grams of DHA daily for six weeks, there was an improvement in mania, depression, and global functioning[121]. A similar, eight-week trial, also showed a modest improvement in mania among younger children with BPD[122]. It takes several weeks for red blood cell membranes to reflect the change in dietary fatty acids. It may take considerably longer to have a turnover of the lipid membrane of neurons sufficient to normalize affect and behavior. Mitochondrial membranes would be expected to have a faster turnover rate, and thus, changes in mitochondrial behavior may manifest more quickly.

Oxidative Stress

Older adults with higher BDNF levels have better cognitive function than adults with lower BDNF levels[123]. Likewise, a study of old, cognitively-impaired dogs showed a significant decrease in BDNF in the temporal cortex when compared with young animals. Dogs treated with either environmental enrichment or an antioxidant diet, responded with increased BDNF levels, and those receiving both the enriched environment and antioxidant diet had BDNF close to those of young animals[124]. Animals that were given blueberries, which are rich in antioxidant flavonoids, as part of the diet were found to have improved spatial memory and increased BDNF levels in the hippocampus[125].

Exercise induces culling of inefficient mitochondria and thus reduces production of reactive oxygen species and oxidative stress. Exercise increases the synthesis of BDNF[126], and thus, induces the formation of new neurons and increases the survival of mature neurons in the hippocampus.

Alcohol decreases BDNF level in the hippocampus of lab animals and induces depressive-like behaviors[127]. Alcohol also lowers NGF, and alcohol's deleterious effects on fetal brain development are due in part to a reduction of NGF and BDNF. Some of alcohol's effects are the result of oxidative stress. Red wine, which has antioxidant phenolic compounds, curtails some of the effect upon NGF but does not prevent the deleterious effect of alcohol on BDNF[128].

Glutathione and melatonin are among the most important antioxidants in the central, enteric, and autonomic nervous systems. Glutathione is not absorbed intact from the diet but rather formed by the body from its component amino acids. The supplement N-acetyl cysteine helps form glutathione, and several B vitamins help recycle SAMe reduce glutathione to its antioxidant form. Melatonin and r-alpha-lipoic acid (r-ALA) also important antioxidants for the CNS. ALA helps mitigate cellular stress and H_2O_2 induced activation of acid SMase.

Vitamin D₃

Several lines of evidence implicate vitamin D deficiency in the pathogenesis of mood disorders including depression, seasonal affective disorder, post-partum depression and BPD. Vitamin D receptors and enzymes for converting vitamin D into its active form are present in the amygdala[129], indicating that "inactive" 25-OHD3, previtamin D, formed in the skin, has direct action in the brain. This may be a reason that sunshine feels so good.

In a population study of eight thousand Americans, individuals with vitamin D₃ levels lower than 50 nmol/L were 85 percent more likely to meet the criteria for depression than those with levels above 75 nmol/L[130]. In a study of over 3000 middle-aged European men, lower levels of vitamin D were associated with a 70 percent increased probability of depression[131]. Vitamin D₃ supplementation has been found to improve depressive symptoms and other symptoms, including those of carbohydrate craving, hypersomnia, and lethargy in Seasonal Affective Disorder[132, 133]. Serum vitamin D levels have been found to be inversely related to post-partum depression scores[134].

Vitamin D₃ may interact with dietary n-3 fats. Figure 20-2 in Chapter 20; illustrates a relationship between low n-3 fats consumption and coronary disease. It also shows that northern countries have higher coronary disease rates for a given n-3 fat intake, suggesting an interaction between vitamin D deficiency and low n-3 fat intake with high rates of coronary disease. Bipolar disorder has a high comorbidity with coronary artery disease. Figure 31-3 shows BPD rates in various countries by dietary-3 fat consumption, mainly from intake of fish. Countries with higher levels of n-3 fat consumption have lower rates of BPD. Note that the high latitude countries, Norway and New Zealand have higher rates of BPD than other countries for the amount of n-3 fats consumed[135]. This suggests that low solar exposure, with lower vitamin D formation, along with lower dietary intake of n-3 fats raise the risk of developing BPD. Calcitriol, the active form of vitamin D₃, also enhances the formation of S1P, while inhibiting the formation of ceramide-1-phosphate.

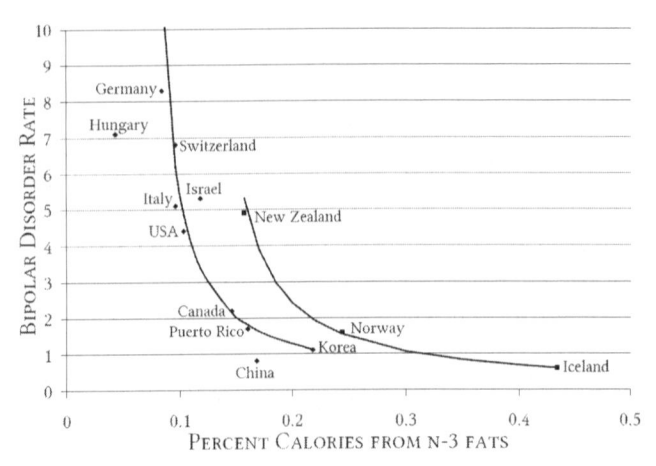

Figure 31-3: Prevalence of Bipolar Disorder by n-3 Fat Intake by Country.

While vitamin D₃ does not affect BDNF transcription, it does help regulate the production of other neurotrophins[136]. NGF is decreased in BPD patients[137]; Vitamin D₃ strongly increases NGF transcription[138]. Conversely, NT-3 and NT-4 are elevated in patients with exacerbations of BPD[139, 140]. Vitamin D₃ up-regulates NT-3 and down-regulates NT-4. As mentioned earlier, vitamin D₃ also inhibits PGE₂.

In an animal model of Alzheimer's disease, utilizing transgenic mice that spontaneously produce β-amyloid plaques, a vitamin D₃ supplemented diet was found to prevent plaque formation as compared to a vitamin D₃-deficient diet. The vitamin D₃ enriched diet was also found to increase NGF[141]. Lower NGF production was found in the brain of normal rats raised on a low vitamin D₃ diet[142].

> While NGF levels are lower than normal in bipolar disorder, NGF levels remain elevated for about one year after falling in love, with levels nearly twice those found in persons in long-term relationships[143]. Early stage romantic love is associated with increased positive mood states, elation, a reduced requirement for of sleep, and improved concentration; comparable to hypomania[144].

Folate, Vitamin B₆, B₁₂, and Betaine

The principal function of folic acid (vitamin B₉) is that it acts as a methyl donor, adding carbon atoms to molecules. One of the important functions of vitamin B₁₂ is to recycle folate into its active form so that folate can continue to do its job. During this process, methionine is recycled from homocysteine and then into S-adenosylmethionine (SAMe). If these vitamins are deficient, levels of the toxic metabolite, homocysteine, can rise. The principal toxic action of HCY, as noted above, is through its induction of acid SMase.

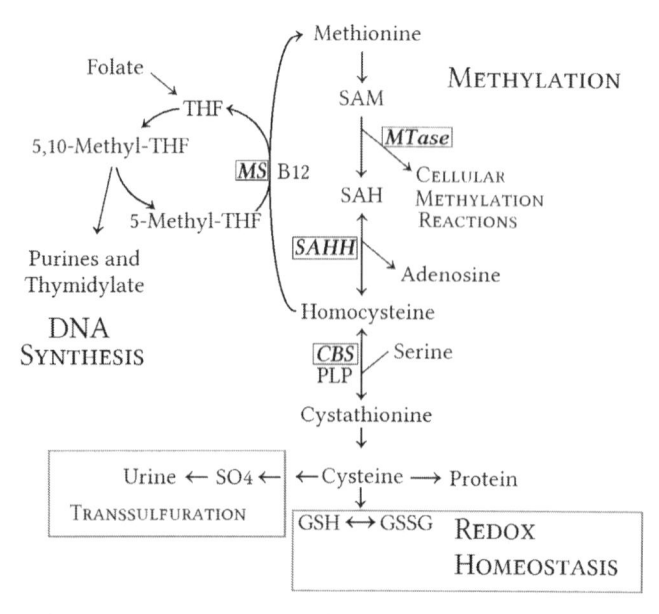

Figure 31-4: Methionine/ Homocysteine/ Cysteine Pathways: MS: methionine synthase, **SAHH:** S-Adenosyl-L-homocysteine hydro-lase, **CBS:** Cystathionine-β-synthase, **MTase:** methionine S-methyltransferase. B12 is vitamin B₁₂, and PLP is pyridoxal-5-phosphate, the active form of vitamin B₆.

Twelve hours after lab animals are injected with homocysteine; they had impairments in short- and long-term memories and reduced hippocampal BDNF levels. Pretreatment with folic acid prevents both the memory deficits and the reduction in the BDNF in these animals[145]. A study of patients having their first psychotic episode of schizophrenia, who had not been previously treated, were found to have low levels of folate, vitamin B[12,] and DHA, but increased levels of cortisol and homocysteine when compared to controls[146].

In rat pups exposed to high folic acid with deficient vitamin B[12], NGF and BDNF were found to be low in comparison to control pups. The addition of the fatty acid DHA prevented the negative effects on NGF but did not prevent them for BDNF[147]. Excess folic acid was found to induce oxidative stress that lowered DHA levels[148]. Excess folate with deficient vitamin B[12] was also associated with increased methylation of BDNF DNA, thus altering gene expression. *Sufficient DHA prevented excessive methylation.*

In adult rats, vitamin B[12] deficiency provokes increased NGF production along with increased TNF-α in the spinal cord, which, in combination, promote the development of spinal cord white matter lesions leading to peripheral neuropathy. Use of anti-NGF-antibody treatment in these animals prevented the myelinolytic spinal cord lesions[149]. NGF and TNF-α activate NF-κB, and this up-regulates immune response[150]. NGF stimulates microglia to repair nerve injuries, however, in the presence of inflammatory cytokines, NGF may stimulate aggressive remodeling and removal of viable neurons. This may also help explain how elevated BDNF and NGF levels found in patients with fibromyalgia[151, 152] contribute to its pathology.

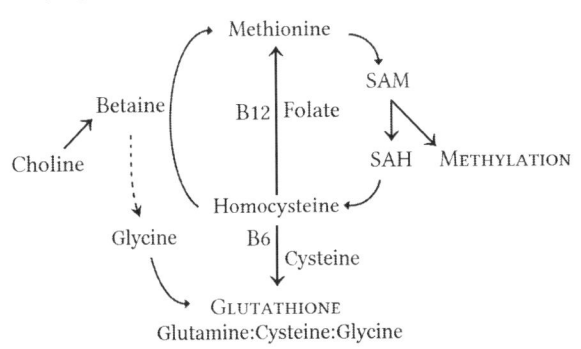

Figure 31-5: Betaine in Homocysteine Methylation

A few small studies have found a beneficial effect of folate or S-Adenosylmethionine (SAMe) for in the treatment of depression, usually as an adjunct to antidepressant medication[153]. Trimethylglycine (TMG, aka betaine) acts as a secondary pathway for recycling homocysteine to methionine. This is particularly importance when folate activity is blocked by inhibition of methionine synthase by the presence of acetaldehyde toxicity, as occurs with alcohol consumption[154]. TMG also supplies glycine to the mitochondria that helps prevent the production of reactive oxygen species. Additionally, TMG also supplies glycine for the production of the tripeptide antioxidant glutathione. Betaine is further discussed in Chapters 30 and 40.

The active form of vitamin B6, pyridoxine-5-phosphate (PLP) is an essential cofactor in the formation of the NMDA antagonist, kynurenic acid, and for the removal of toxic metabolites of kynurenine. PLP is also a cofactor for S1P lyase, the enzyme that destroys S1P. Additionally PLP helps convert HCY to cysteine, both removing a toxic metabolite and supplying an amino acid for the formation of glutathione.

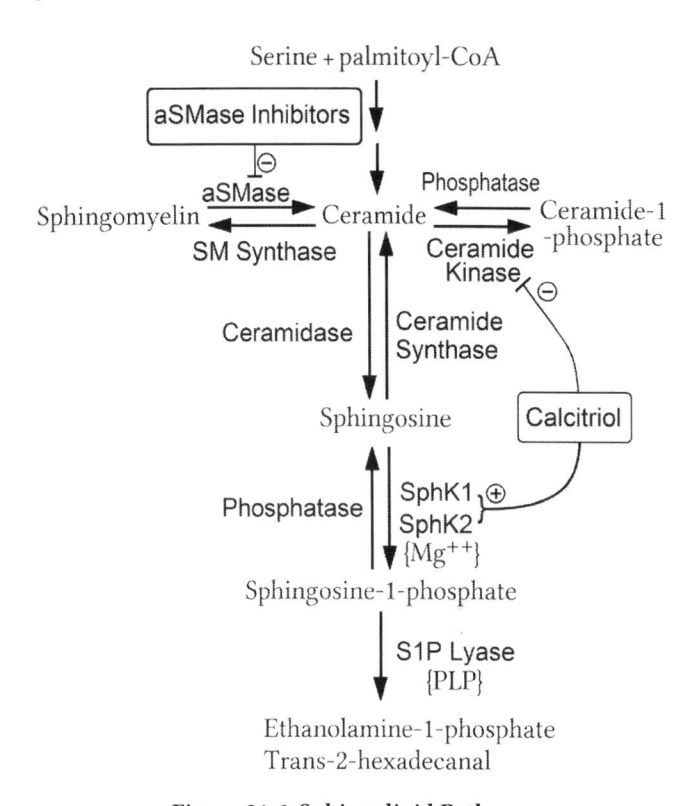

Figure 31-6: Sphingolipid Pathway

Retinoic Acid, Vitamin A

Retinoic acid (RA) receptors are found in the midbrain area, and RA agonists increase tissue level of BDNF mRNA[155]. RA induces expression of the tyrosine kinase receptor B (TrkB), the receptor for neurotrophins[156]. RA provides an essential signal for GDNF (Glial cell-derived neurotrophic factor) associated cellular migration for the enteric nervous system and RA may play a similar role in the CNS[157].

In an experiment, mice were fed a vitamin A and zinc-deficient diet for three months, followed by 2 months on either a high-vitamin A, low-zinc diet or a normal-vitamin A, low-zinc diet. Mice on the high-vitamin A diet had high BDNF and NGF levels; while mice on the low-zinc, normal-vitamin A diet had low levels of these neurotrophins. Thus, vitamin A appears to be essential for normal production of BDNF and NGF[158]. Excess vitamin A, however, results in decreased BDNF and changes in CNS metabolism production in lab animals, which may explain cognitive disturbances caused by vitamin A toxicity[159].

Zinc and the Brain

There is a high prevalence of depression among individuals with acne (Chapter 37). Two nutrients often deficient in acne patients are vitamin A and zinc. Multiple studies have shown an association between depression in humans and depressive-type behaviors in animals with low zinc levels.

Zinc supplements have been found be helpful in several studies of depression[160]. Zinc supplements prevent or improve anxiety, depression and learning impairments in animal models of traumatic brain injury[161]. In a study of dialysis patients, in whom depression is highly prevalent, serum zinc levels were significantly lower in the depressed, compared to non-depressed, dialysis patients[162]. In a study of highly stressed adults, dietary zinc intake was inversely correlated with the level of depression[163]. Chronic unpredictable stress lowers both BDNF and zinc levels in animals[164].

Zinc deficiency is common. It results from low dietary intake of zinc; wasting, from malabsorption; alcohol use, and as a result of stress. Low zinc levels are associated with elevated serum corticosteroid levels and increased activity of the hypothalamic-pituitary-adrenal (HPA) axis. Chronic stress is associated with reduced zinc and BDNF levels[165].

Feeding mice a low vitamin A, low zinc diet provoked low BDNF and NGF levels, and this effect was reversed by supplementing the mice with vitamin A and zinc[166]. Zinc alone increased NGF expression but did not improve memory in vitamin A deficiency[167]. Animal studies suggest that zinc deficiency leads to increased corticosteroids levels, resulting in a fall in BDNF levels. This may explain in part why low zinc levels promote depression[168]. Zinc may be a cofactor for BDNF expression and potentiate the BDNF-TrkB signaling pathway that converts pro-BDNF to mature BDNF[169].

Zinc is a cofactor for many enzymes and also a structural component of many proteins. About 90 percent of the zinc in the brain exists in the form of metalloproteins. Only a tiny fraction of zinc in the brain is extracellular. A small, but essential portion of the zinc in the brain in held in presynaptic vesicles in axon terminals. Zinc is relatively concentrated in the hippocampus and the amygdala. Glutamatergic (zincergic) neurons from these areas release zinc as ions into the extracellular neuronal clefts[170]. These zinc ions modulate the ionotropic glutamate receptors (NMDA, AMPA and kainate receptors). Ionotropic glutamate receptors are excitatory ion channels which open in the presence of glutamate and glycine, allowing the influx of calcium that acts as a second messenger in the target neuron. Zinc acts in place of calcium and limits the entrance of calcium[171]. Zinc thus mitigates glutamate excitotoxicity; a process active in the pathology of Alzheimer's disease, autism, Parkinson's disease, the development of schizophrenia and other neurodegenerative conditions. This suggests that zinc not only acts on neurotrophic factors, but also decreases the effect of quinolinic acid from the kynurenine pathway on the NMDA receptors. Zinc also affects inhibits TLR2 expression[172], and thus, has anti-inflammatory effects.

Similar to zinc, one of lithium's actions is the inhibition of calcium flux through the NMDA receptor[173]. There is some evidence indicating that magnesium may have a similar beneficial effect in the treatment of depression[174].

High dose zinc, however, can induce a hippocampal zinc deficiency, and decreases hippocampal BDNF level and TrkB neurotrophic signaling, and impairs learning[169]. High-dose zinc supplements should usually be avoided, and daily supplemental dose limited to 10 to 20 mg daily.

CREB is a DNA transcription factor that specifically regulates several proteins, including BDNF and several neuropeptides. Sleep deprivation prevents induction of CREB and thus inhibits the protein transcription of BDNF; this may help explain how sleep deprivation prevents memory consolidation. Use of caffeine may protect the formation of CREB and BDNF in sleep deprivation[175]. Coffee consumption has been found to decrease the risk of depression. Women who drink two to three cups of coffee a day have a 15% lower rate of depression; it was 20% lower for those drinking 4 or 5 cups a day. Drinking decaffeinated coffee does not decrease the risk of depression[176].

Coffee and other stimulants may increase the risk of mania in patients with bipolar disorder. Patients with bipolar disorder typically have a circadian sleep drive dysfunction. Circadian sleep drive is one of the two sleep drives, the other being homeostatic sleep drive. In BPD, homeostatic sleep drive (HSD) may still function. HSD relies on the accumulation of adenosine during wakefulness, which causes the feeling of being tired and needing sleep. Sleep drive is discussed in Chapter 41.

Caffeine blocks adenosine receptors in the brain and thus, enhances wakefulness. Caffeine should be used with caution in patients with bipolar disorder as it can trigger mania. Theobromine from chocolate can also block adenosine receptors.

In Chapter 9, it was described how rising uric acid levels end hibernation, acting as a stimulant, similar to caffeine. Elevated uric acid levels may also trigger mania in bipolar patients. Uric acid has been found to be elevated during mania and to correlate with mania assessment scores[177]. Allopurinol, which lowers uric acid levels, has been found to be an effective treatment for acute mania[178]. Uric acid levels tend to be even higher in schizophrenic patients, but lower than normal in depressed patients[179].

In mice, a diet deficient in tryptophan for two weeks decreased hippocampal levels of NGF but did not affect levels of BDNF or NT-3. BDNF, however, was significantly lower in the cerebral cortex on the tryptophan deficient diet, while the levels of NGF and NT-3 were unchanged in this brain region. Supplemental tryptophan, in excess of the normal dietary levels, did not affect neurotrophin levels[180].

Exercise, novel experiences, and play help maintain youthful BDNF levels and keep our minds young. Exercise causes an acute increase in inflammatory cytokines including IL-6 and TNF-α[181], and thus triggers a short-term rise in kynurenine levels. Like corticosteroid, this burst of inflammation may cause an increase in BDNF. Short-term elevations in corticosteroids induce BDNF while chronic exposure exhausts hippocampal BDNF levels and may induce long-term, epigenetic reduction in BDNF production. A short-term, burst of inflammatory cytokines, as occurs with exercise, lowers chronic inflammatory cytokine levels. Note, in Figure 31-2, that the kynurenine metabolite, anthranilic acid, provides a negative feedback to IDO. Thus, a short burst of proinflammatory cytokine exposure may induce a negative feedback or kynurenine production. Note also that the enzymes for this feedback process require adequate pyridoxal-5-phosphate (PLP), as does the conversion of tryptophan to neuroprotective compound, kynurenic acid, and the calming neurotransmitter, serotonin.

Fatigue, Myalgia, and INF-γ

Fatigue, poverty of motion, myalgia and somatization are common features of MDD. These signs and symptoms may be caused by elevations of interferon, particularly, INF-γ. INF-γ is elevated during viral or other intracellular infections and helps explain how the flu makes us feel awful. Flu-like symptoms often accompany interferon treatment of hepatitis C. Neopterin, an indicator of macrophage activity and INF-γ production, is often elevated in MDD. Microglia produce INF-γ in response to IL-12 and IL-18[182]. In the CNS, INF-γ activates other microglia and impairs the viability of neural progenitor cells[183]. In the spinal cord, INF-γ produces long-lasting allodynia to innocuous stimuli[184].

INF-γ is an essential part of the immune defense against intracellular infection important for macrophage activity in both innate and adaptive immunity. INF-γ is produced principally by natural killer cells after antigen-specific immunity develops. However, it also can cause illness behavior and symptoms. Thus, pathological elevations of INF-γ should be avoided by identifying and treating the underlying cause.

Table 31-5: Factors Affecting Interferon-γ Production

Increase INF-γ	Examples
Intracellular Infections	*Toxoplasmosis gondii, Yersinia, Chlamydia, Cryptococcus*
Granulomatous Disease	Tuberculosis, Crohn's disease, sarcoidosis, coccidioidomycosis,
Alcohol[185]	
Decrease INF-γ	
Flavonoids	Quercetin[185]
Medications	Milk thistle (*Silybum marianum*)[186]
Xylo-oligosaccharides[187]	Short-chain xylose polysaccharides formed by fermentation in the gut

Schizophrenia

Schizophrenia is a devastating disease, characterized by psychosis, delusions, hallucinations, disorganized thinking, depression, and disability. It is also associated with a 20- to 25-year reduction in life expectancy. It is associated with high rates of homelessness, cardiovascular disease, substance abuse and suicide[188]. Much of the loss in life expectancy results from adverse behaviors, poor choices, and poverty: poor diet, tobacco, alcohol, and drug abuse, and the inability these individuals to properly care for themselves. In the United States, about one-third of the homeless population has schizophrenia or BPD, and 20% of those in jail or prison have schizophrenia[189].

Table 31-6: Major Symptoms of Schizophrenia

Symptoms	Examples
Positive	Delusions, hallucinations, bizarre behavior: responds to dopamine receptor 2 antagonists
Negative	Poverty of speech, anhedonia, avolition, apathy, flat affect. Negative symptoms do not respond to antipsychotic medications.
Cognitive Dysfunction	Inattention, slow mental processing, deficits in executive functioning, impaired memory, and language deviations: a major cause of disability
Mood	Anxiety and depression: another cause of disability

Schizophrenia is a chronic disease which begins long before symptoms manifest. An animal model of schizophrenia can be induced by prenatal immune challenge[190]. In humans, there is a premorbid state, usually during early adolescence, during which neurologic damage occurs. This also occurs in bipolar disorder. These diseases have similar prodromal symptoms which typically manifest in late adolescence. Loss of gray matter in the brain during this time has been documented in schizophrenia[191]. The similar prodromal and early clinical manifestations of these two diseases make them difficult to differentiate early in their courses. The elevations in proinflammatory cytokines present in schizophrenia and bipolar disorder are also similar.

Prodromal symptoms may be followed by frank disease and a psychotic event, at which point treatment usually begins. In schizophrenia, treatment with antipsychotic agents often provides recovery from the positive symptoms; however, the patient lives with the residual symptoms of the disease. Most patients have difficulty living independently.

There is hope that early treatment of schizophrenia and BPD during the prodromal stage can halt the development of these diseases. One difficulty is identifying those at highest risk. It is inappropriate to treat low-risk individuals with drugs, which have side effects, who would not go on to develop the disease. Even with screening, only about one in six of those in the ultra-high risk group develops schizophrenia[192]. To date, only one intervention has worked consistently to prevent progression of prodrome disease to schizophrenia, and that treatment is n-3 fatty acids[193].

Table 31-7: Prodromic Feature Comparison[194, 195]

Feature	Schizophrenia	Bipolar Disorder
Age at Prodrome Identification	17.1 ± 2.7	15.9 ± 1.8
Age at Disease Onset	18.4 ± 2.3	18.4 ± 3.1
Premorbid IQ	102.4 ± 15.7	103.1 ± 14.5
IQ at Diagnosis	96.3 ± 12.5	94.5 ± 23.2
Irritability and Anger	39%	35%
Decreased Academic Performance	42%	64%
Social Isolation	57%	44%
Anxiety	25%	33%
Anhedonia	33%	44%
Obsession or Compulsion	5%	29%*
Mood Swings	9%	30%*
Difficulty Thinking or Communicating	18%	40%*
Suicidal Ideation	7%	31%*
Physical Agitation	17%	40%*
Depression	16%	47%*
Decreased Concentration	25%	52%*
Fatigue or Lack of Energy	12%	31%*
Increased Energy		48%*
Grandiosity		20%*
Strange Ideas	53%*	18%

* The prevalence is statistically greater than in the other disease

Since the 1970's, the treatment of schizophrenia has focused on excess dopamine activity. Dopaminergic drugs, such as amphetamines and PCP, cause psychosis; drugs that block D_2 receptors decreased psychosis. D_2 antipsychotic medications, however, only treat the positive symptoms of schizophrenia. Recent understanding indicates that the multiple symptoms of schizophrenia arise from hypoactivity of glutaminergic neurons, and dopaminergic (DA) hyperactivity occurs as a result of the loss of glutaminergic (or GABAergic) activity[196].

There is mounting evidence that both schizophrenia and bipolar disorder are inflammatory diseases. These diseases may be caused by excitotoxic damage to glutaminergic neurons. Cytokines, such as IL-1β, IL-6, and TNF-α, can affect the glial cells in the CNS, promoting excitatory response. LPS, from enteric bacteria, in the presence of INF-γ, stimulates the immune activation of microglia, the production of NO and TNF-α, and cytotoxicity in the CNS[197]. This inflammatory process may better explain the pathogenesis of schizophrenia as well that of several other neurologic diseases.

IL-1β, IL-6, and TGF-β are usually elevated in patients with schizophrenia at the time of diagnosis. IL-12, IFN-γ, TNF-α, and soluble IL-2 receptor (sIL-2R) are elevated during acute exacerbations and may remain high following antipsychotic treatment[198]. IL-18, which promotes INF-γ production, has also been found to be elevated in patients with newly diagnosed schizophrenia[199]. IL-2, which is important for immune memory, and NGF have been found to be low in these patients[200]. Some atypical antipsychotics, such as clozapine, suppress TNF-α and IL-6, and up-regulated IL-10[201]. This may be an important aspect of their therapeutic efficacy.

LPS from the cell walls of anaerobic bacteria activates cell membrane TLR-4 on WBC's and other cells, activating transcription factors for inflammatory cytokines and growth factors for immune cells and microglia. Most opiates act as TLR-4 agonists while tricyclic antidepressants antagonize TLR-4 activation. Vitamin D_3, zinc, and betaine also down-regulate TLR-4 expression (Figure 32-4). Certain bacteria, fungi, parasites, and viruses activate TLR-2. Minocycline and doxycycline block inflammatory transcription factor activation and thus act as anti-inflammatory agents (See Table 30-5) Minocycline, which crosses the blood-brain barrier, has shown efficacy in the treatment of schizophrenia[202] and bipolar depression[203], usually at a dose of 150 to 200 mg per day[204].

Minocycline and doxycycline also have antidepressant effects. They prevent and reverse LPS-induced increases in IL-1β and declines in hippocampal BDNF levels[205]. Since it is thought that doxycycline does not cross the blood-brain barrier, this reinforces the role of peripheral inflammatory factors in the genesis of depression.

Clearly, these are inflammatory diseases, and preventive treatment, including secondary prevention, should focus on treating inflammation. Neuroinflammatory disease is best identified and treated early, to preventive the loss of neural and glial cells. CNS immunoexcitotoxicity will be discussed in further detail in Chapter 31.

Schizophrenia, Toxoplasmosis, and Prions

On traditional small farms, cats were kept in barns to keep the rodent population down. Rodents are naturally adverse to cat odors, and thus avoid areas with cats. Rats infected with *T. gondii*, however, are sexually aroused by the smell of cats[206]. This fatal attraction is an implicit part of the parasite's life cycle, as it is the means by which cats, the definitive host of this disease, are infected; the rat delivers itself as a meal, containing *T. gondii* cysts. Infected cats, through their scats, can infect sheep, goats, pigs and cattle by contaminating the animals' feeding area parasite eggs.

One-third of humanity is infected with *Toxoplasmosis gondii*. Humans acquire *T. gondii* infection most often from contact with infected cats and their feces, but also from poorly cooked meat from infected farm animals.

Sea otters, apparently infected by cat feces contamination of water from shore, are more likely to die from shark attacks than are unaffected otters. Humans with *T. gondii* are more likely to be in auto accidents[207]. This is likely a result of the slowed reaction times[208] and more aggressive, risky behaviors; perhaps in part, resulting from higher testosterone levels[209]; male students with this infection are taller and have more masculine faces[210]. Another behavioral oddity is that it is not only infected rats that like the smell of cats. It appears that affected humans do as well[211], which may give rise to cat hoarding.

The causal mechanism for these distinctive behavioral changes may be explained by enzymes T. gondii produces in its hosts. In addition to testicular steroidogenesis, this intracellular parasite produces aromatic hydroxylases, analogous to tyrosine hydroxylase and phosphatidylserine decarboxylase[212]. Tyrosine hydroxylase (TH) increases dopamine biosynthesis in the brain and increases production of ROS. Elevated levels of dopamine release have been found in rodents infected with T. gondii[213]. T. gondii infects microglia and increases production of kynurenine and its metabolites in the brain[214].

This increase in dopamine may also explain the increased risk of schizophrenia among those infected with this T. gondii. At least 40 studies have shown an increased risk for schizophrenia among individuals with antibodies to Toxoplasmosis gondii. Infected individuals are about 2.7 times more likely to developing schizophrenia than unaffected persons[215]. Further, schizophrenic patients appear to have impaired CD8+ cell immunity, required for fighting this infection[216].

Toxoplasmosis gondii infection has also been associated with increased risk of suicide, bipolar disorder, migraines, obsessive-compulsive disorder, Parkinson's disease, and Alzheimer's disease[211]. Phosphatidylserine decarboxylase's main product is phosphatidylethanolamine, which affects the membrane structure, and can alter the folding of proteins, including causing the induction of prions[217]. T. gondii infection is common in among goats, sheep, cattle[218], mink, and cats; animals that are susceptible to prion diseases such as scrapie and bovine spongiform encephalopathy (Mad Cow Disease).

The most common prion disease in humans is the invariably fatal Creutzfeldt–Jakob (CJD) disease, which fortunately, is nearly as rare as it is terrifying. It is responsible for about 1 death per million in the U.S. An epidemic, variant form of the disease occurred in Great Britain in the 1990's, as a result of eating beef that had been given feed containing rendered animal protein from sheep with scrapie. CJD can be transmitted through consumption of affected meat, from contaminated surgical instruments, or from brain or optical tissue. Most cases, however, or arise spontaneously.

In Alzheimer's disease (AD), alterations in protein folding cause an accumulation of β-amyloid plaques. AD patients were found to have T. gondii antibodies nearly twice as often as age-matched controls[219]. While alterations in protein folding may be associated with this disease, the very similar relative risks T. gondii confers on Parkinson's disease[220], OCD[221], and migraine[222], and autoimmune disorders, including rheumatoid arthritis and inflammatory bowel disease[223], suggest a similar, immunoexcitotoxicity mechanism among these diseases. In both bipolar disorder[224] and schizophrenia[225], T. gondii antibodies are highly correlated with antibodies to foods (antergies) and to ASCA (yeast). T. gondii infection greatly increases IgG response to gluten in experimental animals[226]. This parasite appears to induce antergies and promote enteroimmune disease.

In a murine model, T. gondii infection appears to promote enteric biofilm proliferation from normally commensal E. coli, thus triggering the inflammatory response, through the production of LPS and activation via TLR-4 receptors[227]. As an intracellular infection, T. gondii would be expected to increase INF-γ production, and its increase in TH would increase oxidative stress in the CNS.

Unless data becomes available that proscribes it, T. gondii infection should be treated in prodromal and new-onset schizophrenia and bipolar disorder as there is active, and likely irreparable, inflammatory damage to postmitotic cells in the CNS. Research is needed in the area of prevention and on the efficacy of treatment of toxoplasmosis during the different phases of these diseases. Clearly, the greatest benefit is expected from treatment prior to damage to the CNS. Treatment late in the disease is unlikely to do much.

To prevent T. gondii infections, cats, and their litter boxes should be kept out of the kitchen and dining areas. Hand washing should be done after handling cats and before meals. Meat should be fully cooked to destroy paracytic cysts in meat. Cooking does not destroy or inactivate the prions. To prevent contraction of prion disease, consumption of brain and other neurological tissue should be foresworn.

Estrogen appears to be protective against schizophrenia. Women have a lower incidence, later onset, and less debilitating disease; however, the disease worsens in women after menopause. Estrogen therapy has been shown to be effective adjuvant therapy for schizophrenia in women[228], and use of selective estrogen receptor modulators, which would avoid feminization, has been suggested for men with schizophrenia[229].

Here, I suggest the use of boron supplements as adjunctive therapy for schizophrenia. Boron helps stabilize estrogen and raises the estrogen/testosterone ratio. Boron is discussed in Chapter 37.

Summary

Inflammation plays a central role in the causation of affective disease and thought disorders. Systemic inflammation can arise from enteroimmunopathy, with the production of LPS from intestinal bacteria. This and other immune activities which elicit inflammatory cytokines may adversely stimulate kynurenine and impair neurotrophin production. LPS and inflammatory cytokines, such as IL-1β, IL-6, INF-γ and TNF-α, induce IDO and the kynurenine pathway and a fall in BDNF from the hippocampus. These cytokines activate glial inflammatory activity producing oxidative and neuroexcitotoxic damage. LPS[230] and chronic stress raise corticosterone levels, and thereby, impair neurotrophin production.

In an animal model in which anxiety behavior is induced by mild to moderate colonic inflammation, two mechanisms for anxiety were observed: activation of the kynurenic pathway and a decline in BDNF. Certain anti-inflammatory treatments including steroids were able to normalize behavior, but as would be expected, steroids did not to normalize the BDNF levels. Probiotic bacteria were able to normalize behavior and BDNF levels but did not normalize the kynurenic pathway[231]. This suggests that both pathways contribute to depressive and anxiety behaviors; each resulting from different aspects of inflammation.

Depression and other affective disorders, and thought disorders, such as schizophrenia are neuroinflammatory diseases. Treatment that addresses the inflammatory underpinnings is essential to successful treatment. Emotional, physical, and oxidative stress, and sleep deprivation can induce inflammatory cytokines, promote IDO and impair BDNF production.

Acute, high levels of cytokines, released during intensive exercise, downregulate the kynurenic pathway and acute stress increases BDNF. Play and novel situations, such as travel and exploration, provide positive short-term stimulus which give "acute stress" a beneficial effect on BDNF. Low BDNF is associated with depression and anxiety, and may affect memory and learning. GDNF and other neurotrophic factors likely have similar influences in other CNS diseases.

Inappropriately high levels of neurotrophic factors may also cause disease. Dysregulation of neurotrophic factors, where levels are excessive, perhaps resulting from a rebound from low levels or induced by repeated injury/repair cycles, may damage the nervous system. Multiple sclerosis may be an example of this.

The n-3 fatty acids EPA and DHA decrease inflammation. DHA increases the production of BDNF and helps prevent hypermethylation during the perinatal period.

Chronic stress can cause the methylation of DNA, and thus, chronic, epigenetic downregulation of BDNF transcription in the hippocampus. During embryogenesis, epigenetic setttings are erased; the epigenic settings are restored to normal, allowing reprogramming of BDNF and other stress adaptors, so that the offspring can better adapt to their environment. Although slow, cellular replacement may also allow an opportunity to undo epigenetic imprinting.

The antidepressant imipramine has been demonstrated to reverse methylation of BDNF DNA with chronic treatment, to restore normal BDNF production. Some non-toxic components of the diet can also reverse DNA methylation. These compounds may also lower risk of cancer and are further discussed in Chapter 41. Of course, it is only beneficial to reset epigenetic reprogramming during times of health and in a favorable environment; not during times of chronic stress, where the outcome would be an adaptation to adversity, increased stress and risk of disease.

Dietary factors that can help reset epigenetic programming are outlined in table 29-2.

> Medications for depression are among those most commonly prescribed. The commonly used, second-generation antidepressants have, at best, about 50% response rate[232]. The information provided in this chapter is not intended to dissuade appropriate use of these medications, but rather, to explain secondary prevention of mood disorders.

Prevention and Remediation of Depression, Mood, and Thought Disorders

1. Avoid Inflammation
2. Avoid Oxidative Stress
3. Avoid Chronic Stress.
4. Avoid Sleep Deprivation.
5. Avoid Alcohol.
6. Avoid intestinal dysbiosis, leaky gut, and malabsorption.
7. Test for and avoid food immunogens.
8. Treat nutrient deficiencies.
9. Reduce n-6 fats in the diet, and increase n-3 fats.
10. Engage in short-term stress and novel experiences. Play, exercise and have fun!
11. Use interdiction in the inflammatory pathway (Chapter 32)
12. Test for and treat *Toxoplasmosis* or chronic intracellular infections.

2. Avoid Oxidative Stress. Prevention of oxidative stress is discussed in Chapter 21. Adding antioxidants, however, does not repair existing oxidative damage and is not as effective as a healthy diet in preventing oxidative damage. Supplements may be helpful when there are nutritional deficits, but a healthful diet contains a diverse mix of antioxidants phenolic compounds not likely to be found in supplements. Polyphenol compounds that are not absorbed help keep food fresh, and may act as antioxidants and as quorum sensing inhibitors in the intestine.

Glutathione is the major antioxidant in the nervous system. N-acetyl cysteine may be useful to replenish glutathione. Alpha-lipoic acid reduces H_2O_2, and thus, prevents activation of acid SMase by hydrogen peroxide, created during cellular stress. Betaine (trimethylglycine) supplies glycine for glutathione, and thus helps prevents oxidative damage. Betaine helps recycle homocysteine into SAMe and lowers HCY toxicity. It also down-regulates inflammatory TLR expression. Additionally, betaine is a source of glycine for the neuron, which helps regulate glutaminergic activity.

Consume a balanced diet high in antioxidants. Carotenoids (including lutein, β-carotene, and zeaxanthin), vitamins E, vitamin C, selenium, and PQQ. It also includes multiple antioxidant polyphenols from fruits, seeds, and vegetables. It is nearly impossible to get adequate amounts of these antioxidants when the diet derives most of its calories from refined or manufactured foods.

3. Avoid Chronic Stress: Stress is often self-induced, and stress reactions largely result from our response to situations. Depressed individuals are more likely to have strong stress reactions to moderately stressful situations and crisis reactions to worse ones. Stress can thus snowball. Avoiding stressors, such as sleep deprivation, alcohol, and hunger can make life's daily stresses wield less impact. Chapter 29 contains a section on stress reduction. In Chapter 32, the first section under mitigation and treatment has additional information on stress mitigation.

In-utero stress and stress during infancy may induce lifelong hyperreactivity to stress through epigenetic modification in the expression of stress hormones, thus increasing susceptibility to chronic stress reactions. As in adults, an active, enriched environment, exercise, and play act as short-term stress and lower stress response.

Stress that has induced epigenetic basis is difficult to correct, but can be rectified, as is discussed in Chapter 29.

3. Maintain a Normal Sleep Cycle and Avoid Sleep Deprivation: Circadian disturbances are common in depression, premenstrual dysphoric syndrome, and bipolar disorder. Individuals with bipolar disorder should avoid stimulants, including caffeine and theobromine, as well as avoiding elevations in uric acid level. Sleep deprivation increases levels of proinflammatory cytokines. Chapter 41 provides an in-depth discussion of sleep.

5. Avoid Alcohol: Consumption of more than moderate amounts of alcohol greatly increases the risk for depression. Moderate consumption of alcohol does not. Moderate consumption, limiting consumption to no more than the equivalent of one ounce of red wine per day per 30 pounds of ideal body weight, is not a risk for most adults (other than pregnant women or women with a family history of breast cancer). This level of alcohol consumption also does not cause intoxication. Health benefits and risks from alcohol are further discussed in Chapters 17 and 40.

6. Avoid malabsorption, dysbiosis, SIBO and leaky gut: Proteins that are incompletely digested ferment in the colon, promote bacterial overgrowth, dysbiosis and production of LPS and other toxins. LPS induces IDO and kynurenine production. Prevention and treatment of dysbiosis are covered in Chapter 23; SIBO in Chapter 24; and leaky gut in Chapter 25. Elevation in fecal chymotrypsin levels may be used as an indicator of poor protein absorption. Diet with a high diversity of vegetables and fruit provides for a healthy, diverse colonic biome, less likely to promote biofilm and LPS production.

7. Test for and avoid food immunogens: Depression, mood, and thought disorders are inflammatory conditions, and the intestine is the most common source of peripheral inflammatory cytokines. The intestinal mucosa houses half the immune cells in the body and can produce significant inflammation without localizing symptoms. Intestinal mucosal hyperpermeability allows the immune system to be confronted with proteins and peptides from foods, and greater absorption of LPS and other toxins. Repeated immune confrontation by food proteins and peptides promotes mast cell hypertrophy and up-regulates T_H17 immune function. *Elimination of food antergens and allergens often provides rapid relief in mood, behavioral, and thought disorders.* Testing and treatment of antergies is discussed in Chapter 19. Elevated levels of antibodies to foods, including yeasts (ASCA) are found in patients with bipolar disorder and in schizophrenia. Mast cell activation can also trigger inflammation and oxidative stress in the brain. See Chapter 12.

8. Treat nutrient deficiencies: Supplements are unlikely to provide many benefits to those with good nutrition and a healthy gastrointestinal system. Inflammatory disease, however, usually indicates there are nutritional problems. SIBO, malabsorption, and alcohol use all cause loss of zinc and other nutrients. The fat-soluble vitamins (A, D, E, and K), folate, vitamin B_{12}, magnesium, and tryptophan are easily lost in malabsorption. Of these, only vitamin K was not discussed as a factor in depression in this chapter; however, its anti-inflammatory effects in the CNS are in Chapters 31. Essential to the treatment of nutrient deficiencies is the treatment of the underlying cause: poor diet, malabsorption or dysbiosis of the gut being the usual suspects.

Vitamin D_3 helps to modulate the immune response and likely interacts with n-3 fats in disease prevention. Adequate Vitamin D_3 should be assured (See Chapter 20). It may take 6000 IU daily, over several months, to reach a target 25-OHD_3 treatment level of 100 nmol/L[233]. Thus, if vitamin D levels are low, an oral loading dose of up to 300,000 units may be appropriate. Vitamin D treatment requires follow-up to verify that it has been effective. See Chapter 20.

Magnesium (Mg) is essential in minimizing CNS inflammation and downregulated neuroglial inflammatory activity. Several studies have shown that Mg supplements to have synergistic effects with SSRI's in treating depression, and Mg supplementation improves symptoms of depression in major depression, postpartum depression, premenstrual syndrome, and chronic fatigue syndrome[234].

Mg decreases sphingolipid and kynurenine toxicity. Mg and vitamin D are most common nutritional deficits for those consuming Western diets. An organic Mg salt, such as Mg citrate, at 300 mg daily is usually appropriate. The B vitamins, especially those involved in the formation of SAMe; folate, PLP, B12, and betaine are important nutrients in the prevention and treatment of mood and thought disorders. Recommendations for Vitamin A (provitamin A) and zinc are given in Chapter 36, on acne. Vitamin K2 (menatetrenone) 5 mg daily can be helpful to decrease chronic CNS inflammation.

9. Reduce saturated, n-6 fats in the diet. Increase n-3 fat intake: Depression and other diseases that respond to n-3 fatty acid supplements are not caused just by dietary deficits of α-linolenic acid and its metabolite EPA, but rather, more commonly, due to excesses of arachidonic acid-derived eicosanoids resulting from excess linoleic acid (LA) in the western diet. A low-fat diet, with less vegetable oil and less corn-fed animal protein, contains less LA and more α-linolenic acid. Nuts are a good source of α-linolenic acid, and fish is an excellent source of EPA and DHA. It may be especially important to avoid medium chain saturated fats. 16:0, 18:0, and 20:0 fatty acids and ceramides give rise to inflammatory sphingolipids associated with CNS inflammation and depression.

A reasonable dose for the treatment of depression, based on treatment trials, is one gram of EPA twice daily. A four ounce serving of Atlantic herring contains about one gram of EPA. A four ounce serving of Atlantic salmon has about one-third of this amount[235]. Although fish are an excellent source of EPA, it would be difficult to get this amount of EPA from the diet. Treatment of BPD or schizophrenia should provide both DHA and EPA, one gram twice daily.

α-linolenic acid or EPA and DHA supplements may have therapeutic effects; however, just adding n-3 fat supplements is not as efficient as is replacing excess dietary LA. A change in the food supply to a healthier content and balance of fatty acids should be the goal of individuals and for society as a whole. A food supply which prevents an epidemic of depression, other mood disorders, and inflammatory diseases, is an essential goal for a sustainable society. The oceans cannot feed the world's population with several pounds of fish per person per week.

An appropriate goal is to reduce the amount of n-6 fatty acids in the food supply and reduce excess fructose. Corn subsidies create market conditions where feed corn, corn oil and corn syrup make food cheap. However, we pay for this with a disease burden which ruins lives and consumes 17% of the gross domestic product.

10. Play, exercise and have fun! Play is good for the brain at every age. Remember to have fun. Adults in our society should not expect to have sufficient fun, without planning and reserving time for it. Do something different. Novelty, visiting new places, and doing new activities increase the formation of BDNF in the brain.

BDNF is induced by exercise[236] and new experiences. Earlier, I suggested the evolutionary role of BDNF in foraging. This involved exercise: walking, or running during a hunt or while exploring new places. Foragers often had the reward of an antioxidant food. Recreate this in your life. Visit new places, and engage in activities that include walking and foraging. Even if it is only trying a new food store, or taking a walk in a different park, inviting a friend for a meal, or trying a different eatery; step out of routines and do new things. I suggest keeping a log, keeping notes of activities: dates, persons, place, motive, and results, helps stimulate memory formation. BDNF is required for antidepressants to work.

BDNF is also required for new place memory; thus, going to new places stimulates its production. Different types of experiences and learning and development of different skills induces the production of different neurotrophic factors. BDNF appears important in depression; other neurotrophic factors may help in the recovery from other neurologic diseases. The frontal lobe is important for judgment, discrimination, and impulse control. For example, tasks or games which require sorting based on varying criteria may induce neurotrophic factors that induce growth in this area. BDNF only promotes growth when in the presence of anti-inflammatory cytokines. In an inflammatory milieu, there is greater neuronal loss.

Exercise: For exercise to be effective in lowering oxidative stress, it needs to be intense enough to provoke mitophagy – the removal of old, inefficient mitochondria. The muscles need to get warmed up and export lactate. Ten minutes of vigorous exercise a day may be a minimum requirement. Exercise is further discussed in Chapter 21. Lactate is used as fuel by the brain during exercise and may help to stimulate the turnover of mitochondria in the CNS as well as in the muscles.

Additional Treatment Concerns for Bipolar Disorder and Schizophrenia

Patients with bipolar disorder should avoid caffeine and theobromine as they can disrupt the homeostatic sleep drive. Uric acid can also have this effect, and elevated levels may also worsen symptoms in schizophrenia. Bipolar and schizophrenia patients should be monitored and treated to keep uric acid levels within the optimal range. Uric acidemia should be checked especially during episodes of mania. These patients should be advised to limit high fructose diets and alcohol to prevent elevated serum uric acid levels. Optimal ranges for uric acid and preventive treatment are given in Chapter 9.

Vitamin D levels (Chapter 20) should also be optimized for these patients and a low n-6: n-3 fat ratio maintained in their diet: they should have at least one gram of n-3 fats in the daily diet.

Mitigation of LPS, TNF-α, INF-γ, and other inflammatory cytokines is especially important in the secondary prevention of BPD and schizophrenia. TNF-α mitigation is discussed in Chapter 31.

Medications and supplements may also be used to prevent the transcription of inflammatory cytokines. Vitamin D and betaine down-regulated TLR-2 and TLR-4 expression. DHA and PQQ activate PPAR-γ, and thus, inhibit TLR inflammatory signaling. Many plant polyphenols, tricyclic antidepressants, and minocycline inhibit transcription of inflammatory cytokines and thus, may be useful in the treatment of BP disorder and schizophrenia and other inflammatory disorders. See chapters 31 and 42 for further discussion and references.

PQQ, N-acetyl cysteine, and melatonin are antioxidant in the CNS that may be useful in the secondary prevention of BP disorder and schizophrenia. N-acetylcysteine also indirectly stimulates presynaptic metabotropic glutamate receptors and has demonstrated clinical efficacy in the treatment of schizophrenia two randomized, double-blinded trials[237]. Lipoic acid, as an antioxidant, helps prevent liberation of ceramide from sphingomyelin in the cell membrane as a result of acid SMase activity, which can induce apoptosis, or be converted to C1P and S1P, which induce inflammation and microglial activation. TNF-α and IL-1β also induce S1P, and should be mitigated.

Melatonin, SAMe, and DHA modulate epigenetic imprinting that can increase the lifetime risk for depression. Epigenetic imprinting is discussed in Chapter 29.

As nutritional supplements, N-acetyl cysteine and trimethylglycine should be thought of as amino acid supplements. They are used in gram doses rather than milligram or microgram doses.

Boron, as amino acid chelates, may be helpful in schizophrenia. For men, I suggest starting with 10 – 12 mg daily, and then reducing the dose after a few weeks to 6 mg daily, and 6 mg daily for women.

Schizophrenia and BPD should be considered urgent medical conditions, in which delayed treatment is associated with progressive, irreversible, neurologic damage. Use of benign dietary supplements should not be withheld awaiting a response from either dietary modification nor from pharmacologic interventions.

Testing for and treating *T. gondii* in prodromal or newly diagnosed schizophrenia, BPD or depression may provide benefit.

The following list is an example of daily starting supplements for the treatment of schizophrenia. Doses may be split (E.g.: half in A.M. and half in P.M.):

Pyridoxine – 5 mg
Riboflavin – 15 mg
EPA + DHA - 1000 mg
R-alpha-lipoic acid: Use R–lipoic acid sodium – 100 mg*
Quercetin – 1000 mg
Vitamin D3[†] (10-day loading dose) – 30,000 IU
N-Acetyl Cysteine – 2000 mg
Betaine – 3000 mg
Magnesium citrate or Mg Malate – 400 mg
Boron: – 12 mg
Vitamin K2 (Menatetrenone MK4): – 5 mg[‡]
Melatonin – 3 mg at bedtime

* See Lipoic acid supplementation in Chapter 40.

† Vitamin D3, if documented to be low, can be administered as a loading dose, as discussed in Chapter 20. Here, 30,000 can be given daily for 10 days, before lowering the amount to the maintenance dose of about 6000 IU per day.

‡ If malabsorption is considered to be a contributing factor to disease causation, Vitamin K2 (Menatetrenone) should be added. Menatetrenone inhibits inflammation by inhibiting NF-κB activation[238].

[1] Prevalence, severity, and comorbidity of 12-month DSM-IV disorders in the National Comorbidity Survey Replication. Kessler RC, Chiu WT, Demler O, Merikangas KR, Walters EE. Arch Gen Psychiatry. 2005 Jun;62(6):617-27. PMID:15939839

[2] Depressive-like parameters in sepsis survivor rats. Comim CM, Cassol-Jr OJ, Constantino LC, et al. Neurotox Res. 2010 Apr;17(3):279-86. PMID:19705213

[3] Overweight, obesity, and depression: a systematic review and meta-analysis of longitudinal studies. Luppino FS, de Wit LM, Bouvy PF, et al. Arch Gen Psychiatry. 2010 Mar;67(3):220-9. PMID:20194822

[4] Circulating long-chain ω-3 fatty acids and incidence of congestive heart failure in older adults: the cardiovascular health study: a cohort study. Mozaffarian D, Lemaitre RN, King IB, et al. Ann Intern Med. 2011 Aug 2;155(3):160-70. PMID:21810709

[5] Low levels of the omega-3 index are associated with sudden cardiac arrest and remain stable in survivors in the subacute phase. Aarsetoey H, Aarsetoey R, Lindner T, Staines H, Harris WS, Nilsen DW. Lipids. 2011 Feb;46(2):151-61. PMID:21234696

[6] Dietary intake of α-linolenic acid and low ratio of n-6:n-3 PUFA are associated with decreased exhaled NO and improved asthma control. Barros R, Moreira A, Fonseca J, Delgado L, Castel-Branco MG, Haahtela T, Lopes C, Moreira P. Br J Nutr. 2011 Aug;106(3):441-50. PMID:21443816

[7] Dietary conjugated linoleic acid and n-3 polyunsaturated fatty acids in inflammatory bowel disease. Bassaganya-Riera J, Hontecillas R. Curr Opin Clin Nutr Metab Care. 2010 Sep;13(5):569-73. PMID:20508519

[8] Acne vulgaris, mental health and omega-3 fatty acids: a report of cases. Rubin MG, Kim K, Logan AC. Lipids Health Dis. 2008 Oct 13;7:36. PMID:18851733

[9] Meta-analysis of the effects of eicosapentaenoic acid (EPA) in clinical trials in depression. Sublette ME, Ellis SP, Geant AL, Mann JJ. J Clin Psychiatry. 2011 Sep 6. PMID:21939614

[10] Cognitive and emotional alterations are related to hippocampal inflammation in a mouse model of metabolic syndrome. Dinel AL, André C, Aubert A, Ferreira G, Layé S, Castanon N. PLoS One. 2011;6(9):e24325. PMID:21949705

[11] Antidepressant drug effects and depression severity: a patient-level meta-analysis. Fournier JC, DeRubeis RJ, Hollon SD, et al. JAMA. 2010 Jan 6;303(1):47-53. PMID:20051569

[12] Indoleamine 2,3-dioxygenase in intestinal immunity and inflammation. Cherayil BJ. Inflamm Bowel Dis. 2009 Sep;15(9):1391-6. Review.PMID: 19322906

[13] Predictors of mood response to acute tryptophan depletion. A reanalysis. Booij L, Van der Does W, Benkelfat C, et al. Neuropsychopharmacology. 2002 Nov;27(5):852-61.PMID: 12431859

[14] Low-dose tryptophan depletion in recovered depressed women induces impairments in autobiographical memory specificity. Haddad AD, Williams JM, McTavish SF, Harmer CJ. Psychopharmacology (Berl). 2009 Dec;207(3):499-508. PMID:19813003

[15] Effects of acute tryptophan depletion on mood and cognitive functioning in older recovered depressed subjects. Porter RJ, Phipps AJ, Gallagher P, Scott A, Stevenson PS, O'Brien JT. Am J Geriatr Psychiatry. 2005 Jul;13(7):607-15. PMID:16009737

[16] A double dissociation in the roles of serotonin and mood in healthy subjects. Robinson OJ, Sahakian BJ. Biol Psychiatry. 2009 Jan 1;65(1):89-92. PMID:18996509

[17] Effects of acute tryptophan depletion in serotonin reuptake inhibitor-remitted patients with generalized anxiety disorder. Hood SD, Hince DA, Davies SJ, et al. Psychopharmacology (Berl). 2010 Feb;208(2):223-32. PMID:19936713

[18] The effects of high-dose and low-dose tryptophan depletion on mood and cognitive functions of remitted depressed patients. Booij L, Van der Does AJ, Haffmans PM, et al. J Psychopharmacol. 2005 May;19(3):267-75. PMID:15888512

[19] The effects of experimentally lowered serotonin function on emotional information processing and memory in remitted depressed patients. Merens W, Booij L, Haffmans PJ, van der Does A. J Psychopharmacol. 2008 Aug;22(6):653-62. PMID:18308809

[20] Low-dose tryptophan depletion in recovered depressed women induces impairments in autobiographical memory specificity. Haddad AD, Williams JM, McTavish SF, Harmer CJ. Psychopharmacology (Berl). 2009 Dec;207(3):499-508. PMID:19813003

[21] Thirty four years since the discovery of gastrointestinal melatonin. Bubenik GA. J Physiol Pharmacol. 2008 Aug;59 Suppl 2:33-51. PMID:18812627

[22] Melatonin and serotonin effects on gastrointestinal motility. Thor PJ, Krolczyk G, Gil K, Zurowski D, Nowak L. J Physiol Pharmacol. 2007 Dec;58 Suppl 6:97-103. PMID:18212403

[23] Fructose malabsorption is associated with decreased plasma tryptophan. Ledochowski M, Widner B, Murr C, Sperner-Unterweger B, Fuchs D. Scand J Gastroenterol. 2001 Apr;36(4):367-71.PMID: 11336160

[24] Tryptophan degradation in irritable bowel syndrome: evidence of indoleamine 2,3-dioxygenase activation in a male cohort. Clarke G, Fitzgerald P, Cryan JF, Cassidy EM, Quigley EM, Dinan TG. BMC Gastroenterol. 2009 Jan 20;9:6.PMID: 19154614

[25] Effects of normal meals rich in carbohydrates or proteins on plasma tryptophan and tyrosine ratios. Wurtman RJ, Wurtman JJ, Regan MM, McDermott JM, Tsay RH, Breu JJ. Am J Clin Nutr. 2003 Jan;77(1):128-32. PMID:12499331

[26] High-glycemic-index carbohydrate meals shorten sleep onset. Afaghi A, O'Connor H, Chow CM. Am J Clin Nutr. 2007 Feb;85(2):426-30. Erratum in: Am J Clin Nutr. 2007 Sep;86(3):809. PMID:17284739

[27] Human tryptophan dioxygenase: a comparison to indoleamine 2,3-dioxygenase. Batabyal D, Yeh SR. J Am Chem Soc. 2007 Dec 19;129(50):15690-701. PMID:18027945

[28] Substrate stereo-specificity in tryptophan dioxygenase and indoleamine 2,3-dioxygenase. Capece L, Arrar M, Roitberg AE, Yeh SR, Marti MA, Estrin DA. Proteins. 2010 Nov 1;78(14):2961-72. PMID:20715188

[29] The first step of the dioxygenation reaction carried out by tryptophan dioxygenase and indoleamine 2,3-dioxygenase as revealed by quantum mechanical/molecular mechanical studies. Capece L, Lewis-Ballester A, Batabyal D, et al. J Biol Inorg Chem. 2010 Aug;15(6):811-23. PMID:20361220

[30] Enhanced indoleamine 2,3-dioxygenase activity in patients with severe sepsis and septic shock. Tattevin P, Monnier D, Tribut O, et al. J Infect Dis. 2010 Mar 15;201(6):956-66. PMID:20151841

[31] Localization of indoleamine 2,3-dioxygenase in human female reproductive organs and the placenta. Sedlmayr P, Blaschitz A, Wintersteiger R, et al. Mol Hum Reprod. 2002 Apr;8(4):385-91.PMID: 11912287

[32] Effects of 25-hydroxyvitamin D3 and 1,25-dihydroxyvitamin D3 on cytokine production by human decidual cells. Evans KN, Nguyen L, Chan J, Innes BA, Bulmer JN, Kilby MD, Hewison M. Biol Reprod. 2006 Dec;75(6):816-22. PMID:16957024

[33] Vitamin D-mediated immune regulation in multiple sclerosis. Correale J, Ysrraelit MC, Gaitán MI. J Neurol Sci. 2011 Dec 15;311(1-2):23-31. PMID:21723567

[34] Pharmacological manipulation of kynurenic acid: potential in the treatment of psychiatric disorders. Erhardt S, Olsson SK, Engberg G. CNS Drugs. 2009;23(2):91-101. doi: 10.2165/00023210-200923020-00001. PMID: 19173370

[35] Tryptophan catabolism by indoleamine 2,3-dioxygenase 1 alters the balance of TH17 to regulatory T cells in HIV disease. Favre D, Mold J, Hunt PW, et al. Sci Transl Med. 2010 May 19;2(32):32ra36. PMID:20484731

[36] An interaction between kynurenine and the aryl hydrocarbon receptor can generate regulatory T cells. Mezrich JD, Fechner JH, Zhang X, Johnson BP, Burlingham WJ, Bradfield CA. J Immunol. 2010 Sep 15;185(6):3190-8. PMID:20720200

[37] A biological pathway linking inflammation and depression: activation of indoleamine 2,3-dioxygenase. Christmas DM, Potokar J, Davies SJ. Neuropsychiatr Dis Treat. 2011;7:431-9. PMID:21792309

[38] Elevated levels of kynurenic acid in the cerebrospinal fluid of patients with bipolar disorder. Olsson SK, Samuelsson M, Saetre P, et al. J Psychiatry Neurosci. 2010 May;35(3):195-9.PMID: 20420770

[39] Depressive and anxiety symptoms in the early puerperium are related to increased degradation of tryptophan into kynurenine, a phenomenon which is related to immune activation. Maes M, Verkerk R, Bonaccorso S, Ombelet W, Bosmans E, Scharpé S. Life Sci. 2002 Sep 6;71(16):1837-48.PMID: 12175700

[40] Somatization, but not depression, is characterized by disorders in the tryptophan catabolite (TRYCAT) pathway, indicating increased indoleamine 2,3-dioxygenase and lowered kynurenine aminotransferase activity. Maes M, Galecki P, Verkerk R, Rief W. Neuro Endocrinol Lett. 2011;32(3):264-73. PMID:21712776

[41] Immunoexcitotoxicity as a central mechanism in chronic traumatic encephalopathy-A unifying hypothesis. Blaylock RL, Maroon J. Surg Neurol Int. 2011;2:107. PMID:21886880

[42] Tryptophan metabolites and brain disorders. Stone TW, Mackay GM, Forrest CM, Clark CJ, Darlington LG. Clin Chem Lab Med. 2003 Jul;41(7):852-9. PMID: 12940508

[43] The gut-brain barrier in major depression: intestinal mucosal dysfunction with an increased translocation of LPS from gram negative enterobacteria (leaky gut) plays a role in the inflammatory pathophysiology of depression. Maes M, Kubera M, Leunis JC. Neuro Endocrinol Lett. 2008 Feb;29(1):117-24. PMID:18283240

[44] COX-2 inhibitors as antidepressants and antipsychotics: clinical evidence. Müller N. Curr Opin Investig Drugs. 2010 Jan;11(1):31-42. Review.PMID: 20047157

[45] The impact of neuroimmune dysregulation on neuroprotection and neurotoxicity in psychiatric disorders--relation to drug treatment. Müller N, Myint AM, Schwarz MJ. Dialogues Clin Neurosci. 2009;11(3):319-32. Review.PMID: 19877499

[46] IL-17 and therapeutic kynurenines in pathogenic inflammation to fungi. Romani L, Zelante T, De Luca A, Fallarino F, Puccetti P. J Immunol. 2008 Apr 15;180(8):5157-62. PMID:18390695

[47] Dietary vitamin B6 intake modulates colonic inflammation in the IL10-/- model of inflammatory bowel disease. Selhub J, Byun A, Liu Z, Mason JB, Bronson RT, Crott JW. J Nutr Biochem. 2013 Dec;24(12):2138-43. PMID:24183308

[48] Low plasma vitamin B-6 status affects metabolism through the kynurenine pathway in cardiovascular patients with systemic inflammation. Midttun O, Ulvik A, Ringdal Pedersen E, et al. J Nutr. 2011 Apr 1;141(4):611-7. PMID:21310866

[49] Psychobiological aspects of somatization syndromes: contributions of inflammatory cytokines and neopterin. Euteneuer F, Schwarz MJ, Hennings A, et al. Psychiatry Res. 2012 Jan 30;195(1-2):60-5. PMID:21864915

[50] Activation of cell-mediated immunity in depression: association with inflammation, melancholia, clinical staging and the fatigue and somatic symptom cluster of depression. Maes M, Mihaylova I, Kubera M, Ringel K. Prog Neuropsychopharmacol Biol Psychiatry. 2012 Jan 10;36(1):169-75. PMID:21945535

[51] Reduction of high-fat diet-induced obesity after chronic administration of brain-derived neurotrophic factor in the hypothalamic ventromedial nucleus. Godar R, Dai Y, Bainter H, Billington C, Kotz CM, Wang CF. Neuroscience. 2011 Oct 27;194:36-52. PMID:21856381

[52] Sustained hippocampal chromatin regulation in a mouse model of depression and antidepressant action. Tsankova NM, Berton O, Renthal W, Kumar A, Neve RL, Nestler EJ. Nat Neurosci. 2006 Apr;9(4):519-25. PMID:16501568

[53] DNA methylation profiles of the brain-derived neurotrophic factor (BDNF) gene as a potent diagnostic biomarker in major depression. Fuchikami M, Morinobu S, Segawa M et al. PLoS One. 2011;6(8):e23881. PMID:21912609

[54] Maternal deprivation induces depressive-like behaviour and alters neurotrophin levels in the rat brain. Réus GZ, Stringari RB, Ribeiro KF, et al. Neurochem Res. 2011 Mar;36(3):460-6. PMID:21161589

[55] Imipramine reverses alterations in cytokines and BDNF levels induced by maternal deprivation in adult rats. Réus GZ, Dos Santos MA, Abelaira HM, et al. Behav Brain Res. 2013 Apr 1;242:40-6. PMID:23238043

56 Antidepressant-like effect induced by systemic and intra-hippocampal administration of DNA methylation inhibitors. Sales AJ, Biojone C, Terceti MS, Guimarães FS, Gomes MV, Joca SR. Br J Pharmacol. 2011 Nov;164(6):1711-21. PMID:21585346

57 Eicosapentaenoic acid demethylates a single CpG that mediates expression of tumor suppressor CCAAT/enhancer-binding protein delta in U937 leukemia cells. Ceccarelli V, Racanicchi S, Martelli MP, et al. J Biol Chem. 2011 Aug 5;286(31):27092-102. PMID:21659508

58 Prescription n-3 fatty acids, but not eicosapentaenoic acid alone, improve reference memory-related learning ability by increasing brain-derived neurotrophic factor levels in SHR.Cg-Lepr(cp)/NDmcr rats, a metabolic syndrome model. Hashimoto M, Inoue T, Katakura M, Tanabe Y, Hossain S, Tsuchikura S, Shido O. Neurochem Res. 2013 Oct;38(10):2124-35. PMID:23963508

59 Serum levels of brain-derived neurotrophic factor in major depressive disorder: state-trait issues, clinical features and pharmacological treatment. Molendijk ML, Bus BA, Spinhoven P, et al. Mol Psychiatry. 2010 Sep 21. PMID:20856249

60 Action control is mediated by prefrontal BDNF and glucocorticoid receptor binding. Gourley SL, Swanson AM, Jacobs AM, et al. Proc Natl Acad Sci U S A. 2012 Dec 11;109(50):20714-9. PMID:23185000

61 BDNF overexpression in mouse hippocampal astrocytes promotes local neurogenesis and elicits anxiolytic-like activities. Quesseveur G, David DJ, Gaillard MC, et al. Transl Psychiatry. 2013 Apr 30;3:e253. PMID:23632457

62 Serum BDNF levels before treatment predict SSRI response in depression. Wolkowitz OM, Wolf J, Shelly W, et al. Prog Neuropsychopharmacol Biol Psychiatry. 2011 Aug 15;35(7):1623-30. PMID:21749907

63 Psychotropic drugs on in vitro brain-derived neurotrophic factor production in whole blood cell cultures from healthy subjects. Lee BH, Myint AM, Kim YK. J Clin Psychopharmacol. 2010 Oct;30(5):623-7. PMID: 20814321

64 Serum levels of brain-derived neurotrophic factor in major depressive disorder: state-trait issues, clinical features and pharmacological treatment. Molendijk ML, Bus BA, Spinhoven P, et al. Mol Psychiatry. 2011 Nov;16(11):1088-95. PMID:20856249

65 Molecular evidence for BDNF- and GABA-related dysfunctions in the amygdala of female subjects with major depression. Guilloux JP, Douillard-Guilloux G, Kota R, et al. Mol Psychiatry. 2011 Sep 13. PMID:21912391

66 Inhibition of the Function of TRPV1-Expressing Nociceptive Sensory Neurons by Somatostatin 4 Receptor Agonism: Mechanism and Therapeutical Implications. Szolcsányi J, Pintér E, Helyes Z, Pethő G. Curr Top Med Chem. 2011;11(17):2253-2263. PMID:21671870

67 Activity-dependent brain-derived neurotrophic factor expression regulates cortistatin-interneurons and sleep behavior. Martinowich K, Schloesser RJ, Jimenez DV, Weinberger DR, Lu B. Mol Brain. 2011 Mar 9;4:11. PMID:21388527

68 Antidepressant drugs transactivate TrkB neurotrophin receptors in the adult rodent brain independently of BDNF and monoamine transporter blockade. Rantamäki T, Vesa L, Antila H, Di Lieto A, Tammela P, Schmitt A, Lesch KP, Rios M, Castrén E. PLoS One. 2011;6(6):e20567. PMID:21666748

69 Acute BDNF treatment upregulates GluR1-SAP97 and GluR2-GRIP1 interactions: implications for sustained AMPA receptor expression. Jourdi H, Kabbaj M. PLoS One. 2013;8(2):e57124. 27. PMID:23460828

70 Antidepressant interactions with the NMDA NR1-1b subunit. Raabe R, Gentile L. J Biophys. 2008;2008:474205. PMID:20107576

71 Altered expression of neurotrophic factors in patients with major depression. Otsuki K, Uchida S, Watanuki T, et al. J Psychiatr Res. 2008 Oct;42(14):1145-53. PMID:18313696

72 Methylation at SLC6A4 is linked to family history of child abuse: an examination of the Iowa Adoptee sample. Beach SR, Brody GH, Todorov AA, Gunter TD, Philibert RA. Am J Med Genet B Neuropsychiatr Genet. 2010 Mar 5;153B(2):710-3. PMID:19739105

73 Methylation at 5HTT mediates the impact of child sex abuse on women's antisocial behavior: an examination of the Iowa adoptee sample. Beach SR, Brody GH, Todorov AA, Gunter TD, Philibert RA. Psychosom Med. 2011 Jan;73(1):83-7. PMID:20947778

74 Altered production of brain-derived neurotrophic factor by peripheral blood immune cells in multiple sclerosis. Yoshimura S, Ochi H, Isobe N, et al. Mult Scler. 2010 Oct;16(10):1178-88 PMID:20656764

75 Dysregulated neurotrophin mRNA production by immune cells of patients with relapsing remitting multiple sclerosis. Urshansky N, Mausner-Fainberg K, Auriel E, Regev K, Farhum F, Karni A. J Neurol Sci. 2010 Aug 15;295(1-2):31-7. PMID:20541775

76 Elevated plasma ceramides in depression. Gracia-Garcia P, Rao V, Haughey NJ, et al. J Neuropsychiatry Clin Neurosci. 2011 Spring;23(2):215-8. PMID:21677254

77 Plasma phosphatidylcholine and sphingomyelin concentrations are associated with depression and anxiety symptoms in a Dutch family-based lipidomics study. Demirkan A, Isaacs A, Ugocsai P, et al. J Psychiatr Res. 2013 Mar;47(3):357-62. PMID:23207112

78 Acid sphingomyelinase-ceramide system mediates effects of antidepressant drugs. Gulbins E, Palmada M, Reichel M, et al. Nat Med. 2013 Jul;19(7):934-8. PMID:23770692

79 A new take on ceramide: starving cells by cutting off the nutrient supply. Guenther GG, Edinger AL. Cell Cycle. 2009 Apr 15;8(8):1122-6. PMID:19282666

80 The role of ceramide in major depressive disorder. Kornhuber J, Reichel M, Tripal P, et al. Eur Arch Psychiatry Clin Neurosci. 2009 Nov;259 Suppl 2:S199-204. PMID:19876679

81 Anger attacks in major depressive disorder and serum levels of homocysteine. Fraguas R Jr, Papakostas GI, Mischoulon D, et al. Biol Psychiatry. 2006 Aug 1;60(3):270-4. PMID:16325154

82 Homocysteine and B vitamins relate to brain volume and white-matter changes in geriatric patients with psychiatric disorders. Scott TM, Tucker KL, Bhadelia A, Bet al. Am J Geriatr Psychiatry. 2004 Nov-Dec;12(6):631-8.PMID:15545331

83 Homocysteine induces cerebral endothelial cell death by activating the acid sphingomyelinase ceramide pathway. Lee JT,

Peng GS, Chen SY, Hsu CH, Lin CC, Cheng CA, Hsu YD, Lin JC. Prog Neuropsychopharmacol Biol Psychiatry. 2013 Aug 1;45:21-7. PMID:23665108

[84] Sphingosine kinase and sphingosine-1-phosphate: regulators in autoimmune and inflammatory disease. Snider AJ. Int J Clin Rheumtol. 2013 Aug 1;8(4). PMID:24416079

[85] Brain Aging: Models, Methods, and Mechanisms. Chapter 13Stress and Glucocorticoid Contributions to Normal and Pathological Aging. Ki A. Goosens and Robert M. Sapolsky Boca Raton (FL): CRC Press; 2007.

[86] Effects of increasing durations of immobilization stress on plasma corticosterone level, learning and memory and hippocampal BDNF gene expression in rats. Nooshinfar E, Akbarzadeh-Baghban A, Meisami E. Neurosci Lett. 2011 Aug 1;500(1):63-6. PMID:21683767

[87] Stress-mediated decreases in brain-derived neurotrophic factor as potential confounding factor for acute tryptophan depletion-induced neurochemical effects. van Donkelaar EL, van den Hove DL, Blokland A, Steinbusch HW, Prickaerts J. Eur Neuropsychopharmacol. 2009 Nov;19(11):812-21. PMID:19640687

[88] High dose hydrocortisone immediately after trauma may alter the trajectory of PTSD: Interplay between clinical and animal studies. Zohar J, Yahalom H, Kozlovsky N, et al. Eur Neuropsychopharmacol. 2011 Nov;21(11):796-809. PMID:21741804

[89] Hippocampal neurogenesis as a target for the treatment of mental illness: a critical evaluation. DeCarolis NA, Eisch AJ. Neuropharmacology. 2010 May;58(6):884-93. PMID:20060007

[90] BDNF function as a potential mediator of bipolar disorder and post-traumatic stress disorder comorbidity. Rakofsky JJ, Ressler KJ, Dunlop BW. Mol Psychiatry. 2012 Jan;17(1):22-35. PMID:21931317

[91] Stress and inflammation reduce brain-derived neurotrophic factor expression in first-episode psychosis: a pathway to smaller hippocampal volume. Mondelli V, Cattaneo A, Murri MB, et al. J Clin Psychiatry. 2011 May 18. PMID:21672499

[92] Pro- and anti-inflammatory cytokines expression in rat's brain and spleen exposed to chronic mild stress: Involvement in depression. You Z, Luo C, Zhang W, Chen Y, He J, Zhao Q, Zuo R, Wu Y. Behav Brain Res. 2011 Nov 20;225(1):135-41. PMID:21767575

[93] Stress and inflammation reduce brain-derived neurotrophic factor expression in first-episode psychosis: a pathway to smaller hippocampal volume. Mondelli V, Cattaneo A, Murri MB, Di Forti et al. J Clin Psychiatry. 2011 May 18. PMID:21672499

[94] Depressive symptoms following interferon-α therapy: mediated by immune-induced reductions in brain-derived neurotrophic factor? Kenis G, Prickaerts J, van Os J, Koek GH, Robaeys G, Steinbusch HW, Wichers M. Int J Neuropsychopharmacol. 2011 Mar;14(2):247-53. PMID:20667172

[95] Reductions of acetylcholine release and nerve growth factor expression are correlated with memory impairment induced by interleukin-1beta administrations: effects of omega-3 fatty acid EPA treatment. Taepavarapruk P, Song C. J Neurochem. 2010 Feb;112(4):1054-64. PMID:19968753

[96] Pro- and anti-inflammatory cytokines expression in rat's brain and spleen exposed to chronic mild stress: Involvement in depression. You Z, Luo C, Zhang W, Chen Y, He J, Zhao Q, Zuo R, Wu Y. Behav Brain Res. 2011 Nov 20;225(1):135-41. PMID:21767575

[97] Curcumin reverses corticosterone-induced depressive-like behavior and decrease in brain BDNF levels in rats. Huang Z, Zhong XM, Li ZY, Feng CR, Pan AJ, Mao QQ. Neurosci Lett. 2011 Apr 15;493(3):145-8. PMID:21334417

[98] Curcumin reverses corticosterone-induced depressive-like behavior and decrease in brain BDNF levels in rats. Huang Z, Zhong XM, Li ZY, et al. Neurosci Lett. 2011 Apr 15;493(3):145-8. PMID:21334417

[99] Curcumin reverses impaired hippocampal neurogenesis and increases serotonin receptor 1A mRNA and brain-derived neurotrophic factor expression in chronically stressed rats. Xu Y, Ku B, Cui L, Li X, Barish PA, Foster TC, Ogle WO. Brain Res. 2007 Aug 8;1162:9-18. PMID:17617388

[100] Curcumin, an antioxidant and anti-inflammatory agent, induces heme oxygenase-1 and protects endothelial cells against oxidative stress. Motterlini R, Foresti R, Bassi R, Green CJ. Free Radic Biol Med. 2000 Apr 15;28(8):1303-12. PMID:10889462

[101] Curcumin reverses the effects of chronic stress on behavior, the HPA axis, BDNF expression and phosphorylation of CREB. Xu Y, Ku B, Tie L, Yao H, Jiang W, Ma X, Li X. Brain Res. 2006 Nov 29;1122(1):56-64. PMID:17022948

[102] The total flavonoids extracted from Xiaobuxin-Tang up-regulate the decreased hippocampal neurogenesis and neurotrophic molecules expression in chronically stressed rats. An L, Zhang YZ, Yu NJ, et al. Prog Neuropsychopharmacol Biol Psychiatry. 2008 Aug 1;32(6):1484-90. PMID:18547700

[103] Effects of olive polyphenols administration on nerve growth factor and brain-derived neurotrophic factor in the mouse brain. De Nicoló S, Tarani L, Ceccanti M, et al. Nutrition. 2013 Apr;29(4):681-7. PMID:23466052

[104] Rutin activates the MAPK pathway and BDNF gene expression on beta-amyloid induced neurotoxicity in rats. Moghbelinejad S, Nassiri-Asl M, Farivar TN, et al. Toxicol Lett. 2014 Jan 3;224(1):108-13. PMID:24148604

[105] Cocoa powder triggers neuroprotective and preventive effects in a human Alzheimer's disease model by modulating BDNF signaling pathway. Cimini A, Gentile R, D'Angelo B, et al. J Cell Biochem. 2013 Oct;114(10):2209-20. PMID:23554028

[106] A high-fat diet impairs neurogenesis: involvement of lipid peroxidation and brain-derived neurotrophic factor. Park HR, Park M, Choi J, Park KY, Chung HY, Lee J. Neurosci Lett. 2010 Oct 4;482(3):235-9. PMID:20670674

[107] A high cholesterol diet elevates hippocampal cytokine expression in an age and estrogen-dependent manner in female rats. Lewis DK, Bake S, Thomas K, Jezierski MK, Sohrabji F. J Neuroimmunol. 2010 Jun;223(1-2):31-8.PMID: 20435353

[108] The interplay between oxidative stress and brain-derived neurotrophic factor modulates the outcome of a saturated fat diet on synaptic plasticity and cognition. Wu A, Ying Z, Gomez-Pinilla F. Eur J Neurosci. 2004 Apr;19(7):1699-707. PMID:15078544

[109] The effects of energy-rich diets on discrimination reversal learning and on BDNF in the hippocampus and prefrontal cortex of the rat. Kanoski SE, Meisel RL, Mullins AJ, Davidson TL. Behav Brain Res. 2007 Aug 22;182(1):57-66. PMID:17590450

[110] Prostanoids, not reactive oxygen species, mediate COX-2-dependent neurotoxicity. Manabe Y, Anrather J, Kawano T, Niwa K, Zhou P, Ross ME, Iadecola C. Ann Neurol. 2004 May;55(5):668-75.PMID: 15122707

[111] Phospholipase A2 and cyclooxygenase 2 genes influence the risk of interferon-alpha-induced depression by regulating polyunsaturated fatty acids levels. Su KP, Huang SY, Peng CY, Lai HC, Huang CL, Chen YC, Aitchison KJ, Pariante CM. Biol Psychiatry. 2010 Mar 15;67(6):550-7. PMID:20034614

[112] EPA but not DHA appears to be responsible for the efficacy of omega-3 long chain polyunsaturated fatty acid supplementation in depression: evidence from a meta-analysis of randomized controlled trials. Martins JG. J Am Coll Nutr. 2009 Oct;28(5):525-42.PMID: 20439549

[113] Omega-3 fatty acid eicosapentaenoic acid. A new treatment for psychiatric and neurodegenerative diseases: a review of clinical investigations. Song C, Zhao S. Expert Opin Investig Drugs. 2007 Oct;16(10):1627-38. Review.PMID: 17922626

[114] EPA but not DHA appears to be responsible for the efficacy of omega-3 long chain polyunsaturated fatty acid supplementation in depression: evidence from a meta-analysis of randomized controlled trials.Martins JG. J Am Coll Nutr. 2009 Oct;28(5):525-42. PMID:20439549

[115] Therapeutic use of omega-3 fatty acids in bipolar disorder. Balanzá-Martínez V, Fries GR, Colpo GD, Silveira PP, Portella AK, Tabarés-Seisdedos R, Kapczinski F. Expert Rev Neurother. 2011 Jul;11(7):1029-47. PMID:21721919

[116] Cross-national comparisons of seafood consumption and rates of bipolar disorders. Noaghiul S, Hibbeln JR. Am J Psychiatry. 2003 Dec;160(12):2222-7. PMID:14638594

[117] Deficits in docosahexaenoic acid and associated elevations in the metabolism of arachidonic acid and saturated fatty acids in the postmortem orbitofrontal cortex of patients with bipolar disorder. McNamara RK, Jandacek R, Rider T, Tso P, Stanford KE, Hahn CG, Richtand NM. Psychiatry Res. 2008 Sep 30;160(3):285-99. PMID:18715653

[118] Deficits in docosahexaenoic acid and associated elevations in the metabolism of arachidonic acid and saturated fatty acids in the postmortem orbitofrontal cortex of patients with bipolar disorder. McNamara RK, Jandacek R, Rider T, Tso P, Stanford KE, Hahn CG, Richtand NM. Psychiatry Res. 2008 Sep 30;160(3):285-99. PMID:18715653

[119] Regional differences of the mouse brain in response to an α-linolenic acid-restricted diet: Neurotrophin content and protein kinase activity. Miyazawa D, Yasui Y, Yamada K, Ohara N, Okuyama H. Life Sci. 2010 Oct 9;87(15-16):490-4. PMID:20837030

[120] Dietary n-3 fatty acid deficiency decreases nerve growth factor content in rat hippocampus. Ikemoto A, Nitta A, Furukawa S, Ohishi M, Nakamura A, Fujii Y, Okuyama H. Neurosci Lett. 2000 May 12;285(2):99-102. PMID:10793236

[121] Reduced mania and depression in juvenile bipolar disorder associated with long-chain omega-3 polyunsaturated fatty acid supplementation. Clayton EH, Hanstock TL, Hirneth SJ, Kable CJ, Garg ML, Hazell PL. Eur J Clin Nutr. 2009 Aug;63(8):1037-40. PMID:19156158

[122] Omega-3 fatty acid monotherapy for pediatric bipolar disorder: a prospective open-label trial. Wozniak J, Biederman J, Mick E, et al. Eur Neuropsychopharmacol. 2007 May-Jun;17(6-7):440-7. PMID:17258897

[123] Serum brain-derived neurotrophic factor is associated with cognitive function in healthy older adults. Gunstad J, Benitez A, Smith J, et al. J Geriatr Psychiatry Neurol. 2008 Sep;21(3):166-70. PMID:18503034

[124] BDNF increases with behavioral enrichment and an antioxidant diet in the aged dog. Fahnestock M, Marchese M, Head Eet al. Neurobiol Aging. 2010 May 4. PMID:20447733

[125] Blueberry-induced changes in spatial working memory correlate with changes in hippocampal CREB phosphorylation and brain-derived neurotrophic factor (BDNF) levels. Williams CM, El Mohsen MA, Vauzour D, et al Free Radic Biol Med. 2008 Aug 1;45(3):295-305. PMID:18457678

[126] Exercise-induced improvement in cognitive performance after traumatic brain injury in rats is dependent on BDNF activation. Griesbach GS, Hovda DA, Gomez-Pinilla F. Brain Res. 2009 Sep 8;1288:105-15. PMID:19555673

[127] Alcohol induced depressive-like behavior is associated with a reduction in hippocampal BDNF. Hauser SR, Getachew B, Taylor RE, Tizabi Y. Pharmacol Biochem Behav. 2011 Sep 10;100(2):253-258. PMID:21930150

[128] Early exposure to ethanol or red wine and long-lasting effects in aged mice. A study on nerve growth factor, brain-derived neurotrophic factor, hepatocyte growth factor, and vascular endothelial growth factor. Ceccanti M, Mancinelli R, Tirassa P, Laviola G, Rossi S, Romeo M, Fiore M. Neurobiol Aging. 2010 Apr 9. PMID:20382450

[129] Distribution of 1,25-dihydroxyvitamin D3 receptor immunoreactivity in the limbic system of the rat. Walbert T, Jirikowski GF, Prüfer K. Horm Metab Res. 2001 Sep;33(9):525-31. PMID:11561211

[130] Serum vitamin D concentrations are related to depression in young adult US population: the Third National Health and Nutrition Examination Survey. Ganji V, Milone C, Cody MM, McCarty F, Wang YT. Int Arch Med. 2010 Nov 11;3:29. PMID:21067618

[131] Lower vitamin D levels are associated with depression among community-dwelling European men. Lee DM, Tajar A, O'Neill TW, O'Connor DB, et al. J Psychopharmacol. 2010 Sep 7. PMID:20823081

[132] Vitamin D vs broad spectrum phototherapy in the treatment of seasonal affective disorder. Gloth FM 3rd, Alam W, Hollis B. J Nutr Health Aging. 1999;3(1):5-7. PMID:10888476

[133] Vitamin D3 enhances mood in healthy subjects during winter. Lansdowne AT, Provost SC. Psychopharmacology (Berl). 1998 Feb;135(4):319-23. PMID:9539254

[134] An exploratory study of postpartum depression and vitamin D. Murphy PK, Mueller M, Hulsey TC, Ebeling MD, Wagner CL. J Am Psychiatr Nurses Assoc. 2010 May;16(3):170-7. PMID:21659271

[135] Healthy intakes of n-3 and n-6 fatty acids: estimations considering worldwide diversity. Hibbeln JR, Nieminen LR, Blasbalg TL, Riggs JA, Lands WE. Am J Clin Nutr. 2006 Jun;83(6 Suppl):1483S-1493S. PMID:16841858

[136] 1,25-dihydroxyvitamin D3 regulates NT-3, NT-4 but not BDNF mRNA in astrocytes. Neveu I, Naveilhan P, Baudet C, Brachet P, Metsis M. Neuroreport. 1994 Dec 30;6(1):124-6. PMID:7703399

[137] Impaired nerve growth factor homeostasis in patients with bipolar disorder. Barbosa IG, Huguet RB, Neves FS, Reis HJ, Bauer ME, Janka Z, Palotás A, Teixeira AL. World J Biol Psychiatry. 2011 Apr;12(3):228-32. PMID:20923384

[138] 1,25-Dihydroxyvitamin D3 regulates the expression of VDR and NGF gene in Schwann cells in vitro. Cornet A, Baudet C, Neveu I, Baron-Van Evercooren A, Brachet P, Naveilhan P. J Neurosci Res. 1998 Sep 15;53(6):742-6. PMID:9753201

[139] Increased neurotrophin-3 in drug-free subjects with bipolar disorder during manic and depressive episodes. Fernandes BS, Gama CS, Walz JC, et al. J Psychiatr Res. 2010 Jul;44(9):561-5. PMID:20060128

[140] Increased serum neurotrophin-4/5 levels in bipolar disorder. Walz JC, Magalhães PV, Giglio LM, Cunha AB, Stertz L, Fries GR, Andreazza AC, Kapczinski F. J Psychiatr Res. 2009 Apr;43(7):721-3. PMID:19081579

[141] Vitamin D3-enriched diet correlates with a decrease of amyloid plaques in the brain of AβPP transgenic mice. Yu J, Gattoni-Celli M, Zhu H, Bhat NR, Sambamurti K, Gattoni-Celli S, Kindy MS. J Alzheimers Dis. 2011;25(2):295-307. PMID:21422528

[142] Developmental Vitamin D3 deficiency alters the adult rat brain. Féron F, Burne TH, Brown J, Smith E, McGrath JJ, Mackay-Sim A, Eyles DW. Brain Res Bull. 2005 Mar 15;65(2):141-8. PMID:15763180

[143] Raised plasma nerve growth factor levels associated with early-stage romantic love. Emanuele E, Politi P, Bianchi M, Minoretti P, Bertona M, Geroldi D. Psychoneuroendocrinology. 2006 Apr;31(3):288-94. PMID:16289361

[144] Romantic love, hypomania, and sleep pattern in adolescents. Brand S, Luethi M, von Planta A, Hatzinger M, Holsboer-Trachsler E. J Adolesc Health. 2007 Jul;41(1):69-76. PMID:17577536

[145] Acute homocysteine administration impairs memory consolidation on inhibitory avoidance task and decreases hippocampal brain-derived neurotrophic factor immunocontent: prevention by folic acid treatment. Matté C, Pereira LO, Dos Santos TM, Mackedanz V, Cunha AA, Netto CA, Wyse AT. Neuroscience. 2009 Nov 10;163(4):1039-45. PMID:19619620

[146] Reduced folic acid, vitamin B12 and docosahexaenoic acid and increased homocysteine and cortisol in never-medicated schizophrenia patients: implications for altered one-carbon metabolism. Kale A, Naphade N, Sapkale S, et al. Psychiatry Res. 2010 Jan 30;175(1-2):47-53. PMID:19969375

[147] Altered brain neurotrophins at birth: consequence of imbalance in maternal folic acid and vitamin B_{12} metabolism. Sable P, Dangat K, Kale A, Joshi S. Neuroscience. 2011 Sep 8;190:127-34. PMID:21640168

[148] Effects of altered maternal folic acid, vitamin B12 and docosahexaenoic acid on placental global DNA methylation patterns in Wistar rats. Kulkarni A, Dangat K, Kale A, Sable P, Chavan-Gautam P, Joshi S. PLoS One. 2011 Mar 10;6(3):e17706. PMID:21423696

[149] Increased spinal cord NGF levels in rats with cobalamin (vitamin B12) deficiency. Scalabrino G, Mutti E, Veber D, et al. Neurosci Lett. 2006 Mar 27;396(2):153-8. PMID:16352395

[150] Indirect down-regulation of nuclear NF-kappaB levels by cobalamin in the spinal cord and liver of the rat. Veber D, Mutti E, Tacchini L, Gammella E, Tredici G, Scalabrino G. J Neurosci Res. 2008 May 1;86(6):1380-7. PMID:18183619

[151] Increased levels of neurotrophins are not specific for chronic migraine: evidence from primary fibromyalgia syndrome. Sarchielli P, Mancini ML, Floridi A, et al. J Pain. 2007 Sep;8(9):737-45. PMID:17611164

[152] Increased plasma levels of brain derived neurotrophic factor (BDNF) in patients with fibromyalgia. Haas L, Portela LV, Böhmer AE, Oses JP, Lara DR. Neurochem Res. 2010 May;35(5):830-4. PMID:20119637

[153] Complementary and alternative medicine for the treatment of major depressive disorder. Nahas R, Sheikh O. Can Fam Physician. 2011 Jun;57(6):659-63.PMID:21673208

[154] The effect of ethanol and its metabolites upon methionine synthase activity in vitro. Kenyon SH, Nicolaou A, Gibbons WA. Alcohol. 1998 May;15(4):305-9.PMID:9590515

[155] Retinoic acid receptor stimulation protects midbrain dopaminergic neurons from inflammatory degeneration via BDNF-mediated signaling. Katsuki H, Kurimoto E, Takemori S, Kurauchi Y, Hisatsune A, Isohama Y, Izumi Y, Kume T, Shudo K, Akaike A. J Neurochem. 2009 Jul;110(2):707-18. PMID:19457078

[156] Increased processing of APLP2 and APP with concomitant formation of APP intracellular domains in BDNF and retinoic acid-differentiated human neuroblastoma cells. Holback S, Adlerz L, Iverfeldt K. J Neurochem. 2005 Nov;95(4):1059-68. PMID:16150056

[157] Vitamin A facilitates enteric nervous system precursor migration by reducing Pten accumulation. Fu M, Sato Y, Lyons-Warren A, Zhang B, Kane MA, Napoli JL, Heuckeroth RO. Development. 2010 Feb;137(4):631-40. PMID:20110328

[158] High-dose dietary supplementation of vitamin A induces brain-derived neurotrophic factor and nerve growth factor production in mice with simultaneous deficiency of vitamin A and zinc. Kheirvari S, Uezu K, Yamamoto S, Nakaya Y. Nutr Neurosci. 2008 Oct;11(5):228-34. PMID:18782483

[159] Total and mitochondrial nitrosative stress, decreased brain-derived neurotrophic factor (BDNF) levels and glutamate uptake, and evidence of endoplasmic reticulum stress in the hippocampus of vitamin A-treated rats. de Oliveira MR, da Rocha RF, Stertz L, Fries GR, de Oliveira DL, Kapczinski F, Moreira JC. Neurochem Res. 2011 Mar;36(3):506-17. PMID:21188516

[160] The efficacy of zinc supplementation in depression: Systematic review of randomised controlled trials. Lai J, Moxey A, Nowak G, Vashum K, Bailey K, McEvoy M. J Affect Disord. 2011 Jul 26. PMID:21798601

[161] Zinc supplementation provides behavioral resiliency in a rat model of traumatic brain injury. Cope EC, Morris DR, Scrimgeour

AG, Vanlandingham JW, Levenson CW. Physiol Behav. 2011 Oct 24;104(5):942-7. PMID:21699908

[162] Association of zinc deficiency and depression in the patients with end-stage renal disease on hemodialysis. Roozbeh J, Sharifian M, Ghanizadeh A, Sahraian A, Sagheb MM, Shabani S, Hamidian Jahromi A, Kashfi M, Afshariani R. J Ren Nutr. 2011 Mar;21(2):184-7. PMID:21093288

[163] Dietary Intake of Zinc was Inversely Associated with Depression. Yary T, Aazami S. Biol Trace Elem Res. 2011 Sep 20. PMID:21932045

[164] Chronic unpredictable stress-induced reduction in the hippocampal brain-derived neurotrophic factor (BDNF) gene expression is antagonized by zinc treatment. Cieślik K, Sowa-Kućma M, Ossowska G, et al. Pharmacol Rep. 2011;63(2):537-43. PMID:21602609

[165] Chronic unpredictable stress-induced reduction in the hippocampal brain-derived neurotrophic factor (BDNF) gene expression is antagonized by zinc treatment. Cieślik K, Sowa-Kućma M, Ossowska G, Legutko B, Wolak M, Opoka W, Nowak G. Pharmacol Rep. 2011 Mar-Apr;63(2):537-43. PMID:21602609

[166] High-dose dietary supplementation of vitamin A induces brain-derived neurotrophic factor and nerve growth factor production in mice with simultaneous deficiency of vitamin A and zinc. Kheirvari S, Uezu K, Yamamoto S, Nakaya Y. Nutr Neurosci. 2008 Oct;11(5):228-34. PMID:18782483

[167] Increased nerve growth factor by zinc supplementation with concurrent vitamin A deficiency does not improve memory performance in mice. Kheirvari S, Uezu K, Sakai T, Nakamori M, Alizadeh M, Sarukura N, Yamamoto S. J Nutr Sci Vitaminol (Tokyo). 2006 Dec;52(6):421-7. PMID:17330505

[168] Significance of serum glucocorticoid and chelatable zinc in depression and cognition in zinc deficiency. Takeda A, Tamano H, Ogawa T, Takada S, Ando M, Oku N, Watanabe M. Behav Brain Res. 2011 Sep 19. PMID:21946308

[169] High dose zinc supplementation induces hippocampal zinc deficiency and memory impairment with inhibition of BDNF signaling. Yang Y, Jing XP, Zhang SP, et al. PLoS One. 2013;8(1):e55384. PMID:23383172

[170] Zinc signaling in the hippocampus and its relation to pathogenesis of depression. Takeda A. Mol Neurobiol. 2011 Oct;44(2):166-74. PMID:21161611

[171] Insight into glutamate excitotoxicity from synaptic zinc homeostasis. Takeda A. Int J Alzheimers Dis. 2010 Dec 20;2011:491597. PMID:21234391

[172] Zinc salts inhibit in vitro Toll-like receptor 2 surface expression by keratinocytes. Jarrousse V, Castex-Rizzi N, Khammari A, Charveron M, Dréno B. Eur J Dermatol. 2007 Nov-Dec;17(6):492-6. PMID:17951128

[173] Neuroprotective action of lithium in disorders of the central nervous system. Chiu CT, Chuang DM. Zhong Nan Da Xue Xue Bao Yi Xue Ban. 2011 Jun;36(6):461-76. PMID:21743136

[174] Magnesium for treatment-resistant depression: a review and hypothesis. Eby GA 3rd, Eby KL. Med Hypotheses. 2010 Apr;74(4):649-60. PMID:19944540

[175] Sleep deprivation prevents stimulation-induced increases of levels of P-CREB and BDNF: protection by caffeine. Alhaider IA, Aleisa AM, Tran TT, Alkadhi KA. Mol Cell Neurosci. 2011 Apr;46(4):742-51. PMID:21338685

[176] Coffee, caffeine, and risk of depression among women. Lucas M, Mirzaei F, Pan A, Okereke OI, Willett WC, O'Reilly EJ, Koenen K, Ascherio A. Arch Intern Med. 2011 Sep 26;171(17):1571-8. PMID:21949167

[177] Evaluation of plasma antioxidant levels during different phases of illness in adult patients with bipolar disorder. De Berardis D, Conti CM, Campanella D, et al. J Biol Regul Homeost Agents. 2008 Jul-Sep;22(3):195-200. PMID:18842173

[178] A double-blind, randomized, placebo-controlled 4-week study on the efficacy and safety of the purinergic agents allopurinol and dipyridamole adjunctive to lithium in acute bipolar mania. Machado-Vieira R, Soares JC, Lara DR, Luckenbaugh DA, Busnello JV, Marca G, Cunha A, Souza DO, Zarate CA Jr, Kapczinski F. J Clin Psychiatry. 2008 Aug;69(8):1237-45. PMID:18681754

[179] Serum uric acid levels and the clinical characteristics of depression. Wen S, Cheng M, Wang H, Yue J, Wang H, Li G, Zheng L, Zhong Z, Peng F. Clin Biochem. 2012 Jan;45(1-2):49-53. PMID:22040815

[180] Decrease in the levels of NGF and BDNF in brains of mice fed a tryptophan-deficient diet. Lee DR, Semba R, Kondo H, Goto S, Nakano K. Biosci Biotechnol Biochem. 1999 Feb;63(2):337-40. PMID:10192916

[181] Heat stress, cytokines, and the immune response to exercise. Starkie RL, Hargreaves M, Rolland J, Febbraio MA. Brain Behav Immun. 2005 Sep;19(5):404-12. PMID:16061150

[182] Production of interferon-gamma by microglia. Kawanokuchi J, Mizuno T, Takeuchi H, et al. Mult Scler. 2006 Oct;12(5):558-64. PMID:17086900

[183] Interferon-gamma produced by microglia and the neuropeptide PACAP have opposite effects on the viability of neural progenitor cells. Mäkelä J, Koivuniemi R, Korhonen L, Lindholm D. PLoS One. 2010 Jun 14;5(6):e11091. PMID:20559421

[184] IFN-gamma receptor signaling mediates spinal microglia activation driving neuropathic pain. Tsuda M, Masuda T, Kitano J, et al. Proc Natl Acad Sci U S A. 2009 May 12;106(19):8032-7. PMID:19380717

[185] The protective effect of quercetin on long-term alcohol consumption-induced oxidative stress. Kahraman A, Çakar H, Köken T. Mol Biol Rep. 2012 Mar;39(3):2789-94. PMID:21674185

[186] Biochemical and immunological basis of silymarin effect, a milk thistle (Silybum marianum) against ethanol-induced oxidative damage. Das SK, Mukherjee S. Toxicol Mech Methods. 2012 Jun;22(5):409-13. PMID:22409310

[187] Dietary xylooligosaccharide downregulates IFN-γ and the low-grade inflammatory cytokine IL-1β systemically in mice. Hansen CH, Frøkiær H, Christensen AG, et al. J Nutr. 2013 Apr;143(4):533-40. PMID:23427328

[188] Congruencies in increased mortality rates, years of potential life lost, and causes of death among public mental health clients in eight states. Colton CW, Manderscheid RW. Prev Chronic Dis. 2006 Apr;3(2):A42. PMID:16539783

[189] http://www.schizophrenia.com/poverty.htm 12/20/2012

[190] Animal models of prenatal immune challenge and their contribution to the study of schizophrenia: a systematic review. Macêdo DS, Araújo DP, Sampaio LR, et al. Braz J Med Biol Res. 2012 Mar;45(3):179-86. PMID:22392187

[191] The staging model in schizophrenia, and its clinical implications. Agius M, Goh C, Ulhaq S, McGorry P. Psychiatr Danub. 2010 Jun;22(2):211-20. PMID:20562749

[192] Attenuated psychosis and the schizophrenia prodrome: current status of risk identification and psychosis prevention. Tandon N, Shah J, Keshavan MS, Tandon R. Neuropsychiatry (London). 2012;2(4):345-353. PMID:23125875

[193] Managing the prodrome of schizophrenia. Fleischhacker WW, Simma AM. Handb Exp Pharmacol. 2012;(212):125-34. PMID:23129330

[194] Comparing clinical and neurocognitive features of the schizophrenia prodrome to the bipolar prodrome. Olvet DM, Stearns WH, McLaughlin D, Auther AM, Correll CU, Cornblatt BA. Schizophr Res. 2010 Oct;123(1):59-63. PMID:20716479

[195] Differentiation in the preonset phases of schizophrenia and mood disorders: evidence in support of a bipolar mania prodrome. Correll CU, Penzner JB, Frederickson AM, et al. Schizophr Bull. 2007 May;33(3):703-14. PMID:17478437

[196] Glutamate neurocircuitry: theoretical underpinnings in schizophrenia. Schwartz TL, Sachdeva S, Stahl SM. Front Pharmacol. 2012;3:195. PMID:23189055

[197] A carbon monoxide-releasing molecule (CORM-3) attenuates lipopolysaccharide- and interferon-gamma-induced inflammation in microglia. Bani-Hani MG, Greenstein D, Mann BE, Green CJ, Motterlini R. Pharmacol Rep. 2006;58 Suppl:132-44. PMID:17332683

[198] Meta-analysis of cytokine alterations in schizophrenia: clinical status and antipsychotic effects. Miller BJ, Buckley P, Seabolt W, Mellor A, Kirkpatrick B. Biol Psychiatry. 2011 Oct 1;70(7):663-71. PMID:21641581

[199] Elevated interleukin-18 serum levels in chronic schizophrenia: Association with psychopathology. Xiu MH, Chen da C, Wang D, et al. J Psychiatr Res. 2012 Aug;46(8):1093-8. PMID:22647522

[200] The role of NGF and IL-2 serum level in assisting the diagnosis in first episode schizophrenia. Xiong P, Zeng Y, Wan J, Xiaohan DH, Tan D, Lu J, Xu F, Li HY, Zhu Z, Ma M. Psychiatry Res. 2011 Aug 30;189(1):72-6. PMID:21277636

[201] Atypical antipsychotics suppress production of proinflammatory cytokines and up-regulate interleukin-10 in lipopolysaccharide-treated mice. Sugino H, Futamura T, Mitsumoto Y, Maeda K, Marunaka Y. Prog Neuropsychopharmacol Biol Psychiatry. 2009 Mar 17;33(2):303-7. PMID:19138716

[202] A double-blind, randomized study of minocycline for the treatment of negative and cognitive symptoms in early-phase schizophrenia. Levkovitz Y, Mendlovich S, Riwkes S, Braw Y, Levkovitch-Verbin H, Gal G, Fennig S, Treves I, Kron S. J Clin Psychiatry. 2010 Feb;71(2):138-49. PMID:19895780

[203] Minocycline as adjunctive therapy for patients with unipolar psychotic depression: an open-label study. Miyaoka T, Wake R, Furuya M, et al. Prog Neuropsychopharmacol Biol Psychiatry. 2012 Jun 1;37(2):222-6. PMID:22349578

[204] Minocycline supplementation for treatment of negative symptoms in early-phase schizophrenia: a double blind, randomized, controlled trial. Liu F, Guo X, Wu R, et al. Schizophr Res. 2014 Mar;153(1-3):169-76. PMID:24503176

[205] Effects of doxycycline on depressive-like behavior in mice after lipopolysaccharide (LPS) administration. Mello BS, Monte AS, McIntyre RS, et al. J Psychiatr Res. 2013 Oct;47(10):1521-9. PMID:23835040

[206] Predator cat odors activate sexual arousal pathways in brains of Toxoplasma gondii infected rats. House PK, Vyas A, Sapolsky R. PLoS One. 2011;6(8):e23277. PMID:21858053

[207] Increased incidence of traffic accidents in Toxoplasma-infected military drivers and protective effect RhD molecule revealed by a large-scale prospective cohort study. Flegr J, Klose J, Novotná M, Berenreitterová M, Havlícek J. BMC Infect Dis. 2009 May 26;9:72. PMID:19470165

[208] Decrease of psychomotor performance in subjects with latent 'asymptomatic' toxoplasmosis. Havlícek J, Gasová ZG, Smith AP, Zvára K, Flegr J. Parasitology. 2001 May;122(Pt 5):515-20. PMID:11393824

[209] Toxoplasma gondii infection enhances testicular steroidogenesis in rats. Lim A, Kumar V, Hari Dass SA, Vyas A. Mol Ecol. 2013 Jan;22(1):102-10. PMID:23190313

[210] Influence of latent Toxoplasma infection on human personality, physiology and morphology: pros and cons of the Toxoplasma-human model in studying the manipulation hypothesis. Flegr J. J Exp Biol. 2013 Jan 1;216(Pt 1):127-33. PMID:23225875

[211] Toxoplasma gondii infection, from predation to schizophrenia: can animal behaviour help us understand human behaviour? Webster JP, Kaushik M, Bristow GC, McConkey GA. J Exp Biol. 2013 Jan 1;216(Pt 1):99-112. PMID:23225872

[212] The obligate intracellular parasite Toxoplasma gondii secretes a soluble phosphatidylserine decarboxylase. Gupta N, Hartmann A, Lucius R, Voelker DR. J Biol Chem. 2012 Jun 29;287(27):22938-47. PMID:22563079

[213] The neurotropic parasite Toxoplasma gondii increases dopamine metabolism. Prandovszky E, Gaskell E, Martin H, Dubey JP, Webster JP, McConkey GA. PLoS One. 2011;6(9):e23866. PMID:21957440

[214] Evaluation of kynurenine pathway metabolism in Toxoplasma gondii-infected mice: Implications for schizophrenia. Notarangelo FM, Wilson EH, Horning KJ, Thomas MA, Harris TH, Fang Q, Hunter CA, Schwarcz R. Schizophr Res. 2014 Jan;152(1):261-7. PMID:24345671

[215] Toxoplasma gondii and other risk factors for schizophrenia: an update. Torrey EF, Bartko JJ, Yolken RH. Schizophr Bull. 2012 May;38(3):642-7. PMID:22446566

[216] Psychiatric disorders in toxoplasma seropositive patients--the CD8 connection. Bhadra R, Cobb DA, Weiss LM, Khan IA. Schizophr Bull. 2013 May;39(3):485-9. PMID:23427221

[217] Isolation of phosphatidylethanolamine as a solitary cofactor for prion formation in the absence of nucleic acids. Deleault NR, Piro JR, Walsh DJ, Wang F, Ma J, Geoghegan JC, Supattapone S. Proc Natl Acad Sci U S A. 2012 May 29;109(22):8546-51. PMID:22586108

[218] Toxoplasma gondii in animals used for human consumption. Tenter AM. Mem Inst Oswaldo Cruz. 2009 Mar;104(2):364-9. PMID:19430665

[219] Could Toxoplasma gondii have any role in Alzheimer disease? Kusbeci OY, Miman O, Yaman M, Aktepe OC, Yazar S. Alzheimer Dis Assoc Disord. 2011 Jan-Mar;25(1):1-3. PMID:20921875

[220] The probable relation between Toxoplasma gondii and Parkinson's disease. Miman O, Kusbeci OY, Aktepe OC, Cetinkaya Z. Neurosci Lett. 2010 May 21;475(3):129-31. PMID:20350582

[221] Is there any role of Toxoplasma gondii in the etiology of obsessive-compulsive disorder? Miman O, Mutlu EA, Ozcan O, Atambay M, Karlidag R, Unal S. Psychiatry Res. 2010 May 15;177(1-2):263-5. PMID:20106536

[222] Is Toxoplasma gondii a causal agent in migraine? Koseoglu E, Yazar S, Koc I. Am J Med Sci. 2009 Aug;338(2):120-2. PMID:19564786

[223] Prevalence of anti-Toxoplasma antibodies in patients with autoimmune diseases. Shapira Y, Agmon-Levin N, Selmi C, et al. J Autoimmun. 2012 Aug;39(1-2):112-6. PMID:2229714

[224] Seroreactive marker for inflammatory bowel disease and associations with antibodies to dietary proteins in bipolar disorder. Severance EG, Gressitt KL, Yang S, et al. Bipolar Disord. 2013 Dec 6. PMID:24313887

[225] Gastrointestinal inflammation and associated immune activation in schizophrenia. Severance EG, Alaedini A, Yang S, et al. Schizophr Res. 2012 Jun;138(1):48-53. PMID:22446142

[226] Anti-gluten immune response following Toxoplasma gondii infection in mice. Severance EG, Kannan G, Gressitt KL, et al. PLoS One. 2012;7(11):e50991. PMID:23209841

[227] Exacerbation of murine ileitis by Toll-like receptor 4 mediated sensing of lipopolysaccharide from commensal Escherichia coli. Heimesaat MM, Fischer A, Jahn HK, et al. Gut. 2007 Jul;56(7):941-8. PMID:17255219

[228] Estradiol for treatment-resistant schizophrenia: a large-scale randomized-controlled trial in women of child-bearing age. Kulkarni J, Gavrilidis E, Wang W, et al. Mol Psychiatry. 2014 Apr 15. PMID:24732671

[229] The Role of Estrogen in the Treatment of Men with Schizophrenia. Kulkarni J, Gavrilidis E, Worsley R, Van Rheenen T, Hayes E. Int J Endocrinol Metab. 2013 Summer;11(3):129-136. PMID:24348584

[230] LPS Exposure Increases Maternal Corticosterone Levels, Causes Placental Injury and Increases IL-1B Levels in Adult Rat Offspring: Relevance to Autism. Kirsten TB, Lippi LL, Bevilacqua E, Bernardi MM. PLoS One. 2013 Dec 2;8(12):e82244. PMID:24312647

[231] Chronic gastrointestinal inflammation induces anxiety-like behavior and alters central nervous system biochemistry in mice. Bercik P, Verdu EF, Foster JA, et al. Gastroenterology. 2010 Dec;139(6):2102-2112.e1. PMID:20600016

[232] Comparative efficacy and acceptability of 12 new-generation antidepressants: a multiple-treatments meta-analysis. Cipriani A, Furukawa TA, Salanti G, et al. Lancet. 2009 Feb 28;373(9665):746-58. PMID:19185342

[233] Therapeutic effect of vitamin d supplementation in a pilot study of Crohn's patients. Yang L, Weaver V, Smith JP, et al. Clin Transl Gastroenterol. 2013 Apr 18;4:e33. PMID:23594800

[234] Magnesium in depression. Serefko A, Szopa A, Wlaź P, et al. Pharmacol Rep. 2013;65(3):547-54. PMID:23950577

[235] USDA Food Nutrient Report: NDB 15040, NDB 15076. USDA Food Search, Nutrient Data Laboratory, Beltsville MD

[236] Exercise training increases size of hippocampus and improves memory. Erickson KI, Voss MW, Prakash RS, et al. Proc Natl Acad Sci U S A. 2011 Feb 15;108(7):3017-22. PMID:21282661

[237] N-Acetylcysteine and metabotropic glutamate receptors: implications for the treatment of schizophrenia: a literature review. Zavodnick AD, Ali R. Psychiatr Q. 2014 Jun;85(2):177-85. PMID:24390716

[238] The role of PKC isoforms in the inhibition of NF-κB activation by vitamin K2 in human hepatocellular carcinoma cells. Xia J, Matsuhashi S, Hamajima H, et al. J Nutr Biochem. 2012 Dec;23(12):1668-75. PMID:22475810

32. Fibromyalgia Syndrome, Pain Sensitization, Chronic Fatigue and Anxiety

In Fibromyalgia Syndrome (FMS) there is widespread pain and tenderness at distinct areas of the body without visible lesions. It is often accompanied by depression, irritable bowel syndrome, chronic urticaria, morning stiffness and other comorbidities. FMS is common, affecting about 6% of American women, but is only about one-tenth as common in men. Although this diagnosis is rare in children, patients commonly report chronic pain or trauma during childhood.

Pathological findings were elusive in FMS for many years; it had no diagnostic clinical laboratory tests, no alterations on x-rays, no signs visible on physical exam, and no visible alterations under a microscope. Until recently, many physicians considered it a functional (psychiatric) disorder[1]. While FMS includes psychological morbidity, there is now ample evidence that it is a physical disease with systemic pathology.

Frustrating to both patient and physician, FMS remains resistant to therapy. Medications currently approved for the treatment of FMS are effective in providing relief in only about 30 percent of patients. A medication that may be effective for one patient can be ineffective for others. The variance in efficacy among treatments likely stems from the multifactorial causation of this syndrome. It is through understanding causation that a rational treatment can be designed.

Diagnostic Criteria for FMS

- Pain over the past week in several areas of the body, including a number of the areas shown in Figure 31-1,
- Fatigue and non-restorative sleep,
- Cognitive problems (memory and thought,
- Associated conditions and symptoms (Tables 32-1),
- The condition enduring at least three months,
- Not having another condition that would explain the pain and other symptoms.

In FMS, the pain is found on both sides of the body and both in the upper and lower body. The pain can be provoked with a 4-kg force. Note that the symptoms listed in Tables 32-1 are quite similar to those for mast cell activation syndrome given in Table 12-1.

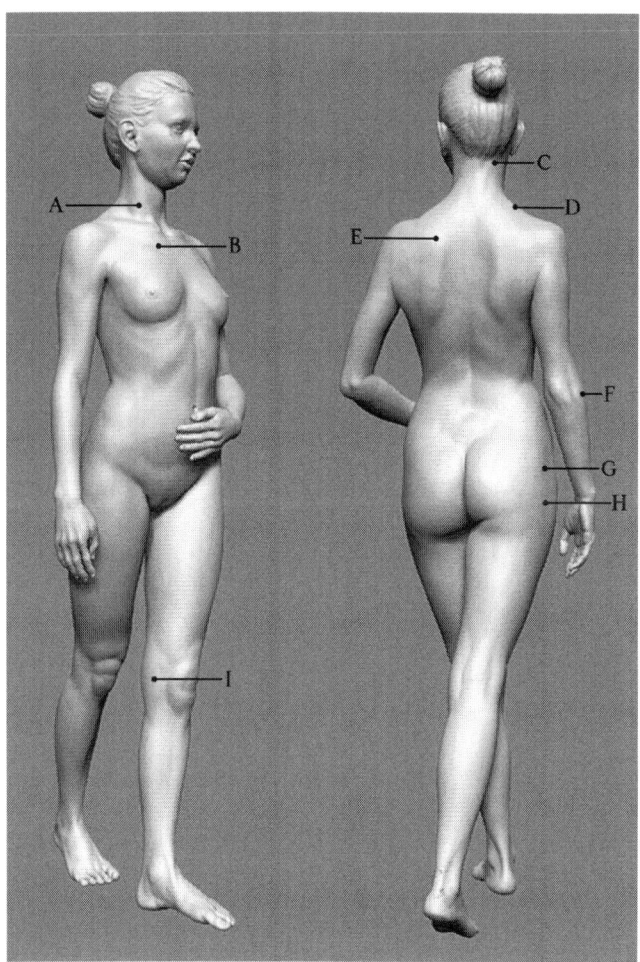

Figure 32-1: Tender points in FMS
Digital sculpture by Selwy

A. Low cervical: at the anterior aspect of the interspaces between the transverse processes of C5–C7
B. Second rib: just lateral to the second costochondral junctions
C. Occipital: at the insertions of one or more of the following muscles: trapezius, sternocleidomastoid, splenius capitus, and semispinalis capitus
D. Trapezius: at the midpoint of the upper border
E. Supraspinatus: above the scapular spine near the medial border
F. Lateral epicondyle: 2 cm distal to the lateral epicondyle
G. Gluteal: at the upper outer quadrant of the buttocks at the anterior edge of the gluteus maximus muscle
H. Greater trochanter: posterior to the prominence of the greater trochanter
I. Knee: at the medial fat pad proximal to the joint line.

Table 32-1A: Conditions Associated with FMS

• Rheumatoid Arthritis
• Bipolar disorder (especially mania)[2]
• Major Depression, Anxiety
• Irritable Bowel Syndrome (IBS)
• Interstitial cystitis, (frequency, bladder spasm)
• Reynaud's phenomenon

Table 32-1B: Symptoms in FMS

- Fatigue, insomnia, non-restorative sleep
- Difficulty with memory and concentration; commonly referred to "Fibro fog."
- Headaches, seizures
- Tinnitus, hearing difficulties, dizziness
- Blurred vision, dry eyes
- Dry mouth, change in taste, loss of appetite
- Aphthous ulcers
- Esophagitis, chest pain
- Shortness of breath, wheezing
- Morning stiffness, muscle weakness, and myalgia
- Painful menstruation
- Restless legs syndrome
- Sensitivity to heat and cold, noise or bright lights
- Constipation, abdominal cramping, nausea, diarrhea
- Paresthesias; numbness or tingling of the extremities
- Chronic urticaria, easy bruising, hair loss, rash
- Sun sensitivity

Differential Diagnosis: Since fibromyalgia (FM) is a clinical diagnosis and one of exclusion, it is critical to assure that other diseases with similar presentation are excluded.

Osteomalacia, another common disease, is frequently misdiagnosed as FM. Osteomalacia, caused by vitamin D deficiency, can have similar symptoms of generalized pain, tenderness, and fatigue. Osteomalacia can often be distinguished from FMS on physical exam by finding tenderness to palpation over the sternum and tibia; these are not expected in FM. Care should be used to distinguish tenderness to the sternum from costochondritis, in which there is tenderness at the joints of the sternum and ribs.

Vitamin D deficiency is common in FM, with only 30% of patients having vitamin D levels within the normal range. FMS patients with insufficient vitamin D are at increased risk for anxiety and depression[3]. Individuals diagnosed with FMS should be tested for vitamin D level, and treated if OHD3 levels are less than optimal (see Chapter 20). Individuals with fibromyalgia are at increased risk for osteomalacia and treatment of deficiency provides benefit. Osteoporosis and other osteoimmune disorders are discussed in Chapter 42.

A less common disease misdiagnosed as fibromyalgia is Myotonic Dystrophy type 2 (MD2). This condition presents with muscle pain, stiffness, fatigue, and muscular weakness, especially in the neck, shoulders, hips, and upper legs. This genetic disease occurs in about one of 2000 Europeans[4]. Also, like FM, there can be poor quality sleep, daytime sleepiness, fatigue, difficulty with concentration and organizing thoughts, and restless leg syndrome[5,6]. This mild form of muscular dystrophy is an autosomal dominant genetic disease; it affects about half of the offspring of affected parents without gender predilection. MD2 often has a mild presentation, with limited symptoms during youth. Disability may be delayed into late adulthood.

In a study of female fibromyalgia patients, three percent of those (2 of 59) who had been diagnosed as having FMS had MD2, while the gene defect was not found in any of the 200 asymptomatic persons tested[7]. Fibromyalgia is much less common among men than in women; while MD2 affects both genders equally. Based on the population prevalence of these two diseases it can be estimated that about one in eleven men with FM-like symptoms has MD2. Thus, MD2 should be considered as a potential diagnosis in patients who present with FM, especially in men and when there is a family history consistent with MD2.

Causation

Fibromyalgia is, in part, a chronic pain syndrome resulting from central sensitization of pain. In this syndrome, the brain becomes abnormally sensitive to stimuli so that low level, non-harmful stimuli become painful. Functional MRI studies show that trivial somatic stimulation in these patients can induce activity in multiple areas of the brain that are indistinguishable from that which occurs in normal individuals with very painful stimuli[8]. Fibromyalgia (FM) is one of several chronic central sensitization syndromes (CSS) in which the spinal cord and brain are sensitized to pain. Other conditions include IBS, interstitial cystitis, tension headaches, endometriosis, post-surgical pain, some cancer and post-cancer pain, and some chronic low back pain.

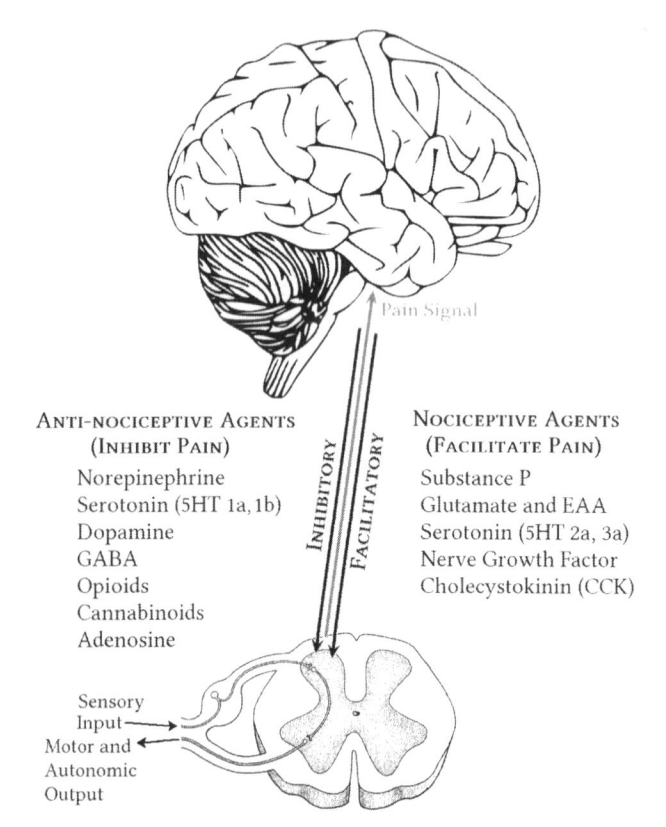

Figure 32-2: Facilitation and inhibition of pain signals from the spinal cord by various neurotransmitters[9].

Central sensitization syndromes arise when there is the loss of inhibition or facilitation of pain signaling between the dorsal horn of the spinal cord and the brain. Multiple neurotransmitters affect pain transmission. INF-γ, IL-6, and IL-8 can also sensitize the spinal cord to pain. CSS should be understood, and treatment targeted, through understanding physiologic processes affecting them.

In fibromyalgia, NE, serotonin, dopamine, and GABA levels are low in the cerebral spinal fluid. Meanwhile, substance P, glutamate, Nerve Growth Factor (NGF) and endogenous opiate levels are elevated. Magnetic resonance spectroscopy has shown the excitatory neurotransmitter, glutamate, to be elevated in the brains of patients with FM[10, 11], and other neuropathic pain syndromes.

Pain Facilitation in Central Sensitization

Several neurotransmitters facilitate the pain signals in the spinal cord. These include substance P, NGF, CCK, and neurotransmitters stimulating the serotonin 2a and 3a receptors, and most importantly, glutamate. Elevated central TNF-α is associated with neuropathic pain.

Glutamate

Glutamate is the most abundant excitatory neurotransmitter in the CNS. It acts through multiple receptors including NMDA, kainate, AMPA, and at least eight glutamate metabotropic receptors. Glutamate is stored in vesicles in nerve endings, and released when the nerve fires. Glutamate stimulation enhances attention, learning, memory, and alertness. Glutamate also is utilized, along with glucose and lactate, as fuel for the production of ATP by the mitochondria of the neurons.

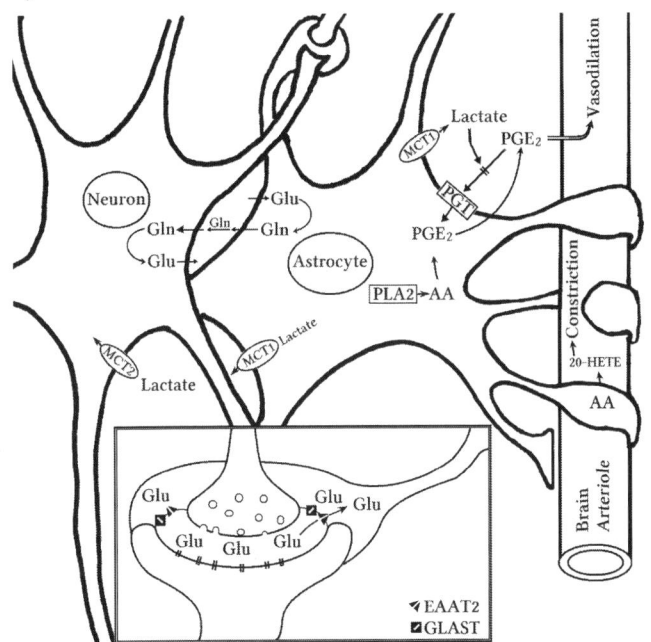

Figure 32-3: Neuron and perivascular astrocyte. Glu; glutamate, Gln; Glutamine. PLA2 Phospholipase A2, AA; arachidonic acid, PGT; prostaglandin transporter. MCT; lactate transporter.

Glial cells, such as astrocytes, serve as support cells for the neurons. Glial cells also help regulate neuroexcitatory activity by moving glutamate out the synaptic clefts via glutamate transporters, such as EAAT, and GLAST. This transport prevents excessive neuroexcitation.

The astrocytes metabolize glutamate into glutamine, which is then available for re-uptake and reutilization by the neurons. Perivascular astrocytes also regulate blood flow to the nervous system. Depending on oxygenation level, lactate, and other factors, perivascular astrocytes produce PLA2, which releases arachidonic acid (AA) from the cell membrane that is converted to the vasoconstrictor 20-HETE. COX1 (PTGS1) also converts AA into PGE2; that acts as a vasodilator. When lactate levels are sufficient, such as in during hypoxia, acidosis or produced by muscles during vigorous exercise, reuptake of PGE2 by prostaglandin transporter PGT, is inhibited; allowing for increase blood flow to that region of the nervous system. This also occurs under the stimulus of the sympathetic nervous system. This increases regional blood flow to the brain and enhances neuroexcitation during fight or flight reactions; allowing animals to have better vision and faster response to perceived threats.

Excessive glutamate stimulus is excitotoxic. It allows excess calcium influx; resulting in HCY and ROS formation that can lead to neuronal damage and promote to a cascade resulting in nerve cell apoptosis.

Excitotoxicity is a pathway for neurological damage in TBI, Alzheimer's disease, Parkinson's disease, Amyotrophic Lateral Sclerosis, alcohol withdrawal, and in ischemia-reperfusion injury, such as from a stroke. In these conditions, astrocyte glutamate transporters fail to remove glutamate from extracellular space synaptic clefts; allowing excessive glutamic stimulus and calcium influx. If not taken up by astrocytes, glutamate cannot be converted to the neuroinhibitor, GABA, or into glutamine.

Glutathione (GSH) is the principal antioxidant of the CNS. Under excitotoxic stress, GSH becomes oxidized to GS:SG. Excess glutamate also prevents the absorption of cysteine by the neuron that is required for the formation of GSH; thus contributing to GSH depletion[12]. Oxidative damage to the CNS, associated with low GSH, has been found in patients with major depressive disorder, bipolar disorder, and schizophrenia[13]. Low GSH increases acid SMase activity, and formation of ceramide. Thus, glutamate, an excitatory neurotransmitter, important in attention and alertness, not only increases transmission of pain signaling, but also causes the excitotoxic neuronal damage that underlies multiple CNS diseases.

GABA

Gamma-aminobutyric acid is chiefly an inhibitory neurotransmitter that activates $GABA_A$ receptors. These receptors are chloride ion channels that, in general, decrease polarization; thus inhibiting nerve transmission. In FMS, there may be disequilibrium between glutamate and GABA in the brain, resulting in excess glutamate activity. GABA helps to activate the transition to parasympathetic dominance of the autonomic nervous system at night[14]; this may fail to occur in FMS patients.

GABA does not cross the blood-brain barrier, but instead, is formed in the CNS from glutamate by glutamate decarboxylase. Pyridoxal-5-phosphate, the active form of vitamin B_6, is a required coenzyme for this enzyme. See Table 28-4. The herbs, valerian and gotu kola, also increase glutamate decarboxylase activity. GABA availability may also be enhanced by decreasing the activity of the enzyme 4-aminobutyrate aminotransferase which converts GABA to glutamate. The seizure medication valproic acid and the herb, lemon balm, decrease the activity of this enzyme.

Cholecystokinin (CCK)

Cholecystokinin, the satiation peptide, also acts in pain transmission. CCK helps create avoidance memory and increases transmission of visceral pain via the vagal nerve[15]. CCK increases pain by increasing the release of PGE2 and 5-hydroxyindoleacetic acid (5-HIAA), which is a 5-HT$_3$ serotonin agonist[16]. As shown in Figure 31-2, the same cytokines and inflammatory compounds that induce kynurenine, induce IDO to convert serotonin into 5-HIAA, a modulator of pain. CCK also augments pain transmission through the endocannabinoid system by inhibiting GABAergic transmission[17], favoring glutamate activity.

CCK released after a consumption of fermented protein, such as that present in putrid meat, high in polyamines, causes nausea, pain, especially visceral pain, and heightens avoidance memory. CCK is synthesized as a preprohormone that is converted into several isoforms. The CCK-4 isoform induces unpleasant anxiety and fear. Injection of CCK-4 reproduces panic attacks, in patients subject to them, with no other stimulus[18].

There are several cannabinoid receptors. CB1 receptors are found primarily in the central and peripheral nervous system; THC, found in marijuana, is a ligand for CB1. CB2 receptors are present primarily in immune cells, and microglia, but not in neurons. CB2 receptors are up-regulated in the dorsal root ganglion of the spinal cord, in animal models of neuropathic pain, and CB2 agonists have potential as therapeutic agents[19]. CB1 may prevent presynaptic CCK release.

Norepinephrine (NE) /Sympathetic Stimulus

Sympathetic stimulation of the reticular activating system of the brain enhances vigilance and diverts resources from cognitive processing in the prefrontal cortex. This helps disengage emotional and judgmental processing during fight or flight reactions that might impair optimal physical coordination and response[20]. NE also disengages pain, during the response to acute stress, when it could impair defensive or aggressive behaviors. Thus, NE inhibits pain transmission, as illustrated in figure 32-2. This rerouting of cognitive processing enhances survival for the individual but is not so kind for those around them. Social danger created by NE during stress is discussed in Chapter 37.

Chronic sympathetic stimulus, however, has an inverse effect; it increases pain sensitivity. In fibromyalgia, there is little diurnal variation in sympathetic tone. Normally there is a decrease in sympathetic tone and predominance of parasympathetic activity during sleep, but this is lacking in patients with FMS[21]. FMS patients also have higher TNF-α and IL-6 levels, with a lack of the normal diurnal variation[22]. FMS patients also have a decreased sympathetic activation in response to physical activity and mental stress[23] and lower levels of NPY. Additionally, these patients have a lower ACTH response to exercise[24]. Patients with posttraumatic stress disorder (PTSD) also show a blunted sympathetic response to mental stress[25] and lower levels of NPY. Together, this suggests chronic sympathetic overstimulation and lack of adaptive response.

Induced bioamine depletion can be used as an animal model for FMS[26]. FMS patients have increased adrenergic activity and increased sensitivity to pain. Certain alleles for adrenergic receptors have been associated with fibromyalgia risk, which explains their increased sensitivity to pain[27], as well as some other symptoms of the disease.

FMS and PTSD are often precipitated by deeply troubling traumatic events. The most frequently cited events triggering FMS include emotional trauma and chronic stress. Acute illness, physical injuries, surgery, and motor vehicle accidents are also cited. Many patients attribute the onset of FMS to emotional abuse as a child or as an adult[28]. The trauma may induce alterations in gene transcription, consistent with epigenetic changes found in these patients.

We become alert and ready to react when we are about to walk across a busy intersection with traffic coming from different directions, but relax our attention once safely across the street. The increase in alertness allows us react more quickly to unexpected potential danger; a busy intersection is expected to be a place of high risk. Imagine how it might feel to enter such an intersection if you had been severely injured or witnessed a loved one killed in such an intersection. Now imagine being trapped in that intersection 24 hours a day. It is easy to imagine that one might be on guard and unable to relax following a traumatic event. FMS and PSTD are more likely to follow traumatic incidents which occur in what should be the safest place; the home, and at the hands of parents or lovers, or when the trauma occurred as an unpredictable event. Events that initiate FMS and PTSD are often devastating because they leave no safe place; no place for the victim to relax their guard. The individual thus remains on a continuous level of high vigilance. The chronic sympathetic activity can also prevent useful and adaptive emotional processing after traumatic events. During chronic stress, instead of increasing the anti-inflammatory effect of cortisol, the sympathetic response increases the production of inflammatory cytokines by immune cells.

Acute sympathetic activity lowers generalized immune response, but chronic stimulus increases specific areas of immune function. Chronic adrenergic activity stimulates the growth of sympathetic nerve endings in areas of the lymph nodes populated by T cells[29]. This chronic β-adrenergic stimulus increases TGF-β, IL-6 and IL-8 production[30]. The presence of TGF-β and IL-6 together promotes the transformation of naïve T helper 4+ cells into T_H17 cells[31] and down-regulates T_H1 cell production, by increasing production of INF-γ and decreasing production of INF-β. The sympathetic system also innervates the intestinal immune system[30] and increases the activity of T_H17 cells; increasing the risk of immune reactivity to foods and commensal bacterial. Sympathetic blood flow diminution to the intestine may impair digestion of nutrients and mucous production, favoring biofilm formation. This would increase production of LPS, and thereby, TNF-α, IL-1β, and other inflammatory cytokines[32], further enhancing excitotoxic kynurenine and 5-HIAA levels. Chronic stress also increases glutaminergic activity.

Sympathetic activity can boost regional immunity through IL-1β, TNF-α, and IL-8 production[30], leading to regional vasodilation and central pain sensitization which helps to immobilize the affected area. This immobility may help with healing after an acute injury, but creates disability in chronic pain. Substance P stimulates the production of IL-8 that increases sympathetic pain.

Adrenergic stimulation of the muscles increases calcium influx and strengthens contractions. Sustained sympathetic activity can cause muscle fatigue. In the heart, prolonged adrenergic stress is associated increased production of reactive oxygen species, development of heart failure and cardiac arrhythmias[33]. Chronic adrenergic stimulation of the skeletal muscles also promotes oxidative stress. Oxidative stress in the carotid bodies, in turn, increases sympathetic activity; a similar, central, positive feedback mechanism is probable[34].

CSS is often accompanied by catastrophizing and undo fear of harm[35], illness behaviors that increase sympathetic stress. Successful treatment of FMS and CSS may depend on the patient understanding that most chronic CSS pain is not associated with harm. Once this is understood, the patient is more likely to exercise and stretch, activities that are helpful for relieving pain.

Opiates

Opiates are used in the treatment of severe pain and can be quite effective in treating acute pain. Opiates, however, are not effective for chronic treatment of FMS or CSS. In FM, levels of endogenous opiates in the CSF are elevated. Opiates increase sensitivity to chronic pain.

Mu-receptor expression is quickly downregulated by most opiates[36]. Tachyphylaxis occurs, along with upregulation of glutamate activity, thereby increasing the transmission of pain[37]. Opiate use increases synaptic plasticity, favoring the development of opiate tolerance, pain sensitization, and relapse to addiction[38]. Even years after ending chronic opiate use, pain sensitivity remains elevated in patients who have used long-term opiates. Additionally, opiates are agonists for TLR4; and thus increases the transcription of inflammatory cytokines, such as TNF-α and IL-1β, contribute to addiction, and prevents apoptosis of inflammatory cells as a result of NF-κB activation; thus opiates enhance and maintain inflammation[39].

Some tricyclic medications block the same activation area (MD2) on TLR 2 and TLR4 that is activated by opiates. Of eight tricyclics tested, amitriptyline was the most potent inhibitor of TLR2 and TLR4 signaling[40]. Tricyclic antidepressants are useful in the treatment of chronic pain, may prevent inflammation including CNS inflammation and may help in the treatment of opiate addiction.

Assessing Pain

Studies among various races, performed on difference continents, have revealed that people from every race studied, estimate the pain level being experienced by persons of other races to be lower than that for the same injury in patients of their own race; our estimate of pain being experienced by other relies on empathy. This can be measured by functional MRI in the observer's cingulate cortex[41,42]. Studies of medical professionals have shown that we are no different in this bias.

Kindling, from repeated pain, increases sensitivity to it; we do not become inured to pain, but rather more sensitive and more adept at feeling pain with the experience of it. Timely and adequate treatment of pain, thus, helps prevent its amplification and chronicity.

Many patients who claim to have high thresholds for pain, in fact, have the reverse; with repeated or chronic pain, they have become more sensitized to it. Often, those claiming to have high thresholds for pain are rather reporting chronic stoicism in the face of unrelenting pain.

Tumor Necrosis Factor-α

Radicular pain is often provoked by nerve root compression by a herniated disk. Many patients, however, have chronic pain and paresthesias even when nerve compression is absent. Spinal trauma can induce inflammation activation and pain without nerve compression. Exogenous application of TNF-α duplicates nerve damage pain. Etanercept (Enbrel) a medication that acts as a soluble decoy receptor for TNF-α, has provided a remarkable, long-lasting relief of chronic discogenic pain within minutes of a paraspinal injection[43]. Administration of TNF-α into the cerebral spinal fluid (CSF) of animals provokes anxiety and depressive behaviors[44]. TNF-α antibody blocks this effect[45]. In FMS, the mix of peripheral cytokines is mainly anti-inflammatory with relatively low levels of TNF-α and IL-1β[46]. But while peripheral levels of inflammatory cytokines are low in FMS, levels in the CNS can be elevated. In the CNS TNF-α, via TNF-R1, also activation of acid SMase, production of ceramide, HCY, and oxidative stress.

Fog and Fatigue

FMS is more than central pain sensitization. Fatigue and brain "fog" might be dismissed as pain induced sleep deprivation, which in itself raise cytokine levels, but FMS has a wide array of comorbid conditions. Many of these are similar to Mast Cell Activation Syndrome, suggesting a common cause or at lease common pathological pathways and treatment. FMS also shares much in common with chronic fatigue syndrome.

Chronic Fatigue Syndrome (CFS)

CFS is characterized by profound exhaustion, cognitive slowness, sleep difficulties, joint and muscle pain, and disabling fatigue, sometimes with sudden onset. Similar to fibromyalgia, CFS is a chronic inflammatory disease with widespread neuroinflammation and activation of microglia. In CFS, the level of microglial activation in the amygdala, thalamus, and midbrain, demonstrated by PET scan imaging, correlate with cognitive impairment[47]. CFS is also associated with bilateral white matter atrophy, including loss of right arcuate fasciculus mass, which may cause conductive aphasia, and atrophy of the right inferior longitudinal fasciculus among right-handed individuals[48], which may impair recognition of facial expression.

Serum IgA and IgM to gram-negative bacteria LPS levels correlate with CSF symptoms, and remission of CFS symptoms accompanies normalization of LPS translocation from the intestine. LPS induces NF-κB, TNF-α, and microglia activation. Elevated IgA and IgM to LPS is also found in major depressive disorder and highly associated with irritable bowel symptoms, and illness behaviors, including fatigue, subjective experience of infection, and difficulty with memory[49]. CFS is an enteroimmune disease associated with leaky gut syndrome.

Patients with FMS have elevated levels of the cytokines TNF-α, IL-8, and IL-10 in many studies IL-17A, IL-6 and IL1β are also elevated.

IL-10 down-regulates T_H1 development and NF-κB activity; while IL-17A stimulates T_H17 cell maturation[50]. This suggests that there is immune activation against colonic bacteria in FMS, thus, FMS too, is an enteroimmune disease. IL-10 can directly activate the HPA axis, culminating in the release of cortisol by the adrenal glands, which stimulates the production of IL-6. Cortisol increases somatostatin production, resulting in decreased release of growth hormone and IGF-1 that are important for healing and nerve growth and repair. Chronic elevation of IL-6 is associated with a low threshold for pain, fatigue and depression[51].

IL-8 is produced in response to oxidative stress. IL-8, produced by smooth muscle, promotes local vasodilation and angiogenesis, IL-8 produced by white blood cells promotes chemotaxis and phagocytosis. Pain recovery in successful FMS treatment is highly correlated with a fall in IL-8 levels[52].

The oxidative stress that induces IL-8 may be generated via the sphingomyelinase (SMase) and kynurenine pathways. SMase mediates cell death or proliferation in inflammation. Ceramide promotes apoptosis, but can be converted to S1P (sphingosine-1-phosphate) which induces proliferation and activation of WBS's. Ceramide inhibits cystathionine β-synthase; increasing HCY and preventing the production of glutathione, the principal antioxidant of the CNS. HCY triggers production ROS via NADPH oxidase activity[53].

Ceramide induces sickness behavior, neurotoxicity and impairs muscular strength, including that of the diaphragm, causing fatigue[54]. Acid SMase, the principal form in the CNS, is induced by activation of the TNF-R1 receptor by TNF or other activating ligands. LPS induced oxidative stress in the endoplasmic reticulum can be inhibited by blocking acid SMase[55], thus, TLR4 contributes to SMase activation. TNF-α, via ceramide, can stimulate pericytes to release MMP-9, damaging the blood-brain barrier[56].

Further toxicity may be induced through the kynurenine pathway (Chapter 31) through activation of IDO by LPS, or TNF-α plus IL-1 or IL-6. IL-1β in the CNS stimulates the release of TNF-α. IL-1β and TNF-α promote damage to endothelial cells, neurons, and glial cell.

Mast Cell Activation

Seventy percent of patients with chronic urticaria were found to have fibromyalgia[57]. In a study of 63 FMS patients, every patient had an elevated number of activated mast cells on skin biopsy, while they were rare in control patients[58], This suggests mast cell degranulation into the dermis and mast cell activation or hyperplasia in this condition. Irritable bowel syndrome (IBS) is also a mast cell activation disorder.

IBS, interstitial cystitis (IC/BPS), and chronic urticaria are common comorbidities of FM. Clonal mast cell activation may result from the unbalanced T_H17 activity from chronic adrenergic stimulus, and lack of apoptosis of these immune cells, which are sustained by IL-10 and IL-17A, and sympathetic stimulus present in FM. Increased CRH production and elevated T_H17 activity, present in FMS and PTSD, increases intestinal paracellular permeability, proclivity to form food anterges, and increased bacterial transmigration.

Patients with myalgic encephalomyelitis/chronic fatigue syndrome have higher IBS symptom scores and have been found to have increased levels of TNF-α, IL-1, neopterin, and IgA antibodies to LPS of commensal bacteria, indicating bacterial overgrowth and translocation. IL-1, TNF-α, and neopterin levels correlate with fatigue, flu-like malaise, irritability, sadness and autonomic and neurocognitive symptoms[59]. Increased paracellular permeability of the intestine allows greater absorption of LPS, resulting in increased CNS TNF-α. Anterges may trigger other symptoms and behaviors including depression, irritability, and rage; see Chapters 30 and 37.

Depression in FM

In depression, there is hypersecretion of CRH and cortisone. In FMS and PTSD, there is CRH hypersecretion, but blunted ACTH responses. BDNF and NGF levels are also elevated[60,61]. NGF facilitates pain transmission. In PTSD, the cortisol levels are subnormal despite elevated CRH[62]. Patients with FMS have an elevated sympathetic tone with decreased diurnal variance. Increased sympathetic tone increases CRH output and decreases serum DHEA sulfate levels[63]. Ceramide and oxidative stress inhibit BDNF supported neuronal growth.

Genetic linkage studies, while unable to explain the majority of FM, do provide insight. One of the gene allele variants associated with FMS in such studies is COMT. In mice bred to be COMT deficient, male and female mice have different behavioral changes; the males, if housed together, are consistently aggressive to each other; the females show anxiety behavior, and are reluctant to come out of a dark box into the light. COMT deficient females take nine times as long to come out into the light, and when they do, they roam less than do normal COMT mice. COMT deficient males have higher than normal frontal cortex dopamine activity, but it is below normal in COMT deficient females. Norepinephrine and serotonin were unchanged in the frontal cortex of the male mice, but both were lower the females[64]. An analogous deficiency of COMT in the frontal cortex in humans would be expected to reduce forebrain activity; impairing forethought and promoting impulsive behavior in men, and promoting anxiety, depression and diminished activity in women.

Ghrelin is principally a neuromodulatory hormone produced by the stomach that signals hunger when the stomach is empty. Ghrelin also protects against depression that can occur in hostile environments and chronic stress[65]. It is hypothesized that ghrelin supports hunter-gatherer behavior in humans and other animals, encouraging them to venture forth and seek food, even though the meal may lie in hostile territory. Lab animals with low ghrelin became easily depressed when exposed to social stress, such as bullying. Ghrelin has been found to be low in patients with fibromyalgia.

Patients with FMS (mostly female) with low COMT and low ghrelin levels would be expected to avoid venturing out and being physically active. With diminished physical activity, the mollycoddled mitochondrial become lazy, leaky, and effete. FMS patients have fewer and less efficient mitochondria. The male response to low COMT, however, would be expected to promote more aggressive behavior and preserve muscular activity, and thus, maintain mitochondrial efficiency.

Indeed, gender differences are found in depression. Men with depression men are more irritable, have less impulse control, have a higher frequency of outbursts of rage, and are more likely to exhibit hyperactive behavior; whereas women suffer more from hypersomnia and often complain of leaden paralysis, where limbs seem too heavy and difficult to move[66]. Anger is a common complaint among individuals with FM[28], and without a clear definition, the anger which is reported by FMS patients may actually represent rage, a condition that has considerable causal overlap with FMS (See Chapter 36).

In depression, there is a loss of brain volume; there is apoptosis of neural and glial cells. The same underlying pathology may occur in FM, may trigger depression, irritable bowel syndrome, pain, and paresthesias. SMase and ceramide are important causes of depression and oxidative stress.

Alzheimer's Disease

Fibrillar amyloid-beta (Aβ) peptides are central to the pathology of Alzheimer's disease (AD). Aβ activates both TLR2 and TLR4[67] signaling in microglia. TLR4 activates NF-κB transcription of COX2 (PTGS2)[68], iNOS, TNF-α and IL-1β, and TLR2 increases transcription of IL-6 and activates microglia[69,70]. Furthermore, TNF-α increases the expression of TLR2 receptors on microglia[71].

The inflammatory cytokines, TNF-α, IL-1β, IL6, and INF-γ[72,73], in turn, increase the production of Aβ, at least in part through the production of quinolinic acid as part of the kynurenine pathway (Chapter 31). This creates a positive feedback loop for continued production of Aβ, activated microglia, and inflammatory cytokines, and activation of the kynurenine pathway, furthering CNS damage in Alzheimer's' disease.

TNF-α is elevated in the cerebral spinal fluid of patients with Alzheimer's disease (AD), with levels 25 times the normal level. TNF-α acts as a glial-transmitter in neuro-inflammatory disorders, via its induction of the kynurenine and acid SMase pathways. TNF-α in the CNS increases glutamate and decreases GABA. Paraspinal injection of etanercept, absorbed and distributed into the cerebral spinal fluid, slows the cognitive decline in AD. Similar to the rapid response to this treatment to discogenic pain, family members have reported improved cognition within minutes of etanercept treatment in some studies[74].

In experimental autoimmune encephalomyelitis, an animal model multiple sclerosis (MS), anxiety behavior becomes apparent before motor defects are seen. Etanercept injected into the CSF prevents this anxiety behavior. This suggests that TNF-α activates anxiety-behavior associated with neuroinflammation[75].

The damage caused by the inflammatory cytokines is due, in part, to oxidative damage[76]. Antioxidants, including soy isoflavones, which also inhibit TNF-α production, protect the mitochondria from oxidative stress induced by Aβ[77]. These isoflavones have been demonstrated to decrease the inflammatory response and improve memory and learning in animals who's CNS has been exposed to Aβ[78]. Co-administration of folate significantly potentiated the antioxidant effects of the isoflavones in their protection against Aβ induced neurotoxicity[79].

LPS from the cell walls of gram-negative bacteria activates TLR4. Lipoteichoic acid, from the walls of gram-positive bacteria, and cell wall components from certain other pathogens activate TLR2 in microglia and other immune cells in an analogous manner[80] (Table 42-4.) Betaine and vitamin D down-regulate TLR2 and TLR4 production. Some flavonoid compounds appear to offer protection from neuroinflammation. Caffeic acid inhibits the upregulation of TLR2 by TNF-α[71]. Several phenolic compounds that have been documented to inhibit TNF-α activity are listed in Table 32-2.

Minocycline (which crosses the blood brain barrier) and doxycycline inhibit at least some of the transcription factors activated by TLR2. Some tricyclic medications inhibit TLR2 and TLR4 activity. These medications have shown benefit in the treatment some CNS diseases and may help in the treatment of Alzheimer's disease and other CNS and spinal cord inflammatory disorders.

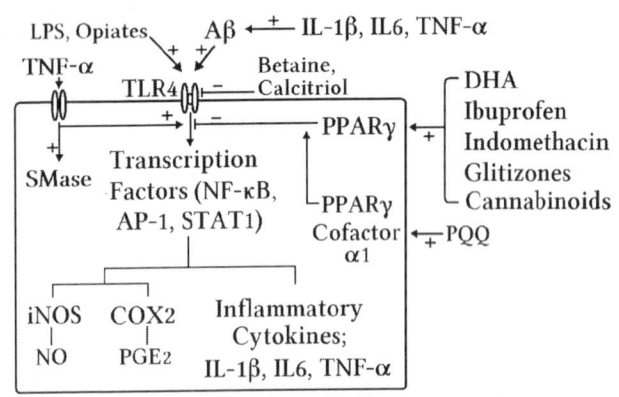

Figure 32-4: TLR4 Induction of Inflammatory Agents

Oxidative Stress and Nerve Damage

Weak, inefficient mitochondria leak energy in the form of free radicals. The primary radical is the superoxide anion, which creates many secondary radical species, including peroxynitrite and its toxic and dangerous oxidation products. The superoxide anion induces the production and release of cytokines including IL-6 and IL-8 at the spinal ganglion. IL-6 sensitizes nerves to pain and increases CRH release from the hypothalamus. The release of ACTH is, however, somewhat delayed in FMS patients[81], likely because of increased circulating CRH binding protein[82]. Oxygen radicals also increase the activity of IDO and the conversion of tryptophan in the kynurenine pathway and serotonin to 5-HIAA, which can increase pain. Oxidative stress also increases PLA2 that releases arachidonic acid that under the influence of COX2 forms PGE2. TNF-α stimulates SMase, converting sphingomyelin into ceramide, thus inducing oxidative stress via HCY and GSH deficits.

Superoxide also causes pain through direct peripheral sensitization. Although FMS is principally a CSS, FMS also causes increased sensitivity to peripheral pain. Mitochondrial dysfunction and oxidative stress affect unmyelinated nerves in the dermis, decreasing the threshold for pain, and, and can damage or destroy postmitotic peripheral neurons. It might be expected that when nerve cells, which transmit pain, do not function correctly, there would be less pain; however, the reverse occurs. A loss of these nerve fibers causes a decrease in cortical inhibition. The brain then amplifies the signal.

In IBS, experimental balloon distension of the bowel causes pain, where the same distension, in normal persons, does not. IBS may also have loss of nerve fibers in the bowel, causing poorly-coordinated peristalsis, resulting in constipation or diarrhea. In a similar situation, normal bladder distension may cause bladder pain in interstitial cystitis/bladder pain syndrome (IC/BPS).

Electron microscopy shows ballooning of the Schwann cells on the unmyelinated axons in the skin of patients with fibromyalgia[83]. Schwann cells surround the nerves to shield and protect them. The mitochondria of patients with FMS have been found to have higher superoxide levels, increased oxidative stress, more lipid peroxidation, and lower membrane potentials and co-enzyme Q10 than controls[84]. Muscle cells of patients with fibromyalgia have fewer mitochondria, accumulation of glycogen, and fragmentation of nuclear DNA[85]. The mitochondria that remain are large and irregular, and poorly functioning. Patients with FMS have been found to have lower levels of CoQ10 in their WBC's, and a high correlation between TNF-α and ROS in these cells. Increased levels of lipid oxidation were found, which correlated with headache scores[86]. CoQ10 supplements provided significant improvements in FMS symptoms[87].

In a systemic review of pharmacologic agents used in the treatment of painful diabetic neuropathy, the antioxidant alpha-lipoic acid (ALA) was found to be more effective than gabapentin, amitriptyline, marijuana extract, topiramate, or fluoxetine[88]. ALA improves motor nerve conduction velocity in diabetic neuropathy and raises the levels of reduced glutathione (GSH). ALA is a potent, lipophilic free-radical scavenger for the peripheral nerves and protects them from ischemia-reperfusion damage[89]. In patients with diabetic peripheral neuropathy, both motor and sensory nerve conduction velocity improved with ALA. ALA prevents the oxidative stress mediated induction of acid SMase that increases ceramide and S1P levels. Activation of S1P receptors on neurons increases the perception of pain[90]. ALA treatment is enhanced by the coadministration of (vitamin B$_{12}$) methylcobalamin[91].

Among NSAIDS, only ibuprofen use has been provided neuroprotection in observational studies[92]; however, treatment benefits do not necessarily outweigh the risks associated with treatment. Ibuprofen may also act through other mechanisms[93], including downregulation of NOS[94].

Tricyclic antidepressant medications, particularly low-dose amitriptyline, provides pain relief for neuropathic pain as a functional inhibitor of acid SMase. It also inhibits the activation of TLR2 and TLR4, and thus, may reduce the production of IL-1β and IL-6, TNF-α[95]. The nutrient betaine (TMG) and vitamin D3 inhibit the expression of the TLR4 and thereby prevents the downstream events, including the production of TNF-α and other inflammatory cytokines[96]. Betaine also prevents the formation of HCY.

The nutrient PQQ decreases pain in animal models of nerve injury and decreases the production of TNF-α[97] by inducing PPAR-γ cofactor α-1. PQQ reduces the size of spinal cord injury in lab animals and diminishes the induction of iNOS, thus, further moderating pain and nerve damage[98], and stimulates the generation of new mitochondria.

Summary

FMS is a complex disease which includes central pain sensitization and chronic sympathetic activation. Chronic sympathetic stress results in dysregulation of the neuro-endocrine-immune system and increased levels of peripheral and CNS inflammatory cytokines. These cytokines induce excitotoxic glutamic activity and increase transmission of pain, and activate SMase and IDO producing ROS and toxins. These factors can lead to both central and peripheral nerve damage. Especially in women, chronic stress promotes depression and inactivity, followed by mitochondrial dysfunction and oxidative damage.

FMS is a disease syndrome characterized by multiple dysfunctional positive feedback loops. Pain, leading to a paucity of muscular activity in FMS allows the survival of inefficient mitochondria that leak free radicals and increase oxidative stress. Mast cell activation disorder, common in FM, may occur as a secondary reaction to chronic sympathetic activity and be sustained by inflammatory cytokines. Mast Cell Activation Syndrome causes secondary symptoms, such as chronic urticaria and IBS. T_H17 immune activation. and increased CRH production that raises the propensity to form IgG anteries to food, and promotes the development of sustained disease.

Mitigation and Treatment

1. Chronic Stress mitigation: Treatment of the stress should be addressed. If the stressor remains in the patient's environment, such as physical or emotional abuse, it needs to be eliminated. If the patient has a chronic stress reaction from past events or if the source cannot be elucidated, the chronic stress reaction should be treated. EMDR has been helpful in PTSD and is discussed below. Massage has also been found to be helpful for FM[28]. Chapter 29 discusses stress reduction. Appendix D contains a tool for assessing domestic violence, Appendix G a tool for assessing the reaction to past traumatic events, and Appendix K a tool for assessing traumatic brain injury, but can be used to assess CNS inflammatory activation in FMS.

FMS patients tend to catastrophize and anticipate excessive harm[30]. The pain is real, and it is essential to acknowledge the reality of their pain. However, the patient's assessment of risk and calamity are often excessive. Overcoming or controlling fears and anxieties can reduce chronic emotional, sympathetic and HPA stress reactions. Even after mitigation of traumatic events and conditions, chronic stress reaction may continue due to epigenetic changes in gene expression. Adequate folate, vitamin B_{12}, DHA, melatonin, and phenolic compounds found in foods may help reset the epigenetically maintained stress response. This may help normalize DNA transcription in response to stress. Epigenetic "reset" is discussed in Chapter 29, and foods and supplements which may be effective are summarized in Table 29-2. Alcohol use should be avoided.

2. Treatment of Pain: Excessive glutamate activity is present in most CSS. Glutamate activity is enhanced by TNF-α. Reducing TNF-α induction curtails glutaminergic and SMase activity. Vitamin D_3 and betaine down-regulates TLR4, thus decreasing TNF-α. Vitamin D_3 has been found to be helpful in chronic pain[99], and in FM. Docosahexaenoic acid (DHA, from fish oil) may help protect the brain from glutamate hyperexcitability through activation of PPAR-γ. PQQ facilitates the activity of PPAR-γ and decreases neuropathic pain. Lipoic acid (best as R-lipoic acid sodium) is an effective treatment of diabetic neuropathic pain. PPAR-γ agonists reduce lesion size, motor dysfunction, and neuropathic pain after spinal cord injury[100]. Magnesium blocks glutaminergic NMDA ion channels[101] and has been found to reduce post-operative pain[102].

Table 32-2: Factors that Decrease TNF-α levels

Factor	Chapter
Melatonin	9
Exercise	12
Chocolate	17
Betaine (TMG)	Herein
Docosahexaenoic acid (DHA)	Herein
Pyrroloquinoline quinone (PQQ)	Herein
Calcitrol (Vitamin D_3)	Herein
Ibuprofen	Herein
Tricyclic antidepressants	Herein
Dietary flavonoids	Table 32-2

Table 32-3: Flavonoids that Decrease TNF-α levels[103, 104, 105, 106]

Flavonoid	Major Dietary Sources[107]
Apigenin	Sage, rosemary, oregano, marjoram, virgin olive oil
Caffeic Acid[71]	Black chokeberry, sunflower seeds, herbs, and spices
Curcumin*	Tumeric
Diosmetin	Peppermint leaves, citrus juice
Epigallocatechin gallate	Green tea, oolong tea, pecans
Quercetin	Capers, chocolate, elderberries
Hydroxytyrosol	Olives
Tyrosol	Olives, sherry, red wine
Oleuropein	Olives
Naringin and Hesperidin	Citrus fruit, parsley
Oligomeric procyanidins	Cocoa, nectarines, broad beans, apples, red wine, plums,
Resveratrol	Loganberries, cranberries, wine
p-hydroxycinnamic acid	Dates, peanuts green olives
Soy isoflavones[78]	Soy
Luteolin[108]	Artichoke, sage, thyme

* Curcumin is a phenolic compound but is not a flavonoid.

Several dietary flavonoid compounds decrease TNF-α levels and by inhibiting the TNF-α signaled release of NF-κB from IKK. These flavonoids, including those in chocolate, have been found to decrease pain. In Chapter 23, Table 23-1 lists several factors to avoid that *increase* TNF-α.

Magnesium supplements can decrease neuropathic pain[109], [110]. In a double-blinded study, a six-week program of Mg supplementation diminished neuropathic pain and increased spinal range of motion at six-month follow-up assessment. The anti-inflammatory effects of Mg are discussed in Chapter 30.

Co-enzyme Q10 has been successfully used in the treatment of FMS using a dose of 300 mg daily[111]. Rather than providing CoQ10, which is very poorly absorbed, or SAMe that can have toxic effects, B vitamins that help produce these compounds (folate, B_6, B_{12}, and betaine) are recommended. Vitamin B12 supplements are very poorly absorbed when swallowed whole. They should be chewed or allowed to melt in the mouth so that the vitamin can be protected from stomach acid by haptocorrin in the saliva. A weekly dose of 500 micrograms should suffice if allowed to melt in the mouth. Vitamin B_{12} can be given as an injection, to assure rapid absorption. Pyridoxine may also be helpful in the treatment of neuropathic pain. Pyridoxal-5-phosphate (PLP), the active form of vitamin B_6 may be required, rarely, some patients do not convert pyridoxine to the active form efficiently. PLP helps process tryptophan into non-toxic kynurenine, serotonin, and melatonin. PLP also is required for the enzymatic conversion of glutamate to GABA.

CSS and other forms of neuropathic pain may be helped with tricyclic or SNRI antidepressants medications and certain anticonvulsant medications. Of the anticonvulsants, topiramate appears to be particularly effective in PTSD[112], likely as a result its effects on AMPA and kainate receptors. Nevertheless, nutrient supplements appear just as effective, without toxicity or side effects.

Table 32-4: Nutrients for Neuropathic Pain

Factor	Recommended Daily Dose
R-α-lipoic acid (sodium)	50 to 100 mg
Vitamin B_{12}	500 μg*
Magnesium Organic Salt	100 mg (Elemental)
Betaine (TMG)	1000 -2000 mg
EPA and DHA n-3 fatty acids[113]	1000 to 2000 mg
Calcitrol (Vitamin D_3)	See Chapter 20
Zinc	10 mg
Vitamin B_6 (pyridoxine HCL)	25 mg
Folate	400 μg
Riboflavin	5 mg
Vitamin K_2 Menatetrenone	5 mg
N-acetyl cysteine	500 – 1000 mg
Pyrroloquinoline quinone (PQQ)	10 mg
Dietary flavonoids	
PPAR-γ Agonists (n-3 fatty acids)	See Chapter 30

Patient with FMS and CSS are subject to unrelated peripheral pain and somatic pain. Peripheral pain will accelerate central pain; thus, it should address, and the underlying causes removed or treated. Trigger point injections can be helpful (see Appendix J.)

Opiates have no therapeutic role in chronic pain management and worsen CSS. Low dose (10 to 25 mg) amitriptyline[114] may be helpful. It inhibits TLR signaling and helps with sleep. At higher doses, however, is associated with significant weight gain, can cause drowsiness although problems are unusual at the 10 mg. It is quite toxic in overdose; thus, it should be avoided in patients with suicidal ideation. Even so, a month supply of 10 mg tablets is unlikely to be fatal to an adult.

3. Treat Leaky Gut Syndrome, SIBO, and Biofilms: Avoid Production of LPS. LPS is a potent stimulator of TLR4 and also activates mast cells. LPS may be controlled by controlling biofilm formation as discussed in Chapter 23- 25. In some conditions, CCK is responsible for pain and nausea. Trypsin inhibits CCK release; thus trypsin inhibitors may also increase CCK levels. Cooking denatures most trypsin inhibitors found in food; however, those in potatoes remain active. Some trypsin inhibitors are present in foods that may be eaten raw. A list of foods containing in trypsin inhibitors is given in Table 23-3. Foods high in polyamines increase the release of CCK. If the enteric mucosa is functioning properly, most polyamines are metabolized prior to absorption. Avoidance of dietary polyamines may be helpful. Polyamines are discussed in Chapter 13.

Probiotics that have been used to relieve chronic stress behavior in animal models have been called "psychobiotics[115]." Use of *Lactobacillus* and *Bifidobacterium* species has been demonstrated to help relieve chronic stress behavior and its psychological sequelae that have been caused by stress-induced leaky gut syndrome[116]. Overgrowth of clostridia causes similar stress behavior. Although some researchers focus on which strain of probiotic bacteria will be most effective in modulating human behavior[117], the term psychobiotic may be misleading; the goal of treatment is normalization of the enteric biome for comprehensive health. The use of probiotics without a change in diet, including and prebiotics and prevention of malabsorption is unlikely to provide long-term improvements in health.

4. Modulate Excessive Sympathetic Activity: Sympathetic tone can be evaluated by heart rate variability (HRV). A 24 or 48 hour Holter monitor, with HRV assessment, may be helpful in diagnosing and documenting chronic sympathetic dysregulation.

Maintaining normal, light-entrained sleeping and eating cycles, and getting adequate exercise may help restore sympathetic/parasympathetic diurnal cycling. Exercise sufficient to cause short-term increases in lactic acid are probably required to down-regulate sympathetic activity.

Both clonidine and prazosin have been found to be useful in the treatment of PTSD[118] and are especially useful for nightmares that disturb sleep. Clonidine acts by stimulating α₂-adrenergic receptors in the brain, which helps to down-regulate sympathetic activity. Prazosin acts as a α₁-antagonist in the brain, which has a similar effect. β-blockers are sometimes used to treat chronic adrenergic hyperactivity in PTSD. Although there are no published trials using α₁-antagonist or α₂-agonist in FM, these agents may be helpful when used at bedtime as they are for PTSD.

5. Melatonin sensitizes opiate receptors, potentiates GABA, is a neural antioxidant, inhibits inflammatory eicosanoids, helps with sleep, and decreases sympathetic activity at night. Melatonin is helpful to many patients with FM, as well as in IBS and chronic fatigue syndrome[119]. Melatonin is also a neuromodulator in the GI system, and important for helping the GI system move into the "sleep mode" at night, lowering appetite and helping to heal the mucosa. The dose required in most trials of melatonin for FMS is 3 mg in the evening. My recommendation is 3 to 5 mg of timed released melatonin taken about 30 minutes before bedtime[120]. An additional 0.3 to 0.5 mg of sublingual melatonin at bedtime can be helpful if there is delayed sleep onset. If medications are used in the treatment of FMS or CSS, those causing drowsiness; such as tricyclic antidepressants, and those that decrease sympathetic activity, should be taken at bedtime, to help with sleep.

Bright light, fluorescent light (which has a considerable amount of blue light) and TV or computer screens should be avoided or at least one hour and preferably two hours before bedtime. It is blue light (around 480 nm) which suppresses the pituitary from making melatonin[121]. Light/Dark entrainment and melatonin may also help to down-regulate sympathetic activity and increase parasympathetic dominance during sleep.

Sleep disorders and sleep hygiene are covered in chapter 43. Restoration of diurnal metabolic rhythms is also discussed in Chapter 29.

6. Prevent Inflammatory Signaling: TLR4 (and TLR2) are activated by LPS and other several other microbial compounds (Table 10-7), and most opiates. TLR2 and TLR4 activation increase the transcription of inflammatory cytokines, eicosanoids, growth factors and other mediators of inflammation and oxidative stress. Figures 31-4 and 42-4 show several factors that affect this signaling. Addressing prevention using multiple approaches allows the use of natural, non-toxic compounds and low doses of medication such as amitriptyline or minocycline, which can lower the risk of side effects.

Vitamin D₃ and betaine decrease the expression of TLR4 receptors and Vitamin D₃ and zinc decrease the expression of TLR2 receptors, thus decreasing inflammatory reactivity. Vitamin K₂ and flavonoids decrease the production of transcription factors for NF-κB release, as described in Chapter 42, and thus decrease TNF-α production. Antioxidants decrease the production of inflammatory cytokines. Use supplements that increase PPARγ activity, such as the n-3 fatty acid DHA decrease other inflammatory transcription factors, and inflammatory cytokines. Preventing intestinal biofilm formation avoids production of LPS by microbes in the intestine, which can trigger TLR activation. IL-1β increases NF-κB activation; factors that increase IL-1β include sleep deprivation, chronic stress, mast cell activation, high-fat diet, leptin, and LPS. NF-κB activation increases IL-1β, TNF-α, COX2 and NOS transcription.

Individual patients may respond differently to different aspects of inflammatory signaling inhibition. Use of various supplements to target various aspects of inflammatory signaling gives a better chance of response with very low risk.

Phenolic compounds such as curcumin or flavonoids are helpful in pain and inflammation. Curcumin from turmeric has been found to be as effective as ibuprofen for the treatment of osteoarthritis[122].

7. Mitochondrial Rehabilitation and Oxidative Stress: FMS treatment can benefit from culling of the weak, ineffective mitochondria and develop new ones. Aerobic exercise causes inefficient mitochondria to be eliminated and selects healthiest ones to reproduce to fill the demand for energy.

FMS patients are typically severely fatigued, and movement is painful. These patients avoid exercise. Jacuzzi's, warm baths, and warm (90°F+) swimming pool exercise give some benefits similar to exercise. Once feeling better, patients with FMS should begin a progressive exercise routine. Gentle exercise in a warm pool and walking are good starting points. Eventually, the goal of exercise is to sustain an elevated heart rate for at least 10 minutes at a time, daily as this appears to be required for recovery. Exercise can include stretching, strength training, and aerobic exercises. It is essential to start with a low level and progressively increase activity. Hot baths are one of the most effective non-pharmacologic treatments of fibromyalgia[123].

Overly aggressive exercise by a motivated patient early in recovery may increase pain and deter further attempts. It may also trigger a wave of apoptosis of neurons (Chapter 21). It is far better to proceed gracefully, slowly increasing activity over two to three months.

Part of the success derived from exercise therapy depends on the cognitive understanding that the exercise is not harmful. Patients logically associate hurting with harm. In CSS, however, most of the pain experienced is not associated with harm. When patients understand this, they become less resistant to exercise, have less muscular guarding, and begin to move more normally.

Glutathione is the principal antioxidant of the CNS. While the diet contains GSH, it is poorly absorbed. GSH is a tripeptide consisting of glycine, glutamate, and cysteine. Cysteine is the rate-limiting factor and scarce in the diet.

The dietary supplement *N*-acetylcysteine is a well-absorbed source of cysteine for the production of GSH. Cysteine is principally formed from HCY in a two-step process requiring vitamin B_6 (PLP). SAMe may also help in the formation of GSH; however, folate and vitamin B_{12} or betaine are safer routes for SAMe recycling. ALA helps reduce oxidized cystine to cysteine, a required step in the production of GSH[124]. A daily dose of 50 to 100 mg of sodium stabilized r-ALA offers optimal benefit without undesirable side effects in most patients[125]. Co-administration of vitamin B12 may enhance the efficacy of ALA treatment of peripheral neuropathy.

The antioxidant Coenzyme Q10 is discussed in the previous section. PQQ is another important antioxidant, which also helps activate PPAR-γ and generate new mitochondria.

Vitamin D induces the production of enzymes required for GSH production. Malabsorption of the fat-soluble vitamins may occur in FMS. FMS symptoms may be caused by low vitamin D levels. Vitamin D should be tested in all patients with FMS, and treated if low. (See Chapter 20.) Because malabsorption is common, it is important to test 25OHD3 levels to make sure that the patient is absorbing and retaining the vitamin.

Chapter 21 covers mitochondrial health, exercise, foods and supplements which may help rehabilitate mitochondria and antioxidants which may prevent oxidative stress. A patient questionnaire for assessing physical activity is provided in Appendix E.

8. Sleep Disorders: Sleep disturbances, which have overlapping symptoms with FMS, are common in this disease. FMS patients commonly report adequate time in bed but have poor sleep efficiency. Some of this may be secondary to pain, or it may worsen the pain.

In healthy individuals, the sympathetic nervous system dominates during the day and at night the parasympathetic system dominates the autonomic nervous system (ANS). This provides for activity in the day and vegetative functions at night when the body temperature drops, heart rate slows, and blood pressure drops. The diurnal control over the ANS is mediated in the suprachiasmatic nucleus of the brain that sets its cycle by the influence of light[126]. In FMS, the sympathetic nervous system looses its diurnal rhythm and is constantly activated. Eventually, this leads to system fatigue. Many of the symptoms of FMS are consistent with non-restorative sleep. Exercise in the AM and a regular sleep and eating cycle may be helpful.

9. Mast Cell Activation Disorder: It should be assumed that patients with FMS have MCAS. The elevated CRH in FMS and PTSD increases both mast cell activation and paracellular permeability. MCAS and their treatments are discussed in Chapter 12. Treatment of paracellular hyperpermeability is covered in chapter 25.

10. Food Antergies: Sympathetic activity increases the activation of T_H17 immune function in the gut, increasing the risk of immune reactions to food. These reactions increase the production of IL-17 and promote the development of secondary disease manifestations commonly seen in FM. It is often helpful to test and treat FMS patients for IgG food antergens. Details are given in Chapter 19. FMS patients should additionally be tested for food allergies they believe they may have.

11. Comorbidities: Several comorbid conditions, common in FMS, are covered in other chapters in this text, including IBS, depression, rage, and mitochondrial dysfunction.

12. Cannabinoids: CB2 receptor agonists may provide benefit in pain management. Medical marijuana has some utility; however, its prominent CB1 activity affects cognition and function, limiting its value. Little is known about its long-term value in pain management. The herb, echinacea, has CB2 agonistic activity, and it may have some, probably short-term, efficacy in pain management. It, however, is antigenic, and allergies or antergies may develop to it. Cannabidiol, which act mostly as a CB1 and CB2 antagonist, may have medical utility.

PTSD

PSTD, like FMS, is caused by chronic sympathetic hyperactivity. Treatment of PTSD is similar to that for sympathetic over activity in FMS but should also include the treatment recommended for rage and sleep disorders. PTSD often a comorbidity of injuries causing traumatic brain injury; thus, TBI should also be treated (Chapter 30). PTSD, however, is less likely to have IBS and other comorbidities associated with mitochondrial dysfunction; thus may not require treatment for those conditions. Rage and anger are addressed in Chapter 36; anxiety treatment below.

Anxiety

Stressed mice with anxiety have been found to have high levels of ROS in their neurons and granulocytes; the neurons of the cerebral cortex and hippocampus had seven times the level of ROS levels as did non-anxious mice. ROS levels were four times higher in the granulocytes of anxious mice compared to non-anxious ones. When normal mice were subjected to a compound that caused oxidative stress that depleted glutathione, it caused stress behavior[127].

Oxidative stress can induce the production of inflammatory cytokines, induce prostaglandin synthesis, increase the activity of sphingomyelinase and production of ceramide, and cause neuronal apoptosis. It should be no surprise that it can cause anxiety, or create an ambiance in which anxiety is prone to develop.

Anxiety, in PSTD and other conditions, is a learned condition. Even though an oxidative stress milieu or traumatic event may have caused the anxiety, once learned, the reaction to stimuli that cause anxiety, continue to cause anxiety reactions or aggressive defensive response.

Extinction learning is a paradigm for the treatment of anxiety in which the subject is repeatedly exposed to an aversive stimulus until the fear response to that stimulus is inhibited. The individual learns that the anxiety associated stimulus, in itself, is not a danger. For example, not all spiders are dangerous, not all exposure to spiders warrants a panic attack. While the "learning" portion of extinction learning is accurate, at least a considerable part of "extinction" is better described as "supervision."

Children rely on "gut-level" responses to dangerous situations to keep them safe as they lack sufficient experience and knowledge to make informed decisions on risk and its management. As adults, risk can be evaluated more cognitively. With experience and information, the management of risk stimuli can be transferred from the hypothalamic and midbrain emotional reaction to supervision of response by the prefrontal and frontal areas of the brain that control emotional response and provide judgment of risk (Chapter 36.)

A therapeutic technique, Eye Movement Desensitization and Reprocessing (EMDR), is an effective treatment for PTSD[128] and for others who have experienced trauma. The lack of explanation for mechanistic action has hampered its acceptance, despite its high success rate. Recent studies have demonstrated that EMDR shifts emotional processing of disturbing memory to cognitive processing[129], providing relief from negative emotional experiences. In part, EMDR may act through cognitive discordance; the scanning eye movement simulates a state of vigilance, as would occur in an exposed situation, and the traumatic event is reviewed; however, the patient realizes that they are in a safe setting. This allows the patient to disconnect the visceral reactions from the memory, view it more dispassionately, and respond to environmental stimuli at a more functional level of vigilance. Additionally, these eye movements may reproduce the walking/searching activities that stimulate BNDF production in the hypothalamus. BNDF promotes neuronal growth and enhances place memory and learning.

Both anxiety and the dismissal of anxiety are learned, and both are associated with feeding behavior. Finding foods in the wild is risky business; hunger is associated with lower levels of anxiety, and this helps animals go out to seek food. Satiation is associated with increased anxiety; you may want to lie down and nap after a meal, but this is not a great idea if predators are about. Hunger and fearlessness; and satiation and anxiety; and learning and memory; are controlled by neurohormones and neurotransmitters.

Anxiety is a visceral reaction; the gut hormone, CCK, helps create avoidance memory. CCK promotes satiety after a meal and increases anxiety learning. CCK helps create avoidance memory. In contrast, NPY helps extinguish aversion memory. FMS and PTSD patients have lower baseline plasma NPY levels than do healthy individuals. NPY increases feeding behavior by increasing hunger and decreasing anxiety. NPY blunts the fear response and aids in learning to dismiss aversion and anxiety that has been learned.

Table 32-5: Learning, Feeding, and Anxiety[18]

Mediator	Effects
CRH	↑ Fear learning, threat recognition
CCK-4	↑ Avoidance memory, panic, fear, satiation
NPY	Aversion memory extinction ↑ Hunger and feeding
Glutamate	Attention, alertness, memory consolidation[130]
Histamine H_2R[131, 132]	↑ Vigilance ↑ Attention Inhibitory avoidance memory consolidation Fear extinction consolidation ↓ Feeding, ↑ Object recognition memory[133]
BDNF	Increased plasticity, enhances extinction[134]
Magnesium	Increased plasticity, enhances extinction[135]
CB1	Prevents the release of CCK, ↑ Feeding ↓ Object recognition memory

The excitatory neurotransmitter, glutamate is essential for learning and the creation of memory. It stimulates alertness and attention and triggers the calcium channel mediated transcription of proteins used in developing new memory, principally, through stimulation of ionotropic NMDA receptors. Histamine increases glutaminergic neuronal excitability and facilitates NMDA glutamatergic receptor-mediated responses, especially when Mg^{2+} levels are high. Histamine causes a lasting potentiation of neuronal excitability that is mediated mainly by H_2 receptor activation[136].

EMRD, cognitive behavioral therapy (CBT), and Acceptance Based Therapy (Chapter 29) are all similarly effective treatments for anxiety. They all rely on "extinction learning," wherein the prefrontal and frontal areas learn to supervise the midbrain emotional response. This shift relies on learning and "rewriting" the traumatic memories while the patient is in a low-threat internal and external milieu. Treatment for the ablation of anxiety should, thus, be performed while the subject awake, alert, and calm, and with an appetite; before a meal; when NPY is high, and CCK is low.

The environment should be relaxed and non-threatening. The subject should be well rested if possible, and pretreated with antioxidants and supplements to repeat glutathione levels (Chapter 21). Factors that augment BDNF formation, such as walking, low-dose zinc and beta-carotene are discussed in Chapter 31. Magnesium enhances anxiety extinction learning, and supplements should be used daily as Mg^{2+} absorption is limited, and it may take a couple of weeks to normalize low Mg levels (Chapter 30). Immune activation that increases CRH should be avoided (Chapters 18 and 19.)

Sympathetic activation impairs frontal lobe activity in favor of fight or flight, and thus, anxiety ablation learning is best done when the patient is calm. An hour after exercise or a hot bath, both which increases sympathetic tone, may help lower it activity in patients with chronically elevated sympathetic tone.

Theanine is a non-protein amino acid occurring in tea (*Camellia sinensis*). It has anti-anxiety properties, yet increases memory and learning[137]. It induces BNDF and is an NMDA agonist[138], however, it also protects neurons from excitotoxicity[139]. A dose of 50 to 100 mg of theanine, given 30 minutes prior to learning, including therapeutic relearning, may provide benefit.

Antihistamines; especially H_2 blockers, and medications that antagonize histamine should be avoided during learning, such as during aversion memory extinction as they can impair memory consolidation[140]. CB1 agonists, such as marijuana, may decrease anxiety and increase feeding, but impair learning.

Phosphodiesterase inhibitors slow disease progression in Alzheimer's disease. They likely act through muscarinic induction of endocannabinoids. Activation of presynaptic cannabinoid CB1 receptors inhibits both glutamate and GABA nerve transmission[141]. This anti-glutaminergic action may prevent neuronal excitotoxicity injury. Stimulation of cannabinoid CB1 receptors mitigates the action of TNF-α [142].

The story of the patient's trauma should be reviewed and verbalized in detail; describing both the internal and external environment; what they saw, heard, felt, and thought as the event unfolded. The goal is to re-remember relearn and recode the event, in a calm, controlled, safe, internal and external environment.

Writing things down is useful for creating organized, informational memory, but also helps move concerns out of the active actionable memory pool. When we write a grocery list, we can stop running the list through our minds in our attempts to make sure we are not forgetting anything. Writing down the traumatic event, in a calm, therapeutic milieu, can help relearn it as a less emotional and less traumatizing memory.

Alzheimer's Disease

Alzheimer's disease is a neuroinflammatory disease in which TLRs activate microglia. There is mounting evidence that this inflammation can be controlled by inhibiting TLR2 and TLR4 mediated transcription of inflammatory mediators, cytokines and growth factors. A diet rich in plant phenols would be expected decrease the production of TNF-α. Vitamin D, betaine, folic acid, and the N-3 fatty acid DHA promote the down-regulation of TLR2 and TLR4 mediated inflammation. Magnesium increases PI3K/Akt signaling and supports microglia repair rather than inflammatory activities, and along with PLP helps prevention excitotoxicity, AD is also discussed in Chapter 31. Free copper may be central to AD disease progression, and lowering them with low dose zinc has been shown to slow disease progression[143]. Preventive treatment of Alzheimer's disease will have a better outcome than attempts to reverse it late in its course.

Phenolic Foods Compounds

Over 500 different plant polyphenols are found in food. Although best known as antioxidants, they have other metabolic effects, and most of these effects are beneficial.

Resveratrol, kaempferol, quercetin, and luteolin have been shown to induce autophagy – the process of breaking down cellular organelles for recycling[144]. Various polyphenols possess anti-inflammatory, anti-oxidant, anti-allergic, hepatoprotective, anti-thrombotic, anti-viral and anti-carcinogenic activities. They act by interfering with a large number and variety of mammalian enzymes[145].

Over a dozen polyphenols have been demonstrated to be potent inhibitors of 5-alpha-reductase, the enzyme that converts testosterone into the more active androgen, dihydrotestosterone (DHT)[146]. DHT is the most potent androgen, and the one thought to promote acne. The phenolic compound rutin blocks the enzyme AKR1C3 that helps metabolizes androgens and prostaglandins PGD_2, PGH_2 into $PGF_{2\alpha}$. Quercetin and rutin and some other flavonoids block the enzyme CBR1 that converts PGE_2 to $PGF_{2\alpha}$ and also prevents toxicity of certain chemotherapy agents[147].

Green tea polyphenols may decrease the risk of breast cancer and prostate cancer[148,149]. Green tea polyphenols inhibit VEGF, MMP-2 and MMP-9, proteins involved in metastasis. Certain polyphenols appear to block intracellular signaling involved in early metastasis[150].

Certain flavonoids inhibit 5-lipoxygenase (ALOX-5) and thus may prevent the inflammatory conversion of AA in the keratinocytes into leukotrienes.

A diet with a mix of polyphenols from a wide selection of fruits and vegetables is recommended for health. Too little is known about these compounds to recommend high doses of any single polyphenols, or a single food source of polyphenols to maintain health; green tea polyphenols, for example, can affect multiple enzymes, and thus may have unintended consequences at high doses. Specific polyphenols may be useful as medications to target specific diseases.

Dietary phenolic compounds decrease the proliferation of toxin-producing bacteria in the colon, likely acting as quorum sensing inhibitors (See Chapter 23).

Polyphenol supplements, beyond those that are part of a healthy diet, should be avoided during pregnancy. Many of the enzymes and intracellular signaling which are activated in cancer are present in the cells because they are required in embryogenesis. Phenolic compounds found in the diet with diverse fruits, herbs and vegetables are safe during pregnancy.

[1] Developments in the scientific and clinical understanding of fibromyalgia. Buskila D. Arthritis Res Ther. 2009;11(5):242. PMID:19835639

[2] Comorbidity of fibromyalgia and psychiatric disorders. Arnold LM, Hudson JI, Keck PE, Auchenbach MB, Javaras KN, Hess EV. J Clin Psychiatry. 2006 Aug;67(8):1219-25. PMID:16965199

[3] Vitamin D deficiency is associated with anxiety and depression in fibromyalgia. Armstrong DJ, Meenagh GK, Bickle I, et al. Clin Rheumatol. 2007 Apr;26(4):551-4. PMID:16850115

[4] Population frequency of myotonic dystrophy: higher than expected frequency of myotonic dystrophy type 2 (DM2) mutation in Finland. Suominen T, Bachinski LL, Auvinen S, et al. Eur J Hum Genet. 2011 Jul;19(7):776-82. PMID:21364698

[5] Poor sleep quality and fatigue but no excessive daytime sleepiness in myotonic dystrophy type 2. Tieleman AA, Knoop H, van de Logt AE, et al. J Neurol Neurosurg Psychiatry. 2010 Sep;81(9):963-7. PMID:20798200

[6] Restless legs syndrome and daytime sleepiness are prominent in myotonic dystrophy type 2. Lam EM, Shepard PW, St Louis EK, et al. Neurology. 2013 Jul 9;81(2):157-64. PMID:23749798

[7] Myotonic dystrophy type 2 found in two of sixty-three persons diagnosed as having fibromyalgia. Auvinen S, Suominen T, Hannonen P, et al. Arthritis Rheum. 2008 Nov;58(11):3627-31. PMID: 18975316

[8] Temporal summation of second pain and its maintenance are useful for characterizing widespread central sensitization of fibromyalgia patients. Staud R, Robinson ME, Price DD. J Pain. 2007 Nov;8(11):893-901. PMID:17681887

[9] The role of the central nervous system in the generation and maintenance of chronic pain in rheumatoid arthritis, osteoarthritis and fibromyalgia. Lee YC, Nassikas NJ, Clauw DJ. Arthritis Res Ther. 2011 Apr 28;13(2):211. PMID:21542893

[10] Metabolic abnormalities in pain-processing regions of patients with fibromyalgia: a 3T MR spectroscopy study. Feraco P, Bacci A, Pedrabissi F, et al. AJNR Am J Neuroradiol. 2011 Oct;32(9):1585-90. PMID: 21799042

[11] Elevated insular glutamate in fibromyalgia is associated with experimental pain. Harris RE, Sundgren PC, Craig AD, et al. Arthritis Rheum. 2009 Oct;60(10):3146-52. PMID:19790053

[12] Oxidative glutamate toxicity involves mitochondrial dysfunction and perturbation of intracellular Ca^{2+} homeostasis. Pereira CF, Oliveira CR. Neurosci Res. 2000 Jul;37(3):227-36. PMID: 10940457

[13] Decreased levels of glutathione, the major brain antioxidant, in post-mortem prefrontal cortex from patients with psychiatric disorders. Gawryluk JW, Wang JF, Andreazza AC, Shao L. Int J Neuropsychopharmacol. 2011 Feb;14(1):123-30. PMID:20633320

[14] The biological clock tunes the organs of the body: timing by hormones and the autonomic nervous system. Buijs RM, van Eden CG, Goncharuk VD, Kalsbeek A. J Endocrinol. 2003 Apr;177(1):17-26. PMID:12697033

[15] Vagus nerve stimulation modulates visceral pain-related affective memory. Zhang X, Cao B, Yan N, Liu J, Wang J, Tung VO, Li Y. Behav Brain Res. 2013 Jan 1;236(1):8-15. PMID:22940455

[16] Activation of descending pain-facilitatory pathways from the rostral ventromedial medulla by cholecystokinin elicits release of prostaglandin-E2 in the spinal cord. Marshall TM, Herman DS, Largent-Milnes TM, et al. Pain. 2012 Jan;153(1):86-94. PMID:22030324

[17] Cholecystokinin exerts an effect via the endocannabinoid system to inhibit GABAergic transmission in midbrain periaqueductal gray.Mitchell VA, Jeong HJ, Drew GM, Vaughan CW. Neuropsychopharmacology. 2011 Aug;36(9):1801-10. PMID:21525858

[18] Neuropeptide regulation of fear and anxiety: Implications of cholecystokinin, endogenous opioids, and neuropeptide Y. Bowers ME, Choi DC, Ressler KJ. Physiol Behav. 2012 Dec 5;107(5):699-710. PMID:22429904

[19] Central and peripheral sites of action for CB2 receptor mediated analgesic activity in chronic inflammatory and neuropathic pain models in rats. Hsieh GC, Pai M, Chandran P, et al. Br J Pharmacol. 2011 Jan;162(2):428-40. PMID:20880025

[20] The reticular-activating hypofrontality (RAH) model of acute exercise. Dietrich A, Audiffren M. Neurosci Biobehav Rev. 2011 May;35(6):1305-25. PMID:21315758

[21] Objective measures of disordered sleep in fibromyalgia. Chervin RD, Teodorescu M, Kushwaha R, et al. J Rheumatol. 2009 Sep;36(9):2009-16. PMID:19684146

[22] Lack of Circadian Pattern of Serum TNF-α and IL-6 in Patients with Fibromyalgia Syndrome. Fatima G, Mahdi AA, Das SK, Anjum B, Verma NS, Kumar P, Shrivastava R. Indian J Clin Biochem. 2012 Oct;27(4):340-3. PMID:24082457

[23] Stress and autonomic dysregulation in patients with fibromyalgia syndrome. Friederich HC, Schellberg D, Mueller K, et al. 2005 Jun;19(3):185-8, 190-2, 194. PMID:15138868

[24] Evidence of reduced sympatho-adrenal and hypothalamic-pituitary activity during static muscular work in patients with fibromyalgia. Kadetoff D, Kosek E. J Rehabil Med. 2010 Sep;42(8):765-72. PMID:20809059

[25] Autonomic and respiratory characteristics of posttraumatic stress disorder and panic disorder. Blechert J, Michael T, Grossman P, Lajtman M, Wilhelm FH. Psychosom Med. 2007 Dec;69(9):935-43. PMID:17991823

[26] Biogenic amine depletion causes chronic muscular pain and tactile allodynia accompanied by depression: A putative animal model of fibromyalgia. Nagakura Y, Oe T, Aoki T, Matsuoka N. Pain. 2009 Nov;146(1-2):26-33. PMID:19646816

[27] Association of adrenergic receptor gene polymorphisms with different fibromyalgia syndrome domains. Vargas-Alarcón G, Fragoso JM, Cruz-Robles D, et al. Arthritis Rheum. 2009 Jul;60(7):2169-73.PMID: 19565482

[28] An internet survey of 2,596 people with fibromyalgia. Bennett RM, Jones J, Turk DC, Russell IJ, Matallana L. BMC Musculoskelet Disord. 2007 Mar 9;8:27. PMID:17349056

[29] Autonomic innervation and regulation of the immune system (1987-2007). Nance DM, Sanders VM. Brain Behav Immun. 2007 Aug;21(6):736-45 PMID:17467231

[30] The sympathetic nerve--an integrative interface between two supersystems: the brain and the immune system. Elenkov IJ, Wilder RL, Chrousos GP, Vizi ES. Pharmacol Rev. 2000 Dec;52(4):595-638. PMID:11121511

[31] Th17 cells: from precursors to players in inflammation and infection. Awasthi A, Kuchroo VK. Int Immunol. 2009 May;21(5):489-98. PMID:19261692

[32] Increased IgA responses to the LPS of commensal bacteria is associated with inflammation and activation of cell-mediated immunity in chronic fatigue syndrome. Maes M, Twisk FN, Kubera M, et al. J Affect Disord. 2012 Feb;136(3):909-17. PMID:21967891

[33] Mitochondrial production of reactive oxygen species contributes to the β-adrenergic stimulation of mouse cardiomycytes. Andersson DC, Fauconnier J, Yamada T, Lacampagne A, Zhang SJ, Katz A, Westerblad H. J Physiol. 2011 Apr 1;589(Pt 7):1791-801. PMID:21486840

[34] Elevated mitochondrial superoxide contributes to enhanced chemoreflex in heart failure rabbits. Ding Y, Li YL, Zimmerman MC, Schultz HD. Am J Physiol Regul Integr Comp Physiol. 2010 Feb;298(2):R303-11. PMID:19923358

[35] Cerebral activation and catastrophizing during pain anticipation in patients with fibromyalgia. Burgmer M, Petzke F, Giesecke T, et al. Psychosom Med. 2011 Nov-Dec;73(9):751-9. PMID:22048836

[36] Opioids and clonidine modulate cytokine production and opioid receptor expression in neonatal immune cells. Chavez-Valdez R, Kovell L, Ahlawat R, McLemore GL, Wills-Karp M, Gauda EB. J Perinatol. 2012 PMID:23047422

[37] Mechanisms underlying morphine analgesic tolerance and dependence. Ueda H, Ueda M. Front Biosci. 2009 Jun 1;14:5260-72. PMID:19482614

[38] Regulation of the extrinsic and intrinsic apoptotic pathways in the prefrontal cortex of short- and long-term human opiate abusers. García-Fuster MJ, Ramos-Miguel A, Rivero G, et al. Neuroscience. 2008 Nov 11;157(1):105-19. PMID:18834930

[39] Opioid activation of toll-like receptor 4 contributes to drug reinforcement. Hutchinson MR, Northcutt AL, Hiranita T, et al. Neurosci. 2012 Aug 15;32(33):11187-200. PMID:22895704

[40] Evidence that tricyclic small molecules may possess toll-like receptor and myeloid differentiation protein 2 activity. Hutchinson MR, Loram LC, Zhang Y, et al. Neuroscience. 2010 Jun 30;168(2):551-63. PMID:20381591

[41] Do you feel my pain? Racial group membership modulates empathic neural responses. Xu X, Zuo X, Wang X, Han S. J Neurosci. 2009 Jul 1;29(26):8525-9. PMID:19571143

[42] Their pain is not our pain: brain and autonomic correlates of empathic resonance with the pain of same and different race individuals. Azevedo RT, Macaluso E, Avenanti A, et al. Hum Brain Mapp. 2013 Dec;34(12):3168-81. PMID:22807311

[43] Perispinal etanercept: a new therapeutic paradigm in neurology. Tobinick E. Expert Rev Neurother. 2010 Jun;10(6):985-1002. PMID:20518613

[44] Depressive-like behavior induced by tumor necrosis factor-α in mice. Kaster MP, Gadotti VM, Calixto JB, Santos AR, Rodrigues AL. Neuropharmacology. 2012 Jan;62(1):419-26. PMID:21867719

[45] Chronic Administration of Infliximab (TNF-Alpha Inhibitor) Decreases Depression and Anxiety-like Behaviour in Rat Model of Chronic Mild Stress. Karson A, Demirtaş T, Bayramgürler D, Balcı F. Basic Clin Pharmacol Toxicol. 2012 Nov 20. PMID:23167806

[45] Preliminary Evidence of Increased Pain and Elevated Cytokines in Fibromyalgia Patients with Defective Growth Hormone Response to Exercise. Ross RL, Jones KD, Bennett RM, Ward RL, Druker BJ, Wood LJ. Open Immunol J. 2010;3:9-18. PMID:20467575

[46] Plasma cytokine fluctuations over time in healthy controls and patients with fibromyalgia. Togo F, Natelson BH, Adler GK, et al. Exp Biol Med (Maywood). 2009 Feb;234(2):232-40. PMID:19064941

[47] Neuroinflammation in Patients with Chronic Fatigue Syndrome/Myalgic Encephalomyelitis: An 11C-(R)-PK11195 PET Study. Nakatomi Y, Mizuno K, Ishii A, et al. J Nucl Med. 2014 Mar 24;55(6):945-950. PMID:24665088

[48] Right Arcuate Fasciculus Abnormality in Chronic Fatigue Syndrome. Zeineh MM, Kang J, Atlas SW, et al. Radiology. 2014 Oct 29:141079. PMID:25353054

[49] The gut-brain barrier in major depression: intestinal mucosal dysfunction with an increased translocation of LPS from gram negative enterobacteria (leaky gut) plays a role in the inflammatory pathophysiology of depression. Maes M, Kubera M, Leunis JC. Neuro Endocrinol Lett. 2008 Feb;29(1):117-24. PMID:18283240

[50] Increased levels of IL-17A in patients with fibromyalgia. Pernambuco AP, Schetino LP, Alvim CC, Murad CM, Viana RS, Carvalho LS, Reis DÁ. Clin Exp Rheumatol. 2013 Nov-Dec;31(6 Suppl 79):S60-3. PMID:24021410

[51] Cytokines play an aetiopathogenetic role in fibromyalgia: a hypothesis and pilot study. Wallace DJ, Linker-Israeli M, Hallegua D, Silverman S, Silver D, Weisman MH. Rheumatology (Oxford). 2001 Jul;40(7):743-9. PMID:11477278

[52] Circulating cytokine levels compared to pain in patients with fibromyalgia -- a prospective longitudinal study over 6 months. Wang H, Moser M, Schiltenwolf M, Buchner M. J Rheumatol. 2008 Jul;35(7):1366-70. PMID:18528959

[53] Inhibition of ceramide-redox signaling pathway blocks glomerular injury in hyperhomocysteinemic rats. Yi F, Zhang AY, Li N, Muh RW, Fillet M, Renert AF, Li PL. Kidney Int. 2006 Jul;70(1):88-96. PMID:16688115

[54] Sphingomyelinase stimulates oxidant signaling to weaken skeletal muscle and promote fatigue. Ferreira LF, Moylan JS, Gilliam LA, et al. Am J Physiol Cell Physiol. 2010 Sep;299(3):C552-60. PMID:20519448

[55] ASMase is required for chronic alcohol induced hepatic endoplasmic reticulum stress and mitochondrial cholesterol loading. Fernandez A, Matias N, Fucho R, et al. J Hepatol. 2013 Oct;59(4):805-13. PMID:23707365

[56] Brain pericytes among cells constituting the blood-brain barrier are highly sensitive to tumor necrosis factor-α, releasing matrix metalloproteinase-9 and migrating in vitro. Takata F, Dohgu S, Matsumoto J, et al. J Neuroinflammation. 2011 Aug 26;8:106. PMID:21867555

[57] Chronic urticaria is usually associated with fibromyalgia syndrome. Torresani C, Bellafiore S, De Panfilis G. Acta Derm Venereol. 2009;89(4):389-92.PMID: 19688152

[58] Abnormal overexpression of mastocytes in skin biopsies of fibromyalgia patients. Blanco I, Béritze N, Argüelles M, et al. Clin Rheumatol. 2010 Dec;29(12):1403-12. PMID:20428906

[59] Increased IgA responses to the LPS of commensal bacteria is associated with inflammation and activation of cell-mediated immunity in chronic fatigue syndrome. Maes M, Twisk FN, Kubera M, Ringel K, Leunis JC, Geffard M. J Affect Disord. 2012 Feb;136(3):909-17. PMID:21967891

[60] Increased levels of neurotrophins are not specific for chronic migraine: evidence from primary fibromyalgia syndrome.

Sarchielli P, Mancini ML, Floridi A, et al.. J Pain. 2007 Sep;8(9):737-45. PMID:17611164

[61] Increased plasma levels of brain derived neurotrophic factor (BDNF) in patients with fibromyalgia. Haas L, Portela LV, Böhmer AE, et al. Neurochem Res. 2010 May;35(5):830-4. PMID:20119637

[62] Returning from war with invisible wounds. (CME course)2010 Prime Education , Inc. www.priminc.org

[63] During a corticotropin-releasing hormone test in healthy subjects, administration of a beta-adrenergic antagonist induced secretion of cortisol and dehydroepiandrosterone sulfate and inhibited secretion of ACTH. Kizildere S, Glück T, Zietz B, Schölmerich J, Straub RH. Eur J Endocrinol. 2003 Jan;148(1):45-53. PMID:12534357

[64] Catechol-O-methyltransferase-deficient mice exhibit sexually dimorphic changes in catecholamine levels and behavior. Gogos JA, Morgan M, Luine V, Santha M, Ogawa S, Pfaff D, Karayiorgou M. Proc Natl Acad Sci U S A. 1998 Aug 18;95(17):9991-6.PMID: 9707588

[65] The orexigenic hormone ghrelin defends against depressive symptoms of chronic stress. Lutter M, Sakata I, Osborne-Lawrence et al. Nat Neurosci. 2008 Jul;11(7):752-3..PMID: 18552842

[66] Anger attacks in depression--evidence for a male depressive syndrome. Winkler D, Pjrek E, Kasper S. Psychother Psychosom. 2005;74(5):303-7.PMID:16088268

[67] Soybean isoflavone alleviates β-amyloid 1-42 induced inflammatory response to improve learning and memory ability by down regulation of Toll-like receptor 4 expression and nuclear factor-κB activity in rats. Ding BJ, Ma WW, He LL, et al. Int J Dev Neurosci. 2011 Aug;29(5):537-42. PMID:21515354

[68] Oligomers of β-amyloid protein (Aβ1-42) induce the activation of cyclooxygenase-2 in astrocytes via an interaction with interleukin-1β, tumour necrosis factor-α, and a nuclear factor κ-B mechanism in the rat brain. Carrero I, Gonzalo MR, Martin B, et al. Exp Neurol. 2012 Aug;236(2):215-27. PMID:22617488

[69] Pattern recognition receptors involved in the inflammatory attenuating effects of soybean isoflavone in β-amyloid peptides 1-42 treated rats. Yuan L, Zhou X, Li D, Ma W, Yu H, Xi Y, Xiao R. Neurosci Lett. 2012 Jan 11;506(2):266-70. PMID:22133809

[70] Fibrillar amyloid-beta peptides activate microglia via TLR2: implications for Alzheimer's disease. Jana M, Palencia CA, Pahan K. J Immunol. 2008 Nov 15;181(10):7254-62. PMID:18981147

[71] Tumor necrosis factor-alpha (TNF-alpha) regulates Toll-like receptor 2 (TLR2) expression in microglia. Syed MM, Phulwani NK, Kielian T. J Neurochem. 2007 Nov;103(4):1461-71. PMID: 17961202

[72] A review: inflammatory process in Alzheimer's disease, role of cytokines. Rubio-Perez JM, Morillas-Ruiz JM. Scientific World Journal. 2012;2012:756357. PMID:22566778

[73] Ibuprofen decreases cytokine-induced amyloid beta production in neuronal cells. Blasko I, Apochal A, Boeck G, et al. Neurobiol Dis. 2001 Dec;8(6):1094-101. PMID:11741404

[74] Rapid cognitive improvement in Alzheimer's disease following perispinal etanercept administration. Tobinick EL, Gross H. J Neuroinflammation. 2008 Jan 9;5:2. PMID:18184433

[75] TNF-α-mediated anxiety in a mouse model of multiple sclerosis. Haji N, Mandolesi G, Gentile A, et al. Exp Neurol. 2012 Oct;237(2):296-303 PMID:22836148

[76] Antagonizing effects of soybean isoflavones on β-amyloid peptide-induced oxidative damage in neuron mitochondria of rats. Feng JF, He LL, Li D, et al. Basic Clin Pharmacol Toxicol. 2012 Oct;111(4):248-53. PMID:22551092

[77] Soy isoflavone attenuates brain mitochondrial oxidative stress induced by beta-amyloid peptides 1-42 injection in lateral cerebral ventricle. Ding J, Yu HL, Ma WW, et al. J Neurosci Res. 2013 Apr;91(4):562-7. PMID:23239252

[78] Soybean isoflavone alleviates β-amyloid 1-42 induced inflammatory response to improve learning and memory ability by down regulation of Toll-like receptor 4 expression and nuclear factor-κB activity in rats. Ding BJ, Ma WW, He LL, et al. Int J Dev Neurosci. 2011 Aug;29(5):537-42. PMID:21515354

[79] Neuroprotection of soyabean isoflavone co-administration with folic acid against beta-amyloid 1-40-induced neurotoxicity in rats. Ma WW, Xiang L, Yu HL, Yuan LH, Guo AM, Xiao YX, Li L, Xiao R. Br J Nutr. 2009 Aug;102(4):502-5. PMID:19534845

[80] Highly purified lipoteichoic acid induced pro-inflammatory signalling in primary culture of rat microglia through Toll-like receptor 2: selective potentiation of nitric oxide production by muramyl dipeptide. Kinsner A, Boveri M, Hareng L, et al. J Neurochem. 2006 Oct;99(2):596-607. PMID:16879708

[81] Responses of the sympathetic nervous system and the hypothalamic-pituitary-adrenal axis to interleukin-6: a pilot study in fibromyalgia. Torpy DJ, Papanicolaou DA, Lotsikas AJ, Wilder RL, Chrousos GP, Pillemer SR. Arthritis Rheum. 2000 Apr;43(4):872-80. PMID:10765933

[82] Blunted ACTH and cortisol responses to systemic injection of corticotropin-releasing hormone (CRH) in fibromyalgia: role of somatostatin and CRH-binding protein. Riedel W, Schlapp U, Leck S, Netter P, Neeck G. Ann N Y Acad Sci. 2002 Jun;966:483-90. PMID:12114308

[83] Characteristic electron microscopic findings in the skin of patients with fibromyalgia--preliminary study. Kim SH, Kim DH, Oh DH, Clauw DJ. Clin Rheumatol. 2008 Mar;27(3):407-11.PMID: 18323007

[84] Mitochondrial dysfunction and mitophagy activation in blood mononuclear cells of fibromyalgia patients: implications in the pathogenesis of the disease. Cordero MD, De Miguel M, Moreno Fernández AM, et al. Arthritis Res Ther. 2010;12(1):R17. PMID:20109177

[85] Increased DNA fragmentation and ultrastructural changes in fibromyalgic muscle fibres. Sprott H, Salemi S, Gay RE, et al. Ann Rheum Dis. 2004 Mar;63(3):245-51. PMID:14962957

[86] Oxidative stress correlates with headache symptoms in fibromyalgia: coenzyme Q10 effect on clinical improvement. Cordero MD, Cano-García FJ, Alcocer-Gómez E, De Miguel M, Sánchez-Alcázar JA. PLoS One. 2012;7(4):e35677. PMID:22532869

[87] Is inflammation a mitochondrial dysfunction-dependent event in Fibromyalgia? Cordero MD, Díaz-Parrado E, Carrión AM, et al. Antioxid Redox Signal. 2012 Sep 3. PMID:22938055

[88] Systematic review and meta-analysis of pharmacological therapies for painful diabetic peripheral neuropathy. Snedecor SJ, Sudharshan L, Cappelleri JC, Sadosky A, Mehta S, Botteman M. Pain Pract. 2014 Feb;14(2):167-84. PMID:23534696

[89] Alpha-lipoic Acid and diabetic neuropathy. Vallianou N, Evangelopoulos A, Koutalas P. Rev Diabet Stud. 2009 Winter;6(4):230-6. PMID:20043035

[90] An update on the biology of sphingosine 1-phosphate receptors. Blaho VA, Hla T. J Lipid Res. 2014 Jan 23. PMID:24459205

[91] Meta-analysis of methylcobalamin alone and in combination with lipoic acid in patients with diabetic peripheral neuropathy. Xu Q, Pan J, Yu J, et al. Diabetes Res Clin Pract. 2013 Aug;101(2):99-105. PMID:23664235

[92] Non-steroidal anti-inflammatory drugs as disease-modifying agents for Parkinson's disease: evidence from observational studies. Rees K, Stowe R, Patel S, Ives N, Breen K. Cochrane Database Syst Rev. 2011 Nov 9;(11):CD008454. PMID:22071848

[93] Ibuprofen and lipoic acid codrug 1 control Alzheimer's disease progression by down-regulating protein kinase C ε-mediated metalloproteinase 2 and 9 levels in β-amyloid infused Alzheimer's disease rat model. Zara S, Rapino M, Sozio P, Di Stefano A, Nasuti C, Cataldi A. Brain Res. 2011 Sep 15;1412:79-87. PMID:21820649

[94] Ibuprofen attenuates oxidative damage through NOX2 inhibition in Alzheimer's disease. Wilkinson BL, Cramer PE, Varvel NH, Reed-Geaghan E, Jiang Q, Szabo A, Herrup K, Lamb BT, Neurobiol Aging. 2012 Jan;33(1):197.e21-32. PMID:20696495

[95] A study on the mechanisms involving the anti-inflammatory effect of amitriptyline in carrageenan-induced paw edema in rats. Sadeghi H, Hajhashemi V, Minaiyan M, Movahedian A, Talebi A. Eur J Pharmacol. 2011 Sep 30;667(1-3):396-401. PMID:21645506

[96] Betaine inhibits toll-like receptor 4 expression in rats with ethanol-induced liver injury. Shi QZ, Wang LW, Zhang W, Gong ZJ. World J Gastroenterol. 2010 Feb 21;16(7):897-903. PMID:20143470

[97] Effect of pyrroloquinoline quinone on neuropathic pain following chronic constriction injury of the sciatic nerve in rats. Gong D, Geng C, Jiang L, Aoki Y, Nakano M, Zhong L. Eur J Pharmacol. 2012 Dec 15;697(1-3):53-8. PMID:23063836

[98] Pyrroloquinoline quinone attenuates iNOS gene expression in the injured spinal cord. Hirakawa A, Shimizu K, Fukumitsu H, Furukawa S.Biochem Biophys Res Commun. 2009 Jan 9;378(2):308-12. PMID:19026989

[99] Improvement of pain, sleep, and quality of life in chronic pain patients with vitamin D supplementation. Huang W, Shah S, Long Q, et al. Clin J Pain. 2013 Apr;29(4):341-7. PMID:22699141

[100] Mechanisms of anti-inflammatory and neuroprotective actions of PPAR-gamma agonists. Kapadia R, Yi JH, Vemuganti R. Front Biosci. 2008 Jan 1;13:1813-26. PMID:17981670

[101] Magnesium sulfate protects against the bioenergetic consequences of chronic glutamate receptor stimulation. Clerc P, Young CA, Bordt EA, et al. PLoS One. 2013 Nov 13;8(11):e79982. PMID:24236167

[102] Magnesium Can Decrease Postoperative Physiological Ileus and Postoperative Pain in Major non Laparoscopic Gastrointestinal Surgeries: A Randomized Controlled Trial. Shariat Moharari R, Motalebi M, Najafi A, et al. Anesth Pain Med. 2013 Dec 6;4(1):e12750. PMID:24660146

[103] Effects of plant-derived polyphenols on TNF-alpha and nitric oxide production induced by advanced glycation endproducts. Chandler D, Woldu A, Rahmadi A, et al. Mol Nutr Food Res. 2010 Jul;54 Suppl 2:S141-50. PMID:20540146

[104] Effects of antioxidant polyphenols on TNF-alpha-related diseases. Kawaguchi K, Matsumoto T, Kumazawa Y. Curr Top Med Chem. 2011;11(14):1767-79. PMID:21506932

[105] The bone anabolic carotenoid p-hydroxycinnamic acid promotes osteoblast mineralization and suppresses osteoclast differentiation by antagonizing NF-κB activation. Yamaguchi M, Weitzmann MN. Int J Mol Med. 2012 Sep;30(3):708-12. PMID:22751682

[106] Scientific evidence and rationale for the development of curcumin and resveratrol as nutraceutricals for joint health. Mobasheri A, Henrotin Y, Biesalski HK, Shakibaei M. Int J Mol Sci. 2012;13(4):4202-32. PMID:22605974

[107] Phenol Explorer: http://www.phenol-explorer.eu

[108] Luteolin downregulates TLR4, TLR5, NF-κB and p-p38MAPK expression, upregulates the p-ERK expression, and protects rat brains against focal ischemia. Qiao H, Zhang X, Zhu C, et al. Brain Res. 2012 Apr 11;1448:71-81. PMID:22377454

[109] Efficacy of intravenous magnesium in neuropathic pain. Brill S, Sedgwick PM, Hamann W, Di Vadi PP. Br J Anaesth. 2002 Nov;89(5):711-4. PMID:12393768

[110] Relief of neuropathic pain with intravenous magnesium. Tanaka M, Shimizu S, Nishimura W, et al. Masui. 1998 Sep;47(9):1109-13. PMID:9785788

[111] Coenzyme Q10 in salivary cells correlate with blood cells in Fibromyalgia: improvement in clinical and biochemical parameter after oral treatment. Cordero MD, Santos-García R, Bermejo-Jover D, et al. Clin Biochem. 2012 Apr;45(6):509-11. PMID:22342824

[112] Meta-analysis of the efficacy of treatments for posttraumatic stress disorder. Watts BV, Schnurr PP, Mayo L, et al. J Clin Psychiatry. 2013 Jun;74(6):e541-50. PMID:23842024

[113] Omega-3 fatty acids for neuropathic pain: case series. Ko GD, Nowacki NB, Arseneau L, Eitel M, Hum A. Clin J Pain. 2010 Feb;26(2):168-72. PMID:20090445

[114] Treatment chronic pain with amitriptyline. A double-blind dosage study with determination of serum levels. Brenne E, van der Hagen K, Maehlum E, et al. 1997 Oct 10;117(24):3491-4. PMID:9411906

[115] Microbiota, the immune system, black moods and the brain-melancholia updated. Smythies LE, Smythies JR. Front Hum Neurosci. 2014 Sep 15;8:720. PMID:25309394

[116] Prevention of gut leakiness by a probiotic treatment leads to attenuated HPA response to an acute psychological stress in rats. Ait-Belgnaoui A, Durand H, Cartier C, et al. Psychoneuro-endocrinology. 2012 Nov;37(11):1885-95. PMID:22541937

[117] Targeting the microbiota-gut-brain axis to modulate behavior: which bacterial strain will translate best to humans? McLean PG, Bergonzelli GE, Collins SM, Bercik P. Proc Natl Acad Sci U S A. 2012 Jan 24;109(4):E174; author reply E176. PMID:22247294

[118] Pharmacologic reduction of CNS noradrenergic activity in PTSD: the case for clonidine and prazosin. Boehnlein JK, Kinzie JD. J Psychiatr Pract. 2007 Mar;13(2):72-8. PMID:17414682

[119] Clinical uses of melatonin: evaluation of human trials. Sánchez-Barceló EJ, Mediavilla MD, Tan DX, Reiter RJ. Curr Med Chem. 2010;17(19):2070-95. PMID:20423309

[120] Adjuvant use of melatonin for treatment of fibromyalgia. Hussain SA, Al-Khalifa II, Jasim NA, Gorial FI. J Pineal Res. 2011 Apr;50(3):267-71. PMID:21158908

[121] A "melanopic" spectral efficiency function predicts the sensitivity of melanopsin photoreceptors to polychromatic lights.

Enezi JA, Revell V, Brown T, Wynne J, Schlangen L, Lucas R. J Biol Rhythms. 2011 Aug;26(4):314-23. PMID:21775290

[122] Efficacy and safety of Curcuma domestica extracts in patients with knee osteoarthritis. Kuptniratsaikul V, Thanakhumtorn S, Chinswangwatanakul P, Wattanamongkonsil L, Thamlikitkul V. J Altern Complement Med. 2009 Aug;15(8):891-7. PMID:19678780

[123] Complementary and alternative medicine in the treatment of pain in fibromyalgia: a systematic review of randomized controlled trials. Terhorst L, Schneider MJ, Kim KH, et al. J Manipulative Physiol Ther. 2011 Sep;34(7):483-96. PMID:21875523

[124] Alpha-lipoic acid as a dietary supplement: molecular mechanisms and therapeutic potential. Shay KP, Moreau RF, Smith EJ, Smith AR, Hagen TM. Biochim Biophys Acta. 2009 Oct;1790(10):1149-60. PMID:19664690

[125] Oral treatment with alpha-lipoic acid improves symptomatic diabetic polyneuropathy: the SYDNEY 2 trial. Ziegler D, Ametov A, Barinov A, et al. Diabetes Care. 2006 Nov;29(11):2365-70. PMID:17065669

[126] Coordinated regulation of circadian rhythms and homeostasis by the suprachiasmatic nucleus. Nakagawa H, Okumura N. Proc Jpn Acad Ser B Phys Biol Sci. 2010;86(4):391-409. PMID:20431263

[127] Oxidative stress and anxiety: relationship and cellular pathways. Bouayed J, Rammal H, Soulimani R. Oxid Med Cell Longev. 2009 Apr-Jun;2(2):63-7. PMID:20357926

[128] School-based intervention programs for PTSD symptoms: a review and meta-analysis. Rolfsnes ES, Idsoe T. J Trauma Stress. 2011 Apr;24(2):155-65. PMID:21425191

[129] Neurobiological correlates of EMDR monitoring - an EEG study. Pagani M, Di Lorenzo G, Verardo AR, et al. PLoS One. 2012;7(9):e45753. PMID:23049852

[130] Histamine enhances inhibitory avoidance memory consolidation through a H2 receptor-dependent mechanism. da Silva WC, Bonini JS, Bevilaqua LR, Izquierdo I, Cammarota M. Neurobiol Learn Mem. 2006 Jul;86(1):100-6. PMID:16488163

[131] Histamine enhances inhibitory avoidance memory consolidation through a H2 receptor-dependent mechanism. da Silva WC, Bonini JS, Bevilaqua LR, Izquierdo I, Cammarota M. Neurobiol Learn Mem. 2006 Jul;86(1):100-6. PMID:16488163

[132] Histamine facilitates consolidation of fear extinction. Bonini JS, Da Silva WC, Da Silveira CK, Köhler CA, Izquierdo I, Cammarota M. Int J Neuropsychopharmacol. 2011 Oct;14(9):1209-17. PMID:21211106

[133] The role of histamine receptors in the consolidation of object recognition memory. da Silveira CK, Furini CR, Benetti F, Monteiro Sda C, Izquierdo I. Neurobiol Learn Mem. 2013 Jul;103:64-71 PMID:23583502

[134] Fear extinction and BDNF: translating animal models of PTSD to the clinic. Andero R, Ressler KJ. Genes Brain Behav. 2012 Jul;11(5):503-12. PMID:22530815

[135] Effects of elevation of brain magnesium on fear conditioning, fear extinction, and synaptic plasticity in the infralimbic prefrontal cortex and lateral amygdala. Abumaria N, Yin B, Zhang L, Li XY, et al. J Neurosci. 2011 Oct 19;31(42):14871-81. PMID:22016520

[136] Histaminergic mechanisms for modulation of memory systems. Köhler CA, da Silva WC, Benetti F, Bonini JS. Neural Plast. 2011;2011:328602. PMID:21876818

[137] Assessing the effects of caffeine and theanine on the maintenance of vigilance during a sustained attention task. Foxe JJ, Morie KP, Laud PJ, Rowson MJ, de Bruin EA, Kelly SP. Neuropharmacology. 2012 Jun;62(7):2320-7. PMID:2232694

[138] Behavioral and molecular evidence for psychotropic effects in L-theanine. Wakabayashi C, Numakawa T, Ninomiya M, et al. Psychopharmacology (Berl). 2012 Feb;219(4):1099-109. PMID: 21861094

[139] L-theanine administration results in neuroprotection and prevents glutamate receptor agonist-mediated injury in the rat model of cerebral ischemia-reperfusion. Zukhurova M, Prosvirnina M, Daineko A, et al. Phytother Res. 2013 Sep;27(9):1282-7. PMID:23097345

[140] Impairment of fear memory consolidation and expression by antihistamines. Nonaka A, Masuda F, Nomura H, Matsuki N. Brain Res. 2013 Feb 1;1493:19-26. PMID:23178698

[141] Muscarinic modulation of synaptic transmission via endocannabinoid signalling in the rat midbrain periaqueductal gray. Lau BK, Vaughan CW. Mol Pharmacol. 2008 Nov;74(5):1392-8. PMID:18678620

[142] Cannabinoid CB1 receptors regulate neuronal TNF-α effects in experimental autoimmune encephalomyelitis. Rossi S, Furlan R, De Chiara V, et al. Brain Behav Immun. 2011 Aug;25(6):1242-8. PMID:21473912

[143] Zinc deficiency and zinc therapy efficacy with reduction of serum free copper in Alzheimer's disease. Brewer GJ, Kaur S. Int J Alzheimers Dis. 2013;2013:586365. PMID:24224111

[144] Concurrent detection of autolysosome formation and lysosomal degradation by flow cytometry in a high-content screen for inducers of autophagy. Hundeshagen P, Hamacher-Brady A, Eils R, Brady NR. BMC Biol. 2011 Jun 2;9:38. PMID:21635740

[145] The dietary bioflavonoid quercetin synergizes with epigallocathechin gallate (EGCG) to inhibit prostate cancer stem cell characteristics, invasion, migration and epithelial-mesenchymal transition. Tang SN, Singh C, Nall D, et al. J Mol Signal. 2010 Aug 18;5:14. PMID:20718984

[146] Structure-activity relationships for inhibition of human 5alpha-reductases by polyphenols. Hiipakka RA, Zhang HZ, Dai W, et al. Biochem Pharmacol. 2002 Mar 15;63(6):1165-76. PMID:11931850

[147] Flavonoids as inhibitors of human carbonyl reductase 1. Carlquist M, Frejd T, Gorwa-Grauslund MF. Chem Biol Interact. 2008 Jul 30;174(2):98-108. PMID:18579125

[148] Green tea polyphenol and epigallocatechin gallate induce apoptosis and inhibit invasion in human breast cancer cells. Thangapazham RL, Passi N, Maheshwari RK. Cancer Biol Ther. 2007 Dec;6(12):1938-43. PMID:18059161

[149] Molecular targets for green tea in prostate cancer prevention. Adhami VM, Ahmad N, Mukhtar H. J Nutr. 2003 Jul;133(7 Suppl):2417S-2424S. PMID:12840218

[150] The dietary bioflavonoid quercetin synergizes with epigallocathechin gallate (EGCG) to inhibit prostate cancer stem cell characteristics, invasion, migration and epithelial-mesenchymal transition. Tang SN, Singh C, Nall D, et al. J Mol Signal. 2010 Aug 18;5:14. PMID:20718984

33. Autoimmune Disease

Table 33-1: Some T_H17 Related Autoimmune Diseases

- Systemic Lupus Erythematosus (SLE)[3]
- Rheumatoid Arthritis (RA)[19]
- Multiple Sclerosis (MS)
- Crohn's Disease (CrD)
- Systemic Sclerosis[4]
- Celiac Disease[5]
- Psoriasis
- Uveitis[6]
- Autism[7]
- Behçet's Disease[8]
- Ankylosing Spondylitis[9]
- Hashimoto's Thyroiditis[10]
- Sjögren's syndrome (SS)[11]
- Type 1 Diabetes (DM1)

Naïve T helper cells differentiate into T_H1, T_H2, T_H17 or T_{REG} cell lineages, in accordance with the influence of cytokines and sphingolipids. γδTCR T cells migrate into the intestinal epithelium from the thymus in the absence of pathogenic stimulus. These cells produce IL-17, which stimulates naïve T cells to develop into T_H17 cells; the dominant and native T cells of the intestinal mucosa. αβTCR T cells, which are the more common form distributed to most other lymphatic tissue, migrate to the intestinal epithelium only under the influence of S1P, as a reaction to stress or infection.

T_H17 are critical in preventing invasion and infection from the gram-negative, enteric bacteria and fungi that are the normal residents of the colon. T_H17 cells induce B cell production of antibodies, primarily of the sIgA class. In the intestine; sIgA neutralizes pathogenic bacteria, preventing them from adhering to the mucosal surface. IgG, and particularly IgG_1, is also produced.

While not needed for γδTCR T cell migration, S1P induces development and proliferation of T_H17 cells. IL-17 stimulates reinforces T_H17 proliferation and induces these cells to produce several proinflammatory cytokines, including IL-1β, IL-6, TNF-α; chemokines; and induces nitric oxide synthase (NOS-2). In addition, T_H17 cells produce other interleukin cytokines than other T helper cells, including IL-17_A, IL-17_F, IL-21, and IL-22. IL-17 also further enhances T_H17 cell production. The cytokines produced by T_H17 cells can induce massive tissue reaction due to the broad distribution of cytokine receptors in various tissues[1].

Understanding of the role of T_H17 cells in health and disease has progressed dramatically in recent years. Previous to the year 2000, autoimmune diseases, such as multiple sclerosis, were attributed to immune activity of T_H1 cells. However, T_H17 cells are the clear ringleaders in cell-mediated autoimmune disease[2]. Linking T_H17 cells to the pathology of autoimmune disease establishes a direct connection in the pathology of autoimmune disease with the lymphatic epithelium of the intestines.

Mast cells also participate in the pathogenesis of autoimmune disease. IL-6 from T cells can induce mast cell proliferation. S1P emanating from the intestine induces migration of mast cells to the lamina propria of the intestine. Mast cells have Fcγ receptors for IgG, and activation by this ligand induces the release of TNF, IL-1β, and IL-17[12]. IL-1β increases the production of IL-6, other inflammatory cytokines, and PGE_2.

The action of mast cells in the immune system is not restricted to degranulation and the release of inflammatory mediators. Mast cells activate autoreactive T cells in autoimmune disease[13]. Mast cells are essential to the pathogenesis of rheumatoid arthritis, multiple sclerosis, glomerulonephritis[14], systemic sclerosis[15], and inflammatory bowel disease[16].

An example of an autoimmune disease associated with T_H17 and diet is Rheumatoid Arthritis (RA). While RA principally affects synovial joints, it is a systemic disease which also affects the lungs, eyes, heart, kidneys and other organs. Not only is it a multi-organ disease, multiple immune mechanisms are active in this disease. A principal pathological component in RA is the formation of immune complexes, which form in, or gain entry into, the joint spaces. Here, they trigger activation of the complement system, activating the inflammatory reaction that damages the joints. Additionally, RA affects the lungs, where it forms granuloma. The granuloma, composed largely of macrophages, which produces INF-γ and numerous other cytokines, chemokines and inflammatory mediators that further inflict malaise, fatigue, and other disease behaviors.

Although the intestines are not a common target of RA, there is evidence that it may be a source of the disease. The gut is the largest lymphoid organ in the body. RA has been successfully treated with the nonabsorbable anti-inflammatory medication sulfasalazine. This medication reduces IL-6 levels and lowers IgA, IgG and IgM rheumatoid factor and anti-gliadin antibodies, in patients with RA[17]. IgA, IgG, and IgM antibodies to foods have been found to be elevated in patients with RA[18]. More recently an association between RA and T$_H$17 cells has been recognized[19], thus implicating the enteric immune system as a mediator of this disease.

Several studies have used an elemental diet, consisting of simple amino acids, carbohydrates, and fats, for the treatment of RA; thus eliminating proteins and peptides from the diet, and eliminating dietary immunogens. Elemental diets were found to give superior relief when compared to RA treatment with prednisone[20]. While these trials show improvements in RA symptoms, elemental diets are not palatable, and this limits the duration of such trials. Changes in blood markers of the disease have not been observed using elemental diets; however, such short-term trials do not allow time for resolution of blood markers of the chronic immune reaction underlying this disease. RA symptoms returned with the return to the patients' regular diets[21, 22].

Immune reactions to certain food proteins can cross-react with MHC alleles in some individuals, putting them at risk for the disease. The most notorious of these proteins are gluten; which provokes celiac disease, and proteins in cow's milk; which can induce type 1 diabetes in children[23].

A specific food protein cross-reaction with an individual's HLA type is not required for T$_H$17 immune response to food to cause autoimmune disease. In multiple sclerosis (MS), certain HLA types are associated with the disease condition; HLA class II haplotypes DR2/DQ6, DR3/DQ2, and DR4/DQ8 show the strongest association with the disease. Having one of these types gives the individual susceptibility to the disease but does not, in itself, cause disease. The cytokine IL-17 exacerbates MS in at least those carrying the DQ8 genotype[24]. Any immune reactions which increase IL-17 may activate this disease in susceptible individuals. Bowel infections and immune reactions to foods that stimulate T$_H$17 activity increase IL-17 levels.

Sphingolipids and Autoimmune Disease

Acid sphingomyelinase, (aSMase) is a lysosomal, zinc-dependent enzyme. Activated during cellular stress, it cleaves sphingomyelin into ceramide and sphingosine. These signaling molecules can, depending on the cellular milieu, promote apoptosis and upregulate immune cell activity, including microglial activation. Under favorable conditions, these signaling molecules are phosphorylated, whereupon they act to signal repair and regrowth support functions from the neuroglia.

Sphingosine-1-phosphate (S1P) promotes inhibition of apoptosis via induction of ERK and AKT phosphorylation. In the CNS, sphingomyelin from damaged neurons and neurites can activate the oligodendrocytes and prevents their apoptosis, maintaining their activity.

There are five S1PR G-protein coupled membrane receptors for S1P. They are present in many immune cells and modulate many immune activities.

The medication fingaloid (Gilenya) is used in the treatment of MS, preventing disease relapses by about 50%. This medication promotes the degradation of S1P1 receptors on immune cells, which preventing egress of lymphocytes from lymph nodes and Peyer's patches. Circulating T cells periodically reenter the lymphatic tissue, and S1P is also needed for their re-release back into the lymph and then to the bloodstream. Thus, inhibiting S1P activity reduces the population of autoaggressive T$_H$17 cells, particularly central memory T cells[25], in the circulation, and prevents their migration to the CNS and to peripheral nerves, where they can promote demyelinating neuropathy. In the CNS, fingaloid also down-modulates S1P1 induced S1P activated neural cells and astrocytes, reducing astrogliosis[26]. Fluoxetine, a functional inhibitor of acid SMase (FIASMA) has been shown to have a beneficial effect on the course of MS[27].

The S1P4 S1P receptor is also involved in autoimmune disease. Although T cells have few S1P4 receptors, this receptor is present on dendritic cells and has profound affects DC cell migration and cytokine secretion that enhance TH17 cell differentiation. In a mouse model of IBD, knocking out the S1P4 receptors diminished disease intensity[28].

Sphingosine kinase (SphK) converts sphingosine to S1P. Lipopolysaccharide toxin (LPS) from enteric bacterial cell walls enhances SphK expression and activity, down-regulating IL-12p70 and favoring immune activation of T$_H$17 and T$_H$2 cells[29].

The immune cell membrane receptor S1P1 activates inflammation through JAK→STAT3, via IL-6. In MS, IL-17 mediated somatic inflammation stimulates production of IL-17 expressing CD4+ T-cells, which become TH17 cells that can infiltrate the CNS. Here they exacerbate autoimmune neuroinflammation[30].

Treatment and Prevention

Cytokines produced by T$_H$17 cells, including IL-17$_F$ and IL-23, activate and maintain cytotoxic autoimmune responses. IL-17 and its receptors are current targets in the development of pharmaceutical treatment of these diseases. Monoclonal antibodies, which bind to and inactivate IL-17, or which block these cytokine receptors have been developed for the treatment of autoimmune disease. These medications are, however, not free of serious risks and are not effective in all patients.

Foods are an antigenic exposure that stimulates and maintains T$_H$17 cell inflammatory response. Their reactions can often be quickly quelled by eliminating these antigenic exposures. Antigens from infectious agents, such as enteric bacterial biofilm antigens and *Candida,* also stimulate LPS, and thus, T$_H$17, IgG, and mast cell and activity. SIBO, intestinal dysbiosis, biofilm formation, and dietary gliadins can set the stage for hyperpermeability and amplify the presentation of food antigens to dendritic cells. An intestinal milieu which activates bacteria into pathogenic activity can create a large antigenic load, and their toxins can increase absorption of LPS, flagellin and other ligands for toll-like receptor activation. Elimination of reactive foods, normalization of the enteric mucosa, and treatment of dysbiosis can mitigate the excess production of IL-23 by dendritic cells in the intestine that stimulates T_H17 adaptive response and the cytokines it induces. This, in turn, allows the autoimmune process to remit, the sphingolipid pathway to diminish its activity, mast cells and other immune cells stimulated by these cytokines to undergo apoptosis, and enterocytes to function normally.

Immunoglobulins to multiple foods have been documented in RA[6], CrD[31], DM1[32] and other diseases (Chapter 19). These immune reactions set the stage for autoimmune disease. Treatment of autoimmune diseases thus should include testing for anterges and elimination of active antigens. It is essential to remove as many reactive antigens as possible so that T_H17 cytokine production decline, thus limiting support for excessive inflammatory immune cells survival.

The most sensitive test for T_H17 immune response to food is sIgA testing of intestinal aspirate[18]. In health, there is no obvious adaptive advantage to forming sIgA to food. Food should not be perceived by the immune system as a threat. It is rarely alive by the time its meets the small intestine, and not likely to mount an invasion. Formation of sIgA to foods indicates the immune presentation of food peptides and proteins to the lymphocytes of the Peyer's patches and immune response. Formation of IgM and IgG suggests repeated exposure and intestinal hyperpermeability. IgG, helps mediates the intestinal mast cell immune response to food antigens.

SIBO and colonic dysbiosis, with biofilm formation, boost the production and absorption of LPS and other bacterial and fungal toxins, in addition to bacterial, fungal and food antigens. These toxins and antigens can increase the absorption and immune presentation of these compounds.

Mast cells in the synovial lining of the joint are required for the destructive immune reactions in rheumatoid arthritis. Fcγ receptors on mast cells in the synovial are activated by IgG or IgG immune complexes. Testing for serum IgG reactivity to foods is useful for identifying anterges which promoting the immune response.

Sympathetic activity from chronic stress can also promote the induction of T_H17 immune cells and the growth of nerve fibers to the lymph nodes. These nerve fibers are maintained by nerve growth factors. Normalizing autonomic tone, with normal diurnal variance, should be a goal of treatment.

Vitamin D_3 deficiency has been found to increase the risk for MS, and high doses of vitamin D_3 can help induce remission of this disease. MS patients with higher vitamin D_3 levels are more likely to stay in remission; while those with lower levels are at higher risk of disease reactivation. Vitamin D_3 has multiple actions, including enhancing the development of antiinflammatory IL-10 producing cells and reducing the number of proinflammatory IL-6 and IL-17 secreting cells[33].

Autoimmune Disease Remission

The goal of treatment is to decrease the T_H17 immune response to a normal level of activity.

1. Food Reactive Antigen Elimination: Patients with autoimmune disorders should be tested for IgG food anterges, and eliminate reactive foods from their diet. A wide panel of tests is required, both to eliminate as many reactive foods as possible and to give as many non-reacting foods as possible, as alternative choices to replace foods eliminated from the diet. The goal is to remove all reacting foods so that the inflammatory reaction remits.

A correctly implemented elimination diet (comprehensive elimination of reactive immunogens from the diet), the patient's symptoms should diminish within several days. Food immunogenicity can be retested after several months, and patients may be able to reintroduce some foods, but may also have new foods that require elimination. Younger patients can often reintroduce foods after a few months, however, older patients and patients with more severe pathology, often take more time foe anterges to specific foods to fade. Certain foods, wheat, for example in patients with celiac disease, are best avoided permanently. Food immunogenicity is discussed in Chapter 19. If it is suspected that IgE reactions to foods are present, these too should be tested for and eliminated. IgE food allergies tend to be fixed and often can never be reintroduced in an adult's diet. Small children, however, often outgrow food allergies. (See Chapter 11.)

There is a very high prevalence of autoimmune diseases among patients with gluten disease. Given the ubiquity of wheat in the Western diet, all patients presenting with autoimmune disease should be tested for tissue transglutaminase antibodies and anti-gliadin antibodies. (See Chapter 22.)

2. Alleviate Intestinal Dysbiosis: Enteric bacterial biofilms can produce LPS and other toxins which impair the mucosal barrier and allow antigenic exposure. LPS also support IL-17 production and T_H17 transformation. LPS helps induce SphK and the formation of S1P. Prebiotics, probiotics, and anti-biofilm polyphenols can help prevent intestinal dysbiosis and biofilm formation. Treatment of dysbiosis is discussed in Chapters 4, 23, 24, and 25. Patients with an autoimmune disease may benefit from testing for fecal chymotrypsin levels, stool fat, or other tests to determine if they have adequate formation and activation of pancreatic enzymes. Those with low levels may benefit from treatment with pancreatic enzyme supplements, and avoidance of trypsin inhibitors, as described in Chapter 23. Limiting protein intake to easily digested proteins, and amounts required for adequate nutrition may also be helpful.

3. Improve Mucosal Barrier: Antigenic reactions occur as a result of the passage of food and microbial antigens into the lamina propria where they can be presented to immune cells. This can result as a failure of the mucosal barrier, increased intracellular permeability, and from loss of sIgA, which neutralizes antigens and bacteria in the lumen of the intestine. Alcohol, toxins, infections and nutritional deficiencies can also impair the mucosal barrier. Successful treatment requires an intact mucosal barrier. Chapter 24 details treatment of mucosal hyperpermeability.

4. Vitamin D: Vitamin D promotes the development of IL-10 producing cells and reduces the number of IL-6 and IL-17 secreting cells, thus promoting T_{REG} cells and down-regulation of T_H17 hyperactivity. T cells can metabolize 25OHD3 into active 1,25OHD3[33]. High doses, (often as high as 10,000 units of vitamin D_3 daily) are used in the treatment of MS[34]. A target level target level of 125 nmol/L of 25OHD3 is reasonable for most people, with the goal of keeping serum 25OHD3 levels between 100 and 150 nmol/L. Most adults do not get sufficient sun exposure and thus require about 4000 IU supplementation of vitamin D_3 daily. (Vitamin D is discussed in Chapter 20). Malabsorption causes loss of vitamin D, thus testing 25OHD3 levels is important to assure adequate response to treatment.

5. Avoid Sphingosine-1-Phosphate activation. Acid SMase is induced by inflammation and exposure to free radicals. Avoiding cellular stress, and use of antioxidants, perhaps particularly, alpha-lipoic acid, may decrease activation of this enzyme. Certain medications, including a few anti-depressants, are functional inhibitors of aSMase. The most potent of these are amitriptyline, sertraline, and fluoxetine (Chapter 30) Tomatidine, a compound found in tomatoes and especially green tomatoes, is an acid sphingomyelinase inhibitor[35] that also supports muscle growth[36]. S1P is inactivated by S1P lyase, an enzyme requiring PLP, an active form vitamin B_6.

In addition to LPS, TNF-α and Il-1β induce S1P production, by the inducing sphingosine kinase[37],[38]. The activation of this enzyme by LPS, TNF-α, and Il-1β is coincidental with the activation of IDO, the enzyme that sends tryptophan down the kynurenine pathway (Figure 31-2). Avoiding LPS formation is discussed above. Avoiding sphingosine kinase activation is discussed at the end of Chapter 34.

5. Restoration Autonomic Balance: Sympathetic dominance of the autonomic nervous system up-regulates and maintains T_H17 activity. Restoration of autonomic balance requires normalization of circadian cycles. Normal sleep and meal cycles should be encouraged. Melatonin may help to restore the sleep cycle. Vigorous exercise and other short-term stressors can help restore the normal variability in the autonomic response.

6. Stress Reduction: Stress, including social stress, stimulates the transformation of T_H0 cells into T_H17 cells through the action of chronic sympathetic stimulus. Additionally, CRH (corticotropin releasing hormone) from the HPA Axis causes increased intracellular hyperpermeability. Reduction of chronic stress is an essential component of treatment. Without the abatement of chronic stress, remission should not be anticipated, but rather, continued formation of new antergies and thus, hyperreactivity and dominance of T_H17 immunity. Hypothalamic pituitary axes function may require normalization. The effects of stress and its management are covered in Chapter 29. Treatment of excessive sympathetic activity from stress is further discussed in the treatment section of Chapter 32.

7. Melatonin Supplementation: Melatonin levels have been found to be low in MS patients and may partially explain the depression associated with this disease[39]. Melatonin has an anti-inflammatory effect on the brain[40] and in the gut[41] and helps maintain the mucosal barrier, critical to avoiding immune reactions to dietary antigens. Melatonin may also help sleep disturbances. A dose of 3 to 5 mg of timed released melatonin taken about 30 minutes before bedtime[42] may be considered for patients with autoimmune disorders. An additional 0.3 to 0.5 mg of sublingual melatonin at bedtime may be helpful if there is delayed sleep onset.

8. Get Sufficient Sleep: Sleep disturbances should be treated, as they are associated with elevated IL-6, and thus promote T_H17 activation. (Chapter 42) A regular, normal diurnal sleep cycle should be maintained.

9. N-3 Dietary Fatty Acids: DHA and EPA may be helpful. A high n-6 to n-3 ratio promotes an inflammatory milieu while DHA promotes PPARγ activity, which limits inflammatory cytokine production. DHA and EPA may help autoimmune disease into remission.

10. Mast Cell Activation Disorders: Many autoimmune diseases are associated with an increase in mast cell number, in the affected tissues, or have aberrant mast cell behavior. Mast Cell Activation Disorder treatment is outlined in Chapter 12.

11. Magnesium: Magnesium promotes the downregulation of destructive inflammatory processes and supports repair and regrowth. Magnesium supplements are appropriate in most patients with autoimmune disease,

12. Prevent and Treat Chronic Infections: As discussed in Chapter 31, Toxoplasmosis is a risk factor for autoimmune disorders, including rheumatoid arthritis, inflammatory bowel disease[43], and perhaps especially for MS[44] and may induce antergies[45]. It should be tested for and treated if present. Other chronic infections should also be eliminated when possible.

[1] IL-17 and Th17 Cells. Korn T, Bettelli E, Oukka M, Kuchroo VK. Annu Rev Immunol. 2009;27:485-517. PMID:19132915

[2] IL-33 is a crucial amplifier of innate rather than acquired immunity. Oboki K, Ohno T, Kajiwara N, Arae K, Morita H, Ishii A, Nambu A, Abe T, Kiyonari H, Matsumoto K, Sudo K, Okumura K, Saito H, Nakae S. Proc Natl Acad Sci U S A. 2010 Oct 26;107(43):18581-6. Epub 2010 Oct 11. PMID:20937871

[3] Expression of interleukin-17 is correlated with interferon-α expression in cutaneous lesions of lupus erythematosus. Oh SH, Roh HJ, Kwon JE, Lee SH, Kim JY, Choi HJ, Lim BJ. Clin Exp Dermatol. 2011 Jul;36(5):512-20 PMID:21631571

[4] Th17 peripheral cells are increased in diffuse cutaneous systemic sclerosis compared with limited illness: a cross-sectional study. Rodríguez-Reyna TS, Furuzawa-Carballeda J, Cabiedes J, Fajardo-Hermosillo LD, Martínez-Reyes C, Díaz-Zamudio M, Llorente L. Rheumatol Int. 2011 Jul 26. PMID:21789610

[5] Differential mucosal IL-17 expression in two gliadin-induced disorders: gluten sensitivity and the autoimmune enteropathy celiac disease. Sapone A, Lammers KM, Mazzarella G, Mikhailenko I, Carteni M, Casolaro V, Fasano A. Int Arch Allergy Immunol. 2010;152(1):75-80. PMID:19940509

[6] Involvement of Th17 cells and the effect of anti-IL-6 therapy in autoimmune uveitis. Yoshimura T, Sonoda KH, Ohguro N, Ohsugi Y, Ishibashi T, Cua DJ, Kobayashi T, Yoshida H, Yoshimura A. Rheumatology (Oxford). 2009 Apr;48(4):347-54. PMID:19164426

[7] Plasma cytokine profiles in subjects with high-functioning autism spectrum disorders. Suzuki K, Matsuzaki H, Iwata K, Kameno Y, Shimmura C, Kawai S, Yoshihara Y, Wakuda T, Takebayashi K, Takagai S, Matsumoto K, Tsuchiya KJ, Iwata Y, Nakamura K, Tsujii M, Sugiyama T, Mori N. PLoS One. 2011;6(5):e20470. PMID:21647375

[8] Expression of Th-17 and RORγt mRNA in Behçet's Disease. Hamzaoui K, Bouali E, Ghorbel I, Khanfir M, Houman H, Hamzaoui A. Med Sci Monit. 2011 Apr;17(4):CR227-34. PMID:21455110

[9] Increased serum IL-17 and IL-23 in the patient with ankylosing spondylitis. Mei Y, Pan F, Gao J, Ge R, Duan Z, Zeng Z, Liao F, Xia G, Wang S, Xu S, Xu J, Zhang L, Ye D. Clin Rheumatol. 2011 Feb;30(2):269-73. PMID:21161669

[10] Increased circulating pro-inflammatory cytokines and Th17 lymphocytes in Hashimoto's thyroiditis. Figueroa-Vega N, Alfonso-Pérez M, Benedicto I, Sánchez-Madrid F, González-Amaro R, Marazuela M. J Clin Endocrinol Metab. 2010 Feb;95(2):953-62. PMID:20016049

[11] Systemic and local interleukin-17 and linked cytokines associated with Sjögren's syndrome immunopathogenesis. Katsifis GE, Rekka S, Moutsopoulos NM, Pillemer S, Wahl SM. Am J Pathol. 2009 Sep;175(3):1167-77. PMID:19700754

[12] JNK1 controls mast cell degranulation and IL-1{beta} production in inflammatory arthritis. Guma M, Kashiwakura J, Crain B, Kawakami Y, Beutler B, Firestein GS, Kawakami T, Karin M, Corr M. Proc Natl Acad Sci U S A. 2010 Dec 21;107(51):22122-7. PMID:21135226

[13] MASTering the immune response: mast cells in autoimmunity. Gregory GD, Bickford A, Robbie-Ryan M, Tanzola M, Brown MA. Novartis Found Symp. 2005;271:215-25; discussion 225-31. PMID:16605138

[14] The mast cell IgG receptors and their roles in tissue inflammation. Malbec O, Daëron M. Immunol Rev. 2007 Jun;217:206-21. PMID:17498061

[15] Involvement of mast cells in systemic sclerosis. Yukawa S, Yamaoka K, Sawamukai N, Shimajiri S, Saito K, Tanaka Y. Nihon Rinsho Meneki Gakkai Kaishi. 2010;33(2):81-6. PMID:20453443

[16] Fc gamma receptor signaling in mast cells links microbial stimulation to mucosal immune inflammation in the intestine. Chen X, Feng BS, Zheng PY, Liao XQ, Chong J, Tang SG, Yang PC. Am J Pathol. 2008 Dec;173(6):1647-56. PMID:18974296

[17] Evidence for differential effects of sulphasalazine on systemic and mucosal immunity in rheumatoid arthritis. Kanerud L, Engström GN, Tarkowski A. Ann Rheum Dis. 1995 Apr;54(4):256-62. PMID: 7763101

[18] The gut-joint axis: cross reactive food antibodies in rheumatoid arthritis. Hvatum M, Kanerud L, Hällgren R, Brandtzaeg P. Gut. 2006 Sep;55(9):1240-7. PMID:16484508

[19] The potential role of Th17 in mediating the transition from acute to chronic autoimmune inflammation: rheumatoid arthritis as a model. Ferraccioli G, Zizzo G. Discov Med. 2011 May;11(60):413-24. PMID:21616040

[20] Is rheumatoid arthritis a disease that starts in the intestine? A pilot study comparing an elemental diet with oral prednisolone. Podas T, Nightingale JM, Oldham R, Roy S, Sheehan NJ, Mayberry JF. Postgrad Med J. 2007 Feb;83(976):128-31. PMID: 17308218

[21] A pilot study of the effect of an elemental diet in the management of rheumatoid arthritis. Haugen MA, Kjeldsen-Kragh J, Førre O. Clin Exp Rheumatol. 1994 May-Jun;12(3):275-9. PMID: 8070160

[22] The effects of elemental diet and subsequent food reintroduction on rheumatoid arthritis. Kavanaghi R, Workman E, Nash P, Smith M, Hazleman BL, Hunter JO. Br J Rheumatol. 1995 Mar;34(3):270-3. PMID: 7728405

[23] Dietary intervention in infancy and later signs of beta-cell autoimmunity. Knip M, Virtanen SM, Seppä K, Ilonen J, Savilahti E, Vaarala O, Reunanen A, Teramo K, Hämäläinen AM, Paronen J, Dosch HM, Hakulinen T, Akerblom HK; Finnish TRIGR Study Group. N Engl J Med. 2010 Nov 11;363(20):1900-8. PMID:21067382

[24] Role of HLA class II genes in susceptibility and resistance to multiple sclerosis: Studies using HLA transgenic mice. Luckey D, Bastakoty D, Mangalam AK. J Autoimmun. 2011 May 30. PMID:21632210

[25] Th17 central memory T cells are reduced by FTY720 in patients with multiple sclerosis. Mehling M, Lindberg R, Raulf F, et al. Neurology. 2010 Aug 3;75(5):403-10. PMID:20592255

[26] FTY720 (fingolimod) in Multiple Sclerosis: therapeutic effects in the immune and the central nervous system. Brinkmann V. Br J Pharmacol. 2009 Nov;158(5):1173-82. PMID:19814729

[27] Functional inhibitors of acid sphingomyelinase (FIASMAs). Kornhuber J, Tripal P, Gulbins E, Muehlbacher M. Handb Exp Pharmacol. 2013;(215):169-86. PMID:23579455

[28] Sphingosine-1-phospate receptor 4 (S1P$_4$) deficiency profoundly affects dendritic cell function and TH17-cell differentiation in a murine model. Schulze T, Golfier S, Tabeling C, et al. FASEB J. 2011 Nov;25(11):4024-36. PMID:21825036

[29] The sphingosine kinase 1 and S1P1 axis specifically counteracts LPS-induced IL-12p70 production in immune cells of the spleen. Schröder M, Richter C, Juan MH, et al. Mol Immunol. 2011 May;48(9-10):1139-48. PMID:21435724

[30] Defective sphingosine 1-phosphate receptor 1 (S1P1) phosphorylation exacerbates TH17-mediated autoimmune neuroinflammation. Garris CS, Wu L, Acharya S, et al. Nat Immunol. 2013 Nov;14(11):1166-72. PMID:24076635

[31] Antibody (IgG, IgA, and IgM) to baker's yeast (Saccharomyces cerevisiae), yeast mannan, gliadin, ovalbumin and betalactoglobulin in monozygotic twins with inflammatory bowel disease. Lindberg E, Magnusson KE, Tysk C, Järnerot G. Gut. 1992 Jul;33(7):909-13.PMID: 1644330

[32] Enhanced levels of cow's milk antibodies in infancy in children who develop type 1 diabetes later in childhood. Luopajärvi K, Savilahti E, Virtanen SM, et al. Pediatr Diabetes. 2008 Oct;9(5):434-41. Epub 2008 May 21. PMID:18503496

[33] Vitamin D-mediated immune regulation in Multiple Sclerosis.. Correale J, Ysrraelit MC, Gaitán MI. J Neurol Sci. 2011 Jul 1. PMID:21723567

[34] Safety of vitamin D3 in adults with multiple sclerosis. Kimball SM, Ursell MR, O'Connor P, Vieth R. Am J Clin Nutr. 2007 Sep;86(3):645-51.PMID: 17823429

[35] Identification of novel functional inhibitors of acid sphingomyelinase. Kornhuber J, Muehlbacher M, Trapp S, et al. PLoS One. 2011;6(8):e23852. PMID:21909365

[36] http://now.uiowa.edu/2014/04/green-good Accessed May 2014 http://www.jbc.org/content/early/2014/04/09/jbc.M114.556241.abstract.

[37] Activation of sphingosine kinase by tumor necrosis factor-alpha inhibits apoptosis in human endothelial cells. Xia P, Wang L, Gamble JR, Vadas MA. J Biol Chem. 1999 Nov 26;274(48):34499-505. PMID:10567432

[38] Sphingosine kinase and sphingosine-1-phosphate: regulators in autoimmune and inflammatory disease. Snider AJ. Int J Clin Rheumtol. 2013 Aug 1;8(4). PMID:24416079

[39] The association of nocturnal serum melatonin levels with major depression in patients with acute multiple sclerosis. Akpinar Z, Tokgöz S, Gökbel H, Okudan N, Uğuz F, Yilmaz G. Psychiatry Res. 2008 Nov 30;161(2):253-7. PMID:18848732

[40] Antiinflammatory activity of melatonin in central nervous system. Esposito E, Cuzzocrea S. Curr Neuropharmacol. 2010 Sep;8(3):228-42. PMID:21358973

[41] Gut clock: implication of circadian rhythms in the gastrointestinal tract. Konturek PC, Brzozowski T, Konturek SJ. J Physiol Pharmacol. 2011 Apr;62(2):139-50. PMID:21673361

[42] Adjuvant use of melatonin for treatment of fibromyalgia. Hussain SA, Al-Khalifa II, Jasim NA, Gorial FI. J Pineal Res. 2011 Apr;50(3):267-71. PMID:21158908

[43] Prevalence of anti-Toxoplasma antibodies in patients with autoimmune diseases. Shapira Y, Agmon-Levin N, Selmi C, et al. J Autoimmun. 2012 Aug;39(1-2):112-6. PMID:2229714

[44] Toxoplasmosis and Polygenic Disease Susceptibility Genes: Extensive Toxoplasma gondii Host/Pathogen Interactome Enrichment in Nine Psychiatric or Neurological Disorders. Carter CJ. J Pathog. 2013;2013:965046. PMID:23533776

[45] Anti-gluten immune response following Toxoplasma gondii infection in mice. Severance EG, Kannan G, Gressitt KL, et al. PLoS One. 2012;7(11):e50991. PMID:23209841

34. Inflammatory Bowel Disease

Inflammatory bowel disease (IBD) refers to several diseases with chronic, inflammatory diseases of the GI track which typically cause chronic diarrhea, inflammation, and injury to the intestines. IBD has severe morbidity, and can cause death; IBS confers a high risk for intestinal lymphoma and colon cancer[1,2]. The morbidity from IBD is not limited to the gut; these diseases disrupt the patient's social and work life, and certain forms of IBD are accompanied with inflammatory arthritis and other extra-intestinal manifestations.

IBD is often accompanied by psychological problems. It was long assumed that the pain, discomfort, and social impact of the disease on the patient's life were the source of the psychological impact. Almost 20% of patients with Crohn's disease meet the diagnostic criteria for post-traumatic stress disorder[3]. The psychological comorbidity prevalent in IBD had been attributed to the impact that the bowel dysfunction has on the activities of daily living including social and career limitations patients confront living with this disease. However, is likely that the disease directly affects the mind. Depression, bipolar disorder, and schizophrenia are also enteroimmune diseases, as discussed in Chapter 31. Chapter 36 reviews aspects of the pathology of autism, a disease of the gut with the most obvious manifestations being behavior and cognition. Altered absorption of nutrients and toxins from the gut may allow absorption of bacterial toxins, biogenic amines, lipids and peptides which affect the cognition and behavior. Conversely, neurohormonal influences may exacerbate the intestinal manifestations of these diseases.

Two severe and prevalent forms of IBD are Crohn's disease (aka regional enteritis), and ulcerative colitis (UC). These are distinct diseases with different causes, but with overlapping manifestations. Crohn's disease (CrD) can affect the entire gastrointestinal tract from the mouth to the anus; while UC is usually limited to the colon. In CrD, inflammation is patchy, deep and can penetrate the wall of the intestines; meanwhile, in UC usually presents as a shallow continuous ulcer, confined to the colon.

Genetic factors account for far more risk in CrD than for UC. Nevertheless, concordance for IBD in various twin studies appears to have fallen over the last 50 years. The concordance rate for CrD in monozygotic twins, ranges from below 35% to over 90%[4,5,6], but is less than 10% in UC in most studies. The risk of UC is 3.5 times higher in first-degree relatives of patients with CrD than in the general population[7], suggesting overlapping risks. It also shows that both UC and CrD can appear in the same family.

Gastrointestinal infections is a risk factor for developing IBD's. Among discordant twins, the sibling with IBD has spent more time with animals than the unaffected sibling[8]. This may be explained by the increased risk for IBD associated with the presence of toxoplasmosis gondii antibodies[9]; discussed in Chapter 31. Bacterial enteritis often precedes IBD.

Crohn's Disease

Crohn's disease is a T_H17 mediated autoimmune disorder, as are multiple sclerosis, rheumatoid arthritis and several other diseases, as discussed in Chapter 33. Crohn's disease responds to eliminations diets, and to eliminating foods to which the patient has elevated IgG_4 antibodies[10]. As many as 80% of Crohn's disease patients have antibodies to baker's yeast (*Saccharomyces cerevisiae*), although they may not be detectable in the serum[11]. In contrast, these characteristics are uncommon in UC, a T_H2 related disease.

Similar to rheumatoid arthritis, IgA and IgM levels are more sensitive than IgG levels in detecting elevation in Anti-Saccharomyces cerevisiae antibodies (ASCA)[11,12]. ASCA, however, is not unique to CrD; it is can commonly be found in patients with UC, Celiac disease[13], and intestinal tuberculosis but is unusual in healthy persons[14].

Yeast

The yeast, *Candida albicans*, is a normal commensal organism the in the gastrointestinal tract; it is present in about 80% of the human population. Nevertheless, it is also the most common fungal pathogen in humans, and can cause both mucosal and systemic infections, especially in immune-compromised patients[15].

Candida are polymorphic; they usually grow as ovoid single cells, that split and form two daughter cells. This is the commensal form of *Candida*. Under certain stimuli, however, *Candida* can transform into pseudohyphae or true hyphae; multicellular organisms[16]. Hyphae formation appears to be critical for epithelial invasion. When hyphae are induced, different genes are expressed which allow this ordinarily commensal organism to become pathogenic.

Similar to bacterial biofilms, hyphae can produce proteins that allow pathogenesis, while the lone, single-cell organisms cannot. In its pathogenic form, *Candida* can invade epithelial cells by inducing endocytosis or by active penetration of the enterocytes or other cells[17]. Once *Candida* enters the cells, most often epithelial cells, it acts as an intracellular pathogen. Here, it reproduces causes systemic disease. *Candida albicans* can be inducted into the hyphal form by exposure to hemoglobin that acts as a signaling molecule that alters gene expression. This allows the hyphal adhesion to several extracellular matrix proteins[18]. Hypoxia may also help induce the hyphal form[19]. The fungus also uses hemoglobin as an iron source for growth.

Around 75% of patients with Crohn's disease have anti-

Saccharomyces cerevisiae antibodies (ASCA), and the ASCA test is used as a diagnostic test for this disease. Additionally, about 15 percent of patients with ulcerative colitis and 5% of the general population have elevated ASCA titers. This organism, however, is not a human pathogen. Different cultivated strains of *Saccharomyces cerevisiae* include brewer's yeast and baker's yeast.

The ASCA associated antigen is oligomannan; a four mannose chain polymer found in the cell wall of yeasts. Mannan from *Candida* is also recognized by this antibody. It is likely that the ASCA antigen is a component of the hyphae form of *Candida*, and thus, antibodies to it represent a reaction to the pathogenic form of *Candida*, but not to the commensal, budding form of this fungus.

An important element in the body's innate immune system is Mannose-Binding Lectin (MBL). This protein is an acute-phase reactant produced by the liver. It recognizes and binds to particular mannose sugar chains which are found on some yeasts, bacteria, and viruses. Once bound, it can activate complement, and cause lysis of many pathogens. MBL also promotes phagocytosis by neutrophils and macrophages. MBL defends the body against several bacterial infections including *Mycobacterium*, *Salmonella*, *Listeria*, and *Neisseria*. Fungal pathogens, such as *Candida albicans* and *Cryptococcus neoformans*, and some viruses are also bound by MBL.

There are genetic variations in MBL alleles that affect how much MBL is present in the blood. Children with low MBL levels are subject to frequent and severe infections. Low levels are also associated with risk of contracting HIV infection and tuberculosis (TB), although high levels are also associated with intracellular diseases, such as HIV. Low levels impede the body's ability to prevent the infections. High levels increase the likelihood of a strong immune response; which can be destructive, especially in diseases, such as TB, and in HIV. MBL induces the uptake of intracellular pathogens into white blood cells; if not destroyed there, the pathogen may reproduce.

In Crohn's disease, low MBL levels are associated with increased risk for stricture, penetrating disease, and high ASCA levels, as compared to patients with uncomplicated forms of the disease[20]. Although ASCA cross-reacts with other yeast, *Candida* appears able to induce both ASCA antibodies and mucosal inflammation[21]. CrD patients and their family members have increased the risk for invasive *Candida* infections[22].

Some *Mycobacterium* antigens cross-react with ASCA; therefore, some non-tuberculosis *Mycobacterium* have been suspected as etiologic factors for CrD[23]. Hepatitis C is also more common in IBD. These infections, however, may represent secondary opportunistic infection in susceptible hosts, rather than acting being causal agents of Crohn's disease. ASCA antibody levels have been found to be correlated with IgG antibodies to foods (antergies) and to *T. gondii* antibody levels. *T gondii* activates immune inflammation in the intestine. ASCA antibodies are associated with bipolar disorder; these patients are four times more likely to have ACSA antibodies than are control subjects[24]. A similar association between ASCA, food antibodies and T gondii has been found in schizophrenia[25].

While MBL is controlled in part by genetics, it is induced by certain infections and levels are regulated by hormones. Thyroid hormones (T_3 and less so T_4) and growth hormone (GH) both induced MBL RNA, with a higher induction when T_3 and GH are combined[26]. These two hormones are simultaneously released during the first hours of sleep; thus, regular sleep cycles help control infection and prevent CrD progression.

As hemoglobin promotes *Candidal* transformation into the pathogenic form, patients that are positive for ASCA should be checked for blood in the stool and for H. pylori infection. Any source of intestinal bleeding should be treated.

IgG Antibodies to Yeast: IgG antibodies to yeast (*Saccharomyces cerevisiae*) are common in individuals with food immunogenicities. It is the most common food reactant seen with IgG testing for antergies[27]. In a study of irritable bowel syndrome, baker's yeast was the most the most common reactive food antigen, testing positive in 85% of patients[28], and in another study, 87% of patients with IBS has elevated IgG to baker's and brewer's yeast combined[29]. In migraine patients, 38% of the patients, as compared to 4% of controls, had IgG to baker's yeast[30].

For testing, yeast antigens are prepared by making a homogenate from baker's or brewer's yeast. Budding yeast may have hundreds of different antigens, and a patient may form antibodies to one or more of these. Formation of antibodies to dietary yeast proteins does not indicate that the patient has had a pathological growth of *Saccharomyces cerevisiae*, or of *Candida*. Rather, it indicates that the intestinal mucosal barrier is incompetent and that immune cells of the intestine have been exposed to *Saccharomyces cerevisiae* antigens from food.

Treatment for immunogenicity to baker's or brewer's yeast should include avoidance of foods and beverages made with yeast until IgG levels have dropped, and intestinal permeability has been treated (Chapter 25). Presence of IgG antibodies to baker's or brewer's yeast does not determine need for pharmacological treatment of *Candida* infection but does suggest that ASCA testing may be indicated.

Diagnostic Markers

IBD is characterized by inflammatory activity. Several markers for WBC's can be found in the stool and are useful in the differential diagnosis and follow-up IBD activity, as the markers fall with effective treatment. The selection of markers may have more to do with protein stability in the stool sample and ease of testing than its biological activity in causing or reflecting the disease process. Additionally, plasma citrulline less than 20 µmol/L indicates insufficient small intestinal enterocyte mass as can occur in CrD[31].

Table 34-1: Testing in IBD [32,33,34,35,36]

Test	Ulcerative Colitis	Crohn's disease	Lymphocytic Colitis	MCE / IBS-D
Fecal Calprotectin	↑ (@ 90%)	↑ (@ 90%)	↑ (in 75%)	<15% *
Fecal ECP	↑ with disease activity	↑ with disease activity	↑ (in 92%)	Normal
Fecal EPX	↑ with disease activity	↑ with disease activity	↑ (in 67%)	<15% *
Fecal Tryptase			↑ (in 50%)	↑ (in 55%)
ASCA / pANCA	rare / 52%	60% / 10%		6% / rare
Calgranulin C	↑ (@ 90%)	↑ (@ 90%)		< 4% *
Endoscopy	Colon – shallow ulcers	Entire GI tract Deep ulcers	Grossly normal ↑ Lymphocytes	Grossly normal ↑ Mast cell activity

ECP = eosinophil cationic protein; EPX = eosinophil protein X; Calgranulin C = S100A12. Lymphocytic colitis (LC) includes collagenous colitis. MCE = Mast Cell Enterocolitis. * Positive tests in MCE suggest a diagnosis of LC or other IBD. See **Appendix C** for test availability.

Neutrophil Markers: Calprotectin (CP) levels are elevated in UC, CrD and often in LC. Sixty percent of the granule protein mass in neutrophils is CP, and it thus is a marker of neutrophil activity. CP binds Zn^{++} and Mn^{++}, required for bacterial and fungal growth. Manganese and zinc sequestration may participate in the IBD disease process. Patients need to be off proton pump inhibitors before testing to prevent false positive tests. CP is elevated in about 90% of patients with UC or CrD. Calgranulin C (S100A12) (CC), a calcium sequestrant protein, is even more specific for neutrophils than in CP that is also produced by monocytes. There are fewer studies on CC than CP, but CC has a higher predictive value for UC and CrD does than CP. Lactoferrin, an iron-binding protein, also has very high sensitivity and specificity. CP, however, responds to treatment more quickly and thus can be used as a marker of treatment success. CP testing is also commonly available.

Eosinophil Markers: Eosinophil Cationic Protein (ECP) and Eosinophil Protein X (EPX) are granulocytic proteins from eosinophils. Their presence thus can indicate allergic or parasitic activity[37]. Fecal ECP (and tryptase) levels increase with food challenges and correlate to symptoms. Fecal ECP is elevated in lymphocytic colitis (LC), but not in MCE. ECP degranulation is stimulated by peptidoglycan[38] from gram-positive bacteria, such as *Clostridia* proliferation.

Mast Cell Marker: Fecal tryptase is elevated in MCE and LC. Fecal tryptase testing is not commercially available, and few studies have been published on it. In lymphocytic colitis, both ECP and tryptase rise with exposure to IgE food allergens. In IBS, there is reactivity to IgG food sensitivities (antergies) and increase in tryptase, but ECP and EPX are normal. IBS-D should be considered "mast cell enterocolitis"[39]. Although mast cell number is usually elevated in MCE, it is abnormal mast cell activity and behavior, much more than mast cell number, responsible for the disease. See Chapter 26 for more on IBS-D.

ASCA/p-ANCA antibodies: Serum Anti-Saccharomyces cerevisiae antibodies (ASCA) tests are usually positive in CrD but not in UC or IBS. Perinuclear anti-neutrophil cytoplasmic antibodies (p-ANCA) form to myeloperoxidase, but occasionally to lactoferrin, elastase or other protein. This test is commonly positive in UC. These tests may be helpful in distinguishing UC from CrD when it is not clear from endoscopy. Although ASCA is rarely positive in IBS, IgG reactivity to food yeast is very common in IBS.

Lymphocytic and Collagenous Colitis

Collagenous colitis (CC), lymphocytic colitis (LC), and mast cell enterocolitis (MCE) and Behçet's disease are other forms of IBD. LC and CC are usually referred to as Microscopic Colitis (MC) as changes are seen on biopsy but not on colonoscopy. MCE accounts for most IBS-D and is also a "microscopic colitis" as the intestines appear normal on colonoscopy. In CC, in addition to colonic mucosal infiltration with T cell lymphocytes, there is accumulation of collagen fibers in the mucosa. CC and LC are clinically indistinguishable, and likely have common causality, thus herein both are referred to as lymphocytic colitis (LC).

The occurrence of LC increases greatly after the age of 40 and accounts for 15 to 20% of cases of chronic watery diarrhea. LC has many similarities to MCE/ IBS-D. Similar to post infectious-IBS, LC often occurs after an enteric infection with *Yersinia enterocolitica, Campylobacter jejuni, Clostridium difficile* or in food-related epidemics outbreaks. It's time course is similar to Pi-IBS, resolving, on average, after five years. Similar to IBS, bile acid malabsorption is found in up to 60% of LC cases, and there is an increase in paracellular permeability. Also similar to IBS, LC is more common in those with autoimmune arthritis, diabetes, thyroid disease, and celiac disease[40].

Even though T cell infiltration is the predominant feature of LC, the symptomatic disease is likely due eosinophilic activation. As with MCE, it is the state of activation of eosinophils, rather than the cell count that is relevant. Fecal ECP correlates with disease activity, and treatment success with a fall in eosinophils. Mast cell activation may also be present in LC, but eosinophilic activation is unusual in MCE. Lymphocytes elute cytokines that induce the development of eosinophils and chemokines that bring them into the colonic mucosa. In LC, there is a greatly increased production of nitric oxide by colonic epithelial cells, secondary to induction of iNOS by NF-κB. This may explain the increase in paracellular permeability and increased fluid losses.

Diet and Crohn's Disease

Elemental Diets: It has long been understood that food impacts IBD. Most patients with Crohn's disease go into remission when placed on total parenteral nutrition (feeding an elemental diet through the vein), or with an oral elemental diet, made up of simple amino acids without peptides or proteins[41]. "Bowel rest" is successful in most patients. Other studies have shown that a diet limited to small peptides may work as well as one using simple amino acids in achieving remission of CrD[42]. However, enteral or parenteral feeding is neither inexpensive nor pleasant, and elemental diets are, at best, barely palatable. Thus, these treatments are impractical for long-term treatment.

Exclusion Diets: Exclusion diets can provide benefit in CrD and MCE. In an exclusion diet, the patient starts with an elemental diet or enteral nutrition and then sequentially adds one food item at a time, to determine which items cause problems. Exclusion diets can be very effective in some patients[43]; however, patients may have difficulty in identifying food triggers[44]. Thus, simple exclusion diets may not be practical, especially if not preceded with an elemental diet and a period of remission so that there is a change in symptoms when an aggravating food is added.

Effective exclusion diets succeed with the reintroduction of individual foods no more often than once a day; if the food consumption was associated with diarrhea or abdominal pain, that food was excluded from the diet. The most common problem foods include cereals, dairy, and yeast. While exclusion diets work in many CrD patients, who may stay in remission for long periods without the use of medication, others patients feel that flare-ups are unrelated to diet, or choose not to comply with the regimen.

As with other autoimmune diseases, it is not specific foods that are associated with disease exacerbation, but rather idiosyncratic antergic reactions associated with T_H17 activation of the enteric immune system. Although dietary yeasts are a particularly common antigen in CrD and IBS, testing for a wide array of IgG reactive foods helps identify the usually multiple food antergies, typical in these patients that maintain enteroimmune activity.

Vitamin D and Crohn's Disease

CrD disease activity is inversely related to vitamin D levels; in a study CrD patients in remission, with mild or moderately active disease, average 25-OHD3 levels were 64, 49 and 21 nmol/L[45]. Vitamin D levels of the anti-inflammatory cytokine, IL-10, have been found to be lower in CrD patients with inadequate vitamin D levels[46].

Several studies have shown that CrD is a risk factor for lower vitamin D levels[47, 48, 49], especially with small intestinal involvement[50], because of pancreatic enzyme deficiency and poor intestinal reabsorption during enterohepatic recycling. Malabsorption can cause loss of vitamin D. Vitamin K levels are also low in CrD patients[51], caused by malabsorption. In a study in which CrD patients were supplied with progressive amounts of supplemental vitamin D_3, beginning with 1000 IU a day, and increasing to a maximum of 5000 IU daily, over 75% of the patients required the full 5000 IU dose, and still, half the patients had 25-OHD3 levels below the 100 nmol/L target.

In this population, vitamin D supplementation was associated with a decrease in disease activity score by more than half. Ninety-four percent of the CrD patients had lower disease activity scores after 24 weeks of vitamin D supplements; two-thirds of patients treated with vitamin D went into remission[52]. Thus, CrD activity lowers 25-OHD3 blood levels, and low 25-OHD3 levels exacerbate the disease.

25-OHD3 is provitamin D_3 that must be converted to active 1, 25-OHD3 by the kidneys. TNF-α, which is elevated in active CrD, suppresses parathyroid hormone (PTH) synthesis, and thus, inhibits 1-α-hydroxylase activity in the kidneys, suppressing the conversion of provitamin D_3 to active vitamin D_3[53]. Thus, inflammation prevents activation of vitamin D, even when levels are adequate. Vitamin D therapy for an inflammatory disease should coincide with TNF-α mitigation (Tables 23-1, 32-1 and 32-2).

Ulcerative Colitis

Ulcerative Colitis has a different causal mechanism than CrD. UC does not respond to bowel rest or elimination diets as do CrD, LC or MCE. UC is, thus, unlikely to go into remission in response to food elimination diets.

UC, however, is associated with the "Western Diet," characterized by a high n6:n3 fatty acid ratio, high protein content, the consumption of potatoes, and diets with low intake of vegetables. N-6 fats are associated with the formation of inflammatory prostaglandins and leukotrienes. Sulfite consumption can cause oxidative stress and induce mast cell degranulation. Potatoes may inhibit proteolysis and digested proteins promote dysbiosis and production of ammonia in the colon. Sulfites are also associated with inflammatory scoring on sigmoidoscopy in UC[54]. UC may also be associated with leukotriene associated hypersensitivity[55] (Chapter 15). A genetic polymorphism, with limited AOC1 activity in the colon, has been found among patients with severe UC, who require immunosuppressive drugs[56]. In these patients, histamine and other biogenic amines that are normally degraded by this enzyme, remain active. (See Chapter 13).

Potatoes and IBD

While IgG formation to foods is idiosyncratic, potatoes seem to be particularly troublesome for patients with IBD. It has been observed that IBD is highest in countries with the highest consumption of potatoes, and potatoes have been noted by many UC patients to exacerbate their disease.

Potatoes contain 5-lipoxygenase, which may increase leukotriene A_4. When arachidonic acid is the prevalent substrate, leukotrienes are proinflammatory and may increase inflammation in the intestine. Potatoes lectin can bind to IgE on Mast cells and trigger mast cell degranulation[57], and thus can act as a nonspecific immunogen in atrophic individuals or individuals with mast cell activation disorders. (See Chapter 14).

Potatoes contain protease inhibitors (trypsin kallikrein, enterokinase, and carboxypeptidase inhibitors) that inhibit some digestive protein enzymes, especially if consumed raw. Potato lectin (solanum tuberosa agglutinin) survives cooking, inhibits trypsin and impairs protein digestion. Undigested proteins are more likely to provoke an immune response as they travel through the small intestine.

In UC, there is an abnormal distribution of bacterial populations living in the colon and dysfunction of the mucous lining the colon. This may result from the presence of undigested proteins. Proteins that arrive in the colon are the fermented into ammonia and bioactive amines. Bioamine production can especially problematic for patients with UC; as many of these patients have reduced AOC1 enzymatic activity (Chapter 13). Ammonia is toxic to colonocytes and can disrupt the mucous barrier which isolates the colonocytes from direct contact with bacteria and toxins in the colon. Undigested proteins in the colon support the growth of *Clostridia*. Animals fed high proportion of potatoes as a food source had increased the growth of *Clostridium perfringens*, higher levels of its toxins, and a high incidence of necrotic enteritis[58, 59].

Trypsin inhibitors curtail alkaline SMase activity in the lumen of the intestine, especially in the colon, which relies on alkaline SMase formed in the proximal intestine; thus trypsin inhibitors limit colonic inflammatory cell apoptosis, and may increase the risk of colorectal cancer. Potatoes also contain a protease inhibitor, which increase the release of CCK[60], facilitating transmission of visceral pain[61]. Potatoes can also induce mast cell degranulation in individuals with mast cell hypertrophy or mast cell activation syndromes.

Potatoes Glycoalkaloids: Potatoes contain glycoalkaloids, in, and just below, the skin that protects them from being eaten by insects and animals. These toxic glycoalkaloids, mainly solanine and chaconine, induce changes to the mucosal membrane integrity of the intestine[62]. Mice fed high glycoalkaloid potatoes had elevated levels of the inflammatory cytokines IFN-γ, TNF-α and IL-17 in the colon, and increased colonic permeability. These results occurred in mice with either a genetic susceptibility to IBD or in a model where dextran sodium sulfate was used to disrupt the mucous layer that normally coats the large bowel and protected the colonocytes from bacterial in the colon[63]. Thus, individuals with genetic susceptibility to IBD or preexisting damage to the intestinal mucosa would have an increased susceptibility to these toxins.

Potato alkaloids are not destroyed by cooking temperatures. Fried potatoes have higher levels than boiled potatoes do; the toxin is water soluble, and when the potatoes are boiled, some of the toxins diffuse into the water, which is usually discarded. Peeling the potato will decrease the glycoalkaloid content, but will not decrease the level of anti-nutritional potato lectins that can trigger degranulation in susceptible individuals.

The amount of glycoalkaloids present in potatoes depends upon potato variety, the season of growth, and weather conditions; with higher levels produced in cooler, moist climates. Injury to the tuber during harvest can also increase the production of toxins. If the tuber is exposed to light, it produces higher amounts of these bitter toxins. This dissuades insects and other animals from browsed on them. This increase in toxins can occur while the potato is in the ground, or during storage. Although a greenish tint in the potato skin is from chlorophyll, it indicates exposure to light and usually correlates with higher amounts of these toxins. Sprouting, green, or bitter tasting potatoes should not be eaten.

Intestinal Alkaline Sphingomyelinase

Alkaline SMase is a brush border enzyme that acts on sphingomyelin in the alkaline environment of the intestine. Its production is greatest in the mid-jejunum and decreases further along the intestine. However, alkaline SMase is not deactivated; so it accumulates, and its activity increases along its path into the colon. Alkaline SMase is present on enterocytes, but it also acts as an ectoenzyme with even greater activity after being cleaved from the mucosa by the enzyme trypsin. Trypsin inhibitors prevent the freeing of alkaline SMase from the mucosa[64], preventing it from acting in the colon. In the intestinal lumen, alkaline SMase acts on dietary sphingomyelins in addition to those from sloughed enterocytes and other cells. Acid and neutral SMases are also present in the intestinal cells; however, they are structurally unrelated to alkaline SMase[65] and are inactivated by trypsin. Alkaline SMase activity is also dependent on bile acids[66], perhaps also by helping free it from the mucosa[67], particularly by the taurine conjugated bile salts, taurocholate and tauro-chenodeoxycholate and ursodeoxycholic acid[68].

Alkaline SMase protein expression, and thus its activity, is affected by the diet; less is produced with a high-fat diet. These fats are less avidly recovered when there is surplus fat consumption. More alkaline SMase in produced with high-fiber diets. Alkaline SMase production is also inversely associated with cholesterol absorption.

Sphingomyelin is present in the cell membranes of animals, thus, is present in the diet, mostly in eggs, milk and meat, including fish and fowl[69]. From two to 20 percent of the cell membrane of mammals is composed of sphingolipids.

Sphingomyelin is not absorbed intact. Sphingolipids are phospholipids, and thus as polar molecules do not cross the cell membrane. Sphingomyelin, for example, is composed sphingosine, an 18-carbon amino alcohol; a long chain fatty acid; and phosphocholine. Other sphingolipids have phosphoethanolamine as the phospho-nitrogen group. When phosphocholine is enzymatically cleaved from sphingomyelin by SMase, the remaining sphingosine-fatty acid molecule is known as ceramide. At the brush border membrane, ceramide is further hydrolyzed by ceramidase into sphingosine and a free fatty acid, and the three components can be absorbed.

Both phosphocholine and ceramide are immune modulators. Phosphocholine may trigger complement activation[70], and ceramide acts to stimulate apoptosis of senescent colonic mucosal cells, helping prevent colon cancer[71] and regulates mucosal growth[72]. Dietary sphingomyelin inhibits cholesterol absorption[73], likely via the effects of ceramide[74]. Alkaline SMase additionally inactivates the immune signaling activator, platelet-activating-factor (PAF). This inhibition of PAH activity further decreases the risk of colon cancer[75], and likely decreases the destructive activity modulated by PAF in the inflammatory cascade that occurs in Crohn's disease and ulcerative colitis[76,77].

Thus, the lower cholesterol absorption and lower colon cancer incidence, which has been observed among those consuming low-fat, high-fiber diets, may be the result of alkaline SMase activity. Conversely, high cholesterol diets impede the absorption of sphingolipids[78] and may interfere with sphingosine-1-phosphate (S1P) mediated immune functions.

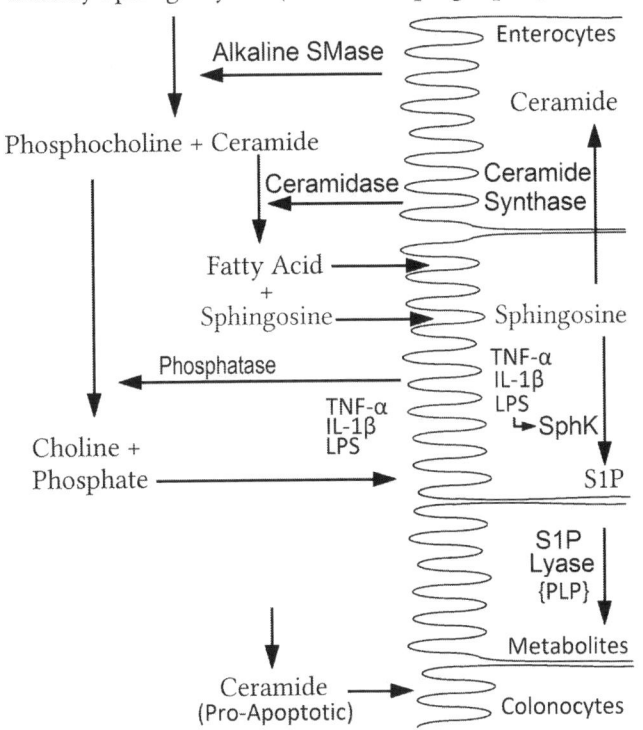

Figure 34-1: Sphingolipid Digestion

Sphingolipid activity is modulated by cytokines and other mediators of the immune response. TNF-α and IL-1β induce S1P production by inducing sphingosine kinase[79,80]. S1P activates NF-κB, promoting the transcription of inflammatory cytokines, and induces production of PGE2, NO, ROS, chemoattractants and adhesion molecules that promote neutrophil migration into the intestinal wall. S1P further enhances the survival of neutrophils by preventing their apoptosis. In an animal model of UC, neutrophil infiltration, cytokine production, and inflammation were greatly inhibited through chronic suppression of the enzyme sphingosine kinase[81].

Sphingosine, once absorbed by enterocytes and passed to the immune cells of the lamina propria, can be rapidly phosphorylated into the immune regulator sphingosine-1-phosphate (S1P), by the enzyme sphingosine kinase (Figure 33-1). The lamina propria is not limited to sphingosine directly absorbed from dietary sources, but by the same measure, it is exposed to sphingosine even when it is not liberated by activation of SMase due to oxidative or cellular stress, as occurs in other areas of the body.

In contrast to the activity of S1P, ceramide promotes apoptosis, autophagy and regulates growth. Not all ceramides are created equal, and they may not provide the same stimulus. There are six ceramide synthase isomers. Their activity is fairly specific to the length of the fatty acid chain in the ceramide molecule[82]. Ceramide synthase (CerS) activity modulates cell growth, apoptosis, and autophagy. Ceramide 16:0 is the most common and is produced by CerS5 and CerS6. CerS1 predominantly produces Cer18:0, while CerS4 produces mostly Cer18:0 and 20:0 ceramides. CerS2 produces a broad range of very long chain ceramides, which are often monounsaturated, the most abundant of which is Cer24:1[83]. CerS3 can produce very long chain polyunsaturated ceramides, with chain lengths of 28 to 32 with five or six double bonds, which are required for spermiogenesis[84]. Long chain fatty acids in the diet are a required substrate for CerS3, as they may also be for CerS2. A balance between short and long chain sphingolipids appears to be required for normal physiologic function and maintaining a balance between immune cell proliferation and apoptosis[85]; providing a balance between protection from microbial infection and the development of enteroimmunopathies and autoimmune disease; between growth and development and proliferation of cancer cells.

Treatment of UC and other forms of IBD should include targeting of the sphingolipid inflammatory pathway. This includes reducing TNF-α induction of S1P production, and thus, reducing intracellular sphingosine kinase (SphK) activity. Betaine and R-α-lipoic acid may be helpful here in addition to avoidance of TNF-α and LPS. Additionally, S1P lyase activity may be enhanced with vitamin B_6 (pyridoxine) if levels are sub-optimal.

TNF-α is a reasonable target. Curcumin, a flavonoid-like compound, increases ceramide synthase activity and promote apoptosis[86]. Curcumin and perhaps flavonoids may increase ceramide synthase activity; they are also known to reduce TNF-α (Table 32-2). These measures may decrease the auto-immune destruction seen in these diseases and their associated risk for colon cancer.

Preventive Therapy for Inflammatory Bowel Disease

CrD, MCE, and LC: Elimination of dietary antergens usually gives quick benefit to many patients with IBD. CrD is an enteroimmunopathic disease involving T_H17, and MCE and about half of LC are mast cell activation disorders, and should be treated as such.

Ulcerative Colitis: Antergies are not as important in UC; testing for food immunogens, however, may be helpful to prevent immune diversion.

Especially in UC, avoidance of preformed bioamines in the diet and fermentation of amino acids in the large intestine can be helpful. Some patients, especially with more severe UC, have low levels of the intestinal enzyme, AOC1, which catabolizes histamine and other diamines. Coenzymes for AOC1 and enzyme cofactors that aid in the catabolism of bioamines are shown in Table 13-4. These cofactors may be helpful as nutritional supplements. UC patients may respond to AOC1 supplementation, using the over-the-counter supplement, Histame. Histamine blockers may also help. Alcohol impairs the breakdown of bioamines in the intestine, which is particularly an issue for UC, and thus should be avoided. (See Chapter 13 on Bioamines)

LC: Standard therapy is budesonide (9 mg daily for 6-8 weeks, followed by 3-6 mg for six months) to controls symptoms, but relapse is common if medication is stopped. Treatment for BAM with bile acid sequestrants is often helpful. Mesalazine (which may act as quorum sensing inhibitor) often results in long-term remission. Like IBS, LC patients should have stools tested for parasites and be tested for food allergies using ImmunoCAP testing (Chapter 11). Mast cell activation may also be present.

Additional Therapeutics for IBD

1. Test and treat nutrient deficiencies: Vitamins A, D, E, K, folate, vitamin B_{12}, magnesium, and zinc, are easily lost in malabsorption, and may be low in patients with IBD, and especially if the small intestine is affected. Additionally, WBC proteins that sequester minerals to prevent bacterial growth (e.g.: Lactoferrin – Fe^{++}, CP – Zn^{++} and Mn^{++}, Calgranulin - Ca^{++}) may cause deficiencies. Inadequate zinc causes increased paracellular permeability that can worsen the disease. It should be assumed that these deficiencies are present in patients with IBD and malabsorption syndromes until testing shows otherwise. Test, treat, and test again to assure that treatment have been sufficient.

LPS from colonic bacterial biofilms activates TLR-4. Vitamin D down-regulates TLR-4 that is stimulated by LPS from bacterial biofilms. *TLR4 activation promotes NF-κB activity and transcription of inflammatory mediators such as NO and cytokines and prevents apoptosis of inflammatory WBC's in the mucosa, thus maintaining disease activity.* Vitamins K_2 and flavonoids also curtail NF-κB activation, by interfering with TNF-α signaling.

Treatment of vitamin D deficiency should be accompanied by mitigation of TNF-α (Tables 23-1, 32-1 and 32-2). Doses of vitamin D_3 at 6000 IU a day for several months are often required to assure that sufficient levels (100 to 200 nmol/L, (40 to 80 ng/ml) are reached. A loading dose may help move the patient into remission more quickly; use of up to 300,000 IU of vitamin D_3 may be appropriate, preferably given over ten days. See Chapter 20.

2. Screen for and treat bone loss: As a result of malabsorption, and treatment with steroids, 50% of CrD patients develop osteopenia, and one in eight develops osteoporosis. Twenty percent of men with CrD were found to have vertebral compression fractures, even among those with normal bone density and those not using steroids. The increased risk for elevated parathyroid hormone in these patients[87] suggests insufficient vitamin D levels, which would be expected with small bowel malabsorption and vitamin D and vitamin K loss. Osteopenia and osteoimmunity are discussed in Chapter 43.

2. S1P mitigation: S1P activity helps maintain neutrophil infiltration of the intestinal wall and maintain antergies. Pyridoxine supplements of 25 mg daily should be sufficient to provide sufficient PLP for most patients for S1P lyase activity.

THI (2-acetyl-4-Tetrahydroxybutylimidazole), a component of caramel food colorant III (e150c) used in food products, inhibits the enzyme S1P lyase and thus caramel food coloring should be avoided. Caramel color III is used to color some beers, soy and other sauces, balsamic vinegar, soups, and confectionery[88].

Mitigation of TNF-α can be done by consuming foods high in flavonoids. Table 32-2 lists several such foods. Table 23-1 list factors which increase TNF-α, and Table 32-1 factors that lower it. Curcumin, and perhaps flavonoids, also increase the activity of ceramide synthase, and thus, these may additionally act to downregulated intestinal inflammation.

S1P acts at least largely through activation of NF-κB. Thus, mitigation of NF-κB, may be helpful. Intervention, however, would have to be at, or upstream of the point at which TNF-α acts. Vitamin K and flavonoids may be helpful. Additionally, factors that activate PPARγ or PI3K, such as magnesium, may help down regulate inflammation and promote repair. As sphingosine, the precursor for S1P, is absorbed directly from the intestine, avoidance of foods high in sphingolipids may be helpful for patients with CrD.

3. Sleep: Sleep deprivation increases inflammation and should be avoided. Additionally, a regular sleep cycle is needed for the diurnal intestinal cycle. Sleep is also needed for T_3 and growth hormone induced production of MBL.

4. Pancreatic Enzyme Insufficiency (PEI): PEI is common in IBD affecting the small intestine. Low fecal pancreatic elastase-1, chymotrypsin or high fecal fat indicate pancreatic exocrine insufficiency and inadequate enzymes for protein digestion that increase fermentation of protein in the colon. Unabsorbed amino acids and proteins that enter the colon are fermented; producing ammonia and bioamines, including histamine. These proteins promote dysbiosis, with an increase in growth of *Clostridia*, toxin production, and ammonia. Ammonia disrupts the colon's protective mucous layer, essential in preventing access of bacteria to the colonocytes. Pancreatic enzyme insufficiency and treatment are covered in Chapter 8.

Biofilm inhibiting foods: Include biofilm inhibiting foods in the diet that are tolerated. See Table 23-2 and 23-4.

Avoid Trypsin Inhibitors: Table 23-3 lists several foods that contain trypsin inhibitors. Most trypsin inhibitors, other than those in potatoes, are denatured by normal cooking temperatures.

Avoid Nutrients Malabsorption: Avoid consumption of sugars and proteins that are poorly absorbed, and thus, promote bacterial overgrowth. Poorly absorbed sugar can greatly decrease oral cecal transit time and carry peptides and amino acids into the colon that have not had a chance to be digested and absorbed. Poorly absorbed sugars are discussed in Chapter 5.

Avoid Raw Foods: Many plant proteins are difficult to digest. This is especially true for raw or lightly cooked plant proteins. Thorough cooking of proteins in water can partially hydrolyze some proteins, and lower their antigenicity. Many plants used as foods contain lectins that are toxic if not denatured by cooking. Lectins are discussed in Chapter 7. Pressure cooking hydrolyzes some proteins, lowering their antigenicity.

Limit Dietary Protein Intake: Limiting the amount of dietary protein to amounts required for proper nutrition may help avoid passage of protein into the colon where it is fermented. The WHO promulgates a daily intake of 0.45 grams of protein per kilogram of ideal body weight in adults. This is considerably less than the amount consumed in the typical Western diet. Limiting protein intake to easily absorbed, properly cooked foods may help with protein absorption.

Prebiotics: Lactulose, used as a prebiotic, may alter the intestinal microbiota and prevent the formation of ammonia. Both prebiotics and probiotics may be helpful to change the balance of bacteria in the colon. Foods high in fructose oligosaccharides should be included in the diet, to help archive a eubiotic intestinal biota. The gradual introduction of fiber is more comfortable for the patient and helps with compliance. Prebiotics are discussed in Chapter 4.

Avoid Potatoes: Potatoes should be avoided in patients with IBD especially if the disease is active. Potatoes contain proteolytic enzyme inhibitors, some which are not inactivated by cooking. If potatoes cannot be avoided, the risk of exposure to glycoalkaloids toxins may be lowered by using freshly harvested potatoes grown in warm climates, such as Mexico, peeling the potatoes and discarding the skins, and boiling rather frying the potatoes. Peeling potatoes will not prevent the effects of lectins or release of CCK. Potatoes that are peeled and cut should be immediately put into water as oxidation of the cut surfaces may increase adverse reactions to potatoes.

5. ASCA Positive: If the ASCA test is positive the stool can be cultured for *Candida* and treated with antifungal agents. The stool should also be tested for blood, a growth factor for invasive yeast growth. Additionally, these individuals should be tested for IgG antibodies to dietary yeasts, and yeast products (bread, yeast flavoring, such as marmite, and fermented products) should be avoided. Long-term treatment depends on the prevention of pathologic biofilms in the intestine that induce quorum sensing for *Candida*. *Candida* biofilm can act as a quorum sensing agent for bacteria and thus induce bacterial biofilm. The stool should be tested for hemoglobin and parasites.

6. Biomarker ECP or EPX Positive: These tests are indicative of eosinophil activity; thus the patient should be evaluated for parasitic infestation and ImmunoCAP testing for IgE food allergies. There also may be an association with leukotriene associated hypersensitivity. (See Chapters 11 and 15). ECP may also reflect gram-positive bacteria biofilm and peptidoglycan from their cell wall.

7. Neutrophil Markers: Fecal CP and other neutrophil markers suggest biofilm formation and the presence of high levels of LPS a TLR-4 activator or flagellin, a TLR-5 activator. Treatment of Biofilms is covered in Chapter 23. Calgranin C is a stimulating ligand for TLR-4.

8. Investigate possible MCAS in IBD Patients: Mast cell activation is common in IBD and underlies MCE. Fecal tryptase testing can guide treatment if available. Assess and treat IBD patients, especially MCE and LC for MCAS as described in Chapter 12. Avoid triggers for mast cell degranulation (Chapter 14).

9. Bile acid Malabsorption (BAM). BAM is common in IBD, especially when the ileum is affected, as in CrD, LC, and MCE/IBS-D and is an important cause of diarrhea. Treatment can give quick benefit to patients. BAM, BAD, and its treatment are covered in Chapter 26

10. Glycine: Glycine is the principal fuel for enterocytes in the ilium, and thus aid digestion for nutrient and bile absorption. Trimethyl-glycine (**betaine**) may be an effective way of delivering glycine to these cells, promotes glutathione production and prevents the formation of homocysteine that promotes acid SMase activity.

Suggested Daily Supplements in IBD:

Vitamin D_3 – 6000 IU
Vitamin K_2 (menatetraenone) – 5 mg
R-α-lipoic acid (sodium stabilized) – 100 mg
Betaine - 1200 mg
Pyridoxine (Vitamin B_6) – 25 mg
Vitamin B_{12} – 250 mcg;
    (sublingually or dissolved in the mouth).
Folate – 400 mg
Magnesium (citrate or another organic salt) – 600 mg
Zinc – 10 mg
Turmeric, quercetin, or other flavonoids – 1 gram
Biofilm inhibiting foods (See Chapter 23).

Treat with pancreatic enzymes when indicated.

[1] Meta-analysis: colorectal and small bowel cancer risk in patients with Crohn's disease. Canavan C, Abrams KR, Mayberry J. Aliment Pharmacol Ther. 2006 Apr 15;23(8):1097-104. PMID:16611269

[2] Risk of colorectal high-grade dysplasia and cancer in a prospective observational cohort of patients with inflammatory bowel disease. Beaugerie L, Svrcek M, Seksik P, et al; CESAME Study Group. Gastroenterology. 2013 Jul;145(1):166-175.e8. PMID:23541909

[3] Post-traumatic stress in Crohn's disease and its association with disease activity. Camara RFA, Gander ML, Berge S, vonKanel R. Frontline Gastroenterol doi:10.1136/fg.2010.002733

[4] Concordance for IBD among twins compared to ordinary siblings--a Norwegian population-based study. Bengtson MB, Aamodt G, Vatn MH, Harris JR. J Crohns Colitis. 2010 Sep;4(3):312-8. PMID:21122520

[5] Inflammatory bowel disease in a Swedish twin cohort: a long-term follow-up of concordance and clinical characteristics. Halfvarson J, Bodin L, Tysk C, Lindberg E, Järnerot G, et al. Gastroenterology. 2003 Jun;124(7):1767-73. PMID:12806610

[6] Concordance of inflammatory bowel disease among Danish twins. Results of a nationwide study. Orholm M, Binder V, Sørensen TI, Rasmussen LP, Kyvik KO. Scand J Gastroenterol. 2000 Oct;35(10):1075-81. PMID:11099061

[7] Inflammatory bowel disease. An epidemiological and genetic study. Monsén U. Acta Chir Scand Suppl. 1990;559:1-42. PMID:2092567

[8] Role of genetic and environmental factors in British twins with inflammatory bowel disease. Ng SC, Woodrow S, Patel N, et al. Inflamm Bowel Dis. 2012 Apr;18(4):725-36. PMID:21557397

[9] Infectious serologies and autoantibodies in inflammatory bowel disease: insinuations at a true pathogenic role. Lidar M, Langevitz P, Barzilai et al. Ann N Y Acad Sci. 2009 Sep;1173:640-8. PMID:19758210

[10] Food specific IgG4 -guided exclusion diets improve symptoms in Crohn's disease: A pilot study. Rajendran N, Kumar D. Colorectal Dis. 2010 Jul 7. PMID: 20626437

[11] Targeting tissular immune response improves diagnostic performance of anti-Saccharomyces cerevisiae antibodies (ASCA) in Crohn's disease. Bertin D, Grimaud JC, Lesavre N, et al. PLoS One. 2013 Nov 26;8(11):e80433. PMID:24303014

[12] Clinical relevance of IgG antibodies against food antigens in Crohn's disease: a double-blind cross-over diet intervention study. Bentz S, Hausmann M, Piberger H, et al. Digestion. 2010;81(4):252-64. Epub 2010 Jan 30.PMID: 20130407

[13] Antibodies anti-Saccharomyces cerevisiae (ASCA) do not differentiate Crohn's disease from celiac disease. Kotze LM, Nisihara RM, Utiyama et al. Arq Gastroenterol. 2010 Sep;47(3):242-5.PMID: 21140083

[14] Anti-Saccharomyces cerevisiae antibody does not differentiate between Crohn's disease and intestinal tuberculosis. Makharia GK, Sachdev V, Gupta R, Lal S, Pandey RM. Dig Dis Sci. 2007 Jan;52(1):33-9. Epub 2006 Dec 8. PMID:17160471

[15] Genetics and molecular biology in Candida albicans. Hernday AD, Noble SM, Mitrovich QM, Johnson AD. Methods Enzymol. 2010;470:737-58. Epub 2010 Mar 1. PMID:20946834

[16] Dynamic expression of cell-surface antigens probed with Candida albicans-specific monoclonal antibodies. Deslauriers N, Michaud J, Carré B, Léveillée C. Microbiology. 1996 May;142 (Pt 5):1239-48. PMID:8704964

[17] From attachment to damage: defined genes of Candida albicans mediate adhesion, invasion and damage during interaction with oral epithelial cells. Wächtler B, Wilson D, Haedicke K, Dalle F, Hube B. PLoS One. 2011 Feb 23;6(2):e17046. PMID:21407800

[18] Hemoglobin is an effective inducer of hyphal differentiation in Candida albicans. Pendrak ML, Roberts DD. Med Mycol. 2007 Feb;45(1):61-71. PMID:17325946

[19] Transcriptional response of Candida albicans to hypoxia: linkage of oxygen sensing and Efg1p-regulatory networks. Setiadi ER, Doedt T, Cottier F, Noffz C, Ernst JF. J Mol Biol. 2006 Aug 18;361(3):399-411. PMID:16854431

[20] Low Mannan-binding lectin serum levels are associated with complicated Crohn's disease and reactivity to oligomannan (ASCA). Schoepfer AM, Flogerzi B, Seibold-Schmid B, et al. Am J Gastroenterol. 2009 Oct;104(10):2508-16. PMID:19532127

[21] Anti-Saccharomyces cerevisiae mannan antibodies (ASCA) of Crohn's patients crossreact with mannan from other yeast strains, and murine ASCA IgM can be experimentally induced with Candida albicans. Schaffer T, Müller S, Flogerzi B, et al. Inflamm Bowel Dis. 2007 Nov;13(11):1339-46. PMID:17636567

[22] Candida albicans colonization and ASCA in familial Crohn's disease. Standaert-Vitse A, Sendid B, Joossens M, et al. Am J Gastroenterol. 2009 Jul;104(7):1745-53. PMID:19471251

[23] Partial overlap of anti-mycobacterial, and anti-Saccharomyces cerevisiae mannan antibodies in Crohn's disease. Müller S, Schaffer T, Schoepfer AM, Hilty A, Bodmer T, Seibold F. World J Gastroenterol. 2008 Jun 21;14(23):3650-61. PMID:18595132

[24] Seroreactive marker for inflammatory bowel disease and associations with antibodies to dietary proteins in bipolar disorder. Severance EG, Gressitt KL, Yang S, et al. Bipolar Disord. 2013 Dec 6. PMID:24313887

[25] Gastrointestinal inflammation and associated immune activation in schizophrenia. Severance EG, Alaedini A, Yang S, et al. Schizophr Res. 2012 Jun;138(1):48-53. PMID:22446142

[26] Hormonal regulation of mannan-binding lectin synthesis in hepatocytes. Sørensen CM, Hansen TK, Steffensen R, Jensenius JC, Thiel S. Clin Exp Immunol. 2006 Jul;145(1):173-82. PMID:16792688

[27] Personal communication with Dr. Emil Schandl, M.D., lab director at Immuno Laboratories, Ft. Lauderdale, FL, June 2011.

[28] Treating irritable bowel syndrome with a food elimination diet followed by food challenge and probiotics. Drisko J, Bischoff B, Hall M,etal. J Am Coll Nutr. 2006 Dec;25(6):514-22.PMID:17229899

[29] Food elimination based on IgG antibodies in irritable bowel syndrome: a randomised controlled trial. Atkinson W, Sheldon TA, Shaath N, et al. Gut. 2004 Oct;53(10):1459-64.PMID: 15361495

[30] Food allergy mediated by IgG antibodies associated with migraine in adults. Arroyave Hernández CM, Echavarría Pinto M, Hernández Montiel HL. Rev Alerg Mex. 2007 Sep-Oct;54(5):162-8. Erratum in: Rev Alerg Mex. 2010 Mar-Apr;57(2):49. PMID:18693538

[31] Citrulline as a biomarker of intestinal failure due to enterocyte mass reduction. Crenn P, Messing B, Cynober L. Clin Nutr. 2008 Jun;27(3):328-39. PMID:18440672

[32] Antibodies to flagellin indicate reactivity to bacterial antigens in IBS patients. Schoepfer AM, Schaffer T, Seibold-Schmid B, et al. Neurogastroenterol Motil. 2008 Oct;20(10):1110-8. PMID:18694443

[33] Detection of inflammatory markers in stools from patients with irritable bowel syndrome and collagenous colitis. Lettesjö H, Hansson T, Peterson C, et al. Scand J Gastroenterol. 2006 Jan;41(1):54-9. PMID:16373277

[34] Diagnostic utility of faecal biomarkers in patients with irritable bowel syndrome. Däbritz J, Musci J, Foell D. World J Gastroenterol. 2014 Jan 14;20(2):363-75. PMID:24574706

[35] Detection of local mast-cell activity in patients with food hypersensitivity. Peterson CG, Hansson T, Skott A, et al. J Investig Allergol Clin Immunol. 2007;17(5):314-20. PMID:17982924

[36] Clinical value of serum eosinophilic cationic protein assessment in children with inflammatory bowel disease. Wędrychowicz A, Tomasik P, Pieczarkowski S, et al. Arch Med Sci. 2014 Dec 22;10(6):1142-6. PMID:25624851

[37] Measurements of eosinophil activation before and after food challenges in adults with food hypersensitivity. van Odijk J, Peterson CG, Ahlstedt S, et al. Int Arch Allergy Immunol. 2006;140(4):334-41. PMID:16757922

[38] Intracellular signaling mechanisms regulating toll-like receptor-mediated activation of eosinophils. Wong CK, Cheung PF, Ip WK, et al. Am J Resp Cell Mol Biol. 2007 Jul;37(1):85-96. PMID:17332440

[39] A clinicopathologic study of 24 cases of systemic mastocytosis involving the gastrointestinal tract and assessment of mucosal mast cell density in irritable bowel syndrome and asymptomatic patients. Doyle LA, Sepehr GJ, Hamilton MJ, Akin C, et al. Am J Surg Pathol. 2014 Jun;38(6):832-43. PMID:24618605

[40] Recent advances in diagnosis and treatment of microscopic colitis. Tysk C, Wickbom A, Nyhlin N, Eriksson S, Bohr J. Ann Gastroenterol. 2011;24(4):253-262. PMID:24713787

[41] Has total bowel rest a beneficial effect in the treatment of Crohn's disease? Lochs H, Meryn S, Marosi L, Ferenci P, Hörtnagl H. Clin Nutr. 1983 Apr;2(1):61-4.PMID: 16829411

[42] Randomized controlled trial of amino acid based diet versus oligopeptide based diet in enteral nutritional therapy of active Crohn's disease. Ueki M, Matsui T, Yamada M, et al. 1994 Sep;91(9):1415-25. PMID: 7933639

[43] Comparison of total parenteral nutrition and elemental diet in induction of remission of Crohn's disease. Long-term maintenance of remission by personalized food exclusion diets. Jones VA. Dig Dis Sci. 1987 Dec;32(12 Suppl):100S-107S.PMID: 3121268

[44] Long-term effects of elemental and exclusion diets for Crohn's disease. Giaffer MH, Cann P, Holdsworth CD. Aliment Pharmacol Ther. 1991 Apr;5(2):115-25.PMID: 1909583

[45] Active Crohn's disease is associated with low vitamin D levels. Jørgensen SP, Hvas CL, Agnholt J, et al. J Crohns Colitis. 2013 Nov 1;7(10):e407-13. PMID:23403039

[46] Vitamin D status and cytokine levels in patients with Crohn's disease. Kelly P, Suibhne TN, O'Morain C, O'Sullivan M. Int J Vitam Nutr Res. 2011 Jul;81(4):205-10. PMID:22237768

[47] Risk factors for vitamin D deficiency in patients with Crohn's disease. Tajika M, Matsuura A, Nakamura T, et al. J Gastroenterol. 2004 Jun;39(6):527-33. PMID:15235869

[48] Determinants of vitamin D status in adult Crohn's disease patients, with particular emphasis on supplemental vitamin D use. Gilman J, Shanahan F, Cashman KD. Eur J Clin Nutr. 2006 Jul;60(7):889-96.. PMID:16493452

[49] Vitamin D deficiency in Crohn's disease and healthy controls: A prospective case-control study in the Netherlands. de Bruyn JR, van Heeckeren R, Ponsioen CY, et al. J Crohns Colitis. 2014 Mar 22. pii: S1873-9946(14)00099-3. PMID:24666975

[50] 25 (OH) vitamin D level in Crohn's disease: association with sun exposure & disease activity. Joseph AJ, George B, Pulimood AB, et al. Indian J Med Res. 2009 Aug;130(2):133-7. PMID:19797809

[51] Low serum and bone vitamin K status in patients with longstanding Crohn's disease: another pathogenetic factor of osteoporosis in Crohn's disease? Schoon EJ, Müller MC, Vermeer C, et al. Gut. 2001 Apr;48(4):473-7. PMID:11247890

[52] Therapeutic effect of vitamin d supplementation in a pilot study of Crohn's patients. Yang L, Weaver V, Smith JP, et al. Clin Transl Gastroenterol. 2013 Apr 18;4:e33. PMID:23594800

[53] Changes in Vitamin D-Related Mineral Metabolism Following Induction with Anti-Tumor Necrosis Factor-α Therapy in Crohn's Disease. Augustine MV, Leonard MB, Thayu M, et al. J Clin Endocrinol Metab. 2014 Mar 11:jc20133846. PMID:24617709

[54] Associations between diet and disease activity in ulcerative colitis patients using a novel method of data analysis. Magee EA, Edmond LM, Tasker SM, Kong SC, Curno R, Cummings JH. Nutr J. 2005 Feb 10;4:7. PMID:15705205

[55] Significance of salicylate intolerance in diseases of the lower gastrointestinal tract. Raithel M, Baenkler HW, et al. J Physiol Pharmacol. 2005 Sep;56 Suppl 5:89-102.PMID: 16247191

[56] Severity of ulcerative colitis is associated with a polymorphism at diamine oxidase gene but not at histamine N-methyltransferase gene. García-Martín E, Mendoza JL, Martínez C, et al. World J Gastroenterol. 2006 Jan 28;12(4):615-20. PMID:16489678

[57] Potato lectin activates basophils and mast cells of atopic subjects by its interaction with core chitobiose of cell-bound non-specific immunoglobulin E. Pramod SN, Venkatesh YP, Mahesh PA. Clin Exp Immunol. 2007 Jun;148(3):391-401. PMID:17362264

[58] Effect of dietary protein concentrates on the incidence of subclinical necrotic enteritis and growth performance of broiler chickens. Palliyeguru MW, Rose SP, Mackenzie AM. Poult Sci. 2010 Jan;89(1):34-43. PMID:20008800

[59] Effect of diets containing potato protein or soya bean meal on the incidence of spontaneously-occurring subclinical necrotic enteritis and the physiological response in broiler chickens. Fernando PS, Rose SP, Mackenzie AM, Silva SS. Br Poult Sci. 2011 Feb;52(1):106-14. PMID:21337205

[60] Potato protease inhibitors inhibit food intake and increase circulating cholecystokinin levels by a trypsin-dependent mechanism. Komarnytsky S, Cook A, Raskin I. Int J Obes (Lond). 2011 Feb;35(2):236-43. Epub 2010 Sep 7. PMID: 20820171

[61] Activation of descending pain-facilitatory pathways from the rostral ventromedial medulla by cholecystokinin elicits release of prostaglandin-E2 in the spinal cord. Marshall TM, Herman DS, Largent-Milnes TM, Badghisi H, Zuber K, Holt SC, Lai J, Porreca F, Vanderah TW. Pain. 2012 Jan;153(1):86-94. PMID:22030324

[62] Potato glycoalkaloids adversely affect intestinal permeability and aggravate inflammatory bowel disease. Patel B, Schutte R, Sporns P, Doyle J, Jewel L, Fedorak RN. Inflamm Bowel Dis. 2002 Sep;8(5):340-6. PMID:12479649

[63] Naturally occurring glycoalkaloids in potatoes aggravate intestinal inflammation in two mouse models of inflammatory bowel disease. Iablokov V, Sydora BC, Foshaug R, et al. Dig Dis Sci. 2010 Nov;55(11):3078-85. PMID:20198430

[64] Pancreatic trypsin cleaves intestinal alkaline sphingomyelinase from mucosa and enhances the sphingomyelinase activity. Wu J, Liu F, Nilsson A, Duan RD. Am J Physiol Gastrointest Liver Physiol. 2004 Nov;287(5):G967-73. PMID:15205117

[65] Alkaline sphingomyelinase: an old enzyme with novel implications. Duan RD. Biochim Biophys Acta. 2006 Mar;1761(3):281-91. PMID:16631405

[66] Effects of bile diversion in rats on intestinal sphingomyelinases and ceramidase. Duan RD, Verkade HJ, Cheng Y, et al. Biochim Biophys Acta. 2007 Feb;1771(2):196-201. PMID:17204455

[67] Psyllium and fat in diets differentially affect the activities and expressions of colonic sphingomyelinases and caspase in mice. Cheng Y, Ohlsson L, Duan RD. Br J Nutr. 2004 May;91(5):715-23. PMID:15137923

[68] Ursodeoxycholic acid increases the activities of alkaline sphingomyelinase and caspase-3 in the rat colon. Cheng Y, Tauschel HD, Nilsson A, Duan RD. Scand J Gastroenterol. 1999 Sep;34(9):915-20. PMID:10522612

[69] Meats and fish consumed in the American diet contain substantial amounts of ether-linked phospholipids. Blank ML, Cress EA, Smith ZL, Snyder F. J Nutr. 1992 Aug;122(8):1656-61. PMID:1640259

[70] The physiological structure of human C-reactive protein and its complex with phosphocholine. Thompson D, Pepys MB, Wood SP. Structure. 1999 Feb 15;7(2):169-77. PMID:10368284

[71] Dietary sphingomyelin inhibits colonic tumorigenesis with an up-regulation of alkaline sphingomyelinase expression in ICR mice. Zhang P, Li B, Gao S, Duan RD. Anticancer Res. 2008 Nov-Dec;28(6A):3631-5. PMID:19189644

[72] Crucial role of alkaline sphingomyelinase in sphingomyelin digestion: a study on enzyme knockout mice. Zhang Y, Cheng Y, Hansen GH, et al. J Lipid Res. 2011 Apr;52(4):771-81. PMID:21177474

[73] Milk sphingomyelin is more effective than egg sphingomyelin in inhibiting intestinal absorption of cholesterol and fat in rats. Noh SK, Koo SI. J Nutr. 2004 Oct;134(10):2611-6. PMID:15465755

[74] Generating ceramide from sphingomyelin by alkaline sphingomyelinase in the gut enhances sphingomyelin-induced inhibition of cholesterol uptake in Caco-2 cells. Feng D, Ohlsson L, Ling W, Nilsson A, Duan RD. Dig Dis Sci. 2010 Dec;55(12):3377-83. PMID:20393874

[75] Intestinal alkaline sphingomyelinase hydrolyses and inactivates platelet-activating factor by a phospholipase C activity. Wu J, Nilsson A, Jönsson BA, Stenstad H, Agace W, Cheng Y, Duan RD. Biochem J. 2006 Feb 15;394(Pt 1):299-308. PMID:16255717

[76] Platelet activating factor in stool from patients with ulcerative colitis and Crohn's disease. Hocke M, Richter L, Bosseckert H, Eitner K. Hepatogastroenterology. 1999 Jul-Aug;46(28):2333-7. PMID:10521992

[77] The platelet activating factor (PAF) signaling cascade in systemic inflammatory responses. Yost CC, Weyrich AS, Zimmerman GA. Biochimie. 2010 Jun;92(6):692-7. PMID:20167241

[78] A mutual inhibitory effect on absorption of sphingomyelin and cholesterol. Nyberg L, Duan RD, Nilsson A. J Nutr Biochem. 2000 May;11(5):244-9. PMID:10876096

[79] Activation of sphingosine kinase by tumor necrosis factor-alpha inhibits apoptosis in human endothelial cells. Xia P, Wang L, Gamble JR, Vadas MA. J Biol Chem. 1999 Nov 26;274(48):34499-505. PMID:10567432

[80] Sphingosine kinase and sphingosine-1-phosphate: regulators in autoimmune and inflammatory disease. Snider AJ. Int J Clin Rheumtol. 2013 Aug 1;8(4). PMID:24416079

[81] Suppression of ulcerative colitis in mice by orally available inhibitors of sphingosine kinase. Maines LW, Fitzpatrick LR, French KJ, Zhuang Y, Xia Z, Keller SN, Upson JJ, Smith CD et al. Dig Dis Sci. 2008 Apr;53(4):997-1012. PMID:18058233

[82] The equilibrium between long and very long chain ceramides is important for the fate of the cell and can be influenced by co-expression of CerS. Hartmann D, Wegner MS, Wanger RA, et al. Int J Biochem Cell Biol. 2013 Jul;45(7):1195-203. PMID:23538298

[83] Selective knockdown of ceramide synthases reveals complex interregulation of sphingolipid metabolism. Mullen TD, Spassieva S, Jenkins RW, et al. J Lipid Res. 2011 Jan;52(1):68-77. PMID:20940143

[84] Male germ cells require polyenoic sphingolipids with complex glycosylation for completion of meiosis: a link to ceramide synthase-3. Rabionet M, van der Spoel AC, Chuang CC, et al. J Biol Chem. 2008 May 9;283(19):13357-69. PMID:18308723

[85] Long chain ceramides and very long chain ceramides have opposite effects on human breast and colon cancer cell growth. Hartmann D, Lucks J, Fuchs S, et al. Int J Biochem Cell Biol. 2012 Apr;44(4):620-8. PMID:22230369

[86] Modulation of ceramide synthase activity via dimerization. Laviad EL, Kelly S, Merrill AH Jr, Futerman AH. J Biol Chem. 2012 Jun 15;287(25):21025-33. PMID:22539345

[87] Vertebral fractures and role of low bone mineral density in Crohn's disease. Siffledeen JS, Siminoski K, Jen H, Fedorak RN. Clin Gastroenterol Hepatol. 2007 Jun;5(6):721-8. PMID:17482522

[88] Effects of the colour additive caramel colour III on the immune system: a study with human volunteers. Houben GF, Abma PM, van den Berg H, vet al. Food Chem Toxicol. 1992 Sep;30(9):749-57. PMID:1427513

35. Autism

Autism is not a single disease, and it does not have a single cause. Autism is a syndrome in which there are two main findings; a deficit in social behavior and restricted, repetitive behaviors[1]. These changes may reflect injury to or deficits in, specific areas, and cognitive circuits that control these behaviors. Often, especially in mild disease, however, there is little evidence of brain injury or metabolic malfunction. Essential to understanding autism is that the critical point of injury to the CNS is *the point in time* in a child's development when the injury occurs, or development fails to occur.

There are numerous developmental milestones in children's emotional, intellectual and neurological development; these are timed fairly consistently in healthy children. The brain is programmed to learn different tasks at different ages, and perhaps in a particular sequential order. For example, language is best acquired before the age of four. By the age of six, a child should be able to carry on adult-like conversations; learn five to ten words a day; have a vocabulary of 10,000–14,000 words and use appropriate verb tenses, word order, and sentence structure. It is not impossible to become fluent after the age of six, but it is considerably more difficult. Few people become "native speakers" of a language, without an accent, if the language is learned after about the age of 14; it is much less difficult if the language is learned before the age of ten.

These opportune times for learning may not represent the only time to learn an ability, but these windows of opportunity are the easiest times and are periods of time when acquiring the skill is nearly effortless.

While the inclination for social interaction is inherent, it may be discarded if not reinforced. Infants who are later diagnosed with autism have normal eye fixation to their mother's face in the first month of life, however, this gazing at their mother's eyes declines between two and six months of age in the affected children[2]. This has been attributed to a failure in the dopamine reward system; the infant fails to feel pleasure in seeing the mother's eyes; thus, there is a lack of reinforcement for learning interpretation of facial expression and social interaction. Facial orienting, however, is normal in adults with autism[3]. It is not a CNS lesion, nor inability to focus attention, but rather that this part of social interaction was not learned nor reinforced during its native period for learning.

One of the essential windows for learning those skills affected by autism occurs around 10 to 12 months of age; this is the time most children begin to recognize and interpret the emotional content of facial expression and language; they learn to recognize other people's emotions through tone of voice and expression. This helps them to recognize their own emotional states. These abilities are typically limited in autistic individuals.

Other social developments that manifest during this age period include:

- Self-recognition as apart from their mother
- Demonstration of affection, humor, guilt and playfulness
- Seeking to engage in interaction with adults

The social deficits which typify autism, involve several behaviors that normally develop during the ages of 10 – 12 months. This suggests that the pathological process has been initiated by this age or begins soon enough afterward to prevent the consolidation of these skills.

Clearly, some patients with autistic behaviors have CNS dysfunction, caused by injury or metabolic disorders, but for most, there are no apparent CNS lesions. Transient neurologic conditions, which prevent learning and maturation at critical stages of development, may later resolve, leaving developmental deficits. Milestone can be missed, as a result of infection or other disease, which later resolve. Inflammatory conditions that last an extended period may affect multiple milestones. Can remediation be done at a later date when the impairment has healed? Certainly the answer is yes, but the individual may never become a "native speaker." They are unlikely to ever attain the fluency for these skills comparable to someone that attained them at the time the brain was primed to learn them as native skills.

Thus, even a temporary impediment to learning, if it occurs between two and fourteen months of age, may impair these aspects of social behavior development. A temporary disease state, during this period, may cause mild Asperger syndrome but longer lasting impairment of development would be expected to provoke a more pervasive deficit with broader and more severe sequelae.

Thus, different pathologies may result in similar appearing developmental disorders if children are exposed at similar developmental stages. Likewise, a specific pathologic condition may provoke different developmental disorders depending on the age at which a child is exposed. In some developmental disorders, the pathologic condition causing the disorder may have resolved even before the diagnosis is made, leaving little evidence for understanding the disease or how to prevent it.

Regressive Autism

Regressive autism describes autistic children that have lost social and motor skills they had previously acquired. Children may become quiet, and stop trying to talk; they may find it more difficult to walk, and become less social. Some children appeared to have had normal development before the onset of regression. Occasionally the onset of regression may be well defined, and the parents of the affected children often attribute the onset to an infectious disease, treatment with antibiotics, to vaccination or another event.

> In 1998, the journal Lancet published a study of 12 children that suggested a link between the MMR vaccine and autism. The lead author, Wakefield, was later found guilty of fraud. He had fudged the data. He was being paid by lawyers who were suing vaccine makers, and he was applying for a patent on a new vaccine.
>
> Since that time, there have been over 20 high-quality studies involving over half a million children to assess whether there is an association between the MMR vaccine and autism. No association has been found[4].
>
> This red herring has diverted enormous research efforts into a black hole. This research and funding could have been used for proactive research for prevention and treatment of autism. The unbridled greed of a few individuals has harmed vast numbers; children, at risk of disease because of avoided vaccines; vaccine makers who have left the vaccine market; making existing and new vaccines less available, raising health care costs, and by misdirecting scarce resources for preventing or curing autism. Further, this lie continues to harm public health as many parents have an unbalanced sense of risk from vaccines and mistrust scientists.

Causation

Only about 10 percent of cases of autism are explained by single gene defects; however, familial occurrence is very common. The probability of a boy being diagnosed with autism is one in four if his older sibling has autism; while the risk is about one in 12 for girls with an affected older sibling[5]. This suggests genetic susceptibility, where risks factors and exposures which would not provoke any harm in most individuals can trigger autism in those susceptible families.

A frequently observed biochemical marker found in autism is a low fecal chymotrypsin level[6]. About seventy percent of children with autism have been found to have this marker. A low chymotrypsin level is indicative of low pancreatic enzyme release into the duodenum.

Another finding in autism is an elevated level of certain inflammatory cytokines[7], with IL-17 being the most elevated, at over two times the levels found among controls[8]. The high IL-17 levels suggest T_H17 mediated inflammation in the intestine. In a separate study (which did not test for IL-17), IL-1β, IL-6, IL-8 and IL12p40 subunit were elevated in patients with regressive autism[7]. In a mouse model, immune response to food antigens (cow's milk protein) shortly after weaning induced autistic-like behavioral changes; reduced social behavior and repetitive behaviors. These behaviors were accompanied by reduced dopaminergic activity in the prefrontal cortex and the paraventricular nucleus of the hypothalamus[9].

Family members of autism patients have been found to have increased incidence of elevated intestinal paracellular permeability compared to a normal population[10]. High permeability increases the risk of immune reactions to dietary proteins and absorption of bacterial toxins. Disaccharidase deficiency is also prevalent in autism[11].

A subset of children with autism has been shown to have elevated antibodies to mitochondrial DNA. The source of the mitochondria has been suggested to be from activated neutrophils or mast cells in the gut[12]. Mast cell activation is common in children with autism[13]. Neurotensin (NT), which increases the paracellular permeability of the intestinal mucosal, can trigger the release of mitochondrial DNA from mast cells. Elevated levels of NT have been found in both the brain and in the intestines of children with autism[14]. These findings suggest that enteroimmune inflammation underlies the pathogenesis for most patients with autistic disorders.

Kynurenine

Pancreatic enzymes have direct antibacterial effects which help keep a low bacterial count in the upper intestine. Additionally, pancreatic and brush border enzymes prevent small intestinal bacterial overgrowth (SIBO) and small and large bowel dysbiosis by aiding in digestion of nutrients so that they are effectively absorbed. Unabsorbed nutrients support the growth of pathogenic bacteria and biofilm formation, and thus the production bacterial lipopolysaccharides (LPS)[15] and other toxins and virulence factors produced by biofilms. LPS and TNF-α (with IL-1 or IL-6) from biofilm induces inflammatory shifts in the tryptophan metabolic pathway via IDO towards production of kynurenic acid and metabolites including 3-HK and quinolinic acid, an agonist for NMDA receptors and, a neuroexcitotoxin. This also shifts tryptophan away from the generation of serotonin that is calming; and melatonin, an antioxidant that protects the brain. The kynurenine pathway is implicated in the causation of schizophrenia[16], Alzheimer's disease[17], seizures and other neurodegenerative diseases. (See Chapters 31 and 32).

Mast Cell Activation

Deficient pancreatic enzyme activity of proteases allows for increased passage of proteins and peptides into the small intestine where they can act as antigens. If these antigens gain access to the immune cells in the intestinal lamina propria, they can cause immune reactions and mast cell activation. Autism patients and their families have been found to have increased intestinal paracellular permeability (IPP) which increases the risk both for immune reactions to foods and for mast cell activation. Mast cell activation may contribute to GI and blood-brain barrier hyperpermeability and increase the risk of inflammation in the brain. Children with autism are many times more likely to have mastocytosis than are other children[18].

Neurotensin is released by N cells in the jejunum and ileum by the presence of fat in the chyme; NT increases the release of bile acids from the gallbladder. Elevated NT, seen in autism, may be a feedback reaction to insufficient lipase activity. NT also increases intestinal paracellular permeability. If pancreatic lipase is deficient, bile micelles pass into the cecum and colon where they are fermented into secondary bile acids. These secondary bile acids may damage the intestinal mucosa and increase risk of immune reactions to foods. A lipase deficit also increases the loss of fat-soluble vitamins: A, D, E, and K, and other nutrients.

Histamine release from mast cells may affect learning. At high levels, histamine, through its effects on the H_3 receptor, increases aversion memory, anxiety and impulsivity but decreases learning, judgment, and memory acquisition[19]. Cytokines and other inflammatory mediators from mast cells may also impact the memory and learning.

Colonic Dysbiosis

Deficient pancreatic enzyme activity prevents protein degradation, as well as impairing lipid and carbohydrate absorption. Unabsorbed nutrients are passed into the colon where they are fermented by bacteria. Fermentation of protein and other non-absorbed nutrients change the colonic environment favoring an altered array of microbiota in the cecum and colon, and biofilm formation.

Infants with SIBO are more susceptible to intestinal paracellular hyperpermeability, blood stream infections and have elevated inflammatory cytokine levels[20]. SIBO and colonic biofilms supported by malabsorption would be expected to support the production of toxins including LPS, and virulence factors by pathogenic bacteria.

A study of children with autism found nine species of *Clostridia* as components of the colonic microbiota, which were not found in control subjects[21]. Other studies have confirmed an increased abundance of certain *Clostridia* in children with autism[22,23]. Treatment with oral vancomycin, an antibiotic that *Clostridia* are susceptible to, may lead to temporary improvement in some cases of regressive autism. Many *Clostridia* species produce toxins, including neurotoxins. A *Clostridium* produced compound, HPHPA, has been found to be elevated in urine samples of children with autism. A schizophrenic patient with an extremely high HPHPA level responded to vancomycin treatment with resolution of the acute psychotic episode[24]. However, *Clostridia* are a spore-forming bacterium, and these spores are resistance to antibiotics. Thus, these bacteria recover and cause a relapse soon after antibiotic treatment[25].

The pathogenic bacteria *Clostridia perfringens*, for example, lacks enzymes for the formation of most amino acids and thus relies on the environment or host cells for nutrients it requires for reproduction and toxin production[26]. Normally a mucus layer in the large intestine prevents bacteria from directly contacting the colonocytes. Injury or compounds which disrupt the mucous layer can allow direct contact with the cells and can allow production of toxins by *Clostridia*[27]. Protein malabsorption resulting in colonic protein fermentation supports the growth of *Clostridia* and the formation of their toxins[28]. Fermentation of most amino acids causes the production of ammonia that damages the mucous layer in the colon.

Desulfovibrio is another genus of toxin-producing bacteria that have been found to be more common in autism[29]. Both *Clostridia* and *Desulfovibrio* are spore-forming and thus resistant to elimination by antibiotics. Antibiotic treatment of children, for infections such as for earaches, easily disrupts the commensal microbiota balance of the gut. Use of antibiotics favors the survival and growth of spore-forming bacteria whose spores survive the treatment. This may explain the onset of regressive autism following antibiotic treatment that has been observed by some parents.

Ammonia

Unlike carbohydrates and fats, the body does not store amino acids, but rather continually builds and breaks proteins down. Excess dietary protein or that broken down into amino acids during stress, starvation, injury or infection is metabolized into ammonia (NH3). Deficient pancreatic enzyme activity of proteases increases the passage of proteins and peptides into the colon where they are fermented by bacteria and also form NH3 that get absorbed into the blood stream. NH3 is then converted in the urea cycle to urea that is disposed of in the urine. If the body cannot rid itself of NH3 because of a metabolic defect, levels rise, and it is highly toxic to the CNS. Some excess NH3 can be converted into glutamine and then into orotic acid. Serum glutamine levels may rise in advance to NH3 levels, and urinary orotic acid levels also rise. Infants with hyperammonemia often require immediate hemodialysis to avoid or minimize irreversible CNS damage.

Hepatic Encephalopathy

The liver is the only site of the complete urea cycle. In chronic alcoholism, liver damage which impairs its ability to convert NH3 created by fermentation of protein in the colon into nontoxic urea, which can be metabolized into other metabolites or be eliminated in the urine. The onset of hepatic encephalopathy (HE) is usually precipitated by factors that increase NH3 levels, such as constipation, high protein intake, or a GI bleed. Ammonia crosses the blood-brain barrier where it causes swelling of the astrocytes, the support cells for neurons. HE causes intellectual dysfunction with deficits in attention, impaired speech, delirium, spatial and temporal disorientation, impaired memory and other deficits. There are sleep disturbances, alterations in muscle tone and asterixis (flapping). It is hypothesized that changes in the glutamate–NO–cGMP pathway resulting from exposure of the brain to ammonia may lead to the observed impairment of learning and impaired intellectual function observed in HE[30].

Although most amino acids from dietary protein form ammonia when fermented, histidine forms bioamines and tryptophan forms indolamines. Bioamines and indolamines produced in the colon may affect the brain. Bioamines are discussed in Chapter 13. Indolamines produced by bacterial fermentation of the amino acid tryptophan in the colon may have CNS effects. Indolamines include serotonin and melatonin, but also include LSD and other hallucinogens.

Ammonia is quite toxic to the CNS, affecting energy metabolism, NO synthesis, axonal and dendritic growth, and other aspects of CNS function. The brain does not metabolize ammonia to urea as does the liver. Instead, in astrocytes glutamine synthetase converts ammonia and glutamate into glutamine. Glutamine is then utilized along with lactate as the principal fuel for the neuron using the lactate-alanine shuttle[31]. Ammonia's toxic effects on the brain act through several mechanisms[32]:

1. Ammonia induces the formation of quinolinic acid (see kynurenine above and in Chapter 31).
2. Ammonia induces both neuronal nitric oxide synthase (nNOS) in neurons and inducible NOS (iNOS) in astrocytes, increasing NO production. NO creates oxidative stress and free radical generation in the neurons that can provoke cell dysfunction and death.
3. Excess NO in astrocytes, also blocks glutamine synthase, the enzyme that converts ammonia and glutamate to glutamine, thus blocking detoxification of ammonia. Glutamine normally diffuses from astrocytes to neurons for use in the lactate-alanine shuttle, thus by impairing this process; ammonia also starves the neuron of a fuel source.
4. Ammonia impairs the glutamate transporter on astrocytes allowing increased glutamatergic activity. Excess glutamate can cause hyperexcitability and act as an excitotoxin.
5. Ammonia is toxic to the mitochondria in the neurons and astrocytes, creating energy deficits that can lead to cell death.
6. Ammonia has toxic effects on glial cells, impairing axonal growth.
7. Ammonia impairs transport of aromatic amino acids across the blood-brain barrier, leading to increased production of the neurotransmitters, octopamine and phenylethylamine, which function as "false neurotransmitters"[33] by displacing the classic monoamines neurotransmitters from their storage pools.
8. Hyperammonemia down-regulates claudin-12, suggesting that ammonia toxicity can affect tight junction integrity and increases the permeability of the blood-brain barrier[34].
9. Extracellular accumulation of cyclic GMP (cGMP) arising from stimulation of nitric oxide (NO) synthesis leads to impaired learning and memory[35].

Infants and small children are more easily susceptible to ammonia toxicity as the immature liver has limited ability to metabolize it into urea. Furthermore, the developing brain is more susceptible to toxicity from ammonia than is an adult's brain. The effects of exposure depend on the magnitude, duration and timing of the ammonia exposure. In newborns, hyperammonemia can cause cortical atrophy, enlargements of the ventricles, and demyelination. Ammonia toxicity can cause cognitive impairment, seizures, and cerebral palsy if exposure occurs during the neonatal period[36]. In a study of 100 children with autism, ammonia levels were found to be elevated along with alanine levels while pyruvate and carnitine levels were found to be low[37].

Inflammation

One of the biomarkers found to be elevated in regressive autism was the IL-12 subunit p40[7]. IL-12p40 is elevated Experimental Autoimmune Neuritis (EAN), an animal model for Guillain-Barré syndrome of humans, and the p40 segment is also elevated and provokes demyelination and glial cell activation in Experimental Allergic Encephalomyelitis (EAE), an animal model for multiple sclerosis. IL-12 appears to be required for fighting intracellular pathogens, such as salmonella. Antigen presenting cells produce the p40 subunit of IL-12. It is also produced by macrophages and dendritic cells, which produce IL-23 to stimulate T_H17 cell induction.

The p40 subunit of IL-12 and IL-23 causes activation of microglia cells in the brain. This activation may be pivotal in the pathophysiological processes leading to several neurodegenerative diseases. The p40 subunit from peripheral inflammation may cause over-activation of microglia in autism. Intestinal immune reactions to foods or infectious agents may stimulate the production of IL-12 or IL-23 and the p40 subunit.

IL-17 is also elevated in autism, that suggesting elevated intestinal immune activity. IL-17 induces the production of many inflammatory cytokines by T_H17 cells, including IL-1β, IL-6, TNF-α; chemokines including IL-8; and eicosanoids (prostaglandins) which can induce inflammatory reactions and stimulate further immune and inflammatory signaling through induction of the sphingosine-1-phospahate, kynurenine, and other pathways.

Opiate Hypothesis

There are several food proteins that include peptide sequences that have opiate-like activity; these include casomorphin from cow's milk and gliadorphin in wheat[38], as well as ones in spinach and blood sausage. Cow milk proteins are those most common in an infant's diet. If there is incomplete digestion of these peptides, they can act as opiates, and activate TLR2 and TLR4, and promote immune activation in the CNS (Chapter 30). These peptides may impair neurological development in infants[39].

Enteric Management for Autism

There are successful treatments for autism, including physical and occupational therapy, which can provide great benefit to affected children. This section is focused solely on prevention of the underlying causes of intestinal disease, which is present in a majority of patients with autism. Testing for biomarkers of intestinal dysfunction is recommended, as treatment is unlikely to be productive if underlying pathology outlined in the chapter is not present.

Even if causal conditions no longer exist or if the dysfunction was secondary to traumatic or other brain injury, supplements recommended for TBI in Chapter 30 may still be of benefit to the individual.

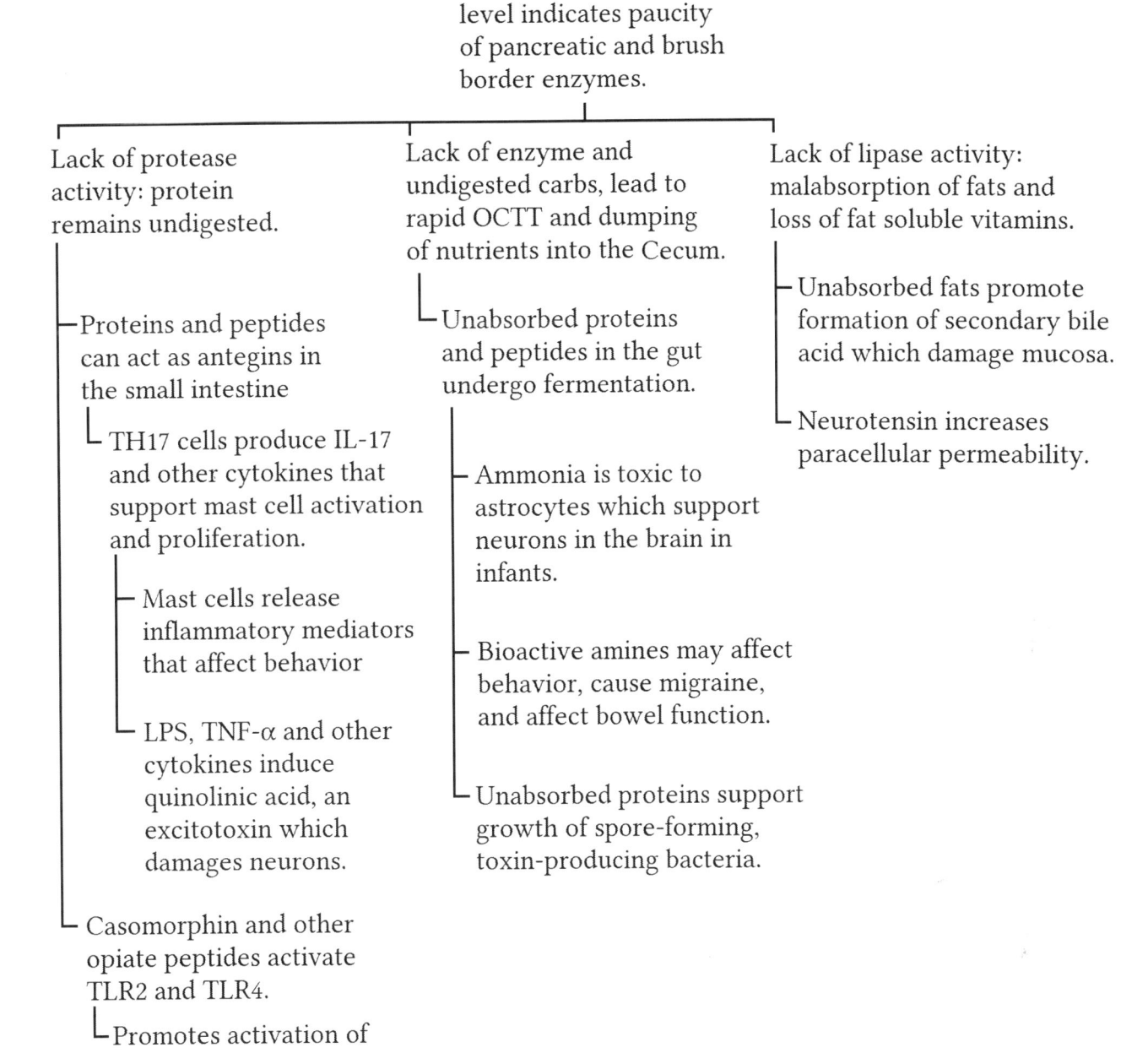

```
                    Low fecal chymotrypsin
                    level indicates paucity
                    of pancreatic and brush
                    border enzymes.
    ┌───────────────────────┼───────────────────────┐
Lack of protease        Lack of enzyme and      Lack of lipase activity:
activity: protein       undigested carbs, lead to malabsorption of fats and
remains undigested.     rapid OCTT and dumping   loss of fat soluble vitamins.
                        of nutrients into the Cecum.
                                                  ├─ Unabsorbed fats promote
 ├─ Proteins and peptides  └─ Unabsorbed proteins    formation of secondary bile
 │  can act as antegins in    and peptides in the gut acid which damage mucosa.
 │  the small intestine       undergo fermentation.
 │  └ TH17 cells produce IL-17                    └─ Neurotensin increases
 │    and other cytokines that                       paracellular permeability.
 │    support mast cell activation
 │    and proliferation.    ├─ Ammonia is toxic to
 │      ├─ Mast cells release  astrocytes which support
 │      │  inflammatory mediators neurons in the brain in
 │      │  that affect behavior   infants.
 │      │
 │      └ LPS, TNF-α and other ├─ Bioactive amines may affect
 │        cytokines induce       behavior, cause migraine,
 │        quinolinic acid, an    and affect bowel function.
 │        excitotoxin which
 │        damages neurons.     └ Unabsorbed proteins support
 │                                growth of spore-forming,
 └─ Casomorphin and other         toxin-producing bacteria.
    opiate peptides activate
    TLR2 and TLR4.
    └ Promotes activation of
      inflammatory neuroglia.
```

Figure 35-1: Diagram illustrating possible contributing causality in autism from intestinal malabsorption.

Testing for Enteroimmune Causation in Autism:

Stool Enzymes: Fecal elastase-1 (FE1) is well accepted as a test for pancreatic enzyme insufficiency; it is highly specific, and reproducible due to its stability in the stool; it can be stored at room temperature for days without degrading, making storage during transport easy. Fecal Chymotrypsin (FC) degrades at room temperature, and thus, false positive tests can occur if the stool is not collected and transported correctly. FC has been best documented as an indicator of digestive dysfunction among autistic children, and perhaps is a more sensitive test for postcibal asynchrony. Both tests should be done if possible, as low FC may be an indicator of more than just pancreatic exocrine insufficiency.

Other Tests: The same markers used in IBD and IBS that show activation of immune cells in the intestine may be helpful in directing treatment for autism. Fecal ECP, for example, may be elevated if there is a proliferation of gram positive bacteria such as *Clostridia*. Cultures may be done. Fecal fat may reveal steatorrhea. See the list in Appendix C. IL-17, IL-23 and markers for mast cell elevation may be elevated (Chapter 12). Citrulline levels may be abnormal. Blood collection in autistic children can be traumatic for the child, and should be done as infrequently as possible; favoring the use of stool studies. Ammonia can be measured in the breath. The carbon-13 breath test with mixed-chain-triglycerides (MCT) might be an ideal test for this population, but this has not been clinically evaluated.

Enteroimmune Management in Autism

Prevent Dysbiosis and *Clostridia* Growth: Dietary intervention to prevent malabsorption that leads to *Clostridia* growth in the colon should be implemented.

Fructose and lactose intake may need to be curtailed, especially in children with signs of malabsorption (i.e.; excessive foul-smelling flatulence), as these and other poorly absorbed sugars induce rapid oral cecal transit time, and delivery of unabsorbed nutrients to the cecum and colon; thus promoting dysbiosis. (Chapters 5 and 24) Prebiotics, such as fructose oligosaccharides, which prevent biofilm formation, should be included in the diet (Chapter 5). Prebiotics are fermented in the proximal large intestine; while protein is mainly fermented in the distal colon. Prebiotics alter the milieu of the colon, in part by decreasing ammonia production, and in doing so, create an environment less favorable for toxic biofilm formation. Lactulose acts as a prebiotic, supporting bacteria in the left colon that consume amino acids, and thereby, prevent the proliferation of *Clostridia* in the distal colon. Prevention of biofilms that produce toxins and virulence factors is discussed in Chapters 23.

Pancreatic Enzymes: Low levels of chymotrypsin or elastase-1 in the stool suggest poor digestion of protein that which can support overgrowth of *Clostridia*. If fecal pancreatic enzyme levels are low, the child should be treated with pancreatic enzymes until a cause for the low enzyme level can be identified and reversed. Pancreatic enzymes can also be helpful in the treatment and prevention of hepatic encephalopathy and other diseases where protein malabsorption induces toxin-producing biofilms in the colon. Dosing is given in Chapter 8.

Potatoes contain trypsin and chymotrypsin inhibitors and thus impede protein digestion. This inhibitor is only fractionally denatured by normal cooking methods for potatoes[40]. Potatoes should be avoided as food for children under the age of two. (See the section on potatoes in Chapter 33) Soy and other beans also contain trypsin inhibitors; however, about 90% of these proteins are irreversibly deactivated by boiling for 20 minutes[41]. Table 23-3 in Chapter 23 lists some foods that have trypsin/chymotrypsin inhibiting activity. As some of these are typically consumed raw, they can be especially problematic.

> The most resistant soy trypsin inhibitors are a class of smaller proteins that also inhibit chymotrypsin, referred to as Bowman-Birk Inhibitors (BBI). BBI are not easily fermented in the colon and do not cause alterations in the microbiota or increase the growth of *Clostridia*[42]. BBI from legumes have anticarcinogenic properties and have anti-inflammatory actions, delaying the migration of T_H17 cells from the intestine to the CNS[43]. A diet including BBI was found to delay the onset of experimental autoimmune encephalitis, an animal model of multiple sclerosis[44].

Colonic bacteria can be treated with antibiotics, such as vancomycin, as a temporary measure, or as a therapeutic trial. Long-term success will require changing the milieu of the colon and elimination of undigested protein. This requires normalization of protease enzyme activity by supplementation, or by reversing the cause of the deficiency. Pancreatic enzyme therapy for children with autism who have low fecal chymotrypsin levels is being tested in a stage-three clinical trial at the time of this writing in 2015[45]. Prebiotics help support the growth of commensal bacteria that inhibit the proliferation of Clostridia.

Treatment of dysbiosis and LPS production are also discussed in Chapters 4 and 23 and 33.

2: SIBO: SIBO is usually the result of impaired or disorganized enteric motility. SIBO may be aggravated by irregular meal and sleep times. This is especially true in children, as they are not in control of when meals are given. Sufficient, real food should be provided at meal and snack times to provide sustenance to the child through to their next meal. Sweets, which temporarily alleviate hunger, should be avoided as they may disrupt the migrating motor complex. Treatment of SIBO and infantile colic are discussed in Chapter 24.

3: Intestinal Hyperpermeability: Hyperpermeability of the intestine (leaky gut) is common in autism. Preventive treatment for this is covered in Chapter 25.

4: Ammonia: (This section applies to subclinical NH3 excess, not severe toxicity.) Ammonia creates oxidative stress and mitochondrial damage. Avoiding ammonia toxicity includes similar strategies to those for avoiding clostridial overgrowth, as outlined above; they include avoidance of protein malabsorption and the inclusion of prebiotics in the diet.

A. Maintain a healthy enteric biome: Antibiotic use should be avoided unless their use is clearly indicated. Probiotics have been shown to decrease hepatic encephalopathy[46]. Probiotics are more effective when used along with prebiotics to supporting a diverse colonic biome.

B. Avoid Constipation: As noted above, in adults, hepatic encephalopathy may be triggered by constipation. Constipation is common in children with autism. Lactulose not only treats constipation, but is a prebiotic that prevents ammonia production. Fructose oligosaccharides should be included in the diet. Mother's milk contains galactose oligosaccharides that have this effect (Chapter 5).

Inadequate dietary magnesium (Mg) may be the most significant common causes of functional constipation in preschool age children, followed by under-consumption fruit and vegetable fiber[47]. In a study of young women with low fiber intake, low water, and low Mg intake were the associated with constipation[48]. Foods high in Mg include vegetables, fruits, nuts, and legumes, including soy and soy products and whole grains, thus supplying both Mg and fiber. Additionally, magnesium is a cofactor for glutamate-ammonia ligase, which converts ammonia and the potentially excitotoxic neurotransmitter glutamate into glutamine (Table 28-4).

GI bleeds can also trigger hepatic encephalopathy. Stool testing for occult blood is appropriate in children with gastrointestinal disorders including autism.

C. Creatinine, acetyl-L-carnitine, taurine, l-citrulline: Creatine[32], acetyl-L-carnitine[32,49], and taurine[50,51] have all been proposed to help prevent ammonia caused damage to astrocytes and neurons. Creatine and acetyl-L-carnitine likely act as alternative energy sources for mitochondria during ammonia toxicity. Taurine may prevent activation of excitatory NDMA receptors and prevent the generation of free radicals by ammonia[52].

Of these three, only acetyl-L-carnitine has undergone sufficient clinical trials to make a recommendation for its use for treatment of ammonia toxicity. Acetyl-L-carnitine improves functioning in patients with both mild[53] and severe[54] hepatic encephalopathy. These trials showed improvements in cognitive deficits, a general improvement in the quality of life, and a reduction of anxiety and depression in these patients.

Both creatine and taurine have been shown, in laboratory conditions, to improve function in neuronal tissue exposed to ammonia[55,56]. Creatine has been demonstrated to protect developing brain cells from some toxic effects of ammonia, including preventing axonal growth impairment[57]. Supplements of creatine and taurine may be appropriate if their levels are demonstrated to below that expected.

Taurine and hypotaurine can act as endogenous neurotransmitters. Taurine and hypotaurine are made in the body from L-cystine. Their production may be impaired if cofactors for their formation are in short supply. The cofactors include iron, NAD (niacin), and pyridoxal-5-phosphate (Vitamin B_6).

A rare genetic disorder, AGAT deficiency, causes creatine deficiency that causes mental retardation, language disorders, autistic-like behaviors and movement disorders[58]. Creatine is contained in muscle, so eating meat can supply it, or creatine supplements can be used. Creatine is not an essential nutrient, however as it is formed in the body in the following enzymatic steps:

Table 35-1: Creatine Formation

Enzyme	Substrates	Products
L-Arginine: glycine amidinotransferase (AGAT)	L-arginine + glycine	L-ornithine + guanidinoacetate
Guanidinoacetate N-methyltransferase (GMAT)	S-adenosyl-L-methionine + guanidinoacetate	S-adenosyl-L-homocysteine + creatine

Supplementation of arginine and SAMe may facilitate creatine formation. SAMe has potential toxicity, so supplementing cofactors for SAMe recycling is recommended. These cofactors include folate, vitamin B_{12}, pyridoxine, and betaine. L-Legumes (beans) in the diet supply canavanine, or l-citrulline may be used in the place of arginine. In genetic condition affecting the urea cycle, OTC deficiency causes NH3 accumulation, causing CNS damage. Here too arginine and l-citrulline are helpful.

5. Kynurenine/S1P: The most important cofactor in the kynurenine pathway is pyridoxal-5-phosphate. Vitamin B_6 (PLP) is also the nutritional supplement that parents of children with autism most commonly report provides benefit. Adequate PLP should be assured. Pyridoxine HCl at 3 mg a day is sufficient for most adults to ensure adequate PLP levels.

LPS and other inflammatory mediators can increase the production of kynurenine metabolites. Thus, bacterial overgrowth should be prevented. LPS acts by through its action on TLR4 receptors, which stimulate the production of iNOS, COX2, and production of TNF-α and other inflammatory cytokines. Factors that act through TLR2 may also be causal in autism. Mitigation of the effects of LPS on TLR4 receptors is discussed in Chapter 31. TLR2 and factors which affect it are discussed in Chapters 30 and 42. Prevention of toxic kynurenine products is also further discussed in Chapter 30

Mitigation of the proinflammatory cytokine TNF-α, another factor in the pathogenesis of autism, is discussed at the end of Chapter 34 in the section on S1P mitigation. Many of the compounds that mediate toxic kynurenine metabolism also affect mediate S1P formation; these metabolites participate in neuroinflammation and sustaining inflammatory cells in the intestine.

6. Mast Cell Activation and Inflammation: Children with autism have been found to have an increased prevalence of mast cell activation[59]. Children diagnosed with autism should be screened for mast cell activation disorders, at least looking for skin lesions. Treatment of Mast cell activation is detailed in Chapter 12.

7. Inflammation: When inflammation is mediated by T_H17 lymphocytes, as it is in autism, it should be assumed that the intestine is the source of the inflammatory process. T_H17 mediated diseases should include avoidance of foods that the patient reacts to. Patients should be tested for and treated for antergies, by avoidance and supplements which help with normalizing the intestine milieu (Chapter 19). If food allergies are suspected, they should also be tested for, and reacting foods removed from the diet.

Antioxidants may help prevent neurotoxicity induced by ammonia and other sources of oxidative stress. Neuroprotectin D1 is an eicosanoid formed from the n-3 fatty acid, docosahexaenoic acid (DHA). Neuroprotectin D1 is anti-apoptotic, anti-inflammatory and neuroprotective[60] for nerve cells under oxidative stress[61]. Neuroprotectin D1 may also protect the brain against excitotoxins[62]. DHA supplementation is discussed in Chapter 9. Neuroprotectin D1 and melatonin are discussed in Chapter 21.

Nutritional deficiencies caused by malabsorption should be treated. Lipid soluble vitamin levels may be assessed and supplemented. Folate, PLP and vitamins B_{12}, D_3 and K_2 levels may be low in malabsorption syndromes. Magnesium and zinc levels are also compromised by malabsorption.

8. Melatonin and N-Acetyl Cysteine: Melatonin may also be used as an antioxidant that protects both the brain and the GI tract. Melatonin has been found to be helpful, in several clinical trials, for sleep problems in autism. The doses used in most trials were similar to those used in adults. Even small, physiologic doses of melatonin (0.1 to 0.3 mg) are helpful for sleep problems in children, and often most effective when given 30 minutes before bedtime[63], although sublingual melatonin which is rapidly absorbed through the buccal mucosa can be given at bedtime.

N-Acetyl Cysteine supplies cysteine for the formation of glutathione, the major CNS antioxidant.

Pediatric Dosing of Supplements:

Demand for nutrients is determined by metabolic activity, which is not linearly associated with body weight. For most nutrients and supplements, body surface area will give an estimate of nutritional needs. Additionally, children may have a higher nutrient demand to support growth. Direct conversion of supplement dose by the kilogram from adult to a child would generally underestimate the nutrient requirement.

Suggested adult doses in this text generally assume a 60 kg male, with a body surface area (BSA) of 1.6 square meters.

A simple calculation for BSA[64] in square meters equals

$$BSA\ (m^2) = \sqrt{([Height\ in\ cm \times Weight\ in\ kg]/\ 3600)}$$

---

8. Scheduling: Maintaining regular sleep times, dim lights in the evening and dark at night help to maintain the circadian cycle and natural production of melatonin. The GI system also has a circadian cycle and melatonin production. Regular meal times and avoidance of late meals before bedtime help to maintain and restore gastrointestinal motility. (See Chapter 24 on SIBO). The circadian genes play a role in the regulation of intestinal permeability[65], and thus maintenance of a regular circadian sleep, meal, and gastrointestinal cycle help maintain the intestinal membrane. Melatonin may help with this. Inadequate sleep increases IL-6 level, which increases glial activation, and inflammatory activity.

9. Recovery: The brain has two main periods of growth; early childhood and early adolescence. Early adolescence is a critical window of opportunity for recovery and growth of the brain. The best time, however, to initiate recovery is today, as today is the only day in which progress can be made. Removing the underlying causation of autism may provide an opportunity for recovery. Chapter 30 on mood disorders discusses neurotrophic growth factors and how to enhance their production. These steps may also be applied to recovery of other autism and other neurologic conditions.

Life Hack: Learning new skills can be difficult and frustrating. However, it may take much less time and effort to achieve basic fluency to develop useful skill levels than one might expect.

Basic fluency is a level of skill at which an individual has the ability to use the skills to accomplish purposeful tasks, to self-monitor, to continue to develop the skill through applied use, and to derive positive internal feedback from use. This applies to a wide range of skills, including foreign language, music, or juggling.

Basic fluency for most skills takes a total of about 20 hours (1200 minutes) of well focused, appropriate, intentional progressive practice. The skill to be learned should be broken down into small achievable components to be learned and practiced. Understanding that it often only takes 20 hours to get past the frustrating part, may help the learner stay on course.

---

[1] The Autism Diagnostic Observation Schedule: revised algorithms for improved diagnostic validity. Gotham K, Risi S, Pickles A, Lord C. J Autism Dev Disord. 2007 Apr;37(4):613-27. PMID:17180459

[2] Attention to eyes is present but in decline in 2-6-month-old infants later diagnosed with autism. Jones W, Klin A. Nature. 2013 Dec 19;504(7480):427-31. PMID:24196715

[3] Robust orienting to protofacial stimuli in autism. Shah P, Gaule A, Bird G, Cook R. Curr Biol. 2013 Dec 16;23(24):R1087-8. PMID:24355781

[4] The autism-vaccine story: fiction and deception? Allan GM, Ivers N. Can Fam Physician. 2010 Oct;56(10):1013. PMID:20944043

[5] Recurrence Risk for Autism Spectrum Disorders: A Baby Siblings Research Consortium Study. Ozonoff S, Young GS, Carter A, et al. Pediatrics. 2011 Aug 15. PMID:21844053

[6] Method for confirming a diagnosis of autism. Joan Fallon. US Patent Application 20090197289. 08/06/2009

[7] Elevated plasma cytokines in autism spectrum disorders provide evidence of immune dysfunction and are associated with impaired behavioral outcome. Ashwood P, Krakowiak P, Hertz-Picciotto I, et al. Brain Behav Immun. 2011 Jan;25(1):40-5. PMID:20705131

[8] Plasma cytokine profiles in subjects with high-functioning autism spectrum disorders. Suzuki K, Matsuzaki H, Iwata K, et al. PLoS One. 2011;6(5):e20470. PMID:21647375

[9] Autistic-like behavioural and neurochemical changes in a mouse model of food allergy. de Theije CG, Wu J, Koelink PJ, et al. Behav Brain Res. 2014 Mar 15;261:265-74. PMID: 24333575

[10] Alterations of the intestinal barrier in patients with autism spectrum disorders and in their first-degree relatives. de Magistris L, Familiari V, Pascotto A, et al. J Pediatr Gastroenterol Nutr. 2010 Oct;51(4):418-24. PMID:20683204

[11] Intestinal disaccharidase activity in patients with autism: effect of age, gender, and intestinal inflammation. Kushak RI, Lauwers GY, Winter HS, Buie TM. Autism. 2011 May;15(3):285-94. PMID:21415091

[12] Mitochondrial DNA and anti-mitochondrial antibodies in serum of autistic children. Zhang B, Angelidou A, Alysandratos KD, et al. J Neuroinflammation. 2010 Nov 17;7:80. PMID:21083929

[13] Autism spectrum disorders and mastocytosis. Theoharides TC. Int J Immunopathol Pharmacol. 2009 Oct-Dec;22(4):859-65. PMID:20074449

[14] Neurotensin is increased in serum of young children with autistic disorder. Angelidou A, Francis K, Vasiadi M, et al. J Neuroinflammation. 2010 Aug 23;7:48. PMID:20731814

[15] Small intestinal bacterial overgrowth in nonalcoholic steatohepatitis: association with toll-like receptor 4 expression and plasma levels of interleukin 8. Shanab AA, Scully P, Crosbie O, et al. Dig Dis Sci. 2011 May;56(5):1524-34. PMID:21046243

[16] Downregulated kynurenine 3-monooxygenase gene expression and enzyme activity in schizophrenia and genetic association with schizophrenia endophenotypes. Wonodi I, Stine OC, Sathyasaikumar KV, et al. Arch Gen Psychiatry. 2011 Jul;68(7):665-74. PMID:21727251

[17] Kynurenine and its metabolites in Alzheimer's disease patients. Gulaj E, Pawlak K, Bien B, Pawlak D. Adv Med Sci. 2010 Dec 30;55(2):204-11. PMID:20639188

[18] Autism spectrum disorders and mastocytosis. Theoharides TC. Int J Immunopathol Pharmacol. 2009 Oct-Dec;22(4):859-65. PMID:20074449

[19] Histaminergic mechanisms for modulation of memory systems. Köhler CA, da Silva WC, Benetti F, Bonini JS. Neural Plast. 2011;2011:328602. PMID:21876818

[20] The rate of bloodstream infection is high in infants with short bowel syndrome: relationship with small bowel bacterial overgrowth, enteral feeding, and inflammatory and immune responses. Cole CR, Frem JC, Schmotzer B, et al. J Pediatr. 2010 Jun;156(6):941-7, 947.e1. PMID:20171649

[21] Gastrointestinal microflora studies in late-onset autism. Finegold SM, Molitoris D, Song Y, et al. Clin Infect Dis. 2002 Sep 1;35(Suppl 1):S6-S16. PMID:12173102

[22] Differences between the gut microflora of children with autistic spectrum disorders and that of healthy children. Parracho HM, Bingham MO, Gibson GR, McCartney AL. J Med Microbiol. 2005 Oct;54(Pt 10):987-91. PMID:16157555

[23] Real-time PCR quantitation of clostridia in feces of autistic children. Song Y, Liu C, Finegold SM. Appl Environ Microbiol. 2004 Nov;70(11):6459-65. PMID:15528506

[24] Increased urinary excretion of a 3-(3-hydroxyphenyl)-3-hydroxypropionic acid (HPHPA), an abnormal phenylalanine metabolite of Clostridia spp. in the gastrointestinal tract, in urine samples from patients with autism and schizophrenia. Shaw W. Nutr Neurosci. 2010 Jun;13(3):135-43. PMID:20423563

[25] Therapy and epidemiology of autism--clostridial spores as key elements. Finegold SM. Med Hypotheses. 2008;70(3):508-11. PMID:17904761

[26] Virulence gene regulation by the agr system in Clostridium perfringens. Ohtani K, Yuan Y, Hassan S, Wang R, Wang Y, Shimizu T. J Bacteriol. 2009 Jun;191(12):3919-27. PMID:19363118

[27] Contact with enterocyte-like Caco-2 cells induces rapid upregulation of toxin production by Clostridium perfringens type C isolates. Vidal JE, Ohtani K, Shimizu T, McClane BA. Cell Microbiol. 2009 Sep;11(9):1306-28. PMID:19438515

[28] Effect of diets containing potato protein or soya bean meal on the incidence of spontaneously-occurring subclinical necrotic enteritis and the physiological response in broiler chickens. Fernando PS, Rose SP, Mackenzie AM, Silva SS. Br Poult Sci. 2011 Feb;52(1):106-14. PMID:21337205

[29] Desulfovibrio species are potentially important in regressive autism. Finegold SM. Med Hypotheses. 2011 Aug;77(2):270-4. PMID:21592674

[30] Pharmacological manipulation of cyclic GMP levels in brain restores learning ability in animal models of hepatic encephalopathy: therapeutic implications. Rodrigo R, Monfort P, Cauli O, Erceg S, Felipo V. Neuropsychiatr Dis Treat. 2006 Mar;2(1):53-63. PMID:19412446

[31] Lactate metabolism: a new paradigm for the third millennium. Gladden LB. J Physiol. 2004 Jul 1;558(Pt 1):5-30. PMID:15131240

[32] Hyperammonemia-induced toxicity for the developing central nervous system. Cagnon L, Braissant O. Brain Res Rev. 2007 Nov;56(1):183-97. PMID:17881060

[33] Alterations of Blood Brain Barrier Function in Hyperammonemia: An Overview. Skowrońska M, Albrecht J. Neurotox Res. 2011 Aug 27. PMID:21874372

[34] Hyperammonemia induces transport of taurine and creatine and suppresses claudin-12 gene expression in brain capillary endothelial cells in vitro. Bélanger M, Asashima T, Ohtsuki S, et al. Neurochem Int. 2007 Jan;50(1):95-101. PMID:16956696

[35] Taurine reduces ammonia- and N-methyl-D-aspartate-induced accumulation of cyclic GMP and hydroxyl radicals in microdialysates of the rat striatum. Hilgier W, Anderzhanova E, Oja SS, Saransaari P, Albrecht J. Eur J Pharmacol. 2003 May 2;468(1):21-5. PMID:12729839

[36] Ammonia toxicity to the brain: effects on creatine metabolism and transport and protective roles of creatine. Braissant O. Mol Genet Metab. 2010;100 Suppl 1:S53-8. PMID:20227315

[37] Relative carnitine deficiency in autism. Filipek PA, Juranek J, Nguyen MT, Cummings C, Gargus JJ. J Autism Dev Disord. 2004 Dec;34(6):615-23. PMID:15679182

[38] Opioid receptor ligands derived from food proteins. Teschemacher H. Curr Pharm Des. 2003;9(16):1331-44. PMID:12769741

[39] Beta-casomorphins-7 in infants on different type of feeding and different levels of psychomotor development. Kost NV, Sokolov OY, Kurasova OB, et al. Peptides. 2009 Oct;30(10):1854-60. PMID:19576256

[40] Chymotrypsin inhibitor I from potatoes. Large scale preparation and characterization of its subunit components. Melville JC, Ryan CA. J Biol Chem. 1972 Jun 10;247(11):3445-53. PMID:4624116

[41] Inactivation of soybean trypsin inhibitors with ascorbic acid plus copper. Sessa DJ, Haney JK, Nelsen TC. J of Agric & Food Chem, July 1990, 1469-1474

[42] Anti-carcinogenic soyabean Bowman-Birk inhibitors survive faecal fermentation in their active form and do not affect the microbiota composition in vitro. Marín-Manzano MC, Ruiz R, Jiménez E, Rubio LA, Clemente A. Br J Nutr. 2009 Apr;101(7):967-71. PMID:19353764

[43] Bowman-Birk inhibitor attenuates experimental autoimmune encephalomyelitis by delaying infiltration of inflammatory cells into the CNS. Dai H, Ciric B, Zhang GX, Rostami A. Immunol Res. 2011 Dec;51(2-3):145-52. PMID: 22095543

[44] Bowman-Birk inhibitor suppresses autoimmune inflammation and neuronal loss in a mouse model of multiple sclerosis. Touil T, Ciric B, Ventura E, Shindler KS, Gran B, Rostami A. J Neurol Sci. 2008 Aug 15;271(1-2):191-202. PMID:18544456

[45] A Trial of CM-AT in Children With Autism – Open Label Extension Study. NCT00912691 Curemark. www.clinicaltrials.gov

[46] Probiotics prevent hepatic encephalopathy in patients with cirrhosis: a randomized controlled trial. Lunia MK, Sharma BC, Sharma P, et al. Clin Gastroenterol Hepatol. 2014 Jun;12(6):1003-8.e1. PMID: 24246768

[47] Increased prevalence of constipation in pre-school children is attributable to under-consumption of plant foods: A community-based study. Lee WT, Ip KS, Chan JS, Lui NW, Young BW. J Paediatr Child Health. 2008 Apr;44(4):170-5. PMID:17854410

[48] Association between dietary fiber, water and magnesium intake and functional constipation among young Japanese women. Murakami K, Sasaki S, Okubo H, et al. Eur J Clin Nutr. 2007 May;61(5):616-22. PMID:17151587

[49] Ammonia-mediated LTP inhibition: effects of NMDA receptor antagonists and L-carnitine. Izumi Y, Izumi M, Matsukawa M, Funatsu M, Zorumski CF. Neurobiol Dis. 2005 Nov;20(2):615-24. PMID:15935684

[50] Taurine prevents ammonia-induced accumulation of cyclic GMP in rat striatum by interaction with GABAA and glycine receptors. Hilgier W, Oja SS, Saransaari P, Albrecht J. Brain Res. 2005 May 10;1043(1-2):242-6. PMID:15862540

[51] Taurine rescues hippocampal long-term potentiation from ammonia-induced impairment. Chepkova AN, Sergeeva OA, Haas HL. Neurobiol Dis. 2006 Sep;23(3):512-21. PMID:16766203

[52] Endogenous neuro-protectants in ammonia toxicity in the central nervous system: facts and hypotheses. Albrecht J, Wegrzynowicz M. Metab Brain Dis. 2005 Dec;20(4):253-63. PMID:16382336

[53] Acetyl-L-carnitine reduces depression and improves quality of life in patients with minimal hepatic encephalopathy. Malaguarnera M, Bella R, Vacante M, et al. Scand J Gastroenterol. 2011 Jun;46(6):750-9. PMID:21443422

[54] Acetyl-L-carnitine improves cognitive functions in severe hepatic encephalopathy: a randomized and controlled clinical trial. Malaguarnera M, Vacante M, Motta M, et al. Metab Brain Dis. 2011 Aug 26. PMID:21870121

[55] Ammonia-mediated LTP inhibition: effects of NMDA receptor antagonists and L-carnitine. Izumi Y, Izumi M, Matsukawa M, et al. Neurobiol Dis. 2005 Nov;20(2):615-24. PMID:15935684

[56] Taurine rescues hippocampal long-term potentiation from ammonia-induced impairment. Chepkova AN, Sergeeva OA, Haas HL. Neurobiol Dis. 2006 Sep;23(3):512-21. PMID:16766203

[57] Ammonia toxicity to the brain: effects on creatine metabolism and transport and protective roles of creatine. Braissant O.Mol Genet Metab. 2010;100 Suppl 1:S53-8. PMID:20227315

[58] Guanidinoacetate and creatine plus creatinine assessment in physiologic fluids: an effective diagnostic tool for the biochemical diagnosis of arginine:glycine amidinotransferase and guanidinoacetate methyltransferase deficiencies. Carducci C, Birarelli M, Leuzzi V, Carducci C, Battini R, Cioni G, Antonozzi I. Clin Chem. 2002 Oct;48(10):1772-8. PMID:12324495

[59] Mast cell activation and autism. Theoharides TC, Angelidou A, Alysandratos KD, Zhang B, Asadi S, Francis K, Toniato E, Kalogeromitros D.Biochim Biophys Acta. 2012 Jan;1822(1):34-41. PMID:21193035

[60] Omega-3 fatty acids, pro-inflammatory signaling and neuroprotection. Bazan NG. Curr Opin Clin Nutr Metab Care. 2007 Mar;10(2):136-41. PMID:17285000

[61] Neuroprotectin D1 modulates the induction of pro-inflammatory signaling and promotes retinal pigment epithelial cell survival during oxidative stress. Calandria JM, Bazan NG. Adv Exp Med Biol. 2010;664:663-70. PMID:2023807

[62] The omega-3 fatty acid-derived neuroprotectin D1 limits hippocampal hyperexcitability and seizure susceptibility in kindling epileptogenesis. Musto AE, Gjorstrup P, Bazan NG. Epilepsia. 2011 May 13. PMID:21569016

[63] Clinical uses of melatonin in pediatrics. Sánchez-Barceló EJ, Mediavilla MD, Reiter RJ. Int J Pediatr. 2011;2011:892624. PMID:21760817

[64] Simplified calculation of body-surface area. Mosteller RD. N Engl J Med. 1987 Oct 22;317(17):1098. PMID:3657876

[65] Role of intestinal circadian genes in alcohol-induced gut leakiness. Swanson G, Forsyth CB, Tang Y, et al. Alcohol Clin Exp Res. 2011 Jul;35(7):1305-14. PMID:21463335

36. RAGE

Irritability and rage are scourges to the soul and upon the family. They are part of a pathologic process that injures the host and those they love. Rage is not anger. Anger is brewed in a dark kettle that can simmer, stew, and steam for seasons. Rage can unexpectedly detonate like a bolt of blue-sky lightning. Angry people believe themselves to be rational in their fantasies and plots of revenge.

An angry person needs to forgive and forgive themselves (as there is often repressed guilt) in order to live free. They poison their lives with their anger while the person they hate is often unaware that they are blamed for any injury.

During a rage, the hosts may watch themselves in abhorrence as they explode into an attack. Although they may be able to control their actions, they can no more turn off the boiling rage than a person with a migraine or having a panic attack can just turn them off. Explosive rage, in fact, has many parallels with migraines and seizures.

In animals, including humans, predatory attack, and defensive rage have different neurologic mechanisms[1]. Predation requires activation of the lateral hypothalamus and involves the cerebral cortex – thinking, plotting, and strategic planning. This planning takes time, and some humans plan aggressive attacks for months or years waiting for an advantageous moment.

Rage is activated by real or perceived threat. It is associated with marked sympathetic nervous system output, in contrast to the calculated predatory attack. Defensive rage does not allow the luxury of time or wisdom and avails impulsivity. There is little involvement of the forebrain, and even less forethought. Its actions principally rely on the reptilian brain with limited cortical involvement.

Irritability is typically the bed in which rage rests. I trained my office staff to recognize and alert me if a patient in the waiting room was acting irritable; as they were a danger to themselves and those around them, including staff and me. Pacing, grimacing, clenching of the fists, with shoulders tight, are all signs of imminent danger.

Defensive rage is an outburst of aggressive behavior that is the fighting portion of the flight or fight survival reaction. If cornered and unable to flee, an animal will fight to survive. Under the right scenario, rage aids in survival, if not for the hunted, at least for its kind, as the predator may reconsider the next time he thinks that one of these animals is an easy snack. But the animal that had the rage usually does not come out unscathed. Rage has a high cost; emotional, physical, and social.

Normally, rage is reserved for extreme situations. But for some, rage is the result of altered brain chemistry. "Anger Attacks" are frequent in major depression, especially in men[2], seasonal affective disorder (SAD)[3] and in bipolar disorder[4]. About 30 percent of individuals with depression, about 40 percent of patients with SAD, and 62 percent with bipolar syndrome have "anger attacks." In SAD the average number of "anger attacks" is 18 per month while only about four occur during non-seasonal depression. Outbursts of rage also occur in many patients with PTSD, fibromyalgia, autism, and other diseases that effect affect, and in which inflammatory cytokines are elevated.

These "anger attacks" are usually accompanied by palpitations or tachycardia, sweating, feelings of panic or anxiety, shaking or trembling, shortness of breath or heavy breathing, light-headedness, and muscle tension. The person usually feels out control, feels that their actions are uncharacteristic of their ideal self; they usually regret their behavior and feel guilt afterwards[3].

The term "Anger Attack" is used to describe outbursts of rage in the some of the medical and psychological literature. The term "explosive disorder," and my favorite, IED (Intermittent Explosive Disorder) are also employed. Herein, the term rage is preferred to distinguish it from the cognitive process of anger, and to highlight rage as an instinctually programmed behavior which is elicited by stress and perceived danger. Using animal models of rage, allows understanding and the potential for controlling it.

Table 36-1: Rage Questionnaire[5]

Overreaction to minor annoyances	Over the past six months, do you feel that you have overreacted with rage or anger to minor annoyances or trivial issues?
Episodes of inappropriate rage or anger	Over the past six months, have you had episodes where you would become angry and enraged with other people or things, in a way that you realize was excessive or inappropriate to the situation?"
If either or both are answered in the affirmative, it indicates a rage disorder.	

Rage is not easily controlled. However, if it can be recognized before it hits its flashpoint; it may be diffused and avoided. To avoiding rage, it is essential to preventing the irritability that sets the stage for it.

Three different behavioral provocations trigger rage:

1. Pestering: This response can occur with repeated low-level challenges or annoyances. The archetypal response is a snap like a bitch might nip at her puppy if it is pestering her. The aggression is not intended to inflict serious harm, but to end the annoyance, create space, and teach respect.

2. Alpha-Challenge: This occurs when the alpha dominant individual's status is challenged. This trigger is more likely to provoke a feigned or incomplete rage reaction, and less likely to trigger actual aggressive attack and violence. If violence occurs, it is likely to be a very short burst of aggression unless the challenger does not back down. A dog may roll on its back, exposing its neck, to show submission in this situation to stop the attack.

3. Cornering: This is the archetypal trigger for defensive rage. This is the reaction of a threatened animal backed into a corner without an escape route. It is the instinctual defend or die reaction, and may be an all out defensive attack, which can pose a serious risk to the animal perceived to be threatening. Rage resulting from cornering is much more than a nip or ruffled feathers. It is a potential life and death situation.

We can see these behaviors in cats and dogs. We have also seen them in humans. Pestering can lead to a snap, an outburst of unkind words or flick of the wrist. It can occur as an almost automated response, which can surprise the pestered as much as the pesterer.

It's easy to step into an alpha-challenge situation unexpectedly, and it is helpful in life to recognize when you made an unwitting alpha-challenge, so that you back down quickly and keep it from accelerating into something more than a display of force. When the retaliatory action is directed at you, assume violence may follow if you fail to back down. The alpha-challenge in society is often triggered by a challenge to authority, or over turf. It can come from a person with no real authority, who is playing a role of authority, (the 5th-grade hall monitor) so it can surprise you that they think they are the top dog. In any case, it is not usually worth the confrontation, and polite apologies are recommended.

Apologies

I have instructed and hope my children have learned to apologize, even when they believe they have done nothing wrong. Apologies must appear sincere for them to diffuse tension, so saying something you don't believe is likely to come out sounding sarcastic, and thus, not helpful. I also taught my children not to incriminate themselves, especially when they are not at fault.

The trick is to tell the truth and have that truth be that you regret the other person's suffering. "I'm sorry that your feelings got hurt" takes no blame. Looking at the floor may also help. "I'm so sorry that you got hurt" is something a friend may say, who had no part in its causation.

"I want to apologize…" is a strong preamble to soothe feelings, and can also be used without accepting blame. For example; "I want to apologize, I didn't mean to offend you" or "I want to apologize, I didn't see you coming."

An apology can relieve the tension, and give a chance for a new start. "I want to apologize" is a phase worth practicing, as so many of us find those words so difficult to pronounce. Enemies consume a lot of energy; apologies can be free.

Animal Model of Rage

Animals give us a useful model for rage that can occur during cornering. Here is what rage looks like in cats and some analogous behaviors in humans

Table 36-2: Rage in Cat and Man

Cats	Humans
Hissing	Growling, spewing expletives
Crouching and arching of the back	Shoulders tight and rolled forward, contraction of upper back muscles. Head forward. (Muscles: trapezius, sternocleidomastoid, and triceps tensed)
Extension of the claws	Clenching of the fists
Retraction of the ears and piloerection	
Fangs bared, mouth half open	Teeth bared, mouth half open (snarling)
Eyes half shut	Eyelids half shut
Tail lashing	Pacing
Striking with the forepaw	Pounding, smashing

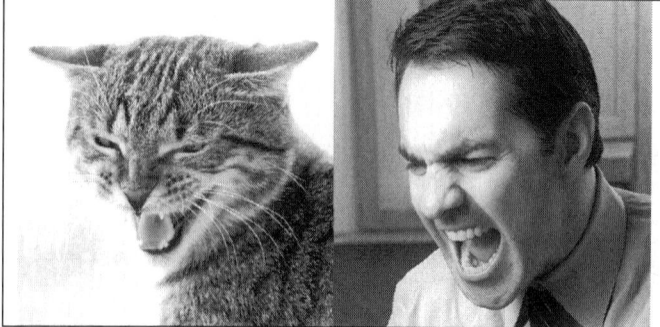

(Stock photos; the man is an actor)

The medial hypothalamus and the dorsal and lateral aspects of the periaqueductal gray area (PAG) are two brain areas which interact to trigger the rage reaction. A more modern feature, the ventral prefrontal area (PFA) of the brain controls the automated responses. The PFA acts like a brake that allows individuals to slow down as they find themselves careening out of control down a treacherous incline. When one puts on the brakes, the vehicle should come out of gear so that you can stop accelerating. The frontal lobe has the job of discrimination between real threat or not; friend or foe and make deliberations and judgments: What are the consequences of action? Is the action ethical? What is the appropriate response to the situation? Do I really want to do this? The PFA allows the luxury of decision-making, to act on the primal rage impulse or not. The PFA gives some control over rage.

Defensive rage reactions can be reliably elicited in animals by electrical stimulation to the medial hypothalamus or periaqueductal gray midbrain area. This gives a reproducible model for studying rage. Multiple studies have used this type of electrical stimulus in the brains of cats to study rage behavior. By using different amounts of chemical neuromodulators and differing amounts of electrical current, the effects and interactions of these agents on triggering rage reactions have been studied.

In nature, it is not electrical wires implanted deep within the skull that control primal, instinctual behavior, but rather neuromodulators, such as neurotransmitters, cytokines, hormones and toxins that act on various target tissues. A simplified model[6] that compartmentalizes these target tissues is illustrated in Figure 36-1. An expanded list of neuromodulators is given in Table 36-3.

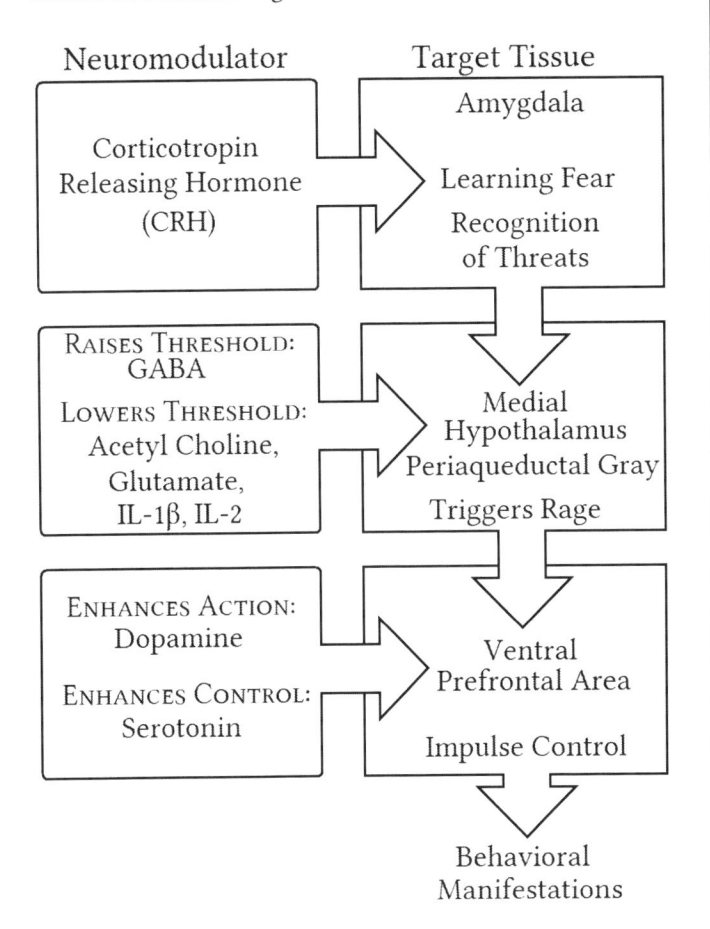

Figure 36-1: Model for Rage Behavior

Neuromodulator → Target Tissue

- Corticotropin Releasing Hormone (CRH) → Amygdala: Learning Fear, Recognition of Threats
- RAISES THRESHOLD: GABA; LOWERS THRESHOLD: Acetyl Choline, Glutamate, IL-1β, IL-2 → Medial Hypothalamus, Periaqueductal Gray: Triggers Rage
- ENHANCES ACTION: Dopamine; ENHANCES CONTROL: Serotonin → Ventral Prefrontal Area: Impulse Control

→ Behavioral Manifestations

The Amygdala: Perception of Danger

The amygdala alerts us to danger. For example, if we are dining in a group and someone at the table starts vomiting, we may also vomit. This is adaptive, as it can help us from being poisoned by tainted food. The purpose of making and reading facial expression is that it allows us to take cues from our social group. A bitter expression shows that the food is bitter, warning us not to eat it as it may contain toxic compounds, such as glycoalkaloids. A fearful expression shows that there is something to be afraid of, and an angry expression means we might want to back off.

Non-cognitive learning: CRH stimulates recognition of environmental cues as potential threats. CRH levels are elevated in individuals with fibromyalgia PTSD and depression. CHR promotes the perception that persons, places or events in the environment represent a threat or danger. Tryptophan depletion increases recognition of negative facial expressions[7]. These alterations in perception and learning not need be rational, and often we are not even conscious of them. CCK also increases fear and anxiety learning (Table 32-5).

Humans gained a survival advantage when they lost facial hair, as this allowed better reading of facial expression. Women do not grow beards, and this allows small children, who throughout primate evolution have spent more time with adult females, to learn to understand facial expression better.

Teenagers are poor at reading adult facial expression. They are in a state of flux from the more automatic (amygdala) reading by children with visceral (gut-level) reactions to the more experiential facial expression reading by adults. Teenagers are also egocentric; they tend to assume that others people's emotional content is all about them. Thus, fatigue, worry, or pain revealed in an adult's facial expression is often assumed by teenagers to be anger or disappointment directed towards them.

Perception of danger (amygdala) strengthens the response of the Reticular Activating System (RAS) of the brain. Chronic exposure to danger or unexpected attack in what is a trusted, safe environment can cause long term up-regulation of this system with vigilance and a lower threshold for perceived danger. In post-traumatic stress disorder (PTSD) the RAS is over-activated. The sufferer can no longer trust their environment, and they become chronically vigilant. This occurs especially after repeated contact with dangers, especially when unexpected, or when it occurs in what is supposed to be a safe environment, as occurs in domestic violence.

The Hypothalamus and Periaqueductal Grey: The Trigger

The medial hypothalamus (MH) and the PAG hold the trigger to rage. When stimulated, the individual is irritable, and rage can much more easily occur. There are numerous neuromodulators that can lower the threshold for rage; some of these modulate the Glutamate/GABA balance in specific brain areas. Glutamate lowers the threshold and thus lowers the required stimulus to trigger rage while GABA increases the threshold, thus requiring a stronger threat stimulus to trigger rage. Kynurenine shifts this balance away from glutamate, but its toxic metabolites, 3-HK and quinolinic acid enhance glutaminergic activity.

The Chase: During exercise, working skeletal muscles release more lactate into the bloodstream than it absorbs. Lactate can then be utilized as the preferential fuel by the myocardium; accounting for as much as 60% of the heart's energy needs. Under sympathetic stimulation, the brain also utilizes lactate as its preferred fuel. Lactate is also a substrate for production of the excitatory neurotransmitter glutamate[8].

Sympathetic stimulation during a chase or escape run switches the Glutamate/GABA balance in the brain towards glutamate production and readies the body for a fight.

> Sympathetic stimulus by norepinephrine (NE) facilitates the rage reaction. This may help explain rage reactions in fibromyalgia and PTSD patients, who have chronic sympathetic activation.
>
> Unfortunately, this instinctual aggression can manifest in inexperienced police officers at the end of the chase, especially when more than one officer is involved in the chase; beatings or other excessive use of force can occur as a result of this primitive instinctual behavior.

One of the most influential factors in lowering the threshold for rage is Interleukin-1β (IL-1β)[1,2]. IL-1β also greatly lowers the threshold for seizures[9,10], although the mechanism for IL-1β actions differs in these two conditions. This proinflammatory cytokine is produced by monocytes, macrophages, dendritic cells, fibroblasts, and by glial cells in the brain. It has a role in fighting infections, causing fever and regulating the production of new immune cells. However, when the medial hypothalamus and midbrain periaqueductal gray matter are exposed to high levels of IL-1β, rage is facilitated. This means that sick and injured animals are more likely to have rage reactions.

In experiments where IL-1β is injected into these brain areas, it takes 1 to 3 hours for this facilitation to peak. Thus, IL-1β itself does not trigger rage, but rather lowers the threshold for it[11]. This slow reaction of interleukin in the brain is likely mediated by the induction of cyclooxygenase and the subsequent synthesis and release of prostaglandin E2 mediated through 5-HT$_2$ induction.

Interleukin 2, an anti-inflammatory cytokine, modulates the rage response. It can raise of lower the threshold depending on its location.

Interleukin-1β mediates the rage reaction by its effect on the 5-HT$_{1A}$ and 5-HT$_{2C}$ serotonin receptors in the medial hypothalamus and the PAG. Serotonin does not trigger a reaction, but it may set the sensitivity. These receptors are for excitatory responses. Serotonin stimulation is usually anti-anxiolytic; however, it can increase anxiety and aggression by stimulating 5-HT$_{1A}$ receptors in the hypothalamus. This can occur when the receptors are influenced by certain neuromodulators, such as IL-1β, neurokinin-1 (NK1), and Substance P.

Repetitive triggering of defensive rage in laboratory animals facilitates rage reactions; the behavior becomes progressively more automatic. This facilitation of the rage process is called kindling.

Table 36-3: Neuromodulators and neurotransmitters affecting Defensive Rage[12]

Mediator	Target tissue	Receptor	Effect
			Up-Regulation
Interleukin-1β (IL-1β)	Medial hypothalamus	5-HT$_{2A\ and\ 2C}$	Lowers rage threshold; promotes prostaglandin E2
IL-1β[13]	Periaqueductal Grey	5-HT$_{2A\ and\ 2C}$	Lowers rage threshold; promotes prostaglandin E2
Interleukin-2 (IL-2)	Periaqueductal Grey	NK1	Lowers rage threshold
Substance P	Periaqueductal Grey	NK1	↑ Defensive rage
Prostaglandin E2 + Lipopolysaccharide	Medial hypothalamus	EP1	Loss of impulse behavior control via the dopaminergic system[14]
Prostaglandin E2 + Lipopolysaccharide	Periaqueductal Grey	EP1	Loss of impulse behavior control via the dopaminergic system[14]
Cholecystokinin		CCK$_B$	↑ Defensive Rage
Dopamine	Ventral tegmentum projecting to the Ventral Prefrontal cortex	D$_1$-like receptors?	Increases impulsivity; Increases aggressive behavior
Glutamate	Periaqueductal Grey	NMDA	↑ Defensive rage
Acetylcholine		Muscarinic	↑ Defensive rage
Norepinephrine	Locus ceruleus	α$_2$	↑ Defensive rage
Nitric Oxide Synthase (NOS)	Anterior cingulate cortex		↓ Activity; associated with impulsivity, hyperactivity, and aggressive behaviors[15]
Vasopressin			↑ Aggression
Histamine	Prefrontal area	H$_3$	↑ Impulsivity and anxiety
			Down-Regulation
IL-2	Medial Hypothalamus	GABA$_A$	Raises rage threshold; ↓ Aggression
Serotonin	Ventral Prefrontal cortex	5-HT$_{1A}$	Raises the threshold for rage, decreases impulsivity; Decreases anxiety
Prostaglandin E2	Ventral Prefrontal cortex	EP1	Impulse behavior control through control of the dopaminergic system[14]
Opiate Peptides	Periaqueductal Grey	μ	↓ Defensive rage
GABA	Medial hypothalamus	GABA$_A$	↓ Aggression

↓: Decreased, ↑: Increased

The Prefrontal Area: The Gatekeeper

Serotonin and dopamine are neurotransmitters that affect impulsivity and aggression. Previously, the action of the prefrontal area was compared to the brakes on a vehicle. That is the effect of serotonin on the PFA. Dopamine acts like a gas pedal in the PFA, increasing impulsivity; action before thought. Deficient serotonergic, excessive dopaminergic activity; or a combination of these can result in hyperactivity, which may promote impulsive behavior. This seems to be particularly important in the prefrontal area of the brain. In a study of murderers, those whose crime was impulsive had lower activity in the ventral prefrontal cortex and increased activity in the subcortical areas; while those who planned the murder had normal levels[16].

Prefrontal dysfunction with low serotonin and high dopaminergic activity is associated with: impulsivity, substance abuse, depression, suicide, murder, and Type II alcoholism (early onset alcoholism, poor impulse control, risk taking and antisocial behavior). It may be that rage from the hypothalamus and PAG is limited to smashing dishes and spewing explicatives when the ventral prefrontal cortex (PFC) is functioning properly. The PFC acts like the brakes on the range of behavior. However, without the judgment and restraint of a functioning prefrontal area violence can occur. Thus, the PFA performs the function of gatekeeper, controlling behavior, acting as a brake to keep things in check. If the gates are open or, the brakes do not work, disaster can occur. Sympathetic activity shunts blood flow away from the prefrontal areas; impeding judgment and cognition during excitation.

PGE2 in the prefrontal cortex helps control impulsive behavior. However, PGE2 in the presence of LPS produced by gram-negative bacterial infection or intestinal biofilm cause loss of impulse control (Table 36-3).

Nurture, Nature, Rage, and Violence

Two genes that are important in personality and behavioral variation are the MAO_A gene and the SERT gene. Monoamine oxidase A (MAO_A) is a key enzyme responsible for degrading serotonin, and SERT is the serotonin transporter gene, which moves serotonin out of the synaptic area. Both these genes lower the availability of serotonin. There is allelic variation in the activity of these genes within the population. Individuals, who have lower functioning phenotypes, have more serotonin activity.

Men with the high MAO_A activity gene, the typical form, who are raised in an abusive environment as children are about twice as likely to be violent adults as those raised in non-abusive environments. Men who carry a genetic variant for MAO_A, which has lower activity, sometimes called the "Warrior Gene" in the popular media, are 9.8 times as likely to be convicted for violent offenses if they were abused as children. However, they have about half the normal risk of violent behavior compared to those with the high MAO_A gene if raised in a non-abusive environment[17].

Thus, the so-called warrior gene can be *protective against* developing a violent disposition if the child is raised in a non-threatening environment. Having the lower MAO_A activity gene and being raised in a non-abusive environment is also very protective against the promotion of antisocial personality disorder, while it increases the risk in an abusive environment. Thus, the low activity MAO_A gene makes an individual more adaptive to epigenetic imprinting from their environment while the high MAO_A activity gene confers less variability in response to childhood environments.

A loving and caring environment aids in the formation of frontal lobe judgment, compassion and discernment.

Serotonin is an important neurotrophic growth factor beginning early in fetal development. In mice, excessive serotonin in the first trimester promotes depressive behavior, and excess in the third trimester causes anxious behavior. Inhibition of MAO_A in during fetal development in mice causes aggressive behavior[18]. Alcohol exposure inhibits MAO. Even at low exposure levels, third-trimester exposure to alcohol is associated with aggressive behavior (See Chapter 17.) Thus, polymorphisms of these genes and other influences that affect serotonin levels can have a large effect on the developing brain, with the effect of exposure to serotonin during development being paradoxical to its general effect later in life.

In the brain, the amygdala modulates learning emotional responses to fearful and possibly dangerous situations. The amygdala is the site for gut-level reactions, which interpret a situation as dangerous. This is important especially for children who do not have the experiential repertoire to make informational-based judgments of danger or trust. Individuals with lower activity MAO_A and SERT gene alleles have increased activation of the amygdala to fearful facial expression, and thus have a stronger reaction to this type of stimuli.

MAO_A variants with lower activity have been associated with depression, anxiety, alcoholism and impulsivity. These effects also have a gender predisposition in the manner in which individuals react to early, higher level exposure to serotonin. Females tend to develop depressive disorders, anxiety disorders, and posttraumatic stress syndrome; while males are more susceptible to ADHD, alcoholism, drug dependence and antisocial behavior. In males, the central theme is impulsivity; in females, it is fearfulness.

Another gene allele variant is that for inducible nitric oxide synthase (iNOS). Individuals with decreased transcriptional activity for this enzyme tend to be more impulsive, hyperactive and aggressive. It is associated with hypo-activation of the anterior cingulate cortex, which is involved in the processing of emotion and reward in behavioral control. A gene variant of iNOS with lower activity is seen more commonly in families with ADHD, suicide attempts and among criminal offenders.

Corticotropin Releasing Hormone

CRH levels are elevated during chronic stress. CRH activates the amygdala to recognize situations as threatening. This hormone is anxiogenic and also increases paracellular hyperpermeability. It can trigger mast cell degranulation. It is best mitigated by reducing stress and avoiding hypersensitivity reactions, such as those that release histamine and antergies to foods. CRH is further discussed in Chapter 29.

Foods, Fear, Irritability, and Rage: Histamine and other Biogenic Amines

Histamine has both CNS and peripheral effects. Histamine released during allergic reactions can cause a sense of doom and foreboding as a result of activation of the H_3 receptor, and it can trigger panic attacks. This compels us to avoid foods we are allergic to and foods with high histamine content, such as certain spoiled fish. Table 13-4 lists effects of histamine. It can be understood that foods containing large amounts of histamine, such as scombroid seafood poisoning or allergic reactions, which cause the release of endogenous histamine, can affect the thinking machine. Histamines reaction on the brain can:

- Increase vigilance and perception of danger
- Creation of linking: people, places, objects to danger (which, of course, may be false associations)

Table 36-4: CNS effects of Histamine

Receptor	Effects
H_1 receptors	↑ Vigilance and wakefulness ↑ Attention ↓ Feeding
H_2 receptors	↑ Relational Associations (Working Memory)
H_3 receptors	CNS: arousal, circadian rhythm ↑ Aversion memory, anxiety and impulsivity ↓ Learning, judgment, and memory acquisition ↑ Neuropathic pain

Histamine increases the activity and duration of excitatory glutaminergic activity. It increases vigilance memory and learning. It also increases danger warnings signals in the brain and increase irritability and the potential for rage reactions. Higher levels of histamine also affect the frontal lobe; increasing impulsivity and decreasing learning and judgment, mediated through the H_3 receptors. Thus, histamine can get in the way of the normal PFA cognitive brakes that control a rage reaction.

Mast cells are important in the healing process[19], and it is histamine that causes itching in healing wounds and burns. Use of antihistamines after abdominal surgery is associated with higher risk of abscess formation[20] because they prevent histamine from helping wounds to heal. Foods that contain high levels of histamine as a toxin can increase fear and aversion learning. Food allergies that cause the release of histamine can also do this.

However, in food allergies, antergies, and in mast cell activation disorders (MCAD) degranulation of mast cells in does more than cause histamine release. CRH can also provoke mast cell degranulation in the brain and other areas. Both histamine and CRH increases recognition of stimuli as dangers. However, mast cells also release immune mediators released during degranulation that decrease threshold for rage over the following 12 to 36 hours with the transcription and promotion of PGE2, IL-1β, and other inflammatory mediators.

Agents that provoke mast cell degranulation, allergic reactions, antergic reactions and foods with high levels of histamine or other bioamines that interfere with histamine degradation, can all increase the risk of rage reactions. (See chapters, 11, 15, 19 and 25). Cofactors for enzymatic degradation of histamine are shown in Table 13-6 in chapter 13.

Other foods containing biogenic amines may also provoke irritability. Since this is a threshold reaction, small amounts from food may not cause a noticeable reaction when used alone, but in combination with other foods with small amounts may lower the threshold sufficiently to have a reaction, much like seizures or migraines.

In a healthy gut, dietary (and locally produced) biogenic amines are degraded by diamine oxidase (DAO) and by histamine-N-methyltransferase (HNMT) in the colon. In inflammatory or neoplastic bowel disease, such as Crohn's disease, ulcerative colitis, food allergies, enteropathies and colorectal neoplasm, there is a reduction of DAO and HNMT in the gut[21], which not only plays a role in these diseases, but allows for systemic absorption and biogenic amines. Alcohol inhibits the activity of DAO.

Injured animals have elevated circulating histamine levels. Wounds contaminated by enteric bacterial, as may occur with bites, are expected to have a T_H17 response, and increase in IL-6. Stress increases CRH release. Thus, animals recovering from an injury may be irritable. An immobilized animal is, in essence, cornered; they cannot flee, and rage reactions may protect them.

CRH also increases paracellular permeability in the gut, increasing the passage of LPS into the body. LPS interacts with PGE2 to decrease impulse control. Thus, bacterial biofilm formation also increases the risk of rage behavior.

Cytokines: Inflammatory Mediators

Cytokines are small proteins secreted by cells of the immune system that have effects on other cells, sometimes cells distant from the site of the immune reaction, thus, acting as hormones. Table 36-3 summarizes the effects of IL-1β and IL-2 on the medial hypothalamus and the PAG.

Several markers of inflammation found in the blood have been shown to be associated with hostility[22], including C-reactive protein (CRP) and IL-6. CRP may activate stress pathways in the brain, or perhaps, it is simply a correlate of general inflammation, with no direct action on behavior. IL-1β has been established to lower the threshold for rage and seizures.

Elevated homocysteine (HCY) promotes rage (anger attacks)[23] and is toxic to cerebral endothelial cells and can induce white matter and vascular lesions in the brain[24]. The effect of HCY is most likely mediated through its activation of acid sphingomyelinase. Acid SMase promotes intracellular ceramide accumulation[25] and the production of S1P. S1P activates neuroglia, production of pro-inflammatory cytokines and inflammatory mediators. Acid SMAse activity is also triggered by H_2O_2 and other ROS, and can be mitigated by antioxidants such as alpha-lipoic acid. Control of HCY is discussed in chapter 31, (see Figures 31-4 and 31-5).

IL-6 becomes elevated with sleep deprivation[26]. IL-1, which is elevated in infections and skin conditions, such as urticaria, inhibits REM sleep and thus, prevents its restorative actions. Restorative sleep is an important aspect of mental health and avoidance of irritability. The relationship of foods and sleep is discussed in chapter 43. Chronic stress also raises CRH, IL-1β, IL-6 and other inflammatory cytokine levels[27] (Chapter 29).

N3 and N6 Fatty Acids

N3 and n6 fatty acids influence inflammation and prostaglandin synthesis and induction of inflammatory cytokines, and thus affect mood and rage reactions. The n-3 fatty acids may have their effect through elevation of PPAR-γ and its inhibitory effect of NF-κB its transcription of IL-1β, TNF-α, and COX2. N-3 fatty acids also decrease the promotion of the series 2-prostaglandins in favor of series 3-prostaglandins and series 4-leukotrienes in favor of series 5-leukotrienes, which are less inflammatory. (Figure 6-5). Homicide rates are lower in countries with lower n-6 fat intake and higher n-3 fat intake[28]. N-3 fatty acid supplements were found to lower hostility and suicidal ideation[29]. See figure 31-4.

Glutamate and GABA

The balance between GABA and Glutamate is important in controlling the tone of the hippocampus. Many antiseizure medications act by raising the activity of GABA, and some of these medications may help control rage reactions as well.

Glutamate is the source of GABA. GABA is formed from glutamate by the enzyme L-glutamate decarboxylase, which requires pyridoxal-5-phosphate (PLP) as a co-enzyme. PLP is a phosphated form of the B vitamin pyridoxine. Deficiencies in pyridoxine or its metabolism can cause anemia, seizures, nerve damage, skin and oral lesions. PLP is also required for formation monoamine neurotransmitters; serotonin, dopamine, norepinephrine and epinephrine, and for the metabolism of kynurenine compounds that impact glutamate activity and metabolizing sphinophosphates to less immunostimulating forms. Table 28-4 in Chapter 28 provides a list of some of the enzymes and cofactors that help in GABA and Glutamate metabolism.

Lead and Violence:

As much as 90% of the variance in aggravated assault between cities may be explained by the amount of lead dust released into the local environment 22 years earlier[30] mainly from vehicle exhaust fumes. Children's brains are extremely susceptible to this toxin, and the violent behavior culminates when they reach adulthood. Lead is toxic to multiple enzymes. It may aggravate violent behavior by its effect on the development of the hippocampus, on DNA expression, and it interferes with the release of glutamate and blocks NMDA receptors[31]

Serotonin: Putting on the Brakes

Serotonin is calming and helps put the brakes on impulsivity; while dopamine is activating and increases impulsivity. Serotonin reuptake inhibitors used as antidepressants increase the availability of serotonin. MAO_A catabolizes serotonin, and medications that block this enzyme increase the availability of serotonin. Normal diets usually have sufficient tryptophan for the formation of serotonin, but some vegetarian diets can be lacking. PLP is also required for conversion of tryptophan to serotonin. See Table 28-3 in chapter 28 for the pathway and coenzymes required for serotonin metabolism.

Nitric Oxide Synthase (NOS)

Low activity of the enzyme inducible nitric oxide synthase (iNOS: NOS3) is associated with aggressive behavior. Assuring a supply of iNOS substrates and cofactors may be helpful. These include NADPH, which requires niacin, and Arginine. Aspirin inhibits expression and function of this enzyme. Inducible NOS forms NO upon stimulation with INF-γ, produced in association with T_H1 activity. Excessive diversion of T-cells towards T_H17 activity may decrease NOS activity.

NOS in the brain (NOS1) also uses arginine as a substrate and requires NADPH but additionally requires Heme, FAD, FMN, tetrahydrobiopterin (BH4) and calcium as cofactors. Thus arginine, riboflavin, niacin, folate, iron, and calcium need to be sufficiently available for efficient generation of NO.

Arginine supplementation to increase NO production is not helpful, as arginine is mostly converted into urea by the liver upon absorption. Citrulline bypasses metabolism by the liver during absorption and is later converted to arginine by the kidney. L-citrulline is thus a better supplement for use in increasing NO production.

Summary

The goal of avoiding irritability and rage can be approached by avoiding inflammation that increases the release of CRH and inflammatory cytokines and by improving the function of the frontal areas of the brain that control judgment.

1. Learn about the world in a safe, non-threatening environment. Lower stress (Chapter 29)
2. Raise the threshold for triggering rage. This involves lowering the irritability of the medial hypothalamus and PAG and raising the threshold for perception of danger.
3. Control impulsivity by improving the functioning of the prefrontal area.

Rage is an instinctual reaction to perceived threat; nevertheless, an inflammatory milieu lowers the threshold at which rage is triggered. This threshold is often low in chronic inflammatory disorders including seasonal affective disorder, PTSD, and fibromyalgia. Repeated rage episodes of rage may cause kindling, facilitating, and thus making rage be more easily triggered.

Outbursts of rage may be prevented by the treatment of inflammatory conditions which facilitate it. It is also useful to avoid it to avoid kindling. Patients should be taught to recognize their reactions to acute stress, and the physical manifestations of stress in their bodies, such as clenching, pacing and crouching postures, when explosive behaviors are eminent, and be taught to remove themselves from the aggravating stimulus, before they react. The earlier they can recognize their internal stress response, the more successful they will be at avoiding rage reactions.

1. Inflammation: Inflammation associated with infections, immune reactions, oxidative stress, chronic emotional stress and sleep deprivation can decrease the threshold for rage. Inflammation can tie up pyridoxal-5-phosphate and make it unavailable for tryptophan metabolism, GABA production, S1P lyase, and other processes.

PGE_2 production in the brain increases propensity for rage: PGE_2 is elevated in diets high in n-6 fatty acids. Treatment should include avoidance of a pro-inflammatory diet; maintaining a low n-6 intake and sufficient n-3 fat intake to prevent excess inflammatory prostaglandin production and maintain PPAR-γ production. Vitamin D, tocotrienols, and some flavonoids decrease production of PGE_2. Flavonoids and other phenolic antioxidants in the diet may increase the threshold for rage. See Chapters 6, 15, 20 and 40.

The inflammatory cytokine IL-1β decreases the threshold for rage. IL-1β may be elevated through TLR4 and NF-κB, via LPS, by TLR2, by sleep deprivation or chronic social stress, as examples. Each is additive. A multifactorial approach to lowering inflammatory cytokines and reducing stress is most likely to raise the threshold and prevent rage reactions. IL-1β also increases the production of TNF-α and other inflammatory factors.

LPS increases the production of iNOS, COX2, and TNF-α through activation of NF-κB, via TLR4. COX2 increases PGE2 production. LPS from biofilm formation in the gut increases toxic kynurenines, activates TLR4, and may lower the threshold for rage through direct effects on the PAG. Lung or other infection can also produce sufficient LPS to lower the threshold for rage. SIBO, dysbiosis, and intestinal biofilm overgrowth should be investigated and treated if present. (Chapters 4, 5, 7, 23, 24, and 25) Nutritional and medicinal control of the LPS → TLR4 inflammatory pathway is discussed in Chapter 31.

S1P, acid SMAse inhibitors, and ALA are discussed in Chapters 10, 31, 32 and 34. Medications that are functional inhibitors of acid SMAse (FIASMA) (Appendix M) may be helpful in the treatment of rage.

2. Avoid Antergens: Enteroimmune sources of inflammation often are the major ones lowering the threshold for rage. Antergies increase the release of CRH and inflammatory cytokines and histamine. Antergen elimination often effectively controls rages and explosive disorder. Seizure patients, too, should be tested for IgG food antergies, and these foods eliminated from the diet. (See Chapters 11 and 19.)

Mast cell activation syndrome and food allergies should also be considered and treated. Histamine may increase impulsivity and anxiety by increasing glutaminergic response. Allergic reactions, mast cell activation, and biogenic amines increase histamine levels. MAO and DAO assist in the catabolism of histamine. Assure adequate nutritional cofactors for histamine and bioamine catabolism. See Chapters 11, 12,13, 14 and 17.

3. Corticotropin Releasing Hormone: CRH triggers the amygdala to recognize threats. CHR is elevated during stress and disruption of circadian rhythms. Avoid chronic stress. Avoid stress during pregnancy and avoid stressing infants and children. Distress during these developmental stages can affect a child's response to stress for their entire lifetime. See chapters 29 and 41. Stress and immune reactions also release CRH. Avoid and prevent these.

4. GABA/Glutamate: GABA decreases the threshold for rage reactions; while glutamate and IL-1β, decrease the threshold. See chapters 28 and 31. TNF-α increases glutaminergic activity, at least in part, through stimulation of the kynurenic acid pathway. Serotonin increases frontal control over behavioral reaction to rage while dopamine increases impulsivity. LPS and inflammatory cytokines shift tryptophan from serotonin production into kynurenine production.

5. Frontal Lobe Function: Rage is a frequent comorbidity of chronic traumatic encephalopathy (CTE). Treat traumatic brain injury, PTSD, fibromyalgia, Seasonal Affective Disorder, bipolar disorder or depression when present. See Chapters 30, 31 and 32.

6. Sleep. Sufficient restorative sleep is essential. See Chapter 43.

[1] Understanding human aggression: New insights from neuroscience. Siegel A, Victoroff J. Int J Law Psychiatry. 2009 Jul-Aug;32(4):209-15. PMID: 19596153

[2] Anger attacks in depression--evidence for a male depressive syndrome. Winkler D, Pjrek E, Kasper S. Psychother Psychosom. 2005;74(5):303-7. PMID:16088268

[3] Anger attacks in seasonal affective disorder. Winkler D, Pjrek E, Konstantinidis A, et al. Int J Neuropsychopharmacol. 2006 Apr;9(2):215-9. PMID:16004620

[4] The prevalence and clinical correlates of anger attacks during depressive episodes in bipolar disorder. Perlis RH, Smoller JW, Fava M, et al. J Affect Disord. 2004 Apr;79(1-3):291-5. PMID:15023510

[5] Validation of a simplified definition of anger attacks. Winkler D, Pjrek E, Kindler J, Heiden A, Kasper S. Psychother Psychosom. 2006;75(2):103-6. PMID:16508345

[6] Neurobiology of aggression and violence. Siever LJ. Am J Psychiatry. 2008 Apr;165(4):429-42. PMID: 18346997

[7] The effects of experimentally lowered serotonin function on emotional information processing and memory in remitted depressed patients. Merens W, Booij L, Haffmans PJ, van der Does A. J Psychopharmacol. 2008 Aug;22(6):653-62. PMID:18308809

[8] Lactate metabolism: a new paradigm for the third millennium. Gladden LB. J Physiol. 2004 Jul 1;558(Pt 1):5-30. May 6. PMID: 15131240

[9] A novel non-transcriptional pathway mediates the proconvulsive effects of interleukin-1beta. Balosso S, Maroso M, Sanchez-Alavez M, Ravizza T, Frasca A, Bartfai T, Vezzani A. Brain. 2008 Dec;131(Pt 12):3256-65. Oct 24.PMID: 18952671

[10] The role of interleukin-1beta in febrile seizures. Heida JG, Moshé SL, Pittman QJ. Brain Dev. 2009 May;31(5):388-93. PMID: 19217733

[11] Role of IL-1 beta and 5-HT2 receptors in midbrain periaqueductal gray (PAG) in potentiating defensive rage behavior in cat. Bhatt S, Bhatt R, Zalcman SS, Siegel A. Brain Behav Immun. 2008 Feb;22(2):224-33. Sep 24.PMID: 17890051

[12] The neurobiological bases for development of pharmacological treatments of aggressive disorders. Siegel A, Bhatt S, Bhatt R, Zalcman SS. Curr Neuropharmacol. 2007;5(2):135-47.PMID: 18615178

[13] Role of IL-1 beta and 5-HT2 receptors in midbrain periaqueductal gray (PAG) in potentiating defensive rage behavior in cat. Bhatt S, Bhatt R, Zalcman SS, Siegel A. Brain Behav Immun. 2008 Feb;22(2):224-33. PMID:17890051

[14] Prostaglandin E receptor EP1 controls impulsive behavior under stress. Matsuoka Y, Furuyashiki T, Yamada K, et al. Proc Natl Acad Sci U S A. 2005 Nov 1;102(44):16066-71. PMID: 16247016

[15] Influence of functional variant of neuronal nitric oxide synthase on impulsive behaviors in humans. Reif A, Jacob CP, Rujescu D, etal. Arch Gen Psychiatry. 2009 Jan;66(1):41-50.PMID: 19124687

[16] Role of Serotonin and Dopamine System Interactions in the Neurobiology of Impulsive Aggression and its Comorbidity with other Clinical Disorders. Seo D, Patrick CJ, Kennealy PJ. Aggress Violent Behav. 2008 Oct;13(5):383-395.PMID: 19802333

[17] Role of genotype in the cycle of violence in maltreated children. Caspi A, McClay J, Moffitt TE, Mill J, Martin J, Craig IW, Taylor A, Poulton R. Science. 2002 Aug 2;297(5582):851-4.PMID:12161658

[18] Serotonin, genetic variability, behaviour, and psychiatric disorders--a review. Nordquist N, Oreland L. Ups J Med Sci. 2010 Feb;115(1):2-10. PMID:20187845

[19] Mast cells are required for normal healing of skin wounds in mice. Weller K, Foitzik K, Paus R, Syska W, Maurer M. FASEB J. 2006 Nov;20(13):2366-8. PMID:16966487

[20] Influence of histamine receptor antagonists on the outcome of perforated appendicitis: analysis from a prospective trial. St Peter SD, Sharp SW, Ostlie DJ. Arch Surg. 2010 Feb;145(2):143-6. PMID:20157081

[21] Histamine and histamine intolerance. Maintz L, Novak N. Am J Clin Nutr. 2007 May;85(5):1185-96. PMID:17490952

[22] Antagonistic characteristics are positively associated with inflammatory markers independently of trait negative emotionality. Marsland AL, Prather AA, Petersen KL, Cohen S, Manuck SB. Brain Behav Immun. 2008 Jul;22(5):753-61. PMID: 18226879

[23] Anger attacks in major depressive disorder and serum levels of homocysteine. Fraguas R Jr, Papakostas GI, Mischoulon D, et al. Biol Psychiatry. 2006 Aug 1;60(3):270-4. PMID:16325154

[24] Homocysteine and B vitamins relate to brain volume and white-matter changes in geriatric patients with psychiatric disorders. Scott TM, Tucker KL, Bhadelia A, Bet al. Am J Geriatr Psychiatry. 2004 Nov-Dec;12(6):631-8.PMID:15545331

[25] Homocysteine induces cerebral endothelial cell death by activating the acid sphingomyelinase ceramide pathway. Lee JT, Peng GS, Chen SY, et al. Prog Neuropsychopharmacol Biol Psychiatry. 2013 Aug 1;45:21-7. PMID:23665108

[26] Sleep loss activates cellular markers of inflammation: sex differences. Irwin MR, Carrillo C, Olmstead R. Brain Behav Immun. 2010 Jan;24(1):54-7. PMID: 19520155

[27] Pro- and anti-inflammatory cytokines expression in rat's brain and spleen exposed to chronic mild stress: Involvement in depression. You Z, Luo C, Zhang W, et al. Behav Brain Res. 2011 Nov 20;225(1):135-41. PMID:21767575

[28] Healthy intakes of n-3 and n-6 fatty acids: estimations considering worldwide diversity. Hibbeln JR, Nieminen LR, Blasbalg TL, Riggs JA, Lands WE. Am J Clin Nutr. 2006 Jun;83(6 Suppl):1483S-1493S. PMID:16841858

[29] Omega-3 fatty acid supplementation in patients with recurrent self-harm. Single-centre double-blind randomised controlled trial. Hallahan B, Hibbeln JR, Davis JM, Garland MR. Br J Psychiatry. 2007 Feb;190:118-22. PMID:17267927

[30] The urban rise and fall of air lead (Pb) and the latent surge and retreat of societal violence. Mielke HW, Zahran S. Environ Int. 2012 Aug;43:48-55. PMID:22484219

[31] The function of the amino terminal domain in NMDA receptor modulation. Huggins DJ, Grant GH. J Mol Graph Model. 2005 Jan;23(4):381-8. PMID:15670959

37. ACNE

Acne, a nasty little disease, even has vulgar right in the name; "acne vulgaris." It is a Western disease, associated with the Western diet and lifestyle; in our society, acne affects over 80% of teenagers and afflicts men and women into middle age; 54% of women and 40 percent of men between the ages of 25 and 44 have acne[1], and about 6% of those 50 to 59 years of age still get acne lesions[2]. Meanwhile, acne is absent in hunter-gatherer cultures[3]. Inuit peoples and Africans in Zambia did not experience acne until they started eating western foods[4].

Acne is not just a skin disease. It is associated with anxiety, depression and risk of suicide. Adolescents with acne are 2.3 times more likely to have anxiety, twice as likely to suffer from depression, and 50 percent more likely to attempt suicide than their peers without acne[5]. The longer the duration of acne, the more severe the psychosocial impact is, especially among females[6]. It is also associated with anger[7].

In adults, acne is associated with poorer quality of life[8] and social impairment. In a study of insurance claims data, the diagnosis of depression was 2 to 3 times higher in patients with acne than in other patients; about 11 percent of female patients with acne suffer from clinical derepression while about 5% of male patients do. The majority of the acne patients who are using antidepressants are in the 36-64 age group[9]. Mental distress is correlated with the severity of acne; adolescents whose mental distress scores are higher, rate their current level of acne as more severe than do other adolescents. The odds ratio for suffering mental distress is 1.7 times higher among adolescent boys and 2.0 times higher among girls with acne[10].

Chicken or the Egg?

Acne is clearly correlated with negative affect, including anxiety and depression, but does acne cause emotional morbidity, or does stress cause acne? The most plausible models are:

1. **Acne causes emotional morbidity:**
   a. Acne, being an ugly and repugnant disease, causes loss of self-esteem, degrades self-image and causes real or feared or ostracization by peers and rejection by potential mates. This leads to anxiety and depression.
   b. Acne lesions produce inflammatory mediators that affect the CNS causing anxiety, depression and anger.
2. **Emotional disorders cause acne**: In this scenario, anxiety and depression trigger a metabolic cascade that increases the risk for acne.
3. **Something causes both:** A causal process increases the risk of both acne and anxiety/depression.

Premise 1: Acne Causes Emotional Morbidity

It has been observed that the association between acne and depression is stronger in females[10], in whom appearance is more closely related to social status. This would support the hypothesis that affective response to acne causes depression. However, this study did not have an objective rating of acne; thus, the young women studied may have rated their acne to be more severe if they were distressed. Women with psychosocial impairment tend to overrate the severity of their acne as compared to women with better self-esteem with the same degree of acne. After nine months of treatment with oral contraceptives and considerable improvement in acne, the psychosocial impairment did not change for the women with low self-esteem[11]. Recall, from the chapter on depression, that while tryptophan depletion does not have a significant effect on mood, it does promote a reduction in personal and positive memory, increased attention to neutral information[12], and increases recognition of negative facial expressions[13].

Isotretinoin (Accutane), an oral medication used for the treatment of severe cystic acne, carries a black box warning related to the risk of depression, suicide, and psychosis[14]. Patients who were prescribed isotretinoin were 2.7 times more likely to be hospitalized for depression in the following months than control patients were[15]. However, this might be explained by the correlation of acne to depression. In follow-up studies, the emotional status of patients with acne either stayed the same or improved slightly with successful isotretinoin treatment[16,17,18,19,20].

Several studies have reported improvement in depression with the use of topical or systemic treatment for acne[16]. Just the use of makeup that concealed acne was found to improve emotional status rapidly[21]. This topical treatment would not be expected to have a systemic effect on anxiety or depression; thus, this would support the role of improved self-perception, stress relief, and social interaction in emotional well-being. Emotional status appears to improve with the amelioration of acne. In a study in which women were taught to care for their skin and supplied with non-comedogenic makeup, both acne and emotional status improved[21].

Even though acne may cause emotional morbidity, this morbidity may not be purely, or even predominantly, psychological. Significant inflammatory lesions in the skin may provoke the release of cytokines and other inflammatory mediators that trigger anxiety, depression and anger.

Premise 2: Anxiety and Depression Provoke Acne

Patients often cite stress as a trigger for an outbreak of acne[10,22]. If anxiety and depression cause acne, then successful treatment of these conditions would be expected to be associated resolution of acne. However, this does not appear to be the usual case. Many patients complain of worsening acne when placed on treatment for depression, and acne is listed as a possible side effect of sertraline (Zoloft)[23], bupropion (Wellbutrin)[24], and other antidepressants. In one brief report of a series of seven patients, paroxetine (Paxil) appeared to help clear acne; although other anti-depressants did not[25]. This effect, if real, may represent a unique property of paroxetine that is likely unrelated to its efficacy as an antidepressant.

> While the medical literature, in general, does not suggest that serotonin reuptake inhibitors help acne, antidepressant medications are useful in the treatment of neurotic or compulsive "acne excoriée," a condition in which patients, mostly females, pick on themselves, causing skin damage. Acne excoriée is common; it is estimated to make up about two percent of all referrals to dermatologists[26].

Premise 3: Acne and Depression Share Causality

It may be that acne and depression are caused by shared risk factors. Antioxidants may help prevent both. Diets high in n-6 fatty acids, especially when accompanied by low n-3 fatty acid intake, provokes an inflammatory milieu that is hypothesized to increase the risk for acne and emotional morbidity. In one small trial with fish oil with other supplements, improvements were seen in mental, emotional and social well-being as well as a decrease in the number and severity of acne lesions[27].

Lack of sleep has been associated with worsening acne in several[28,29,30] but not all studies[31]. Lack of sleep is associated with inflammatory cytokines that may increase the risk for acne and depression. Academic examination stress is associated with outbreaks of acne[31,32]; however, change in both sleep and dietary habits, which may occur around exam times, are associated with acne outbreaks. Several of the nutritional risk factors (discussed below) are common for both acne and depression. Other stressors that are sometimes associated with acne are smoking and alcohol consumption[22,10]. Stress, poor diet and lack of sleep can be expected to have a negative effect on emotional well-being.

Of these three associations, the third premise is the most appealing in that it suggests that finding and eliminating risk factors for either of these diseases will likely help ameliorate the other.

The Pathogenesis of Acne

Four main processes come into play in the development of acne:

1. With the onset of puberty, there is an increase in sebum production under stimulation of androgens.

2. The pilosebaceous unit becomes colonized by the bacteria *Propionibacterium acnes*.

3. Keratinocytes from the hair follicle associated with the sebaceous glands form a plug that obstructs the pilosebaceous unit, forming a comedo.

4. The sebum is oxidized, resulting in the triggering of an inflammatory cascade resulting in the rupture of the pilosebaceous unit into the surrounding tissue, causing a more severe inflammatory reaction.

Sebum Production

With adolescence, there is an increased production of androgens. Dihydrotestosterone, the most active androgen, not only stimulates the production of sebum in the skin but also stimulates induction of the inflammatory cytokines IL-6 and TNF-α[33]. Women with acne or polycystic ovary syndrome have high serum levels of the androgen dehydroepiandrosterone sulfate[34]. When compared to other androgens in the blood, serum dehydroepiandrosterone levels were found to be those most closely correlated with the number of acne lesions[35].

In health, sebum combines with lipids from keratinocytes to form skin surface lipids (SSL). This lipid layer protects the skin; it is a lubricant that helps prevent abrasion and skin tears, a sunscreen that helps protect the skin from actinic damage from UV radiation and prevents aging, and moisturizer that prevents dryness. The SSL of humans is unusual in that it contains large amounts of squalene, a precursor of cholesterol. Squalene decreases water loss through the skin, acts as a barrier to many chemicals and has anti-carcinogenic properties[36].

Humans are the only primate with squalene in the SSL. Most mammals with squalene in the SSL are aquatic; beavers and otters, for example. Humans lack hair to give protection from UV radiation and squalene acts as an efficient quencher of free radicals created by UV radiation.

Table 37-1: Skin Surface Lipids

Typical Lipid Content of Human Sebum[37]	Percent
Triglycerides	32
Free fatty acids	25
Wax esters	25
Squalene	13
Cholesterol	2
Other compounds	3

Individuals with acne have been found to have twice the squalene levels of unaffected individuals. Stabilization of squalene depends on antioxidants in the SSL, including coenzyme Q_{10} and vitamin E, to protect it from oxidation[37]. Oxidative stress increases the potential for squalene to be peroxidized. Peroxidation products of squalene induce sebaceous gland hyperplasia and hyperkeratosis. They are comedogenic and promote the release of inflammatory mediators, such as cytokines. Application of UV-irradiated squalene to rabbit ears produces comedones; the more strongly peroxidized the squalene is, the larger the comedos elicited are[36].

Squalene peroxidation products can also promote activation of peroxisome proliferators-activated receptors (PPARs)[38]. PPAR-δ is the PPAR receptor most active in the sebaceous gland[39]. Although acting as transcription factors for anti-inflammatory proteins, one of the functions of PPARs is to induce the transcription of enzymes involved in lipid catabolism. PPAR-δ can also promote apoptosis of the sebocytes. This may provide additional nutrients for bacteria colonizing the follicle.

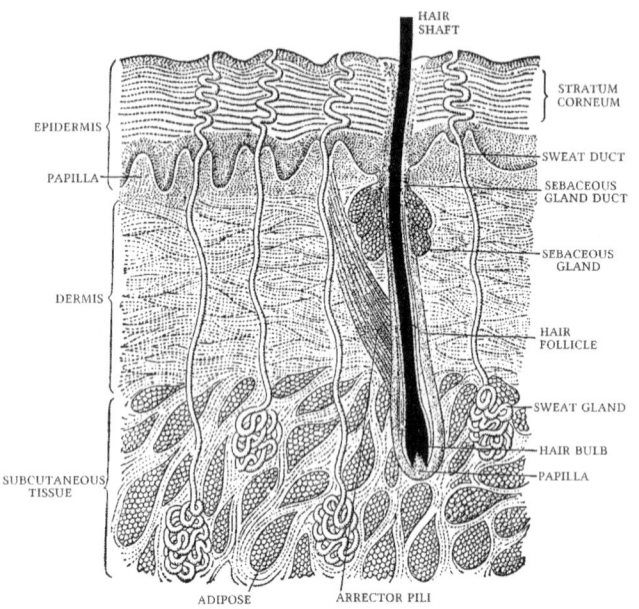

Figure 37-1: The Pilosebaceous Unit

Bacteria

In normal sebaceous glands, the bacterial count is low. In acne, however, there is colonization of the pilosebaceous unit by the bacteria *Propionibacterium acnes* (*P. acnes*). When there is a high density of *Propionibacterium acnes* in the pilosebaceous unit, bacterial quorum signals initiate biofilm formation, and the bacteria switch to the sessile phenotype. *P. acnes* have usually been considered to trigger acne; however, colonization by this bacteria is dependent upon oxidative stress. Oxidized squalene in the sebum provides the microaerophilic microenvironment that allows these bacteria to flourish[40].

The sessile form of *P. acnes* is more resistant to antibiotic agents than its planktic form[41]. *P. acnes* can produce the quorum sensing molecule autoinducer-2, which induces the sessile form, and under which *P. acnes* produce virulence factors including extracellular lipases[42], which can free fatty acids from triglycerides in the sebum. These bacteria use fatty acids as a fuel source. Arachidonic acid (AA), present in the fats is freed and available for generation of inflammatory eicosanoids. AA is also available in the cell membranes of shed keratinocytes in the sebum. AA can stimulate 5-lipoxygenase and thus the formation LTB_4 and interleukin-6 by sebocytes. LTB_4 can additionally act as a ligand for activating PPAR. Zileuton, a medication which blocks the activity of 5-lipoxygenase, has been found to be effective in the treatment of acne[43].

Surface proteins from *P. acnes* stimulate IL-8 production by the keratinocytes, through toll-like receptor signaling, and stimulate superoxide anions production via CD36 receptors. Following this, over the next several hours, superoxide anions combine with NO to produce peroxynitrite, and in turn, hydrogen peroxide. These reactive oxygen species help eliminate the bacteria, but also generate inflammation. IL-8 acts as a chemotactic agent that brings neutrophils to the area. These cells release lysosomal enzymes that produce more ROS, causing further damage to the follicular epithelium[44]. This process depletes antioxidants, leading to further oxidation of squalene.

Central to its role in causing acne, the *P. acnes* biofilm produces a glycocalyx polymer that acts as a biologic glue. This allows the bacteria to adhere to follicular walls. Additionally, this polymer mixes with sebum and acts as cement for keratinocytes that have been shed, forming concretions that plug the follicles, creating comedones[45].

Keratinocytes and Inflammation

Keratinocytes are short-lived cells that make up most of the outer layers of skin. These cells are constantly growing and being replaced. In their afterlife, they compose most of the cells in the stratum corneum, the outermost layer of skin, which is slowly shed while being replaced from below.

Keratinocytes are more than just a scaly barrier providing protection. They are part of the skin's immune defense. They hold the Langerhans cells (antigen presenting cells) and lymphocytes in place in the skin, and they help modulate inflammation. Keratinocytes can produce the anti-inflammatory factors IL-10, TGF-β and neutral endopeptidase (NEP). NEP is a cell surface enzyme that degrades several neuropeptides thereby terminating their biologic actions. *P. acnes* are one of the few gram-negative bacteria species known to produce antigens that activate TLR2. TLR2 and TLR4 activation elicit transcription of the inflammatory cytokines TNF-α, IL-1β, and chemokines in keratinocytes, which activate white blood cells and keep them from leaving the area[46,47]. Thus, keratinocytes act as immune regulators in the dermis. Keratinocytes are also shed into the pilosebaceous unit and help to form the sebum, which protects the skin from damage and infection. When cemented together by biofilm glycocalyx, these shed cells can plug in the pilosebaceous unit.

Initially, an acne lesion begins as a non-inflammatory comedo. Bacterial cell walls compounds, bacterial metabolic wastes, byproducts of sebum fermentation, and oxidation products, including oxidized squalene, induce the keratinocytes and other local cells to produce inflammatory cytokines and chemokines. These activate mast cells and draw monocytes to the area, activating them. If the comedo ruptures into the dermis, further inflammation results and a pustule or papule forms.

The neuropeptide, Substance P (SP), has several effects on the skin and sebaceous gland. It stimulates the production of IL-1, IL-6, and TNF-α, all which are proinflammatory. SP also stimulates the production of NEP and PPAR-γ in the sebaceous gland[48], which can thus act as a feedback mechanism to down-regulate inflammation. In acne, however, NEP, which is normally a cell surface enzyme, is limited to the Golgi apparatus of the cells[49]; it does not make its way to the surface, and thus not down regulate neuropeptide-induced inflammation.

In normal, healthy skin, the sebaceous glands are not innervated; they are not under the control of the central or peripheral nervous system. Patients with acne, however, have many fine nerve fibers around the sebaceous glands. Innervation likely results under the influence of nerve growth factor (NGF); induced by IL-6. Recall from Chapter 29 that in chronic stress, such as social stress, NGF stimulates the development of sympathetic innervation to the paracortex area of lymph nodes. Patients with acne have a high density of mast cells in their skin that can release inflammatory mediators, including proinflammatory cytokines and eicosanoids.

During stress, local nerve endings in the skin release CRH[50] and SP[46]; both trigger mast cell degranulation. Individuals with acne have a higher concentration of mast cells in affected areas than do individuals without acne. Additionally, CRH increases the production of melanocortin, which stimulates the production of sebum from the sebaceous gland[51]. The melanocortin, α-MSH, not only induces sebum production but also decreases glutathione, increasing oxidative potential. Patients with acne were found to have lower levels of glutathione in biopsies of normal areas of their skin[52].

Acne is not just a local disease of the skin. Peripheral blood mononuclear cells from patients with acne have lower levels of the anti-inflammatory cytokine IL-10 and elevated levels of IL-8[53], INF-γ, and IL-12p40[54]. Acne is, thus, a systemic inflammatory disease.

Table 36-2 shows several enzymes and vitamins important to control of oxidative stress in patients with acne. The enzymes SOD, glutathione peroxidase, catalase and MAO were all found to be lower in patients with acne. Platelet MAO is considered to correlate well with MAO in the central nervous system and thus suggest cerebral oxidative stress, as well. The anti-oxidant vitamins C, E and β-carotene were all lower in acne patients than controls, and

Table 37-2: Antioxidants and Acne

Compound or Enzyme	Tissue	Levels in Acne Patients as Compared to Controls
Superoxide dismutase (SOD)[55]	Neutrophils	45% lower
Glutathione peroxidase[56]	Unaffected skin	Lower
Xanthine oxidase[57]	Blood	Higher
Superoxide dismutase	Blood	Lower
Catalase (CAT)	Blood	38% lower
Vitamin A[58]	Serum	33% lower
β-Carotene	Serum	64% lower
Vitamin C	Serum	40% lower
Vitamin E	Serum	46% lower
Malondialdehyde[57]	Blood	86% higher
Malondialdehyde	Serum	230% higher
Monoamine Oxidase (MAO)[56]	Platelet	50% lower
Zinc[59]	Serum	Lower

β-carotene levels were depressed further than vitamin A levels in the same set of patients. In a separate study, zinc levels were lower in acne patients. Malondialdehyde is the end-product of oxidation and is considered a good indicator of oxidative stress. It has been found to be elevated in several studies of acne.

In these studies of acne, antioxidant vitamin levels were found to be low. Acne affects over 80% of the age-susceptible population consuming a Western diet. Thus, serum antioxidant vitamin levels, which are considered normal in this population, appear by this measure to be inadequate to prevent acne or provide optimal health.

Antioxidants are important for the prevention of acne as they prevent the peroxidation of squalene. Oxidative stress is also seen in depression[60], and thus, may explain the association of acne with depression.

Treatments Without Scientific Basis

An extensive literature review performed in 2004 found a lack of scientific basis for several often recommended treatments for acne[61]:

Soap and scrubs: Although chlorhexidine soap does improve acne lesions, other soap and scrubs have not been shown to provide benefit. Some commonly used soaps and shampoos have been found to be comedogenic when applied to rabbit ears. Detergents or abrasives may traumatize the skin and exacerbate acne. Cleansing the skin to avoid acne is somewhat like thinking that toilet paper use will prevent stool formation.

Sun or UV-Exposure: There is no medical literature demonstrating that UV therapy or sunlight is beneficial as a treatment for acne. There is a seasonal effect with less acne in the summer months for most patients; however, this could be the effect of vitamin D or seasonal variances in diet, such as the availability of fresh fruits and vegetables, changes in exercise or other factors. Sufficient sun exposure for vitamin D formation (15 minutes a day in the summer) to the torso and legs can be recommended; even then, it is best to avoid sun exposure to the face and other chronically exposed areas to avoid aging and UV exposure. UV light in lab animals tends to be comedogenic as it acts as an oxidant. Sun or UV exposure sufficient to produce redness or sunburn should be avoided anywhere on the body.

Note: Many sunscreens, especially waterproof sunscreens, are comedogenic. Non-comedogenic sunscreens should be used on the face or other areas subject to acne in those prone to comedones or acne.

Avoiding Makeup: Many of the oily compounds that have been used in makeup are comedogenic[62,63]. These include natural ingredients, such as cocoa butter and lanolin. The cosmetic industry has improved in its use of non-comedogenic ingredients over recent years, but not all companies are careful. Well formulated makeup should not increase the risk of acne[21]. A list of comedogenic compounds used in cosmetics is given at the end of this chapter.

The Influence of Diet on Acne

In the 1950's, dermatology textbooks recommended diets and provided food avoidance lists to mitigate acne. These were based only on conventional wisdom, however, and these recommendations were later removed, as they lacked a scientific validation. A few small studies on the effect of food on acne were conducted in the late 1960's, followed by 40 years of neglect on this issue. There have been a few studies on the relationship of certain foods with acne; however, most are not especially useful. Here are some findings: Skim milk[64], potato chips, and diets low in raw vegetables cause acne[10], fried fish and chocolate, desserts and fruit juice may cause acne[65]. This short list of specific foods does not explain but does give clues to how foods might affect acne.

Chocolate and Acne

Chocolate does not cause acne, except when it does. When consumption of dairy free chocolate bars was compared to an equivalent "white chocolate" bar with the same ingredients, other than leaving out the cocoa, white chocolate bars were equally comedogenic[66]. It is not the cocoa. It is other components, perhaps the cocoa butter, which are comedogenic[67].

Milk: The best documented association between food and acne is milk. Milk consumption is associated with increased risk for acne in adolescents. Teenage boys who consumed more than two glasses of whole milk a day were about 10 percent more likely to have acne than those who drank less than one glass a day, but 19 percent more likely if they drank skim milk[68]. Data from the Nurses Health Study similarly found that whole milk consumption was associated with about 12 percent increase in the incidence of severe acne, but that skim milk consumption was associated with a 44 percent increase in risk. Other dairy products, including instant breakfast drink, cottage cheese, and cream cheese, were also positively associated with acne[64]. Skim milk is two to four times more likely to cause acne than whole milk; this might suggest that milk fat (butter) is protective against acne. However, the finding that cream cheese is associated with acne contradicts this. Meanwhile, lactoferrin, a protein in milk whey has been used successfully as at treatment for acne; decreasing the number of inflammatory lesions by 39%[69]. A possible explanation for why whole milk is less comedogenic than skim milk is that butterfat slows gastric emptying. This would slow the rate that milk enters the small intestine, and may limit lactose malabsorption.

Lactose intolerance and lactose overload increase risk for rapid oral-cecal transit time and fermentation of this sugar and other nutrients, resulting in dysbiosis. This can trigger T_H17 dominated immune response that may directly or indirectly increase the risk for acne. In SIBO, there is an increase of mast cells in the intestinal mucosa, paralleling the increase of mast cells in the skin of patients with acne. SIBO also increases circulating inflammatory cytokines.

Lactose intolerance, itself, may be caused by damage to the enterocytes and can be associated with malabsorption of other nutrients. These may include loss of essential nutrients, particularly the fat-soluble vitamins (A, D, E, and K), magnesium, zinc, folate, vitamin B_{12} and other nutrients. At least three, and probably all four, fat-soluble vitamins protect against acne. SIBO is often associated with malabsorption of vitamins and minerals and is associated with depression[70]. Malabsorption can also cause loss of steroid hormones, which normally undergo enterohepatic circulation, and thus may cause imbalances in sex hormones. Fruit juices may also be associated with carbohydrate (fructose) malabsorption, which can increase the risk for SIBO and nutrient loss. In a study of over 13,000 adolescents, sebaceous gland disorders, including acne and rosacea were highly correlated with gastrointestinal symptoms including halitosis, gastric reflux, abdominal bloating and constipation[71].

Few studies have explored the relationship of acne to intestinal pathology. Reactivity to the bacterial endotoxin LPS from E. coli was found in 65% of patients with acne but was rare in controls[72]. LPS reactivity suggests increased intestinal paracellular permeability. Dysbiosis has been found in the majority of patients with acne[73]. Probiotics have been found to be helpful in acne[69].

IgG Immunogenicity and acne: No studies have yet been conducted to assess the relationship of IgG immunogenicity to foods and acne. However, I have had patients with known IgG antergens to foods report flares of acne after consuming known antergens.

> **EYE MITES: Blepharitis and Rosacea**
>
> Propionibacterium is not the only organism to live in the pilosebaceous unit. There are parasitic tiny mites: microscopic arthropods, related to ticks, also like to live on sebum in the hair follicles and meibomian glands. These are *Demodex*; two species that live in the follicles and on the eyelids. About 20 percent of human adults have these bugs living in their skin[74].
>
> One species lives in the eyelash follicle and causes chronic blepharitis, causing reddened lid margins and crusting. The other lives in the meibomian gland on the inner edge of the eyelid and can cause posterior blepharitis and dry eyes, leading to keratoconjunctivitis[75]. These creepy creatures crawl out of the follicles, have sex on your eyelashes, right in front of your eyes while you sleep at night, and then return into the follicle to lay eggs and feed on sebum. *Demodex* induce an inflammatory reaction that increases cytokine levels in the tear film[76]. The immune response to this parasite behaves more like a reaction to enteric bacteria, with an elevated IL-17 level, rather than that expected from an arthropod. Indeed, it may represent an inflammatory response to the bacteria that *Demodex* carries in its gut and to the excrement it deposits in the follicle, rather than to the parasite itself[75,77,78].
>
> *Demodex* mites are also a cause of acne rosacea[79]. Small intestinal bacterial overgrowth (SIBO) is found in nearly half of patients with rosacea; about nine times more frequently than in control patients[80]. Immune activity in patients with SIBO would be expected to be dominated by T_H17 cells in these patients, which may explain a heightened IL-17 immune response to *Demodex* infestation.
>
> Tea tree oil (5%) has been used to eliminate Demodex in rosacea[81] and for blepharitis; this treatment of blepharitis caused a decline in IL-17 and IL-1β in the tear film[82]. Tea tree oil is also helpful in acne vulgaris[83].
>
> GI immune function may prime the sebaceous glands for an inflammatory response to *Demodex* in blepharitis and rosacea. Blepharitis and rosacea should be considered to be enteroimmunopathies and investigated as such.

N-6/N-3 Fatty Acids

Another clue food is potato chips. Perhaps no other food has such a high ratio of saturated and trans fats to total calories. Potato chips usually are made with vegetable fats high in linoleic acid, an n-6 fatty acid. But who eats chips alone? Other high caloric, fatty foods and high fructose beverages usually accompany them in.

The finding that zileuton treats and prevents acne reinforces the observation that acne is prevalent in populations that consume a high n-6 fat diet. Dietary N-6 fats, mainly linoleic acid (LA), are converted into AA acid and incorporated into triglycerides and phospholipids in the cell membranes. Dietary n-3 fats, α-linolenic acid (ALA), EPA and DHA are incorporated into triglycerides and phospholipids, which also end up in the sebum. In natural diets, there are both lesser amounts of n-6 fats and lower n-6:n-3 fat ratios; this decreases the inflammatory reaction in response to the liberation of fatty acids. The ratio of n-6 to n-3 fatty acid consumption is about 10:1 in the typical American diet[84] while a ratio less than 2.5:1 would have been found in most pre-industrialized diets. As explained in Chapters 6 and 10, it is not just the ratio, but also the amount of n-6 fat consumed that determines the production of AA and the sphingolipids formed by the body. As a corollary to acne, women who consume higher amounts of ALA (n-3) and lower amounts of LA (n-6) are less likely to suffer from depression[85].

The n-3 fatty acids ALA and EPA are precursors for eicosatetraenoic acid (20:4 n-3) which competes with AA for the formation of eicosanoids. The eicosatetraenoic acid eicosanoid products are non-inflammatory, in contrast to those made from AA. In an eight-week trial, an EPA supplement combination (1000 mg EPA per day) decreased both the number and severity of acne lesions[27]. AA promoted inflammatory eicosanoids; n-3 fatty acids do not. (See Chapter 6, Figure 6-3). The effect of zileuton on acne is a clear indication of the role of AA in acnes pathogenesis.

Vitamin A and β-Carotene

Vitamin A deficiency is associated with night blindness due to the incorporation of retinal in visual pigment. Vitamin A deficiency also causes hyperkeratosis. In the eye, glands that normally produce mucus, to lubricate the eye, produce keratinized epithelium in vitamin A deficiency. In the place of a lubricant, keratin debris enters the eye, causing dry eyes, and eventually, corneal erosions. A similar process can also occur along the mucous membranes. Vitamin A deficiency causes hyperkeratosis in the sebaceous gland, which contributes to plugging and comedo formation. Retinoic acid regulates over 300 genes in the keratinocyte including those involved in the cell cycle and apoptosis[86].

Retinoids; analogs of vitamin A, are among the most effective medications for acne. These drugs are not without toxic side effects, but neither is vitamin A, which is too toxic for use a medication at doses effective for acne[87]. Synthetic analogs of retinoids are also more stable, and thus, longer acting, may be easier to dose, less toxic, and may be less expensive[88]. Retinoic acid, retinol, and the synthetic analog isotretinoin block the production of IL-8 by keratinocytes and decrease their production of ROS[89].

No other vitamin has such a narrow range of normal levels between that required to avoid deficiency and that which causes toxicity, as does vitamin A. Excess vitamin A can easily induce teratogenic effects on embryos, including major alterations in organogenesis. It may be more practical to consider β-carotene as the vitamin and the retinols as hormones. The body converts dietary β-carotene into vitamin A, and this feedback mechanism limits the amount of vitamin A produced[90].

β-carotene absorption requires bile acid and active transport by SCARB1, a brush border surface membrane protein. In the enterocyte, β-carotene is then enzymatically cleaved into two molecules of retinal (vitamin A$_1$), and then to retinol, and to retinyl ester by the enzyme lecithin retinol acyltransferase. The enterocyte also produces retinal binding protein-2. Retinyl ester is then packaged into chylomicrons with the other fat-soluble vitamins (D, E and K), and released from the enterocyte by exocytosis for transport through the bloodstream to different parts of the body for usage and storage[91]. β-carotene requires intact enterocytes for absorption.

Although preformed vitamin A is more easily absorbed and potentially toxic in the stable retinyl ester form, it requires pancreatic lipase and phospholipase for absorption.

Zinc

Zinc is required for absorption of vitamin A. Low serum zinc levels increase the severity of vitamin A deficiency. Zinc is also a required cofactor for the enzyme ALDH, which converts retinol into the hormone retinoic acid (RA). RA is the active hormone form of vitamin A that is responsible for most of its actions. The enzyme ALDH also prevents excess accumulation of vitamin A[92]. Zinc is thus needed for vitamin A to act efficiently.

Zinc deficiency has been found to be associated with acne, particularly with severe acne[93]. Zinc supplements have been found to decrease the number of lesions and decrease the number of inflammatory nodules, with improvement seen within 21 days, using 30 mg of zinc in the form of zinc gluconate[94, 95]. Topical zinc has also been shown to help in the treatment of acne. Although several studies show good results with zinc, some patients respond more than others[95]. This variance likely results from differences in the underlying pathology; if the zinc is provided to individuals with acne and zinc deficiency; the treatment is much more likely to be effective. It usually requires only about four weeks of treatment to normalize zinc levels[96]. Low zinc (and magnesium) levels are highly correlated with mood disorders[97].

Zinc is known to be a cofactor for nearly 300 enzymes and helps to stabilize the 3-dimensional structures of hundreds of proteins. Zinc modulates antibody synthesis, activation of T-cells and is required by proteins in the tight junctions of the intestinal mucosa. Zinc decreases the expression of Toll-like receptor 2 (TLR2) in keratinocytes, which is induced by P. acnes[98, 99]. TLR2 activates the inflammatory mediator IL-8. Nicotinamide, a form of vitamin B$_3$, inhibits TLR2 induced activation of IL-8[100] and may be helpful in the treatment of acne. The antioxidant α-lipoic acid decreases the transcription of TLR2 and decreases the activation of NF-κB in keratinocytes[101]. Glucocorticoids, in contrast, increase the expression of TLR2 in keratinocytes[102].

Zinc deficits may increase intestinal hyperpermeability, another possible risk factor for acne.

Boron

Boron is an essential trace nutrient which affects the metabolism of steroid hormones, including vitamin D. Boron is required for the conversion of estrogen to its most potent form, 17-beta-estradiol, and boron raises the estradiol/testosterone ratio[103]. Additionally, it increases free testosterone levels and the levels of the active form of vitamin D; 1,25-OH D$_3$[104]. Boron may help stabilize cis-diol forms of steroid molecules[105]. This suggests that estrogen would be favored over estrone, and Δ5-androstenediol, a precursor of testosterone, would be favored over dehydroepiandrosterone in the presence of sufficient boron. Dehydroepiandrosterone is associated with acne and polycystic ovary syndrome[34]. Adequate boron is known to increase testosterone levels. Nevertheless, boron also favors the conversion of DHT, the most potent androgen, into the estrogenic metabolite 3β-androstenediol and perhaps into the inactive metabolites 3α-androstenediol. Consumption of adequate dietary boron may prevent acne lesion as it helps normalize steroid hormone activity with decreased androgenic effect through enhanced elimination of DHT and by increasing vitamin D activity.

In a cross-over study of postmenopausal women given first a low boron diet (0.25 mg/day), followed by one with adequate boron (3.25 mg/day) there was a 36% reduction in urinary calcium excretion, a 43% reduction in urinary magnesium excretion, and serum 17β-estradiol and serum testosterone levels more than doubled[106].

In lab animals, dietary boron improves the absorption of calcium, phosphorus, and magnesium, likely an indirect effect, secondary to its effect on the steroid hormones[107]. Boron also increased bone strength in animals[108]. Boron increased insulin sensitivity in an animal model[109] and prevented oxidative damage caused by some heavy metals in vitro[110].

The boron content in food depends on the boron content of the soil in which the plants are grown. The best dietary sources of boron include fruits, tubers, and legumes. Avocados, peanuts, prunes, grapes, pecans, raisins, and cocoa are among best sources. Potatoes and coffee also contain boron, but grains, oils, animal flesh, and sweets have minimal amounts. Milk and milk products have moderate amounts of boron. Vegetarians usually have higher intakes of boron. With the exception of dairy; plants are the principal source of boron in the diet[111]. An appropriate dietary intake of boron is about 2 mg for every 1000 kcal.

The upper tolerable intake of boron is 20 mg per day in adults who are not lactating or pregnant, 17 mg/day for adolescents and women who are pregnant or breastfeeding female and one mg per day per year of age for children 1 to 14[112].

Other Micronutrients

The levels of antioxidant vitamins C and E levels have been found to be low in patients with acne. Vitamin D may be comedolytic. Vitamin D helps regulate the sebaceous gland and keratinocyte differentiation[113], protects the skin from UV damage, modulates inflammation, and may play a role in the prevention of acne[114]. PQQ is a powerful dietary antioxidant found in vegetables and fruit. (See chapter 28 for more on PQQ.) Carotenoids, such as lutein and zeaxanthin, also protect the skin from UV damage.

Several polyphenol compounds have been demonstrated to have efficacy in reducing acne: salicylic acid[115], green tea extract[116], resveratrol[117], kaempferol, and quercetin[118].

The sphingolipid phytosphingosine is present in the skin. Here, it stimulates the differentiation of keratinocytes[119] and has anti-acne[120] and anti-inflammatory[121] effects. Dietary sources of phytosphingosine and phytoceramide include fruits, vegetables, and fungi. Phytosphingosine and phytoceramide were discussed in Chapter 9, as they decrease serum cholesterol, improve glucose tolerance, stimulate PPARγ, help regulate heat shock protein induction of ubiquitination, and have an anti-inflammatory effect by inhibiting NF-κB signaling.

Summary

Acne is highly prevalent in industrialized societies, but rare in pre-industrialized societies. It has been associated with consumption of a palatable, low-fiber diet, high in refined carbohydrates and fats. It may not be so much what is eaten, rather than what is not. It is unlikely for a refined diet to provide the diversity and content of micronutrients found in a healthy diet.

Fruits and vegetables contain micronutrients, such as boron, PQQ, polyphenols and other nutritional compounds that are unlikely to be found in a vitamin tablet. Prebiotics that support healthful intestinal microbiota are often scarce in the palatable and high-fat Western diet. It is difficult to get sufficient micronutrients in the diet when a majority of the caloric intake is from fat and refined sugars. Perhaps most importantly, the western diet also contains high levels of n-6 fats that are proinflammatory, and which contribute to the formation of LTB_4.

Sympathetic activation promotes innervation of the pilosebaceous unit and associated mast and other immune cells in the skin. Stress can trigger an inflammatory reaction and a new crop of acne lesions. Biofilm formation is required for the formation of the comedo. Androgens increase the production of sebum, and dihydrotestosterone supports the formation of an inflammatory response with increased production of TNF-α and IL-6.

Dysbiosis and T_H17 gastrointestinal immune function may also help explain acne. Oxidative stress results from immune reactions in the skin and elsewhere in the body, depleting antioxidants. Polyphenols, carotenoids, PQQ, vitamins C, and vitamin E are dietary antioxidants that help protect the sebum from oxidative stress and the ensuing inflammation. Vitamin A is helpful in acne but is easily toxic. With appropriate zinc and β-carotene intake, there should be adequate conversion provision of retinoic acid. Malabsorption of sugars and intestinal fermentation of nutrients can easily cause loss of availability of micronutrients and may alter the body's balance of steroid hormones.

Acne and depression share at least oxidative stress, high n-3 fats, and inflammation as etiological influences. Acne is a microcosm of health worn on the face. If there is acne on the outside, there is likely inflammation and oxidative stress elsewhere. Anxiety, depression, and anger, gastrointestinal symptoms and polycystic ovary syndrome are common comorbidities of acne. They have common etiologies and share preventive treatments.

Secondary Treatment of Acne

1. Treat intestinal dysbiosis and avoid poorly absorbed sugars: Malabsorption should be investigated, at least in those individuals with acne who have symptoms consistent with GI disturbances or food sensitivities. Avoid the consumption of sweet beverages, including soda pop, fruit juices, and skin milk. Sugar malabsorption is discussed in Chapter 5. Intestinal dysbiosis is discussed in Chapter 23.

Biofilm in the pilosebaceous unit depends upon the oxidation of sebum and squalene in the SSL. Biofilm development can be prevented with certain antibiotics (erythromycin) but also with salicylic acid, both which are used to treat acne.

2. Consume a diet high in vegetables and fruits: Vegetables and fruits are likely to provide adequate minerals and micronutrients including boron, zinc, PQQ, tocotrienols and vitamin C. Flavonoids, which have been demonstrated to inhibit ALOX-5 are listed in Tables 15-4 and 15-6 in Chapter 15. Many plant phenols inhibit TNF-α and other inflammatory cytokines (Table 31-2).

3. Avoid Inflammation and Oxidative stress: While mitochondrial dysfunction seems unlikely in the prime ages for acne, there is certainly sufficient evidence that this is a disease of oxidative stress. This suggests the dietary deficiencies may be present although increased demand from increased oxidative damage may also play a role. Antioxidant vitamins and supplements, such as N-acetyl cysteine and r-α-lipoic acid may be helpful, especially if the diet is deficient or there is inflammatory stress. Sub-antimicrobial dose doxycycline, which blocks TLR2 signaling, may be helpful (See Chapter 43).

Food immunogenicities may increase inflammatory cytokines, and increase mast cell activation in the skin. IgG testing for food immunogens that cause antergies may be helpful (Chapter 19).

4: Stress and sleep deprivation: Sleep deprivation and stress are triggers for inflammatory acne lesions. These factors increase inflammatory cytokines. Chapter 29 discusses stress reduction; Chapter 42 discusses sleep.

5. Limit n-6 fat intake: Increase intake of EPA and DHA (see Chapter 9)

6. Treat vitamin and mineral deficiencies. Deficiencies may arise as a result of:

- Inadequate dietary intake,
- Loss through malabsorption, or
- Depletion, as in the case of antioxidants from acute of chronic inflammation
- Insufficient sun exposure to form vitamin D

Supplements can be helpful over a short term, especially to speed recovery, but underlying causes should be addressed.

Vitamin C:	60 to 100 mg/day
Vitamin E:	10 mg/day (as mixed-tocotrienols)
Zinc:	10 to 15 mg/day
Boron:	6 mg/day
Vitamin D:	5000 IU/day
β-Carotene	6000 μg/day in oil (10,000 units)
R-α- lipoic acid	50 - 100 mg/day
N-acetyl cysteine	500 mg/day

Vitamin A supplements are not advised for the treatment acne, as vitamin A has a narrow therapeutic range and is toxic at high doses. Vitamin A supplements should not be used in individuals taking retinoid analogs, such as isotretinoin (Accutane) or similar medications. See Chapter 39 on supplements for vitamin A cautions and data on other supplements.

7. Avoid topical creams and cosmetics that are comedogenic.

The rabbit external ear canal has been used as a model to test chemicals that may cause comedo formation on topical application. Some of the tested ingredients are in currently used in topically applied formulations.

Comedogenic compounds used in cosmetics[62, 63]:

1. isopropyl palmitate
2. isopropyl myristate
3. butyl stearate
4. isopropyl isostearate
5. decyl oleate
6. isostearyl neopentanoate
7. isocetyl stearate
8. myristyl myristate
9. cocoa butter
10. octyl stearate
11. octyl palmitate
12. propylene glycol-2 (PPG-2)
13. lanolin

D&C Red dyes (xanthenes (D&C Red 19, 22, 27, 28, 40), monoazoanilines (D&C Red 4, 6, 7, 8, 9, 31.33, 34, 36), fluorans (D&C Red 21, 27), and indigoids D&C 30)

[1] Prevalence of facial acne in adults. Goulden V, Stables GI, Cunliffe WJ. J Am Acad Dermatol. 1999 Oct;41(4):577-80. PMID:10495379

[2] Prevalence of facial acne vulgaris in late adolescence and in adults. Cunliffe WJ, Gould DJ. Br Med J. 1979 Apr 28;1(6171):1109-10. PMID:156054

[3] Acne vulgaris: a disease of Western civilization. Cordain L, Lindeberg S, Hurtado M, Hill K, Eaton SB, Brand-Miller J. Arch Dermatol. 2002 Dec;138(12):1584-90. PMID:12472346

[4] Acne and diet: truth or myth? Costa A, Lage D, Moisés TA. An Bras Dermatol. 2010 Jun;85(3):346-53. PMID:20676468

[5] Acne, anxiety, depression and suicide in teenagers: a cross-sectional survey of New Zealand secondary school students. Purvis D, Robinson E, Merry S, Watson P. J Paediatr Child Health. 2006 Dec;42(12):793-6. PMID:17096715

[6] Psychosocial Aspects of Acne Vulgaris: A Community-based Study with Korean Adolescents. Do JE, Cho SM, In SI, Lim KY, Lee S, Lee ES. Ann Dermatol. 2009 May;21(2):125-9. PMID:20523769

[7] Anger and acne: implications for quality of life, patient satisfaction and clinical care. Rapp DA, Brenes GA, Feldman SR, Fleischer AB Jr, Graham GF, Dailey M, Rapp SR. Br J Dermatol. 2004 Jul;151(1):183-9. PMID:15270889

[8] Social sensitivity and acne: the role of personality in negative social consequences and quality of life. Krejci-Manwaring J, Kerchner K, Feldman SR, Rapp DA, Rapp SR. Int J Psychiatry Med. 2006;36(1):121-30. PMID:16927583

[9] Acne vulgaris and depression: a retrospective examination. Uhlenhake E, Yentzer BA, Feldman SR. J Cosmet Dermatol. 2010 Mar;9(1):59-63. PMID:20367674

[10] Is the association between acne and mental distress influenced by diet? Results from a cross-sectional population study among 3775 late adolescents in Oslo, Norway. Halvorsen JA, Dalgard F, Thoresen M, Bjertness E, Lien L. BMC Public Health. 2009 Sep 16;9:340. PMID:19758425

[11] Psychosocial impact of acne vulgaris; evaluation of the relation between a change in clinical acne severity and psychosocial state. Mulder MM, Sigurdsson V, van Zuuren EJ, et al. Dermatology. 2001;203(2):124-30. PMID:11586010

[12] The effects of high-dose and low-dose tryptophan depletion on mood and cognitive functions of remitted depressed patients. Booij L, Van der Does AJ, Haffmans PM, et al. J Psychopharmacol. 2005 May;19(3):267-75. PMID:15888512

[13] The effects of experimentally lowered serotonin function on emotional information processing and memory in remitted depressed patients. Merens W, Booij L, Haffmans PJ, van der Does A. J Psychopharmacol. 2008 Aug;22(6):653-62. PMID:18308809

[14] Retinoic acid and affective disorders: the evidence for an association. Bremner JD, Shearer KD, McCaffery PJ. J Clin Psychiatry. 2011 Aug 23. PMID:21903028

[15] Isotretinoin and the risk of depression in patients with acne vulgaris: a case-crossover study. Azoulay L, Blais L, Koren G, LeLorier J, Bérard A. J Clin Psychiatry. 2008 Apr;69(4):526-32. PMID:18363422

[16] Isotretinoin has no negative effect on attention, executive function and mood. Ergun T, Seckin D, Ozaydin N, et al. J Eur Acad Dermatol Venereol. 2011 May 4. PMID:21545542

[17] Comparison of depression, anxiety and life quality in acne vulgaris patients who were treated with either isotretinoin or topical agents. Kaymak Y, Taner E, Taner Y. Int J Dermatol. 2009 Jan;48(1):41-6. PMID:19126049

[18] No association found between patients receiving isotretinoin for acne and the development of depression in a Canadian prospective cohort. Cohen J, Adams S, Patten S. Can J Clin Pharmacol. 2007 Summer;14(2):e227-33. PMID:17556790

[19] Comparison of depression, anxiety and life quality in acne vulgaris patients who were treated with either isotretinoin or topical agents. Kaymak Y, Taner E, Taner Y. Int J Dermatol. 2009 Jan;48(1):41-6. PMID:19126049

[20] Depression and suicidal behavior in acne patients treated with isotretinoin: a systematic review. Marqueling AL, Zane LT. Semin Cutan Med Surg. 2007 Dec;26(4):210-20. PMID:1839566

[21] Make-up improves the quality of life of acne patients without aggravating acne eruptions during treatments. Hayashi N, Imori M, Yanagisawa M, Seto Y, Nagata O, Kawashima M. Eur J Dermatol. 2005 Jul-Aug;15(4):284-7. PMID:16048760

[22] A multicenter epidemiological study of acne vulgaris in Korea. Suh DH, Kim BY, Min SU, et al. Int J Dermatol. 2011 Jun;50(6):673-81. PMID:21595660

[23] Zoloft Prescribing Information: http://labeling.pfizer.com/ShowLabeling.aspx?id=517

[24] Wellbutrin SR Prescribing Information: http://us.gsk.com/products/assets/us_wellbutrinSR.pdf

[25] Improvement of acne in depressed patients treated with paroxetine. Moussavian H. J Am Acad Child Adolesc Psychiatry. 2001 May;40(5):505-6. PMID:11349692

[26] Psychogenic excoriation responding to fluoxetine: a case report. Sharma H. J Indian Med Assoc. 2008 Apr;106(4):245, 262. PMID:18828345

[27] Acne vulgaris, mental health and omega-3 fatty acids: a report of cases. Rubin MG, Kim K, Logan AC. Lipids Health Dis. 2008 Oct 13;7:36. PMID:18851733

[28] Community-based epidemiological study of psychosocial effects of acne in Japanese adolescents. Kubota Y, Shirahige Y, Nakai K, et al. J Dermatol. 2010 Jul;37(7):617-22. PMID:20629827

[29] Prevalence and risk factors of facial acne vulgaris among Chinese adolescents. Wu TQ, Mei SQ, Zhang JX, et al. Int J Adolesc Med Health. 2007 Oct-Dec;19(4):407-12. PMID:18348416

[30] Coping with acne: beliefs and perceptions in a sample of secondary school Greek pupils. Rigopoulos D, Gregoriou S, Ifandi A, et al. J Eur Acad Dermatol Venereol. 2007 Jul;21(6):806-10. PMID:17567312

[31] The response of skin disease to stress: changes in the severity of acne vulgaris as affected by examination stress. Chiu A, Chon SY, Kimball AB. Arch Dermatol. 2003 Jul;139(7):897-900. PMID:12873885

[32] Pre-examination stress in second year medical students in a government college. Rizvi AH, Awaiz M, Ghanghro Z, Jafferi MA, Aziz S. J Ayub Med Coll Abbottabad. 2010 Apr-Jun;22(2):152-5. PMID:21702291

[33] Effect of dihydrotestosterone on the upregulation of inflammatory cytokines in cultured sebocytes. Lee WJ, Jung HD, Chi SG, Kim BS, Lee SJ, Kim do W, Kim MK, Kim JC. Arch Dermatol Res. 2010 Aug;302(6):429-33. PMID:20043171

[34] High serum dehydroepiandrosterone sulfate is associated with phenotypic acne and a reduced risk of abdominal obesity in women with polycystic ovary syndrome. Chen MJ, Chen CD, Yang JH, et al. Hum Reprod. 2011 Jan;26(1):227-34. PMID:21088016

[35] Correlation between serum levels of insulin-like growth factor 1, dehydroepiandrosterone sulfate, and dihydrotestosterone and acne lesion counts in adult women. Cappel M, Mauger D, Thiboutot D. Arch Dermatol. 2005 Mar;141(3):333-8. PMID:15781674

[36] Biological and pharmacological activities of squalene and related compounds: potential uses in cosmetic dermatology. Huang ZR, Lin YK, Fang JY. Molecules. 2009 Jan 23;14(1):540-54. PMID:19169201

[37] Surface lipids as multifunctional mediators of skin responses to environmental stimuli. De Luca C, Valacchi G. Mediators Inflamm. 2010;2010:321494. PMID:20981292

[38] Lipid mediators in acne. Ottaviani M, Camera E, Picardo M. Mediators Inflamm. 2010;2010. pii: 858176. PMID:20871834

[39] Peroxisome proliferator-activated receptor activators protect sebocytes from apoptosis: a new treatment modality for acne? Schuster M, Zouboulis CC, Ochsendorf F, et al. Br J Dermatol. 2011 Jan;164(1):182-6. PMID:21091942

[40] A possible role for squalene in the pathogenesis of acne. II. In vivo study of squalene oxides in skin surface and intra-comedonal lipids of acne patients. Saint-Leger D, Bague A, Lefebvre E, Cohen E, Chivot M. Br J Dermatol. 1986 May;114(5):543-52. PMID:2941050

[41] Biofilms in skin infections: Propionibacterium acnes and acne vulgaris. Coenye T, Honraet K, Rossel B, Nelis HJ. Infect Disord Drug Targets. 2008 Sep;8(3):156-9. PMID:18782032

[42] Biofilm formation by Propionibacterium acnes is associated with increased resistance to antimicrobial agents and increased production of putative virulence factors. Coenye T, Peeters E, Nelis HJ. Res Microbiol. 2007 May;158(4):386-92. PMID:17399956

[43] Zileuton, a new efficient and safe systemic anti-acne drug. Zouboulis CC. Dermatoendocrinol. 2009 May;1(3):188-92. PMID:20436887

[44] Production of superoxide anions by keratinocytes initiates P. acnes-induced inflammation of the skin. Grange PA, Chéreau C, Raingeaud J, Nicco C, Weill B, Dupin N, Batteux F. PLoS Pathog. 2009 Jul;5(7):e1000527. PMID:19629174

[45] Expanding the microcomedone theory and acne therapeutics: Propionibacterium acnes biofilm produces biological glue that holds corneocytes together to form plug. Burkhart CG, Burkhart CN. J Am Acad Dermatol. 2007 Oct;57(4):722-4. PMID:17870436

[46] Neuropeptides and sebaceous glands. Toyoda M, Nakamura M, Morohashi M. Eur J Dermatol. 2002 Sep-Oct;12(5):422-7. PMID:12370127

[47] Induction of toll-like receptors by Propionibacterium acnes. Jugeau S, Tenaud I, Knol AC, et al. Br J Dermatol. 2005 Dec;153(6):1105-13. PMID:16307644

[48] Influence of substance-P on cultured sebocytes. Lee WJ, Jung HD, Lee HJ, Kim BS, Lee SJ, Kim do W. Arch Dermatol Res. 2008 Jul;300(6):311-6. Epub 2008 Apr 22. PMID:18427822

[49] Sebaceous glands in acne patients express high levels of neutral endopeptidase. Toyoda M, Nakamura M, Makino T, Kagoura M, Morohashi M. Exp Dermatol. 2002 Jun;11(3):241-7. PMID:12102663

[50] Acne and sebaceous gland function. Zouboulis CC. Clin Dermatol. 2004 Sep-Oct;22(5):360-6. PMID:15556719

[51] Melanocortin-5 receptor and sebogenesis. Zhang L, Li WH, Anthonavage M, Pappas A, Rossetti D, Cavender D, Seiberg M, Eisinger M. Eur J Pharmacol. 2011 Jun 11;660(1):202-6. PMID:21215742

[52] Decrease in glutathione may be involved in pathogenesis of acne vulgaris. Ikeno H, Tochio T, Tanaka H, Nakata S. J Cosmet Dermatol. 2011 Sep;10(3):240-4. PMID:21896138

[53] Interleukin-10 secretion from CD14+ peripheral blood mononuclear cells is downregulated in patients with acne vulgaris. Caillon F, O'Connell M, Eady EA, et al. Br J Dermatol. 2010 Feb 1;162(2):296-303. PMID:19796181

[54] Increased interferon-gamma, interleukin-12p40 and IL-8 production in Propionibacterium acnes-treated peripheral blood mononuclear cells from patient with acne vulgaris: host response but not bacterial species is the determinant factor of the disease. Sugisaki H, Yamanaka K, Kakeda M, et al. J Dermatol Sci. 2009 Jul;55(1):47-52. PMID:19375895

[55] Superoxide dismutase and myeloperoxidase activities in polymorphonuclear leukocytes in acne vulgaris. Kurutas EB, Arican O, Sasmaz S. Acta Dermatovenerol Alp Panonica Adriat. 2005 Jun;14(2):39-42. PMID: 16001098

[56] The role of the antioxidative defense system in papulopustular acne. Basak PY, Gultekin F, Kilinc I. J Dermatol. 2001 Mar;28(3):123-7. PMID:11349462

[57] Oxidative stress in acne vulgaris. Sarici G, Cinar S, Armutcu F, Altinyazar C, Koca R, Tekin NS. J Eur Acad Dermatol Venereol. 2010 Jul;24(7):763-7. PMID:19943837

[58] Oxidant/antioxidant status in obese adolescent females with acne vulgaris. Abulnaja KO. Indian J Dermatol. 2009;54(1):36-40. PMID:20049267

[59] Serum zinc in acne vulgaris. Amer M, Bahgat MR, Tosson Z, Abdel Mowla MY, Amer K. Int J Dermatol. 1982 Oct;21(8):481-4. PMID:6217164

[60] Major depressive disorder is accompanied with oxidative stress: short-term antidepressant treatment does not alter oxidative-antioxidative systems. Sarandol A, Sarandol E, Eker SS, et al. Hum Psychopharmacol. 2007 Mar;22(2):67-73. PMID:17299810

[61] A systematic review of the evidence for 'myths and misconceptions' in acne management: diet, face-washing and

sunlight. Magin P, Pond D, Smith W, Watson A. Fam Pract. 2005 Feb;22(1):62-70. PMID:15644386

[62] Comedogenicity of current therapeutic products, cosmetics, and ingredients in the rabbit ear. Fulton JE Jr, Pay SR, Fulton JE 3rd. J Am Acad Dermatol. 1984 Jan;10(1):96-105. PMID:6229554

[63] Comedogenicity in rabbit: some cosmetic ingredients/vehicles. Nguyen SH, Dang TP, Maibach HI. Cutan Ocul Toxicol. 2007;26(4):287-92. PMID:18058303

[64] High school dietary dairy intake and teenage acne. Adebamowo CA, Spiegelman D, Danby FW, Frazier AL, Willett WC, Holmes MD. J Am Acad Dermatol. 2005 Feb;52(2):207-14. PMID:15692464

[65] An investigation of the association between diet and occurrence of acne: a rational approach from a traditional Chinese medicine perspective. Law MP, Chuh AA, Molinari N, Lee A. Clin Exp Dermatol. 2010 Jan;35(1):31-5. PMID:19549242

[66] Effect of chocolate on acne vulgaris. Fulton JE Jr, Plewig G, Kligman AM. JAMA. 1969 Dec 15;210(11):2071-4. PMID:4243053

[67] Comedogenicity in rabbit: some cosmetic ingredients/vehicles. Nguyen SH, Dang TP, Maibach HI. Cutan Ocul Toxicol. 2007;26(4):287-92. PMID:18058303

[68] Milk consumption and acne in teenaged boys. Adebamowo CA, Spiegelman D, Berkey CS, et al. J Am Acad Dermatol. 2008 May;58(5):787-93. PMID:18194824

[69] Dietary effect of lactoferrin-enriched fermented milk on skin surface lipid and clinical improvement of acne vulgaris. Kim J, Ko Y, Park YK, et al. Nutrition. 2010 Sep;26(9):902-9. PMID:20692602

[70] State and trait anxiety and depression in patients affected by gastrointestinal diseases: psychometric evaluation of 1641 patients referred to an internal medicine outpatient setting. Addolorato G, Mirijello A, D'Angelo C, et al. Int J Clin Pract. 2008 Jul;62(7):1063-9. PMID:18422970

[71] Risk factors for sebaceous gland diseases and their relationship to gastrointestinal dysfunction in Han adolescents. Zhang H, Liao W, Chao W, Chen Q, Zeng H, Wu C, Wu S, Ho HI. J Dermatol. 2008 Sep;35(9):555-61. PMID:18837699

[72] Acne vulgaris, probiotics and the gut-brain-skin axis - back to the future? Bowe WP, Logan AC. Gut Pathog. 2011 Jan 31;3(1):1. PMID:21281494

[73] [Impact of the impaired intestinal microflora on the course of acne vulgaris]. Volkova LA, Khalif IL, Kabanova IN. Klin Med (Mosk). 2001;79(6):39-41. Russian. PMID:11525176

[74] Risk factors and prevalence of Demodex mites in young adults. Horváth A, Neubrandt DM, Ghidán Á, Nagy K. Acta Microbiol Immunol Hung. 2011 Jun;58(2):145-55. PMID:21715284

[75] Pathogenic role of Demodex mites in blepharitis. Liu J, Sheha H, Tseng SC. Curr Opin Allergy Clin Immunol. 2010 Oct;10(5):505-10. PMID:20689407

[76] Tear cytokines and chemokines in patients with Demodex blepharitis. Kim JT, Lee SH, Chun YS, Kim JC. Cytokine. 2011 Jan;53(1):94-9. PMID:21050771

[77] Correlation between ocular Demodex infestation and serum immunoreactivity to Bacillus proteins in patients with Facial rosacea. Li J, O'Reilly N, Sheha H, Katz R, Raju VK, Kavanagh K, Tseng SC. Ophthalmology. 2010 May;117(5):870-877.e1. PMID:20079929

[78] What is the importance of Demodex folliculorum in Behçet's disease? Emre S, Aycan OM, Atambay M, Bilak S, Daldal N, Karincaoglu Y. Turkiye Parazitol Derg. 2009;33(2):158-61. PMID:19598094

[79] Retrospective analysis of the association between Demodex infestation and rosacea. Zhao YE, Wu LP, Peng Y, Cheng H. Arch Dermatol. 2010 Aug;146(8):896-902. PMID:20713824

[80] Small intestinal bacterial overgrowth in rosacea: clinical effectiveness of its eradication. Parodi A, Paolino S, Greco A, et al. Clin Gastroenterol Hepatol. 2008 Jul;6(7):759-64. PMID:18456568

[81] Pathogenic role of Demodex mites in blepharitis. Liu J, Sheha H, Tseng SC. Curr Opin Allergy Clin Immunol. 2010 Oct;10(5):505-10. PMID:20689407

[82] Clinical and immunological responses in ocular demodecosis. Kim JH, Chun YS, Kim JC. J Korean Med Sci. 2011 Sep;26(9):1231-7. PMID:21935281

[83] The efficacy of 5% topical tea tree oil gel in mild to moderate acne vulgaris: a randomized, double-blind placebo-controlled study. Enshaieh S, Jooya A, Siadat AH, Iraji F. Indian J Dermatol Venereol Leprol. 2007 Jan-Feb;73(1):22-5. PMID:17314442

[84] Polyunsaturated fatty acids in the food chain in the United States. Kris-Etherton PM, Taylor DS, Yu-Poth S, et al. Am J Clin Nutr. 2000 Jan;71(1 Suppl):179S-88S. PMID:10617969

[85] Dietary intake of n-3 and n-6 fatty acids and the risk of clinical depression in women: a 10-y prospective follow-up study. Lucas M, Mirzaei F, O'Reilly EJ, et al. Am J Clin Nutr. 2011 Jun;93(6):1337-43. PMID:21471279

[86] Retinoid-responsive transcriptional changes in epidermal keratinocytes. Lee DD, Stojadinovic O, Krzyzanowska A, et al. J Cell Physiol. 2009 Aug;220(2):427-39. PMID:19388012

[87] Vitamin A and vitamin E in dermatology. Menni S, Piccinno R. Acta Vitaminol Enzymol. 1985;7 Suppl:55-60. PMID:3916047

[88] Retinoid receptors and keratinocytes. Fisher C, Blumenberg M, Tomić-Canić M. Crit Rev Oral Biol Med. 1995;6(4):284-301. PMID:8664420

[89] Production of superoxide anions by keratinocytes initiates P. acnes-induced inflammation of the skin. Grange PA, Chéreau C, Raingeaud J, Nicco C, Weill B, Dupin N, Batteux F. PLoS Pathog. 2009 Jul;5(7):e1000527. PMID:19629174

[90] Regulation of bile acid synthesis by fat-soluble vitamins A and D. Schmidt DR, Holmstrom SR, Fon Tacer K, Bookout AL, Kliewer SA, Mangelsdorf DJ. J Biol Chem. 2010 May 7;285(19):14486-94. PMID:20233723

[91] KEGG Pathway Vitamin Digestion and Absorption; accessed September 2011. http://www.genome.jp/kegg-bin/show_pathway?hsa04977+949

[92] Retinoic acid synthesis and signaling during early organogenesis. Duester G. Cell. 2008 Sep 19;134(6):921-31. PMID:18805086

[93] Serum zinc in acne vulgaris. Amer M, Bahgat MR, Tosson Z, Abdel Mowla MY, Amer K. Int J Dermatol. 1982 Oct;21(8):481-4. PMID:6217164

[94] Efficacy and safety study of two zinc gluconate regimens in the treatment of inflammatory acne. Meynadier J. Eur J Dermatol. 2000 Jun;10(4):269-73. PMID:10846252

[95] Effect of zinc gluconate on propionibacterium acnes resistance to erythromycin in patients with inflammatory acne: in vitro and in vivo study. Dreno B, Foulc P, Reynaud A, et al. Eur J Dermatol. 2005 May-Jun;15(3):152-5. PMID:15908296

[96] Acne treatment with oral zinc and vitamin A: effects on the serum levels of zinc and retinol binding protein (RBP). Vahlquist A, Michaëlsson G, Juhlin L. Acta Derm Venereol. 1978;58(5):437-42. PMID:82355

[97] Nutrient intakes are correlated with overall psychiatric functioning in adults with mood disorders. Davison KM, Kaplan BJ. Can J Psychiatry. 2012 Feb;57(2):85-92. PMID:22340148

[98] Zinc salts inhibit in vitro Toll-like receptor 2 surface expression by keratinocytes. Jarrousse V, Castex-Rizzi N, Khammari A, et al. Eur J Dermatol. 2007 Nov-Dec;17(6):492-6. PMID:17951128

[99] Induction of toll-like receptors by Propionibacterium acnes. Jugeau S, Tenaud I, Knol AC, et al. Br J Dermatol. 2005 Dec;153(6):1105-13. PMID:16307644

[100] Nicotinamide inhibits Propionibacterium acnes-induced IL-8 production in keratinocytes through the NF-kappaB and MAPK pathways. Grange PA, Raingeaud J, Calvez V, Dupin N. J Dermatol Sci. 2009 Nov;56(2):106-12. PMID:19726162

[101] Micronutrient modulation of NF-κB in oral keratinocytes exposed to periodontal bacteria. Milward MR, Chapple IL, Carter K, et al. Innate Immun. 2012 Aug 13. PMID:22890546

[102] Glucocorticoids enhance Toll-like receptor 2 expression in human keratinocytes stimulated with Propionibacterium acnes or proinflammatory cytokines. Shibata M, Katsuyama M, Onodera T, et al. J Invest Dermatol. 2009 Feb;129(2):375-82. PMID:18704103

[103] The significance of dietary boron, with particular reference to athletes. Naghii MR. Nutr Health. 1999;13(1):31-7. PMID:10376277

[104] The nutritional and metabolic effects of boron in humans and animals. Samman S, Naghii MR, Lyons Wall PM, Verus AP. Biol Trace Elem Res. 1998 Winter;66(1-3):227-35. PMID:10050922

[105] Why boron? Bolaños L, Lukaszewski K, Bonilla I, Blevins D. Plant Physiol Biochem. 2004 Dec;42(11):907-12. PMID:15694285

[106] Effect of dietary boron on mineral, estrogen, and testosterone metabolism in postmenopausal women. Nielsen FH, Hunt CD, Mullen LM, Hunt JR. FASEB J. 1987 Nov;1(5):394-7. PMID:3678698

[107] Dietary boron supplementation enhances the effects of estrogen on bone mineral balance in ovariectomized rats. Sheng MH, Taper LJ, Veit H, Thomas EA, Ritchey SJ, Lau KH. Biol Trace Elem Res. 2001 Jul;81(1):29-45. PMID:11508330

[108] The effects of dietary boric acid on bone strength in rats. Chapin RE, Ku WW, Kenney MA, McCoy H. Biol Trace Elem Res. 1998 Winter;66(1-3):395-9. PMID:10050932

[109] Dietary boron decreases peak pancreatic in situ insulin release in chicks and plasma insulin concentrations in rats regardless of vitamin D or magnesium status. Bakken NA, Hunt CD. J Nutr. 2003 Nov;133(11):3577-83. PMID:14608076

[110] The effects of some boron compounds against heavy metal toxicity in human blood. Turkez H, Geyikoglu F, Tatar A, Keles MS, Kaplan I. Exp Toxicol Pathol. 2010 Jul 19. PMID:20663653

[111] Dietary Reference Intakes for Vitamin A, Vitamin K, Arsenic, Boron, Chromium, Copper, Iodine, Iron, Manganese, Molybdenum, Nickel, Silicon, Vanadium, and Zinc. Chapter 13. National Academy press, 2001 Institute of Medicine. Food and Nutrition Board.

[112] WEBMD http://www.webmd.com/vitamins-supplements/ingredientmono-894-BORON.aspx?activeIngredientId=894&activeIngredientName=BORON&source=3 accessed September 2011

[113] Comedolytic effect of topically applied active vitamin D3 analogue on pseudocomedones in the rhino mouse. Hayashi N, Watanabe H, Yasukawa H et al. Br J Dermatol. 2006 Nov;155(5):895-901. PMID:17034516

[114] Vitamin D and the skin: an ancient friend, revisited. Reichrath J. Exp Dermatol. 2007 Jul;16(7):618-25. PMID:17576242

[115] Management strategies for acne vulgaris. Whitney KM, Ditre CM. Clin Cosmet Investig Dermatol. 2011;4:41-53. Epub 2011 Apr 26. PMID:21691566

[116] The efficacy of topical 2% green tea lotion in mild-to-moderate acne vulgaris. Elsaie ML, Abdelhamid MF, Elsaaiee LT, Emam HM. J Drugs Dermatol. 2009 Apr;8(4):358-64. PMID:19363854

[117] Resveratrol-containing gel for the treatment of acne vulgaris: a single-blind, vehicle-controlled, pilot study. Fabbrocini G, Staibano S, De Rosa G, et al. Am J Clin Dermatol. 2011 Apr 1;12(2):133-41 PMID:21348544

[118] In vitro activity of kaempferol isolated from the Impatiens balsamina alone and in combination with erythromycin or clindamycin against Propionibacterium acnes. Lim YH, Kim IH, Seo JJ. J Microbiol. 2007 Oct;45(5):473-7. PMID:17978809

[119] Phytosphingosine stimulates the differentiation of human keratinocytes and inhibits TPA-induced inflammatory epidermal hyperplasia in hairless mouse skin. Kim S, Hong I, Hwang JS, et al. Mol Med. 2006 Jan-Mar;12(1-3):17-24. PMID:16838068

[120] Anti-microbial and -inflammatory activity and efficacy of phytosphingosine: an in vitro and in vivo study addressing acne vulgaris. Pavicic T, Wollenweber U, Farwick M, Korting HC. Int J Cosmet Sci. 2007 Jun;29(3):181-90. PMID:18489348

[121] Phytosphingosine derivatives ameliorate skin inflammation by inhibiting NF-κB and JAK/STAT signaling in keratinocytes and mice. Kim BH, Lee JM, Jung YG, et al. J Invest Dermatol. 2014 Apr;134(4):1023-32. PMID:24177187

38. Sexual Dysfunction and Male Infertility

Sexual dysfunction is so closely tied to psychological issues, social inhibitions, religious inculcation, cultural taboos, and history of emotional, physical or sexual abuse, that it is hard to imagine that psychological issues are not the primary cause of its pathogenesis. Nevertheless, the prevalence of female sexual dysfunction (FSD) is so high among women with migraine, irritable bowel syndrome, fibromyalgia, depression, interstitial cystitis, and related disorders that these cases account for a large majority of FSD cases in the population. Many physicians and psychologists consider FSD to be somatization disorders, which often follows sexual or other abuse. However, even if abuse plays a role in FSD, it is only part of the story must be understood for successful treatment and healing.

Women with fibromyalgia report decreased sexual desire and arousal, decreased experience of orgasm, and increased pain with intercourse[1]. About forty-three percent of both men and women with IBS report sexual dysfunction[2]. Eighty-eight percent of women with interstitial cystitis report sexual dysfunction[3]. Thirty-four percent of men with chronic prostatitis/painful bladder syndrome have erectile dysfunction, and 55% have ejaculatory dysfunction[4]. Sexual dysfunction is reported in forty to seventy-four percent of women with multiple sclerosis[5]. Migraineurs have an increased frequency of sexual dysfunction and pain on intercourse[6].

About one in four women, in the general population, report having been sexually assaulted[7]. A very similar proportion of women with IBS report being victims of sexual assault[8]. This suggests that it may not be the event, but rather, the reaction to the event associated with the dysfunction. Many soldiers are exposed to trauma; some develop PTSD; others do not. One difference is that those with PTSD have elevated CRH levels compared to soldiers who have been traumatized, but who do not have PTSD[9]. CRH elevation can disrupt the hypothalamic-pituitary-adrenal axis and the hypothalamic-pituitary-gonadal axis, as well as increase paracellular hyperpermeability that promotes enteroimmune hyperreactivity. The difference in an individual's hormonal and immune responses to a stressor may account for why some women develop FSD and other stress-related diseases while others do not. (See Epigenetics box in Chapter 29)

Chronic stress affects the hypothalamic-pituitary-gonadal axis, decreasing fertility and sexual receptivity. Decreased fertility and sexual desire are a functional response to famine and stress; times when fertility could put the mother at risk and conditions which might bring a newborn into a high-risk environment.

Depression has a negative effect on sexuality. Depressed women have less hypothalamic activity after watching an erotic film than other women[10]. Disrupted HPA axis function, during chronic stress, lowers the level of proopiomelanocortin (POMC). POMC protein is cleaved to form both ACTH and melanocortin. ACTH is responsible for stimulating cortisol production and release. Melanocortin plays an important role in sexual arousal and genital engorgement[11]. Additionally, agouti-related protein (AgRP), which has a long-term effect on increasing appetite, may be elevated by stress[12]. AgRP is a melanocortin receptor inverse agonist[13] which, therefore, blocks its activity. Sleep disturbances may decrease the output of luteinizing hormone (LH)[14], thus decreasing the production of sex hormones.

Rather than being a somatic disorder, FSD likely results from immune dysfunction, often enteroimmune dysfunction, which is hormonally mediated. Trauma and abuse can be profound stressors, and stress increases enteric hyperpermeability and proinflammatory cytokine production. Although stress abatement is a necessary part of treatment, ignoring the immune disturbances and comorbidities would make successful treatment unlikely.

Fertility and Intimacy

Smell is important to intimacy. A common complaint heard by marriage counselors is that one partner cannot stand the smell of the other[15]. HLA types play an important role in mate selection through their influence on women's selection of a mate. Women naturally seek a mate that has a genetically determined HLA imparted body smell different than her own (to prevent inbreeding) but genetically close enough to assure that the offspring look similar to her own family[16]. Women who marry a man whose HLA type is too similar to her own have less attraction to their spouse and more extra-marital sexual partners[17].

Women's behavior changes during the fertile portion of the menstrual cycle. They dress more attractively and more revealingly[18]; their voices change pitch[19], and they are more interested in other men than in their mate[20]. Furthermore, men are more attracted to women when they are ovulating[21], but this does not occur if women are using oral contraceptive medications. Men guard their spouses more carefully during the woman's fertile period[22]. Thus, a woman's fertility affects sexual behavior of both the woman and men she is in contact with. Changes in the HPG axis can easily alter not only a woman's fertility, but also her behaviors and those of the men around her.

Exposure, to the semen of a female's mate, activates T$_{REG}$ cells that downregulate the woman's immune response to paternal autoantigens; helping to prevent a woman's immune system from recognizing the mate's antigens, in the fetus as foreign. HLA type is so closely tied to survival that a pregnant female mouse will have an immune-mediated, spontaneous abortion if exposed to the smell of the urine of an unfamiliar male mouse[23]. Continued exposure to the paternal autoantigens in semen may decrease the risk of miscarriage and preeclampsia[24].

Women who have vaginal contact with their mate's sperm are less likely to be depressed than women where the man uses a condom[25]. Nevertheless, casual sexual encounters increase the risk of depression[26], especially when condoms are not used[27]. Regular exposure to the mate's semen supports immune desensitization to him and may support fertility and maintenance of a happy relationship.

Sperm is allergenic and can promote and promote an immune response in woman when the sperms donor is not a genetic match to her. This means that a woman's immune system is disposed to attack and destroy the sperm, and to a lesser extent, the fetus that bears the donor's antigens. Additionally, a woman may suffer dangerous autoimmune reactions that result in preeclampsia or eclampsia.

In a way, it makes survival sense. A one-time donor from another tribe is much less likely to help raise the offspring; the sperm donor might be an enemy invader or rapist. Meanwhile, the frequent immune contact with the child's father would suggest someone who might stick around. The repeated contact with the father's antigens may help sustain a pregnancy and aid in the child's survival as exposure of his sperm with the vaginal mucosa downregulates the immune reaction to the sperm and to the fetal MHC antigens.

While mucosal (vaginal) exposure is effective, intestinal exposure is even more efficient at downregulating the immune response. The oral route of exposure to sperm may be an even more efficient route for immune regulation to decrease the risk that the mother's immune system will attack the fetus, and lowers the risk of preeclampsia for the mother[28, 29, 30, 31].

Treatment of Female Sexual Dysfunction

1. Treat associated diseases: Treatment should begin with treatment of any associated disease, such as migraine (Chapter 28) IBS (Chapter 26), interstitial cystitis (Chapter 27) and fibromyalgia (Chapter 32). $T_H 17$ immune activation and Mast Cell Activation are common to all of these conditions, and thus, a diagnostic workup for IgG food antergy and mast cell activation is appropriate for most patients with sexual dysfunction.

2. Normalize the Hypothalamic- Pituitary (HP) End Organ Axes: Dysregulation of the HP Adrenal, HP Gonadal, and other HP axes affect sexual function and fertility. Restoration of the circadian cycle is essential for this. Meal and sleep times should be regular. A short course of very low dose cortisol taken daily at 8:00 a.m. may help entrain the HPA axis. Chapter 41 discusses sleep. Melatonin, taken at bedtime, may aid in the restoration of the circadian cycle.

3. Stress Management: Stress is likely an underlying cause of the immune dysfunction in FSD, and stress should be treated. PSTD is common in women with a history of abuse and should be treated. Treatment of stress is discussed in Chapter 29. Chapter 32 includes a discussion on PSTD and treatment of sympathetic hyperactivity.

4. Avoid Alcohol Prior to Intercourse: Alcohol inhibits the release of oxytocin and extinguishes the positive reinforcement of intimacy. See Chapter 17.

Irregular menses in a woman of reproductive age should be investigated. This topic is beyond the scope of this discussion; however, women with very low body fat may have irregular or missed menses and low estrogen production placing them at risk of osteoporosis. Women with features of masculinization may produce excess testosterone. Such conditions warrant treatment. Oral contraceptive cycling may be helpful to entrain the HPG axis in women with irregular menses.

Boron for Estrogen Regulation

Boron helps stabilize estrogen and certain steroid hormones, lowers the production, and increase catabolism, of androgens. Boron supplements (may be helpful for treatment of menopausal symptoms and is often helpful in the treatment of hot flashes and night sweats. Young women with dysmenorrhea with had significant reductions in menstrual pain severity and duration when taking 10 mg of boron on five peri-menstrual days a month[32]. This mineral supplement may also be helpful for polycystic ovary syndrome and androgen associated alopecia (male pattern baldness) in women.

Six milligrams of chelated boron daily is a typical effective dose. Boron should be accompanied by vitamin D to be most effective. Boron and its effects on sex hormones are discussed in Chapter 37.

Male infertility

Sperm can be viewed as a package of DNA with a motor and propeller attached. That motor is driven by energy from mitochondria. A common finding in infertility is oxidative damage. Oxidative damage can cause DNA fragmentation in the sperm. In as many as one-third of infertile couples, DNA fragmentation in the sperm has been found to be severe enough to prevent conception[33]. Oxidative damage can also cause problems with sperm motility[34]. This may be for the best, as delivering abnormal DNA to fertilize an egg can have quite undesirable outcomes. There is also increased apoptosis of sperm with oxidative damage[35], which can cause a low sperm count.

The source of oxidative stress is not restricted to dietary causes, but also from environmental exposures.

Studies of sperm in infertile men have shown lower levels of vitamin C[36] and of zinc[37], both which act as antioxidants. Coenzyme Q_{10} levels are also lower in infertile men, and CoQ_{10} supplementation has been found to increase viable sperm count in men in which levels had been low[38]. Smoking[39] appears to be associated with DNA fragmentation of the sperm, as does increasing age[40].

Male infertility is common among men with severe celiac disease.

Although less prevalent, male sexual dysfunction is not uncommon. It should be approached, in the same way, as is FSD.

Treatment of Idiopathic Male Infertility

1. Oxidative Stress: Male infertility can be caused by oxidative stress and poorly functioning mitochondria. Treat mitochondria as described in Chapter 21, with increased exercise, flavonol phenols and avoidance of oxidants, alcohol, and ionizing radiation. Supplements including alpha-lipoic acid, n-acetylcysteine, vitamin C, zinc and CoQ_{10} supplements may be helpful. Men planning on fathering should avoid anything more than light alcohol use during the 90 days prior to conception, to avoid oxidative damage to the sperm, and to prevent abnormal DNA methylation and conveyance of epigenetic disease to the offspring.

2. Gluten Disease Associated Infertility: Patients with celiac disease, gluten enteropathy or dermatitis herpetiformis, who have impaired infertility, should eliminate gluten from the diet. Infertility in these patients should include treatment for gluten disease as described in Chapter 22. Anti-transglutaminase antibody testing may be helpful when other causes of infertility have been excluded.

---

[1] Association between fibromyalgia and sexual dysfunction in women. Kalichman L. Clin Rheumatol. 2009 Apr;28(4):365-9. PMID:19165555

[2] Sexual dysfunction in patients with irritable bowel syndrome and non-ulcer dyspepsia. Fass R, Fullerton S, Naliboff B, Hirsh T, Mayer EA. Digestion. 1998;59(1):79-85. PMID:9468103

[3] Prevalence and correlates of sexual dysfunction among women with bladder pain syndrome/interstitial cystitis. Bogart LM, Suttorp MJ, Elliott MN, Clemens JQ, Berry SH. Urology. 2011 Mar;77(3):576-80. PMID:21215432

[4] Prevalence of sexual dysfunction in men with chronic prostatitis/chronic pelvic pain syndrome. Trinchieri A, Magri V, Cariani L, Bonamore R, Restelli A, Garlaschi MC, Perletti G. Arch Ital Urol Androl. 2007 Jun;79(2):67-70. PMID:17695411

[5] Female sexuality in multiple sclerosis: the multidimensional nature of the problem and the intervention. Bronner G, Elran E, Golomb J, Korczyn AD. Acta Neurol Scand. 2010 May;121(5):289-301. Epub 2010 Jan 12. PMID:20070276

[6] Not only headache: higher degree of sexual pain symptoms among migraine sufferers. Ifergane G, Ben-Zion IZ, Plakht Y, Regev K, Wirguin I. J Headache Pain. 2008 Apr;9(2):113-7. PMID:18317864

[7] Sexual abuse history: prevalence, health effects, mediators, and psychological treatment. Leserman J. Psychosom Med. 2005 Nov-Dec;67(6):906-15. PMID:16314595

[8] Reported sexual abuse predicts impaired functioning but a good response to psychological treatments in patients with severe irritable bowel syndrome. Creed F, Guthrie E, Ratcliffe J, Fernandes L, Rigby C, Tomenson B, Read N, Thompson DG. Psychosom Med. 2005 May-Jun;67(3):490-9. PMID:15911915

[9] Elevated plasma corticotrophin-releasing hormone levels in veterans with posttraumatic stress disorder. de Kloet CS, Vermetten E, Geuze E, Lentjes EG, Heijnen CJ, Stalla GK, Westenberg HG. Prog Brain Res. 2008;167:287-91.PMID:18037027

[10] Assessment of cerebrocortical areas associated with sexual arousal in depressive women using functional MR imaging. Yang JC, Park K, Eun SJ, Lee MS, Yoon JS, Shin IS, Kim YK, Chung TW, Kang HK, Jeong GW. J Sex Med. 2008 Mar;5(3):602-9. PMID:18194182

[11] Melanocortins in the treatment of male and female sexual dysfunction. Shadiack AM, Sharma SD, Earle DC, Spana C, Hallam TJ. Curr Top Med Chem. 2007;7(11):1137-44. PMID:17584134

[12] Relation between the hypothalamic-pituitary-thyroid (HPT) axis and the hypothalamic-pituitary-adrenal (HPA) axis during repeated stress. Helmreich DL, Parfitt DB, Lu XY, Akil H, Watson SJ. Neuroendocrinology. 2005;81(3):183-92. PMID:16020927

[13] Receptor-antagonist interactions in the complexes of agouti and agouti-related protein with human melanocortin 1 and 4 receptors. Chai BX, Pogozheva ID, Lai YM, Li JY, Neubig RR, Mosberg HI, Gantz I. Biochemistry. 2005 Mar 8;44(9):3418-31.PMID:15736952

[14] Decreased pituitary-gonadal secretion in men with obstructive sleep apnea. Luboshitzky R, Aviv A, Hefetz A, Herer P, Shen-Orr

Z, Lavie L, Lavie P. J Clin Endocrinol Metab. 2002 Jul;87(7):3394-8. PMID:12107256

[15] Scents and Sensibility. Svoboda, E. Jan 01, 2008 Psychology Today.

[16] MHC-correlated mate choice in humans: a review. Havlicek J, Roberts SC. Psychoneuroendocrinology. 2009 May;34(4):497-512. Epub 2008 Dec 2. PMID:19054623

[17] Major histocompatibility complex alleles, sexual responsivity, and unfaithfulness in romantic couples. Garver-Apgar CE, Gangestad SW, Thornhill R, Miller RD, Olp JJ. Psychol Sci. 2006 Oct;17(10):830-5. PMID:17100780

[18] Changes in women's choice of dress across the ovulatory cycle: naturalistic and laboratory task-based evidence. Durante KM, Li NP, Haselton MG. Pers Soc Psychol Bull. 2008 Nov;34(11):1451-60. Epub 2008 Aug 21. PMID:18719219

[19] Vocal cues of ovulation in human females. Bryant GA, Haselton MG. Biol Lett. 2009 Feb 23;5(1):12-5. PMID:18845518

[20] Changes in women's mate preferences across the ovulatory cycle. Gangestad SW, Garver-Apgar CE, Simpson JA, Cousins AJ. J Pers Soc Psychol. 2007 Jan;92(1):151-63. PMID:17201549

[21] Ovulation as a male mating prime: subtle signs of women's fertility influence men's mating cognition and behavior. Miller SL, Maner JK. J Pers Soc Psychol. 2011 Feb;100(2):295-308. PMID:20822287

[22] Conditional expression of women's desires and men's mate guarding across the ovulatory cycle. Haselton MG, Gangestad SW. Horm Behav. 2006 Apr;49(4):509-18. Epub 2006 Jan 3.PMID:16403409

[23] Reserpine: inhibition of olfactory blockage of pregnancy in mice. Dominic CJ. Science. 1966 Jun 24;152(730):1764-5. PMID:594934

[24] Activating T regulatory cells for tolerance in early pregnancy - the contribution of seminal fluid. Robertson SA, Guerin LR, Moldenhauer LM, Hayball JD. J Reprod Immunol. 2009 Dec;83(1-2):109-16. Epub 2009 Oct 28. PMID:19875178

[25] Does semen have antidepressant properties? Gallup GG Jr, Burch RL, Platek SM. Arch Sex Behav. 2002 Jun;31(3):289-93. PMID:12049024

[26] No strings attached: the nature of casual sex in college students. Welsh DP, Grello CM, Harper MS. J Sex Res. 2006 Aug;43(3):255-67. PMID:17599248

[27] Depressive symptoms and condom use with clients among female sex workers in China. Hong Y, Li X, Fang X, Zhao R. Sex Health. 2007 Jun;4(2):99-104. PMID:17524287

[28] Activating T regulatory cells for tolerance in early pregnancy - the contribution of seminal fluid. Robertson SA, Guerin LR, Moldenhauer LM, Hayball JD. J Reprod Immunol. 2009 Dec;83(1-2):109-16. Epub 2009 Oct 28. PMID:19875178

[29] Is the use of donor sperm associated with a higher incidence of preeclampsia in women who achieve pregnancy after intrauterine insemination? Kyrou D, Kolibianakis EM, Devroey P, Fatemi HM. Fertil Steril. 2010 Mar 1;93(4):1124-7. PMID:19232411

[30] Inadequate tolerance induction may induce pre-eclampsia. Saito S, Sakai M, Sasaki Y, Nakashima A, Shiozaki A. J Reprod Immunol. 2007 Dec;76(1-2):30-9. Epub 2007 Nov 1. PMID:17935792

[31] Correlation between oral sex and a low incidence of preeclampsia: a role for soluble HLA in seminal fluid? Koelman CA, Coumans AB, Nijman HW, Doxiadis II, Dekker GA, Claas FH. J Reprod Immunol. 2000 Mar;46(2):155-66. PMID:10706945

[32] Effects of boron supplementation on the severity and duration of pain in primary dysmenorrhea. Nikkhah S, Dolatian M, Naghii MR, et al. Complement Ther Clin Pract. 2015 May;21(2):79-83. PMID:25906949

[33] Sperm DNA damage in men from infertile couples. Erenpreiss J, Elzanaty S, Giwercman A. Asian J Androl. 2008 Sep;10(5):786-90. PMID:18645682

[34] Clinical significance of reactive oxygen species in semen of infertile Indian men. Venkatesh S, Riyaz AM, Shamsi MB, Kumar R, Gupta NP, Mittal S, Malhotra N, Sharma RK, Agarwal A, Dada R. Andrologia. 2009 Aug;41(4):251-6. PMID:19601938

[35] Oxidative stress is associated with increased apoptosis leading to spermatozoa DNA damage in patients with male factor infertility. Wang X, Sharma RK, Sikka SC, Thomas AJ Jr, Falcone T, Agarwal A. Fertil Steril. 2003 Sep;80(3):531-5. PMID:12969693

[36] Relationship between seminal ascorbic acid and sperm DNA integrity in infertile men. Song GJ, Norkus EP, Lewis V. Int J Androl. 2006 Dec;29(6):569-75. PMID:17121654

[37] Zinc levels in seminal plasma are associated with sperm quality in fertile and infertile men. Colagar AH, Marzony ET, Chaichi MJ. Nutr Res. 2009 Feb;29(2):82-8. PMID:19285597

[38] Coenzyme Q10 and male infertility. Balercia G, Mancini A, Paggi F, Tiano L, Pontecorvi A, Boscaro M, Lenzi A, Littarru GP. J Endocrinol Invest. 2009 Jul;32(7):626-32. PMID:19509475

[39] Sperm head defects and disturbances in spermatozoal chromatin and DNA integrities in idiopathic infertile subjects: association with cigarette smoking. Elshal MF, El-Sayed IH, Elsaied MA, El-Masry SA, Kumosani TA. Clin Biochem. 2009 May;42(7-8):589-94. PMID:19094977

[40] Sperm quality decline among men below 60 years of age undergoing IVF or ICSI treatment. Hammiche F, Laven JS, Boxmeer JC, Dohle GR, Steegers EA, Steegers-Theunissen RP. J Androl. 2011 Jan-Feb;32(1):70-6. PMID:20467050

39. Food Additives

Food additives are used for enhancing the color or flavoring of foods to make them more appealing. Additives are also used as preservatives. Often, they are added to processed food to supplement their succulence and savor, but they are also added to foods that are wholesome. Not all additives have deleterious effects, and most people can consume them in the amount found in food with impunity. For others, they may cause problems. Some food additives can cause serious immune reactions.

Food Colorings

There are seven artificial food colorings still in use in the United States. Several others have been removed from the market. These base colors are mixed to get the desired hue for the food. Two additional artificial colorings can be legally used. "Citrus Red No. 2," is allowed only for use in coloring the skins of oranges that will not be used in food[1]. Citrus Red No. 2 is a known carcinogen. "Orange B" which was used to color the casings of frankfurters and sausages was also found to be a carcinogen, while still legal for use, its manufacture in the United States was voluntarily discontinued in 1978.

Most of the artificial food colorants have been shown to cause tumors or cancers in lab animals. The FDA allows the use of artificial colors primarily because of political pressure, and with the understanding that the amounts consumed in food are quite small. Dyeing the skin of oranges with citrus Red No. 2, a known carcinogen, is allowed as it does not seep into the fruit, but obviously, the peels from these oranges should not be used for marmalade or candies.

Orange B is used only in hot dogs and sausage casings. Consumption of hot dogs has been associated with risk of childhood leukemia[2] and brain tumors in children[3], but that risk is usually attributed to N-nitroso compounds, rather than the food colorant.

Allergic reactions have been attributed to Blue No.1, Yellow No.6 and especially to Yellow No. 5, although, as non-proteins, it is more likely that these compound cause pseudoallergic reactions than true allergic reactions. Tartrazine (Yellow No. 5) has been associated behavioral problems in children[4] and with pseudoallergic reactions in individuals with leukotriene associated hypersensitivity (aspirin intolerance). The preservative sodium benzoate can provoke this same reaction (See Chapter 15). The red dyes are comedogenic when used in cosmetics and thus can provoke acne[5].

Food additives, especially food colorings, have been suspected of causing behavioral problems, particularly ADD and ADHD, since the 1970's. This remains an area of controversy, as their effect is difficult to study; there are large numbers of variables involved; different colors and additives are allowed or banned in various countries. Furthermore, these agents only represent a few of the dietary and environmental exposures which affect fluctuating behaviors. The studies that have found that food additives increase hyperactivity have used "cocktails" of food colorings, which included the food preservative sodium benzoate[6,7]. Additionally, these studies included the use of colorants not allowed for use in the United States.

Table 39-1: Artificial Food Colorings Legal for Use in the United States:

Designation	Name	E number	Cancer or Tumors in Rats or Mice	Color
FD&C Blue No. 1	Brilliant Blue FCF	E133		Dark Blue
FD&C Blue No. 2	Indigotine	E132	Brain	Blue
FD&C Green No. 3	Fast Green	E134	Bladder	Turquoise
FD&C Yellow No. 5	Tartrazine	E102		Yellow
FD&C Yellow No. 6	Sunset Yellow FCF	E110	Kidney Bladder	Orange
FD&C Red No. 3	Erythrosine	E127	Thyroid	Pink
FD&C Red No. 40	Allura Red AC	E129		Red
FD&C Orange B				Orange
FD&C Citrus Red No. 2		E121	Yes	Red

Complicating the study of the effects of food additives is that interactions may occur when consumed in combination. Brilliant blue, quinoline yellow color, (which is not allowed to be used in the U.S.A.), L-glutamic acid and the artificial sweetener aspartame, all inhibit nerve-fiber growth in cell cultures. Synergistic interactions between these substances can reduce the concentration required to prevent neurite growth by five times or more. When present in combination, these additives result in nerve cell growth inhibition at greatly reduced concentrations[8], as shown in Table 38-2, Artificial additives which may not induce risk at levels consumed in foods when studied individually may cause injury when combined in a food or when foods are combined in a meal.

Table 39-2: Additive effects of Food Additives on Inhibition of Nerve Growth

Food Additive	Concentration Required to Inhibit Neurite Growth by 50%[8]
Brilliant Blue	51.4 nM
Glutamate	48.7 μM
Brilliant Blue with Glutamate	10 nM with 10 μM
Quinoline Yellow	106 μM
Aspartame	153 μM
Quinoline Yellow with Aspartame	10 μM with 8.06 μM

Some food additives are large, polar (water soluble) molecules, which are not normally absorbed by the intestines, and thus, have limited potential toxicity. Individuals with an impaired intestinal mucosal barrier, however, may absorb them. The brains of infants are not protected by the blood-brain barrier until they are several months old. The enteric nervous system can also then be exposed to artificial food additives that are potential neurotoxins. There is not a nutritional purpose for food coloring other than to make artificial foods more attractive, especially to children. These additives are best avoided.

Table 39-3: Natural Food Colorings Allowed for Use in the United States:

Name	Source	E Number	Color
Chlorophyll	Chlorella algae	E140	Green
Tumeric	Curcuma longa	E100	Yellow, orange
Saffron	Crocus sativus	E160a	Yellow - Red
Annatto	Bixa orellana	E160b	Yellow - Red
Cochineal	Dactylopius coccus	E120	Crimson Red
Betanin	Beetroots; Beta vulgaris		Deep red
Elderberry juice	Sambucus (various species)		Magenta

Although natural food colorants may sound benign, a few are not. Two natural food colorants are of special concern, as they are highly immunogenic. Annatto, (also known as bija, bixa, achiote or roucou) is made from the seed of the *Bixa orellana,* a plant native to South America, where it was used as body paint by native peoples. As a food additive, it can be listed as "natural color," annatto, by the refined chemical names bixin or norbixin, or by the E number E160b, which is used in Europe.

Immunogenic reaction to annatto is a fairly common, and it has been associated with irritable bowel syndrome and behavioral problems. Unfortunately, most labs that test for allergies and antergies do not test for IgE or IgG immunoreactivity to annatto. It is used as a lake, a fat-soluble color, for dairy products including cheese, butter, margarine and ice cream, as well as in some snack foods. Annatto is often hidden in otherwise healthy foods (yellow cheese, butter, vanilla ice cream), not places allergenic food dyes are expected.

Cochineal, (also known as carmine, crimson lake, natural red 4, and E120), is a colorant that gives a crimson red color. As of January 2011, FDA regulations require all foods and cosmetics containing cochineal to label its use in the ingredient list. It is made from the pulverized bodies of *Dactylopius coccus,* an insect that lives on prickly pear cactus. During its colonial period, this dye was Mexico's second-most valuable export, following silver. As it is an insect product, it is not vegetarian, not kosher and is Haraam (forbidden) in Islam.

This colorant may be found in candy, beverages, yogurt or ice cream, to impart a red or berry color. Cochineal is immunogenic, and can cause mild to severe allergic reactions, however, is rarely included in panels for immunogenicity testing. Cochineal is made from tiny beetles; its immunogenicity likely cross-reacts with shrimp, fleas, cockroaches and other arthropods.

Elderberries contain lectins including SNA-III, which is a hemagglutinin[9]. Levels used for food coloring would be too low to cause toxicity, but can be associated with immunoreactivity. Turmeric is high in antioxidants and generally healthful, but too, can be associated with allergy or antergy.

Table 39-4: Caramel Colorings Allowed for Use in the United States:

Caramel Coloring I	Caramelized Sugar, Malt	E150A	Amber - Brown
Caramel Coloring II	Caustic sulfite caramel	E150B	Amber - Brown
Caramel Coloring III	Ammonia caramel	E150C	Amber - Brown
Caramel Coloring IV	Sulfite ammonia caramel	E150D	Amber - Brown

Caramel, the candy, and caramel coloring can be made by the heating of sucrose, causing a Maillard reaction. For commercial food coloring, a carbohydrate, usually a sugar such as fructose, sucrose, dextrose, or maltose is treated with an alkali, acids or/and or salt. Caramel colors I and II have been determined to have the same toxicological properties as those made by heating sugar. Caramel colors I and II likely present little risk.

Caramel colors III and IV, however, made with ammonia contain the carcinogen 4-methyl imidazole (4-MEI)[10]. A daily intake of 30 μg of MEI-4 has been estimated to impart a 1:100,000 risk of developing cancer. This amount is present in as little as 2.5 ounces of *Coca-Cola* sold in Washington, DC. In California, however, where it is regulated, there is less than 1 μg of MEI-4 in this amount of the beverage[11]. The amounts present in colas vary greatly, and even in California may exceed levels requiring warning labels for carcinogens[12].

Caramel color III also contains the compound THI, which inhibits the enzyme S1P lyase, and which thus, may affect immune cell activity, especially in the intestine (Chapter 33). Caramel colors III is used in some beers and confectionery.

The FDA normally restricts food additive carcinogen content to levels below that which imparts a 1:1,000,000 risk of cancer. Use and consumption of Caramel colors III and IV should be abandoned.

Food Preservatives

Included among the relatives of cochineal are scale insects and mealy bugs. Certain scale bugs are cultivated in Southeast Asia on the branches of plants for the production of sticklac. Lac is a resinous secretion left on the plants by these creatures. This product is used to make shellac that is used to coat violins. You can also find it in the fruit aisle of your local grocery store, and as well, in the candy section.

Lac is a product used to polish and shine grocery store apples. It provides a moisture barrier to help keep the fruit fresh. It is also used on other fruits and in some candies; such as jellybeans, some chocolate treats, some coated chewing gums and even on some coffee beans. In candies, it may be listed as shellac or as confectioner's glaze. Contrary to urban legend, M&M's do not use lac. In candies, it is also used as a moisture barrier, here, to keep moisture out and keep the candy hard. Lac also gives these products a desirable sheen.

Lac causes headaches in some individuals. If eating apples causes headache, they can be tried without the skin, or vegan apples, from an organic grower, can be tried.

Waxes and Oils are also used on many fruits and vegetables to help retain moisture and keep them looking fresh. Cucumbers, for example, often have an oily feel to them. These oils and waxes are mostly petroleum based products. They are used as moisture barriers to keep the fruits and vegetables from drying out while on display, to improve their shelf-life and appearance. The waxes and oils are similar to that used in lip gloss. Chocolate candy contains paraffin, used to raise the melting temperature to help maintain the candy's shape. As unappetizing as they may sound, I am unaware of any health related problems arising from the proper use of these products.

Sulfites are used as preservatives as they prevent bacterial growth in food. Most wine contains added sulfites, as do many manufactured foods and dried fruits. Sulfites can trigger mast cell degranulation triggering asthma and other reactions. Most studies report that 3 to 10% of asthmatics are sensitive to dietary exposure to sulfites[13]. Sulfites are discussed in detail in Chapter 14.

Nitrates and Sodium Benzoate are used as food preservatives to prevent bacterial growth, usually in meat products. These preservatives can cause pseudoallergic reactions by increasing leukotriene production as discussed in Chapter 15. Sodium Benzoate may provoke ADHD behavior. Nitrates may be transformed into carcinogens during cooking of meats at high temperatures and are further discussed in Chapter 41.

BHA and BHT: BHA (Butylated hydroxyanisole) and BHT (Butylated hydroxytoluene) are antioxidant food additives. Both are lipid soluble.

BHA is used to prevent oils and fats from becoming rancid and having objectionable odors. BHA is used in meat products, margarine, cereals, baked goods, snack foods, dehydrated potatoes, chewing gum, beer, animal feed, and in cosmetics. BHT is now less frequently used as a food preservative than BHA, however, BHT is still used in food packaging materials, and in shortening. BHA may thus be contained in foods labeled as containing shortening. BHA and BHT are carcinogenic in some animals. The low levels of BHA and BHT found in food are unlikely to cause significant health risks; probably less health risk than the processed foods in which they are found. By preventing oxidation of fats, they likely decrease the risk from eating the processed foods they are contained in.

Other Additives: There are many other food additives, several of which are vitamins and minerals. Most of these do not pose health risks. However, α-tocopherol vitamin E, used as an additive, may be less than helpful, as discussed in Chapter 39.

Guar gum is a polysaccharide used for thickening foods, much as starch does. Moreover, it has the unique ability to work in cold water; making it useful in a wide variety of foods. It is also less expensive than many other starches. Guar gum is made from a bean grown as a food crop in India. There is nothing inherently negative about guar gum. It contains about 10% protein, and like other proteins, it can elicit an immune response. Guar gum, thus, can be a hidden immunogen in food. Individuals with an immune response to soy, or other beans, may react to guar protein.

Fructose is a common food additive used to decrease bacterial growth, increase shelf-length, make food softer, chewier, and sweeter. Its considerable health effects are discussed in Chapter 9.

Table 38-5: Listing of Color Additives Exempt from Certification[14].

Annatto extract
Dehydrated beets (beet powder)
Canthaxanthin
Caramel Coloring
[beta]-Apo-8'-carotenal
[beta]-Carotene
Cochineal extract; carmine   (E120)
Sodium copper chlorophyllin   (E141)
For coloring citrus-based dry beverage mixes
Toasted partially defatted cooked cottonseed flour
Ferrous gluconate
Ferrous lactate   (E585)
For the coloring of ripe olives
Grape color extract
For the coloring of non-beverage food
Grape skin extract (enocianina)
For flavoring beverages
Fruit juice
Vegetable juice
Carrot oil
Paprika
Paprika oleoresin
Riboflavin
Saffron
Titanium dioxide
Tomato lycopene extract; tomato lycopene concentrate
Turmeric
Turmeric oleoresin
Mica-based pearlescent pigments
Synthetic iron oxide
For the coloring of sausage casings

Additives as Animal Feed

Several colorants are used in feedstuffs for fish and animals intended for human consumption. These include colorants that give farmed salmon flesh a deeper red color and that give eggs, from chickens fed mostly grain, a bright yellow yolk.

Table 38-6: Colorants used in Animal Feed

Animal Feed Colorant	Used In
Astaxanthin (E161j)	Salmonid fish
Ultramarine blue	Animal feed
Haematococcus algae meal	Salmonid fish
Dried algae meal	Chicken feed
Tagetes (Aztec marigold) meal and extract	Chicken feed
Corn endosperm oil	Chicken feed
Phaffia yeast	Salmonid fish
Paracoccus pigment	Salmonid fish

---

[1] Code of Federal Regulations Title 21, Section 74. USFDA revised April 1, 2010

[2] Cured and broiled meat consumption in relation to childhood cancer: Denver, Colorado (United States) Sarasua S, Savitz DA. Cancer Causes Control. 1994 Mar;5(2):141-8. PMID: 8167261

[3] Processed meats and risk of childhood leukemia (California, USA). Peters JM, Preston-Martin S, London SJ, Bowman JD, Buckley JD, Thomas DC. Cancer Causes Control. 1994 Mar;5(2):195-202. PMID: 8167267

[4] Synthetic food coloring and behavior: a dose response effect in a double-blind, placebo-controlled, repeated-measures study. Rowe KS, Rowe KJ. J Pediatr. 1994 Nov;125(5 Pt 1):691-8. PMID: 7965420

[5] Comedogenicity of current therapeutic products, cosmetics, and ingredients in the rabbit ear. Fulton JE Jr, Pay SR, Fulton JE 3rd. J Am Acad Dermatol. 1984 Jan;10(1):96-105. PMID:6229554

[6] Food additives and hyperactive behaviour in 3-year-old and 8/9-year-old children in the community: a randomised, double-blinded, placebo-controlled trial. McCann D, Barrett A, Cooper A, Crumpler D, Dalen L, Grimshaw K, Kitchin E, Lok K, Porteous L, Prince E, Sonuga-Barke E, Warner JO, Stevenson J. Lancet. 2007 Nov 3;370(9598):1560-7. Erratum in: Lancet. 2007 Nov 3;370(9598):1542. PMID: 17825405

[7] The effects of a double blind, placebo controlled, artificial food colourings and benzoate preservative challenge on hyperactivity in a general population sample of preschool children. Bateman B, Warner JO, Hutchinson E, Dean T, Rowlandson P, Gant C, Grundy J, Fitzgerald C, Stevenson J. Arch Dis Child. 2004 Jun;89(6):506-11.

[8] Synergistic interactions between commonly used food additives in a developmental neurotoxicity test. Lau K, McLean WG, Williams DP, Howard CV. Toxicol Sci. 2006 Mar;90(1):178-87. PMID:16352620

[9] Purification and partial characterization of a novel lectin from elder (Sambucus nigra L.) fruit. Mach L, Scherf W, Ammann M, Poetsch J, Bertsch W, März L, Glössl J. Biochem J. 1991 Sep 15;278 (Pt 3):667-71. PMID: 1910334

[10] http://monographs.iarc.fr/ENG/Monographs/vol101/mono101-015.pdf

[11] Center for Science in the Public Interest, accessed June , 2014 http://www.cspinet.org/new/201206261.html

[12] Consumer Reports: Too many sodas contain potential carcinogen. CNN Accessed June 2014. http://www.cnn.com/2014/01/23/health/consumer-reports-soda-caramel-coloring/

[13] Clinical effects of sulphite additives. Vally H, Misso NL, Madan V. Clin Exp Allergy. 2009 Nov;39(11):1643-51. Epub 2009 Sep 22. Review. PMID: 19775253

[14] Code of Federal Regulations Title 21, Section 73. USFDA revised April 1, 2010

40. NUTRITIONAL SUPPLEMENTS

As a general rule, vitamins and other supplements only provide benefits if there is a nutritional deficiency. It is like going to an automobile repair shop; if your car has a worn-out part and they have the right replacement part, they can fix it, and you can be on your way.

Once, while driving down a rural highway, I heard a thwack, and my car rolled to a stop. A reverse-threaded nut on a pulley had come undone; I saw the pulley roll off into a ditch in my rear view mirror. My serpentine belt was shredded. I walked a couple miles through a thunderstorm and found a phone and arranged for a ride to an auto parts store in a town 30 miles away to get a new serpentine belt. The reverse threaded nut for the pulley, however, was a specialty part only dealers carry. Without it, the car could not run. It was late on a Saturday afternoon, and I had two small children and my wife with me stuck miles from the nearest hamlet, a hundred miles from home. I would have to wait until Monday to just to order the part if I did not find it. It was a cofactor I could not move without. Proteins and enzymes need all their component amino acids to be built, but also need cofactors to function. Miss one required element and things get stuck.

Most people do not drive around with an extra serpentine belt. Putting an extra serpentine belt on your engine would not make your car better. But if the one on the engine goes bad, your car stops. Nutritional supplements are similar. If you do not have a nutritional deficiency, most nutritional supplements are unlikely to provide any benefit. If an individual has a seizure disorder because of a pyridoxine phosphate (PLP) deficiency, or a rare genetic disorder which increases the requirement for a specific nutrient, supplementing that nutrient may prevent the disease. But when there are sufficient vitamins to get the job done, adding more will not help.

Vitamin and mineral supplements have had a hard time in clinical trials. There is surprisingly little evidence that they provide any benefit for most people, and certainly, there is sufficient data indicating that they cause harm to advise avoiding their use as precautionary treatments.

Antioxidants vitamins have been the object of multiple studies for a wide range of disease prevention for in healthy individuals. For example, a randomized trial for the prevention of prostate cancer among 35,000 men who had been tested for, and found not to have any signs of prostate cancer, were given 400 IU of vitamin E a day for 7 years. The men who received vitamin E during the study had a 17% increase in cancer over those who received the placebo; about 1.6 cases per thousand person-years. Selenium supplement also failed to lower risk in this study[1].

As another example, in an uncontrolled population study, 38,000 older women were interviewed about nutritional supplement intake and followed for about 22 years. Use of multivitamins was associated with a 2.4 percent *increase* in mortality. Other supplements also increased mortality:

Zinc	by 3.0%
Magnesium	by 3.6%
Iron	by 3.9%
Vitamin B6	by 4.1%
Folic acid	by 5.9%
Copper	by 18.0%.

Calcium was associated with a decrease in mortality in this population by 3.8%[2]. In a separate study of men and women with an 11-year follow-up of 182,000 patients, multivitamin use did not affect mortality one way or the other[3].

> **Large Studies of Rare Events**
>
> Studies using large populations are required to assess rare events or to measure small effects. To observe the effect of preventive treatment on mortality, it requires follow-up from health to the end of life. To see the potential to cause cancer requires a very large number of individuals without cancer, and then, to follow them until a sufficiently large number of cancer cases are diagnosed. Some vitamins and other supplements have been shown to increase the risk of cancer by a few percentage points. These studies require very large subject population numbers and observation over many years.

In a meta-analysis of sixty-seven prevention studies using antioxidants involving over 230,000 patients[4]:

- Vitamin A increased mortality by 16%,
- β-carotene increased mortality by 7%,
- Vitamin E increased mortality by 4%,
- Vitamin C and selenium neither raised nor lowered risk of mortality.

In 18 blinded clinical trials including 46,000 patients, those taking synthetic vitamin E had no change in mortality rates, but those taking natural vitamin E had a 13 percent increase in mortality[5]. In a placebo-controlled randomized trial for the prevention of prostate cancer, folic acid supplement or placebo was given over a ten-year follow-up period. Those who received the folic acid had a 9.7% probability of being diagnosed with prostate cancer during the follow-up period while only 3.3% of the placebo group was diagnosed with the disease. However, those individuals who had higher serum folate levels but were not vitamin users at baseline were less likely to get prostate cancer[6]. Thus, dietary folate was not a risk, except when it is used as a supplement.

But don't flush your supplements yet.

In a study of poorly nourished population in China with high gastric and esophageal cancer incidence, multi-vitamins did decrease mortality in some groups. In this study, nearly 30,000 adults were randomized into eight groups and given either a placebo or one or more sets of vitamins for five years and then followed-up again after 10 more years. These supplement sets were:

- Retinol and zinc
- Riboflavin and niacin
- Vitamin C and molybdenum
- Vitamin E, β-carotene, and selenium

Retinol and zinc increased mortality, while vitamin E, β-carotene, and selenium decreased mortality in this population, with most of the risk reduction seen in those below age 55 at the onset of the trial[7].

In a French trial, including about 12,000 individuals, a combination of vitamin C, vitamin E, β-carotene, selenium and zinc failed to lower cancer incidence in women, but did lower cancer risk by 30% in men. Prostate cancer risk was cut in half if the men started the study with a PSA of less than 3.0 μg/L at the beginning of the trial, but increased risk by 54% if their PSA level was above 3.0. PSA is a marker for prostate cancer[8]. High dosages of folic acid prevent the development of new tumors in animal studies but support the growth of pre-existing tumors[9].

These data suggest that administration of these vitamins prevent cancer before it gets started, but promote its growth once it is present.

Use Supplements to Treat Deficiencies

Megadoses of vitamins are unlikely to benefit enzymatic function. But vitamin and mineral supplements can sometimes be used as medicine. Magnesium (oxide) can be used as a laxative. Vitamin C can also be used as an osmotic laxative but may encourage bacterial overgrowth. Megadoses of vitamins are more likely to cause harm than benefit. Some vitamins are outright toxic in high doses.

Tetrahydrobiopterin may be helpful in some types of phenylketonuria. In some diseases, vitamins are poorly absorbed or metabolized, and thus, supplements may help. For most vitamins, these are rare exceptions.

Iron deficiencies, for example, are common, and treatment provides a clear benefit. Iron is also quite toxic. Old-fashion iron tablets were once the number one cause of poisoning deaths in small children, as a single tablet could be a toxic dose for a toddler, and they typically resembled an enticing, shiny, bright red M&M candy.

Iron supplements should not be taken if there is not a deficiency, usually due to blood loss. A healthy diet with dark green vegetables supplies sufficient iron for most people.

Hemochromatosis

Hemochromatosis is the most common genetic disease in the Caucasian population; one in 200 to 250 Caucasians are homozygous for the C282Y allele of the HFE gene. In Native Americans, the rate is about 1/1000 individuals, and most other groups are less commonly affected[10]. In hemochromatosis, the body stores excess iron. Women are somewhat protected, as menstruation lowers iron stores.

This disease is associated with elevated ferritin that reflects iron content in the body. Ferritin levels in CY828Y individuals of greater than 1000 μg per liter are associated with fatigue, arthritis, and development of liver disease[11]. Elevated iron stores can cause bronzing of the skin, diabetes, liver cirrhosis, cardiomyopathy, and hepatocellular carcinoma. The iron overload is treated by having the patient donate blood and thus remove excess iron.

Iron supplements put individuals with the C282Y allele at much greater risk for iron overload and disease. Other alleles of the HFE gene can also confer risk for hemochromatosis, and even individuals with the normal allele are subject to iron overload from iron supplements.

Many Americans don't eat a healthful diet, and deficiencies are not uncommon. When food is refined, for example, when bran is removed from wheat and rice, to improve its storage life, many nutrients are lost. Large amounts of the calories in the western diet come from bleached and processed grains, refined sugars, refined corn syrup, and refined vegetable oils. These foods have only small amounts of vitamins and minerals.

Some nutrient deficiencies are so common in the Western diet that vitamins have been added to the food supply. Folic acid is one of the nutrients that have been added to processed, refined foods. Folate deficiencies are associated with increased risk of cervical cancer, birth defects, and heart disease. Folate comes from foliage; green leaves. For most Americans, the largest source of natural dietary folate comes from orange juice, not because O.J. is such a great source of folate, but rather, because the Western diet contains a paucity of green vegetables. The main source of folate in the American diet is from processed foods fortified with this and other vitamins to make up what has been lost from a natural diet.

Use the Correct Dose and Form

Vitamin B_{12} is a cofactor for the enzyme methionine synthase. This enzyme transfers a methyl group from 5-methyltetrahydrofolate to homocysteine, in order to form methionine for the production of S-adenosylmethionine (SAMe). SAMe is the primary methyl group donor in most biological methylation reactions, including methylation of DNA. It also is required by the CNS for myelination of nerves. If there is insufficient vitamin B_{12} present in the body, high doses of folate can make up for many vitamin B_{12} activities, but this may result in the accumulation of toxic metabolites and increase DNA methylation. This hypermethylation can increase the risk of cancer. Thus, excess folate with vitamin B_{12} deficiency is more likely to cause problems, beyond those of vitamin B_{12} deficiency alone[12]. Even in the presence of adequate vitamin B_{12}, excess folate may increase cancer risk.

Folate and Colon Cancer

Low folate levels are a risk for colon cancer, as they can cause hypomethylation of the p53 tumor suppressor gene. This makes the gene more easily induced, and thus, allows it to be more exposed. This puts the gene at higher risk of breaking, and thus, for mutation. Low folate levels may also impair DNA repair mechanism. About half of human colon cancers have a mutation in the p53 gene[13]. Folate also appears to prevent neuroblastoma, a cancer of infants, as the rates for this disease fell by 60% soon after food folate fortification was initiated. Low folate levels are also associated with the risk of cancers of the colorectum, lungs, breast, pancreas, esophagus, stomach, cervix, ovary, and leukemia[14].

Excess folic acid is also suspected to cause cancer; here, by hypermethylation of the p53 gene, which may suppress its activity in preventing tumor growth. In lab animals that have had tumor cells implanted, high doses of folic acid; ten times the physiologic requirements, show increased tumor cell growth. There is, however, no evidence that natural, food-based folates have this effect[14]. There are several forms of folate; folic acid is the one used in most vitamin tablets and for food fortification and it may not be the least toxic choice. In a trial using 1 mg of folic acid in patients with a history of colonic adenomas, folic acid increased the risk of developing new precancerous lesions[15]. Dietary vitamin B_2 (riboflavin) and B_6 (pyridoxal-5-phosphate) levels, however, were found be to inversely associated with the development of advanced adenomas[16].

In a study of patients with p53 positive colon cancers, both low and high folic acid intake and low vitamin B_6 levels were associated with increased risk. The risk for these patients was lowest when folic acid intake was between 350 and 750 micrograms of folic acid per day. Although not statically significant, the nadir for p53 negative colon cancers was associated with folic acid intakes at these levels. Vitamin B6 intakes of less than 1.5 mg a day were associated with increased risk of p53 colon cancer[13].

In a meta-analysis of vitamin D supplementation, looking at 50 randomized studies including 94,000 elderly women, vitamin D_3 decreased the risk of mortality by six percent while vitamin D_2 had no effect[17]. Vitamin D_2 is a fungal vitamin which has been used as a supplement. Vitamin D_3 is the one our bodies use sunlight to make.

Eat Right; Use Supplements as Medicine

The body is fairly robust in the ability to get dietary requirements from a mixed source of foods. Outside of famine it is unusual for healthy individuals to need supplements if they are eating a reasonable mix of foods and getting enough sunshine. Simple criteria; but scarcely occurring. Most Americans do not consume a nutritionally balanced diet or get sufficient sunshine, and far too few are healthy.

Although deficient nutrient intake is not uncommon for certain nutrients, the more salient source of deficiencies arises from malabsorption syndromes. With malabsorption, diets may be perfectly adequate, but the individual fails to absorb, or loses, critical nutrients. Malabsorption and intestinal pathology can cause the loss of vitamins, other nutrients and hormones from the body.

The fat-soluble vitamins (A, D, E and K) are easily lost in fat malabsorption. Vitamin D is excreted into the bile, as are other steroid hormones and they can be lost if there is malabsorption of fats and bile. Vitamin B_{12} is excreted into the bile and reabsorbed; thus, vitamin B_{12} is an element of the enterohepatic circulation[18]. If there is malabsorption or lack of intrinsic factor Vitamin B_{12} can be wasted. β-carotene, vitamin E, and Vitamin K_1 require bile acid for absorption into the enterocyte.

Each of the water-soluble B vitamins; thiamine, riboflavin, and folic acid, have specific carrier proteins on the enterocyte brush border membrane that transport the vitamins into the cell from the lumen of the intestine. Folate needs to be absorbed and then converted in the liver to its active form. It is then excreted into the bile and must be reabsorbed from the small intestine to be available in its active form. Biotin and pantothenic acid share a membrane transporter.

Iron deficiency is also common, especially in children, menstruating women and the elderly. Iron must first be in the ferrous form (Fe^{2+}) for absorption. The enzyme ferric reductase on the enterocyte brush border reduces dietary iron in the ferric form (Fe^{3+}) to Fe^{2+}. The divalent metal transporter protein (DMT1) can then transport the metal ion into the enterocyte. Once in the enterocyte iron binds to a protein; either apoferritin or ferroportin. The enterocyte can store iron for several days, and it can be utilized if needed. Excess iron gets eliminated from the body when enterocytes end their approximately four- to the ten-day life cycle and are eliminated in the feces.

Generally, five to 35 percent of dietary iron may be absorbed, depending on how avidly the body works to raise iron levels. DMT1 also absorbs other divalent metal ions, including copper, manganese, lead and cadmium. In iron deficiency, DMT1 expression is elevated, and iron and other divalent metal ions, including toxic metals are absorbed more avidly[19]. Thus, iron deficiency increases the risk of toxicity from metals. DMT1 is also present in brain tissues; thus, in iron deficiency there is an increased risk of toxic metal associated neurological disease[20].

All of the vitamins that require a specific enterocyte membrane protein for absorption are subject to malabsorption if the enterocytes are damaged, for example, by infection or gluten enteropathy. The toxic lectin phytohemagglutinin causes rapid growth of enterocytes without promoting a full complement of proteins and enzymes, and thus may preclude absorption of nutrients.

Zinc deficiency is not uncommon. Dietary malnutrition with zinc deficiency is not uncommon in children in poor countries where the diet is limited to low-protein diets with starchy vegetables and leaves. Phytate present in many plants can inhibit zinc and other mineral absorption[21]. In developed countries, zinc deficiency is more often caused by malabsorption. Diarrhea and malabsorption syndromes, including Celiac disease and inflammatory bowel disease, decrease the absorption and increase loss of zinc from the body[22]. Lactose, fructose, and other sugar malabsorption speeds the transit of nutrients through the small intestine and decreases the absorption of some nutrients.

Hypochlorhydria, having low stomach acidity, impairs zinc absorption. Proton pump inhibitors (PPI), such as Prilosec (omeprazole), are in common, long-term use. PPIs lower stomach acid secretion; and not unexpectedly, there use lowers serum zinc levels[23].

GERD: An alternative to PPI may, surprisingly, be zinc! Low-dose $ZnCl_2$ quickly inhibits gastric acid secretion in rats and human stomach tissue after histamine stimulation. $ZnCl_2$ at 0.5 mg/kg/day in rats[24], the allometrically adjusted human adult dose equivalent (see below) would be about 6 mg of $ZnCl_2$ or 3 mg of elemental zinc. About sixty percent of a dose of zinc gluconate or citrate is absorbed[25], so a five mg dose (of elemental zinc) delivers about 3 mg.

Five milligrams of zinc can be combined with three milligrams of melatonin, used at bedtime, for the treatment of gastroesophageal reflux disease. Three milligrams of melatonin at bedtime has been found to be as effective of 20 mg of omeprazole in the treatment of GERD[26]. Melatonin is further discussed in Chapter 43. Adding

Most zinc supplements are labeled giving the elemental dose of zinc. Five mg of zinc supplement daily is sufficient supplement for most individuals. Vegans, those with malabsorption, chronic diarrhea or who are poorly nourished may need more. Long-term supplementation of zinc should not exceed 20 mg, and 10 mg of zinc daily is likely the upper prudent limit for safe daily use[27]. Even in acute dosing to recover from a zinc deficiency, 25 mg daily of elemental zinc should be sufficient. High dose zinc supplementation may explain the increased risk of cancer seen with zinc supplementation.

Alcohol use can also cause the malabsorption of several nutrients. H. pylori infection can cause gastric atrophy and prevent vitamin B_{12} absorption. One in six adults over the age of 65 is at risk of vitamin B_{12} deficiency[31]. Oxidative stress can also deplete antioxidant vitamins. Inflammation can prevent vitamin B_6 activity, and inhibit its function as an enzyme cofactor even when the body has normal levels of this vitamin.

Table 40-1: Common Causes of Nutrient Deficiencies

- Damage to enterocyte membrane
- Pancreatic enzyme deficiencies (especially for fat absorption)
- Carbohydrate malabsorption with rapid small intestinal transit time
- Bile acid loss
- Small intestinal bacterial overgrowth
- Alcohol abuse
- Gastric atrophy from Helicobacter pylori infection
- Paucity of vegetables in the Western diet, lack of sunshine

The most common vitamin deficiencies are the fat soluble vitamins and folate and vitamin B_{12} which also depend on the reabsorption from the bile. Iron, zinc and magnesium, and calcium are also often in short supply in the body. Iron deficiency is most often a result of blood loss.

Vitamin A, vitamin D, and vitamin K_2 are the activated forms of fat-soluble vitamins which are formed in the body from precursor compounds. These activated vitamins are excreted into the bile, and they are unique in that they are reabsorbed across the enterocyte membrane by passive diffusion. Vitamin A, vitamin D, and synthetic vitamin K_3 are toxic at high doses, but their precursors; β-carotene, cholesterol, and vitamin K_1 from plants (phylloquinone) are not toxic.

The precursors of these vitamins and all other vitamins require specific carrier proteins on enterocyte brush border surface for absorption[28]. Thus, vitamin absorption is an active process. Damage to the enterocyte membrane thus prevents absorption of most vitamins.

Malnutrition in the Western Diet

There are some nutritional deficiencies seen even in affluent cultures.

- Vegans often have vitamin B_{12} deficiencies. Vegan mothers that breastfeed can pass this deficiency to their infants. Low vitamin B_{12} levels are common among the elderly.
- The western diet contains excessive n-6 fats. This causes a relative n-3 fat deficiency.
- Most individuals in industrialized temperate climates do not get sufficient sun exposure to have adequate vitamin D formation in their skin.
- Magnesium deficiencies are common, as a result of the paucity of green vegetables in the diet.

Dosing

When studies of nutritional supplements are done, researchers usually start out looking to see if high but tolerable doses have beneficial effects. They want fast answers to big questions. Only after they have established an effect does it make sense to do dosing studies, which are usually harder and much more costly, especially when dealing with chronic diseases. Many times the dose used in the first study becomes a standard dose used in supplements as there was evidence of its efficacy, but no evidence of harm from the often short-term study. An example of this is PQQ supplements (Chapter 28), which often contain 10000 mcg while the normal dietary intake is only about 150 mcg. As can be seen by the increase in cancer rates with vitamin supplements – there is good reason to limit the dose of supplements to physiological needs, and not to exceed them many-fold.

Animals studies are much less costly, exact less risk to human life, and are much more convenient than are human studies. Animals can be kept in cages, where their diets, activities, and exercise can be tightly regulated. It is easier to determine the effect of a single controllable variable, such as a nutrient or drug and eliminate the myriad of exposures humans are exposed to day to day.

Thus, there are numerous nutritional studies on animals with data applicable to mankind. Doses, however, need to be adjusted. When using comparative dosing, such as when extrapolating a dose that is effective in mice to man, allometric conversions should be applied. Allometric conversions adjust dose per kilogram according to the animal's metabolic rate. Thus, the dose is adjusted to metabolic activity. Sometimes body surface area is used as a proxy for metabolic activity.

Table 40-2: Converting Animal Dosage to Humans[29]

Species	Reference Weight	Body Surface Area (M^2)	Standard Conversion
Mouse	20 g	0.007	0.081
Rat	150 g	.025	0.162
Rabbit	1.8	0.15	0.324
Dog	10 kg	0.5	0.541
Human Child	20 kg	0.8	
Human adult	60 kg	1.62	

The conversion is used by multiplying the standard conversion dose, in mg/kg, for example, times the conversion factor to get the human dose per kilogram. Thus, if the effective rat dose is 75 mg/kg per day, an adult human dose would be: 75 x 0.162 = 12.15 mg/kg per day.

The human equivalent dose can also be calculated as:

Animal mg per kg dose x (animal wt kg / human wt kg)$^{0.33}$

Thus, 75 mg/kg dose, for a 200 mg rat, in a 60 kg woman would yield: 75 mg per kg x $(.20/60)^{0.33}$ = 11.42 mg per kg.

Allometric assumptions can fail, especially when used for drug toxicity; aspirin is easily toxic for cats, for example, as cats lack drug glucuronidation capacity. Dogs completely lack, while rats excel at drug-acetylation beyond humans. Humans cannot dine on the untreated acorns relished by squirrels. There are differences membrane transporters. Biliary excretion and hepatic enzyme activity can vary widely between species. Thus, the toxicity of drugs eliminated by biliary excretion or metabolized by the liver may not be comparable between animals; while those excreted in the urine tend to be more equivalent. For these reasons, drug testing in humans usually begins at one tenth the allometrically adjusted animal dose per kilogram[30].

It is not uncommon to find journal articles in which doses of nutrient supplements have proposed or their use abandoned, based upon doses from animal studies, that have not been adjusted for metabolic activity, and which thus provide dose estimates clearly in excess of human nutritional needs and in excess of that which would be consumed in a rational diet. After conversion, however, data provided by many studies suggest that these diseases may be avoided or treated nutritionally. For nutrients, the human equivalent dose of a nutrient, as long as it not in excess of the usual safe, non-toxic dose range, provides an appropriate starting dose for nutritional therapy. This dose will be much smaller than the effective small animal dose per kilogram.

Micronutrients

Vitamin A and Carotenoids

Vitamin A has the narrowest therapeutic range of any vitamin, and it can easily be toxic at levels used as a supplement. Vitamin A supplements are, thus, not recommended for general use.

The retinoic acid (RA) form of vitamin A plays an important role in gene transcription and is tightly regulated. This role in gene transcription may explain why vitamin A supplements promote cancer growth, and why its use is associated with increased mortality, especially in older individuals.

β-carotene has been the subject of cancer prevention trials, based on its antioxidant capacity, but it has had the opposite effect; it promoted cancer growth. Previtamin A (β-carotene) can be converted by the body into various forms of vitamin A. β-carotene is not toxic. This, however, does not prevent RA formed from β-carotene from supporting gene transcription and promoting the growth of tumor cells. This may explain why β-carotene is associated with increased mortality in patients with cancer.

There are several other antioxidant carotenoids besides β-carotene in food. Most of these are not converted to vitamin A, and thus, they would not be expected to increase tumor growth. Lutein and zeaxanthin are antioxidants that protect the retina from blue light hazard. A mix of antioxidant carotenoids from food sources, especially dark green and orange vegetables, is a preferable way to supply antioxidants; these impart little if any risk of cancer.

Previtamin A (β-carotene) at 25,000 units a day is a safe dose while this is not a safe dose for vitamin A (retinyl esters). The recommended daily allowance for vitamin A may be used as the upper limit for a supplement when used for treatment; however, use of β-carotene is preferable.

One REA (Retinol Activity Equivalent) is equal to 1 μg of retinol, 2 μg of β-carotene in oil or 12 μg of dietary β-carotene. Other carotenes that the body can convert to vitamin A, though less efficiently, also count as REA, but at a ratio of 1:24. One REA is equivalent to 3.33 units of Retinol activity.

The recommended daily allowances for vitamin A REA are:

- Children, 9 to 13 years; 600 μg/day (2000 units)
- For women, 14 years and older, 700 μg/day (2300 units)
- For men, 14 years and older is 900 μg/day (3000 units)

Considering that nearly 90% of young people are afflicted with acne, and that low vitamin A is associated with this risk, then it may be appropriate to set the carotene intake goal to the REA intake to the population 90th percentile level.

Table 40-3: Usual Retinol Activity Equivalent Intake

Group	REA Mean Intake	REA 90th-percentile[31]
Males 14 – 19	819	1,333
Males 19 – 30	803	1,292
Females 14 – 19	546	877
Females 19 – 30	583	943

Table 40-4: Retinal Activity Equivalents (REA) in Foods High in Carotene:

Food: Half Cup Serving	Retinol Activity Equivalents (μg)	Units Previtamin A
Carrots	550	1800
Sweet Potato	960	3200
Butternut Squash	570	1900
Spinach	470	1400

The upper limits for safety for preformed vitamin A (Retinyl esters) are:

- 9 to 13 years; 1700 mcg/day (6000 units);
- 14 to 18 years (including pregnancy and lactation); 2800 mcg/day (9000 units);
- Adults age 19 and older (including pregnancy and lactation); 3000 mcg/day (10,000 units).

Do not exceed these levels of intake of preformed Vitamin A (retinyl esters). These limits are for total daily intake, including vitamin A from food sources. Preformed Vitamin A supplements should not be used in individuals taking retinoid analogs, such as isotretinoin (Accutane) or similar medications.

The absorption of carotenes requires bile acids, and thus, carotenes are much better absorbed from food in meals with some fat content, in contrast for example to eating a raw carrot as a snack by itself. This is why β-carotene supplements in oil have an REA number six times higher than does β-carotene in food. Adding butter, a bit of olive oil or sour cream to a baked sweet potato and other vegetables can thus be justified by more than just flavor and palatability. It is likely difficult to get sufficient vitamin A from β-carotene in a vegetarian diet without mixing vegetables with foods containing fats. When consumed with fats, the REA numbers for foods given in Table 39-3 would be several times higher.

The B Vitamins

The B vitamins are a diverse set of compounds, grouped together not by similarity in structure, but rather on the basis that they are water soluble, act as coenzymes, and are largely eliminated in the urine. Most of the B vitamins have low, if any, toxicity.

The Numbered B Vitamins	
Vitamin B$_1$	Thiamine
Vitamin B$_2$	Riboflavin
Vitamin B$_3$	Niacin
Vitamin B$_5$	Pantothenic acid
Vitamin B$_6$	Pyridoxal-5-phosphate
Vitamin B$_7$	Biotin
Vitamin B$_9$	Folates
Vitamin B$_{12}$	Cyanocobalamin

Assessing vitamin sufficiency is not a simple task. The classical definitions for vitamin deficiencies were defined by diseases associated with extreme deficiency states, such as scurvy, beriberi, and pellagra, which occurred from long-term, severe dietary deprivation. These deficiencies occurred when an individual or community were sustained on a very limited diet, such as tea and toast. Beriberi became epidemic in populations that had little more than polished rice to eat while brown rice had been able to sustain them.

Assessing the effects of exposure to low-level deficiencies over long time periods is a different and more difficult task than finding a rare disease in patients with an obviously inadequate diet. It is comparable to the difference between assessing the effects of acute high-dose exposure to a toxin with those of the long-term effects of very low-level exposure to the toxin.

One method for evaluating the health effects of long-term exposure to suboptimal nutrition is to assess metabolic intermediaries associated with disease. This can allow the study of the disease process, rather than wait many years to look for outcomes of suboptimal nutrition.

Homocysteine (HCY) is a metabolic intermediary in single-carbon methylation. High levels have been associated with vascular disease. Homocysteine levels in the blood are inversely related to folate, pyridoxine, and cyanocobalamin levels. Figure 39-1 shows data from a study I co-authored on homocysteine and coronary heart disease[32,33], where levels of homocysteine, folate, and vitamin B_{12} were measured in over 200 middle-aged men.

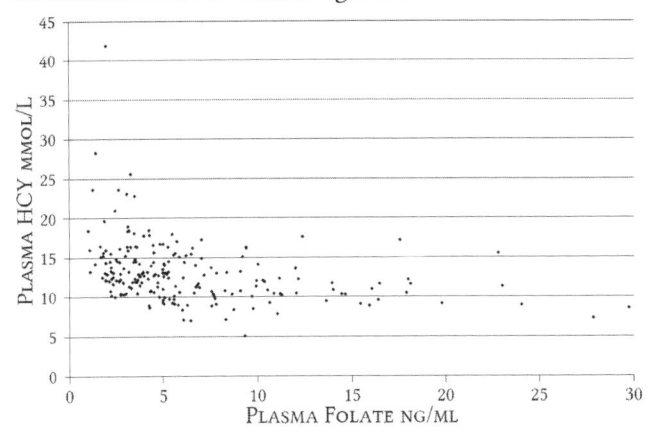

Figure 40-1: Inverse Relation of Folate and Homocysteine

In Figure 39-1, it can be seen that in the case of folates, homocysteine levels fall with rising folate levels until they plateau above 7 ng/ml. HCY is given in µmol/L. There were few individuals with high folate levels. Notice that most of the population studied had levels well below this apparent optimal folate levels of around 8 to 12 ng/ml. This data was collected prior to the fortification of processed foods with folic acid. Population median folate levels have, since, risen from 5.5 ng/ml to 10.5 ng/ml since the onset of fortification in North America[34]. In the U.S., folate fortification became mandatory for flour and breakfast cereals in 1998 and since then, the prevalence of elevated HCY levels have fallen, accompanied by a fall in the incidence of several diseases including neural tube defects. Thus, folate insufficiency, previously common, is now rare in North America, and the occurrence of elevated homocysteine levels has fallen[35].

Similar to folate, HCY levels are inversely associated with vitamin B_{12} levels, up to about 470 pg/ml of the vitamin, above which there is little if any diminution in HCY levels. In the same study as cited above, only about half the population had sufficient vitamin B_{12} levels for optimal HCY metabolism. For both these vitamins much of the population levels were below the apparent metabolic requirement; however, these optimal levels are consistent with, and easily achieved, with the consumption of a healthy diet.

The current reference range for normal folate levels in adults is 5.4 ng/ml (12.2 nmol/L); it is 200 pg/ml (148 pmol/L) for vitamin B_{12}. These data suggest that the current reference ranges for the lower limit of normal folate and vitamin B_{12} are about half of the levels required to maintain low HCY levels. The data presented here suggests a normal reference range for optimal folate to be about 10 ng/ml (@ 22.6 nmol/L) and for vitamin B_{12} to be about 470 pg/ml (@ 350 pmol/L). Data from the National Health and Nutrition Evaluation Survey (NHANES) confirms these results and suggest that plasma vitamin B_{12} levels of at least 500 pg/ml are required to efficiently breakdown HCY and methyl malonic acid (MMA)[36]. Additionally, it has been found that when folate levels are adequate, HCY and MMA concentrations actually increased with serum folate levels when vitamin B_{12} levels are inadequate[37].

Dietary intake of 400 µg of folate is usually adequate to maximize the benefit of folate. However, folate levels may be low in some individuals with sufficient intake because of malabsorption. Nevertheless, folate supplements higher than 500 µg daily should not be used unless vitamin B_{12} levels have been tested to be adequate. If low, vitamin B_{12} should be treated first, and underlying causes for low levels investigated and treated. Adequate n-3 fats may also lower the risks associated with hypermethylation from excess folate in individuals with low vitamin B_{12} levels[12].

Folate and other vitamins are involved in methylation, and nerve injury can deplete resources. After spinal cord or other nerve injury in lab animals, folate is rapidly depleted, and S-adenosylmethionine (SAMe) is converted to S-adenosylhomocysteine (SAH), which further impedes the uptake of folate into the neurons. The lack of SAMe prevents DNA methylation required for growth and repair of neurons[38]. A 10-fold improvement in axon regrowth and functional recovery after CNS injury occurred when mice received 80 µg/kg of folic acid[39]. Using the standard allometric conversion (Table 40-2) yields the adult human equivalent of 6.48 µg/kg, and thus a dose of 454 µg for a 70-kg adult. Thus, even in these conditions, the normal folate supplemental dose should be adequate.

Recommended Dietary Allowances (RDA), are the amount of a nutrient recommended by Institute of Medicine of the National Academy of Sciences to provide an adequate level of nutrients to supply the needs of 97 to 98 percent of the population. Table 39-5 gives RDA levels for adults. The document, <u>Dietary Reference Intakes: Vitamins</u>, contains detailed recommendations for various age groups as well as for pregnant and lactating females. A link to this document in included in Appendix B.

Vitamin B_6

Vitamin B_6 is comprised of six related compounds: pyridoxal, pyridoxine, pyridoxamine, and three more 5'-phosphate compounds (PLP, PNP, PMP). Pyridoxal-5-phosphate (PLP) is the active form of vitamin B_6.

Vitamin B_6 blood levels fall during inflammatory conditions. The vitamin is not lost, but rather becomes tied up, and unavailable. Supplementation may help restore the metabolic pathways which require PLP, during treatment for the underlying cause of inflammation.

In patients with rheumatoid arthritis, supplementation with 50 mg of pyridoxine daily helped restore vitamin B_6 levels and lowered homocysteine levels, but did not resolve inflammation[40]. In cardiovascular patients with systemic inflammation, pyridoxine HCl, at 40 mg/day, greatly lowered levels of the toxic kynurenine metabolite, 3-HK[41]. In another study, risk of recurrent colonic adenomas was diminished in patients who had plasma PLP levels higher than 85 nmol/L; this corresponds to a dietary intake of about 3 mg of vitamin B_6 per day[42]. In a different study, risk of colon cancer was lowest among subjects with a daily intake of vitamin B_6 was between 2 and 5 mg per day[13]. Herein, 3 mg of vitamin B_6 is recommended as an appropriate adult daily intake, although a higher amounts may be required for treatment of inflammatory conditions. Herein, 25 mg, but no more than 50 mg, of pyridoxine HCl is recommended as a therapeutic dose of vitamin B_6 when used in the treatment of disease. Excessive supplementation with vitamin B_6 can have toxic consequences; chronic use of 200 mg daily may result in peripheral neuropathy.

Vitamin B_{12}

To be absorbed, cyanocobalamin (vitamin B_{12}) first binds to haptocorrin, a glycoprotein present in saliva, which protects vitamin B_{12} from being destroyed by stomach acid. In the duodenum, vitamin B12 is released from haptocorrin by pancreatic proteases. Vitamin B_{12} then binds to another glycoprotein, intrinsic factor, which is produced in the stomach. In the ileum, a subset of enterocytes that bear intrinsic factor receptors on their brush border membrane carry the vitamin B_{12}/intrinsic factor complex into the cell, through endocytosis. The complex is then taken up by lysosomes, where the intrinsic factor is removed, and cyanocobalamin is freed.

Vitamin B_{12} levels are very often low, due to defects in one or more steps in this process. Food containing vitamin B_{12} needs to be chewed for it to mix with saliva so that it can bind to, and be protected by, haptocorrin. Pernicious anemia is caused by the autoimmune destruction of gastric parietal cells, leading to atrophic gastritis and loss of intrinsic factor production. Gastric atrophy also results from H. pylori infection, and this too decreases intrinsic factor production. Vitamin B_{12} also enters the enterohepatic circulation where it can be lost in patients with malabsorption. Small bowel overgrowth or damage to the intestinal mucosa may prevent absorption or reabsorption.

Sicca syndrome in Sjögren's syndrome is associated with loss of saliva production. Without saliva, vitamin B_{12} is destroyed by stomach acid. Elderly individuals often have poor dentition or poorly fitting dentures, and thus, may consume a soft diet, which does not require much mastication, thus evading the protection of vitamin B_{12} by haptocorrin.

Vitamin B_{12} deficiency is common among the elderly, mostly due to inadequate absorption. Oral doses of vitamin B_{12} 500 times the RDA or more may be required to normalize blood levels in the elderly[46]. Vitamin B_{12} tablets which are swallowed whole have very low efficacy and thus, require very high doses. Vitamin B_{12} lozenges, sublingual or chewable forms that promote mixing with saliva, give much better vitamin B_{12} absorption. Excessive vitamin B_{12} absorption from lozenges has been reported to cause rashes and acne.

Vitamin B_{12} deficiency is common. It can be considered to be pandemic, occurring in about half the population if the criterion for adequate vitamin B_{12} is set to levels required to maintain normal homocysteine and MMA concentrations. Herein, a normal lower limit for plasma vitamin B_{12} of 500 pg/ml is thus recommended. A daily intake of 6 μg of vitamin B_{12} is sufficient for adults with normal absorption to maintain this level.

Biotin

In biotin deficiency, clinical findings include dermatitis, conjunctivitis, alopecia and central nervous system abnormalities. Biotin deficiency from inadequate dietary intake is rare. One cause is of biotin deficiency is the consumption of raw egg white which contains the protein avidin. Avidin binds to biotin in the intestine and prevents its absorption. Avidin is incompletely destroyed during normal cooking of eggs; however, the risk is considerably lowered. Bacteria also produce biotin in the large intestine, and this supplies much of the body's needs. Overuse of antibiotics or dysbiosis may limit absorption of biotin from commensal bacteria.

Niacin

Niacin may cause flushing and gastrointestinal symptoms with large doses. This does not occur during consumption of foods rich in niacin. Much larger doses of niacin are sometimes used in the treatment of hypercholesterolemia. Large doses of sustained-release niacin have been found to cause fulminant hepatic failure in rare cases[43].

Vitamin C

Vitamin C (ascorbate) is an important antioxidant vitamin. Ascorbate gets concentrated by active transport into white blood cells, wherein, the concentrations may be 80 times higher than in the plasma. In these cells, where there is active production of reactive oxygen species for the breakdown of bacteria, foreign proteins and autophagy; vitamin C provides the cells protection, recycling antioxidants.

Both plasma and neutrophil ascorbate levels rise quickly with increasing dietary intake until they plateau with a daily intake of about 125 mg a day in men. In lactating women, vitamin C content in their milk maximizes with a daily intake of 100 to 200 mg of ascorbate a day. Very little vitamin C is absorbed beyond this level, and excess that is absorbed is eliminated by the kidneys[44]. Larger doses of vitamin C are not absorbed by the intestines.

Vitamin C levels are lower in smokers. Quitting smoking will promote health more than adding a bit of extra vitamin C. Vitamin C levels may also be lower in SIBO or malabsorption syndromes. Less than optimum vitamin C levels should respond to a healthful diet and by resolving the underlying cause of low vitamin C levels.

Table 40-5: B Vitamins

B Vitamin	Deficiency Syndromes	Toxicity
Vitamin B$_1$ Thiamine	Deficiency causes beriberi, Wernicke's encephalopathy, Korsakoff's syndrome. Can cause emotional disturbances, impaired sensory perception, weakness and pain in the limbs, edema, and heart failure. Korsakoff's syndrome in chronic alcoholism can lead to irreversible psychosis with amnesia and confabulation.	None
Vitamin B$_2$ Riboflavin	May cause skin or mucosal lesions. Migraine headaches. Required for FAD and FMN	None
Vitamin B$_3$ Niacin Niacinamide	Deficiency causes pellagra which causes dermatitis, diarrhea, dementia, and can cause death. Deficiency may cause aggression and insomnia. Required for NAD	Large doses of niacin cause flushing and abdominal distress. High doses of slow-release niacin can cause fulminant liver failure.
Vitamin B$_5$ Pantothenic acid	Deficiency only occurs in starvation – may cause acne and paresthesia.	None
Vitamin B$_6$ Pyridoxine	Deficiency causes elevated homocysteine, macrocytic anemia, and mood disorders. Required for tryptophan metabolism and monoamine and GABA neurotransmitter synthesis.	More than 200 mg/day may cause peripheral sensory neuropathy
Vitamin B$_7$ Biotin	Growth disorders in children; usually from an inborn error of metabolism (Multiple carboxylase deficiency)	None
Vitamin B$_9$ Folates	Elevated homocysteine, macrocytic anemia, birth defects cancer risk. Mood disorders; required for the formation of tetrahydrobiopterin – used in monoamine formation (Dopamine, noradrenalin, etc.)	Masks B$_{12}$ deficiency, which may result in permanent neuropathic damage.
Vitamin B$_{12}$ Cyanocobalamin	Elevated homocysteine, macrocytic anemia, peripheral neuropathy, memory loss and other cognitive deficits. Mostly supports folate activity.	Rash or acne. Extremely rare: May cause vision loss in patients with Leber's hereditary optic neuropathy[45].

Table 40-6: Daily Intake Recommendations for the B Vitamins

B Vitamin	RDA Daily	Recommended Supplement Level for Disease Treatment	Upper Tolerable Daily Intake
Vitamin B$_1$ Thiamine	1.2 mg – men 1.1 mg – women	25 mg twice daily	
Vitamin B$_2$ Riboflavin	1.3 mg – men 1.1 mg – women	25 mg twice daily for migraine	
Vitamin B$_3$ Niacin	16 mg – men 14 mg – women	25 mg daily with a meal	35 mg
Vitamin B$_5$ Pantothenic acid	5 mg – men 5 mg – women		
Vitamin B$_6$ Pyridoxal Group	1.3 mg – younger 1.6 mg – older	25 mg once or twice daily	1000 mg
Vitamin B$_7$ Biotin	30 μg		
Vitamin B$_9$ Folates	400 μg	400 μg	1000 μg
Vitamin B$_{12}$ Cobalamin	2.4 μg	1000 – 2000 μg[46] oral dose	
Choline	550 mg – men 425 mg – women	500 mg twice daily for one month	3500 mg

A healthy diet, containing several servings of fruits and vegetables, should easily provide 125 mg of vitamin C a day. If not consuming a healthy diet, a 100 mg supplement will supply sufficient vitamin C. There is little reason to use large doses of vitamin C supplements except as an osmotic stool softener and laxative. It, however, is not an ideal laxative, as it is fermentable and produces bloating, gas formation and diarrhea, and can promote dysbiosis.

Vitamin C and Iron

Vitamin C greatly enhances the absorption of non-heme (non-animal source) dietary iron. Adding 16 mg of ascorbic acid per milligram of iron in a meal nearly triples iron absorption[47]. Taking 50 to 100 mg of vitamin C with meals high in non-heme iron (breakfast with fortified cereal, or meals with dark green vegetables) increases iron absorption and can help prevent iron deficiency, especially among vegetarians.

Vitamin D

Vitamin D is discussed in Chapter 20.

Vitamins E

Overt Vitamin E deficiency is rare, and much of what we know about overt vitamin E deficiency comes through the study of a rare genetic neurodegenerative disease, *ataxia with isolated vitamin E deficiency* (AVED). This disease is caused by a defect in the tocopherol α transfer protein (TTPA) gene, which codes for the protein that transports α-tocopherol into the cells.

There are eight main vitamin E compounds; α, β, δ, and γ tocopherol and α, β, δ, and γ tocotrienol. There are also several different stereoisomeric forms of these compounds, only some of which appear to be active in our bodies. RRR, RSR, RRS, and RSS are active forms of α-tocopherol while SSS, SRR, SRS, and SSR are inactive[44].

Vitamin E requires pancreatic enzymes and bile for absorption. As in β-carotene, it is taken into the enterocyte by the membrane protein, Scavenger Receptor B1. It is packed into chylomicrons in the endoplasmic reticulum and then transported out, into the circulation, through exocytosis. A very small amount of vitamin E is packed into small HDL particles in the enterocyte as well.

The chylomicrons move through the circulation and distribute free fatty acids from the diet to various cells. After most of the fatty acids from the chylomicrons have been removed, the chylomicron, which has an ApoB-48 protein, is taken up by the liver. Here, vitamin E binds to TTPA for inclusion into VLDL or HDL, or it is either excreted into the bile or catabolized and excreted into the urine. TTPA binds most avidly to α-tocopherol, so much so that other forms of vitamin E are quickly eliminated from the bloodstream within a few hours of a meal, leaving α-tocopherol as essentially the only form of vitamin E found in fasting blood samples[48]. As a result of this, it was long believed that R isomers of α-tocopherol were the only active forms of vitamin E.

Without properly functioning TTPA and sufficient intracellular vitamin E, oxidative damage occurs in of axons of large peripheral sensory nerves, leading to peripheral neuropathy. As the disease progresses, spinocerebellar ataxia, skeletal myopathy, pigmented retinopathy and ophthalmoplegia can develop. Since pancreatic lipase and bile are required for the absorption of fats including vitamin E, patients with cystic fibrosis or other severe lipid malabsorption syndromes can also develop vitamin E deficiency with similar signs and symptoms. In overt deficiency with neurologic symptoms, it is important to treat with supplemental vitamin E before irreversible neurologic injury occurs.

High-dose vitamin E supplements have been associated with increased mortally in several studies but decreased mortality in others. One reason is that vitamin E supplementation increases the risk of hemorrhagic stroke by 22 percent, while decreasing the risk of the more frequently occurring ischemic stroke by 10 percent, which thereby cancels out the overall risk of stroke from vitamin E[49]. A-tocopherol lowers the risk of ischemic stroke and thrombosis by decreasing platelet activation, but simultaneously raises the risk of hemorrhagic stroke by increasing the risk of bleeding.

A-tocopherol also increases the activity of cytosolic phospholipase A_2, promoting the release of arachidonic acid (AA) and the formation of eicosanoids. This is especially evident in the presence of IL-1β that increases the activity of cyclooxygenase-2 (prostaglandin-endoperoxide synthase-2)[50]. This results in an increase in prostacyclin, which decreases platelet activity and acts as a vasodilator, thus, increasing blood flow and decreases clotting. Bleeding risk is higher in individuals who have vitamin K deficiencies and who supplement with vitamin E but do not replace vitamin K.

PGE_2 promotes cell proliferation and the development of new blood vessels, which partially explain the increased risk of prostate cancer seen with α-tocopherol supplementation (See chapter 41). When the enhanced cytosolic phospholipase A_2 promoted by α-tocopherol activity occurs in individuals consuming low n-6: n-3 fatty acid diets, it can promote the release of eicosatetraenoic acid and EPA, which would have anti-inflammatory effects. Prostacyclin should have anti-carcinogenic effects as it decreases fibroblast growth and angiogenesis and increases apoptosis. In individuals eating a Western diet with a high n-6: n-3 fatty acid ratio, however, α-tocopherol is inflammatory and increases the proliferation of cancer.

The trials for cancer prevention using vitamin E have used α-tocopherol, as it was assumed to be the only active form of the vitamin, but in cell cultures α-tocopherol does not inhibit cancer cell growth. Nevertheless, several other forms of vitamin E do inhibit cancer cell growth in vitro, the most active forms being δ-tocotrienol and γ-tocotrienol.

The breast cancer medication, tamoxifen, is antagonized by α-tocopherol, whereas tocotrienols, especially δ-tocotrienol and γ-tocotrienol show strong synergistic anticancer effect with tamoxifen[48]. In cell cultures tocotrienol, and specifically γ-tocotrienol, induces apoptosis or impairs the growth of breast cancer[51], prostate cancer[52], and colon cancer cells[53]. Tocotrienols inhibit cyclooxygenase-2 and prevent PGE$_2$ formation.

The tocotrienols are less abundant in food than are the tocopherols. Since tocotrienols bind less avidly to TTPA, selective increase in the intake of α-tocopherol, especially through supplementation with doses exceeding natural dietary intake by a factor of 20, decreases the reabsorption of other forms of vitamin E; and thus, decreases the availability of those forms of vitamin E that are most likely to prevent cancer. Tocotrienols are more lipophilic than tocopherols, which makes them better for dermatologic application and absorption[54]. TTPA is not the only protein which transports vitamin E. Human serum albumin, α-tocopherol associated protein, and P-glycoprotein also transport vitamin E in the blood[54]. All forms of vitamin E can act as antioxidants, but they are not equally effective; rather they act differently upon different species of ROS.

Overt vitamin E deficiency is associated with damage to the large nerve fibers and axons in the cerebellum. Less severe levels of vitamin E deficiency are associated with risk of cancer and arteriosclerosis. In several observational studies of coronary heart disease, dietary vitamin E consumption was inversely associated with risk of disease. In these populations, the favorable outcome occurred when dietary vitamin E consumption was over about 7.5 mg of vitamin E a day[44]. This is the amount of vitamin E found in the average American adult diet. (Data from years prior to the year 2000; beginning in 2000, the NHANES study began calculating only dietary α-tocopherol as it was judged to be the only important vitaminer. Prior to this, NHANES studies provided total vitamin E levels[55].)

Foods with high tocotrienol contents include whole grains, including sweet corn, and also coconut, cabbage, plums, and cranberries[57,56]. The grains with the highest tocotrienols content are oats and barley. Durham wheat has higher tocotrienol levels than soft wheat. Barley and corn contain γ and δ tocotrienol[57]. The oils are richest in tocotrienols are palm oil and rice bran oil.

The Western diet is usually not low in Vitamin E, however because the diet is enriched with α-tocopherol fortified foods. Levels of other E vitaminers, such as γ-tocopherol and the tocotrienols tend to be low. When total vitamin E levels are low, it is usually caused by a malabsorption syndrome, rather than from inadequate vitamin E intake. When levels are low, the underlying condition should be treated. A healthy diet should contain about 12 mg of vitamin E compounds a day with about a quarter of that from tocotrienols. Unfortunately, a large portion of tocotrienols are removed from the grain in processed foods when bran is removed, and replaced in processed foods, such as breakfast cereals with α-tocopherol.

Table 40-7: Properties of Some Vitaminers E

Vitamin E	Properties[54, 58]
α-tocopherol (α-T)	Antioxidant, increases phospholipase A2, thus, increases eicosanoid production.
γ-tocopherol	Is better than α-T at trapping NO and other free radicals. Balances Na+ transport. Inhibits growth of colon cancer cells. Reduces prostaglandin E2 synthesis.
δ-tocopherol	Inhibits the proliferation of prostate cancer cells.
α-tocotrienol	Prevents lipid peroxidation 40 to 60 times more than α-T, and is better at defending cytochrome p-450. Inhibits proliferation of cancer cells
γ-tocotrienol	Inhibits cancer cell growth. Antioxidant.
δ-tocotrienol	Anti-thrombotic, most effective vitamin E to prevent and reduce atherosclerotic plaque. Potent antioxidant. Inhibits the growth and proliferation of cancer cells.

Recommendation: If vitamin E supplementation is desired for general health, I suggest 10 mg of mixed tocotrienols a day, other than for individuals with malabsorption that may require higher doses until the malabsorption has been resolved. The typical American diet is supplemented with α-tocopherol, for example, in breakfast cereals. A healthful diet should contain a mix of natural sources of vitamin E and does not require additional supplements. If treatment is undertaken, a mixed vitamin E with a majority being tocotrienols is recommended.

Vitamins K

Vitamin K$_1$: phylloquinone is found in leafy vegetables, such as cabbage, spinach and some fruits, such as grapes and avocados. Animals convert phylloquinone from plants into vitamin K$_2$: menaquinone-4 (menatetrenone, MK-4), in the cells of the arterial walls, pancreas, and testes. Bacteria, including bacteria in the colon, convert vitamin K$_1$ to various forms of vitamin K$_2$: menaquinone-5 (MK-5) through menaquinone-9 (MK-9). Foods rich in MK-4 include meats, eggs, and dairy products. Bacterial fermented foods, such as cheeses are rich in MK-8 and MK-9 while the fermented soy product, natto is rich in MK-7.

Vitamin K is best known for its role in the coagulation cascade, and severe deficiency can cause bleeding disorders. There appears to be sufficient vitamin K in most diets to prevent bleeding coagulopathy. More modest vitamin K deficiencies are associated with osteoporosis[59], risk for certain malignancies[60] and age-associated cognitive decline[61]. Individuals who are in the upper third of dietary vitamin K$_2$ intake have lower levels of atherosclerosis[62] and cancer[63], and this suggests that much of the population has levels lower than optimum.

Phylloquinone (K$_1$) appears to be the form most active in coagulation; however, high levels of K$_1$ or K$_2$ do not cause pathologic coagulopathy. Vitamins K₁ and K₂ have no known toxicity, and no upper intake level has been set. Synthetic vitamin K3, however, is toxic in high doses and is not sold over-the-counter in the United States. MK-4 is useful for the treatment of osteoporosis, while vitamin K₁ and MK-7 may not be as effective[64]. Vitamin K₂ does not require bile for absorption, and thus, the MK-4 form of vitamin K₂ is useful in the treatment of osteopenia in malabsorption syndromes. MK-4 is anti-inflammatory and prevents coronary artery disease[65], vascular calcification[51], and decreases the risk of cancer[52], while dietary vitamin K₁ does not. MK-4 down-regulates inflammation through inhibition of NF-κB activation and MK-4 thereby, also prevents suppression of apoptosis. (See Chapter 43.)

Vitamin K deficiencies are seen in patients with malabsorption syndromes and intestinal disease. Patients with inflammatory bowel disease have decreased bone mineral density and lower serum vitamin D levels. Patients with Crohn's disease, but not with ulcerative colitis, also have lower serum vitamin K levels[66]. Overt vitamin K deficiency is seen in patients with cystic fibrosis[67]. Women who have undergone bariatric surgery for weight loss have lower vitamin K levels, and their newborn infants can suffer from bleeding and fatal cerebral hemorrhage due to vitamin K deficiency[68]. These infants can also suffer from vitamin A deficiency[69]. Less severe vitamin K deficiency, associated with osteoporosis, can be seen in more modest forms of malabsorption or biliary disease. Bile is required for absorption of vitamin K₁, but not for vitamin K₂[70]. Vitamin K activity is also reduced in obese individuals. Vitamin K is stored in the fat, but in obese individuals it is less available in the blood stream, causing markers for low vitamin K activity (under-carboxylated osteocalcin: ucOC) to be elevated[71].

Plasma levels of vitamin K₁ plateau with dietary phylloquinone intake above about 175 µg per day in adults. These levels of vitamin K₁ were associated with low levels of ucOC. These levels are easily achievable in a healthy diet containing fruits and green vegetables[72]. If supplementation is required, due to malabsorption, a reasonable dose range is to 400 µg of K₂, as it is readily absorbed. Most studies using the MK-4 form of vitamin K₂ have used 45 mg daily. When MK-4 is used as an anti-inflammatory agent, for the treatment of osteoporosis, neurologic conditions or enteroimmune disease, my experience suggests that the use of 5 - 6 mg daily is sufficient. No studies comparing 45 mg to lower effective doses are available. Vitamin K is further discussed in Chapter 43.

Table 40-8: Some Vitamin K Compounds

Vitamin K	Compound	Source
Vitamin K₁	Phylloquinone	Leafy vegetables
Vitamin K₂	Menaquinone: MK-4 MK-7 MK-8, MK-9	Metabolized from phylloquinone: Animal products Fermentation: natto Fermentation: cheese
Vitamin K₃	Menadione	Synthetic

S-Adenosylmethionine and Coenzyme Q₁₀

S-adenosylmethionine (SAMe) is an important single-carbon donor in many metabolic reactions. It is sometimes used as a supplement for various disease states. SAMe appears to be effective for osteoarthritis. It takes about a month before the effects are seen. It has similar efficacy to non-steroidal anti-inflammatory medications[73]. This is in contrast to the supplements glucosamine and chondroitin which fail to show clinical efficacy[74]. SAMe is also helpful for symptomatic relief in some cases of depression[75].

SAMe is unusual as a supplement; it has more toxic side-effects than most supplements, and this limits its utility and desirability. SAMe can cause gastric distress with vomiting, constipation or diarrhea. It can also cause insomnia, anorexia, dizziness, and anxiety. It can cause patients with bipolar disorder to go into mania, and worsen symptoms in patients with Parkinson's disease. It can also interact with medications for depression.

SAMe is formed from methionine and ATP by S-adenosylmethionine synthase isoform type-1 and methionine adenosyl transferase 2, subunit beta. This reaction requires magnesium or cobalt and potassium. SAMe is recycled using the cofactors folate (vitamin B₉) and cyanocobalamin (vitamin B₁₂) or betaine (trimethylglycine). SAMe recycles homocysteine into methionine; without SAMe homocysteine can accumulate, and have toxic effects, at least in part by stimulating the formation of ceramide from sphingomyelin. Vitamin B6 can also detoxify homocysteine, helping to metabolize it into cysteine. (See Figures 31-4 and 31-5) Due to the toxicity of SAMe and its metabolites, it is preferable to assure sufficient SAMe cofactors, rather than to supplement SAMe.

While coenzyme Q₁₀ (CoQ₁₀) has low toxicity and is considered safe, it is a large molecule, and most preparations have very poor bioavailability[76]. Some newer preparations of CoQ₁₀ have been developed which promise better serum levels[77], and this may translate to higher levels in the mitochondria. In spite of studies showing an association of low CoQ₁₀ levels with various disease states, double-blinded clinical trials show the efficacy of treatment is limited[78,79,80], likely due to the poor absorption of CoQ₁₀ supplements.

A more effective approach to promote adequate CoQ₁₀ activity is to ensure an adequate supply of the various nutritional cofactors required for CoQ₁₀'s formation. The biosynthetic pathway of CoQ₁₀ comprises multiple steps including methylations, decarboxylations, hydroxylations and isoprenoid synthesis and transfer[81]. Biosynthesis of CoQ10 depends upon several single-carbon methylation steps each requiring the availability of SAMe and decarboxylases requiring pyridoxal-5-phosphate.

Both SAMe and CoQ₁₀ levels are frequently low in the elderly. Adequate SAMe and CoQ₁₀ and low levels of homocysteine are best assured by assuring adequate vitamin B_{12} levels and eliminating inflammation. Betaine can also be used by the body for the formation of SAMe and may play an important role in CoQ_{10} formation.

Genetic Polymorphisms and Vitamin Deficiencies

Many individuals may be at increased risk for enzyme cofactor, vitamin or mineral deficiency, as a result of genetic polymorphisms. For example, about 10 percent of Americans have an alternate and less active allele compared to the more common form of methylene-tetrahydrofolate reductase (MTHFR). These individuals have increased susceptibility to vascular disease, neural tube defects, colon cancer and acute leukemia. Since this less common allele of MTHFR is less efficient, individuals with this form of the gene require higher levels of folate. This puts these individuals as increase susceptibility to folate deficiency and elevated homocysteine levels[82]. Prior to folate fortification, when much of the population had a borderline deficiency, these individuals were like the canaries in the coal mine – they were the ones at the highest risk, and the population in which much of the low folate associated morbidity. Fortification of processed foods with folic acid has lowered the risk for them and the rest of the population.

There are many other polymorphisms which increase the requirement for nutritional cofactors, and rare individuals may have much higher requirements for certain cofactors. For the vast majority of individuals, maintaining a healthful diet is sufficient. A borderline diet, however, puts one at risk. We should all treat ourselves as if we were the canaries, and keep a margin of safety by eating well.

Breaking the Rules

Most nutrients are present in a natural, balanced diet in adequate amounts to meet optimal physiologic levels. Super-physiologic doses of vitamins and minerals do little good and likely to cause disease. There are situations, such as malabsorption, physiologic stress, and disease, when supplements may be useful but even in these times, the goal is to achieve and maintain the physiologic levels of these nutrients that would be expected in healthy individuals. Nevertheless, there are a few nutrients that may have therapeutic benefits in amounts that are uncommon in this diet.

Menatetrenone: One of the most notable rule breakers is vitamin K_2. There is little evidence that 5 mg of vitamin K_2 daily would be found in a natural diet or made at this level in the body. This dose, however, is useful for decreasing neuroinflammation after brain injury and in secondary prevention of osteoporosis. The 5 or 6 mg effective dose of menatetrenone may be the result of long-term depletion of this fat-soluble vitamin in malabsorption or short-term acute depletion during stress or injury[83]. This dose may represent the amount that can be absorbed and sufficient to replete stores and provide required levels for control of inflammation. Alternatively, vitamin K_2 may be acting as a non-toxic pharmaceutical compound at this dose.

Betaine: Betaine (trimethylglycine) often has therapeutic value at levels that would be difficult to achieve in a natural diet. A discussion of dietary betaine needs to include choline as the body can convert it into betaine. Dietary betaine thus spares choline for other purposes, including the production of the neurotransmitter acetylcholine and membrane phospholipids and sphingomyelin. Choline deficient diets cause fatty liver and damage to the muscles.

Choline is considered to be a vitamin as it is an essential dietary component. Betaine, while a necessary co-enzyme, is not a vitamin, as it can be made from choline in the body. Additionally some betaine is produced by bacteria in the gut from dietary choline and absorbed. The conversion of choline to betaine occurs in a two-step process utilizing the mitochondrial enzyme, choline dehydrogenase, requiring PQQ and $CoQ10^{84}$, followed by cytosol acetaldehyde dehydrogenase, requiring NAD. Choline can also be produced in the body from phosphatidylethanolamine; however, this process cannot supply the bodies needs for choline, and this process comes at high cost; consuming three moles of SAMe for each mole of choline made.

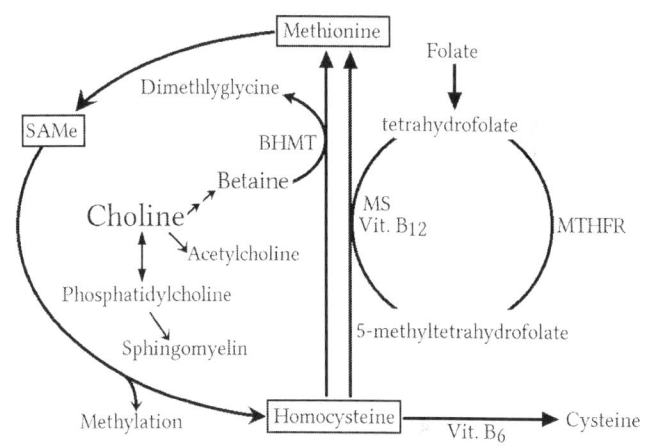

Figure 40-2: Choline and betaine in the methionine cycle.
BHMT: betaine-homocysteine methyltransferase; MS: Methionine synthase; MTHFR: Methylene-tetrahydrofolate reductase.

In middle-aged individuals, high choline to betaine ratios are associated with risk factors for metabolic syndrome and cardiovascular disease[85]. This suggests that mitochondrial enzyme inefficiencies, specifically choline dehydrogenase inefficiency that causes a reduction in the conversion of choline to betaine, adds to this risk. Strenuous activity can reduce the plasma choline concentration by 40 percent, indicating increased conversion and consumption of choline.

The Western diet is deficient in both choline and betaine[86]. According to the Institute of Medicine, an adequate daily intake of choline is estimated to be 550 mg/day of choline for men and 425 mg/day for women. These estimates are based on levels needed to prevent a rise in the liver enzyme ALT[87]. The average choline intake among Americans is about 300 mg for women and about 300 mg for men, and the average betaine intake is about 100 and 120 mg in women and men respectively[88]. In a study of women in New Zealand, only 16% of women consumed the recommended amount of choline[89]. In the Nurse's Health Study, in the United States, less than 5% of women consumed the recommend amount of choline[90].

The foods highest in choline concentration include liver, eggs, salmon, wheat germ, and soy. The foods with the highest concentration of betaine include dark green vegetables, such as spinach, wheat bran, wheat germ, beets, quinoa, and shrimp[91].

Table 40-9: Choline and Betaine per 100 Gram (3.5 oz.) Serving

Food	Betaine	Choline
Spinach	600	23
Beets (canned)	300	6
Wheat Germ	1240	152
Wheat Bran	1340	74
White wheat bread	93	12
Brown Rice	0.4	9
Shrimp	220	70
Eggs	0.5	251
Chicken liver	11	290
Salmon	2	65
Soybean	2	116
Beef liver	6	418

Betaine is particularly concentrated by the liver, kidneys and brain[92] cells by the GABA/betaine transporter (BGT-1). This is one of four GABA membrane transporter proteins, but the only one specific for betaine. Betaine is an osmolyte that maintains cellular hydration and protects protein conformation and aids in the proper folding of new proteins[93].

Betaine decreases the risk of excitotoxicity. BGT-1 is upregulated in astrocytes after excitotoxic injury. Intracellular betaine protects cells against injury by preventing osmotic stress[94] and homocysteine production; both of which increase acid SMAase activity. It also protects intracellular proteins.

Betaine blocks GABA transport by BGT-1, and thus increases the presence of the GABA in the synaptic cleft. Blocking the uptake of GABA, the principal inhibitory neurotransmitter in the CNS, may decrease excitatory activity. In the liver, betaine has been shown to inhibit the expression of TLR-4, otherwise induced by ethanol[95]. Betaine has been shown to downregulates the transcription of TLR-4 and HMGB1, prevent a rise in NF-κB and a fall in HDL-cholesterol caused by high-fat diets in animals[96]. Betaine and SAMe prevented stem cell proliferation in response to liver carcinogens[97] and appeared to reduce the risk of colon and other cancers[98].

Betaine is included with rule-breakers; large doses, exceeding those of a healthy diet, may have therapeutic effects. Doses of 6000 mg of betaine have been used in the treatment of hyperhomocysteinemia due to inborn errors or homocysteine metabolism. Similarly, in the normal population doses from 1,500 to 6000 mg of betaine are useful in lowering homocysteine levels, although very high betaine doses may raise plasma triglyceride levels[99].

Folate or choline deficiencies and certain common polymorphisms for methyl group transfer enzymes raise the risk for neural tube defects, heart disease, fatty liver disease and certain cancers. Common to these is the reduction in the formation of SAMe[100]. Due to genetic variations in the population, many individuals require more choline and betaine for optimal health than is easily available in a balanced, healthy diet.

A therapeutic dose of betaine used for initiating treatment of TBI and schizophrenia is about 3000 mg a day, and 500 to 1000 mg are often useful for long-term supplementation in secondary disease prevention. Large doses of betaine may cause dyspepsia, nausea or diarrhea. It is often formulated with pepsin to prevent this.

N-Acetyl Cysteine: Doses of 500 to 1000 mg of N-acetyl cysteine are useful in supplying cysteine supplementation, for the formation of glutathione. Glutathione, the major antioxidant of the nervous system, is present in the diet, but very poorly absorbed. Cysteine is the rate-limiting amino acid precursor in the production of glutathione. N-acetyl cysteine gives an effective source for this amino acid.

> Average adults make about 120 moles of ATP a day, and this amount may be many times higher under demand. Ball-parking it here; if the mitochondria in a healthy, resting adult, have a one percent leak rate causing the formation of free radicals, 1.2 moles of antioxidants would be required each day to quench them. The molecular mass of glutathione is 307 grams. Thus, these numbers provide a calculated estimate of about 370 grams of glutathione used daily by healthy adults. This amount would be considerably higher with activity, under stress, disease or for individuals with inefficient, leaky mitochondria.
>
> Fortunately, glutathione is recycled and is not the only antioxidant. Nevertheless, a few grams of n-acetylcysteine used to supplement glutathione formation, does not appear to be excessive when a kilogram of glutathione may be consumed daily to quench the oxidative load created by stress, disease and injury, especially when the mitochondria are effete.

Alpha-lipoic acid: ALA is another oddball. It is sold as an antioxidant dietary supplement, and present in the diet, but the actual amount of ALA in the diet, like the amount in the body, is hard to assess; it is bound to protein, and thus, difficult to analyze. Only a small amount of free ALA present in food: levels range from 0.01 to 0.420 mg per 100 grams[101]. The highest concentration is in metabolically active organ meat (kidneys liver, and heart) and in dark green vegetables, (spinach and broccoli). Supplemental ALA is prepared synthetically. It is useful as a supplement, having very low toxicity at effective doses and a reasonably effective absorption[102]. Even absorption is difficult to study, as it quickly disappears, presumably bound by proteins.

The name lipoic acid suggests that is an ionized molecule in water. However, in the body, it is synthesized by lipoyl synthase, (EC 2.8.1.8) from caprylic acid (C8:0), using two molecules of SAMe and of sulfur, directly onto the target protein. Lipoylation is required for the activation of two of the enzymes in the citric acid cycle, as well as in some other enzymes. Lipoylation creates a direct covalent bond with the target proteins, converting them into an active holoproteins[103]. Thus, ALA is not formed as a cytosolic factor, and it may only be free during protein breakdown.

Although ALA is a free radical acceptor, it is not your usual antioxidant. In its reduced form, dihydrolipoic acid, it does scavenge reactive oxygen and nitrogen species. It, however, spends little time in this form. Mostly it is attached to proteins. ALA may exert its anti-oxidative effect indirectly as a messenger, delivering a cellular oxidative stress signal to the nucleus[104]. In animals fed a methionine and choline-deficient diet, ALA protected the animals from oxidative stress; it increased the activity of catalase, SOD, and glutathione in the brain[105]. In the liver, ALA prevents lipid peroxidation and nitrosative stress by increasing SOD and glutathione levels[106]. ALA may act as a stress signal that induces the production of anti-oxidant proteins when lipoylated proteins are damaged by oxidation and scavenged for recycling, oxidized or nitrosylated.

ALA enhances SIRT1 activity and induces the production of enzymes that increase the utilization and disposal of fat[107]. It restored citric acid cycle activity in an animal model of Alzheimer's disease[108]. ALA prevents non-enzymatic glycation of proteins from fructose and prevents the extensive cross-linking of collagen in the skin[109]. It prevents insulin resistance in fructose-fed rats[110]. In rabbits, it inhibited NF-κB activation, decreased T cell content, improved vascular reactivity, and reduced established atherosclerotic plaques, at a dose equivalent to 6.5 mg/kg in man[111]. ALA prevented glomerular injury in diabetic rats at a dose equivalent to 5 mg/kg in man[112].

Most ALA supplements are equal racemic mixtures of the right and left-handed ALA. The right-handed form of ALA (RLA) is made and used by living things. The left-handed form of ALA (SLA) first set foot on the planet Earth in Urbana, Illinois, in 1952, in the lab where it was created. SLA decreases the absorption of RLA, is preferentially eliminated from the body and likely is a competitive inhibitor of RLA activity. Thus, a much higher dose of ALA needs to be taken to get an effective amount to the tissues. Stabilized sodium-R-lipoic acid (RLA-Na) has higher bioavailability either mixed ALA or RLA[113]. Fifty mg of RLA-Na appears to be bioequivalent to about 600 mg of ALA, an amount often used as a therapeutic dose of ALA.

One gram of N-acetyl cysteine, and two grams of betaine, 50 mg of R-lipoic acid (NA), and several mg of vitamin K_2 might not be found in a healthy diet, nevertheless, these supplements in these amounts may be useful for preventing and treating chronic disease. It is for this reason that these rule breakers are useful as supplements; the most effective amounts are more than will be found in the diet.

Summary

Malabsorption and nutrient loss caused by disease are the most common causes of vitamin and mineral deficiencies. Supplements are often helpful to regain health. The goal should be to treat the underlying disorder to restore nutrient absorption and prevent nutrient losses. Supplements may be used as medicine to replace depleted nutrients quickly. A healthful diet should be the mainstay of prevention after recovery.

In mild to moderate TBI, for example, most individuals recover from without apparent sequelae. It may be that only those with impaired metabolic function, with a propensity for inflammation, are in jeopardy. Why take chances when there is little way of knowing who is at risk? Additionally, injuries and healing depletes nutrients. Signs and symptoms of traumatic brain injury (TBI), such as post-traumatic headache, are in themselves evidence of an inflammatory process and compromised nutritional status and inflammatory state.

Concussion, TBI, bipolar disorder and schizophrenia prodromes and psychosis are medical emergencies. These medical emergencies are times to use doses of supplements large enough to ensure that the patient has adequate vitamins, minerals, and antioxidants to prevent disease progression, and to reverse its course where possible.

In the year 2000, the Institute of Medicine of the National Academy of Science, assessing the best scientific evidence available, decided that α-tocopherol was the only form of vitamin E important to health. We now know that animals can live without any tocopherol, using tocotrienols for several generations in good health[114] and that tee tocotrienol forms are important for the prevention of disease. Vitamin bottles should not be relied on for nutrition. Their content and promise is based on limited knowledge. Foods contain thousands of compounds; we understand only a few dozen of these, and our knowledge of them is far from complete. Eating a wide variety of unrefined foods helps assure the consumption of a wide variety of nutrients.

"Covert vitamin deficiencies," those which do not cause overt disease, but increase the risk of chronic disease, are common in the Western diet. Vitamin B_{12}, Vitamin D, K, E and A, magnesium, zinc, levels are low enough to cause chronic disease in a sizable portion of our population. Vitamin and mineral deficiencies among the overfed and obese in industrialized populations may result from the consumption of a refined, industrialized, palatable diet, low in fruits and vegetables. It is too easy to displace real food with lonely calories from manufactured foods and beverages.

Isolated nutrients may increase disease risk. Folic acid alone as a supplement may raise the risk of cancer. This is likely caused by hypermethylation. There is a higher risk of hypermethylation when vitamin B_{12} levels are low and when n-3 fatty acids are in short supply[115], or displaced by excessive consumption of n-6 fatty acids.

But even among the poorly fed, over-nourished, malabsorption, largely from enteroimmune inflammation, is the most prevalent causes of nutrient deficiencies. Malabsorption may be caused by gluten enteropathy, infections, disease, pancreatic deficiencies, biliary disease, bacterial overgrowth, poorly absorbed sugars, or immune damage to the intestine. It is important to diagnose and treat the underlying causes of nutritional deficiencies. Alcohol causes loss of zinc, magnesium, and vitamin A.

Fortification of refined foods is a reasonable approach when the much of the population is at risk from consumption of refined foods and risk from the nutrient is low. Folate supplementation may cause some risk as it increases homocysteine levels and DNA methylation in individuals with low vitamin B_{12} levels. Thus, benefit may be achieved with vitamin B_{12} fortification as well, especially in older individuals who are commonly deficient.

Magnesium deficiency is perhaps the most common nutritional deficiency in the Western diet. (See chapter 31) Like other deficiencies, Mg deficiency results from diets bereft of green vegetables and whole grains, aggravated by malabsorption. Vitamin D insufficiency (Chapter 20) is the most prevalent of vitamin deficiencies. It is caused by lack of exposure to sunlight, exacerbated by intestinal losses. Choline, and thus betaine, inadequacies predominated in those consuming a Western diet.

There are many antioxidants in the diet, and relying on a limited number of them can lead to problems. B-carotene is just one of several dietary antioxidant carotenoids. High doses of β-carotene increase the mortality among individuals with cancer, because it is converted into vitamin A, a growth promoter. Other carotenoids are antioxidants but cannot be converted to vitamin A. and thus, cannot act as growth promoters.

There are multiple forms of vitamin E, and they act differently on different free radicals. Supplements of α-tocopherol increase growth of prostate cancers, probably by displacing other forms of vitamin E that inhibit cancer growth. A natural diet also contains a wide variety of polyphenols, many which act as antioxidants and may have other health effects. *Fat-soluble vitamins β-carotene, E, and K_1 are better absorbed with meals which contain some fat as they require bile for absorption.* This applies to the consumption of vegetables and grains as well as to vitamin supplements.

The rule breakers, betaine, alpha lipoic acid, and N-acetyl cysteine are useful in treating inflammatory disease, even among those consuming a healthful diet. Few adults get enough sunlight exposure to form sufficient vitamin D. Thus, it usually requires supplementation.

Folate, pyridoxine, iron, zinc, copper and magnesium were listed at the top of this chapter as risk factors for increased mortality.

Folate supplements are not recommended for routine use in the U.S., where foods are now fortified with it, and deficiencies are uncommon. The safest forms of folate are the natural ones found in unprocessed foods.

Iron, zinc and copper are pro-oxidants and toxic. Before childproof medicine bottles were available, iron tablets were the most common fatal toxin among children. Hemochromatosis is a common condition; iron should come from food, and should only be used as a supplement for those with deficiencies. Except in small children, where iron deficiency may be nutritional during rapid growth, the cause of the deficiency should be investigated. In adults, it is, usually, from blood loss. Zinc supplements typically come in a dose of 50 mg; many times the appropriate dose. Zinc may accentuate vitamin A activity, and increase the risk of cancer proliferation.

Magnesium supplement's apparent guilt may be secondary to the disease it is used most often to treat; constipation, which is, usually, treated with the poorly absorbed Mg oxide. It may be the underlying causes of constipation, that are the reason for "shortgevity", Supplementation with well-absorbed forms of organic Mg to achieve normal physiologic magnesium levels are unlikely to impose adverse risk.

Note: Utilization of dietary vitamin B_{12} requires that it be protected by the protein haptocorrin from the saliva to prevent it from being destroyed by stomach acid. The dose of vitamin B_{12} required is about 500 times higher when swallowed as a pill than when mixed with sufficient saliva, as occurs while chewing food. This may explain in part why the elderly (with poor dentition and preferring a mechanically soft diet) become B_{12} deficient. Food swallowed whole can be digested, but vitamin B_{12} will be destroyed.

Table 40-10: Some Recommended Supplement Doses

Vitamin or Mineral	Suggested Supplement Dose for Treating Deficiency
Vitamin A:	6000 µg/day β-carotene in oil (10,000 units)
Vitamin B$_6$	3 to 5 mg/day
Vitamin B$_{12}$*	500 mcg, lozenges or chewable forms once a week – especially in vegans.
Vitamin C:	100 mg/day
Vitamin D$_3$:	5000 – 6000 IU/day (See Chapter 12)
Vitamin E:	10 mg/day (as mixed-tocotrienols)
Vitamin K:	400 µg/day. K$_2$ (menaquinone-4) in malabsorption syndromes. As a therapeutic dose for treatment of osteoporosis or acute inflammatory diseases use 5 to 6 mg.
Boron:	6 mg/day; amino acid chelate
Zinc:	5 to 15 mg/day of organic salt, gluconate or citrate organic salt
Magnesium	200 to 300 mg/day of an organic form of Mg, such as Mg citrate.
Calcium	Most Westerners get more than sufficient dietary calcium. Treat the underlying condition. 800 mg/day

*Haptocorrin from the saliva protects vitamin B$_{12}$ from destruction by stomach acid. Much lower doses are required when vitamin B$_{12}$ is mixed with saliva than when swallows as a pill.

Table 40-11: Vitamin E in Food Oils, (mg/100 g product) [116], [117]

Oil	αT	βT	γT	δT	αT3	βT3	γT3	δT3
Canola	10.0-38.6	ND-14.0	18.9-75.3	ND-2.2	ND-0.04	ND	ND	ND
Babassu Palm	ND	ND	ND	ND	2.5-4.6	-	3.2-8.0	0.9-1.0
Coconut	ND-1.7	ND-1.1	ND-1.4	ND-0.6	ND-4.4	0.1	ND-1.9	ND
Corn	2.3-57.3	ND-35.6	26.8-246.8	2.3-7.5	ND-23.9	ND	ND-45.0	ND-2.0
Cottonseed	13.6-67.4	ND-2.9	13.8-74.6	ND-2.1	ND	ND	ND	ND
Grape seed	1.6-3.8	ND-8.9	ND-7.3	ND-0.4	1.8-10.7	-	11.5-20.5	ND-0.3
Olive	11.9	ND	0.7	ND	ND	ND	ND	ND
Palm	0.4-25.6	ND-23.4	ND-52.6	ND-12.3	0.04-33.6	3.2	1.4-71.0	ND-37.7
Palm kernel	ND-6.2	ND-24.8	ND-25.7	ND	ND	ND	ND-6.0	ND
Peanut	4.9-37.3	ND-4.1	8.8-38.9	ND-2.2	ND	ND	ND	ND
Rice Bran	4.9-58.3	ND-4.7	ND-21.2	ND-3.1	ND-62.7	ND	14.2-79.0	ND-5.9
Safflower	23.4-66.0	ND-1.7	ND-7.1	ND	ND	ND	ND-1.2	ND
Sesame	ND-13.6	ND	29.0-98.3	0.4-2.1	ND	ND	ND-2.0	ND
Soy	0.9-35.2	ND-3.6	8.9-230.7	15.4-93.2	ND-6.9	0.1	ND-10.3	ND-0.03
Sunflower	40.3-93.5	ND-4.5	ND-5.1	ND-0.8	ND	ND	ND	ND
Walnut	56.3	ND	59.5	45.0	ND	ND	ND	ND
Wheat germ	133.0	71.0	26.0	27.1	2.6	18.1	ND	ND

Legend: α, β, γ, δ Tocopherols: αT, βT, γT, δT; α, β, γ, δ Tocotrienols: αT3, βT3, γT3, δT3. Ranges are shown as these are natural products, and there is variance in the amount of natural compounds present. Variance may also be due to differences in the analysis method. ND: Not detected. Dashes represent missing data.

[1] Vitamin E and the risk of prostate cancer: the Selenium and Vitamin E Cancer Prevention Trial (SELECT). Klein EA, Thompson IM Jr, Tangen CM, Crowley JJ, Lucia MS, Goodman PJ, et al. JAMA. 2011 Oct 12;306(14):1549-56. PMID:21990298

[2] Dietary Supplements and Mortality Rate in Older Women: The Iowa Women's Health Study. Mursu J, Robien K, Harnack LJ, Park K, Jacobs DR Jr. Arch Intern Med. 2011 Oct 10;171(18):1625-33. PMID:21987192

[3] Multivitamin use and the risk of mortality and cancer incidence: the multiethnic cohort study. Park SY, Murphy SP, Wilkens LR, et al. Am J Epidemiol. 2011 Apr 15;173(8):906-14. PMID:21343248

[4] Antioxidant supplements for prevention of mortality in healthy participants and patients with various diseases. Bjelakovic G, Nikolova D, Gluud LL, Simonetti RG, Gluud C. Cochrane Database Syst Rev. 2008 Apr 16;(2):CD007176. PMID:18425980

[5] Unleashing the untold and misunderstood observations on vitamin E. Gee PT. Genes Nutr. 2011 Feb;6(1):5-16. PMID:21437026

[6] Folic acid and risk of prostate cancer: results from a randomized clinical trial. Figueiredo JC, Grau MV, Haile RW, et al. J Natl Cancer Inst. 2009 Mar 18;101(6):432-5. PMID:19276452

[7] Total and cancer mortality after supplementation with vitamins and minerals: follow-up of the Linxian General Population Nutrition Intervention Trial. Qiao YL, Dawsey SM, Kamangar F, et al. J Natl Cancer Inst. 2009 Apr 1;101(7):507-18. PMID:19318634

[8] The efficacy and safety of multivitamin and mineral supplement use to prevent cancer and chronic disease in adults: a systematic review for a National Institutes of Health state-of-the-science conference. Huang HY, Caballero B, Chang S, et al. Ann Intern Med. 2006 Sep 5;145(5):372-85. PMID:16880453

[9] The mandatory fortification of staple foods with folic acid: a current controversy in Germany. Herrmann W, Obeid R. Dtsch Arztebl Int. 2011 Apr;108(15):249-54. PMID:21556262

[10] Hemochromatosis and iron-overload screening in a racially diverse population. Adams PC, Reboussin DM, Barton JC, et al.; Hemochromatosis and Iron Overload Screening (HEIRS) Study Research Investigators. N Engl J Med. 2005 Apr 28;352(17):1769-78. PMID:15858186

[11] Iron-overload-related disease in HFE hereditary hemochromatosis. Allen KJ, Gurrin LC, Constantine CC,, et al. N Engl J Med. 2008 Jan 17;358(3):221-30. PMID:18199861

[12] Effects of altered maternal folic acid, vitamin B12 and docosahexaenoic acid on placental global DNA methylation patterns in Wistar rats. Kulkarni A, Dangat K, Kale A, et al. PLoS One. 2011 Mar 10;6(3):e17706. PMID:21423696

[13] Folate and vitamin B6 intake and risk of colon cancer in relation to p53 expression. Schernhammer ES, Ogino S, Fuchs CS. Gastroenterology. 2008 Sep;135(3):770-80. PMID:18619459

[14] Will mandatory folic acid fortification prevent or promote cancer? Kim YI. Am J Clin Nutr. 2004 Nov;80(5):1123-8. PMID:15531657

[15] Folic acid for the prevention of colorectal adenomas: a randomized clinical trial. Cole BF, Baron JA, Sandler RS, , etal.; Polyp Prevention Study Group. JAMA. 2007 Jun 6;297(21):2351-9. PMID:17551129

[16] Vitamins B2, B6, and B12 and risk of new colorectal adenomas in a randomized trial of aspirin use and folic acid supplementation. Figueiredo JC, Levine AJ, Grau MV, et al. Cancer Epidemiol Biomarkers Prev. 2008 Aug;17(8):2136-45. PMID:18708408

[17] Vitamin D supplementation for prevention of mortality in adults. Bjelakovic G, Gluud LL, Nikolova D, et al. Cochrane Database Syst Rev. 2011 Jul 6;(7):CD007470. PMID:21735411

[18] Portal and biliary phases of enterohepatic circulation of corrinoids in humans. el Kholty S, Gueant JL, Bressler L, et al. Gastroenterology. 1991 Nov;101(5):1399-408. PMID:1936810

[19] Divalent metal transporter 1 in lead and cadmium transport. Bressler JP, Olivi L, Cheong JH, Kim Y, Bannona D. Ann N Y Acad Sci. 2004 Mar;1012:142-52. PMID:15105261

[20] Involvement of DMT1 +IRE in the transport of lead in an in vitro BBB model. Wang Q, Luo W, Zhang W, Liu M, Song H, Chen J. Toxicol In Vitro. 2011 Jun;25(4):991-8. PMID:19913089

[21] Naturally Occurring Food Toxins. Dolan LC, Matulka RA, Burdock GA. Toxins 2010, 2, 2289-2332.

[22] Zinc: the missing link in combating micronutrient malnutrition in developing countries. Gibson RS. Proc Nutr Soc. 2006 Feb;65(1):51-60. PMID:16441944

[23] Effects of omeprazole consumption on serum levels of trace elements. Joshaghani H, Amiriani T, Vaghari G, et al. J Trace Elem Med Biol. 2012 Oct;26(4):234-7. PMID:22677542

[24] Zinc salts provide a novel, prolonged and rapid inhibition of gastric acid secretion. Kirchhoff P, Socrates T, Sidani S, et al. Am J Gastroenterol. 2011 Jan;106(1):62-70. PMID:20736941

[25] Zinc absorption by young adults from supplemental zinc citrate is comparable with that from zinc gluconate and higher than from zinc oxide. Wegmüller R, Tay F, Zeder C, Brnic M, Hurrell RF. J Nutr. 2014 Feb;144(2):132-6. PMID:24259556

[26] The potential therapeutic effect of melatonin in Gastro-Esophageal Reflux Disease. Kandil TS, Mousa AA, El-Gendy AA, Abbas AM. BMC Gastroenterol. 2010 Jan 18;10:7. PMID:20082715

[27] Zinc requirements and the risks and benefits of zinc supplementation. Maret W, Sandstead HH. J Trace Elem Med Biol. 2006;20(1):3-18. PMID:16632171

[28] Vitamin digestion and absorption - Homo sapiens. KEGG PATHWAY, Kandehisa Laboratories April 2011. http://www.genome.jp/kegg/pathway/hsa/hsa04977.html

[29] Guidance for Industry Estimating the Maximum Safe Starting Dose in Initial Clinical Trials for Therapeutics in in Adult Healthy Volunteers. FDA July 2005. Accessed June 2014 http://www.fda.gov/downloads/Drugs/Guidance/UCM078932.pdf

[30] To scale or not to scale: the principles of dose extrapolation. Sharma V, McNeill JH. Br J Pharmacol. 2009 Jul;157(6):907-21. PMID:19508398

[31] Dietary Reference Intakes for Vitamin A, Vitamin K, Arsenic, Boron, Chromium, Copper, Iodine, Iron, Manganese, Molybdenum, Nickel, Silicon, Vanadium, and Zinc Appendix C. (2001) National Academy of Sciences. Institute of Medicine. Food and Nutrition Board.

[32] Plasma folate adequacy as determined by homocysteine level. Lewis CA, Pancharuniti N, Sauberlich HE. Ann N Y Acad Sci. 1992 Sep 30;669:360-2. PMID:1444047

[33] Plasma homocyst(e)ine, folate, and vitamin B-12 concentrations and risk for early-onset coronary artery disease. Pancharuniti N, Lewis CA, Sauberlich HE, et al. Am J Clin Nutr. 1994 Apr;59(4):940-8. PMID:8147342

[34] Dietary Reference Intakes Research Synthesis: Workshop Summary Carol West Suitor and Linda D. Meyers, Rapporteurs, Planning Committee on Dietary Reference Intakes Research Synthesis. ISBN: 0-309-66627-9, (2006) Chapter 12

[35] Folate and vitamin B-12 biomarkers in NHANES: history of their measurement and use. Yetley EA, Johnson CL. Am J Clin Nutr. 2011 Jul;94(1):322S-331S. PMID:21593508

[36] Tutorial in biostatistics: Analyzing associations between total plasma homocysteine and B vitamins using optimal categorization and segmented regression. Bang H, Mazumdar M, Spence D. Neuroepidemiology. 2006;27(4):188-200. PMID:17035715

[37] In vitamin B12 deficiency, higher serum folate is associated with increased total homocysteine and methylmalonic acid concentrations. Selhub J, Morris MS, Jacques PF. Proc Natl Acad Sci U S A. 2007 Dec 11;104(50):19995-20000. PMID:18056804

[38] Neuronal injury: folate to the rescue? Kronenberg G, Endres M. J Clin Invest. 2010 May;120(5):1383-6. PMID:20424316

[39] Folate regulation of axonal regeneration in the rodent central nervous system through DNA methylation. Iskandar BJ, Rizk E, Meier B, et al. J Clin Invest. 2010 May;120(5):1603-16. PMID:20424322

[40] Pyridoxine supplementation corrects vitamin B6 deficiency but does not improve inflammation in patients with rheumatoid arthritis. Chiang EP, Selhub J, Bagley PJ, Dallal G, Roubenoff R. Arthritis Res Ther. 2005;7(6):R1404-11. PMID:16277693

[41] Low plasma vitamin B-6 status affects metabolism through the kynurenine pathway in cardiovascular patients with systemic inflammation. Midttun O, Ulvik A, Ringdal Pedersen E, et al. J Nutr. 2011 Apr 1;141(4):611-7. PMID:21310866

[42] Vitamins B2, B6, and B12 and risk of new colorectal adenomas in a randomized trial of aspirin use and folic acid supplementation. Figueiredo JC, Levine AJ, Grau MV, et al. Cancer Epidemiol Biomarkers Prev. 2008 Aug;17(8):2136-45. PMID:18708408

[43] Fulminant hepatic failure after ingestion of sustained-release nicotinic acid. Mullin GE, Greenson JK, Mitchell MC. Ann Intern Med. 1989 Aug 1;111(3):253-5. PMID:2665592

[44] Dietary Reference Intakes for Vitamin C, Vitamin E, Selenium, and Carotenoids Panel on Dietary Antioxidants and Related Compounds, Subcommittees on Upper Reference Levels of Nutrients and Interpretation and Uses of DRIs, Standing Committee on the Scientific Evaluation of Dietary Reference Intakes, Food and Nutrition Board, Institute of Medicine. ISBN: 0-309-59719-6, (2000)

[45] Dietary Reference Intakes for Thiamin, Riboflavin, Niacin, Vitamin B6, Folate, Vitamin B12, Pantothenic Acid, Biotin, and Choline (1998) National Academy of Sciences. Institute of Medicine. Food and Nutrition Board. Chapter 9

[46] Response of elevated methylmalonic acid to three dose levels of oral cobalamin in older adults. Rajan S, Wallace JI, Brodkin KI, et al. J Am Geriatr Soc. 2002 Nov;50(11):1789-95. PMID:12410896

[47] Erythorbic acid is a potent enhancer of nonheme-iron absorption. Fidler MC, Davidsson L, Zeder C, Hurrell RF. Am J Clin Nutr. 2004 Jan;79(1):99-102. PMID:14684404

[48] Unleashing the untold and misunderstood observations on vitamin E. Gee PT. Genes Nutr. 2011 Feb;6(1):5-16. PMID:21437026

[49] Effects of vitamin E on stroke subtypes: meta-analysis of randomised controlled trials. Schürks M, Glynn RJ, Rist PM, Tzourio C, Kurth T. BMJ. 2010 Nov 4;341:c5702. PMID:21051774

[50] Vitamin E increases production of vasodilator prostanoids in human aortic endothelial cells through opposing effects on cyclooxygenase-2 and phospholipase A2. Wu D, Liu L, Meydani M, Meydani SN. J Nutr. 2005 Aug;135(8):1847-53. PMID:16046707

[51] Tocotrienols induce apoptosis in breast cancer cell lines via an endoplasmic reticulum stress-dependent increase in extrinsic death receptor signaling. Park SK, Sanders BG, Kline K. Breast Cancer Res Treat. 2010 Nov;124(2):361-75. PMID:20157774

[52] Gamma-tocotrienol induces apoptosis and autophagy in prostate cancer cells by increasing intracellular dihydrosphingosine and dihydroceramide. Jiang Q, Rao X, Kim CY, et al. Int J Cancer. 2011 Mar 11. PMID:21400505

[53] Inhibition of proliferation and induction of apoptosis by gamma-tocotrienol in human colon carcinoma HT-29 cells. Xu WL, Liu JR, Liu HK, Qi GY, Sun XR, Sun WG, Chen BQ. Nutrition. 2009 May;25(5):555-66. PMID:19121919

[54] Towards the interaction mechanism of tocopherols and tocotrienols (vitamin E) with selected metabolizing enzymes. Upadhyay J, Misra K. Bioinformation. 2009 Apr 21;3(8):326-31. PMID:19707294

[55] Estimation of antioxidant intakes from diet and supplements in U.S. adults. Chun OK, Floegel A, Chung SJ, Chung CE, Song WO, Koo SI. J Nutr. 2010 Feb;140(2):317-24. Epub 2009 Dec 23. PMID:20032488

[56] Tocopherol and tocotrienol contents of raw and processed fruits and vegetables in the United States diet. Chuna J, Leeb J, Yea L, Exlerc J, Eitenmiller RR. Journal of Food Composition and Analysis 19 (2006) 196–204

[57] Normal Phase High-Performance Liquid Chromatography; Method for the Determination of Tocopherols and Tocotrienols in Cereals. Panfili G, Fratianni A, Irano M. J. Agric. Food Chem. 2003, 51, 3940-3944

[58] Cancer-preventive activities of tocopherols and tocotrienols. Ju J, Picinich SC, Yang Z, Zhao Y, Suh N, Kong AN, Yang CS. Carcinogenesis. 2010 Apr;31(4):533-42. PMID:19748925

[59] Bone is more susceptible to vitamin K deficiency than liver in the institutionalized elderly. Kuwabara A, Fujii M, Kawai N, Tozawa K, Kido S, Tanaka K. Asia Pac J Clin Nutr. 2011;20(1):50-5. PMID:21393110

[60] Chemoprevention of chemically-induced biliary carcinogenesis in hamsters by vitamin K2. Tsuchida A, Itoi T, Kasuya K, et al. Hepatogastroenterology. 2011 Mar-Apr;58(106):290-7. PMID:21661384

[61] Lifelong low-phylloquinone intake is associated with cognitive impairments in old rats. Carrié I, Bélanger E, Portoukalian J, Rochford J, Ferland G. J Nutr. 2011. Aug;141(8):1495-501. PMID: 21653572

[62] High dietary menaquinone intake is associated with reduced coronary calcification. Beulens JW, Bots ML, Atsma F, et al. Atherosclerosis. 2009 Apr;203(2):489-93. PMID: 18722618

[63] Dietary intake of vitamin K and risk of prostate cancer in the Heidelberg cohort of the European Prospective Investigation into Cancer and Nutrition (EPIC-Heidelberg). Nimptsch K, Rohrmann S, Linseisen J. Am J Clin Nutr. 2008 Apr;87(4):985-92. PMID:18400723

[64] Vitamin K supplementation in postmenopausal women with osteopenia (ECKO trial): a randomized controlled trial. Cheung AM, Tile L, Lee Y, et al. PLoS Med. 2008 Oct 14;5(10):e196. PMID:18922041

[65] A high menaquinone intake reduces the incidence of coronary heart disease. Gast GC, de Roos NM, Sluijs I, et al. Nutr Metab Cardiovasc Dis. 2009 Sep;19(7):504-10. PMID:19179058

[66] Association of vitamin K deficiency with bone metabolism and clinical disease activity in inflammatory bowel disease. Nakajima S, Iijima H, Egawa S, et al. Nutrition. 2011 Oct;27(10):1023-8. PMID:21482072

[67] Late vitamin K deficiency bleeding leading to a diagnosis of cystic fibrosis: a case report. Ngo B, Van Pelt K, Labarque V, Van De Casseye W, Penders J. Acta Clin Belg. 2011 Mar-Apr;66(2):142-3. PMID:21630615

[68] Maternal-neonatal vitamin K deficiency secondary to maternal biliopancreatic diversion. Bersani I, De Carolis MP, Salvi S, et al. Blood Coagul Fibrinolysis. 2011 Jun;22(4):334-6. PMID:21451400

[69] Vitamin A deficiency in a newborn resulting from maternal hypovitaminosis A after biliopancreatic diversion for the treatment of morbid obesity. Huerta S, Rogers LM, Li Z, et al. Am J Clin Nutr. 2002 Aug;76(2):426-9.PMID:12145017

[70] Viability and plasma vitamin K levels in the common bile duct-ligated rats. Akimoto T, Hayashi N, Adachi M, et al. Exp Anim. 2005 Apr;54(2):155-61. PMID:15897625

[71] Adulthood obesity is positively associated with adipose tissue concentrations of vitamin K and inversely associated with circulating indicators of vitamin K status in men and women. Shea MK, Booth SL, Gundberg CM, et al. J Nutr. 2010 May;140(5):1029-34. PMID:20237066

[72] Dietary and nondietary determinants of vitamin K biochemical measures in men and women. McKeown NM, Jacques PF, Gundberg CM, et al. J Nutr. 2002 Jun;132(6):1329-34. PMID:12042454

[73] S-adenosyl methionine (SAMe) versus celecoxib for the treatment of osteoarthritis symptoms: a double-blind cross-over trial.Najm WI, Reinsch S, Hoehler F, Tobis JS, Harvey PW. BMC Musculoskelet Disord. 2004 Feb 26;5:6. PMID:15102339

[74] Effects of glucosamine, chondroitin, or placebo in patients with osteoarthritis of hip or knee: network meta-analysis. Wandel S, Jüni P, Tendal B, et al. BMJ. 2010 Sep 16;341:c4675. PMID:20847017

[75] Evidence for S-adenosyl-L-methionine (SAM-e) for the treatment of major depressive disorder. Papakostas GI. J Clin Psychiatry. 2009;70 Suppl 5:18-22. PMID:19909689

[76] Coenzyme Q10: absorption, tissue uptake, metabolism and pharmacokinetics. Bhagavan HN, Chopra RK. Free Radic Res. 2006 May;40(5):445-53. PMID:16551570

[77] Relative bioavailability comparison of different coenzyme Q10 formulations with a novel delivery system. Liu ZX, Artmann C. Altern Ther Health Med. 2009 Mar-Apr;15(2):42-6. PMID:1928418

[78] Coenzyme Q10 in Parkinson's disease. Symptomatic or neuroprotective effects? Storch A. Nervenarzt. 2007 Dec;78(12):1378-82. PMID:17508194

[79] Blood pressure lowering efficacy of coenzyme Q10 for primary hypertension. Ho MJ, Bellusci A, Wright JM. Cochrane Database Syst Rev. 2009 Oct 7;(4):CD007435. PMID:19821418

[80] A randomized, double-blinded, placebo-controlled, crossover, add-on study of CoEnzyme Q10 in the prevention of pediatric and adolescent migraine. Slater SK, Nelson TD, Kabbouche MA, et al. Cephalalgia. 2011 Jun;31(8):897-905. PMID:21586650

[81] Association between genetic variants in the Coenzyme Q10 metabolism and Coenzyme Q10 status in humans. Fischer A, Schmelzer C, Rimbach G, Niklowitz P, Menke T, Döring F. BMC Res Notes. 2011 Jul 21;4:245. PMID:21774831

[82] Effects of common polymorphisms on the properties of recombinant human methylenetetrahydrofolate reductase. Yamada K, Chen Z, Rozen R, Matthews RG. Proc Natl Acad Sci U S A. 2001 Dec 18;98(26):14853-8. PMID:11742092

[83] Dietary induced subclinical vitamin K deficiency in normal human subjects. Ferland G, Sadowski JA, O'Brien ME. J Clin Invest. 1993 Apr;91(4):1761-8. PMID:8473516

[84] http://www.brenda-enzymes.org/enzyme.php?ecno=1.1.99.1 BRENDA: Accessed Sept 2014

[85] Divergent associations of plasma choline and betaine with components of metabolic syndrome in middle age and elderly men and women. Konstantinova SV, Tell GS, Vollset SE, Nygård O, Bleie Ø, Ueland PM. J Nutr. 2008 May;138(5):914-20. PMID:18424601

[86] Choline and betaine food sources and intakes in Taiwanese. Chu DM, Wahlqvist ML, Chang HY, Yeh NH, Lee MS. Asia Pac J Clin Nutr. 2012;21(4):547-57. PMID:23017313

[87] Institute of Medicine and National Academy of Sciences. USA. Dietary reference intakes for folate, thiamin, riboflavin, niacin, vitamin B12, panthothenic acid, biotin, and choline. Vol. 1. Washington D.C.: National Academy Press; 1998. pp. 390–422. http://www.nap.edu/openbook.php?record_id=6015&page=R1

[88] Dietary choline and betaine intakes in relation to concentrations of inflammatory markers in healthy adults: the ATTICA study. Detopoulou P, Panagiotakos DB, Antonopoulou S, Pitsavos C, Stefanadis C. Am J Clin Nutr. 2008 Feb;87(2):424-30. PMID:18258634

[89] Estimation of usual intake and food sources of choline and betaine in New Zealand reproductive age women. Mygind VL, Evans SE, Peddie MC, Miller JC, Houghton LA. Asia Pac J Clin Nutr. 2013;22(2):319-24. PMID:23635379

[90] The association between betaine and choline intakes and the plasma concentrations of homocysteine in women. Chiuve SE, Giovannucci EL, Hankinson SE, Zeisel SH, Dougherty LW, Willett WC, Rimm EB. Am J Clin Nutr. 2007 Oct;86(4):1073-81. PMID:17921386

[91] Concentrations of choline-containing compounds and betaine in common foods. Zeisel SH, Mar MH, Howe JC, Holden JM. J Nutr. 2003 May;133(5):1302-7. Erratum in: J Nutr. 2003 Sep;133(9):2918. PMID:12730414

[92] The betaine-GABA transporter (BGT1, slc6a12) is predominantly expressed in the liver and at lower levels in the kidneys and at the brain surface. Zhou Y, Holmseth S, Hua R, et al. Am J Physiol Renal Physiol. 2012 Feb 1;302(3):F316-28. PMID: 22071246

[93] Expression of organic osmolyte transporters in cultured rat astrocytes and rat and human cerebral cortex. Oenarto J, Görg B, Moos M, Bidmon HJ, Häussinger D. Arch Biochem Biophys. 2014 Oct 15;560:59-72. PMID:25004465

[94] Changes in GABA transporters in the rat hippocampus after kainate-induced neuronal injury: decrease in GAT-1 and GAT-3 but upregulation of betaine/GABA transporter BGT-1. Zhu XM, Ong WY. J Neurosci Res. 2004 Aug 1;77(3):402-9. PMID:15248296

[95] Betaine inhibits toll-like receptor 4 expression in rats with ethanol-induced liver injury. Shi QZ, Wang LW, Zhang W, Gong ZJ. World J Gastroenterol. 2010 Feb 21;16(7):897-903. PMID:20143470

[96] Betaine protects against high-fat-diet-induced liver injury by inhibition of high-mobility group box 1 and Toll-like receptor 4 expression in rats. Zhang W, Wang LW, Wang LK, Li X, Zhang H, Luo LP, Song JC, Gong ZJ. Dig Dis Sci. 2013 Nov;58(11):3198-206. PMID:23861108

[97] Alcohol, nutrition and liver cancer: role of Toll-like receptor signaling. French SW, Oliva J, French BA, Li J, Bardag-Gorce F. World J Gastroenterol. 2010 Mar 21;16(11):1344-8. PMID:20238401

[98] Plasma methionine, choline, betaine, and dimethylglycine in relation to colorectal cancer risk in the European Prospective Investigation into Cancer and Nutrition (EPIC). Nitter M, Norgård B, de Vogel S, et al. Ann Oncol. 2014 Aug;25(8):1609-15. PMID:24827130

[99] Effects of betaine intake on plasma homocysteine concentrations and consequences for health. Olthof MR, Verhoef P. Curr Drug Metab. 2005 Feb;6(1):15-22. PMID:15720203

[100] Choline: an essential nutrient for public health. Zeisel SH, da Costa KA. Nutr Rev. 2009 Nov;67(11):615-23. PMID: 19906248

[101] Determination of free α-lipoic acid in foodstuffs by HPLC coupled with CEAD and ESI-MS Durrania AI, Schwartza H, Naglb M, Sontaga G. Food Chemistry, 120 (4)1143–1148, 15 June 2010

[102] Age and gender dependent bioavailability of R- and R,S-α-lipoic acid: a pilot study. Keith DJ, Butler JA, Bemer B, et al. Pharmacol Res. 2012 Sep;66(3):199-206. PMID:22609537

[103] http://www.genome.jp/dbget-bin/www_bget?enzyme+2.8.1.8 KEGG: Accessed Sept. 2014

[104] Is alpha-lipoic acid a scavenger of reactive oxygen species in vivo? Evidence for its initiation of stress signaling pathways that promote endogenous antioxidant capacity. Petersen Shay K, Moreau RF, Smith EJ, Hagen TM. IUBMB Life. 2008 Jun;60(6):362-7. PMID:18409172

[105] Alpha-lipoic acid affects the oxidative stress in various brain structures in mice with methionine and choline deficiency. Veskovic M, Mladenovic D, Jorgacevic B, Stevanovic I, de Luka S, Radosavljevic T. Exp Biol Med (Maywood). 2014 Sep 5. pii: 1535370214549521. PMID:25193852

[106] The effects of α-lipoic acid on liver oxidative stress and free fatty acid composition in methionine-choline deficient diet-induced NAFLD. Stanković MN, Mladenović D, Ninković M, et al. J Med Food. 2014 Feb;17(2):254-61. PMID:24325457

[107] α-Lipoic acid regulates lipid metabolism through induction of sirtuin 1 (SIRT1) and activation of AMP-activated protein kinase. Chen WL, Kang CH, Wang SG, Lee HM. Diabetologia. 2012 Jun;55(6):1824-35. PMID:22456698

[108] Reversal of metabolic deficits by lipoic acid in a triple transgenic mouse model of Alzheimer's disease: a 13C NMR study. Sancheti H, Kanamori K, Patil I, et al. J Cereb Blood Flow Metab. 2014 Feb;34(2):288-96. PMID:24220168

[109] Fructose diet-induced skin collagen abnormalities are prevented by lipoic acid. Thirunavukkarasu V, Nandhini AT, Anuradha CV. Exp Diabesity Res. 2004 Oct-Dec;5(4):237-44. PMID:15763937

[110] Lipoic acid prevents liver metabolic changes induced by administration of a fructose-rich diet. Castro MC, Massa ML, Schinella G, Gagliardino JJ, Francini F. Biochim Biophys Acta. 2013 Jan;1830(1):2226-32. PMID:23085069

[111] Lipoic acid effects on established atherosclerosis. Ying Z, Kherada N, Farrar B, et al. Life Sci. 2010 Jan 16;86(3-4):95-102. PMID:19944706

[112] Effects of dietary supplementation of alpha-lipoic acid on early glomerular injury in diabetes mellitus. Melhem MF, Craven PA, Derubertis FR. J Am Soc Nephrol. 2001 Jan;12(1):124-33. PMID:11134258

[113] The plasma pharmacokinetics of R-(+)-lipoic acid administered as sodium R-(+)-lipoate to healthy human subjects. Carlson DA, Smith AR, Fischer SJ, Young KL, Packer L. Altern Med Rev. 2007 Dec;12(4):343-51. PMID:18069903

[114] Delivery of orally supplemented alpha-tocotrienol to vital organs of rats and tocopherol-transport protein deficient mice. Khanna S, Patel V, Rink C, Roy S, Sen CK. Free Radic Biol Med. 2005 Nov 15;39(10):1310-9. PMID:16257640

[115] Effects of altered maternal folic acid, vitamin B12 and docosahexaenoic acid on placental global DNA methylation patterns in Wistar rats. Kulkarni A, Dangat K, Kale A, et al. PLoS One. 2011 Mar 10;6(3):e17706. PMID:21423696

[116] Opinion on mixed tocopherols, tocotrienol tocopherol and tocotrienols as sources for vitamin E added as a nutritional substance in foodsupplements. European Safety Authority The EFSA Journal (2008) 640, 1-34

[117] Codex Standard for Named Vegetable oils, www.codexalimentarius.net/download/standards/336/CXS_210e.pdf CODEX STAN 210-1999

41. Cancer Prevention

One in five Americans die from cancer, but twice that many get cancer during their lives. This does not indicate a 50 percent cure rate; but rather, that many people with cancer die from other causes. For example, 16 percent of men are diagnosed with prostate cancer, and treatment contains the disease in many. A few men are cured. Nevertheless, fewer than three percent of men die from prostate cancer. Since this cancer usually occurs in older men, it is more common for them to succumb to other conditions before prostate cancer can reap its toll.

About six percent of Americans die from lung cancer. If cancers caused by tobacco are separated out, thus removing most lung cancer, the cancers most likely to kill a man are prostate cancer (2.79%), colon and rectal cancers (2.17%), and pancreatic cancer (1.28%). For women, the three most common causes of cancer death other than lung cancer are breast cancer (2.81%), colon and rectal cancers (2.01%), and pancreatic cancer (1.26%)[1].

In 2011, 572,000 Americans were estimated to die from cancer. Thirty percent of those deaths were attributed to tobacco use. If tobacco is removed from the equation, more than half of the remaining cancer deaths can be attributed to diet and nutritional factors and to lack of physical activity[2].

Expert estimates are that seventy percent of cancers are caused by toxic substances in food, alcohol and tobacco. Thus, most cancer risk can be avoided, and most cancers prevented. Other cancers are caused by infectious agents; Human papilloma virus (HPV) causes cervical cancer, and hepatitis B and C cause hepatocellular carcinoma, as examples. Vaccines, which prevent both the disease and associated cancers, are available for two of these three viruses. Furthermore, cancers caused by viruses are affected by nutritional status. Low folate and vitamin B_{12} levels increase the risk of sustained HPV infection[3] and increase the risk of cervical cancer[4]. Alcohol and obesity are risk factors for hepatocellular carcinoma in individuals with chronic infections hepatitis[5,6]. Nutrition, thus, has a large impact on the risk of cancer.

Individuals with Type 2 Diabetes are about one-third more likely to fall victim to cancer[7], with the risk of cancer of the liver, pancreas, and endometrium doubled in these patients.

A portion of this risk is attributable to obesity and lack of physical activity[8]. In Europe, which is less obese than the United States, about 5% of all cancers are attributed to obesity[9]. Among European women, 8.6% of cancers are caused by obesity; 65% of those are cancers of the endometrium, post-menopausal breast, and colorectum[10]. A sedentary lifestyle is an additional risk factor for cancer. Among Canadians, 7.9% of all cancers are attributable to lack of physical activity[11].

Recall, from Chapter 10, that obesity and metabolic syndrome are inflammatory conditions, and from Chapter 21, that exercise helps lower the production of free radicals that can cause DNA damage by culling weak mitochondria.

Tobacco, alcohol, poor nutrition, lack of physical activity, and exposure to toxic chemical cause most cancers, and especially those occurring after the age of 50. Those induced by viral disease, often occur during youth. Most cancer can be avoided, and thus, for most adults, cancer is a choice, or more correctly, a series of unfortunate choices.

Induction of Cancer

Inflammation is necessary for fighting infections and healing wounds; it helps destroy parasites and bacteria and stimulates tissue repair. During inflammation, chemokines concentrate white blood cells in the area of inflammation, and cytokines mediate inflammatory reaction, in part through the production of reactive oxygen species (ROS) which are used for killing bacteria and destroying infected cells.

Mitochondria efficiently produce power for the cell by transferring energy in the form of phosphate bonds to ATP; however, a small amount of energy from the mitochondria leaks out in the form of free radicals. As the mitochondria get worn out, they leak higher amounts of ROS. (See Chapter 21.) Glutathione, vitamin E, vitamin C, uric acid and several other antioxidants are available in the cell, and these quench the free radicals, protecting the cell's proteins and organelles from oxidative damage.

Repetitive or continual oxidative stress can deplete antioxidants and increase the risk of mutations. Deficiencies of dietary antioxidants also increase this risk. Deficiency of folate and vitamin B_{12} can result in hypomethylation of DNA causing certain DNA strands to be more exposed to oxidative damage.

One of the most devastating effects of free radicals is that the radicals can cause breaks in the strands of DNA in the cell's nucleus. The DNA can be repaired, but nucleotide substitutions or deletions errors can occur, which are passed on to daughter cells. These mutational errors can result in conformational changes in the protein encoded by the gene, and the protein may behave differently. Some errors in coding of proteins will keep the cell from functioning properly. Some of these will trigger apoptosis, and the cell will be replaced. We have trillions of cells, and billions are replaced every day. Mistakes are made, but the body is good at recognizing them, fixing the damage through DNA repair, or eliminating cells that are not doing their jobs. Nevertheless, some aberrant cells survive. Accumulation of these errors and the decreased efficiency of metabolism they cause can contribute to aging.

DNA repair errors made on genes that are involved in the regulation of cell proliferation are much more problematic. If the mechanisms responsible for the elimination of cells that function improperly has a mutation that perpetuates the survival and proliferation of aberrant cells, a lineage of cells with unregulated proliferation can ensue. This is how cancer is caused; these mutations cause continual growth or prevent the appropriate apoptosis, or even promote the growth, of unneeded, improperly behaving cells.

Damage to genes, which causes cancer producing changes, is referred to as cancer initiation. Ionizing radiation, X-rays, and UV light, for example, can break the DNA strand, and is a risk factor for cancer initiation.

Certain chemical compounds can covalently bind to the DNA, forming DNA adducts, damaging the DNA either by inducing a mutation resulting from a break and a faulty repair or by binding to the DNA so that the gene can not be transcribed. Inhibiting transcription can cause cancer by preventing a regulatory gene from controlling cell growth. A mutagen is a compound with can break the DNA, prevent its repair, or bind to it so that the gene does not function normally. A mutagen can affect the activity of a protein or enzyme without causing cancer. A compound that can affect regulatory genes and promote unregulated cellular proliferation is a carcinogen.

Table 41-1: Some Mutagenic and Carcinogenic DNA Adducts

Agent	Source
Malondialdehyde	Endogenous lipid peroxidation
Aldehydes	Endogenous alcohol metabolism, present in aged meats
Anthramycin	Chemotherapeutic agent
Cisplatin	Chemotherapeutic agent
Diethylstilbestrol	Medication (A synthetic estrogen)
Heterocyclic Amines (HCA)	Meat cooked at high temperatures
Polycyclic aromatic hydrocarbons (PAH)	Products of combustion; found in tobacco and environmental smoke. Also formed in food, especially charred meat and over toasted foods. Benzo(a)pyrene is a PAH.
Aflatoxin B1	Product of a mold that grows on and contaminates grains, nuts, and other foods.
Metals	Cadmium, lead, arsenic, antimony, manganese, aluminum, strontium, chromium, cobalt, iron

DNA adducts can be exogenous environmental toxins or endogenous products produced by the body. Many adducts are organic compounds; several metals also can be.

Cancer Genes

Mutations in certain genes can greatly increase the lifetime risk for certain cancers. Mutations in the genes BRCA1 or BRCA2 greatly increase the risk for breast, ovarian, prostate, and pancreatic cancers.

BRCA1 is a tumor suppressor gene for a protein that repairs the double-strand breaks in the DNA, or marks it for destruction through ubiquitination. BRCA2 is a different protein but has similar functions. Among various population groups, there are specific mutations of these genes that are heritable, and some of these, especially those of BRCA1 impart high risk for cancer. Without medical intervention, women with BRCA1 mutations only have a 53% survival rate to the age of 70, while 84% of unaffected women do. Those with BRCA2 mutations have a 71% probability of surviving to age 70[12].

While deleterious genes that increase cancer risk are uncommon, cancer is all too common among those with these genes. Less than one percent of the general population carries a mutation in one of the six most common cancer risk genes, including BRCA genes. Among those with cancer, about 10 percent have mutations[13]. The lifetime cancer risk for those with BRCA1 and BRCA2 mutations is as high as:

- 40%-80% for breast cancer
- 11%-40% for ovarian cancer
- 1%-10% for male breast cancer
- Up to 39% for prostate cancer
- 1%-7% for pancreatic cancer

While most cancer is not caused by inherited gene mutations, individuals with these mutations are at high risk. Those with a family or personal history of these cancers should consider genetic screening, and may benefit from preventive treatment. In some persons, this may be frequent cancer screening and pious adherence to a low-risk lifestyle; in some women prophylactic mastectomy and oophorectomy is appropriate. An online decision tool for BRCA1 and BRCA2 carriers is available choosing an informed treatment at http://brcatool.stanford.edu[14].

Promotion of Cancer

In addition to its oxidative activities, chronic inflammation also promotes growth for repair of injured tissue and promotes the survival of inflammatory cells. When the inflammatory signal is downregulated, these inflammatory cells normally undergo apoptosis as they are no longer needed. Unresolved inflammation, however, can maintain the survival of certain cells, including defective cells.

Influences that increase the proliferation of cancer cells are referred to as promoters. For some cells, for example in breast cancer, the female sex hormone progesterone may induce growth. Vitamin A can act as a growth promoter in cancer. The inflammatory process can also act as a growth promoter, by promoting cell division and development of new blood vessels in cancer.

Cancer as an Inflammatory Disease

Non-steroidal anti-inflammatory drugs have been found to decrease the risks for cancers of the esophagus, stomach, and colon as well as for other solid tumors. In a study of patients with Lynch syndrome, which puts patients at very high risk of colorectal cancer, taking 600 mg of aspirin daily for two years decreased the risk of colon cancer by 59 percent at 4½ years of follow-up[15].

In a study using the COX2 inhibitor celecoxib in patients with a history of colonic adenomas, risk of recurrence after three years of treatment was reduced by a third in those taking 200 mg twice a day and by 45% in those taking 400 mg twice a day[16]. About 20 percent of patients, however, had serious side effects from the use of celecoxib, which make the risks associated with the use of this medication higher than its benefits, except perhaps, for those at the highest risk of colon cancer death.

The anti-carcinogenic effects mediated through the action of these medications is through inhibition of the enzyme prostaglandin-endoperoxide synthase 2 (PTGS2), more commonly also known as cyclooxygenase-2 (COX2). These medications prevent the formation of PGE_2 that acts as a cancer promoter by increasing angiogenesis and cell proliferation and decreasing apoptosis. (See Figure 40-1.)

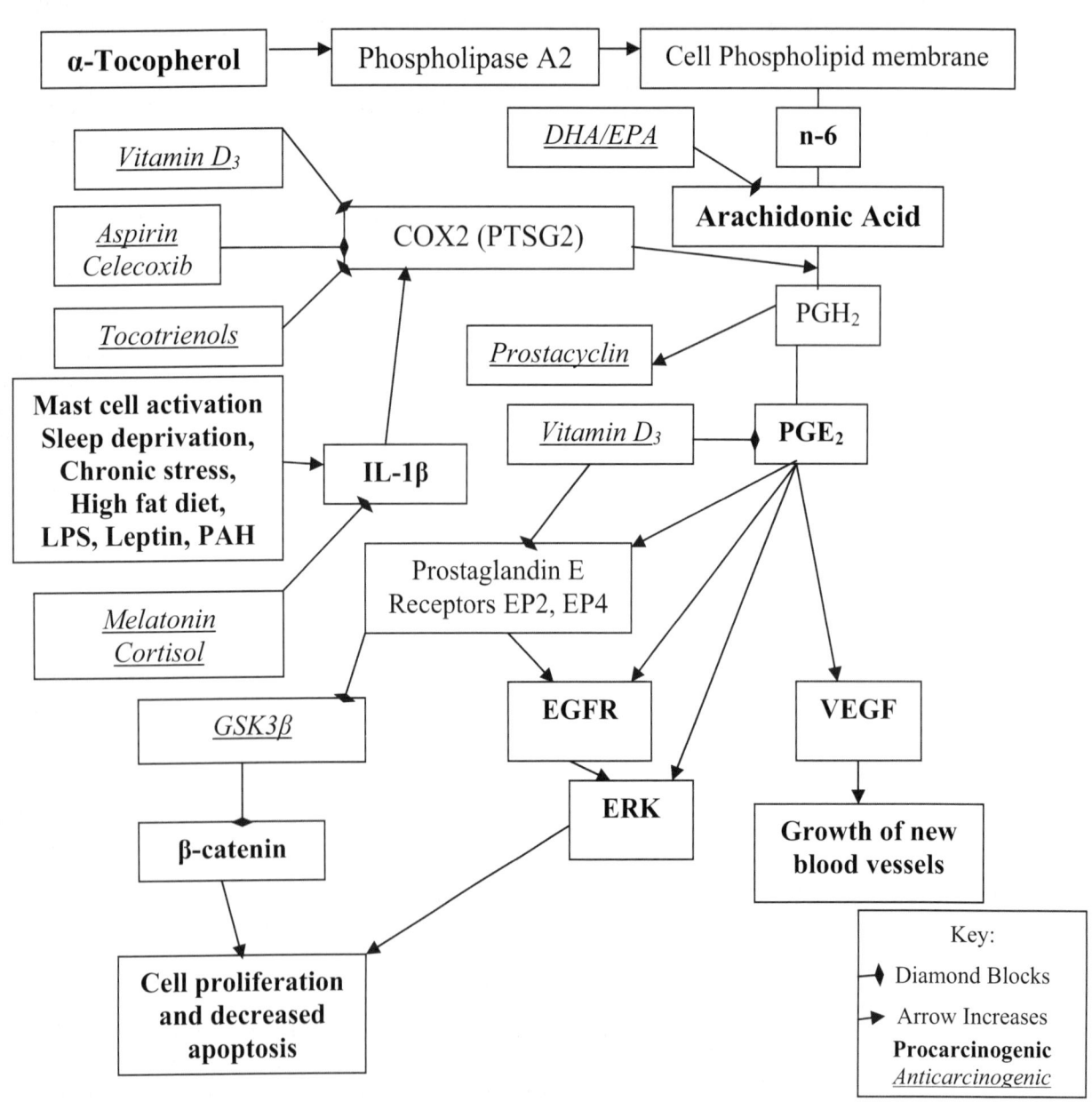

Figure 41-1: The Role of Inflammatory Prostaglandin E2 in Cell Proliferation and Angiogenesis[17].

Phospholipase A2 causes long-chain polyunsaturated acids to be released from the phospholipids cell membrane inner leaf. α-tocopherol increases the activity of phospholipase A2, and thus, can increase the production of PGE$_2$ when there is a high ratio of n-6 to n-3 fats present in the cell membrane[18]. The n-6 fatty acid, arachidonic acid (AA), is converted by PTGS-2 (COX2) into the inflammatory eicosanoid PGE$_2$.

PGE$_2$ increases cell proliferation by activation of β-catenin, by activation of the epidermal growth factor receptor (EGFR) and activation of ERK through a protein kinase C dependent mechanism[19].

β-Catenin is part of a complex of proteins that constitute adherens junctions that bind cells to each other. These proteins maintain adhesion between cells and help to regulate growth. β-catenin anchors the actin cytoskeleton. When β-catenin is not bound to the adherens junction, it acts as a signal indicating that that the cell does not have a full complement of neighboring cells to adhere to and that growth of more cells is required. Free β-catenin thus can act as a signal for cell proliferation[20].

PGE$_2$ activates Prostaglandin E receptors (EP$_2$ and EP$_4$), which phosphorylate glycogen synthase kinase 3 (GSK-3). GSK-3 prevents cell proliferation by acting in a protein complex that destroys free β-catenin. When GSK-3 is phosphorylated, it prevents the destruction of β-catenin, and thus, allows β-catenin to move into the nucleus of the cell where it promotes proliferation and impede apoptotic signaling[21].

EGF receptor stimulation by PGE$_2$ activates ERK (extracellular-signal-regulated kinase). EGF also increases ERK through a separate, protein kinase-C dependent mechanism. ERK is involved in the regulation of mitosis and thus promotes cell division. PGE$_2$ is also a vasodilator and increases VEGF, and thus, it promotes angiogenesis and increases the blood supply to growing tissue[22]. Angiogenesis is needed to support a blood supply for tumor growth. These same signals are helpful for tissue repair after injury; nevertheless, they not beneficial when they promote unregulated growth or cancers.

Aspirin and COX2 inhibitors prevent the proliferation of cancer cells by preventing the formation of PGE$_2$ and its proliferative actions. The cancer risk reduction, however, needs to be weighed against the risk of side effects of these medications. In individuals with a high risk of cancer, aspirin clearly lowers the risk. In those with lower risk, the risk of gastrointestinal bleeding or other side effects of the medication may outweigh risks from cancer. Celecoxib, increases risks of death from heart disease, for example.

PGE$_2$ associated risk for cancer can also be mitigated by vitamin D$_3$[23] and vitamin E tocotrienols[24] and γ-tocopherol[25] through the inhibition of COX2 enzyme activity.

If n-3 fatty acids are present in the lipid membrane, they compete for COX2 activity and produce anti-inflammatory eicosanoids in place of PGE$_2$. Additionally, the n-3 fatty acids eicosapentaenoic acid (EPA) and docosahexaenoic acid (DHA) inhibit the formation of AA. Oleic acid, found in olive oil, also inhibits the formation of AA[26]. In hepatocellular carcinoma cells, DHA and EPA inhibit cancer cell growth. DHA and EPA promote dephosphorylation and, thereby, activation of GSK-3β. This causes degradation of β-catenin in these cancer cells, thus decreasing the cell's viability and ability to avoid apoptosis. Additionally, DHA down-regulates COX2 activity and increases the degradation of PGE$_2$ in these cells[27].

In prostate cancer cells, vitamin D$_3$ was found not only to inhibit the expression of COX2, but it also up-regulated the expression of the enzyme, 15-prostaglandin dehydrogenase, which inactivates prostaglandins. Additionally, vitamin D$_3$ decreased the expression of the prostaglandin receptors EP and FP, which mediate prostaglandin signaling[28].

Several vitamin E compounds downregulate the formation of PGE$_2$. The tocotrienols γ and δ have additional anti-carcinogenic effects. Both γ-tocotrienol and δ-tocotrienol have been found to inhibit the expression β-catenin protein in colon cancer cells[29, 30] and cause apoptosis of these cells. γ-tocotrienol and δ-tocotrienol reduce the activation of ERK and MAP kinase activity in pancreatic cancer cells and induce apoptosis of these cells[31]. These tocotrienols have also been shown to arrest cell growth and cause apoptosis in human melanoma cells[32]. δ-tocotrienol suppresses VEGF-induced angiogenesis while α-tocopherol, the form of vitamin E found in most supplements and food fortification, does not[33]. Rather than having an anti-carcinogenic effect, α-tocopherol inhibits the anti-carcinogenic effect of the tocotrienols by reducing their uptake into the tumor cells[34], and by increasing the activity of phospholipase A2 and the thus formation of eicosanoids.

Prevention of chronic inflammation removes the support for maintenance of cell proliferation of some cancer cell lines. Vitamin D$_3$ and certain forms of vitamin E can help regulate these aspects of inflammation. COX2 inhibitors can also be used to help prevent the proliferation of some cancer cell lineages.

Fatty acid content in the diet also affects the balance of eicosanoids. N-6 fatty acids, which are superabundant in the Western diet, increase the formation of PGE$_2$ while n-3 fatty acids decrease PGE$_2$ and favor the formation of non-inflammatory eicosanoids. Diets high in foods from marine environments would be expected to lower risk for cancer.

Inflammatory Cytokines

T$_1$ helper cells, (T$_H$1 cells) and the cytokines they produce, notably IFN-γ, function as the major anti-tumor immune effector cells. Other cytokines including IL-6, TNF, IL-1β and IL-23 promote tumor growth.

IL-1β is an inflammatory cytokine released from several cell types, including macrophages, dendritic cells, glial cells, smooth muscle and bronchial epithelial cells. IL-1β helps to stimulate and maintain the inflammatory response. One of its functions is to stimulate the induction of COX2 (PTGS2)[35]. IL-6 also promotes cell proliferation and decreases apoptosis through activation of cytokine receptors, induction of Janus kinases (JAK) and Signal Transducers and Activators of Transcription 3 (STAT3)[36], which then down-regulate apoptosis and increase proliferation. (See Figure 40-2.)

TNF-α stimulates apoptosis under certain conditions; however, it promotes proliferation and inhibits apoptosis under other conditions. TNF-α and protein p53 additively promote apoptosis while NF-κB, which can be activated by TNF-α, promotes resistance to apoptosis.

IKKα mediated phosphorylation of CREB binding protein (CBP) changes the CBP binding preference from p53 to NF-κB. This increases NF-κB mediated gene expression and decreases p53-mediated gene expressions, and thus, leads to the promotion of cell proliferation and tumor growth. CBP phosphorylation is inhibited by IL-1β and LPS. LPS activates TLR-4, which stimulates IKKα activity. Both IL-1β and LPS activate NF-κB, and thus, promote cell proliferation in the presence of TNF-α[37]. LPS, from anaerobic biofilms, is thus, a carcinogen. (See Figure 40-2.)

IκBα is bound to NF-κB in the cytosol of the cell, inactivating it. The enzyme IKKα can phosphorylate IκBα, freeing NF-κB, which can then be translocated into the nucleus where gene transcription occurs. Anthocyanins, (blue, red or purple plant pigments) curcumin, resveratrol, and other plant phenolic compounds have been found to prevent phosphorylation of IκBα and thus, these compound inhibit the translocation of NF-κB from cytosol to nucleus[38,39,40]. This explains part of the anti-inflammatory and anticarcinogenic effects of phenolic compounds.

T$_H$17 cells are stimulated by IL-1β. T$_H$17 cells secrete IL-6, TNF-α, IL-1β, and IL-23; these cytokines act as a positive feedback loop which support the generation of more T$_H$17 cells. IL-6 and IL-23 promote cancer. At the same time T$_H$17 cells antagonize the production of T$_H$1 immune cells, and thus, diminish the anti-tumor response[41]. Factors that impact TNF-α level are listed in Tables 23-1, 32-1, and 32-2. Factors that increase IL-6 are given in Table 41-4.

The 2.5 times increased risk of liver cancer observed in obese patients appears to be mediated by IL-6 and TNF, and these cytokines may also explain the increased risk for other cancers seen in obesity[42].

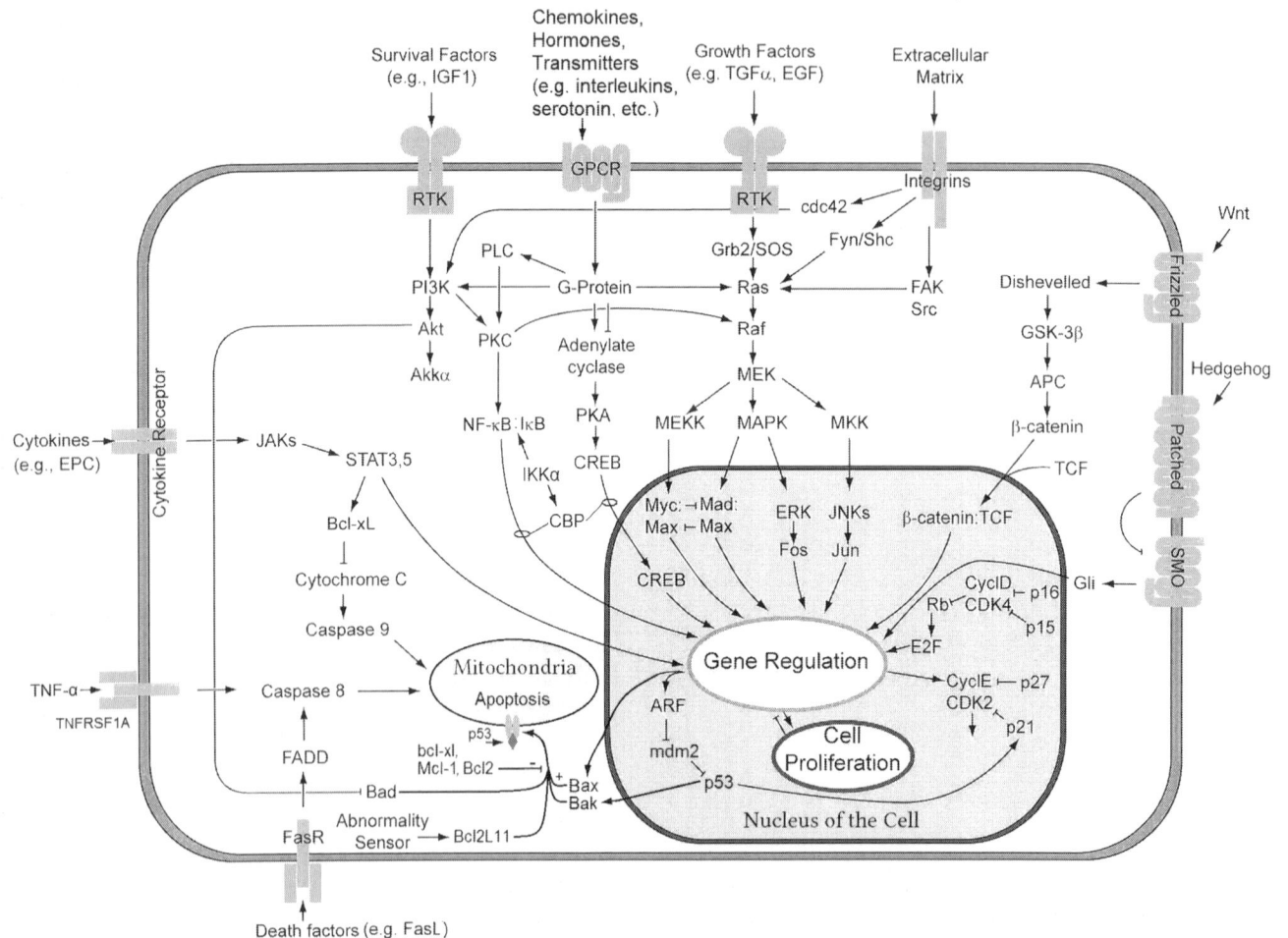

Figure 41-2: Proteins Involved in Cell Proliferation and Apoptosis[43]

Unresolved inflammation should be an early target in the primary and secondary prevention of cancer. IL-6 is elevated in many chronic inflammatory conditions. Sleep deprivation, obesity, and metabolic syndrome increase IL-6 levels. Immune sensitivities to foods are mediated through T_H17 cells, and thus may maintain a pro-carcinogenic milieu. Foods that induce inflammatory reactions should be avoided. Chronic stress also increases IL-6.

Short-term stress (up to a few hours) causes a brief increase in IL-6 that down-regulates IL-6 production over the long term. Play and pleasant adventures serve as short-term stressors that have a beneficial effect and decrease baseline IL-6 levels. Exercise also decreases IL-6 levels, and physical activity has been found to be associated with a decreased risk for colon[44] and other cancers[11]. Even watching an emotive movie (provoking laughter or tears) can act as a short-term stressor with beneficial effect[45]. This would have to act as a novel emotive experience, and while watching several hours of TV daily does not cause a chronic increase IL-6[46], it does increase the risk of cancer and cardiovascular disease through its association with sedimentary behavior[47].

Alcohol

Alcohol increases risk of cancer throughout the length of the alimentary tract. Consumption of alcohol raises the risk for cancers of the mouth, pharynx, esophagus, stomach, colon and rectum[48]. It also raises the risk of cancer of the liver, breast, and prostate. Women, who drink more than three alcohol equivalents on days that they drink, nearly double their risk of colon cancer as compared to those who have one drink on drinking days. Women who drink more frequently have 44% more breast cancer and men who drink more frequently have 55% more prostate cancer[49].

In the Nurses Health Study, binge drinking, drinking at a younger age, or at an older age increased breast cancer risk[50]. This indicates that drinking during breast growth (younger age; before the first pregnancy terminates breast development) can initiate cancer, likely due to alterations in DNA methylation of cell growth regulating genes. Alcohol can also act as a growth promoter once the cancer is present, and thus, consuming alcohol at older age increases risk by a different mechanism[51].

Alcohol is first metabolized into acetaldehyde. Acetaldehyde is mutagenic and carcinogenic as it interferes with DNA synthesis and repair, forms DNA adducts, inhibits normal DNA methylation and induces inflammation. Acetaldehyde is broken down by the enzyme ALDH2, forming acetate as an end product[52]. As mentioned in Chapter 13, ALDH2 is also required for the extracellular catabolism of histamine and other bioamines, and these compete for the availability of this enzyme.

Alcohol can be metabolized into acetaldehyde by several different enzymes. Alcohol is metabolized by alcohol dehydrogenase (ADH) enzymes of which there are at least seven tissue-specific isoenzymes. Isoenzyme ADH1C is active in the intestinal mucosa, and ADH1A is active in the liver. ADH1B is highly expressed in fat cells as well as in the intestinal mucosa and the liver[53].

The ADH1C*2 allele variant, which is common among Caucasians, increases the rate of alcohol metabolism into acetaldehyde by this enzyme by 2.5 times. Individuals who drink heavily and are heterozygotes for ADH1C are eight times as likely to have alcohol induced oral cancer. Those who are homozygous for ADH1C*2 have a risk for oral cancer 40 times higher than ADH1C*1 individuals, as the faster conversion of alcohol into acetaldehyde raises its concentrations and toxicity. The presence of this ADH allele also increases the risk of laryngeal, esophageal, head and neck, breast and liver cancers[52, 54].

The enzyme ALDH2 is responsible for the metabolism of acetaldehyde into acetate. An allelic variant ALDH2*2 is common Asians, with about 35 percent of Asians being heterozygous and about 10% being homozygous for this allele. This allele is less active and thus allows build up of acetaldehyde. Homozygotes rarely consume much alcohol, as it makes them sick. Heterozygotes, however, may drink heavily, and these individuals have ten times the risk of oropharyngeal and laryngeal cancers and 12.5 times the risk of esophageal cancer as those with the usual allele[52].

When consumed in moderate amounts, about 30 percent of the alcohol consumed is metabolized by the inducible cytochrome p450 enzyme CYP2E1. When alcohol is metabolized by this enzyme reactive oxygen species are created; thus, creating oxidative stress. Induction of the CYP2E1 enzyme also increases the metabolism of pro-carcinogenic heterocyclic amines into carcinogens[55].

Alcohol is also metabolized in the mouth and the gastrointestinal tract to acetaldehyde by bacteria. After the use of antibiotics that kill susceptible intestinal bacteria, alcohol metabolism typically slows by about 10 percent. The production of acetaldehyde by bacteria contributes to the development of cancers in mucosal tissues along the gastrointestinal tract from the mouth down[52].

Obesity

Metabolic syndrome, diabetes, and obesity are risk factors for hepatocellular, colorectal, breast[56], prostate[57] and pancreatic cancers[58, 7]. Obesity is not just a risk factor for the development of cancer but is also associated with a poorer response to cancer treatment.

Aspirin has been found to decrease the risk of developing colorectal cancer, and this effect is more pronounced in obese patients[59]. The increased cancer risk may be attributed to the inflammatory nature of abdominal obesity and the increased production of IL-6[42], which induces COX2. Insulin-like growth factor 1 (IGF-1) is also elevated in metabolic syndrome and may promote cell proliferation and survival, by inhibition of apoptosis, via the activation of phosphatidylinositol 3-kinase (PI3K)/Akt signaling pathways[56].

Meat and Cancer

Multiple studies indicate that consumption of red meat is associated with increased risk of cancer, including colorectal[60], breast[61] and brain cancer in children. The good news for carnivores is that it is not the meat; it's how it is prepared that causes cancer. Diets with high intakes of red meat are associated with increased risk of colon cancer. This increased risk is likely associated not with the consumption of the meat per se, but the type of fat (including both visible fat and that contained in the cell membranes of the meat) and the production of carcinogens created in the cooking process.

There are four principal effects by which meat causes cancer:

1. When meats are cooked at high temperatures creatinine and amino acids are transformed into heterocyclic amines (HCA) which are metabolized into mutagenic DNA adducts. Breast cancer is associated with consumption of well-done meat[62]. The risk for colonic polyps is higher among individuals who consume red meat cooked at higher temperatures, which causes the production of HCA[63,64].

2. Processed and preserved meats contain N-nitrosyl compound (NOC) precursors which increase the risk of stomach, colon, rectal and brain cancers.

3. Burning organic material, including food, wood and coal, and tobacco causes the formation of polycyclic aromatic hydrocarbons (PAH), some of which are carcinogens.

4. Most commercially available red meat is from animals fed a diet of corn; and thus, has a high predominance of n-6 fatty acids in the fat and the meats cell membranes. These fatty acids can be converted into arachidonic acid and eicosanoids which are inflammatory, and thus promote cancer. Fats from fish appear to decrease the risk of colon cancer while n-6 fats and diets with high n6:n3 ratios are associated with higher prostate and bowel cancer risk[65,66].

HCA, NOC, and PAH are discussed below. The role n-6 and n-3 fatty acids in cancer were discussed previously in this chapter. Fats are discussed in further detail in Chapter 6.

Heterocyclic Amines

Not all heterocyclic amines are mutagenic or carcinogenic. Two vitamins; niacin and pyridoxine are HCA compounds. There are, however, at least 17 HCA that may be produced during the cooking of muscle tissue, many of these are mutagenic and at least four of these are amino imidazo aza-arenes (AIA) that are human carcinogens.

- 2-amino-3,4-dimethylimidazo[4,5-f]quinoline (MeIQ)
- 2-amino-3,8-dimethylimidazo[4,5-f]quinoxaline (MeIQx)
- 2-amino-3-methylimidazo[4,5-f]quinoline (IQ)
- 2-amino-1-methyl-6-phenyl-imidazo[4,5-b]pyridine (PhIP)

HCA compounds are formed in foods during heating at high temperatures. These compounds are formed from the pyrolization of creatine and amino acids.

The AIA are not quite carcinogenic; they require activation, first, in the liver through via the enzyme cytochrome p450 enzyme CYP1A2 into N-hydroxy AIA, although CYP1A1 and other p450 enzymes can also perform this step. Smoking cigarettes causes cancer, in part, as a result of its induction in CYP1A1 and CYP1A2 activity[67]. Next, the enzyme N-acetyltransferase-1 (NAT-1) and 2 (NAT-2), converts N-hydroxy AIA to form highly reactive N-acetoxy esters that spontaneously hydrolyze into aryl nitrenium ions that form adducts with DNA[68].

An alternative second step in the biotransformation of N-hydroxy AIA can be done by the enzyme: glutathione S-transferase (GST), or one of several other cytosolic enzymes; sulfotransferase, phosphorylase, and prolyl tRNA synthetase. This second-phase metabolism greatly increases the carcinogenic potential of the AIA compounds to bind to DNA.

Individuals with certain polymorphisms of enzymes (*NAT1, NAT2, GSTM1/T1,* and *SULT1A1* genes) that metabolize HCA may be at increased risk for carcinogenesis. Those with a rapid CYP1A1 genotype, rapid NAT1 and NAT2 genotype, are at increased risk of cancer from exposure to AIA HCA compounds. Those that metabolize the AIA via GST more quickly have lower risk, as glutathione S-transferase binds the N-hydroxy AIA to glutathione, forming a conjugate that can be eliminated in the urine.

The increased risk of colorectal cancer associated with HCA from meat cooked at high temperatures appears to be greater in individuals with fast acetylating alleles of the polymorphic enzyme N-acetyltransferase. Fast acetylators may also be at increased risk of colorectal cancer from smoking tobacco[69]. Smokers are at increased risk of colorectal cancer because smoking induces higher levels or cytochrome p450 enzymes which are needed to help eliminate toxins from absorbed from cigarette smoke[70,71]. CYP1A1 is induced by exposure to aromatic hydrocarbons, and individuals with a polymorphism of easily inducible CYP1A1 are at much greater risk of lung cancer than other smokers.

In a study including women with breast cancer, a test meal was given with a known content of AIA. Several hours later the urine was tested for AIA metabolites. Higher levels of carcinogenic metabolites were found in the women with breast cancer These women apparently absorb or metabolize these compounds more actively[72]. Colorectal, breast, prostate and pancreatic cancers appear to be most clearly linked to HCA consumption from meat[71, 73], and red meat consumption is a risk factor for adenocarcinoma and squamous cell carcinoma of the lung, even in individuals who have never smoked[74]. Eventually, these compounds bind to DNA through the formation of N-C bonds at guanine bases in the DNA strands producing DNA adducts.

Rodents fed a diet with HCA developed cancers in several organs, including the colon, breast, and prostate. One HCA produced hepatomas in monkeys. The cells from these cancers exhibited alteration on the genes for several proteins, including Apc, β-catenin, and Ha-ras; all proteins involved in cell growth regulation[75].

CAUTION!

Carcinogenic HCA compounds from consumption of meat cooked at high temperatures can be found in breast milk of rats, and DNA adducts of these carcinogens are found in the organs of their pups[76]. Carcinogenic HCA are also found in human breast milk[77]. More dangerously, carcinogenic HCA cross the placenta, and their DNA adducts can be found in the organs of preborn infant primates[78].

During fetal life and infancy, animals are at greatly increased risk of mutation because of the high rate of cell division during growth. Mice exposed to carcinogenic HCA in the first days of life formed liver cancers at middle age from doses that are a miniscule fraction of the chronic exposure dose required to cause cancer in adult mice[79].

Most of the eggs in a woman's ovaries are formed during her fetal life; before she was born. Thus, exposure to DNA adducts during a pregnancy that results in female offspring can potentially cause mutations that do not appear until the following generation. For males, sperm stem cells develop during early adolescence. Breast development mainly occurs during early adolescence. Thus, these are times of high risk for induction of mutations that can later become cancer. These can may even cause mutations that are passed down to multiple generations.

Pregnancy, infancy, and adolescence are periods when mutagens and carcinogens should be vigilantly avoided. And not just by women. It takes 60 days for sperm to form from stem cells. Those who plan to be fathers should be especially careful to avoid exposure to mutagens and carcinogens during the two months prior to conception. PAH forms DNA adducts in sperm and decreases the number of normal sperm[80]. Men with insufficient seminal vitamin C frequently have sperm DNA damage.[81]. Heavy alcohol exposure can cause DNA methylation in the sperm, and these changes can affect the offspring. Male rats fed a high-fat diet prior to breeding impart a propensity to pancreatic β-cell dysfunction in their daughters, and thus, risk of obesity and diabetes, while their low-fat consuming brethren did not[82].

Creation and Prevention of Carcinogenic HCA

HCA mutagenesis can be avoided by:

- Avoiding their formation during food preparation
- Avoiding their biotransformation from pro-carcinogens to carcinogens
- Consumption of foods that help reverse the damage.

Cooking Meat

Foods: The formation of HCA requires a reaction between creatine (or creatinine) and an amino acid. Muscle contains about 95% of the body's creatine; lower amounts are present in brain, intestinal, and brown adipose tissue and germ cells. Very low levels are found in the lungs, spleen, kidney, liver, and white adipose tissue[83].

The first step in the biosynthesis of creatine in vertebrates occurs in the kidney, with the production of guanidinoacetic acid (GAA) from arginine and glycine. GAA is transported out of the kidney and taken up by the liver and muscles where it is methylated by N-guanidinoacetate methyltransferase to form creatine. Creatine is transported out of the liver into the bloodstream and then is actively transported into the muscles where it is used as an energy source. The biosynthesis of creatine accounts for about 70% of the total utilization of methyl groups in the body[83].

The availability of creatine or creatinine in muscle tissue, along with the presence of free amino acids, makes meat an excellent source of the substrates for the formation of HCA. Most other high-protein foods, such as (milk and cheese, beans, tofu, other plant proteins), do not contain creatine and produce insignificant amounts of mutagenic compounds except during charring, and these are not HCA products[86]. Egg yolk, however, contains creatine and can produce HCA if cooked at high temperatures. Meat sauces, meat and fish stocks and extracts, and gravies are often very potent sources of mutagenic HCA[86]. Organ meats that are low in creatine, such as liver and kidney, produce very low amounts of HCA during cooking. In invertebrates, creatinine is limited to sperm cells[83]. HCA are not formed during the cooking of shellfish. Thus, it may be safe to throw some more shrimp on the barbie.

Temperature: The primary factors that determine the production of mutagens and carcinogens in meat are the temperature and duration the meats are cooked at. HCA content in cooked meat or fish can range from less than 1 ng/g, to over 300 ng/g in well-done, flame-grilled chicken breast. In most studies, the highest association for meat consumption with cancer is for red meats; however, this may reflect how frequently well-done, red meat is eaten in comparison to flame-grilled fish or fowl[84]. Charcoal-grilling, pan-frying or deep-frying chicken or duck produces high HCA levels[85].

Carcinogenic HCA are formed from creatine and amino acids in the presence of heat, moisture and usually a reducing sugar, such as glucose. The first step in the formation of HCA is the conversion of creatine to creatinine. Elevated cooking temperatures cause more rapid conversion of creatine to creatinine[86]. Most of the HCA in cooked food are formed in the first 6 minutes of cooking, and are formed on the surface exposed to the heat, although HCA are formed and also released as volatiles or smoke with further cooking.

The temperature is a major determinant of HCA formation. Under most conditions, HCA will not form below the boiling point of 100°C (212°F). HCA formation in food preparation begins at a temperature of about 150°C (302°F). At medium grilling temperatures of 200°C (392°F) much larger amounts are formed. There is a three-fold increase in the formation of HCA at 250°C (482°F) compared to the amounts formed at 200°C.

Table 41-2: HCA formation and Cooking Methods

Method[87]	Temp °C	Temp °F	HCA formation
Stewing	70 – 80	194	None
Boiling	100	212	None
Pressure cooking, in water	100 – 120	212 – 248	None (high humidity)
Microwave	≤100	≤212	None as long as the meat is not allowed to dry out
Sauté in water-based sauce	≤120	≤248	None or very low as long as not allowed to dry out.
Baking Roasting	100*	212*	Usually, low to intermediate levels
Pan Fry – Sauté in oil	175 – 225	350 – 450	High production
Recommended Deep fat frying	150 – 175	300 – 350	Moderate production
Typical Deep fat frying	190 – 240	374 – 464	High, increases with temperature
Grilling	200 – 260	392 – 500	High, increases with temperature
Charcoal Grill, Barbeque	230 – 270	466 – 518	High, increases with temperature, adds PAH risks and risks from volatiles
Flame Grill	≥430	≥806	Very high; intended to char meat
Searing	≥430	≥806	Very high; intended to char meat

Cooking in water limits the temperature of the food to the boiling point, which under normal conditions, prevents the formation of mutagenic HCA. Baking and roasting, which heat foods through indirect convection, do not reach high temperatures unless allowed to overcook and dry out. If the meat dries out, the temperature can rise and some HCA levels can form, however, if charring does not occur, levels usually remain low. Similarly, microwave cooking will not form HCA unless the meat is overcooked and dries out. Cooking techniques that heat food through radiation or conduction, such as grilling or frying, heat the surface of the meat to very high temperatures, and thus, lead to increased production of mutagenic HCA.

Table 41-3: FDA Recommended Minimum Cooking Temperatures

Meat	Temperature	
Fish	145°F	63°C
Steaks and Roasts	145°F	63°C
Ground Beef	160°F	71°C
Pork	160°F	71°C
Poultry	165°F	74°C

A principal objective in cooking meat is killing bacteria that may be present especially on the surface of the meat, or internally, in the case of hamburger or ground meat. Hamburger, for example, cooked at a grill temperature of 160°C (320°F), and turning the patty once a minute, produces very low HCA levels. In a study of HCA formation during the preparation of hamburger patties, it took 8 minutes to cook 1.5 cm thick patties to an internal temperature of 70°C (158°F). Increasing the grill temperature from 160°C (320°F) to 200°C (392°F) had very little effect on cooking time but tripled HCA formation[88]. (Instructions for cooking hamburger meat are given below.)

The typical temperature recommended by professional chefs for frying foods to obtain optimal flavor, appearance, and texture is 185°C (365°F). At this temperature, there is relatively little HCA formation. These temperatures, however, are easily exceeded when cooking in oils with high smoke point temperatures, such as corn, soy, or canola oil. The high smoke point is what makes them desirable; they withstand higher temperatures, and food can be crisped more quickly, although the cooking time may be little different. A higher temperature, however, tends to overcook the outer layer before the center can be sufficiently heated to kill bacteria and cook the meat.

Creation of smoke or frying at high temperatures creates volatiles that contain HCA and other carcinogenic compounds, such as polycyclic aromatic hydrocarbons (PAH). Inhalation of these compounds increases the risk of lung cancer. When frying or grilling meat indoors, a vent should be used to avoid the inhalation of HCA and PAH volatiles. Smoked fish and meat can have high levels of PAH, which are mutagenic and carcinogenic[89,90].

> Eggs: Egg yolk contains creatine and can form carcinogenic HCA if cooked at high temperatures. Browning of the yolk or lacing during cooking of eggs should be avoided.
>
> The various proteins in eggs coagulate between 63°C° (145 F°) and 80 C° (176 F°). Cooking at higher temperatures makes the egg tough and unpleasant. "Boiled eggs" should not be boiled, but rather simmered between 80°C° (176 F°) to 85 C° (185 F°) for the best results. The ideal open skillet or griddle temperature for cooking an egg is 120 C° (248 F°), a temperature at which water in the butter will sizzle, but at which the butter will not brown[87]. At these temperatures, HCA should not be formed unless the eggs are allowed to overcook. Browning of the egg, especially of the yolk, should be avoided.

Water content: Non-enzymatic browning reactions, called Maillard reactions, are formed most efficiently at water activity levels between 0.6 and 0.7. For example, the browning reaction in milk in the formation of "dulce de leche" only occurs after most of the water has evaporated from the milk. This reaction can be aided by the addition of sugar, which lowers the water activity level.

Likewise, HCA are more efficiently formed when moisture levels in the meat have fallen. Only very low levels of HCA are formed while cooking fish until it has lost over 50 percent of its weight through loss of moisture. When fish is cooked for the same length of time and at the same temperature, uncovered baking, which allows drying of the fish, produces 5 times as much HCA as does covered steaming the fish, which prevents moisture loss. Boiling meat does not produce HCA[101].

Cooking procedures that minimize water loss can also minimize the production of mutagens and carcinogens. This can be as simple as covering the meat while sautéing it so that it cooks in its own steam, or by adding enough moisture to keep the meat from drying. *Poaching and stewing meats does not cause the formation of mutagens.*

Reducing Sugars: The production of HCA also depend on the presence reducing sugars. When heated, the creatine is converted to creatinine. Heating combines creatinine with an amino acid, especially in the presence of a reducing sugar, present at about half the molar concentration of the creatinine or the amino acid. Beef, for example, contains glucose at about 0.07 percent. HCA conversion is most efficient when the reducing sugar (glucose, fructose, and lactose) is present at about 0.15 percent (weight monosaccharide/weight meat). Adding 0.08 percent glucose doubles the production of HCA. This would be equivalent to adding a third of a gram of glucose/pound of meat. Cooking meat with wine, which contains reducing sugars (about 1 gram/liter in red wine, 1.3 grams/liter in white wines), can increase the production of HCA from 60 to 80 percent when wine is added to ground beef[91]. Cooking a steak marinated in a commercial honey barbecue sauce increased the level of HCA by as much as four times[92], likely because of the reducing sugars present in corn syrup. Table sugar (sucrose) is not a reducing sugar and does not have this effect.

Higher concentrations of glucose and other reducing sugars, however, reduce the formation of carcinogenic HCA. At 0.67 percent (w/w), glucose or fructose decrease the production of HCA by about 50%[91]. This would be equivalent to adding 6 grams of glucose per kilogram, or 2.7 grams of glucose per pound of ground beef.

Addition of corn starch to ground beef (15 grams/kg or 7 grams/pound) also reduced the overall mutagenicity of cooked hamburgers[101], perhaps by retaining the meat juices internally and preventing their exposure to the heat of the pan.

Onions have enough sugar (about 14 to 20 grams of reducing sugars per pound) to influence the formation of HCA in beef. Adding a minimum of a half-pound of finely minced onion or 1/3-pound sweet onion to one pound of ground beef decreases the formation of HCA[101], however, adding small amounts of onion (one tablespoon minced onion or onion juice or less, per pound of ground beef), could be expected to increase the formation of HCA.

Meat Pretreatments and HCA

Freezing meat, and especially in a home freezer which is not cold enough for flash freezing causes the formation of large ice crystals that rupture the muscle cells. With commercial freezers, the temperatures are low enough that the ice crystals form more quickly, are smaller, and less likely to rupture the cells. Ruptured muscle cells leak creatine, amino acids, and glucose during cooking, raising the amount of substrates for the formation of HCA.

If meat is allowed to thaw and refreeze, it increases the amount of substrates for HCA production. Processing, such as mechanical tenderization, or grinding beef to make hamburger ruptures or cuts large numbers of cells, greatly increasing the availability of creatinine and amino acids for forming carcinogenic HCA.

HCA production can be greatly diminished by removing extracellular water from the meat, along with the substrates for HCA production; creatine, free amino acids, and glucose. This can be accomplished by microwaving the meat in its ready to cook form (i.e., a hamburger patty) for one-and-a-half to three minutes and discarding the juice which separates prior to grilling the meat. Three-minute, microwave pretreatment of hamburger patties has been demonstrated to reduce the HCA content after grilling at 250°C by nearly 90 percent and decrease mutagenicity by over 95%. Replacing these juices to the hamburger before grilling restored the formation of HCA[93]. Cuts of meat, or meat which has been diced prior to cooking may be rinsed in water and patted dry to remove surface HCA precursors.

The availability of extracellular HCA substrates explains why gravies, stock, extracts, and pan residues can have extremely high HCA contents[94]. Gravies and meat or fish stock should only be made in and from low temperature, high-water content preparation methods.

Marinades: When cooking meat, it is the surfaces that are browned, and this is where the HCA are produced. With hamburger meat, HCA inhibitors can be mixed into the meat before cooking. When cooking non-ground beef, the inhibitors cannot be mixed in as easily. Marinating the meat, however, can greatly reduce the production of HCA[95]. Both beer and red wine decrease the formation of most HCA, although they may increase the concentration of others[96]. Beer does not contain reducing sugars and so does not raise HCA production. Beer also has less effect on the flavor of the cooked meat[97].

In a test of HCA formation using marinades, the liquid for the marinade made from water, soy oil, and vinegar did not lower the production of HCA when grilling steaks. Adding salt and table sugar to the marinade liquid decreased the formation of HCA by half. With the addition of herbs and spices, the production of HCA content in the grilled steak was lowered by as much as 88 percent. The herbs used included rosemary, thyme, and oregano which are high in antioxidant phenolic compounds including carnosic acid, carnosol, and rosmarinic acid[98].

An effective marinade can be made from 30 percent sweet red onion, 30 percent garlic, 15 percent lemon or lime juice[99]. A recipe for a Caribbean style marinade is given at the end of this chapter.

When cooking at high temperatures HCA can also become aerosolized, exposing cooks to airborne carcinogens. Fried bacon produces especially high levels[100]. Baked, roasted and microwave-cooked meat appears to impart little risk, while fried, grilled, and well-done meat do. Different meats may favor the formation of different carcinogenic HCA, but beef, pork, chicken, and fish all will form pro-carcinogenic HCA compounds when cooked at high temperatures.

Antioxidants: Antioxidants can prevent the formation of HCA's. Ascorbic acid (vitamin C) added to 3 grams/kg of ground beef also decreases the production of HCA by 50 percent[101]. At this level, it has little if any noticeable effect on flavor. Many other phenolic antioxidants have also been shown to prevent the formation of HCA. Different antioxidants may act differently to prevent the formation of different HCA[102]. Garlic inhibits the formation of HCA, as does rosemary.

Biotransformation

Cruciferous vegetables (broccoli, Brussels sprouts, cabbage, mustard, watercress, rocket, arugula, and others) have been associated with decreased risk of cancer. Broccoli and cauliflower help prevent progression of prostate cancer[122].

Consumption of turnips and Chinese cabbage lowers the risk of breast cancer in post-menopausal women overall while low intake of cruciferous vegetables doubled the risk of breast cancer in women with the GST_{P1} Val/Val genotype[103]. Consumption of cruciferous vegetables lowers the risk of many types of cancer. Green leafy vegetables and cruciferous vegetables lower the risk of non-Hodgkins lymphoma[104].

Cruciferous vegetables contain isothiocyanates that induce the production and activity of the enzyme glutathione S-transferase (GST). Individuals with the slower GST genotype, appear to be at increased risk for cancer. GST metabolizes N-hydroxylated AIA into conjugated compounds that are easily excreted into the urine. Thus, GST competes with NAT for the metabolism of N-hydroxylated HCA and lowers cancer risk by helping detoxify them and ridding them from the body before they can be transformed into mutagens.

Consumption of cruciferous vegetables appears to decrease the risk of HCA induced carcinogenesis in those with an active GST phenotype, but not in individuals in whom the enzyme is inactive. About half of Americans of European descent and 28 percent of African-Americans have a GST_{M1} genotype which provides no enzyme activity. Eleven percent of European Americans and 23% of African-Americans are homozygous for the GST_{P1} variant with reduced glutathione S-transferase activity, and about 20 percent of Americans have an inactive variant of the GST_{T1} gene[105]. It is those individuals with active GST activity in whom cruciferous vegetables give the greatest reduction in cancer risk[106].

Sulforaphane appears to be isothiocyanate that most actively induces GST activity. Sulforaphane may also act as an anti-carcinogen by inducing the production of pro-apoptotic proteins in the cell[107,108], and by protecting the mitochondria from oxidative stress through the induction of glutathione peroxidase/reductase enzymes[109]. Sulforaphane is not only an anti-carcinogen; it is cardio-protective[110], lowers LDL-cholesterol, and has anti-inflammatory effects[111].

Sulforaphane is, actually, not present in these vegetables. It is rather, its precursor, glucoraphanin. Glucoraphanin is acted upon by the enzyme myrosinase, present in vesicles within the cells in the plant. In intact vegetable tissues, these two compounds are stored in separate vesicles in the cell and only mixed when the cells are crushed or chewed. The purpose of the isothiocyanates is to act as pesticides; so activation only occurs when the plant cell is damaged, as when munched upon by an insect.

Plants that have the myrosinase-glucosinolate defense system include cruciferous vegetables from the mustard family, which includes purple cabbage, red cabbage, and broccoli inflorescences. These, as well as some closely related plants, including radishes, watercress, daikon, and wasabi, are all rich in glucoraphanin[112]. Radishes, radish seed sprouts, and watercress contain glucoraphanin[113]. One advantage of these is that they are usually eaten raw. Radish seedlings and watercress have pleasant spicy flavors.

Enzymatic hydrolysis of glucoraphanin occurs with the cellular disruption that occurs with chewing, cutting, freezing, cooking, and juicing, wherein the enzyme myrosinase and glucoraphanin can mix[114]. Even then, most of the glucoraphanin is converted to sulforaphane nitrile, which is inactive. However, if these cruciferous vegetables are briefly heated to 60°C (140°F) and then crushed (chewed) or liquefied into juice, the amount of sulforaphane produced is greatly increased[115]. Heating to 70°C (158°F) completely inactivates myrosinase and greatly diminishes the amount of sulforaphane available[116,117]. Sulforaphane is also heat labile. It is stable at 50°C (122°F) but destroyed at 90°C (194°F)[118]. Fully cooked cruciferous vegetables have little anti-carcinogenic activity.

> The health benefits of cruciferous vegetables can be maximized by eating them raw. They can also be juiced; preferably after heating them to 60°C (140°F). The juice can then be cooled for later consumption. To prepare cruciferous vegetables for eating cooked, they should be very lightly heated to an internal temperature of 60°C (140°F) and eaten while still warm to maximize sulforaphane availability.
>
> Thus, broccoli can be:
> - Heated in 60°C (140°F) water for 10 minutes
> - Broken into florets and steamed above boiling water for 3 minutes
> - Microwave for 1 minute.

Sulforaphane is not the only compound available in cruciferous vegetables that have anticarcinogenic properties. These vegetables also contain indole-3-carbinol (I3C), which has been shown to suppress the proliferation of various tumors in cells cultures, including breast, prostate, endometrial, and colon cancers and leukemia. IC3 suppresses NF-κB[119] activation and stimulates the cell cycling regulatory proteins p15, p21 and p27 and down-regulates Bcl-2 and Bcl-xL, therefore, arresting tumor growth and promoting apoptosis. It additionally shifts the production of estrogens to forms that less favor estrogen-responsive tumor growth[120]. Cruciferous vegetables, therefore, act not only to decrease the mutagenicity of HCA, but additionally, as anti-carcinogens.

Cruciferous vegetables may also provide benefits for the secondary prevention of cancer. In a study of men diagnosed with prostate cancer, those in the highest quartile of cruciferous vegetable consumption had a 59% decrease in disease progression[121]. A similar decrease in disease progression was found in another study among men with prostate cancer who ate more than one serving a week of broccoli or cauliflower[122].

Primary Prevention

Antioxidant polyphenols prevent carcinogenesis. Treatment of hepatic cells with several phenolic compounds has been shown to attenuate the mutagenic effect of HCA in hepatic cells. Cellular changes induced by HCA in hepatocytes were 75 to 90 percent eliminated by post-treatment with the phenolic compounds vanillin, coumarin, and caffeine[123]. Isothiocyanates, such as in garlic and broccoli, induce the transcription of antioxidant enzymes via activation of Nrf2[124], lowering cancer risk.

N-Nitrosyl Compounds

In addition to the cancer risk imparted by HCA, consumption of red meat and processed meat has been associated in epidemiologic studies with risk of colorectal cancer, whereas white meat did not increase this risk. This risk appears to be associated with the formation of N-nitrosyl compounds (NOC) formed during the digestion of red and processed meats.

Cured meats are a major source of dietary NOC. Hot dogs, sausages, bacon, lunch meats and processed ham contain nitrates and nitrites which are used to preserve color. In the stomach's acidic environment, nitrite from cured meat becomes available to combine with amines and amides derived from foods, and can form NOC. Curing, drying or smoking meats, used to prevent oxidation of fatty acids in food, can cause amines or amides to form in the meat that can then be nitrosated. Several NOC compounds, including nitrosamine, are known carcinogens. They act as DNA adducts and have been shown to induce G to A (guanine to adenine) mutations in the ras gene in exfoliated colonocytes[125]. Some green vegetables also contain significant amounts of nitrites[126]. Since these fresh vegetables also contain antioxidants, they do not readily form NOC. Pickled vegetables, however, such as those frequently consumed in China, are associated with increased cancer risk, specifically esophageal cancer[127].

Polyamines in foods may be converted into carcinogenic NOC, such as N-nitroso-pyrrolidine and N-nitroso-piperidine. This can occur especially in fatty foods, such as bacon when exposed to high cooking temperatures in the presence of water. Putrescine and cadaverine are present in decaying fish and meat and aged cheeses. NOC can also be formed from spermidine that is present in fresh meat when heated at higher cooking temperatures[128].

Red meats contain high quantities of heme, while fish and white meats do not. Heme can also form NOC in the acid environment of the stomach; thus, it is a suspect carcinogen. Processed meats form more, and a wider variety of NOC than do red meats[129]. There is insufficient epidemiologic evidence to support the hypothesis that consequential amounts of carcinogenic NOC are formed from fresh red meat.

NOC forms adducts with DNA that cause alkylation-induced mutations. O(6)-alkyl-guanine is the major carcinogenic lesion in DNA induced by alkylating mutagens. The DNA repair protein O(6)-methylguanine-DNA methyltransferase (MGMT) repairs these mutations, removing this DNA adduct. The liver contains MGMT mRNA levels 30 times higher than other tissues, and thus, it can be presumed to be the major area exposed to these mutagens.

Meta-analysis of studies of red or processed meats consumption reveal either no or very low-risk associations with kidney[130], breast[131], ovarian[132], or prostate[133] cancers. NOC exposure from red or processed meat does not appear to be associated with bladder cancer[134]. An increased risk from the consumption of processed meat has been found in stomach cancer[135] and for colon and rectal cancers[136]. NOC are also associated with risk of esophageal cancer[127]. This suggests that NOC act locally on mucosa but have a low risk of causing systemic carcinogens as do HCA. This is likely because of the body's ability to eliminate these toxins in the liver and to repair DNA damaged caused by NOC.

NOC, however, do cause other cancers. They are a major risk factor for cancers of the brain. In about 12 percent of adults, MGMT protein is not expressed in the brain. These individuals are 4.5 times more likely to develop brain tumors[137]. There is a wide range of MGMT activity in the brain; individuals with lower MGMT activity may also be at increased risk.

There is another population at high risk: preborn infants. MGMT expression develops along with fetal maturity. At 6 to eight weeks post conception, only 25% of fetuses express MGMT in the brain. By 15 to 19 weeks of development, 88% of fetuses have MGMT production in the brain[138]. Thus, NOC exposure during pregnancy is a risk for brain cancer, and the fetus is at highest risk during the first half of pregnancy. This likely explains the pathway for how hotdog consumption during pregnancy increases the risk of brain tumors in children.

An international study of maternal diet during pregnancy and risk of childhood brain tumor was revealing; not only did it show food consumption associated which increased risk of childhood brain cancers, it also showed foods which lowered the risks. Children of mothers who consumed higher levels of cured meats had a 50 percent higher rate of brain cancer, meanwhile, consumption of other meats was not associated with a significant risk. Higher consumption of eggs and dairy products was associated with a 20 percent increased risk. Consumption of higher amounts of fresh fish during pregnancy was associated with a 30 percent reduction in risk of brain cancer in children, yellow-orange vegetables with a 20 percent decrease in risk, and higher intake of grain, with a ten percent decrease in risk. Cruciferous or green leafy vegetables, fruits, and caffeinated beverages did not have significant effects on risk for brain cancer in this population[139].

In studies of adults, higher intake of yellow-orange vegetables was associated with a 30 to 40 percent decreased risk for glioma brain tumors; the decreased risk was associated with carotenoid consumption[140]. In a Chinese study of brain cancer and diet, cancer was inversely associated with consumption of fresh fish, fresh vegetables, especially Chinese cabbage and onions, fresh fruit and poultry. The risk was increased with salted vegetables and salted fish[141].

Although the quantity of nitrates and nitrites added to processed meats has fallen over time[142], consumption of processed meats should be minimized. Processed, smoked and preserved meat consumption should be limited for individuals at high risk for colon and rectal cancers, and the consumption of yellow-orange vegetables encouraged to decrease the risk from NOC. Helicobacter pylori infection is a risk factor for stomach cancer, and thus, should be treated. Sodium ascorbate (vitamin C) used in the processing of meats decreases NOC formation. Pregnant women should be advised to avoid consumption of processed and smoked meats and fish, and be encouraged to eat fresh fish and yellow-orange vegetables to decrease the risk of brain cancer in their children.

Polycyclic Aromatic Hydrocarbons (PAH)

PAH are formed during the burning of organic materials both biomass and fossil fuels. PAH are of concern as several PAH compounds are carcinogens. PAH can form when various foods, especially fats are burned, as can occur when meat is grilled, and the drippings fall on hot coals. The food can be coated with PAH from the smoke which precipitates on the meat or other food being grilled. PAH are also found in air pollution from coal powered power plants, vehicle exhaust, tobacco and wood smoke. Benzo[a]pyrene is found in cigarette smoke and was the first PAH found to be carcinogenic. There are 15 PAH compounds which are known carcinogens. PAH are found in foods cooked at temperatures which cause charring, oil refined at high temperatures (peanut, soy, corn oils) and in smoked foods[126] as well as in air pollution.

Children of women exposed to higher levels of PAH from air pollution during pregnancy had IQ scores 4-5 points lower at age 5 than less heavily exposed children[143]. Prenatal exposure is also associated with lower birth weight[144].

The risks of cancer from food sources of PAH have been difficult to evaluate because of lack of biologic markers. In experimental animals, tumors caused by exposure to PAH generally occur in the area of exposure. The most likely increase in cancer risk from PAH associated with food is lung cancer from inhalation of smoke and volatiles formed during cooking at high temperatures and during barbecuing. A vented hood fan should be used while cooking at high temperatures indoors, or the cooking done out of doors.

Other than perhaps occupational exposure from cooking smoke, most of the exposure to PAH in developed countries is from exposure to tobacco smoke and air pollution[145]. About half of the world' households cook over biomass, including wood, dried dung, grass and agricultural residues, and much of this cooking is done indoors, creating health hazards of respiratory infections and emphysema especially for women and female children[146] in developing countries. Even among these populations, studies of the risk associated with smoke inhalation have attributed the risk of cancer to the use of coal as a fuel or to smoking tobacco[147], rather than to exposure to wood smoke.

Aflatoxin and other Mycotoxins

While certain mushrooms are famously toxic, deaths from these are rare. Another fungus, however, produces a toxin that has a far greater death toll, causing a massive number of deaths. Aflatoxins are naturally occurring fungal toxins produced by several species of Aspergillus. These molds live in the soil and help break down decaying vegetation. When plants are stressed from drought, water soaked soils, insect damage, or poorly adapted to the climate and soil, the plants defenses are weakened, allowing these molds to flourish. These molds can also grow on harvested foods that are stored in warm, humid conditions.

The food crops most commonly affected by *Aspergillus* and contaminated with aflatoxin are peanuts that are affected while still in the ground, and corn that is affected after harvest. Other crops that may be affected include cereals (wheat, rice, sorghum and millet), oil seed plants (soybean, sunflower, cotton, and coconut), tree nuts, peppers, and spices. Aflatoxin is so common in peanuts that in spite of the use of advanced farming practices to prevent it, almost all peanut butter in the United States contains trace amounts of aflatoxin. The FDA sets limits to the amount of aflatoxins in foods that can be sold[148]. While aflatoxin toxicity is not thought to be major carcinogen in the United States, about 5 billion of the 7 billion people on earth are exposed to significant amounts of aflatoxins, especially in warm climates and where food harvest and storage methods do not prevent *Aspergillus* contamination[149]. In a study performed in Texas, the foods associated with the highest aflatoxin intake were rice, corn tortillas, and tree nuts, but not with intake of peanut butter or other corn products[150].

Aflatoxins are acute toxins with high case-fatality rates, usually associated with consumption of corn that has molded. Many outbreaks of acute aflatoxin toxicity have occurred in India and Africa. Acute toxic levels can result in liver necrosis. Chronic lower toxin exposure can result in liver cirrhosis. This toxin crosses the placenta and is associated growth retardation of children in countries where sufficient aflatoxin is found in foods[151].

Aflatoxin has an even greater health impact as a carcinogen, causing DNA alkylation adducts, resulting in liver cancer. Aflatoxin adducts cause mutations in the p53 gene[152], a gene which signals apoptosis, and which helps prevent cells with DNA errors from reproducing. Thus, aflatoxin adducts can promote cancer growth.

Aflatoxin can cause hepatocellular carcinoma (HCC) on its own, or as a co-carcinogen with hepatitis B (HBV) infection. The risk of HCC associated with exposure to aflatoxin is amplified in those with HBV infection. Hepatitis C can also cause hepatocellular carcinoma, but does not appear to interact with aflatoxin. Aflatoxin induced HCC is common in China[153], Taiwan[154], Mexico, and many other regions. HCC is common in China where HBV infection is endemic. Of the 550,000-600,000 incident HCC cases worldwide each year, between 25,000 and 150,000 may be attributable to aflatoxin exposure[155]. Aflatoxin adducts were found in 6 percent of HCC cases in Japan[156], a country with low levels of exposure to these toxins, and in a very small study about 5% of HCC in the US was associated with aflatoxins[157].

Other mycotoxins from molds can also contaminate foods. Fumonisins also contaminate corn, and they have been associated with neural tube defects and esophageal cancers[151].

Universal vaccination of infants against HVB in the United States should decrease the incidence of HCC over time.

Obviously these toxins should be avoided. Mold contaminated food should be discarded; it is not fit for animals as they are also at risk from this toxin. The correlations between aflatoxin urinary metabolites and intake of corn tortillas, rice and tree nuts suggest that the FDA may need to reassess monitoring and permissible levels of aflatoxins for these in foods in the U.S. Green tea polyphenols have been shown to lower biomarkers of aflatoxins by over 40%[158].

Fiber Fruits and Vegetables

Diets high in cruciferous vegetables are associated with lower risk of multiple forms of cancers. Cruciferous vegetables were discussed earlier in this chapter. Other vegetables and fruits also impact the risk of cancer.

In a study of colorectal cancer, cruciferous vegetables, dark yellow vegetables and consumption of apples were associated with decreased cancer risk; meanwhile, fruit juice increased risk[159]. The increased cancer risk from fruit juice may be secondary to induction of decreased oral-cecal transit time associated fructose malabsorption, resulting in lower nutrient absorption in the small intestine, an increase in secondary bile acid formation, and fermentation of protein in the colon, resulting in ammonia and other toxin formation.

Higher levels of dietary fiber intake were associated with a 13% reduction in breast cancer risk. The decreased risk was most clearly related to the intake of soluble fiber from fruit (pectin for example)[160]. Dietary lignans have been associated with increased survival after the diagnosis of breast cancer, specifically, in women with progesterone/estrogen receptor positive tumors. The lignan lariciresinol, which is found in the bran of cereal grains, flax seeds, and sesame seeds, is the lignin most clearly associated with decreased risk[161]. Lariciresinol, however, only decreases the risk for ER+/PR+ breast cancers[162]. Lariciresinol inhibited the tumor growth and tumor angiogenesis and increased apoptosis[163]. Lignans are polyphenol phytoestrogens that appear to act as competitive inhibitors of estrogen[164] and may also act as antioxidants.

Dietary consumption of the polyphenol, quercetin, has been associated with decreased risk of endometrial cancer[165], as is the lignan secoisolariciresinol which is found in high concentration in flaxseed[166].

In studies of colon cancer it does not appear that just any fiber will help, but rather, it is the consumption of whole grains that are associated with decreased colon cancer risk[167, 168]. Eating more than one apple a day also decreases the risk of colon cancer[169]. Fruit fiber appears to decrease the risk of distal colon and rectal cancers. Fruit intake was associated with a decreased risk of gastric cancer that was stronger than the decrease in risk associated with consumption of cruciferous vegetables[170]. Raw vegetables, cruciferous vegetables, and citrus fruits were associated with decreased risk of esophageal cancer[171]. Dietary fiber can bind bile acids[172] that also can decrease the risk of esophageal and colorectal cancers.

Some risk reduction associated with diets higher in fruits and vegetable may be due to differences in dietary patterns; consumption of more of fruits and vegetables may be inversely association with a "meat and fried potato" pattern that may increase risk[173]. Most studies that have evaluated the association of food groups with cancer risk, however, have found that *low fruit and vegetable intake* is the risk factor for cancer[174]. Thus, consumption of fewer than two servings of fruit a day, or cruciferous vegetables less than once week, appears to be the risk factor for cancer. This suggests that a deficiency of compounds contained in fruits and vegetables increases cancer risk. Thus, deficiencies of compounds present in fruits and vegetables increase risk of cancer; much like how vitamin or trace minerals deficiencies cause disease; once there is adequate supply of the compound, adding more likely provides little benefit.
Different fibers act through different mechanisms, with various fibers lowering risk for different types of cancer. A mix of trace minerals, phenolic, and other organic compounds from fruits, vegetables, herbs and spices, supplies hundreds of different nutrients, both for our cells, and those of our internal microbial biome. A diet having a mix of fruits, vegetables, and whole grains is most likely to supply nutritional needs and lower risk of cancer and other diseases.

Vitamin Supplements and Cancer

In cancer, health giving vitamins can feed the disease and accelerate a patient's demise. To recap Chapter 40:

- Vitamin A: Promotes growth of cancers and decreases survival time.
- β-carotene: Lowers risk of cancer, but promotes cancer growth once the cancer is present.
- Folic acid: Lowers the risk of cancer, but once cancer is present decreases survival time.
- α-tocopherol: Increases risk of death from cancer.

Vitamin A promotes the transcription of genes. It does this for cancer cells as well, and thus, helps them grow. β-carotene is an antioxidant that helps prevent cancer, but it is also pre-vitamin A, and thus, helps promote cells growth, including that of tumor cells.

Folic acid promotes the recycling of S-adenosylmethionine, which acts as a methyl group donor. Methylation of DNA helps keep the strands of DNA tied to the histones and helps keep these strands of DNA from being exposed and breaking, thus decreasing the risk of DNA errors and mutations. This activity decreases the risk of cancer.

Folate promotes methylation of the gene for p53 protein, which induces apoptosis of cancer cells. Insufficient folate allows the DNA strand for p53 to be exposed to damage. If it becomes mutated and does not function normally, it increases the risk of cancer. Nevertheless, excessive folate can increase cancer risk by inducing hypermethylation, thus preventing the transcription of p53, and other proteins that help destroy cancer cells. Hypermethylation is more likely to occur when vitamin B_{12} levels are low. The n-3 fatty acid DHA also helps prevent hyper-methylation[175].

The α-tocopherol form of vitamin E increases the risk of cancer; most likely by displacing anti-carcinogenic vitamin E compounds, including γ-tocopherol and tocotrienols. The typical daily dietary intake of tocotrienols is less than 2 mg, and the typical tocopherol intake is about 8 mg. A 300 mg α-tocopherol supplement displaces most other forms of vitamin E and induces their elimination from the body, either through metabolism or excretion. α-tocopherol increases the activity of phospholipase A2, and thus, induces the production of PGE_2, an inflammatory eicosanoid which promotes tumor and inflammatory cell survival, especially in individuals with high n-6 dietary fat intake, as is typical for those eating a Western diet.

Vitamin B_6

Plasma levels of vitamin B_6, pyridoxal-5-phosphate (PLP), are inversely related to colon cancer risk[176, 177]. In men with plasma PLP levels above about 70 pmol/ml (70 nmol/L or 17.5 ng/ml) the risk of colon cancer has been found to be about half as high as for those with lower levels[178]. In a separate study, women with PLP levels lower than about this level were also at increased risk of colon cancer[176].

Low PLP was inversely related to elevated homocysteine and with elevated IL-6 levels in these studies[176, 178]. PLP is also inversely related to toxic kynurenine-metabolite, 3-HK levels[179]. Even though the reference range for normal pyridoxine levels is 20 to 121 nmol/L, vitamin B_6 supplementation may be appropriate for the prevention of cancer risk if levels are less than 70 nmol/L. Three to five milligrams of pyridoxine HCl is sufficient for most people.

Secondary Bile Acids

The secondary bile acid, deoxycholic acid (DCA), is a probable carcinogen; it is thought to increase the risk of gallbladder, bile duct, colorectal, and esophageal cancers. DCA is a topical carcinogen acting on the mucosal surface; in the case of esophageal cancer, it gains access via reflux.

In an experiment where animals had DCA added to their feed, 17 of 18 animals developed colon tumors and ten of these developed colon cancer[180]. Several human studies have found increased risk of colon cancer in individuals with higher DCA levels. In perhaps the largest of these studies, elevated fecal DCA levels more than doubled the risk for colon tumors, and the adjusted odds ratio for large colon tumors was 11.5[181]. Chronic gallbladder infection with the bacterium *Salmonella enterica* (typhoid) promotes the formation of secondary bile acids and induces carcinoma of the gallbladder[182].

Secondary bile acids are formed from primary bile acids by certain enteric bacteria which are commonly found in the colon. Bile acids are recycled through the entero-hepatic circulation; normally, bile acids are absorbed in the small intestine, with only very small amounts of bile acids entering the colon. Malabsorption and rapid small intestinal transit time can increase the passage of bile acids into the cecum. Risks for the formation of the secondary bile acid DCA include malabsorption syndromes, such as carbohydrate malabsorption, fat malabsorption, and high-fat diets[183].

DCA can damage chromosomes through the generation of reactive oxygen species and promotes proliferative signal induction through activation of NF-κB[184].

Secondary bile acids can be removed from the enterohepatic circulation by binding bile acids and eliminating them from the body. The liver then makes new (primary) bile acids to replace them. Bile acid sequestrant medications bind both primary and secondary bile acids. This eliminates them from the body, and thus, promote their replacement with primary bile acids to replenish those removed.

Vegetable fiber also binds bile acids. Steam cooking of green vegetables increases the binding of bile acids. Steamed collard greens, kale, and mustard greens bind 13%; broccoli, 10%; Brussels sprouts and spinach, 8%; green bell pepper, 7%; and cabbage, 5%; these are as effective as is the bile acid sequestrant medication cholestyramine, by dry weight[185]. Rutabaga, green beans, and carrots also bind DCA[172].

Certain polyphenols either prevent the formation of secondary bile acids or aid in their elimination[183]. Antioxidant polyphenols also prevent DCA induced carcinogenesis[180].

Voluntary running in mice nearly doubles bile acid excretion into the feces. This increases cholesterol turnover in the body and formation of new primary bile acids[186] and thus decreases the proportion of secondary bile acids present in the bile[187]. Exercise decreases intestinal cholesterol absorption[188] and decreases the size atherosclerotic lesions in hypercholesterolemic mice[186].

Cancer Prevention

> **Notice:** Primary prevention of cancer; avoiding cancer induction, through diet and avoiding exposure to oxidants, toxins, and ionizing radiation is obvious and well documented. Secondary prevention; the treatment of pre-symptomatic cancer, after the diagnosis, through diets, nutritional supplements and lifestyle has been shown to in some cancers to slow tumor progression and extend survival time. Nevertheless, there are no case-control studies showing cure of cancer using diet or dietary supplements or lifestyle as a primary treatment. Nutritional therapy, supplements and lifestyle can be used as adjunctive treatment, and to reduce the recurrence of tumors and cancer after treatment.
>
> Nothing in this book should be construed to advocate the use of diet or nutritional supplements in place of medical treatment of cancer.

In cancer, our cells grow out of control, invade different tissues, and cause a slow and painful demise. Cancer is difficult to treat successfully – how does one selectively eliminate these aberrant cells without destroying the neighboring, normal ones?

The goal is to provide a milieu in which aberrant cells eliminate themselves through apoptosis. This is the normal process; aberrant cells are created every day in our bodies, and they are eliminated. It is when this process fails that cancer develops.

The inflammatory mediator, PGE_2, favors angiogenesis and prevents the destruction of β-catenin, thus, inhibiting apoptosis. NF-κB mediates inflammation and apoptosis, agents that increase it release, increase the risk of aberrant cell survival. The same mechanisms that sustain chronic inflammatory reactions and survival of inflammatory cells can sustain the survival and growth of aberrant cells. These include certain prostaglandins, sphingolipids, and cytokines and other mediators. An immune defense that concentrates its energies on T_H17 activities diverts cellular immunity away from T_H1 immune activity, thus, diverting immune activity away from the destruction of tumor cells.

It is best to avoid the creation of aberrant cells. Failing that, we want them self-destruct through apoptosis or have the TH1 immune system destroy them before they multiply. Most of the cancer burden in our society can be prevented by avoiding the induction and promotion of cancer.

Avoid

- Consuming meat cooked at high temperatures
- Frequently eating smoked or grilled
- Processed meat, especially during pregnancy
- Mold contaminated foods
- Salt preserved vegetables
- Alcohol intoxication
- Excess n-6 fats
- Formation of secondary bile acids
- Inflammation
- Stress
- Sleep deprivation
- Obesity
- Enteroimmune inflammatory disease
- Vitamin A supplements
- α-tocopherol supplements
- Folic acid supplement beyond 400 μg per day
- Fruit and vegetable deficiencies

Vitamin D₃: Calcitriol down-regulates inflammation by down-regulating COX2, and the prostaglandin E and F receptors and by increasing the breakdown of prostaglandins. Additionally, 1,25 OHD3, the active form of vitamin D, down-regulates estrogen receptor mRNA and estrogen response in breast cancer cells[189]. Vitamin D also decreases TLR4 receptor expression, thus down-regulating the inflammatory response as mediated through NF-κB. A trial using 45 μg (1800 units) of vitamin D₃ once a week and naproxen 375 mg twice daily and showed a slowing of PSA growth, a marker for prostate cancer[190]. This dose of 1800 IU of vitamin D₃ a day was likely far too conservative, yet the trial gave positive results with 75% of the patients showing slowing of tumor growth. Optimal vitamin D levels should be assured to reduce the risk for cancer cell promotion. See Chapter 20 for recommendations on vitamin D dosing.

Vitamin E: The most available form of vitamin E; α-tocopherol does no prevent, but rather increases the risk of cancer promotion, likely through supporting the release of AA from the cellular membrane which can then be converted to PGE_2. In individuals with low n6:n3 ratios, this may not be a problem, but the Western diet supplies high levels of n-6 fats. Other vitamin E compounds, such as γ-tocopherol and tocotrienols, inhibit COX2 more effectively. Moreover, α-tocotrienol is about 60 times more potent as an antioxidant than is α-tocopherol. Both γ-tocotrienol and δ-tocotrienol have shown anti-carcinogenic effects. *α-tocopherol supplements should be avoided.* For primary prevention, small amounts of mixed tocotrienols may be helpful although no human studies have yet been done to confirm this. A diet with 10 -15 mg of vitamin E a day from natural sources is recommended, with at least 20 percent of it consisting of tocotrienols (2 to 4 mg a day).

Vitamin B₆

Individuals on a vitamin B₆ depleting diet exhibited abnormal electroencephalogram patterns when plasma PLP dropped to about 9 nmol/L (2.2 ng/L)[191]. Based on this data, and on population distributions, the plasma PLP level of 20 nmol/L was selected as the lower normal limit for vitamin B₆. Normal reference levels for vitamin B₆ (Plasma PLP) are 20-121 nmol/L (5-30 ng/ml). Levels lower than about 70 nmol/L (17.5 ng/ml) are associated with increased risk for chronic disease. Some individuals may not efficiently convert dietary pyridoxine into the active form PLP. Acetaldehyde, a product of alcohol and histamine catabolism, can decrease PLP formation from dietary pyridoxine.

A total vitamin B₆ intake of 4 mg a day should be a sufficient to maintain low-risk levels for cardiovascular disease[192] and cancer risk[193]. Poultry, fresh fruits, such as banana, vegetables, and whole grains, are good sources of pyridoxine. Most breakfast cereals are fortified with vitamin B₆. Supplementation with vitamin B₆ is appropriate if serum PLP levels are below 70 nmol/L (17.5 ng/ml). About half the population have levels lower than this. Thus, even a small supplement of about 2 mg of pyridoxine a day would be sufficient for most individuals; 5 mg should be sufficient for all, other than those with inborn errors of pyridoxine metabolism.

N-3 Fats: n-3 fats, and especially DHA and EPA decrease inflammation and decrease PGE_2, and, therefore, decrease the risk of cancer cell survival. N-3 fats are discussed in Chapter 9.

Antioxidant Vitamins: Use of antioxidant vitamins and supplements for cancer prevention is discussed in Chapter 40.

Aspirin: 600 mg of aspirin has been found to be effective in reducing the risk of colon cancer in individuals at greatly elevated risk. The most frequent side effects from the use of aspirin are gastritis, gastrointestinal bleeding, and increased risk of hemorrhagic stroke. Aspirin also lowers the risk of thrombotic stroke and myocardial infarction. The higher the risk that an individual has for colon and related cancers (ovarian, breast, and prostate) the more likely the benefits will outweigh these risks. The highest risk individuals are those with family and personal history of these cancers or history of colonic adenomas.

For both those at high and lower risk, fish oil, vitamin D₃ and a diet containing natural tocotrienols should provide multiple benefits without significant risk.

Avoid Inflammatory Fomenting Cytokines

Inflammatory cytokines, particularly IL-1β are involved in the induction of PGE₂ synthesis and directly or indirectly with the promotion of tumor cells and angiogenesis which supports cancer growth. IL-1β promotes NF-κB induced cell proliferation. Conditions and factors which affect the production of these cytokines are discussed throughout this book. These include inflammation, immune reactions to food and bacterial biofilm, but also sleep deprivation, chronic emotional stress, and obesity. Play, exercise, and enjoying a good movie, foods high in plant phenols decrease the production of inflammatory cytokines.

Avoid ROS Production by Mitochondria

Maintenance of an efficient population of mitochondria limits the leaking of protons and the generation of oxygen and nitrosyl radicals. These radicals can damage the DNA and the proteins which repair it. Mitochondrial health, thus, prevents cancer. It is discussed in Chapter 21.

Alcohol

Heavy alcohol consumption is associated with increased risk of multiple forms of cancer. What about light to moderate consumption? Risk of cancer associated with low consumption of alcohol (less than three drinks a week,) appears to slightly lower the risk of cancer, compared to individuals who never drink. Moderate drinking (up to one drink a day for women and up to two drinks a day for men), does not change risk compared to never drinking. A higher consumption of alcohol is associated with increased risk[49]. A drink is equivalent to 5 ounces of wine.

In a study of Chinese women, consumption of less than 15 grams of alcohol a day (equivalent to about 5.5 ounces of wine) decreased the risk of breast cancer by 54% in premenopausal women and by 40% in postmenopausal women compared to women who do not drink any alcohol. Women who consumed less than 5 grams of alcohol a day had even lower breast cancer risk. Consuming more than 15 grams of alcohol a day (more than one drink) was associated with an increased breast cancer risk[194]. In a Swedish study, alcohol consumption over 10 grams a day increased risk of breast cancer, but risk was only seen for estrogen receptor-positive cancer, and especially for estrogen- receptor positive/progesterone-receptor negative (ER+/PR-) breast cancer, where risk was more than doubled[195].

In the Nurses Health Study, consumption of an average of 5 to 9 grams of alcohol a day, equivalent to 3 to 6 drinks a week was associated with a 15 percent increase in risk of breast cancer. Binge drinking was the risk factor at this level of alcohol consumption[50]. It is likely the peak blood alcohol content that confers the cancer risk, through alterations in DNA methylation.

To minimize cancer risk, it is not imprudent to enjoy as much as one ounce of red wine per day/30 pounds of ideal body weight, three times a week. It should be consumed slowly or with a meal to avoid a rapid absorption and high peak alcohol level. This would allow up to 4 ounces of red wine for a 120-pound woman. This amount should have little effect on behavior other than mild relaxation. If the alcohol decreases inhibition gives a sense of euphoria or inhibits concentration, it has likely reached levels that promote carcinogenesis.

Detoxifying Alcohol: Alcohol causes the formation of free radicals. The vitamin-like compound TMG (betaine) recycles SAMe and thereby prevents alcohol-induced damage of the Complex I and III proteins in the mitochondria. TMG also provides a source of glycine for the formation of the antioxidant glutathione. The principle source of dietary TMG is green vegetables.

Supplying sufficient levels of ALDH cofactors magnesium and niacin may help speed catabolism of acetaldehyde. Niacin and zinc are cofactors for alcohol dehydrogenase.

Advice:
- If you drink a small amounts of red wine because you enjoy its flavor, go ahead and enjoy it.
- If you drink alcohol for the phenolic compounds, be aware that there are much safer sources.
- If the people around you can tell you have been drinking by a change in your behavior, you have reached a toxic level.
- If you drink alcohol for the buzz, intoxication is an accurate description.

Caveats: Women with personal or with family history of ER+/PR- breast cancer are at increased risk for alcohol-related breast cancers and should further restrict alcohol intake to less than 1 oz. of red wine per day per 30 pounds of ideal body weight, on days they drink, and the wine should be consumed slowly to avoid high blood levels.

Alcohol should also be completely avoided during pregnancy. Prenatal exposure to alcohol likely increases the risk of breast cancer in the offspring (female or male)[196, 197].

Individuals having fast metabolism of alcohol into acetaldehyde or slow metabolism of acetaldehyde to acetate are at increased risk of cancer. About 40 percent of Asians[42] and Caucasians[43] are at increased risk. Other than genetic testing and family history, the presence of these alcohol-associated risk alleles may be suspected in individuals who get facial flushing easily with alcohol.

The risks and benefits of alcohol consumption are further discussed in Chapter 17.

Eat a Mix of Real Foods: Food contains many compounds that help prevent disease. Nitrites in fresh vegetables do not impose cancer risk, as the vegetables also contain antioxidants, vitamins, minerals, fiber and other compounds which lower disease risks. While there is ample evidence that indole-3-carbinol (I3C) suppresses cancer, high doses IC3 or of capsaicin, which found in hot peppers, promote cancer in some animal experiments[198].

Polyphenols

Several plant phenolic compounds have been shown to have anti-carcinogenic properties. There are hundreds of phenolic compounds present in foods; it should be assumed that the few phenolic compounds which have been evaluated for this property are only ones that provide this benefit. Different polyphenols may act against different DNA adducts. It is prudent to consume a wide range of plant polyphenols in the diet. Table 15-4 in Chapter 15 lists several phenolic compounds and foods that are found in that inhibit the formation of inflammatory prostaglandins and leukotrienes. Table 32-2 list several phenolic compounds and foods they are found in which inhibit the formation of TNF-α.

The phytoestrogen lariciresinol is associated with decreased risk of breast cancer and may also decrease the risk of ovarian cancer[199].

Table 41-4: Foods Rich in Lariciresinol[200]

Foods	Lariciresinol µg/ 100 grams
Sesame Seeds	> 5000
Flax	1000 – 5000
Sunflower seeds, cashews, broccoli	500 – 1000
Whole grain rye bread, granola, cruciferous vegetables, garlic, green beans, sweet peppers, pears, apricots, strawberries, raisins, tomato paste.	100 – 500

Black tea, red wine, and coffee, as well as many other foods, also contain significant levels of lariciresinol. Quercetin is associated with decreased risk of ovarian cancer. Other polyphenols appear to lower the risk of other cancers. A diverse diet with a mix of phenolic compounds from whole foods is recommended.

Meat

"When it's smokin' it's cookin', when it's black it's done."
Recipe for carcinogens

Avoid cooking meats at high temperatures. For example, stewed meat, cooked at a temperature that prevents shrinkage and allows for hydrolysis of collagen and other proteins, (70° to 75°C) gives a better umami flavor, is more easily and completely digested and better satisfies the appetite than meat cooked more quickly at higher temperatures, and does not form carcinogenic HCA.

Hamburger can be cooked at a lower grill temperature, and pre-treated by adding ascorbic acid, glucose, onions, or spices to decrease the formation of HCA. Microwaving a hamburger for 1½ to 3 minutes and draining the free fluid will remove extracellular creatinine and amino acids that form HCA, and thereby decrease HCA formation.

Larger pieces of meats can be roasted in a Dutch-oven to help retain moisture and decrease the formation of HCA. Rinsing and patting dry a cut of meat will remove free creatinine. Meat that is to be grilled can be marinated to decrease the formation of HCA. The liquid remaining in the container after marinating meat should be discarded as it will contain precursors for HCA and will form these if heated and allowed to dehydrate. Pan residues from grilling or pan frying have very high HCA levels and should never be consumed or used for gravy.

Cooking Ground Beef: Ground beef needs to reach a higher center temperature to kill bacteria than that required for intact steaks; in ground meat, surface bacteria have been mixed throughout the meat, whereas properly stored steaks only have bacteria on the outer surface.

More cooking time is thus required to allow heat to transfer into the center of a hamburger patty or meatball. The grill or skillet temperature should be set to 160°C (320°F)[201] and not higher than 180°C (356°F). A higher temperature has little effect on the amount of time it takes to cook the center but increases HCA formation. A grill temperature over 100°C (212°F) gives the hamburger its outer crust.

- Meat needs to be completely thawed before cooking to cook properly. Cooking fish or meat, and especially frozen hamburger paddies which are incompletely thawed, is much more likely to result in an overcooked surface and a raw center; resulting in HCA formation on the surface and live bacteria within.
- Hamburger patties should ideally be about ½ to ¾ inches thick, to be juicy, but no thicker to cook well.
- Do not use a spatula to press the juice out of a hamburger while cooking it; it dries out the patty and supplies more creatine and free amino acids for the formation of HCA.
- Flip the patty once a minute to improve heat transfer to the center of the meat. Frequent flipping cooks the meat more evenly and quickly and avoids HCA formation.
- Expect it to take 9 to 12 minutes to cook, the hamburger, depending on its thickness.
- Cook hamburger meat to an internal temperature of 71°C (160°F), or to 68°C (155°F) for at least 15 seconds.
- A brown center does not guarantee that the interior meat reached a temperature sufficient to kill bacteria.

Frying meat subjects it to high temperatures that can favor the formation of HCA some which are aerosolized and are lung carcinogens. Frying should be done with a hood vent which removes aerosols created by cooking from the building. If meat is to be fried, it can be marinated to decrease the formation of HCA. Using appropriate frying temperatures minimizes HCA formation. The temperature usually recommended by chefs for deep fat frying of meat is 175°C (350°F). The use of higher temperatures over-cooks the outside and leaves the interior undercooked.

Flame grilled, broiled seared, and well-done meat that has visible charring will contain carcinogens including HCA and PAH. Smoke from cooking meat is a lung carcinogen. It should only be done out of doors or under a hood.

The risk of cancer from HCA may be specifically mitigated through consumption of cruciferous vegetables; however, they will do no good if these vegetables are overcooked. They should be eaten raw, juiced or very light steamed and eaten while still warm as described earlier in this chapter.

Secondary Bile Acids

Formation of carcinogenic secondary bile acids can be avoided by limiting the intake of poorly absorbed sugars and avoiding malabsorption that causes bile to pass into the colon where it undergoes transformation by colonic bacteria (discussed in Chapter 24). Bile acid sequestrants may be used to remove bile acids which are then replaced by the liver with primary bile acids. Green leafy vegetables, especially when steamed, also bind bile acids. Exercise increases bile acid excretion and increases fecal bile acid output, causing a preferential decline in secondary bile acids.

Chronic biliary *Salmonella* infection should be treated to avoid risk of biliary cancer.

Anti-androgens for prostate cancer:
Boron, at 6 mg of elemental boron per day, for example in the form of amino acid chelate, acts as an antiandrogen, but also as a pro-estrogen. Thus, boron may slow the growth of prostate cancer but may speed the growth of estrogen-sensitive cancers, such a certain breast cancers.

Several dietary fatty acids, including oleic, palmitoleic, linoleic, α and γ-linolenic acids and DHA inhibit 5-α-reductase and thus inhibit the transformation of testosterone to dihydrotestosterone[202], the most potent androgen. Oleic acid (for example from olive oil) and the n-3 fatty acids (see Chapter 6) do not form series 2 eicosanoids, such as PGE2, which promote tumor proliferation. Thus, these fatty acids would be expected to prevent prostate cancer.

Obesity

Obesity is a risk factor for cancer, and it and its underlying causes should be treated. Obesity is an inflammatory disease and many of the same factors which promote obesity also increase the risk of cancer. When patients were tested for antergens and avoided these foods, they had a rapid loss of excess adiposity. (See Chapter 19.) Chapter 9, on metabolic syndrome and Chapter 8, on satiation, may be helpful for encouraging a normal adiposity.

Table 41-5: Avoiding Exogenous Oxidants

Exogenous Oxidants	Source	What to do
Lipid Peroxides	Rancid polyunsaturated fats; n-3 fats are especially susceptible	Avoid rancid and processed foods, old, ground spices. Use fresh extra virgin olive oil.
Heterocyclic amines	Meat and eggs cooked at temperatures over 350°F	Avoid fried foods, and only use low smoke point oils† for cooking. Avoid charbroiled foods
Nitrosamines	Beer, food preserved with nitrites, decaying fish, tobacco.	Avoid beer and preserved meats: lunch meats, sausage, and smelly fish. Avoid tobacco.
Alcohol[203]	Beer, Liquor, Wine	Avoid alcohol. Consumption of small amounts of red wine containing antioxidants may lower the risk. TMG (Betaine) found in vegetables lowers risk[204]
Smoke	Cigarettes, Fire	Avoid
Air Pollution	Factories, Cars, Power Plants Cleaning Products, Air fresheners	Fire your senators and congressional representatives. Use natural products. Open windows.
Radiation	X-rays, CT scans, alien death rays	Avoid
Pesticides	Bug sprays, Crops	Avoid use in home Wash fruits and vegetables. Buy organic foods

† Extra virgin olive oil has a low smoke point, meaning that it will smoke and can burst into flame at a lower temperature than most oils. This is good and bad. It is good as it tells you that the temperature is too high. It is bad if you don't pay attention and incinerate your home. If food is cooked in olive oil, the temperature must be set lower to avoid smoking, and thus will produce much less carcinogenic heterocyclic amines.

Caribbean Marinade
From: A Taste of Paradise by Susana and Charles Lewis[205]
Ingredients for Criollo Marinade:
20 cloves of garlic peeled (3/4-cups) ½ small sweet red onion (3/4-cups chopped) 1 Tbsp of dry oregano ½ Tbsp dry thyme ½ Tsp coriander seed ½ Tsp rosemary leaves ¼ cup extra virgin olive oil 1 Tsp salt ½-cup of citrus juice (grapefruit or orange)*. 1/2-cup wine (white merlot or white zinfandel for white meat.)
* May use a medium orange peeled, and seeds removed; blend using the pulp.
Preparation: Place the marinade ingredients into a blender and liquefy for 3-5 minutes at high speed.
Notes: Fresh extra virgin olive oil reduces the formation of HCA while year old olive oil does not[101]. Extra virgin olive oil has antioxidants that are destroyed by light, air, contact with metal and time. It is preferable to purchase olive oil in volumes that are expected be to used within two months of opening the container, and storing it in a non-metallic container in a dark cabinet. Red wine may be used for red meats, but darkens white meat.

[1] SEER Cancer Statistics Review 1975-2007. National Cancer Institute.

[2] Cancer Prevention & Early Detection; Facts and Figures 2011. American Cancer Society.

[3] Indian women with higher serum concentrations of folate and vitamin B12 are significantly less likely to be infected with carcinogenic or high-risk (HR) types of human papillomaviruses (HPVs). Piyathilake CJ, Badiga S, Paul P, et al. Int J Womens Health. 2010 Aug 9;2:7-12. PMID:21072292

[4] Common polymorphisms in methylenetetrahydrofolate reductase gene are associated with risks of cervical intraepithelial neoplasia and cervical cancer in women with low serum folate and vitamin B12. Tong SY, Kim MK, Lee JK, et al. Cancer Causes Control. 2011 Jan;22(1):63-72. PMID:21052817

[5] Body mass index is associated with age-at-onset of HCV-infected hepatocellular carcinoma patients. Akiyama T, Mizuta T, Kawazoe S, et al. World J Gastroenterol. 2011 Feb 21;17(7):914-21. PMID:21412500

[6] Hepatocellular Carcinoma Risk Factors and Disease Burden in a European Cohort: A Nested Case-Control Study. Trichopoulos D, Bamia C, Lagiou P, et al. J Natl Cancer Inst. 2011 Oct 21 PMID:22021666

[7] Significantly increased risk of cancer in diabetes mellitus patients: A meta-analysis of epidemiological evidence in Asians and non-Asians. Noto H, Tsujimoto T, Noda M. J Diabetes Investig. 2012 Feb 20;3(1):24-33. PMID:24843541

[8] Diabetes and cancer: is diabetes causally related to cancer? Suh S, Kim KW. Diabetes Metab J. 2011 Jun;35(3):193-8. PMID:21785737

[9] Overweight as an avoidable cause of cancer in Europe. Bergström A, Pisani P, Tenet V, Wolk A, Adami HO. Int J Cancer. 2001 Feb 1;91(3):421-30. PMID:11169969

[10] Incident cancer burden attributable to excess body mass index in 30 European countries. Renehan AG, Soerjomataram I, Tyson M, et al. Int J Cancer. 2010 Feb 1;126(3):692-702. PMID:19645011

[11] Cancer incidence due to excess body weight and leisure-time physical inactivity in Canada: Implications for prevention. Brenner DR. Prev Med. 2014 Jun 23. pii: S0091-7435(14)00219-9. PMID:24967956

[12] Survival analysis of cancer risk reduction strategies for BRCA1/2 mutation carriers. Kurian AW, Sigal BM, Plevritis SK. J Clin Oncol. 2010 Jan 10;28(2):222-31. PMID:19996031

[13] The contribution of deleterious germline mutations in BRCA1, BRCA2 and the mismatch repair genes to ovarian cancer in the population. Song H, Cicek MS, Dicks E, et al. Hum Mol Genet. 2014 Apr 30. PMID:24728189

[14] Online tool to guide decisions for BRCA1/2 mutation carriers. Kurian AW, Munoz DF, Rust P, et al. J Clin Oncol. 2012 Feb 10;30(5):497-506. PMID:22231042

[15] Long-term effect of aspirin on cancer risk in carriers of hereditary colorectal cancer: an analysis from the CAPP2 randomised controlled trial. Burn J, Gerdes AM, Macrae F, et al. Lancet. Oct 28 2011. doi:10.1016/S0140-6736(11)61049-0

[16] Celecoxib for the prevention of sporadic colorectal adenomas. Bertagnolli MM, Eagle CJ, Zauber AG, et al; APC Study Investigators. N Engl J Med. 2006 Aug 31;355(9):873-84. PMID:16943400

[17] Primary prevention of colorectal cancer. Chan AT, Giovannucci EL. Gastroenterology. 2010 Jun;138(6):2029-2043.e10. PMID:20420944

[18] Vitamin E increases production of vasodilator prostanoids in human aortic endothelial cells through opposing effects on cyclooxygenase-2 and phospholipase A2. Wu D, Liu L, Meydani M, Meydani SN. J Nutr. 2005 Aug;135(8):1847-53. PMID:16046707

[19] Cyclooxygenase-2 in tumorigenesis of gastrointestinal cancers: an update on the molecular mechanisms. Wu WK, Sung JJ, Lee CW, Yu J, Cho CH. Cancer Lett. 2010 Sep 1;295(1):7-16. PMID:20381235

[20] CTNNB1 catenin (cadherin-associated protein), beta 1, 88kDa [Homo sapiens] Gene ID: 1499, 23-Oct-2011 NCBI http://www.ncbi.nlm.nih.gov

[21] Mechanical induction of PGE2 in osteocytes blocks glucocorticoid-induced apoptosis through both the β-catenin and PKA pathways. Kitase Y, Barragan L, Qing H, et al. J Bone Miner Res. 2010 Dec;25(12):2657-68. PMID:20578217

[22] PGE2 Stimulates VEGF Production through the EP2 Receptor in Cultured Human Lung Fibroblasts. Nakanishi M, Sato T, Li Y, et al. Am J Respir Cell Mol Biol. 2011 Sep 15 PMID:21921240

[23] Selective inhibition of cyclooxygenase-2 (COX2) by 1alpha,25-dihydroxy-16-ene-23-yne-vitamin D3, a less calcemic vitamin D analog. Aparna R, Subhashini J, Roy KR, et al. J Cell Biochem. 2008 Aug 1;104(5):1832-42. PMID:18348265

[24] Tocotrienols suppress proinflammatory markers and cyclooxygenase-2 expression in RAW264.7 macrophages. Yam ML, Abdul Hafid SR, Cheng HM, Nesaretnam K. Lipids. 2009 Sep;44(9):787-97. PMID:19655189

[25] gamma-tocopherol and its major metabolite, in contrast to alpha-tocopherol, inhibit cyclooxygenase activity in macrophages and epithelial cells. Jiang Q, Elson-Schwab I, Courtemanche C, Ames BN. Proc Natl Acad Sci U S A. 2000 Oct 10;97(21):11494-9. PMID:11005841

[26] Tissue-specific, nutritional, and developmental regulation of rat fatty acid elongases. Wang Y, Botolin D, Christian B, Busik J, Xu J, Jump DB. J Lipid Res. 2005 Apr;46(4):706-15.. PMID:15654130

[27] Omega-3 polyunsaturated fatty acids inhibit hepatocellular carcinoma cell growth through blocking beta-catenin and cyclooxygenase-2. Lim K, Han C, Dai Y, Shen M, Wu T. Mol Cancer Ther. 2009 Nov;8(11):3046-55. PMID:19887546

[28] Inhibition of prostaglandin synthesis and actions contributes to the beneficial effects of calcitriol in prostate cancer. Krishnan AV, Srinivas S, Feldman D. Dermatoendocrinol. 2009 Jan;1(1):7-11. PMID:20046582

[29] γ-Tocotrienol inhibits cell viability through suppression of β-catenin/Tcf signaling in human colon carcinoma HT-29 cells. Xu W, Du M, Zhao Y, Wang Q, Sun W, Chen B. J Nutr Biochem. 2011 Aug 16. PMID:21852086

[30] A paraptosis-like cell death induced by δ-tocotrienol in human colon carcinoma SW620 cells is associated with the suppression of the Wnt signaling pathway. Zhang JS, Li DM, He N, et al. Toxicology. 2011 Jul 11;285(1-2):8-17. PMID:21453743

[31] Tocotrienols inhibit AKT and ERK activation and suppress pancreatic cancer cell proliferation by suppressing the ErbB2 pathway. Shin-Kang S, Ramsauer VP, Lightner J, et al. Free Radic Biol Med. 2011 Sep 15;51(6):1164-74.. PMID:21723941

[32] d-δ-Tocotrienol-mediated cell cycle arrest and apoptosis in human melanoma cells. Fernandes NV, Guntipalli PK, Mo H. Anticancer Res. 2010 Dec;30(12):4937-44. PMID:21187473

[33] delta-Tocotrienol suppresses VEGF induced angiogenesis whereas alpha-tocopherol does not. Shibata A, Nakagawa K, Sookwong P, Tsuduki T, Oikawa S, Miyazawa T. J Agric Food Chem. 2009 Sep 23;57(18):8696-704. PMID:19702331

[34] alpha-Tocopherol attenuates the cytotoxic effect of delta-tocotrienol in human colorectal adenocarcinoma cells. Shibata A, Nakagawa K, Sookwong P, et al. Biochem Biophys Res Commun. 2010 Jun 25;397(2):214-9. PMID:20493172

[35] IL-1β stimulates COX2 dependent PGE$_2$ synthesis and CGRP release in rat trigeminal ganglia cells. Neeb L, Hellen P, Boehnke C, et al. PLoS One. 2011 Mar 4;6(3):e17360. PMID:21394197

[36] STATs in cancer inflammation and immunity: a leading role for STAT3. Yu H, Pardoll D, Jove R. Nat Rev Cancer. 2009 Nov;9(11):798-809. PMID:19851315

[37] Phosphorylation of CBP by IKKalpha promotes cell growth by switching the binding preference of CBP from p53 to NF-kappaB. Huang WC, Ju TK, Hung MC, Chen CC. Mol Cell. 2007 Apr 13;26(1):75-87. PMID:17434128

[38] Anthocyanins From Black Soybean Seed Coat Enhance Wound Healing. Xu L, Choi TH, Kim S, et al. Ann Plast Surg. 2013 Feb 12. PMID:23407247

[39] Curcumin inhibits prostate cancer metastasis in vivo by targeting the inflammatory cytokines CXCL1 and -2. Killian PH, Kronski E, Michalik KM, et al. Carcinogenesis. 2012 Dec;33(12):2507-19. PMID:23042094

[40] Resveratrol mitigates lipopolysaccharide- and Aβ-mediated microglial inflammation by inhibiting the TLR4/NF-κB/STAT signaling cascade. Capiralla H, Vingtdeux V, Zhao H, et al. J Neurochem. 2012 Feb;120(3):461-72. PMID:22118570

[41] Dual roles of immune cells and their factors in cancer development and progression. Zamarron BF, Chen W. Int J Biol Sci. 2011;7(5):651-8. PMID:21647333

[42] Dietary and genetic obesity promote liver inflammation and tumorigenesis by enhancing IL-6 and TNF expression. Park EJ, Lee JH, Yu Gyet al. Cell. 2010 Jan 22;140(2):197-208. PMID:20141834

[43] Signal Transduction by Roadnottaken

[44] Physical activity, obesity, and risk for colon cancer and adenoma in men. Giovannucci E, Ascherio A, Rimm EB, et al. Ann Intern Med. 1995 Mar 1;122(5):327-34. PMID:7847643

[45] Emotion with tears decreases allergic responses to latex in atopic eczema patients with latex allergy. Kimata H. J Psychosom Res. 2006 Jul;61(1):67-9. PMID:16813847

[46] Sedentary Behaviors and Emerging Cardiometabolic Biomarkers in Adolescents. Martinez-Gomez D, Eisenmann JC, Healy GN, et al; AFINOS Study Group. J Pediatr. 2011 Aug 10. PMID:21839464

[47] Television viewing time and mortality: the Australian Diabetes, Obesity and Lifestyle Study (AusDiab). Dunstan DW, Barr EL, Healy GN, et al. Circulation. 2010 Jan 26;121(3):384-91. PMID:20065160

[48] Association between alcohol consumption and cancers in the Chinese population--a systematic review and meta-analysis. Li Y, Yang H, Cao J. PLoS One. 2011 Apr 15;6(4):e18776. PMID:21526212

[49] Prospective Study of Alcohol Consumption Quantity and Frequency and Cancer-Specific Mortality in the US Population. Breslow RA, Chen CM, Graubard BI, Mukamal KJ. Am J Epidemiol. 2011 Nov 1;174(9):1044-53. PMID:21965184

[50] Moderate Alcohol Consumption During Adult Life, Drinking Patterns, and Breast Cancer Risk. Chen CY, Rosner B, Hankinson SE, Colditz GA, Willet WC. JAMA. *2011;306(17):1884-1890.* PMID:22045766

[51] Alcohol consumption in relation to aberrant DNA methylation in breast tumors. Tao MH, Marian C, Shields PG, et al. Alcohol. 2011 Nov;45(7):689-99. PMID:21168302

[52] Acetaldehyde as an underestimated risk factor for cancer development: role of genetics in ethanol metabolism. Seitz HK, Stickel F. Genes Nutr. 2009 Oct 22. PMID:19847467

[53] http://biogps.org (Accessed December 2011)

[54] ADH3 genotype, alcohol intake and breast cancer risk. Terry MB, Gammon MD, Zhang FF, Knight JA, Wang Q, Britton JA, Teitelbaum SL, Neugut AI, Santella RM. Carcinogenesis. 2006 Apr;27(4):840-7. PMID:16344274

[55] CYP2E1 and risk of chemically mediated cancers. Trafalis DT, Panteli ES, Grivas A, Tsigris C, Karamanakos PN. Expert Opin Drug Metab Toxicol. 2010 Mar;6(3):307-19. PMID:20073996

[56] Obesity-induced metabolic stresses in breast and colon cancer. Sung MK, Yeon JY, Park SY, Park JH, Choi MS. Ann N Y Acad Sci. 2011 Jul;1229:61-8. PMID:21793840

[57] The metabolic syndrome and risk of prostate cancer in Italy. Pelucchi C, Serraino D, Negri E, et al. Ann Epidemiol. 2011 Nov;21(11):835-41. PMID:21982487

[58] Metabolic syndrome and pancreatic cancer risk: a case-control study in Italy and meta-analysis. Rosato V, Tavani A, Bosetti C, et al. Metabolism. 2011 Oct;60(10):1372-8. PMID:21550085

[59] Aspirin may be more effective in preventing colorectal adenomas in patients with higher BMI (United States). Kim S, Baron JA, Mott LA, et al. Cancer Causes Control. 2006 Dec;17(10):1299-304. PMID:17111262

[60] Dietary patterns as identified by factor analysis and colorectal cancer among middle-aged Americans. Flood A, Rastogi T, Wirfält et al. Am J Clin Nutr. 2008 Jul;88(1):176-84. PMID:18614739

[61] A review and meta-analysis of red and processed meat consumption and breast cancer. Alexander DD, Morimoto LM, Mink PJ, Cushing CA. Nutr Res Rev. 2010 Dec;23(2):349-65. PMID:21110906

[62] Well-done meat intake and meat-derived mutagen exposures in relation to breast cancer risk: the Nashville Breast Health Study. Fu Z, Deming SL, Fair AM, et al. Breast Cancer Res Treat. 2011 Oct;129(3):919-28. PMID:21537933

[63] Association of meat intake and meat-derived mutagen exposure with the risk of colorectal polyps by histologic type. Fu Z, Shrubsole MJ, Smalley WE, et al. Cancer Prev Res (Phila). 2011 Oct;4(10):1686-97. PMID:21803984

[64] Well-done red meat, metabolic phenotypes and colorectal cancer in Hawaii. Le Marchand L, Hankin JH, Pierce LM, et al. Mutat Res. 2002 Sep 30;506-507:205-14. PMID:12351160

[65] A high ratio of dietary n-6/n-3 polyunsaturated fatty acids is associated with increased risk of prostate cancer. Williams CD, Whitley BM, Hoyo C, Grant DJ, etal. Nutr Res. 2011 Jan;31(1):1-8. PMID:21310299

[66] Intake of polyunsaturated fatty acids and distal large bowel cancer risk in whites and African Americans. Kim S, Sandler DP, Galanko J, et al. Am J Epidemiol. 2010 May 1;171(9):969-79. PMID:20392864

[67] Smoke carcinogens cause bone loss through the aryl hydrocarbon receptor and induction of Cyp1 enzymes. Iqbal J, Sun L, Cao J, rt al. Proc Natl Acad Sci U S A. 2013 Jul 2;110(27):11115-20. PMID:23776235

[68] Modification by N-acetyltransferase 1 genotype on the association between dietary heterocyclic amines and colon cancer in a multiethnic study. Butler LM, Millikan RC, Sinha R, et al. Mutat Res. 2008 Feb 1;638(1-2):162-74. PMID:18022202

[69] Effect of NAT1 and NAT2 genetic polymorphisms on colorectal cancer risk associated with exposure to tobacco smoke and meat consumption. Lilla C, Verla-Tebit E, Risch A, et al. Cancer Epidemiol Biomarkers Prev. 2006 Jan;15(1):99-107. PMID:16434594

[70] DNA adducts of heterocyclic amine food mutagens: implications for mutagenesis and carcinogenesis. Schut HA, Snyderwine EG. Carcinogenesis. 1999 Mar;20(3):353-68. PMID:10190547

[71] Well-done meat intake, heterocyclic amine exposure, and cancer risk. Zheng W, Lee SA. Nutr Cancer. 2009;61(4):437-46. PMID:19838915

[72] Human exposure to heterocyclic amine food mutagens/carcinogens: relevance to breast cancer. Felton JS, Knize MG, Salmon CP, Malfatti MA, Kulp KS. Environ Mol Mutagen. 2002;39(2-3):112-8. PMID:11921178

[73] Meat consumption, cooking practices, meat mutagens, and risk of prostate cancer. John EM, Stern MC, Sinha R, Koo J. Nutr Cancer. 2011 May;63(4):525-37. PMID:21526454

[74] Intakes of red meat, processed meat, and meat mutagens increase lung cancer risk. Lam TK, Cross AJ, Consonni D, Randi G, Bagnardi V, Bertazzi PA, Caporaso NE, Sinha R, Subar AF, Landi MT. Cancer Res. 2009 Feb 1;69(3):932-9. PMID:19141639

[75] Heterocyclic amines: Mutagens/carcinogens produced during cooking of meat and fish. Sugimura T, Wakabayashi K, Nakagama H, Nagao M. Cancer Sci. 2004 Apr;95(4):290-9. PMID:15072585

[76] Metabolism of the food-derived carcinogen 2-amino-1-methyl-6-phenylimidazo[4,5-b]pyridine by lactating Fischer 344 rats and their nursing pups. Davis CD, Ghoshal A, Schut HA, Snyderwine EG. J Natl Cancer Inst. 1994 Jul 20;86(14):1065-70. PMID:8021955

[77] Evidence for the presence of mutagenic arylamines in human breast milk and DNA adducts in exfoliated breast ductal epithelial cells. Thompson PA, DeMarini DM, Kadlubar FF, et al. Environ Mol Mutagen. 2002;39(2-3):134-42. PMID:11921181

[78] DNA adducts of 2-amino-3-methylimidazo[4,5-f]quinoline (IQ) in fetal tissues of patas monkeys after transplacental exposure. Josyula S, Lu LJ, Salazar JJ, et al. Toxicol Appl Pharmacol. 2000 Aug 1;166(3):151-60. PMID:10906279

[79] Comparative carcinogenicity of 4-aminobiphenyl and the food pyrolysates, Glu-P-1, IQ, PhIP, and MeIQx in the neonatal B6C3F1 male mouse. Dooley KL, Von Tungeln LS, Bucci T, Fu PP, Kadlubar FF. Cancer Lett. 1992 Mar 15;62(3):205-9. PMID:1596864

[80] Polycyclic aromatic hydrocarbon-DNA adducts in human sperm as a marker of DNA damage and infertility. Gaspari L, Chang SS, Santella RM, Garte S, Pedotti P, Taioli E. Mutat Res. 2003 Mar 3;535(2):155-60. PMID:12581533

[81] Relationship between seminal ascorbic acid and sperm DNA integrity in infertile men. Song GJ, Norkus EP, Lewis V. Int J Androl. 2006 Dec;29(6):569-75. PMID:17121654

[82] Chronic high-fat diet in fathers programs β-cell dysfunction in female rat offspring. Ng SF, Lin RC, Laybutt DR, Barres R, Owens JA, Morris MJ. Nature. 2010 Oct 21;467(7318):963-6. PMID:20962845

[83] Creatine and creatinine metabolism. Wyss M, Kaddurah-Daouk R. Physiol Rev. 2000 Jul;80(3):1107-213. PMID:10893433

[84] Heterocyclic amines in cooked meat. Vikse R, Reistad R, Steffensen IL, Paulsen JE, Nyholm SH, Alexander J. Tidsskr Nor Laegeforen. 1999 Jan 10;119(1):45-9. PMID:10025205

[85] Effect of cooking methods on the formation of heterocyclic aromatic amines in chicken and duck breast. Liao GZ, Wang GY, Xu XL, Zhou GH. Meat Sci. 2010 May;85(1):149-54. PMID:20374878

[86] Heterocyclic amines: occurrence and prevention in cooked food. Robbana-Barnat S, Rabache M, Rialland E, Fradin J. Environ Health Perspect. 1996 Mar;104(3):280-8. PMID:8919766

[87] On Food and Cooking, the Science and Lore of the Kitchen. Harold McGee.Scribner, New York, 2004

[88] Minimization of heterocyclic amines and thermal inactivation of Escherichia coli in fried ground beef. Salmon CP, Knize MG, Panteleakos FN, Wu RW, Nelson DO, Felton JS. J Natl Cancer Inst. 2000 Nov 1;92(21):1773-8. PMID: 11058620

[89] Mutagenicity of wood smoke condensates in the Salmonella/microsome assay. Asita AO, Matsui M, Nohmi T, et al. Mutat Res. 1991 Sep;264(1):7-14. PMID:1881415

[90] Direct mutagenicity of the polycylic aromatic hydrocarbon-containing fraction of smoked and charcoal-broiled foods treated with nitrite in acid solution. Kangsadalampai K, Butryee C, Manoonphol K. Food Chem Toxicol. 1997 Feb;35(2):213-8. PMID:9146734

[91] Mutagenicity of cooked hamburger is controlled delicately by reducing sugar content in ground beef. Kato T, Michikoshi K, Minowa Y, Kikugawa K. Mutat Res. 2000 Nov 20;471(1-2):1-6. PMID:11080655

[92] Effects of marinating with Asian marinades or western barbecue sauce on PhIP and MeIQx formation in barbecued beef. Nerurkar PV, Le Marchand L, Cooney RV. Nutr Cancer. 1999;34(2):147-52. PMID:10578481

[93] Effect of microwave pretreatment on heterocyclic aromatic amine mutagens/carcinogens in fried beef patties. Felton JS, Fultz E, Dolbeare FA, Knize MG. Food Chem Toxicol. 1994 Oct;32(10):897-903. PMID:7959444

[94] Occurrence of mutagenic/carcinogenic heterocyclic amines in meat and fish products, including pan residues, prepared under domestic conditions. Johansson MA, Jägerstad M. Carcinogenesis. 1994 Aug;15(8):1511-8. PMID:8055627

[95] Effect of marinades on the formation of heterocyclic amines in grilled beef steaks. Smith JS, Ameri F, Gadgil P. J Food Sci. 2008 Aug;73(6):T100-5. PMID:19241593

[96] Effect of red wine marinades on the formation of heterocyclic amines in fried chicken breast. Busquets R, Puignou L, Galceran MT, Skog K. J Agric Food Chem. 2006 Oct 18;54(21):8376-84. PMID:17032054

[97] Effect of beer/red wine marinades on the formation of heterocyclic aromatic amines in pan-fried beef. Melo A, Viegas O, Petisca C, Pinho O, Ferreira IM. J Agric Food Chem. 2008 Nov 26;56(22):10625-32. PMID:18950185

[98] Effect of marinades on the formation of heterocyclic amines in grilled beef steaks. Smith JS, Ameri F, Gadgil P. J Food Sci. 2008 Aug;73(6):T100-5. PMID:19241593

[99] Effect of oil marinades with garlic, onion, and lemon juice on the formation of heterocyclic aromatic amines in fried beef patties. Gibis M. J Agric Food Chem. 2007 Dec 12;55(25):10240-7. PMID:17988088

[100] Airborne mutagens produced by frying beef, pork and a soy-based food. Thiébaud HP, Knize MG, Kuzmicky PA, Hsieh DP, Felton JS. Food Chem Toxicol. 1995 Oct;33(10):821-8. PMID:7590526

[101] Prevention of the formation of mutagenic and/or carcinogenic heterocyclic amines by food factors. Kikugawa K, Hiramoto K, Kato T. Biofactors. 2000;12(1-4):123-7. PMID:11216472

[102] Heterocyclic Amines: 2. Inhibitory Effects of Natural Extracts on the Formation of Polar andNonpolar Heterocyclic Amines in Cooked Beef. Ahn J, Grun IU, J Food Science 70:(4)C263-68, 2005

[103] Cruciferous vegetables, the GSTP1 Ile105Val genetic polymorphism, and breast cancer risk. Lee SA, Fowke JH, Lu W, Ye C, Zheng Y, Cai Q, Gu K, Gao YT, Shu XO, Zheng W. Am J Clin Nutr. 2008 Mar;87(3):753-60. PMID:18326615

[104] Dietary intake of fruit and vegetables and risk of non-Hodgkin lymphoma. Chiu BC, Kwon S, Evens AM, Surawicz T, Smith SM, Weisenburger DD. Cancer Causes Control. 2011 Aug;22(8):1183-95. PMID:21695384

[105] GST polymorphism and excretion of heterocyclic aromatic amine and isothiocyanate metabolites after Brassica consumption. Steck SE, Hebert JR. Environ Mol Mutagen. 2009 Apr;50(3):238-46. PMID:19197987

[106] Cruciferous vegetable consumption and lung cancer risk: a systematic review. Lam TK, Gallicchio L, Lindsley K, Shiels M, Hammond E, Tao XG, Chen L, Robinson KA, Caulfield LE, Herman JG, Guallar E, Alberg AJ. Cancer Epidemiol Biomarkers Prev. 2009 Jan;18(1):184-95. PMID:19124497

[107] Hydrogen sulfide mediates the anti-survival effect of sulforaphane on human prostate cancer cells. Pei Y, Wu B, Cao Q, Wu L, Yang G. Toxicol Appl Pharmacol. 2011 Oct 8. PMID:22005276

[108] D,L-sulforaphane-induced apoptosis in human breast cancer cells is regulated by the adapter protein p66(Shc). Sakao K, Singh SV. J Cell Biochem. 2011 Sep 28. PMID:21956685

[109] Sulforaphane inhibits mitochondrial permeability transition and oxidative stress. Greco T, Shafer J, Fiskum G. Free Radic Biol Med. 2011 Sep 21. PMID:21986339

[110] Comparison of the protective effects of steamed and cooked broccolis on ischaemia-reperfusion-induced cardiac injury. Mukherjee S, Lekli I, Ray D, Gangopadhyay H, Raychaudhuri U, Das DK. Br J Nutr. 2010 Mar;103(6):815-23. PMID:19857366

[111] Sulforophane glucosinolate. Monograph. Altern Med Rev. 2010 Dec;15(4):352-60. PMID:2119425

[112] [Sulforaphane (1-isothiocyanato-4-(methylsulfinyl)-butane) content in cruciferous vegetables]. Campas-Baypoli ON, Bueno-Solano C, Martínez-Ibarra DM, et al. Arch Latinoam Nutr. 2009 Mar;59(1):95-100. PMID:19480351

[113] Bioavailability of Sulforaphane from two broccoli sprout beverages: results of a short-term, cross-over clinical trial in Qidong, China. Egner PA, Chen JG, Wang JB, Wu Y et al. Cancer Prev Res (Phila). 2011 Mar;4(3):384-95. PMID:21372038

[114] The activity of myrosinase from broccoli (Brassica oleracea L. cv. Italica): influence of intrinsic and extrinsic factors. Ludikhuyze L, Rodrigo L, Hendrickx M. J Food Prot. 2000 Mar;63(3):400-3. PMID:10716572

[115] Heating decreases epithiospecifier protein activity and increases sulforaphane formation in broccoli. Matusheski NV, Juvik JA, Jeffery EH. Phytochemistry. 2004 May;65(9):1273-81. PMID:15184012

[116] Effect of meal composition and cooking duration on the fate of sulforaphane following consumption of broccoli by healthy human subjects. Rungapamestry V, Duncan AJ, Fuller Z, Ratcliffe B. Br J Nutr. 2007 Apr;97(4):644-52. PMID:17349076

[117] Changes in glucosinolate concentrations, myrosinase activity, and production of metabolites of glucosinolates in cabbage (Brassica oleracea Var. capitata) cooked for different durations. Rungapamestry V, Duncan AJ, Fuller Z, Ratcliffe B. J Agric Food Chem. 2006 Oct 4;54(20):7628-34. PMID:17002432

[118] Kinetics of the stability of broccoli (Brassica oleracea Cv. Italica) myrosinase and isothiocyanates in broccoli juice during pressure/temperature treatments. Van Eylen D, Oey I, Hendrickx M, Van Loey A. J Agric Food Chem. 2007 Mar 21;55(6):2163-70. Epub 2007 Feb 17. PMID:17305356

[119] Indole-3-carbinol suppresses NF-kappaB and IkappaBalpha kinase activation, causing inhibition of expression of NF-kappaB-regulated antiapoptotic and metastatic gene products and enhancement of apoptosis in myeloid and leukemia cells. Takada Y, Andreeff M, Aggarwal BB. Blood. 2005 Jul 15;106(2):641-9. PMID:15811958

[120] Molecular targets and anticancer potential of indole-3-carbinol and its derivatives. Aggarwal BB, Ichikawa H. Cell Cycle. 2005 Sep;4(9):1201-15. Epub 2005 Sep 6. PMID:16082211

[121] Vegetable and fruit intake after diagnosis and risk of prostate cancer progression. Richman EL, Carroll PR, Chan JM. Int J Cancer. 2011 Aug 5. PMID:21823116

[122] Prospective study of fruit and vegetable intake and risk of prostate cancer. Kirsh VA, Peters U, Mayne ST, et al; Prostate, Lung, Colorectal and Ovarian Cancer Screening Trial. J Natl Cancer Inst. 2007 Aug 1;99(15):1200-9. PMID:17652276

[123] Inhibition of the genotoxic effects of heterocyclic amines in human derived hepatoma cells by dietary bioantimutagens. Sanyal R, Darroudi F, Parzefall W, Nagao M, Knasmüller S. Mutagenesis. 1997 Jul;12(4):297-303. PMID:9237777

[124] Nrf2, a master regulator of detoxification and also antioxidant, anti-inflammatory and other cytoprotective mechanisms, is raised by health promoting factors. Pall ML, Levine S. Sheng Li Xue Bao. 2015 Feb 25;67(1):1-18. PMID:25672622

[125] Effect of processed and red meat on endogenous nitrosation and DNA damage. Joosen AM, Kuhnle GG, Aspinall SM, Barrow TM, Lecommandeur E, Azqueta A, Collins AR, Bingham SA. Carcinogenesis. 2009 Aug;30(8):1402-7. PMID:19498009

[126] Development of a food database of nitrosamines, heterocyclic amines, and polycyclic aromatic hydrocarbons. (Database) Jakszyn P, Agudo A, Ibáñez R, García-Closas R, Pera G, Amiano P, González CA. J Nutr. 2004 Aug;134(8):2011-4. PMID:15284391

[127] Risk factors for esophageal cancer: a case-control study in South-western China. Yang CX, Wang HY, Wang ZM, et al. Asian Pac J Cancer Prev. 2005 Jan-Mar;6(1):48-53. PMID: 15780032

[128] Biogenic amines in meat and fermented meat products. Stadnik J, Dolatowski ZJ. Acta Sci. Pol., Technol. Aliment. 9(3) 2010, 251-263 http://www.food.actapol.net/pub/1_3_2010.pdf

[129] The effect of haem in red and processed meat on the endogenous formation of N-nitroso compounds in the upper gastrointestinal tract. Lunn JC, Kuhnle G, Mai V, et al. Carcinogenesis. 2007 Mar;28(3):685-90. PMID:17052997

[130] Quantitative assessment of red meat or processed meat consumption and kidney cancer. Alexander DD, Cushing CA. Cancer Detect Prev. 2009;32(5-6):340-51. PMID:19303221

[131] A review and meta-analysis of red and processed meat consumption and breast cancer. Alexander DD, Morimoto LM, Mink PJ, Cushing CA. Nutr Res Rev. 2010 Dec;23(2):349-65. PMID:21110906

[132] Red and processed meat consumption and risk of ovarian cancer: a dose-response meta-analysis of prospective studies. Wallin A, Orsini N, Wolk A. Br J Cancer. 2011 Mar 29;104(7):1196-201. PMID:21343939

[133] A review and meta-analysis of prospective studies of red and processed meat intake and prostate cancer. Alexander DD, Mink PJ, Cushing CA, Sceurman B. Nutr J. 2010 Nov 2;9:50. PMID:21044319

[134] Red meat, dietary nitrosamines, and heme iron and risk of bladder cancer in the European Prospective Investigation into Cancer and Nutrition (EPIC). Jakszyn P, González CA, Luján-Barroso L, et al. Cancer Epidemiol Biomarkers Prev. 2011 Mar;20(3):555-9. PMID:21239687

[135] Processed meat consumption and stomach cancer risk: a meta-analysis. Larsson SC, Orsini N, Wolk A. J Natl Cancer Inst. 2006 Aug 2;98(15):1078-87. PMID:16882945

[136] Red and processed meat and colorectal cancer incidence: meta-analysis of prospective studies. Chan DS, Lau R, Aune D, Vieira R, Greenwood DC, Kampman E, Norat T. PLoS One. 2011;6(6):e20456. PMID:21674008

[137] Lack of the DNA repair protein O6-methylguanine-DNA methyltransferase in histologically normal brain adjacent to primary human brain tumors. Silber JR, Blank A, Bobola MS, et al. Proc Natl Acad Sci U S A. 1996 Jul 9;93(14):6941-6. PMID:8692923

[138] O6-methylguanine-DNA methyltransferase deficiency in developing brain: implications for brain tumorigenesis. Bobola MS, Blank A, Berger MS, Silber JR. DNA Repair (Amst). 2007 Aug 1;6(8):1127-33. PMID:17500046

[139] An international case-control study of maternal diet during pregnancy and childhood brain tumor risk: a histology-specific analysis by food group. Pogoda JM, Preston-Martin S, Howe G, et al. Ann Epidemiol. 2009 Mar;19(3):148-60. PMID:19216997

[140] Diet and risk of adult glioma in eastern Nebraska, United States. Chen H, Ward MH, Tucker KL, et al. Cancer Causes Control. 2002 Sep;13(7):647-55. PMID:12296512

[141] Diet and brain cancer in adults: a case-control study in northeast China. Hu J, La Vecchia C, Negri E, et al. Int J Cancer. 1999 Mar 31;81(1):20-3. PMID:10077146

[142] Childhood cancer in relation to cured meat intake: review of the epidemiological evidence. Blot WJ, Henderson BE, Boice JD Jr. Nutr Cancer. 1999;34(1):111-8. PMID:10453449

[143] Prenatal airborne polycyclic aromatic hydrocarbon exposure and child IQ at age 5 years. Perera FP, Li Z, Whyatt R, Hoepner L, Wang S, Camann D, Rauh V. Pediatrics. 2009 Aug;124(2):e195-202. PMID:19620194

[144] Prenatal exposure to airborne polycyclic aromatic hydrocarbons and risk of intrauterine growth restriction. Choi H, Rauh V, Garfinkel R, Tu Y, Perera FP. Environ Health Perspect. 2008 May;116(5):658-65. PMID:18470316

[145] Carcinogenic food contaminants. Abnet CC. Cancer Invest. 2007 Apr-May;25(3):189-96. PMID:17530489

[146] Cooking smoke: a silent killer. Schwela D. People Planet. 1997;6(3):24-5. PMID:12321046

[147] Lung cancer and indoor air pollution in rural china. Kleinerman R, Wang Z, Lubin J, Zhang S, Metayer C, Brenner A. Ann Epidemiol. 2000 Oct 1;10(7):469. PMID:11018397

[148] Guidance for Industry: Action Levels for Poisonous or Deleterious Substances in Human Food and Animal Feed. August 2000. http://www.fda.gov/Food/GuidanceComplianceRegulatoryInformation/GuidanceDocuments/ChemicalContaminantsandPesticides/ucm077969.htm

[149] Costs and efficacy of public health interventions to reduce aflatoxin-induced human disease. Khlangwiset P, Wu F. Food Addit Contam Part A Chem Anal Control Expo Risk Assess. 2010 Jul;27(7):998-1014. PMID:20419532

[150] Aflatoxin and PAH exposure biomarkers in a U.S. population with a high incidence of hepatocellular carcinoma. Johnson NM, Qian G, Xu L, et al. Sci Total Environ. 2010 Nov 1;408(23):6027-31. PMID:20870273

[151] Mycotoxins and human disease: a largely ignored global health issue. Wild CP, Gong YY. Carcinogenesis. 2010 Jan;31(1):71-82. PMID:19875698

[152] Aflatoxin genotoxicity is associated with a defective DNA damage response bypassing p53 activation. Gursoy-Yuzugullu O, Yuzugullu H, Yilmaz M, Ozturk M. Liver Int. 2011 Apr;31(4):561-71. PMID:21382167

[153] Hepatitis B, aflatoxin B(1), and p53 codon 249 mutation in hepatocellular carcinomas from Guangxi, People's Republic of China, and a meta-analysis of existing studies. Stern MC, Umbach DM, Yu MC, et al. Cancer Epidemiol Biomarkers Prev. 2001 Jun;10(6):617-25. PMID:11401911

[154] p53 mutations, chronic hepatitis B virus infection, and aflatoxin exposure in hepatocellular carcinoma in Taiwan. Lunn RM, Zhang YJ, Wang LY, et al. Cancer Res. 1997 Aug 15;57(16):3471-7. PMID:9270015

[155] Global burden of aflatoxin-induced hepatocellular carcinoma: a risk assessment. Liu Y, Wu F. Environ Health Perspect. 2010 Jun;118(6):818-24. PMID:20172840

[156] Hepatic aflatoxin B1-DNA adducts and TP53 mutations in patients with hepatocellular carcinoma despite low exposure to aflatoxin B1 in southern Japan. Shirabe K, Toshima T, Taketomi A, et al. Liver Int. 2011 Jun 28. PMID:21745313

[157] Does aflatoxin B1 play a role in the etiology of hepatocellular carcinoma in the United States? Hoque A, Patt YZ, Yoffe B, et al. Nutr Cancer. 1999;35(1):27-33. PMID:10624703

[158] Modulation of aflatoxin biomarkers in human blood and urine by green tea polyphenols intervention. Tang L, Tang M, Xu L, Luo H, Huang T, Yu J, Zhang L, Gao W, Cox SB, Wang JS. Carcinogenesis. 2008 Feb;29(2):411-7. PMID:18192689

[159] Fruit and vegetable consumption and the risk of proximal colon, distal colon, and rectal cancers in a case-control study in

Western Australia. Annema N, Heyworth JS, McNaughton SA, Iacopetta B, Fritschi L. J Am Diet Assoc. 2011 Oct;111(10):1479-90. PMID:21963014

[160] Dietary fiber intake and risk of breast cancer in postmenopausal women: the National Institutes of Health-AARP Diet and Health Study. Park Y, Brinton LA, Subar AF, Hollenbeck A, Schatzkin A. Am J Clin Nutr. 2009 Sep;90(3):664-71. PMID:19625685

[161] Estimated enterolignans, lignan-rich foods, and fibre in relation to survival after postmenopausal breast cancer. Buck K, Zaineddin AK, Vrieling A, et al. Br J Cancer. 2011 Oct 11;105(8):1151-7. PMID:21915130

[162] Dietary lignan intake and postmenopausal breast cancer risk by estrogen and progesterone receptor status. Touillaud MS, Thiébaut AC, Fournier A, et al. J Natl Cancer Inst. 2007 Mar 21;99(6):475-86. PMID: 17374837

[163] Dietary lariciresinol attenuates mammary tumor growth and reduces blood vessel density in human MCF-7 breast cancer xenografts and carcinogen-induced mammary tumors in rats. Saarinen NM, Wärri A, Dings RP, Airio M, Smeds AI, Mäkelä S. Int J Cancer. 2008 Sep 1;123(5):1196-204. PMID:18528864

[164] Flaxseed and its lignans inhibit estradiol-induced growth, angiogenesis, and secretion of vascular endothelial growth factor in human breast cancer xenografts in vivo. Bergman Jungeström M, Thompson LU, Dabrosin C. Clin Cancer Res. 2007 Feb 1;13(3):1061-7. PMID:17289903

[165] Phytoestrogen consumption and endometrial cancer risk: a population-based case-control study in New Jersey. Bandera EV, Williams MG, Sima C, et al. Cancer Causes Control. 2009 Sep;20(7):1117-27. PMID:9353280

[166] Phytoestrogen intake and endometrial cancer risk. Horn-Ross PL, John EM, Canchola AJ, Stewart SL, Lee MM. J Natl Cancer Inst. 2003 Aug 6;95(15):1158-64. PMID:12902445

[167] Dietary fiber and whole-grain consumption in relation to colorectal cancer in the NIH-AARP Diet and Health Study. Schatzkin A, Mouw T, Park Y, et al. Am J Clin Nutr. 2007 May;85(5):1353-60. PMID:17490973

[168] Intake of dietary fiber, especially from cereal foods, is associated with lower incidence of colon cancer in the HELGA cohort. Hansen L, Skeie G, Landberg R, et al. Int J Cancer. 2011 Aug 22. PMID:21866547

[169] An apple a day may hold colorectal cancer at bay: recent evidence from a case-control study. Jedrychowski W, Maugeri U. Rev Environ Health. 2009 Jan-Mar;24(1):59-74. PMID:19476292

[170] Fruit and vegetable consumption and risk of distal gastric cancer in the Shanghai Women's and Men's Health studies. Epplein M, Shu XO, Xiang YB, et al Am J Epidemiol. 2010 Aug 15;172(4):397-406. PMID:20647333

[171] Vegetables and fruits consumption and risk of esophageal and gastric cancer subtypes in the Netherlands Cohort Study. Steevens J, Schouten LJ, Goldbohm RA, van den Brandt PA. Int J Cancer. 2011 Dec 1;129(11):2681-93 PMID:21960262

[172] Fermentation of vegetable fiber in the intestinal tract of rats and effects on fecal bulking and bile acid excretion. Nyman M, Schweizer TF, Tyrén S, Reimann S, Asp NG. J Nutr. 1990 May;120(5):459-66. PMID:2160526

[173] Dietary patterns and risk of oesophageal cancers: a population-based case-control study. Ibiebele TI, Hughes MC, Whiteman DC, Webb PM. Br J Nutr. 2011 Sep 7:1-10. PMID:21899799

[174] Nonlinear reduction in risk for colorectal cancer by fruit and vegetable intake based on meta-analysis of prospective studies. Aune D, Lau R, Chan DS, Vieira R, Greenwood DC, Kampman E, Norat T. Gastroenterology. 2011 Jul;141(1):106-18. PMID:21600207

[175] Effects of altered maternal folic acid, vitamin B12 and docosahexaenoic acid on placental global DNA methylation patterns in Wistar rats. Kulkarni A, Dangat K, Kale A, et al. PLoS One. 2011 Mar 10;6(3):e17706. PMID:21423696

[176] Plasma vitamin B6 and the risk of colorectal cancer and adenoma in women. Wei EK, Giovannucci E, Selhub J, Fuchs CS, Hankinson SE, Ma J. J Natl Cancer Inst. 2005 May 4;97(9):684-92. PMID:15870439

[177] Vitamin B6 and risk of colorectal cancer: a meta-analysis of prospective studies. Larsson SC, Orsini N, Wolk A. JAMA. 2010 Mar 17;303(11):1077-83. PMID:20233826

[178] Prospective study of plasma vitamin B6 and risk of colorectal cancer in men. Lee JE, Li H, Giovannucci E, Lee IM, Selhub J, Stampfer M, Ma J. Cancer Epidemiol Biomarkers Prev. 2009 Apr;18(4):1197-202. PMID:19336555

[179] Low plasma vitamin B-6 status affects metabolism through the kynurenine pathway in cardiovascular patients with systemic inflammation. Midttun O, Ulvik A, Ringdal Pedersen E, et al. J Nutr. 2011 Apr 1;141(4):611-7. PMID:21310866

[180] Carcinogenicity of deoxycholate, a secondary bile acid. Bernstein C, Holubec H, Bhattacharyya AK, et al. Arch Toxicol. 2011 Aug;85(8):863-71. PMID:21267546

[181] Significance of fecal deoxycholic acid concentration for colorectal tumor enlargement. Kawano A, Ishikawa H, Kamano T, Kanoh M, Sakamoto K, Nakamura T, Otani T, Sakai T, Kono K. Asian Pac J Cancer Prev. 2010;11(6):1541-6. PMID:21338194

[182] Role of bile bacteria in gallbladder carcinoma. Sharma V, Chauhan VS, Nath G, Kumar A, Shukla VK. Hepatogastroenterology. 2007 Sep;54(78):1622-5. PMID:18019679

[183] Consumption of some polyphenols reduces fecal deoxycholic acid and lithocholic acid, the secondary bile acids of risk factors of colon cancer. Han Y, Haraguchi T, Iwanaga S, et al. J Agric Food Chem. 2009 Sep 23;57(18):8587-90. PMID:19711910

[184] The bile acid deoxycholic acid has a non-linear dose response for DNA damage and possibly NF-kappaB activation in oesophageal cells, with a mechanism of action involving ROS. Jenkins GJ, Cronin J, Alhamdani A, et al. Mutagenesis. 2008 Sep;23(5):399-405. PMID:18515815

[185] Steam cooking significantly improves in vitro bile acid binding of collard greens, kale, mustard greens, broccoli, green bell pepper, and cabbage. Kahlon TS, Chiu MC, Chapman MH. Nutr Res. 2008 Jun;28(6):351-7. PMID:19083431

[186] Voluntary wheel running increases bile acid as well as cholesterol excretion and decreases atherosclerosis in hypercholesterolemic mice. Meissner M, Lombardo E, Havinga R, et al. Atherosclerosis. 2011 Oct;218(2):323-9. PMID:21802084

[187] Voluntary wheel running exercise and dietary lactose concomitantly reduce proportion of secondary bile acids in rat feces. Hagio M, Matsumoto M, Yajima T, Hara H, Ishizuka S. J Appl Physiol. 2010 Sep;109(3):663-8. PMID:20616226

[188] Exercise enhances whole-body cholesterol turnover in mice. Meissner M, Havinga R, Boverhof R, Kema I, Groen AK, Kuipers F. Med Sci Sports Exerc. 2010 Aug;42(8):1460-8. PMID:20139791

[189] 1alpha,25-Dihydroxyvitamin D3 down-regulates estrogen receptor abundance and suppresses estrogen actions in MCF-7 human breast cancer cells. Swami S, Krishnan AV, Feldman D. Clin Cancer Res. 2000 Aug;6(8):3371-9. PMID:10955825

[190] Inhibition of prostaglandin synthesis and actions contributes to the beneficial effects of calcitriol in prostate cancer. Krishnan AV, Srinivas S, Feldman D. Dermatoendocrinol. 2009 Jan;1(1):7-11. PMID:20046582

[191] Dietary Reference Intakes for Thiamin, Riboflavin, Niacin, Vitamin B6, Folate, Vitamin B12, Pantothenic Acid, Biotin, and Choline (1998) National Academy of Sciences. Institute of Medicine. Food and Nutrition Board. Chapter 7

[192] Folate and vitamin B6 from diet and supplements in relation to risk of coronary heart disease among women. Rimm EB, Willett WC, Hu FB, Sampson L, Colditz GA, Manson JE, Hennekens C, Stampfer MJ. JAMA. 1998 Feb 4;279(5):359-64. PMID:9459468

[193] Plasma vitamin B6 and the risk of colorectal cancer and adenoma in women. Wei EK, Giovannucci E, Selhub J, Fuchs CS, Hankinson SE, Ma J. J Natl Cancer Inst. 2005 May 4;97(9):684-92. PMID:15870439

[194] Low-to-moderate alcohol intake and breast cancer risk in Chinese women. Zhang M, Holman CD. Br J Cancer. 2011 Sep 27;105(7):1089-95. PMID:21829196

[195] Alcohol and postmenopausal breast cancer risk defined by estrogen and progesterone receptor status: a prospective cohort study. Suzuki R, Ye W, Rylander-Rudqvist T, Saji S, Colditz GA, Wolk A. J Natl Cancer Inst. 2005 Nov 2;97(21):1601-8. PMID:16264180

[196] In utero alcohol exposure increases mammary tumorigenesis in rats. Hilakivi-Clarke L, Cabanes A, de Assis S, et al. Br J Cancer. 2004 Jun 1;90(11):2225-31. PMID:15150620

[197] Fetal alcohol exposure increases mammary tumor susceptibility and alters tumor phenotype in rats. Polanco TA, Crismale-Gann C, Reuhl KR, Sarkar DK, Cohick WS. Alcohol Clin Exp Res. 2010 Nov;34(11):1879-87. PMID:20662802

[198] Beneficial and adverse effects of chemopreventive agents. Lee BM, Park KK. Mutat Res. 2003 Feb-Mar;523-524:265-78. PMID:12628524

[199] Phytoestrogen consumption from foods and supplements and epithelial ovarian cancer risk: a population-based case control study. Bandera EV, King M, Chandran U, et al. BMC Womens Health. 2011 Sep 23;11:40. PMID:21943063

[200] Lignan contents of Dutch plant foods: a database including lariciresinol, pinoresinol, secoisolariciresinol and matairesinol. Milder IE, Arts IC, van de Putte B, Venema DP, Hollman PC. Br J Nutr. 2005 Mar;93(3):393-402. PMID:15877880

[201] Minimization of heterocyclic amines and thermal inactivation of Escherichia coli in fried ground beef. Salmon CP, Knize MG, Panteleakos FN, et al. J Natl Cancer Inst. 2000 Nov 1;92(21):1773-8.

[202] Inhibition of steroid 5 alpha-reductase by specific aliphatic unsaturated fatty acids. Liang T, Liao S. Biochem J. 1992 Jul 15;285 (Pt 2):557-62. PMID:1637346

[203] Alcohol, oxidative stress, and free radical damage. Wu D, Cederbaum AI. Alcohol Res Health. 2003;27(4):277-84. PMID: 15540798

[204] Betaine treatment attenuates chronic ethanol-induced hepatic steatosis and alterations to the mitochondrial respiratory chain proteome. Kharbanda KK, Todero SL, King AL, et al. Int J Hepatol. 2012;2012:962183. PMID:22187660

[205] A Taste of Paradise A Feast of Authentic Caribbean Cuisine and Refreshing Tropical Beverages for Health and Vitality. Lewis SJ, Lewis CA March 2012 ISBN-13: 978-1938318009

42. Osteoimmunology

Although bone is a hard, mineralized structure, it is a dynamic tissue that undergoes continual remodeling. The principal cells that remodel bone are osteoblasts, which deposit new bone material, and osteoclasts, which actively degrade bone. These two cell types coordinate maintenance and repair of bone and the utilization and storage of calcium and other bone minerals. In health, the activity of these cells is balanced. Excess osteoblastic vs. osteoclastic activity causes excessive bone mass as in osteopetrosis that is disabling. Excess osteoclastic vs. osteoblastic activity causes osteopenia and osteoporosis, which increase the risk of fractures. Bone mass peaks in the early twenties.

Osteoblasts: Osteoblasts are specialized fibroblasts that arise from osteoprogenitor cells located in the periosteum and bone marrow. The osteoprogenitor cells differentiate under the stimulus of specific growth factors including bone morphogenetic proteins (BMPs), fibroblast growth factor (FGF), platelet-derived growth factor (PDGF), and transforming growth factor beta (TGF-β). Osteoblasts form new layers of bone by producing osteoid as a bone matrix composed of proteins: Type 1 collagen fibers, chondroitin sulfate and osteocalcin. The osteoblasts also calcify the osteoid protein matrix. After surrounding themselves with new bone, the osteoblasts mature into osteocytes.

Osteoclasts: Osteoclasts are large, multinucleated cells that digest bone. These cells are transformed from monocytes (white blood cells) under the influence of RANKL (Receptor Activator of Nuclear Factor-κβ Ligand), a member of the TNF family, and M-CSF (Macrophage Colony-Stimulating Factor). RANKL binds to RANK, which activates the intracellular protein Nuclear Factor-κβ (NF-κβ), a transcription factor for inflammatory cytokines.

Osteoclasts adhere to the bone and then release hydrogen ions between themselves and the bone. The hydrogen in solution is acid and dissolves the mineralized bone, releasing calcium, phosphate, and bicarbonate into the circulation. The osteoclasts also produce metalloproteinases and Cathepsin K, a cysteine protease, which digests the protein matrix of the bone.

Osteoblasts produce both RANKL and osteoprotegerin (OPG). OPG is a decoy receptor for RANK that prevents its activity. Thus, osteoblasts produce proteins that regulate osteoclast activity. Parathyroid hormone stimulates the expression of RANKL and inhibits the expression of OPG in osteoblasts.

Osteoporosis

Osteoporosis is one of the most prevalent diseases among older adults. The National Osteoporosis Foundation reports that 44 million Americans are affected: half of women and a quarter of all men, over the age of 50, will have a fracture secondary to osteoporosis.

The scanning electron micrograph in figure 42-1 illustrates the trabecular bone mass of a young, healthy man on the left, as compared to a 71-year-old female on the right.

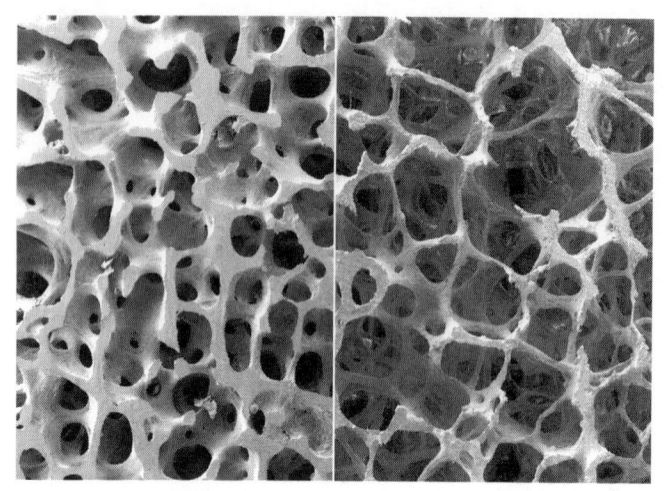

Figure 42-1: Normal and osteoporotic trabecular bone[1].

It was long assumed that osteoporosis resulted from an insufficient dietary intake of calcium; few Americans diets, however, are deficient in calcium. Although dietary factors are critical to the development and maintenance of bone mass, dietary deficiency of calcium and protein cannot explain the prevalence of osteopenia and osteoporosis in America.

Diet does play a pivotal role in osteoporosis. There are three principal components of this risk: insufficient vitamin K, insufficient vitamin D, and enteroimmune processes that cause malabsorption and inflammation. Additionally, vitamin D and vitamin K deficiencies and calcium wasting are often caused or exacerbated by malabsorption resulting from enteroimmune causes.

Vitamin K activates osteocalcin and matrix Gla protein which are critical to the process of laying down new bone. Osteocalcin, additionally, promotes the synthesis of testosterone and the release of insulin. Matrix Gla protein is also found in the heart, kidneys, and lungs. Furthermore, vitamin K prevents bone loss during corticosteroid use by protecting the formation of OPG[2].

Vitamin D helps induce the transcription osteocalcin and matrix Gla protein, and both vitamin D and vitamin K are required for maintenance of a healthy bone mass. Vitamin D also increases the production of the enterocyte calcium pump calbindin-D9k in the intestine, which transports calcium from the intestinal lumen into the body.

When men are diagnosed with osteoporosis, a presumptive diagnosis of gluten enteropathy can be made as it is by far the most common cause of this disease among men. Gluten enteropathy (GE) can be seen as a model that illustrates how enteroimmune disease causes osteoporosis, and thus, how treatment may be approached.

Malabsorption

GE causes osteoporosis, in large part, as a result of malabsorption, with the loss of nutrients into the colon. GE additionally worsens lactose intolerance. Lactose intolerance may not only decrease the absorption of calcium, but additionally, causes individuals with lactose intolerance to avoid dairy products, an important source of dietary calcium, phosphate, and magnesium.

It is not just, nor even primarily, calcium malabsorption that causes osteoporosis. The sex hormones which help to build bone mass undergo excretion in the bile along with vitamin D, vitamin K, folate, and vitamin B_{12}. Normally, these are reabsorbed in the ileum as part of the enterohepatic circulation. These hormones and vitamins are lost in many patients with malabsorption syndromes, and this loss may be central to the depletion of bone mass.

Inflammation

GE and other enteroimmune diseases do not cause osteoporosis solely through malabsorption, but also via inflammation. TNF-α stimulates NF-κB activity; this promotes osteoclast differentiation while impeding osteoblastic development. Endogenous TNF-α, such as that formed in enteroimmune disease or other inflammatory disorders, prevents the development of peak bone mass in young animals[3]. Certain proinflammatory cytokines, including TNF-α, IL-1, and IL-17, are strong inductors of osteoclast activation and bone resorption.

Antergies, through T_H17 activation, promote inflammatory activity. Sessile gram-negative bacteria in the colon form lipopolysaccharides (LPS) which activate Toll-like receptors (TLR). TLR activate transcription factors, such as NF-κB, induce the production of inflammatory cytokines and the transformation of monocytes into osteoclasts.

Vitamin K_2 suppresses the effect of TNF-α, stimulates osteoblasts, and suppresses osteoclastogenesis by increasing the production of the NF-κB inactivation factor IκB, and by antagonizing RANKL activation[4]. Both vitamins D and K suppress inflammation; vitamin D by down-regulating the production of TLR2 and TLR-4. Other cytokines, such as IL-12, IL-18, IL-33, and IFN, suppress osteoclast differentiation and inhibit bone loss[5].

Most of the disease burden of osteoporosis, osteopenia, and osteomalacia is caused by malabsorption and inflammation, rather than from insufficient dietary calcium intake. Treatment of the underlying causes should be the first step in rebuilding bone mass. A healthful diet should contain adequate calcium and vitamin K. Treatment with supplements of vitamins D and K are usually required in the treatment of low bone density. There is little likelihood of building bone mass as long as malabsorption continues. Prevention of osteoporosis requires avoidance of antergens and prevention of intestinal biofilm growth.

Most studies using vitamin D for treatment of osteoporosis have been ineffective in preventing fractures when vitamin D was not accompanied by calcium supplements[6]; however, these studies used tiny doses of vitamin D, usually 400 IU, and only lowered fracture rate by about eight percent. This small dose of vitamin D is insufficient to optimize calcitriol levels or to minimize parathyroid hormone. Parathyroid hormone raises serum calcium levels by increasing RANKL and activating osteoclasts. A daily dose of 4000 IU is required for most adults living in temperate climates during the winter months, and the requirements may be higher in patients with malabsorption. Fracture rates in the elderly decline as 25OHD levels rise, up to at least 115 nmol/L[7]. This is a rational therapeutic target level.

Calcium supplements should not be required in healthy individuals consuming a balanced diet. Supplementation of calcium is appropriate in patients with, or at high risk of, osteoporosis. Calcium is one of few mineral supplements associated with a decrease in mortality[8]. A daily dose of 800 mg of calcium, along with vitamin D, is sufficient to supplement the diet in most at-risk individuals.

Boron (3 to 6 mg) may also be helpful to aid in calcium absorption, and it appears to strengthen bones[9]. Boron, found in leafy green vegetables, helps with calcium and magnesium absorption, likely, as a result of its effect on the conversion of steroid hormones. Boron may also limit NF-κB activation by LPS[10]. Populations with higher dietary boron are at lower risk for osteoarthritis, and use of boron supplements (6 mg per day) improves arthritis pain[11].

Risk Factors

Other risk factors for osteoporosis include smoking, heavy alcohol use, heavy coffee consumption, female gender; especially post-menopause, older age, low body mass, and certain medications; especially long-term corticosteroid therapy. The bone loss associated with certain medications may not be limited to their pharmacologic action, but also be due to the underlying inflammatory disease for which the medications are used. The risk factor, low body mass, may be the result of long-term malabsorption.

Exercise Prevents Osteoporosis

Weight-bearing exercise prevents loss of bone mass density; however, it is not the bearing of weight, but rather the cyclic stimuli of loading and unloading which stimulates the osteoblasts to produce BMP's and other proteins. Standing or lifting weights is not especially effective; however, walking and jogging, in which the weight is applied as a pulsatile stimulus, favors osteoblastic activity. Badminton, with frequent changes in direction, is more effective in building bone mass than the gliding motions of ice hockey[12], and jumping rope is more effective than playing soccer[13].

Even the vibratory shock that occurs during exercise may stimulate an anabolic effect on bone[14]. Mechanical loading of the bones and joints increases the expression of several bone-morphogenetic proteins[15] that promote the deposition of bone. Mechanical loading during exercise may also prevent the formation of osteoclasts that would otherwise be stimulated by IL-1β[16]. Cyclic compressive forces increase activation of RUNX2, a transcription factor for osteoblast differentiation, nevertheless, excessive loads do not[17].

In young animals, exercise at 70% of peak VO2 (Peak oxygen consumption) maximizes bone density, but exercise at 90% of peak VO2 lowers bone density[18]. Treadmill training for 30 minutes a day increases bone density while training for 90 minutes is ineffective[19]. Treadmill training 30 minutes a day, four days a week, builds bone density more than training six days a week[20]. Excessive exercise is associated with microfractures[21].

A link to an online calculator for osteoporosis risk is given in Appendix B. Exercise is an important factor in bone health; still, malabsorption, lack of sufficient vitamin D, vitamin K, and inflammation are the principal risk factors for osteoporosis.

Table 42-1: Medications Associated with Bone Mass Loss[22]

Medication and Associated Disease	Action
Corticosteroids: Inflammatory disorders	Long-term corticosteroid use promotes osteoclastic activity.
Proton pump inhibitors: Peptic ulcer disease	Gastric acid is needed for calcium absorption.
Warfarin: Thrombophlebitis	Prevents recycling of vitamin K.
Anti-epileptics: Seizures	Accelerated vitamin D loss. (Barbiturates, phenytoin).
Thyroxine: Hashimoto's thyroiditis	Overaggressive treatment increases osteoclast activity.
SSRI Medications; Depression	Serotonin may reduce osteoblast activity.
Rosiglitazone: Type 2 diabetes	Increases fat cell formation in the trabecular bone space[23].

Periodontitis

Periodontal disease is an osteoinflammatory condition, in which there is a progressive loss of the alveolar bone which surrounds the teeth, followed by loosening of the teeth, and when severe, results in the loss of the teeth. Periodontal disease is common in the U.S; 31 percent have mild disease, 13 percent moderate, and four percent of the population has advanced periodontal disease[24]. This disease has a high comorbidity with diabetes, coronary artery disease, aortic aneurysms[25], and rheumatoid arthritis[26]. Individuals with high antibody levels to one of the common periodontal pathogens, A. actinomycetemcomitans, are 7.5 times more likely to have coronary artery disease (CAD) than those with low antibody levels[27]. This, however, does not prove that periodontal disease causes CAD but does point to a shared etiology.

Periodontitis is a polymicrobial disease. Biofilm formation, in the form of dental plaque, is associated with the production of LPS, a major component of the outer membrane of gram-negative bacteria. In response to LPS, fibroblasts in the periodontal ligaments (PDL) produce excessive metalloproteinase-8 (MMP-8). MMP-8 is the same protein as neutrophil collagenase.

MMPs are important proteolytic enzymes active in inflammation and tissue repair. MMPs degrade extracellular proteins, including collagen, proteoglycans, elastin, and laminins. There are about 23 human MMPs, which degrade various proteins. MMP- 1, 2, 8, 9, and 13 degrade the triple-helical collagen fibers present in bone, dentin, and cartilage. MMP- 2 and 9 can also degrade Type 4 collagen, and these are referred to as collagenases. MMP- 3, 10, and 11 are stromelysins that can degrade extracellular matrix proteins. The MMPs can be induced by TNF. There are four "tissue inhibitors of metalloproteinases" (TIMPs) which block MMP activity.

In addition to digesting type 1 collagen, MMP-8 activates chemokines that draw white blood cells to the area and cleave other proteins; some into metabolically active toxins and other products[10]. Other MMPs are also elevated in periodontitis; however, MMP-8 predominates.

A bacterial pathogen important in periodontal disease is *Porphyromonas gingivalis*. *P. gingivalis* produces endotoxins that elicit the production of TNF-α from macrophages[28] and IL-6[29] from fibroblasts through the activation of TLR-2 and TLR-4. Smoking tobacco raises the risk of periodontal disease by augmenting *P. gingivalis* biofilm formation[30].

In health, the periodontal ligament (PDL) fibroblasts supply cytokines that participate in communication between cells in order to maintain a balance in osteoblast and osteoclast activity essential for remodeling and growth[31]. Movement of the teeth is required during the growth period in youth, and to maintain proper occlusion throughout life.

In both normal and pathological conditions, TNF-α induces production of NF-κB, which activates osteoclasts. The osteoclasts and their products degrade the alveolar bone and detach the periodontal ligament. OPG inhibits this activity of TNF-α. As in osteoporosis, inflammation elicits excessive production of TNF-α, IL-1β, and other inflammatory cytokines, causing the excessive promotion of osteoclasts. When this occurs, as it does in periodontal disease, cytokines induce the degradation of alveolar bones, of PDL and of the roots of the teeth. LPS from anaerobic bacteria, particularly *P. gingivalis,* elicit this inflammatory response.

Anti-inflammatory cytokines, such as IL-12, IL-18, IL-33 and IFN, decrease osteoclast activity and increase osteoblast activity; stimulating new bone and periodontal ligament formation. When the activity of the osteoblasts and osteoclasts are in balanced, the dentition can respond to the forces of eating and fine-tune their positioning.

Orthodontics

Although orthodontic treatment is not a disease entity, it is a process demanding remodeling and repair of the alveolar bone and periodontal ligaments. There are several common problems faced in orthodontic treatment. The first is dental caries and periodontal inflammation; risk increases because cleaning of the teeth becomes more difficult with braces. Additionally, softer foods, which adhere to the teeth, are eaten to prevent brackets, cemented to the teeth, from being sheared off, adding to the cariogenic risk. The braces also trap food particles and prevent their removal by the tongue.

The second common problem is resorption of the tooth roots. Five to 18 percent of orthodontic patients suffer severe root resorption, and as many as 30 percent lose 3 mm of root in at least one tooth[32]. Among teeth, 56 percent of upper lateral incisors have root shortening, and 94 percent of patients have shortening of at least 1 mm in at least one tooth[33]. The distance the tooth is moved, length of treatment, premolar extraction and continuous rather than intermittent movement, all increase root resorption[34].

A third, nearly ubiquitous, adverse outcome, is a lack of retention; the tendency of teeth to return to their pre-treatment positions. This problem is worsened by resorption of root mass and loss of alveolar bone. Post-treatment tooth mobility can also occur, wherein the teeth lack stability.

The process of moving teeth involves placing unequal pressure on the dental ligaments. As the teeth are pulled, the ligaments are stretched on the apposition-side and compressed towards the bone on the resorption-side.

There are fibroblasts residing among the periodontal ligaments (PDL). The forces applied during treatment cause deformation of these cells. Stretch or compression of the PDL deforms the fibroblast, and these forces elicit the expression of various genes according to the force. In both tension and compression, there is increased production of metalloproteinase enzymes, particularly MMP-8.

Compression of PDL fibroblasts induces COX-2, M-CSF, MMP-1, and RANKL. COX2 increases PGE2 production, which induces NF-κB activation. Compression also decreases the production of OPG[35] and increases production of RANKL[36]. Compression increases the presence of chemokines[37] that draw white blood cells to the area and induce the differentiation of monocytes into osteoclasts. Intrusion of the teeth (compression) causes root resorption, while extrusion does not[38].

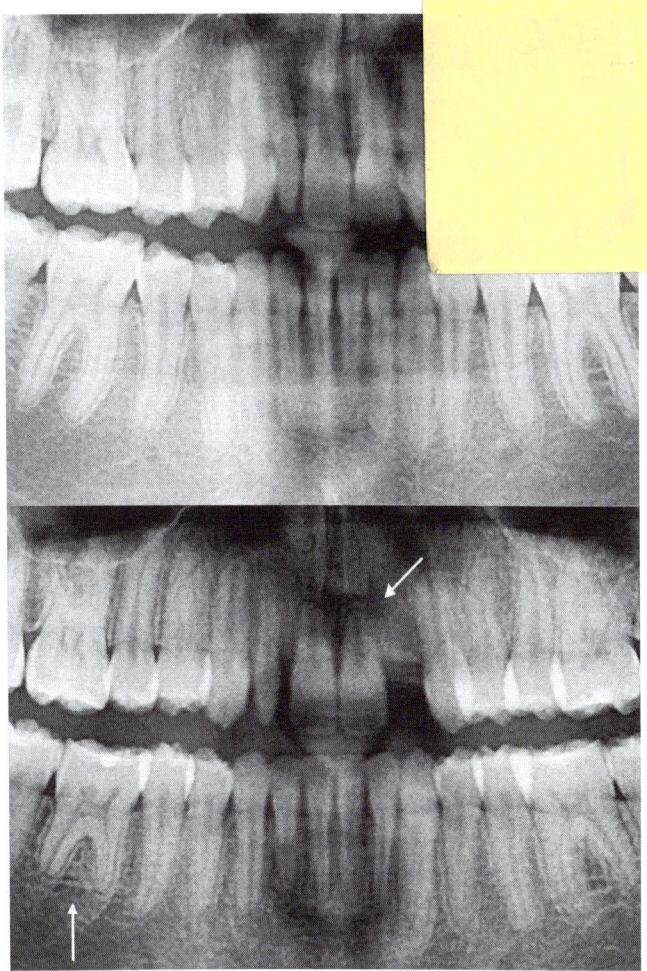

Figure 42-2: Root resorption: before (top) and after orthodontic treatment (below)[39].

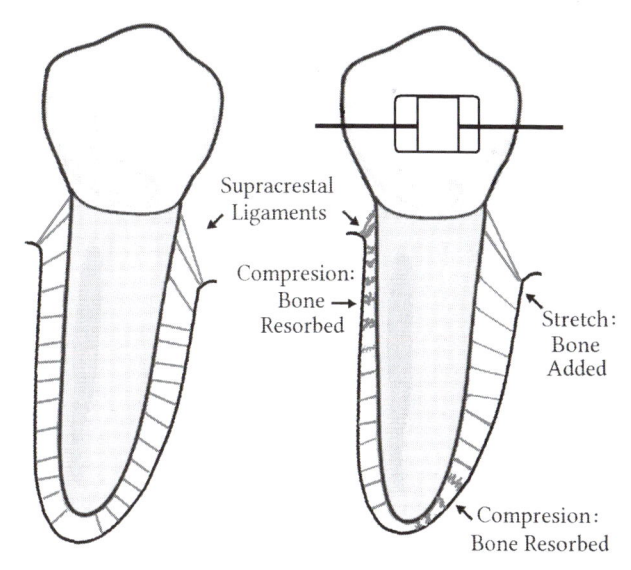

Figure 42-3: Periodontal ligaments prior to treatment on left, and under orthodontic stress on the right.

Tensile force, stretching the fibroblasts, increases the expression of IL-10, OPG, osteocalcin, and TIMP-1[40]. TIMP-1 limits bone resorption by inhibiting MMP's. Stretching the fibroblasts also increases TGF-β[41], thereby decreasing the formation of osteoclasts and increasing the formation of osteoblasts from osteoprogenitor cells.

The tensile and compressive forces promote remodeling of the alveolar bone, with the removal of bone on the compression side and deposition of new bone on the tension side of the tooth. Additionally there is remodeling of the PDL ligaments, at least on the compression side.

Medications and Tooth Movement: Several medications impact the rate of tooth movement during orthodontic treatment. Thyroxin and sustained corticosteroid therapy increase tooth movement by increasing osteoclast activity. These medications are also associated with risk for osteoporosis (Table 42-1).While these medications increase movement of the teeth, there is an increased loss of bone and tooth mass. Vitamin D_3 also facilitates tooth movement[42] and alveolar bone remodeling; it, in contrast, is associated with improved bone mass.

Non-steroidal anti-inflammatory medications slow orthodontic tooth movement, as do bisphosphonates. NSAIDs likely act through the induction of PPAR-γ that prevents activation of NF-κB, and thus, the transcription of inflammatory cytokines.

Orthodontic Retention

Larger tooth movements involving angulation and tooth rotation are at higher risk of regression towards their original position after the completion of orthodontic treatment. This may indicate that the stretched, appositional ligaments, especially the supracrestal ligaments that are not covered with bone, are not replaced during orthodontic treatment. In tooth rotation, it can be understood that there is a tensile force, but little, if any, compressive force. Periodontal ligaments remain stretched and displaced for *at least* seven months after the cessation of orthodontic tooth movement[43]. If these ligaments persist, and there is bone loss subsequent to treatment, as a result of periodontal inflammation or even from normal bone renewal, it allows the teeth to return to their original positions. Circumferential supracrestal fiberotomy, a technique in which the periodontal ligaments above the bone are cut, improves orthodontic retention[44].

The jaw continues to grow into the mid-20's in the area of the lower incisors. This causes loss of orthodontic treatment retention. Movement of the lower incisors after orthodontic treatment occurs in 70 to 90 percent of patients[45]. Orthodontic patients require the use of a retention device, such as a retainer, for at least a year after removal of the braces, and many patients use retainers indefinitely. This is particularly evident in younger patients and for the lower incisors.

Tooth root resorption and loss of alveolar bone support are important risk factors for lack of orthodontic retention[46]. Apical root resorption and alveolar bone loss are common in orthodontic treatment[47]. Root length and health of the periodontal bone and ligaments are also highly correlated to tooth stability and lack of tooth mobility, which can occur years after orthodontic treatment[48].

Root Resorption and Alveolar Bone Loss

Critical to preventing poor outcomes in orthodontic treatment is avoiding the joint effects of inflammation and compression during treatment. COX2 gene expression increases 56-fold, and the RANKL/osteoprotegerin gene expression ratio is 50 times higher when compressive forces and bacterial endotoxins are combined[49]. Thus, even very low levels of periodontal inflammation during orthodontic treatment can synergistically promote excess bone loss and tooth resorption.

Osteoclastic activity may reduce retention, even years after orthodontic treatment if the appositional supracrestal ligaments are retained. Thus, avoidance of LPS and the formation of inflammatory cytokines in the periodontal area, especially in the first years following treatment, is essential for retention. Loss of retention may be prevented in the same ways that periodontitis and osteoporosis can be prevented.

Preventive Treatment for Osteoimmune Disease

Doxycycline: Subantimicrobial-dose doxycycline (SDD) is useful in the treatment of periodontal disease[50,51]. SDD blocks TLR-2 activation of transcription factors AP-1 and C/EBP in neutrophils[52], thus inhibiting the expression of IL-6, IL-8, IL-13, and G-CSF (Figure 42-4). Inhibition of the chemokine IL-8 decreases migration of WBC's, particularly neutrophils, and thus, prevents the production of MMP-8 in the area. Doxycycline, at 100 mg/day, also mitigates inflammatory-mediated aortic aneurysm associated with TLR-2 activation[53], which can be caused by *P. gingivalis*[54]. This mechanism may also explain the anti-inflammatory effect of minocycline, which crosses the blood-brain barrier, on acne, schizophrenia[55], post-herpetic neuralgia[56], multiple sclerosis[57], traumatic brain[58] and spinal cord[59] injuries and rheumatoid arthritis[60]. SDD may help stabilize teeth after the completion of orthodontic movement. SDD may have benefit in other inflammatory diseases activated through TLR-2. (See Table 42-4)

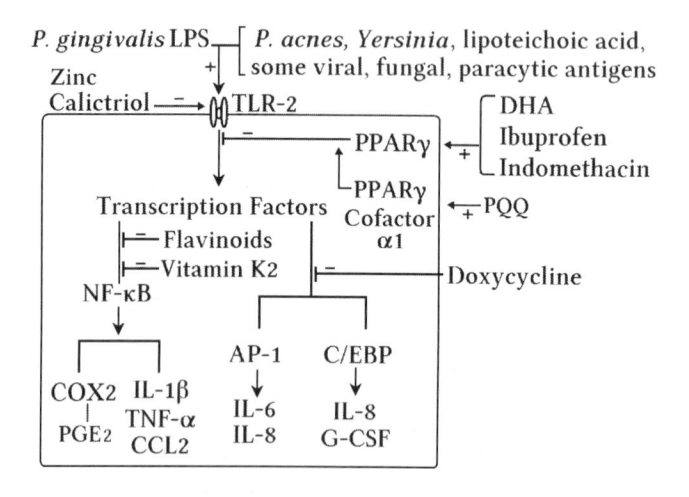

Figure 42-4: TLR-2 activation and inhibition.

Antibiotics: Topical antibiotics, such as metronidazole and chlorhexidine, also have been found useful in the treatment of periodontal disease[61]. Systemic metronidazole has also been shown to be effective[62]. Metronidazole is an antibiotic, specifically active against anaerobic bacteria, which produce LPS. Metronidazole is more effective than most antibiotics for this use, as bacterial resistance develops less readily to it than to most other antibiotics.

Phenolic Compounds: Several studies have shown that the phenolic compounds, flavonoids, exert anti-inflammatory and antibacterial effects in periodontitis. Epigallocatechin-3-gallate, which is found in green tea, prevents the increases in IL-1β, IL-6, TNF-α, RANKL associated with exposure to *P. gingivalis* LPS[63]. The non-flavonoid polyphenols curcumin and resveratrol also inhibit the formation of inflammatory cytokines in the presence of *P. gingivalis*[64, 65]. P-hydroxycinnamic acid promotes calcification of bones and inhibits osteoclast differentiation, by limiting NF-κB activity[66].

Numerous phenolic plant compounds inhibit TNF-α activity. Table 31-2 lists various phenolic compounds that inhibit TNF-α and shows food which are rich in them.

N-3 Fatty Acids: Diets high in n-3 fatty acids prevent alveolar bone loss in animals inoculated with *P. gingivalis*[67]. The n-3 fats DHA and EPA are associated with less expression of the genes for IL-1β, IL-6 and COX2, and higher expression of genes for the antioxidant enzymes catalase and superoxide dismutase, in animals infected with *P. gingivalis*[68].

Vitamin D$_3$: Vitamin D$_3$ lowers serum TNF-α levels, preventing alveolar bone loss. It also down-regulates TLR-4, attenuating the expression of NF-κB and the phosphorylation of Janus family kinase-1 (JAK1) in diabetic periodontitis in animals[69,70]. Vitamin D3 also decreases expression of TLR-2[71].

Bisphosphonates: Bisphosphonates, used for the treatment of osteoporosis, are also effective in slowing the bone loss in periodontal disease. They, however, are associated with a risk of osteonecrosis of the jaw, especially when used as injected medications[72]. Dietary phytates act similarly to bisphosphonates but are not associated with osteonecrosis risk.

Phytate: Phytate is a phosphorus storage compound found in seeds. It binds to zinc, iron, calcium, and magnesium, and thus, prevents absorption of these metal ions from the intestine. In 1949, a study demonstrated that a high phytate diet in puppies resulted in rickets. It was long thought that phytic acid would thus impart risk for osteoporosis. However, recent studies have shown the inverse. Phytic acid in the urine, which correlates with its dietary consumption, is associated with increased bone mass[73]. Dietary phytic acid appears to prevent osteoporosis by inhibiting dissolution of mineralized bone by acid, similar to the mechanism of action for bisphosphonate medications.

Table 42-2 Foods High in Phytates

Tree Nuts:	Legumes:
Almonds	Peanuts
Brazil Nuts	Beans
Walnuts	Soy
Hazelnuts	Tofu
Grains:	Sesame seeds
Brown Rice	Spinach
Wheat (especially bran)	
Oats	

Xylitol: The alcohol sugar xylitol has an antibacterial effect and decreases the production of LPS and IL-1 and TNF-α gene expression in cell culture with P gingivalis[74]. (See Chapter 5.) It may thus be helpful in preventing progression of periodontal disease.

Dental Hygiene: Dental hygiene, including brushing and flossing, can prevent periodontal disease by preventing and treating biofilm (plaque) formation. Although flossing and interdental brushing[75] are helpful, their efficacy is compromised by limited compliance and ineffective technique, such that, in a general population, they provide no statistical benefit[76]. Oral irrigation using a water jet, such as the Waterpik™, while not effective in removing visible plaque, is more effective than flossing in preventing periodontal inflammation[77]. Adolescents with orthodontic braces using water jets formed less plaque and had less bleeding[78]. The benefits provided by water jets likely results through inhibition of biofilm activity, by flushing or diluting quorum sensing agents and endotoxins.

Rotation-oscillation action powered toothbrushes are more effective than manual toothbrushes in removing plaque and preventing bleeding and gingivitis[79] and are more effective than manual brushing plus flossing[80]. However, manual toothbrushes are probably just as effective as powered ones when proper brushing technique is used[81].

Since oral hygiene using manual brushes and flossing is often inadequate, the use of rotation-oscillation action powered toothbrushes and water jets should be encouraged in patients with periodontal disease and those undergoing orthodontic treatment. Effective flossing can be obstructed by braces and other orthodontic devices. It may be counter-productive to teach flossing rather than encouraging the use of water jets when they are accessible.

Summary

1. Osteoclast/Osteoblast Balance: Bone and dental health depend on having a balance of osteoblastic and osteoclastic activity. In health, osteoblasts control the activity of the osteoclasts; however, osteoclastic activity is escalated in inflammation. Osteoclastic activity is mediated mainly by transcription factors for inflammatory cytokines, chemokines, and cell growth factors. Agents which reduce NF-κB, AP-1, C/EBP and other inflammatory transcription factors can prevent osteoclastic differentiation and activity, raise OPG levels and help preserve bone mass, increase orthodontic retention, and reduce tooth root resorption.

Many bacterial products surface antigens are recognized by Toll-like receptors on immune cells. TLR binding with these antigens triggers an inflammatory cascade via NF-κB activation and the transcription of inflammatory mediators, and by preventing apoptosis of inflammatory cells and osteoclasts.

TLR-4 is activated by LPS from the cell walls of most anaerobic gram-negative bacteria. Many opiates are also TRL-4 agonists. Naloxone, however, is a TLR-4 antagonist. Some tricyclic medications, such as amitriptyline, have TLR-4 antagonistic effects. A list of bacterial and viral agents that activate TLR-2 and TLR-4 are given in Table 42-3.

Table 42-3: TLR-2 and TLR-4 Activators

Lipoteichoic acid from:
- Gram-positive bacteria cell walls

Atypical LPS from:
- *Porphyromonas gingivalis* (Periodontitis, CAD)
- *Leptospirosis*

Bacterial Agonists from:
- *Chlamydophila pneumoniae*
- *Borrelia burgdorferi* (Lyme disease)
- *Neisseria meningitidis*
- *Haemophilus influenzae*
- *Propionibacterium acnes* (Acne)
- *Yersinia* (Irritable Bowel Syndrome)
- *Mycobacterium tuberculosis*

Parasite Agonist from:
- *Schistosoma mansoni*
- *Leishmania major*
- *Plasmodium falciparum*

Fungal Agonist from:
- *Saccharomyces cerevisiae*
- *Aspergillus fumigatus*
- *Candida albicans*

Viral Agonist from:
- *Herpes simplex*
- *Varicella zoster*
- *Cytomegalovirus*
- *Measles*

2. Osteoporosis as enteroimmunopathy: The diagnosis of osteopenia and osteoporosis should include prompt an investigation of enteroimmune disease. Loss of bone density is a common result of malabsorption and inflammation. Failure to treat the underlying pathology of the bone loss limits the chances for successful treatment.

3. Phenolic Compounds: Phenolic compounds from many plant sources inhibit NF-κB activity induced by TNF-α. These effects are not limited to periodontal disease, but also have this effect on osteoclasts in the bone. A diet high in phenolic compounds is recommended.

Table 42-4: Agents that down-regulate Osteoclast Activity

Agent	Mechanism of Action
Vitamin D	Down regulates TLR-2 and TLR-4, decreases parathyroid hormone-induced bone resorption.
Vitamin K	Protects osteoprotegerin production. Inhibits NF-κB activation, thus increasing apoptosis of excess osteoclasts.
Boron	Inhibits NF-κB activation.
DHA	Induced PPAR-γ, which prevents activation of NF-κB.
Plant phenolic compounds	Inhibit NF-κB and production of inflammatory cytokines (Table 31-2).
Betaine	Down regulates TLR-4.
NSAIDs	Induced PPAR-γ. Only certain NSAIDs have this effect. (Chapter 31)
PQQ	PPAR-γ cofactor.
α-Lipoic acid	Decreases transcription of TLR2[82].
Zinc	Decreases transcription of TLR2[83].
N-Acetylcysteine	Forms glutathione, which prevents mechanical stress induced SIRT-1 mediated increases in TLR-2 and TLR-4 from PDL fibroblasts[84].
Doxycycline, Minocycline	Inhibits Inflammatory transcription factors AP-1 and C/EPB. Prevents neutrophil chemotaxis.
Metronidazole	Antibiotic prevents LPS formation, which induces NF-κB through TLR-2 and TLR-4.

4. Vitamin K: MK-4 is beneficial in the treatment of osteoporosis. In comparison, other forms of vitamin K, such as vitamin K$_1$ and MK-7, have not been shown to be as effective. In contrast to vitamin K$_1$, vitamin K$_2$ does not require bile for absorption. This makes the MK-4 form of vitamin K$_2$ most appropriate for treatment of osteopenia in patients with malabsorption syndromes. A recommended dose for menaquinone-4 is 5 to 10 mg/day. Other than patients taking warfarin for clotting disorders, vitamin K$_2$ should be considered in the treatment of loss of bone mass, in the treatment of periodontal disease, and for orthodontic patients.

5. Vitamin D$_3$: Vitamin D supplementation should be considered for treatment of patients with osteopenia, osteoporosis, orthodontic patients, patients with malabsorption syndromes, patients with periodontal disease, and for most adults living in temperate climates. A reasonable daily dose for most adults is 5000 IU of vitamin D$_3$. Vitamin D dosage is discussed in Chapter 20.

6. Calcium: Calcium supplements of about 800 mg per day are recommended for the treatment and prevention of osteoporosis and for the treatment of periodontitis.

7. Magnesium: Magnesium deficiency is much more common than is calcium deficiency in the Western diet and is associated with continued inflammation and the lack repair activity after inflammation. Magnesium is also lost in malabsorption syndromes.

Dietary magnesium is found in green leafy vegetables, and seeds such as legumes, nuts and whole grains. Magnesium is discussed in Chapter 30.

8: Dental Hygiene: Biofilm, in the form of plaque, should be prevented using brushing, flossing, and water jet irrigation. Individuals with periodontal disease should be encouraged to use a dental water jet, and those with orthodontia to use a water jet with an orthodontic tip[85]. Use of water jets inhibits biofilm formation and inflammation, which can result in resorption of the roots and poor long-term outcome of treatment. Flossing is especially cumbersome with braces and has too poor compliance in the setting of orthodontics to merit recommendation. Use of rotation-oscillation action powered toothbrushes should be encouraged when brushing technique is inadequate.

8. Antioxidants: The antioxidant glutathione, and its precursor N-acetyl cysteine, decrease alveolar bone loss and likely prevent the loss of tooth root mass and osteoporosis from osteoclastic activity.

9. Exercise: Activity stimulates osteoblastic activity. It is not weight bearing, but cyclic loading and unloading that stimulates bone deposition and remodeling. It is the pressure created during biting and chewing that naturally remodels dental occlusion. Excessive exercise, however, causes microfractures and decreases bone mass, compared to more moderate exercise. Thirty minutes of vigorous exercise three to four times a week is recommended to maximize bone density.

10: Antibiotics: Antibiotics that block the production of LPS are useful the treatment of severe periodontitis but are not relevant to prevention. Bacterial toxins activate TLR-2 and TLR-4, increasing the production of inflammatory mediators. LPS production by enteric bacteria may promote osteoporosis in this way. Prevention of biofilm in the gut may reduce the risk of osteoporosis.

[1] SEM Micrograph: James Weaver and Paul Hansma, UCSB

[2] . Sasaki N, Kusano E, Takahashi H, Ando Y, Yano K, Tsuda E, Asano Y. J Bone Miner Metab. 2005;23(1):41-7. PMID:15616893

[3] Endogenous TNF-alpha lowers maximum peak bone mass and inhibits osteoblastic Smad activation through NF-kappaB. Li Y, Li A, Strait K et al. J Bone Miner Res. 2007 May;22(5):646-55. Erratum in: J Bone Miner Res. 2007 Jun;22(6):949. PMID:17266397

[4] Vitamin K2 stimulates osteoblastogenesis and suppresses osteoclastogenesis by suppressing NF-κB activation. Yamaguchi M, Weitzmann MN. Int J Mol Med. 2011 Jan;27(1):3-14. PMID:21072493

[5] Effects of inflammatory and anti-inflammatory cytokines on the bone. Schett G. Eur J Clin Invest. 2011 Dec;41(12):1361-6. PMID:21615394

[6] Patient level pooled analysis of 68 500 patients from seven major vitamin D fracture trials in US and Europe. DIPART (Vitamin D Individual Patient Analysis of Randomized Trials) Group. BMJ. 2010 Jan 12;340:b5463 PMID: 20068257

[7] Estimation of optimal serum concentrations of 25-hydroxyvitamin D for multiple health outcomes. Bischoff-Ferrari HA, Giovannucci E, Willett WC, Dietrich T, Dawson-Hughes B. Am J Clin Nutr. 2006 Jul;84(1):18-28. PMID: 16825677

[8] Dietary Supplements and Mortality Rate in Older Women: The Iowa Women's Health Study. Mursu J, Robien K, Harnack LJ, et al. Arch Intern Med. 2011 Oct 10;171(18):1625-33. PMID:21987192

[9] Effects of boron and calcium supplementation on mechanical properties of bone in rats. Naghii MR, Torkaman G, Mofid M. Biofactors. 2006;28(3-4):195-201. PMID:17473380

[10] Evidence that boron down-regulates inflammation through the NF-KB pathway. Durick, K.A., Tomita, M., Hunt, C., Bradley, D. 2005. The Federation of American Societies for Experimental Biology Journal. 19(5):A1705.

[11] Essentiality of boron for healthy bones and joints. Newnham RE. Environ Health Perspect. 1994 Nov;102 Suppl 7:83-5. PMID:7889887

[12] Type of physical activity, muscle strength, and pubertal stage as determinants of bone mineral density and bone area in adolescent boys. Nordström P, Pettersson U, Lorentzon R. J Bone Miner Res. 1998 Jul;13(7):1141-8. PMID:9661078

[13] Effect of high impact activity on bone mass and size in adolescent females: A comparative study between two different types of sports. Pettersson U, Nordström P, Alfredson H, et al. Calcif Tissue Int. 2000 Sep;67(3):207-14. PMID:10954774

[14] Low-level accelerations applied in the absence of weight bearing can enhance trabecular bone formation. Garman R, Gaudette G, Donahue LR, Rubin C, Judex S. J Orthop Res. 2007 Jun;25(6):732-40. PMID:17318899

[15] Dynamic regulation of bone morphogenetic proteins in engineered osteochondral constructs by biomechanical stimulation. Nam J, Perera P, Rath B, Agarwal S. Tissue Eng Part A. 2013 Mar;19(5-6):783-92. PMID:23198877

[16] Mechanical loading prevents the stimulating effect of IL-1β on osteocyte-modulated osteoclastogenesis. Kulkarni RN, Bakker AD, Everts V, Klein-Nulend J. Biochem Biophys Res Commun. 2012 Mar 30;420(1):11-6. PMID:22390927

[17] Compressive forces induce osteogenic gene expression in calvarial osteoblasts. Rath B, Nam J, Knobloch TJ, Lannutti JJ, Agarwal S. J Biomech. 2008;41(5):1095-103. PMID:18191137

[18] Different strength intermittent treadmill training of growth period rats and related bone metabolism of the hormone influence. Xie SC, Ma XJ, Guo CJ, eta l. 2012 May;28(3):271-4. PMID:22860434

[19] Running exercise for short duration increases bone mineral density of loaded long bones in young growing rats. Hagihara Y, Nakajima A, Fukuda S, Goto S, Iida H, Yamazaki M. Tohoku J Exp Med. 2009 Oct;219(2):139-43. PMID:19776531

[20] How many days per week should rats undergo running exercise to increase BMD? Hagihara Y, Fukuda S, Goto S, Iida H, et al. J Bone Miner Metab. 2005;23(4):289-94. PMID:15981024

[21] The effects of 10 weeks military training on heel ultrasound and bone turnover. Etherington J, Keeling J, Bramley R, et al. Calcif Tissue Int. 1999 May;64(5):389-93. PMID:10203415

[22] Update on medications with adverse skeletal effects. Pitts CJ, Kearns AE. Mayo Clin Proc. 2011 Apr;86(4):338-43. PMID:21389249

[23] The skeletal effects of thiazolidinedione and metformin on insulin-resistant mice. Wang C, Li H, Chen SG, et al. J Bone Miner Metab. 2012 Nov;30(6):630-7. PMID:22886403

[24] Host-response therapeutics for periodontal diseases. Giannobile WV. J Periodontol. 2008 Aug;79(8 Suppl):1592-600. PMID:18673015

[25] Toll-Like Receptor-2 Plays a Fundamental Role in Periodontal Bacteria-Accelerated Abdominal Aortic Aneurysms. Aoyama N, Suzuki JI, Ogawa M, et al. Circ J. 2013 Feb 13. PMID:23412709

[26] Rheumatoid arthritis and periodontitis - inflammatory and infectious connections. Review of the literature. Rutger Persson G. J Oral Microbiol. 2012;4. PMID:22347541

[27] A common periodontal pathogen has an adverse association with both acute and stable coronary artery disease. Hyvärinen K, Mäntylä P, Buhlin K, Paju S, Nieminen MS, Sinisalo J, Pussinen PJ. Atherosclerosis. 2012 Aug;223(2):478-84. PMID:22704805

[28] Macrophage-Specific TLR2 Signaling Mediates Pathogen-Induced TNF-Dependent Inflammatory Oral Bone Loss. Papadopoulos G, Weinberg EO, Massari P, et al. J Immunol. 2013 Feb 1;190(3):1148-57. PMID:23264656

[29] Stimulation of IL-6 cytokines in fibroblasts by toll-like receptors 2. Souza PP, Palmqvist P, Lundgren I, et al. J Dent Res. 2010 Aug;89(8):802-7. PMID:20505053

[30] Tobacco upregulates P. gingivalis fimbrial proteins which induce TLR2 hyposensitivity. Bagaitkar J, Demuth DR, Daep CA, et al. PLoS One. 2010 May 4;5(5):e9323. PMID:20454607

[31] Effect of metronidazole and modulation of cytokine production on human periodontal ligament cells. Rizzo A, Paolillo R, Guida L, Annunziata M, Bevilacqua N, Tufano MA. Int Immunopharmacol. 2010 Jul;10(7):744-50 PMID:20399284

[32] Biomechanical aspects of external root resorption in orthodontic therapy. Abuabara A. Med Oral Patol Oral Cir Bucal. 2007 Dec 1;12(8):E610-3. PMID:18059250

[33] Apical root resorption during orthodontic treatment. A prospective study using cone beam CT. Lund H, Gröndahl K, Hansen K, Gröndahl HG. Angle Orthod. 2012 May;82(3):480-7. PMID:21919826

[34] Orthodontic and nonorthodontic root resorption: their impact on clinical dental practice. Kokich VG. J Dent Educ. 2008 Aug;72(8):895-902. PMID:18676798

[35] Compressive force induces osteoclast differentiation via prostaglandin E(2) production in MC3T3-E1 cells. Sanuki R, Shionome C, Kuwabara A, et al. Connect Tissue Res. 2010 Apr;51(2):150-8. PMID:20001844

[36] Levels of RANKL and OPG in gingival crevicular fluid during orthodontic tooth movement and effect of compression force on releases from periodontal ligament cells in vitro. Nishijima Y, Yamaguchi M, Kojima T, Aihara N, Nakajima R, Kasai K. Orthod Craniofac Res. 2006 May;9(2):63-70. PMID:16764680

[37] Differential expression of osteoblast and osteoclast chemoattractants in compression and tension sides during orthodontic movement. Garlet TP, Coelho U, Repeke CE, et al. Cytokine. 2008 Jun;42(3):330-5. PMID:18406624

[38] Root resorption after orthodontic intrusion and extrusion: an intraindividual study. Han G, Huang S, Von den Hoff JW, Zeng X, Kuijpers-Jagtman AM. Angle Orthod. 2005 Nov;75(6):912-8. PMID:16448231

[39] Dental x-rays courtesy of Dr. Lucas Stephens, D.O.

[40] Cytokine expression pattern in compression and tension sides of the periodontal ligament during orthodontic tooth movement in humans. Garlet TP, Coelho U, Silva JS, Garlet GP. Eur J Oral Sci. 2007 Oct;115(5):355-62. PMID:17850423

[41] Cyclical tensile force on periodontal ligament cells inhibits osteoclastogenesis through OPG induction. Kanzaki H, Chiba M, Sato A, et al. J Dent Res. 2006 May;85(5):457-62. PMID:16632761

[42] Medication and tooth movement. Kalha AS. Evid Based Dent. 2009;10(2):50-1. PMID:19561581

[43] Clinical and histologic observations on tooth movement during and after orthodontic treatment. Reitan K. Am J Orthod. 1967 Oct;53(10):721-45. PMID:5233926

[44] Orthodontic retention: a systematic review. Littlewood SJ, Millett DT, Doubleday B, Bearn DR, Worthington HV. J Orthod. 2006 Sep;33(3):205-12. PMID:16926314

[45] Retention and relapse. Review of the literature. Kaan M, Madléna M. Fogorv Sz. 2011 Dec;104(4):139-46. PMID:22308954

[46] Orthodontic relapse, apical root resorption, and crestal alveolar bone levels. Sharpe W, Reed B, Subtelny JD, Polson A. Am J Orthod Dentofacial Orthop. 1987 Mar;91(3):252-8. PMID:3469910

[47] Prevalence and severity of apical root resorption and alveolar bone loss in orthodontically treated adults. Lupi JE, Handelman CS, Sadowsky C. Am J Orthod Dentofacial Orthop. 1996 Jan;109(1):28-37. PMID:8540480

[48] Long-term follow-up of tooth mobility in maxillary incisors with orthodontically induced apical root resorption. Jönsson A, Malmgren O, Levander E. Eur J Orthod. 2007 Oct;29(5):482-7. PMID:17974537

[49] Endotoxins potentiate COX-2 and RANKL expression in compressed PDL cells. Römer P, Köstler J, Koretsi V, Proff P. Clin Oral Investig. 2013 Feb 8. PMID:23392729

[50] Clinical studies on the management of periodontal diseases utilizing subantimicrobial dose doxycycline (SDD). Caton J, Ryan ME. Pharmacol Res. 2011 Feb;63(2):114-20. PMID:21182947

[51] Host-response therapeutics for periodontal diseases. Giannobile WV. J Periodontol. 2008 Aug;79(8 Suppl):1592-600. PMID:18673015

[52] Toll-Like Receptor-2 Plays a Fundamental Role in Periodontal Bacteria-Accelerated Abdominal Aortic Aneurysms. Aoyama N, Suzuki JI, Ogawa M, et al. Circ J. 2013 Feb 13. PMID:23412709

[53] Clinical trial of doxycycline for matrix metalloproteinase-9 inhibition in patients with an abdominal aneurysm: doxycycline selectively depletes aortic wall neutrophils and cytotoxic T cells. Lindeman JH, Abdul-Hussien H, van Bockel JH, et al. Circulation. 2009 Apr 28;119(16):2209-16. PMID:19364980

[54] Porphyromonas gingivalis promotes neointimal formation after arterial injury through toll-like receptor 2 signaling. Kobayashi N, Suzuki JI, Ogawa M, Aoyama N, Komuro I, Izumi Y, Isobe M. Heart Vessels. 2013 Sep 4. PMID:24002697

[55] Minocycline benefits negative symptoms in early schizophrenia: a randomised double-blind placebo-controlled clinical trial in patients on standard treatment. Chaudhry IB, Hallak J, Husain N, et al. Psychopharmacol. 2012 Sep;26(9):1185-93. PMID:22526685

[56] Minocycline may attenuate postherpetic neuralgia. Zhang Q, Peng L, Zhang D. Med Hypotheses. 2009 Nov;73(5):744-5. PMID:19467572

[57] The clinical response to minocycline in multiple sclerosis is accompanied by beneficial immune changes: a pilot study. Zabad RK, Metz LM, Todoruk TR, et al. Mult Scler. 2007 May;13(4):517-26. PMID:17463074

[58] Acute minocycline treatment mitigates the symptoms of mild blast-induced traumatic brain injury. Kovesdi E, Kamnaksh A, Wingo D, et al. Front Neurol. 2012 Jul 16;3:111. PMID:22811676

[59] Results of a phase II placebo-controlled randomized trial of minocycline in acute spinal cord injury. Casha S, Zygun D, McGowan MD, Bains I, Yong VW, Hurlbert RJ. Brain. 2012 Apr;135(Pt 4):1224-36. PMID:2250563

[60] Minocycline and doxycycline therapy in community patients with rheumatoid arthritis: prescribing patterns, patient-level determinants of use, and patient-reported side effects. Christopher J Smith, Harlan Sayles, Ted R Mikuls, Kaleb Michaud Arthritis Res Ther. 2011; 13(5): R168. PMID:22008667

[61] Efficacy of chlorhexidine, metronidazole and combination gel in the treatment of gingivitis--a randomized clinical trial. Pradeep AR, Kumari M, Priyanka N, Naik SB. J Int Acad Periodontol. 2012 Oct;14(4):91-6. PMID:23210197

[62] Mechanisms of action of systemic antibiotics used in periodontal treatment and mechanisms of bacterial resistance to

these drugs. Soares GM, Figueiredo LC, Faveri M, et al. J Appl Oral Sci. 2012 May-Jun;20(3):295-309. PMID:22858695

[63] Anti-inflammatory effect of (-)-epigallocatechin-3-gallate on Porphyromonas gingivalis lipopolysaccharide-stimulated fibroblasts and stem cells derived from human periodontal ligament. Jung IH, Lee DE, Yun JH, et al. J Periodontal Implant Sci. 2012 Dec;42(6):185-95. PMID:23346461

[64] Anti-inflammatory activity of curcumin in macrophages stimulated by lipopolysaccharides from Porphyromonas gingivalis. Chen D, Nie M, Fan MW, Bian Z. Pharmacology. 2008;82(4):264-9. PMID:18849645

[65] Effect of resveratrol and modulation of cytokine production on human periodontal ligament cells. Rizzo A, Bevilacqua N, Guida L, et al. Cytokine. 2012 Oct;60(1):197-204. PMID:22749236

[66] The bone anabolic carotenoid p-hydroxycinnamic acid promotes osteoblast mineralization and suppresses osteoclast differentiation by antagonizing NF-κB activation. Yamaguchi M, Weitzmann MN. Int J Mol Med. 2012 Sep;30(3):708-12. PMID:22751682

[67] Omega-3 fatty acid effect on alveolar bone loss in rats. Kesavalu L, Vasudevan B, Raghu B, et al. J Dent Res. 2006 Jul;85(7):648-52. PMID: 16798867

[68] Omega-3 fatty acid regulates inflammatory cytokine/mediator messenger RNA expression in Porphyromonas gingivalis-induced experimental periodontal disease. Kesavalu L, Bakthavatchalu V, Rahman MM, et al. Oral Microbiol Immunol. 2007 Aug;22(4):232-9. PMID:17600534

[69] 25-hydroxyvitamin D(3) ameliorates periodontitis by modulating the expression of inflammation-associated factors in diabetic mice. Li H, Xie H, Fu M, et al. Steroids. 2013 Feb;78(2):115-20. PMID:23138030

[70] 25-Hydroxyvitamin D(3) attenuates experimental periodontitis through downregulation of TLR4 and JAK1/STAT3 signaling in diabetic mice. Wang Q, Li H, Xie H, et al. J Steroid Biochem Mol Biol. 2013 Jan 18;135C:43-50. PMID:23333931

[71] 1-alpha-calcidol modulates major human monocyte antigens and toll-like receptors TLR 2 and TLR4 in vitro. Scherberich JE, Kellermeyer M, Ried C, Hartinger A. Eur J Med Res. 2005 Apr 20;10(4):179-82. PMID:15946915

[72] Increased incidence of osteonecrosis of the jaw after tooth extraction in patients treated with bisphosphonates: a cohort study. Yamazaki T, Yamori M, Ishizaki T, et al. Int J Oral Maxillofac Surg. 2012 Nov;41(11):1397-403. PMID:22840716

[73] The influence of consumption of phytate on the bone mass in posmenopausal women of Mallorca. López-González AA, Grases F, Marí B, et al. Reumatol Clin. 2011 Jul-Aug;7(4):220-3. PMID:21794821

[74] Xylitol inhibits inflammatory cytokine expression induced by lipopolysaccharide from Porphyromonas gingivalis. Han SJ, Jeong SY, Nam YJ, Yang KH, Lim HS, Chung J. Clin Diagn Lab Immunol. 2005 Nov;12(11):1285-91. PMID:16275942

[75] The efficacy of interdental brushes on plaque and parameters of periodontal inflammation: a systematic review. Slot DE, Dörfer CE, Van der Weijden GA. Int J Dent Hyg. 2008 Nov;6(4):253-64. PMID:19138177

[76] The efficacy of dental floss in addition to a toothbrush on plaque and parameters of gingival inflammation: a systematic review. Berchier CE, Slot DE, Haps S, Van der Weijden GA. Int J Dent Hyg. 2008 Nov;6(4):265-79. PMID:19138178

[77] The efficacy of oral irrigation in addition to a toothbrush on plaque and the clinical parameters of periodontal inflammation: a systematic review. Husseini A, Slot DE, Van der Weijden GA. Int J Dent Hyg. 2008 Nov;6(4):304-14. PMID:1913818

[78] Effect of a dental water jet with orthodontic tip on plaque and bleeding in adolescent patients with fixed orthodontic appliances. Sharma NC, Lyle DM, Qaqish JG, et al. Am J Orthod Dentofacial Orthop. 2008 Apr;133(4):565-71; quiz 628.e1-2. PMID:18405821

[79] Manual versus powered toothbrushing for oral health. Robinson PG, Deacon SA, Deery C, et al. Cochrane Database Syst Rev. 2005 Apr 18;(2):CD002281. PMID:15846633

[80] Comparison of the use of different modes of mechanical oral hygiene in prevention of plaque and gingivitis. Rosema NA, Timmerman MF, Versteeg PA, et al. J Periodontol. 2008 Aug;79(8):1386-94. PMID:18672987

[81] A prospective clinical study to evaluate the effect of manual and power toothbrushes on pre-existing gingival recessions. Dorfer CE, Joerss D, Wolff D. J Contemp Dent Pract. 2009 Jul 1;10(4):1-8. PMID:19575048

[82] Micronutrient modulation of NF-κB in oral keratinocytes exposed to periodontal bacteria. Milward MR, Chapple IL, Carter K, Matthews JB, Cooper PR. Innate Immun. 2012 Aug 13. PMID:22890546

[83] Zinc salts inhibit in vitro Toll-like receptor 2 surface expression by keratinocytes. Jarrousse V, Castex-Rizzi N, Khammari A, et al. Eur J Dermatol. 2007 Nov-Dec;17(6):492-6. PMID:17951128

[84] Mechanical stress-activated immune response genes via Sirtuin 1 expression in human periodontal ligament cells. Lee SI, Park KH, Kim SJ, et al. Clin Exp Immunol. 2012 Apr;168(1):113-24. PMID:22385246

[85] Effect of a dental water jet with orthodontic tip on plaque and bleeding in adolescent patients with fixed orthodontic appliances. Sharma NC, Lyle DM, Qaqish JG, et al. Am J Orthod Dentofacial Orthop. 2008 Apr;133(4):565-71. PMID:18405821

43. SLEEP

"And if tonight my soul may find her peace in sleep, and sink in good oblivion, and in the morning wake like a new-opened flower then I have been dipped again in God, and new-created."

D.H. Lawrence

That sleep is essential for health has been evident forever, but it is only recently that scientists have begun to unravel why we need sleep. Nematodes sleep. Sharks have to swim continuously to stay alive, porpoises need to surface to breath, and birds migrate long distances across oceans. These animals, which have to keep moving to stay alive, sleep with one-half of their brains at a time.

Humans sleep about one-third of their life away, or at least we should. With insufficient sleep humans function poorly. Reaction times slow, attention lapses, mood becomes labile, cognition foggy, and memory suffers. Decision-making can become faulty, and logic blurry[1]. If lab rats are prevented from sleeping, they eat more but lose weight, their heart rates accelerate, they develop skin ulcers and die in a few weeks. Excessive wake-time impairs mood, judgment and reaction time. Nineteen hours of sustained wakefulness is associated with a performance deficit equivalent to a blood alcohol level of 0.05%; a level at which it is illegal to operate a motor vehicle in most jurisdictions. After 24 hours of sustained wakefulness, the performance deficit is equivalent to a blood alcohol level of 0.1%[2], a level sufficient to impair reaction times and gross motor control.

Sleep is composed of four different stages which allow for different processes. Three, of these four, sleep stages are cycled throughout a night's sleep:

Table 43-1: Sleep Stages

Stage 1 (N1)	Falling asleep	
Stage 2 (N2)	EEG spindles	
SWS (N3)	Slow Wave Sleep (EEG delta waves)	Deep Sleep
REM	Rapid Eye Movement	Active Dreaming

Stage 1 sleep occurs when first falling to sleep. Sometimes there is the sensation of falling. Stage 1 sleep is a transition stage between wakefulness and sleep. If disturbed during this time, people often deny having been asleep. When a person is sleep deprived, this stage gets shortened from about 30 minutes to about 10 minutes.

Stage 2 sleep is required for feeling refreshed in the morning. Stage 2 sleep is the portion of sleep that is most susceptible to loss during sleep deprivation; this suggests that Stage 2 sleep is less essential for short-term functioning than SWS and REM sleep and that it is sacrificed in favor of them. When getting sufficient sleep, about half the sleep time is spent is in Stage 2 sleep. The largest proportion of the Stage 2 sleep occurs during the second half of the night, after getting sufficient SWS and REM sleep. Stage 2 sleep shows spindles on the electroencephalogram.

Slow wave sleep (SWS), also know as Stage 3 sleep, was for many years, split into stage 3 and Stage 4 sleep but these are now understood to be a single stage. The duration of sleep in this stage is more highly conserved during sleep deprivation than with any other stage, suggesting that SWS is the most essential. About 75 minutes are spent in SWS during a (night's) sleep cycle, even when there is substantial sleep deprivation limiting sleep to only 4 hours. SWS occurs mainly in the first half of the sleep cycle. If woken from the deepest part of SWS, a person will often feel disoriented and groggy.

REM sleep typically has four to five cycles during the night, with the cycles having longer durations during the later part of the sleep cycle. During this time the body is immobilized; this keeps us from acting out our dreams.

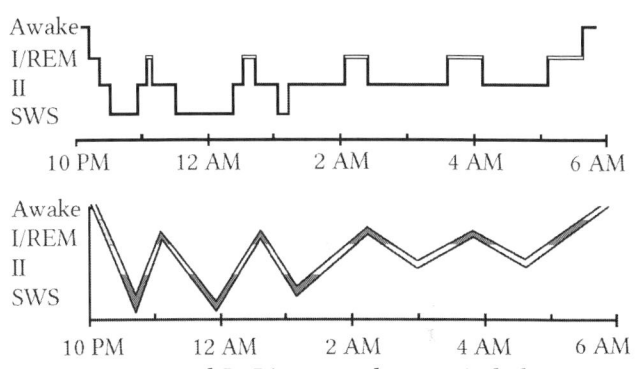

Figures 43-1 A and B: Diagrams show typical sleep stages during one night. Figure 41-1A (above) shows steps while Figure 41-1B illustrates the depth of sleep as a continuum.

Learning and Memory

Sleep enhances in memory consolidation and learning. Learning of visual, auditory, and motor sequence tasks shows improve after sleep, but not after a non-sleep delay. For example, several hours after practicing a piano piece, both technique and the content of the musical piece will have been learned better if some of the time has been spent sleeping, rather than if spent awake. Sleep helps reorganize memories and facilitate automated performance.

Rather than having distinct types of learning associated with different stages of sleep, the sleep stages may be thought of a process that assists learning. In the first part of the sleep cycle, SWS helps to stabilize the memory, and throughout the night REM and Stage 2 sleep help reorganize the content that has been learned.

SWS helps stabilize visual and declarative memory ("Just the facts, ma'am"). Stage 2 sleep helps with learning motor sequencing and automaticity skills, and REM sleep enhances the memory, adds insights, explores interrelationships and helps reorganize information into associative networks[3].

Sleep allows a quiet and undisturbed space for gleaning and interconnecting the relevant and salient information and processes learned during the day while limiting internal and environmental distractions. The repetitive sleep cycles allow for the iterative creation of memory and learning, and for winnowing the salient from the inconsequential. The brain is not relaxing during sleep – it is active and working.

One reason the young people require more sleep is that they are more actively learning. Small children take frequent naps that likely helps them learn motor and language skills more quickly. College students often try to learn more information in a sitting than they can organize and understand and much less integrate. Often the information makes more sense in the morning, and sometimes it takes two to three nights sleep for the information to organize into a gestalt.

Growing and Healing

There is a peak in the release of growth hormone soon after falling asleep in the evening. This triggers the release of Insulin-like growth factor 1 (IGF-1). Thyroid stimulating hormone (TSH) release also peaks after falling asleep, and this is followed by the release of T3 by the thyroid gland. Sleep provides a time to replenish excitatory neurotransmitters. Excitatory neurotransmitters, such as glutamate, associated with activity and alertness, are neurotoxic; sleep may act as an opportunity for the brain to detoxify, replenish antioxidants and repair.

The transcription of genes involved in energy metabolism and for encoding antioxidant proteins is increased during sleep[4]. Thus, at rest, an accounting of energy needs, based on the prior days use, is made and used to plan the accommodation of future energy needs. Sleep may be involved in the regulation of mitochondrial populations. Deprivation of REM sleep can induce loss of neuronal mitochondria through mitophagy[5]. The CLOCK gene, which helps regulate circadian cycles, is involved in the growth and repair of muscles[6]. Melatonin, released from the pineal gland not only helps induce and maintain sleep, but also is an important antioxidant that helps protect neurons[7] in the CNS and in the enteric nervous system. It is little wonder that we feel bad when we are sleep deprived. It also helps explains how non-restorative sleep can cause disease.

How Much Sleep do Adults Need?

Newborn infants require more than 16 hours of sleep daily, and about half of that is REM sleep. Both sleep time and REM time decline with age. Healthy octogenarians may sleep less than 6 hours a day with only 15% of that being REM sleep, but still be getting sufficient sleep. The average healthy young American adult spends about 8.3 hours in bed on weekdays and sleeps about 7.7 hours a night. Americans typically spend an extra hour sleeping on weekends, in part to catch up on missed sleep hours.

> Perhaps octogenarians do not need as much REM sleep as they do little active learning, and perhaps this is by design. After a lifetime of experience, it could be a mistake to overwrite tested habits and behaviors with newer ones. Evolution could not anticipate the rapid changes in culture, technology, and environment that occur today. In previous times, there has been a survival advantage to maintaining a culture; curtailing new learning among elders enhances retention and preservation of culture from one generation to subsequent ones. Older individuals retain skills and historical knowledge and are less likely to abandon them in favor of new and less tested adaptations for survival as they do not learn new things as quickly.

Table 43-2: Hours of Sleep by Age

Age	Typical daily hours of time in bed for sleep
Newborn	16.5
3 months	15
9 months	14
2 years	13
3 years	12
5 years	11
9 years	10
14 years	9
17	9.6
22	8.9
30	8.6
40	8.3
50	8.3
60	8.2
70	9

In a study where sleep time was limited to eight, six or four hours in bed for a two-week period, SWS time did not vary, but there was a reduction in other sleep stages. The effects of sleep loss are cumulative. Daytime sleepiness after one week of sleeping only four hours was equivalent to missing one night's sleep. After two weeks of sleep limited to four hours in bed, sleepiness did not worsen significantly. It took two weeks of sleeping only six hours before volunteers were as sleepy as if they had missed one night's sleep. Participants described the feeling of this amount of sleep deprivation as the difference between "feeling active, vital, alert, or wide awake" and "functioning at high levels, but not at peak, but still able to concentrate"[8].

This study also evaluated reaction time and attention. Here, the decline was also cumulative; it took twice as many days to appear for those sleeping six hours as for those sleeping four hours. After about seven days of being limited to four hours of bedtime, attention scores were equivalent to missing one night's sleep. After 14 days of four hours of bedtime, attention scores were equivalent to staying awake for three full days and nights. It took about 11 days of limiting bed time to six hours to have attention scores fall to the level of missing one night's sleep.

Chronic sleep deprivation usually only causes a mild decline in subjective functioning. Nevertheless, it can cause a severe decline in attention and reaction times. When people are severely and chronically sleep deprived, they do not feel that much worse than if they were only mildly sleep deprived, but their functioning can be seriously impaired. This study demonstrated that the maintenance of peak reaction time requires just over eight hours of sleep each night.

Peak functioning, as measured by attention measurements, depends not on sleep, but rather on avoiding excessive wakefulness. Being awake too long diminishes focus. The effect of time awake is cumulative; being awake an additional hour a day for 8 days in a row diminished the level of focus and attention equivalent to missing one night's sleep; staying awake an extra hour for 16 days in a row will cause the difficulty in focus and attention that missing two night' sleep would. To perform at full attention and focus proscribes being awake more than about 16 hours per day on average[9]; therefore yielding the need for about 8 hours of sleep.

For persons who are actively learning, have creative demands, or require peak attention and reaction times, 8 hours sleep is recommended.

Whether studying Americans, Europeans or Asians, the lowest mortality rates, when assessed by daily sleep duration, are between six and eight hours per night[10,11,12,13,14]. Sleeping less than six hours is associated with a slight increase in mortality, and more than nine hours of sleep at night is associated with an even higher risk. The reason that more sleep is associated with higher risk of mortality among adults is likely due to the reasons they require more sleep time; usually because of low quality or fractured sleep. Retired persons tend to sleep more, perhaps because of less demanding schedules, but this may also be due to poorer health. Even after adjusting for multiple risk factors, five hours of sleep in men and six hours for women appears to be sufficient to prevent an increased risk of mortality when compared to seven or eight hours. Less than four hours of sleep is a risk factor for higher mortality, similar in magnitude to the risk of nine hours.

The optimal sleep time for adults appears to be about 7 hours and 45 minutes. This is about the length of time that adults will sleep if they have no impediments to sleep; a dark, quiet spot, no appointments, no scheduling imperatives, no night-time disturbances. Most people use another 15 minutes for falling asleep and 15 more for lying awake in the morning. This is quite similar to the 7.7 hours average sleep time, and 8.3 hours average time in bed observed in studies of healthy Americans.

Many adults do with much less time without obvious problems. Even if sleep is restricted to only 4 hours a night, most adults will not complain of feeling fatigued or impaired even after two weeks of curtailed sleep. It appears that there are different thresholds for feeling sleep deprived for different individuals[15]. Nonetheless, those who feel well even when sleep is limited are not unimpaired by sleep deprivation; rather they just don't feel tired, but still suffer as much performance deficits as those who do.

Naps: Siestas can be helpful to make up for sleep deficits, and have anti-inflammatory effects; helping to decrease the level of inflammatory IL-6[16]. Napping is an effective sleep supplement that increases vigor and alertness, decrease information overload and boost mental performance and memory.

A "power nap" lasting from six to 30 minutes provides mainly Stage 2 sleep; it is refreshing and improves motor skills and declarative memory[17,18]. Shorter naps, less than 30 minutes, avoid sleep SWS and thus, avoid sleep inertia and grogginess upon awakening, which can last 30 minutes. Nevertheless, longer naps that include SWS provide more sustained cognitive performance than do short naps[19]. Napping for 60 to 90 minutes may allow an entire sleep cycle, thus allowing the napper to awakening from Stage 1/REM, refreshed without sleep inertia. A supine position is better than a seated position for napping[20]. It is best to avoid napping after four P.M. or within six hours of bedtime, to avoid disrupting the nighttime sleep cycle.

Sleep Drivers

There are two main components that drive our sleep cycle: awake time and daytime. After being awake long enough, we get tired, and we recover by sleeping. Without daylight or other external cues, most adults will fall into 25-hour wake-sleep cycles, and sleep about 1/3 of the time. We are also greatly influenced by daylight and night; thus, the circadian cycle gets entrained to the 24-hour day. Having the awake time cycle a bit longer than the 24-hour day is advantageous; as we would be constantly tired if the day were longer than our internal clock. Going to bed exhausted, is more likely to result in waking up tired than going to bed feeling well.

The circadian cycle is entrained by light on the retina, transmitted through the retinohypothalamic tract, to the suprachiasmatic nucleus (SCN) in the brain. Cortisol, aldosterone, testosterone, luteinizing hormone, growth hormone, prolactin, thyroid stimulating hormone and follicle-stimulating hormone all have diurnal variations and are likely controlled by the effect of light. The autonomic nervous system parasympathetic/sympathetic balance is also influenced by through the SCN[21].

Table 43-3: Sleep Drives

Sleep Drive	Length	Effector	Mediator
Homeostatic	25 Hours	Time Awake	Adenosine
Circadian	24 Hour day	Darkness	Melatonin

Hormones and Sleep

The hormone leptin, produced by the adipose tissue, signals that the fat cells have sufficient stores of fat. Leptin down-regulates appetite (over the long term) and helps increase energy use. In contrast, the hormone ghrelin enhances appetite. Short-sleepers, patients with untreated obstructive sleep apnea, sleep-deprived, and obese individuals have a lower circadian peak leptin levels, and higher ghrelin levels.

Sleep deprivation causes increased hunger, especially for fatty and sweet foods. Treatment of sleep apnea with CPAP lowers ghrelin within days and raises leptin within weeks, even without a change in body mass[22], suggesting that sleep loss promotes obesity rather than the obesity causing poor sleep. However, obesity is a strong risk factor for sleep apnea, which then promotes further attenuation of leptin and promotion of ghrelin. These then increase appetite; creating a positive feedback loop of worsening obesity and sleep apnea.

Table 43-4: Hormones Involved with or Affected by Sleep

Hormone	Effects	Notes
Vasoactive intestinal peptide (VIP)	Increased sympathetic activity during daylight.	Released by the SCN
Arginine vasopressin (AVP)	Mediates circadian cycle, blood pressure, water retention, and temperature regulation. Aggression	Released by the SCN[21]
Orexin 1 and 2 [23] (also known as Hypocretin A and B)	Activate histaminergic neurons; promotes wakefulness, increases energy use, increases food intake	Produced by the hypothalamus, Increased food craving. Increased by ghrelin Inhibited by leptin
Leptin	Long term appetite suppression	Produced by adipose tissue, inhibits cortisol release from the adrenal cortex, increases catecholamine release from the adrenal medulla[24]
Ghrelin	Appetite enhancement	Produced by the stomach and pancreas; counteracts leptin's action.
TSH	Controls thyroid hormone output,	Peak output during the first half of the night
T3	Active form of thyroid hormone: metabolic rate, brain growth, protein synthesis regulation, increases serotonin	Released mainly in the first half of the night
T4: thyroxine	Thyroid hormone	Released in the morning
Cholecalciferol[25] (Vitamin D_3)	Numerous proteins regulated	Formed in the skin exposed to UV light from sunlight
Cortisol	Anti-inflammatory hormone, stimulates food intake	Released from adrenal glands with peak about 8 AM
Melatonin	Helps with sleep	Produced by pineal gland, output inhibited by blue light
Growth Hormone	Promotes the release of IGF-1	Output peaks after sleep onset
Insulin-Like Growth Factor 1 (IGF-1)	Mediates growth. Help with sleep. Anti-depression activity	
Interleukin 6	Increases SWS during the second half of the night. Enhances emotional memory consolidation.	Intense release from muscles during exercise. Chronic production by adipocytes.
Prostaglandin D_2 [26]	Stimulates release of adenosine. Protects the brain against excitotoxic injury.	Produced in the brain by lipocalin-type PGD synthase
Adenosine[27]	Induces sleep. Acts on the basal forebrain and the ventrolateral preoptic area	Acts on A2A receptors. Secondary inhibition of histamine release
Prostaglandin E_2	Activate histaminergic neurons; promotes wakefulness	
Histamine	Promotes wakefulness acting on H_1 receptors	Tuberomammillary nucleus, Histaminergic neurons project throughout the brain.

Table 43-5: Effect of Sleep Restriction on Hormones[28] and Cytokines[29]

Hormone	Effect of Sleep Restriction	Effect on Health
Leptin	Lower circadian peak levels. Lower daily leptin production. Likely drives thyroid control (TRH).	Lower levels cause increased hunger, especially for high caloric, soft, palatable foods
Ghrelin	Increased in short sleepers[30]	Stimulates hunger
Orexin (Hypocretin)	Increased in sleep deprivation.	Increases activity
TSH	Loss of circadian nighttime peak. Lower TSH output.	Fatigue, lowered energy use
Cortisol	Decreased circadian cyclic variation. Increase daytime and total cortisol output. Output mirrors (opposite) leptin output.	Increased abdominal obesity.
Sympathovagal balance	Increased sympathetic activity.	Increased resting heart rate, blood pressure, and risk for arrhythmia.
Insulin	Decreased glucose tolerance. Increased insulin resistance.	Increased risk for Type 2 diabetes.
IGF-1[31]	Decreased production.	Decreased healing, increased mortality[32]
Interleukin-6[33]	Proinflammatory cytokine; increased in sleep deprivation May decrease leptin output.	Chronic inflammation
Interleukin-1β	Proinflammatory cytokine	Chronic inflammation, increased T_H17 immune function, decreased T_H1.
Interleukin-17	Proinflammatory cytokine; favors TH17 immune function.	Chronic inflammation, enteroimmune disease.
C-Reactive Protein	An inflammatory marker associated with risk of coronary artery disease.	Increased risk of coronary artery disease.

The Pineal Gland and Melatonin

Melatonin is the hormone most closely associated with sleep; however, it is also an essential antioxidant that protects neurons in the brain and the gut. Melatonin acts through two melatonin receptors, MT_1 and MT_2 in mammals, and additionally, as an antioxidant. It stimulates T4+ and T8+ lymphocyte production, especially when combined with low-dose zinc[34], and helps impart a diurnal rhythm to immune cells, thyroid, testis and other metabolic functions[35]. Melatonin helps with spatial learning and declarative memory consolidation during sleep[36]. The pineal gland may help control the onset of puberty.

The pineal gland is an important site of melatonin production. This tiny gland is only about the size of a grain of rice, and it reaches its complete adult size by the time a child is about two years old. The pineal gland resides within the brain, however; it is not derived from the same embryonic tissues as the brain, and it is not isolated by the blood-brain barrier. The pineal gland is highly perfused, having a tissue blood flow rate second only to that of the kidneys.

The pineal gland tends to calcify with age; most adult's pineal glands have considerable calcification by the late middle age. Even children's pineal glands show calcification. In one study, 39% of those aged 8 to 14 had calcification of the pineal gland, revealed by CT scan[37]. The choroid plexus, which produces cerebral spinal fluid, also calcifies at a rate similar to the pineal gland. Pineal calcification occurs in most mammals as they age, however, calcification is unusual in birds[38].

If calcification of the pineal gland and choroid plexus are near universal, are they physiologic or pathologic? The degree of calcification of the pineal gland correlates with degeneration and herniation of the intervertebral disks[39] and calcification of the abdominal aorta[40]. While calcification may be normal, accelerated calcification certainly is not. The pathologic calcification of the aorta, and presumably the calcification of the pineal gland and choroid plexus, are distinct from that of bone and tooth mineralization. Aortic calcification is unrelated to bone mineral density. Pathologic calcification of vascular tissues, such as the choroid plexus and pineal gland, appears to be mediated by inflammation[41]. Activated, trypsin producing mast cells have been implicated in the calcification of the pineal gland[42]. These cells have also been identified as in the pathology of atherosclerotic plaques in the carotid arteries[43].

Growth-arrest specific gene six (Gas6) prevents apoptosis of vascular smooth muscle cells. Inorganic phosphate (Pi) down-regulates Gas6 and thereby increases smooth muscle cell apoptosis. This may be the how Pi contributes to renal disease[44]. Alpha-lipoic acid has been demonstrated to help improve mitochondrial function and reduce apoptosis of smooth muscle cells in the arteries by restoring Gas6, and thereby, reduces arterial calcification[45]. Taurine[46] and certain statin medications also help up-regulate Gas6 [47]. Elevated blood glucose increases smooth muscle apoptosis through Gas6 signaling[48]. Not unexpectedly, leading a healthy lifestyle, perhaps especially physical activity, is associated with decreased vascular calcification[49]. Arterial calcification and dysfunction may be reversible through aerobic activity[50].

The amount of melatonin that can be detected in the saliva is correlated to the uncalcified mass of the pineal gland as measured by MRI, and this un-calcified mass also correlates with sleep quality and is inversely associated with sleep disturbances[51]. Nevertheless, it is the degree of pineal calcification, rather than its un-calcified mass, which is most highly and inversely correlated with REM sleep, total sleep time and sleep efficiency[52]. This suggests that pineal proteins other than melatonin have additional effects on sleep. In addition to melatonin, pineal proteins induce the production of superoxide dismutase (SOD), ceruloplasmin, and other antioxidants[53].

Melatonin is amphiphilic; both hydrophilic and lipophilic, and thus, easily transported in the blood and CSF, readily enters cells and crosses the BBB. The retina, the cochlea of the ear, hypothalamus and several other areas of the CNS produce the rate-limiting enzyme for melatonin production and thus, also likely produce it. Melatonin is rapidly metabolized in the brain to other products, many of which are metabolically active. Thus, melatonin gains access and acts as an antioxidant in a wide variety of organs, including the heart, liver, kidneys and brain. The pineal gland has additional antioxidant properties. Not only is melatonin an antioxidant, it additionally induces mitochondrial proteins that reduce the production of free radicals[54]. Lab rats, whose circadian cycle is disrupted by exposure to light, suffer from accelerated aging and increased development of tumors. Melatonin administration reduced this aging and tumorigenesis[55]. Thus, melatonin may slow aging and prevent cancer.

Although the pineal gland is the most famous site of melatonin production, it is not the most prodigious. The gastrointestinal tract (GIT) contains more than 400 times as much melatonin as does the pineal gland[56]. Here, it prevents ulcers, reduces the secretion of hydrochloric acid, stimulates immune cells, fosters epithelial regeneration and regulates peristalsis and blood flow to the mucosa. Melatonin is useful in the treatment of stress ulcers[57], irritable bowel syndrome, inflammatory bowel disease[58] and gastroesophageal reflux disease (GERD). Patients with IBD have been found to have elevated levels of homocysteine and lower levels of melatonin[59].

While pineal melatonin output is regulated by light, GIT melatonin is regulated by meals; it is produced when the GIT is at rest[60]; the circadian cycle for melatonin production may be disrupted by irregular meal times or midnight snacks. This suggests that irregular meal times and late meals may be aging and tumorigenic, as is the disruption of the circadian cycle by light.

While the major metabolic end-product of melatonin, 6-sulfatoxymelatonin is simple enough to measure in the urine, this metabolite does not reflect melatonin activity or account for the amount of melatonin produced by the body. Several products created when melatonin is oxidized are metabolically active; cyclic 3-hydroxymelatonin (c3OHM), for example, may be an acetylcholinesterase inhibitor. Some melatonin oxidation products enter the kynurenine pathway; N1-acetyl-N2-formyl-5-methoxykynuramine (AFMK) and N1-acetyl-5-methoxykynuramine (AMK) as examples. AFMK is anti-inflammatory and decreases TNF-α, IL-8, and IL1β production by monocytes. AFMK is also an antioxidant. The melatonin oxidation product AMK protects the mitochondria, down-regulates cyclo-oxygenase, inhibits nitric oxide synthase, and can capture peroxynitrite and other nitrous radicals[61]. Non-oxidative, metabolites of melatonin include 5-methoxytryptomine; a serotonin agonist, and 5-methoxytryptophol that induces sleep.

As a natural product, present in animals and some plants, melatonin is sold a food supplement. Endogenous production of melatonin requires serotonin as a substrate and the B_6 vitamin, pyridoxine-5-phosphate, as a cofactor (Figure 31-2)

Between 0.3 and 1.0 mg of rapidly absorbed, sublingual melatonin at bedtime is a reasonable dose to promote the onset of sleep. Up to 6 mg, usually in slow release form, may be used to maintain sleep, and for use as an antioxidant. For most patients, 1.5 mg is a sufficient dose to help with sleep.

Melatonin is useful in the treatment of many enteroimmune and inflammatory diseases including metabolic syndrome[62], fibromyalgia, IBS[63], GERD[64], migraine[65], cluster headaches[66] and protects against Alzheimer's disease and depression[67].

Inflammation

Sleep deprivation promotes inflammation. It causes increased levels of C-reactive protein, IL-1β, IL-6, and IL-17, The changes in leptin and ghrelin levels observed in sleep deprivation may be the result of changes in these cytokines. IL-6 is typically elevated fibromyalgia syndrome, in which non-restorative sleep is common (Chapter 32). Inflammation caused by sleep deprivation may also explain the increased risk of heart disease in short-sleepers. IL-6 decreases SWS and causes fatigue[68].

Sleep and circadian rhythms have a critical role in the development of immune function. The ROR (retinol-related orphan receptor) genes, which are subject to circadian influence, impact the differentiation of T helper cells into different lineages. Sleep deprivation or disruption of the circadian cycle shifts T helper cell development towards

T_H17 cell development. T_H17 cells are involved in the chronic inflammatory and autoimmune diseases including multiple sclerosis, rheumatoid arthritis, systemic lupus inflammatory bowel disease, psoriasis, and asthma[69] T_H17 cells underlie the development of enteroimmunopathies, and thus sleep deprivation may increase the likelihood of developing antergies to food. Sleep deprivation is also associated with an elevated B lymphocyte and lower NK-cell populations, thus affecting the body's immune response to infection and injury.

Cardiac Dysrhythmias: Sleep deprivation is associated with increased risk of cardiac dysrhythmias. This effect may be the result of inflammation, increased sympathetic tone secondary to leptin's pro-adrenergic effect on the adrenal medulla, dysregulation of thyroid output, the excitatory effect of increased hypocretin, or a combination of these and other factors.

Sleep and Obesity

Short sleepers, those who sleep fewer hours, are more likely to be obese. Children who sleep less than ten hours a day are 1.89 times as likely to be obese than children who get more sleep, and adults who get less than six hours sleep are about 1.55 times as likely to be obese than adults who get more than six hours of sleep[70]. These data result from a meta-analysis of 30 studies carried out on six continents; thus, this effect is not limited to North America or to the Western diet.

Obesity is also associated with longer sleep time; obesity can cause sleep apnea that results in frequent arousals and poor quality of sleep. Thus, patients with sleep apnea may spend more time in bed, and still have sleep deficits.

The effects of sleep deprivation on appetite and satiation and satiety are discussed in Chapter 8.

Insomnia

Occasional insomnia seems ubiquitous. About one-third of all adults in Western countries has difficulty sleeping at least once a week, with women reporting more frequent insomnia than do men. Although insomnia is common, often, it is not benign. Insomnia can have large impacts on health, happiness, behavior, safety, career, and education.

As a group, individuals who suffer from insomnia are at a three times higher risk of death. This is not just from accidents and poor judgment from being sleep deprived, but also from poorer recovery from disease, from hypertension, heart and lung disease[71]. Sleep deprivation is associated with fatigue, mental fog, increased inflammatory cytokines[72], insulin resistance, elevated leptin[73] and cortisol output[74]. Chronic daytime elevations in cortisol can lead to weight gain and adrenal fatigue.

About half of all patients diagnosed with insomnia also have a psychiatric diagnosis. Almost all children with autistic spectrum disorder have sleep disorders[75]; half have insomnia, half have sleep disordered breathing, and a quarter suffer from parasomnias. Early morning insomnia is a common feature of depression and anxiety. Insomnia is a risk factor for later development of depression[76]. Sleep disturbances very often accompany chronic kidney disease. Sleep apnea can cause heart failure and pulmonary hypertension.

So what comes first, insomnia or the disease?

- Lying awake at night occasionally should not be a concern, especially if the individual wakes feeling refreshed.
- Getting insufficient sleep is unpleasant, makes learning more difficult and can damage health.
- Insomnia in itself is not a health risk, but may be caused by conditions that are heath risks.
- Sleep deprivation, which may be caused by insomnia, is a health risk and increases inflammation.
- Sleep deprivation can cause poor cognition, depression and anxiety, disruption of hormonal cycling, promote obesity and other health problems.
- Sleep disorders are often caused by underlying inflammatory conditions.

Thus, sleep deprivation can cause disease, and disease can cause insomnia.

Occasional insomnia is not a health threat. If an adult feels refreshed after getting only five hours of sleep at night, it is not a problem, as long as the sleep can be made up for. To function at their best, adults need about 54 hours of sleep per week, and some sleep time can be made up on following days. Conversely, individuals who feel daytime sleepiness, other than a siesta time dip, are usually chronically sleep deprived, with a sleep deficit that may have accumulated over weeks. If they are getting sufficient sleep time, and still feel tired, it suggests that they have a poor sleep quality. An individual (over the age of about seven) that is often sleepy during the day, regardless of time in bed or perception of insomnia, is not getting enough quality sleep; this is a problem which needs attention.

If an individual complains of excessive insomnia but denies daytime sleepiness, he or she may just require less time in bed. Recent onset of insomnia, however, may be caused by the recent onset of an inflammatory condition or infection.

The Epworth Sleepiness Scale is a simple, but useful test that asks how likely a person is to doze off during the day during eight different sedentary activities. It is scored from zero: (would never doze off) to three: highly likely to doze off). A score of ten is considered sleepy. A score of 18 or more should be regarded as a serious sleep deprivation. A link to the Epworth Sleepiness Scale is given in Appendix B. A link to the Cleveland Adolescent Sleepiness Questionnaire is also provided. Treatment of insomnia is discussed later in this chapter.

On a Personal Note: I consider myself a bit of an expert on insomnia. I used to be very good at it. I spent countless hours lying in bed in the dark, during the wee hours of the night. There was a period of a couple of years where lying awake several hours every night was my norm. I'd like to share a bit of wisdom I gleaned from my experience:

How gravity works: Since the math is rather esoteric, here's the Cliff's notes version: Gravity is entropy of mass; as mass coalesces, time slows; the rotational orbit of electrons along with space shrinks and the environment becomes more conductive and active. $M = E/C^2$: Mass decreases, energy is released, and space: time shrinks. Geothermal energy, for example, is the result of the nuclear entropy of the Earth's molten core. A daily influx of about 200 metric tons of space dust[77] keeps the geothermal engine running.

How not to let insomnia bother me: Don't sweat insomnia. Worrying about being awake only causes frustration and wakefulness. Enjoy the time as personal time for reflection, meditation, or inventing a new story, recipe, device, or outline for a story. Get up and read this book for 20 minutes; it should help you get back to sleep.

One of my first memories is as a toddler; I was two. I was camping in Yosemite valley, laying between my parents in a tent. It was a beautiful, serene night, and the moon had come up, and I could see the heavy timbered picnic table and large ponderosa pines through the open tent flap. Looking out, I watched a large bear lumber into the campsite looking for food. It was just about 20 feet away. I looked over at my dad and then at my mom. Both were sleeping; relaxed and unworried. Using inductive logic, I reasoned that if they weren't worried about the bear, it must not be a problem. I closed my eyes, lying on my favorite red plaid flannel blanket, confident that all was well in my world and fell back asleep.

This is my approach to insomnia: I make my bedroom a comfortable, relaxing sleep environment. Since I have a neighbor up the street that is afraid of the dark and keeps a 68,000-lumen mercury vapor night light on, I put aluminum blinds on my window, and taped over the night-light that lives on the smoke detector in my room, so that my bedroom is an obsidian, Cimmerian oasis. Fresh, cool air, and quiet bathes me as I lay awake, enticing me back to sleep. Once I realized that I would be spending many hours awake in bed, I made one of the best investments; I invested in my bed, putting some cash into my mattress (figuratively). I use high-thread count comfortable sheets and a memory foam pad for my bed. I find that no matter where I get them, pillows are only comfortable for a couple of months, so I buy inexpensive ones and change them several times a year.

Having a luxuriously comfortable bed and a pleasant sleep environment makes lying awake, besides my bride, a pleasure.

Sleep Disorders

There are several common sleep disorders. Each has its own characteristics and should be treated according to the underlying causation. *Initial Insomnia* and *Early Morning Awakening* are the sleep disorders most people associate with insomnia.

Initial Insomnia (II) is a condition in which an individual lies themselves down to sleep, but then just lies awake; sleep just won't come. Sleep latency should be less than 30 minutes. Normally, it should take less than 5 minutes to fall asleep; any more than 30 minutes is considered abnormal. If this is a chronic problem, it may be Circadian Rhythm Disorder, (discussed below) where the day / night sleep cycle is delayed by several hours on both ends.

Table 43-6: Common Sleep Disorders

Sleep Disturbance	Characteristic
Initial Insomnia	Difficulty falling asleep; lying awake more than 30 minutes after going to bed.
Early morning awakening	Waking up, usually around 3-4 AM, and difficulty falling back asleep until near dawn, usually accompanied by rumination.
Primary Sleep Deprivation	Primary Sleep Deprivation refers to intentional wakefulness supplanting sleep time.
Sleep apnea	Cycles of interrupted breathing during sleep followed by brief waking (usually not remembered) repeatedly through the night. Most commonly caused by upper-airway obstruction.
Non-restorative sleep (NRS)	Poor quality sleep, lacking sufficient deep sleep, usually sleep punctuated by near awakenings.
Circadian Rhythm Disorders (CRD)	In CRD, including Delayed Sleep-Phase Syndrome the sleep cycle is out of time with the day / night cycle. Occurs in teenagers, shift-work sleep disorder, SWSD, and with jet-lag.
Parasomnias	Unusual activity associated with sleep; night terrors, sleep walking, periodic limb movement, etc.

Light to moderate exercise in the evenings improves sleep and a sense of well-being upon awakening in the morning[78]. A warm bath or shower (cool in hot weather, warm in cool weather) before sleep can decrease sleep latency[79].

Full spectrum fluorescent lights should be avoided for at least an hour prior to bedtime. Fluorescent lights, televisions, and computer monitors have much more blue light than incandescent lighting does. Blue light (around 446-484 nm) promotes wakefulness by stimulating melanopsin in ganglion cells of the retina[80]. Lower light levels before bedtime (an artificial dusk) helps promote sleep, especially in children. Some compact fluorescent lights have less blue light than others, and usually have much less blue light emission than fluorescent tubes that are used to help keep workers, shoppers and students alert in commercial and school settings.

Sublingual melatonin can be used to help fall asleep. A low dose of about 0.3 mg to 1.0 mg is enough to help many people get to sleep. The sublingual route gives a quick rise in blood melatonin level that helps initiate sleep.

Table 43-7: Common Causes of Initial Insomnia

Causes of Initial Insomnia	Examples	Remedies
Stimulants	Caffeine, i.e.; Coffee, sodas Theobromine (chocolate), nicotine	Avoid stimulants, such as caffeine, for eight hours before bedtime.
Exercise	Vigorous exercise	Avoid vigorous exercise for six hours before bedtime (Evening walks and swimming help sleep)
Light	Bright lighting, especially with light in the blue spectrum prevents the formation of melatonin: Fluorescent lights* (computer monitors, TV) Children are especially susceptible.	Avoid bright lights for two hours before bedtime. Use amber glasses if needed to filter out the blue part of the spectrum.
Anxiety and Excitement	Personal situations and activities. Also virtual excitement: computer games or TV and movies, especially for children	Try to set the evening aside for relaxing, low-stress activities.
Full Bellies	Large meals too close to bedtime	Avoid eating large meal for three hours before bedtime
Discomfort	Uncomfortable bed or room	Make sure bed and bedroom are comfortable dark and quiet.
Early Retirement	Going to bed when not sleepy	Try to maintain a regular sleep time, not to get excessive sleep during the day

Early Morning Awakening (EMA): EMA is a common symptom of depression. It is so common that any person with EMA should be screened for depression. Typically in EMA, the individual wakes between 2 and 4 A.M. and is unable to fall back asleep until about 5:30 A.M. The wakefulness in depression is often accompanied by rumination: recurring worried thoughts. These ruminations often are trivial, extraneous or rubbish.

Depressive Worrying

Worrying and sadness are hallmarks of depression. When depressed, people can find all sorts of things to worry about. I had a patient who was certain that her depression was caused by learning that her cousin had been diagnosed with cancer. I asked if they were close. She had not seen nor talked to that cousin in over 20 years.

In depression, anxiety, and sadness are often attributed to the most proximal cause – whatever reason is at hand. It is similar to what occurs as a person is about to leave their house for a trip and has a feeling that they've forgotten something. This is the functioning of the right side of the brain. The mind goes through a checklist; "doors locked, stove off, keys in hand, have wallet, …." This is the left side of the brain. A normal person goes through the list and checks them off and thinks, "No, got it all", and does not worry any further. A person with obsessive-compulsive disorder will check the doors three times just in case they might have only thought that they had checked the locks.

A depressed or anxious person will do the same thing. The right side of the brain has an alarm go off saying "Oh no! Something is amiss! Watch out!" but the left-side of the brain does not know why the right-side is feeling this way. It may be that the threshold for the alarm is set too low and that almost everything sets it off, even when there is, in fact, no danger. The right side of the brain hears the alarm going off and looks for a reason. It makes up a list and chooses the one that seems to make the most sense, even though there is no real problem, and thus no right answer. Something has to take the blame for the alarm.

In caring for depression or anxiety, patients often want to focus on resolving the identified problem they have identified, often some Freudian issue. The identified issue is often an attribution error, not the source of the disease. The goal should be to get the alarm to trigger at a more appropriate level, and to turn down the trigger point for the alarm system by treating the depression, which usually has an inflammatory basis.

Early morning wakening occurs in some individuals who are not depressed or anxious. The underlying mechanism is likely the same. Non-sedating antidepressants work well for some individuals with EMA even when they do not show signs of depression. Early morning wakening can be caused by inflammation. Histamine and PGE_2 promote wakefulness. Mast cell activation disorders and food antergies can provoke early morning awakening. EMA is a sign of an inflammatory disorder. If no cause can be found, it can be treated as for depression (Chapter 31.)

> During sleep the body temperature falls, from the daytime average of about 37 degrees C (98.6°F) to about 36.3 degrees (96.3°F) during the wee hours of the night. We are adapted to have night time temperatures cooler than during the day.
>
> In some circadian sleep disorders, the body temperature does not fall. Lowering room temperature at night can help entrain the normal fall in body temperature during sleep[81]; this improves sleep and gives an enhanced feeling of refreshment in the morning.

Rebound Insomnia: Another form of insomnia is rebound insomnia. It is similar to EMA but typically occurs earlier in the night. It is often caused by the use of alcohol around bedtime. Alcohol is a depressant sedative with a short half-life. It may help an individual get to sleep, but then, wears off in a couple of hours. The sleeper then awakens and has difficulty getting back to sleep. Alcohol is a poor choice of soporifics.

Primary Sleep Deprivation: The number one cause of primary sleep deprivation in our society is electronic devices. A television, computer or electronic games, the internet, and phones in the bedroom are more enticing than sleep to kids. Parent, who prefer not to add "sleep cop" to their roster of duties, are wise to eliminate electronics from their children's bedrooms. This includes cell phones. Televisions should be banished from the boudoir. If bored; read a book.

> Caution: Close distance visual use (less than 14 inches) just before turning off the lights to sleep may promote myopia. Bed time reading should be followed by focusing the eyes at a distance of at least a few feet for a several minutes before sleep, especially in young persons.

In adults, a major cause of sleep deprivation is working long hours. This was once common in my industry (doctors working long shifts) and in truck drivers. This is less common than in the past, as legislation now limits the duration of some commercial activities as sleep deprivation caused many accidents.

Sleep Apnea

The most prevalent form of sleep apnea is obstructive sleep apnea (OSA), which is epidemic among overweight and obese individuals. In these patients, the pharynx collapses during sleep and obstructs breathing. When this occurs, their oxygen saturation falls, causing them to wake momentarily and take a few catch-up breaths. In OSA, a cycle of apnea and brief awakening may repeatedly occur throughout the night, as many as 20 times an hour. Thus, these patients spend very little time in deep restorative sleep. The upper-airway obstruction causes sonorous breathing. The triad of daytime sleepiness, obesity and snoring is typical in OSA. Individuals, including children that snore and have daytime sleepiness should be evaluated for OSA.

Early treatment of OSA is important, as OSA can lead to congestive heart failure as well as to other morbidities. It is a major cause of industrial and traffic accidents. Lack of sleep from sleep apnea can also cause academic failure and behavioral problems in children. Less recognized is OSA's effect on neurological disease. I have had patients with seizures, intractable migraines, and organic brain syndrome that had a complete or near-complete recovery as soon as they were adequately treated for sleep apnea.

Treatment of obstructive sleep apnea requires treatment of the obstruction. In children, removal of enlarged tonsils is often helpful. Surgical treatment is occasionally helpful in adults; nevertheless, in severe or long-standing OSA, fibrosis of the muscles in the pharynx often prevents much recovery. CPAP treatment is effective in most patients with sleep apnea. Early treatment may prevent the fibrosis of these muscles that occurs with long-standing OSA.

Other than OSA caused by a mechanical blockage from enlarged tonsils, surgical treatment, such as uvulectomy, does not treat the usually underlying cause; obesity. Obesity is the most common and important risk factor for OSA. Sleep disordered breathing is highly correlated with metabolic syndrome and insulin resistance, even after adjusting for body-mass index[82]. Thus, treatment for Metabolic Syndrome (Chapter 9) is appropriate in patients with sleep disordered breathing.

OSA can be provoked by food allergies. Sinus congestion will contribute to snoring and obstruction, and food allergies, and pseudo allergies (Chapters 11, 13, 15, and 19) may contribute to this.

Central sleep apnea is caused by a CNS problem rather than by an airway obstruction.

Non-Restorative Sleep (NRS)

Non-restorative sleep is different from insomnia. An individual can have insomnia (excessive time awake while in bed during sleep time), still get sufficient sleep to function well during the day, and not have symptoms of sleep deprivation. With NRS, an individual can get more than enough hours of sleep, and still feel tired, sluggish, and fatigued. NRS also decreases cognitive performance and increases irritability. While pain can cause NRS, NRS also causes pain, myalgia, sensation of limb heaviness and stiffness[83].

The problem in NRS appears to be a lack of deep sleep; the individual cycles through sleep stages near wakefulness, with brief arousals that are usually not remembered. Sleep is fragmented; similar to the situation in sleep apnea. There is insufficient restorative deep sleep. The treatment of NRS is to treat the underlying condition.

In some cases, a sleep disorder or a circadian disorder is the primary cause. Narcolepsy is thought to be the result of an autoimmune disease which affects hypocretin receptors in the hypothalamus. Bipolar disorder and mood disorders have been linked to genetic variants of the genes involved in the regulation of circadian rhythms[84,85].

Table 43-8: Conditions in which Non-restorative Sleep is Common

Condition	Treatment
Irritable Bowel Syndrome	Chapter 26
Major Stress Event within one year Stress or HPA axis dysrhythmia	Chapter 29
Traumatic Brain Injury	Chapter 30
Depression Anxiety disorders Bipolar disorder Depression	Chapter 31
Fibromyalgia Chronic Fatigue Syndrome	Chapter 32
Rheumatoid Arthritis Systemic Lupus Erythematosus Narcolepsy	Chapter 33
Obstructive Sleep Apnea Periodic Limb Movement Disorder	In this Chapter
Pain	Treat pain and the underlying condition

Circadian Rhythm Disorders (CRD): There are several CRD, one of which is Delayed Sleep-Phase Syndrome (DSPS). These disorders can cause severe disability. Individuals with CRD are sometimes misdiagnosed as having schizophrenia, bipolar disorder, or attention deficit hyperactivity disorder (ADHD). They often perform poorly in school and work situations. Alcohol can induce CRD. Jet lag is another form of CDR, and shift workers usually adaptive DSPS.

Is ADHD primarily a sleep disorder?

Sleep disturbances are common in ADHD. Sleep deprivation can cause hyperactive behavior, especially in children. Sleep disturbances are common is patients with ADHD, including periodic limb movement disorder and disturbed sleep architecture. ADHD-like behavior may be secondary to sleep deprivation from obstructive sleep apnea; insufficient sleep because of delayed bedtime; or from other cause sleep deprivation. As noted above DSPS can mimic ADHD. Iron deficiency (see below) can cause sleep disturbances that manifest as ADHD[86].

Fatigue: Fatigue has a multiplicity of causes, including sleep deprivation from shift work, sleep apnea or other factors. Fatigue is a symptom of many diseases. Table 41-9 provides a list of some common causes of fatigue. Note that many of these conditions are associated with sleep problems. Many of the diseases in which fatigue is common, affect sleep or impede restorative sleep.

Table 43-9 Common Causes of Fatigue

Condition	Effect on Sleep
Fibromyalgia	Associated with pain and non-restorative sleep
Anemia	Iron deficiency is associated with poor sleep
Vitamin B_{12} deficiency	Required for circadian entrainment to light
Depression	Insomnia with early morning wakening is common
Chronic Infections	Inflammatory cytokine IL-6 decreases SWS and causes fatigue
Hypothyroidism	TSH and T3 output should peak during sleep
Nocturia	Disturbs sleep continuity
Caffeine overload	Stimulant can affect sleep Can cause nocturia
Urinary Track Infection or Interstitial cystitis	Nocturia, IL-6
Diabetes	Sleep deprivation can decrease insulin sensitivity. Nocturia may wake patient several times at night.
Heart Failure	Can be caused by sleep apnea Causes orthopnea that disturbs sleep
Food Allergies and Antergies	Increased IL-6 decreases SWS. Histamine and PGE_2 promote alertness preventing sleep
Lack of exercise	Poorer quality sleep
Dehydration	Poorer quality sleep
Skipping meals, Low-quality food, low-protein or High-carbohydrate diet	Poorer quality sleep
Alcohol use	Disrupts sleep and the circadian cycle, causes nocturia and dehydration, depletes glycogen.
Statin Drugs[87]	Exertional fatigue; may be related to lowered vitamin D_3 production.

Delayed Sleep-Phase Syndrome (DSPS): In DSPS, the sleep cycle is out of sync with society's normal daytime-active/ nighttime-sleep cycle. People with DSPS are often considered extreme night owls, with their typical onset of sleep being around 3 AM with wakening about 11 AM.

DSPS is common among teenagers; with a prevalence of about 7 percent It is more common among males. DSPS affects about 0.15% of adults. Attempts at resetting the sleep phase using phototherapy, melatonin, or chronotherapy (sleep-phase time advancement), is often successful, nevertheless, most adults with DSPS return to their usual sleep cycle within a year after discontinuation of treatment. There is some evidence that DSPS may have a genetic component. Clearly, it may be advantageous to the community have a small percent of the population with "night watchman" gene. In a primitive village society, having a couple of teenage boys stay up talking at night, tending the fire, and sounding the alarm if a predator or raiding neighbors shows up, would have survival advantages. However, as a parent, the advantages of having a night owl teenager are limited. It can disrupt school, social and family functions, and increases the risk of the teenager participating in unchaperoned, risky activities.

Even though DSPS in adolescents is not considered to be a pathological condition, treatment is sometimes requested. One treatment for DSPS is a low dose (e.g. 0.3 mg) melatonin, about six hours prior to the desired onset of sleep[88]. Another treatment is to use light to slowly entrain the sleep cycle, delaying sleep by 15 minutes per day until the sleep-wake cycle matches the societal day-awake/night-sleep cycle. Yet another treatment is to progressively delay sleep one-hour each day until the night-sleep cycle matches society's.

Many adults with DSPS simply adapt their schedules to their sleep cycle, selecting jobs that allow them to work at night. Unfortunately, high schools usually do not adapt to adolescents with DSPS, and this creates a situation and environment in which it is difficult for them to do well.

Table 43-10: Delayed Sleep-Phase Syndrome Therapy

Treatment	Details
Low-dose melatonin	0.3 mg daily 6 hours before desired sleep time
Maintain routine bedtime	Maintain the same bedtime every day including weekends, and rise at the same time. Day-wake / night-sleep schedules should be encouraged.
Maintain routine mealtime	Eating at regularly scheduled times helps maintain the normal circadian gastrointestinal motility cycle and melatonin output. Avoid large meals before bedtime.
Avoid Stimulants	Caffeine, Nicotine, Chocolate, others
Light Entrainment	Minimize bright light (UV and Blue light) television, and computer screens use for two hours before desired bedtime. Amber sunglasses may be used. Sleep in a dark room and use artificial dawn if natural light-dark cycle disrupted by city lights.
Avoid Alcohol	No alcoholic beverages

Disturbances in circadian rhythm homeostasis are suspected in the causation of several disease conditions. Some are listed in Table 43-11.

Table 43-11: Disorders with Circadian Disturbances

Bipolar disorder[89]	Chapter 31
Major depression[90]	Chapter 31
Autism[91]	Chapter 35
Premenstrual dysphoric disorder[92]	Treat as for depression

Thus, treatment for these conditions should include management of DSPS to help restore a normal circadian cycle. These conditions should also be treated as inflammatory disorders. Premenstrual dysphoric disorder should also be treated as an inflammatory condition, similar to depression, IBS or rage.

Parasomnias

Parasomnias are sleep disturbances that include unusual movements, perceptions, dreams or emotions that occur in association with sleep; while falling asleep, during or between stages of sleep, or during arousal. These include sleepwalking, night terrors, nightmares, sleep vocalizations, teeth grinding, restless leg syndrome, periodic limb movement, and confusional arousals. These can be disturbing to the patients and family, especially when they involve knives.

Parasomnias are often associated with sleep fragmentation that can be caused or exacerbated, by conditions that affect sleep architecture. Parasomnias should be investigated to look for underlying conditions that are provoking sleep fragmentation.

Table 43-12: Diseases with Increased Prevalence of Parasomnias

Rheumatic Diseases[93],
Pulmonary Hypertension[94],
Atrophic Dermatitis[95]
Heart Failure[96]
Iron Deficiency[97]

Nocturia

Nocturia, on a regular basis, greater than once per sleep period, is usually a sign of either a medical problem that is inadequately treated or of sleep disturbance. Poor health habits, such as caffeinated or alcoholic beverages before bedtime can also contribute to nocturia. Traumatic brain injury/ postconcussion syndrome often causes nocturia, as a result of posterior pituitary injury. In these patients, there is inappropriate secretion of the hormone ADH (SIADH); these patients have diabetes insipidus, which usually resolved after several months[98].

Nocturia disturbs sleep and contributes to sleep deprivation and fatigue. Nocturia should be addressed, treating its underlying causes.

Table 43-12: Causes of Nocturia

Mechanism	Conditions
Increased urine production	Diabetes Diabetes insipidus Polydipsia Diuretic use
Increased nocturnal urine production	Congestive heart failure Nephritic syndrome Obstructive sleep apnea Edema
Bladder disturbances Decreased nocturnal bladder capacity	Urinary tract infection Cystitis Neurogenic bladder Prostatic obstruction
Sleep Disturbances	Patient gets up as they are awake
Bad habits	Alcoholic or caffeinated beverages late in the day.
Mixed causation	Many patients have multiple contributory causes.

Treatment of Sleep Disorders

Sleep disorders should be approached by through understanding the underlying causation and removing those factors when possible. If an adult dedicates eight hours to their pillow and is not getting sufficient quality sleep to wake refreshed, there is a problem, and it should be addressed.

1. Immune Reactions: IgE intolerances are usually easy to identify, as they occur soon after contact with the offending agent. Allergic reactions, with itchy skin, especially will impede sleep. Interleukin-6, abundant in the skin and released in allergic dermatitis, will disturb sleep. Histamine helps maintain wakefulness and is released in allergic reactions. If unidentified food allergies are suspected, ImmunoCAP testing may be helpful to identify foods triggering reactions (Chapter 11).

Pseudo allergies can similarly disturb sleep. They are discussed in chapters 12, 14, 15 and 16.

Mast cell activation disorders (MCAD) are commonly associated with fatigue. Fibromyalgia, IBS, IC/BPS, and autism are mast cell activation disorders which have associated chronic sleep disturbances. MCAD should be considered in the differential diagnosis of chronic sleep disorders. MACD is covered in Chapter 13.

Sleep deprivation induces IL-1β production and favors T_H17 immune activation, thus promoting the development of autoimmune disease and food antergies. Some antergic reactions to food cause insomnia, and if not recognized, this it can cause chronic sleep disturbances. In antergic reactions, cytokines can induce histamine release, production of PGE_2 and IL-6 production in the CNS, with little peripheral symptoms. These IgG food reactions are usually delayed by many hours and thus difficult to associate with their disease manifestations. IgG testing for food antergies can be used to identify foods which may trigger insomnia, autoimmune conditions and mood disorders including depression, mast cell activation, obesity, and other disease conditions that are associated with sleep disturbances. (See Chapter 19).

2. Obesity: Sleep deprivation is an important cause of obesity. Obesity increases the risk of sleep apnea, and thus can worsen the sleep disorder. Treatment of other contributing factors of obesity can also be treated to help break the loop of obesity and sleep deprivation.

3. Iron deficiency: Iron deficiency can cause sleep disturbances, especially in infants and children. In infants, this sleep disturbance can persist long after the iron deficiency is corrected[99]. Iron deficiency in the first six months of infancy not only affects the development of sleep architecture, but delays brain development[100], nerve myelination and affects the activity of neurotransmitters even after the deficiency has been corrected[101]. Sleep disturbances in children with autism improved after correction of the iron deficiency[102]. Iron deficiency also affects sleep in adults. In a study of patients with anemia, heart failure and sleep disturbances, treatment for anemia including iron not only improved heart function, but also caused improvements in sleep deprivation and improved both central and obstructive sleep apnea[103]. Iron deficiency is associated with restless leg syndrome.

If an expectant mother is iron deficient during the pregnancy, the infant will have low iron reserves and can be iron deficient. If the mother is iron deficient during lactation, (as might result from a postpartum hemorrhage) the child will likely become iron deficient. Normally, breast milk has sufficient lactoferrin, which is a highly absorbable form of iron. Iron in baby formula is less well absorbed but formulated to be sufficient. Iron deficiency not severe enough to manifest as anemia can still be severe enough to cause delays in neurodevelopmental milestones[104], thus sleep disturbances in infants and young children should be investigated with blood tests for ferritin. Testing for anemia is not adequately sensitive to rule out iron deficiency severe enough to cause sleep disturbances.

4: Stress Relief: Stress can disrupt circadian hormonal rhythms, and this disruption can continue long after the original stressor has been removed[105]. The resulting disturbance in the circadian cycles can cause sleep deprivation and poorer response to stress. Stress should be treated through identification and elimination or accommodation of stressors. With chronic stress, the initiating stressor may have disappeared while the disrupted feedback loop continues. Chapter 29, on the HPA axis, discusses stress and its treatment.

5. Light and Light Therapy: Fluorescent and LED lights have more energy in the blue end of the spectrum than the incandescent lights previously used in the home. Thus, household lighting in the evening now has more impact on the release of melatonin from the pituitary before bedtime. Use of computer monitors and televisions adds to the exposure of blue light on the retina in the hours before bedtime. Computer monitors are problematic because of their close viewing, and the televisions are increasing in size. This should be expected to raise the incidence of sleep disturbances and circadian disturbance disorders including mood disorders, ADHD, bipolar syndrome and premenstrual dysphoric disorder.

The body responds to light from above the visual horizon, natural light from the sky, to set the circadian cycle. It is thus, the upper visual field, the lower half of the retina, which is most sensitive to the effect of blue light of melanopsin production, and effects on the circadian cycle. Yellow or amber tinted glasses worn in the evenings may help prevent disturbing the circadian cycle especially in individuals with high sensitivity to the effects of blue light. Glasses tinted in the upper visual fields may be clear in the lower half. Computer programs are available that automatically change the screen to diminish blue light from the monitor after dark. A "smart home" should do the same.

Bright light in the mornings and the use of "natural sunrise" can be used to entrain the circadian clock. "Alarm clocks" are available that gently increase light in the room, simulating a natural sunrise.

6. Restoring circadian rhythm: Low dose melatonin (0.3 to 0.5 mg) given several hours prior to sleep has been found helpful to restore circadian rhythms. Low-dose melatonin has also been found to be helpful in preventing "sundowning" delirium in the elderly[106]. Larger doses of slow-release melatonin (3 mg to 6 mg) may be helpful to maintain sleep in patients with early morning wakening, along with the investigation and treatment of the underlying causes.

Vitamin B_{12} is a cofactor that amplifies the response of light in resetting the circadian clock[107]. Vitamin B_{12} is helpful in the treatment for some individuals with circadian rhythm disorders, such as DSPS[108]. Vitamin B_{12} levels should be checked when investigating sleep disturbances.

As noted in Chapter 20 on vitamin D, bipolar disorder is more common in northern and extreme southern countries. Vitamin D may be helpful in the primary and secondary prevention of circadian and other sleep disorders[25]. Vitamin D deficiency may also manifest as osteomalacia and other pain syndromes which impair sleep.
Adequate pyridoxine is needed for the formation of melatonin and kynurenic acid.

Keeping regular meal times helps maintain the gastrointestinal circadian rhythm and helps with regular sleep. This is especially important in small children. Avoid large meals within 3 hours of bedtime. A protein/ carbohydrate/ calcium snack, (ice-cream as an example), an hour before bedtime can induce production of serotonin and melatonin, and help with sleep onset. (See Chapter 30, Box: Tryptophan and Napping).

7. Exercise: Getting sufficient physical activity during the day helps with sleep. Part of this may be the brief rise and subsequent lowering of IL-6 levels that occur with exercise. Vigorous or strenuous exercise, however, should be completed several hours before regular sleep time.

8. Avoid Stimulants: Coffee is a health food for most people. Studies of moderate coffee intake show that coffee drinkers are less depressed, more active and live longer. Moderate amounts of caffeine (200 to 400 mg per day) are associated with longevity and health (about 2 to 5 cups of coffee a day). Caffeine is the world's favorite stimulant; it is used to ward off sleep.

Adenosine is the metabolite that makes us feel tired, as a result of the homeostatic sleep drive. It builds up during wakefulness and is eliminated during sleep. Caffeine blocks the adenosine receptors in the brain and thus enhances wakefulness. Caffeine does not work against the circadian sleep drive. When used in the morning or early enough in the day, caffeine can be used to enhance the homeostatic diurnal drive by helping to time activities to the desired alert- awake/ drowsy-sleep cycle. When used inappropriately caffeine is a major cause of insomnia.

> Bipolar patients often have worsened symptoms when using caffeine. Patients with bipolar disorder have a circadian dysfunction, but the homeostatic sleep drive still functions. Caffeine impairs the homeostatic drive; with neither sleep drive working, sleep dysrhythmia can become severe and incapacitating, and promotes psychosis. Caffeine, theobromine, and other stimulants should be avoided in individuals with bipolar disorder. Serum uric acid (UA) can also block adenosine receptors, and high UA levels are associated with mania. UA levels should be normalized if elevated as discussed in Chapter 31.

Caffeine consumed in the morning is rarely a problem for night sleepers. But it should not be used less than about six hours before bedtime to prevent it from disturbing sleep. Caffeine in the evening is more likely to cause stomach upset. Irritability, fatigue, depression and heart arrhythmias may be associated with disturbed sleep caused by caffeine rather than by caffeine itself. The average half-life of caffeine in the body is about 6 hours. If two cups of coffee are consumed after supper at 7 PM, 63 percent of the caffeine would still present in the system at 11 PM. If the person metabolizes caffeine more slowly than the average person, then even more caffeine would be present.

Caffeine causes habituation and can be associated with headaches if a dose is late or missed. To alter a coffee habit, wean the dose slowly over several days.

Table 43-13: Caffeine Doses

Caffeine Source	Typical amount of Caffeine
Coffee – brewed 8 oz.	100 to 200 mg
Coffee – instant 8 oz.	30 -170 mg
Coffee – instant decaffeinated 8 oz.	2 – 15 mg
Starbucks Espresso 1 oz.	60 – 75 mg
Starbucks Vanilla Latte 16 oz.	150 mg
Black Tea – brewed 8 oz.	40 – 120 mg
Black Tea–decaffeinated 8 oz.	2 – 10 mg
Arizona Green Tea 16 oz.	15 mg
Snapple unsweetened 16 oz.	18 mg
Coca-Cola classic 12 oz. can	35 mg
Mountain Dew 12 oz. can	54 mg
Red Bull 8.3 oz.	76 mg
Coffee Ice cream 8 oz.	50 – 85 mg
NoDoz 1 tablet	200 mg
Excedrin Maximum Strength 1 tablet	200 mg
Chocolate Kisses (9 pieces)	11 mg
Dark Chocolate Kisses (9 pieces)	25 mg

Chocolate: Chocolate contains some caffeine, but much less than coffee. Chocolate also contains the alkaloid theobromine, a molecule similar to caffeine, but at a level several times higher than its caffeine content. Like caffeine, theobromine binds to adenosine receptors and thus promotes wakefulness and can cause insomnia. Caffeine is, in part, metabolized into theobromine. Like caffeine, theobromine has a seven-hour half-life for most individuals and acts similarly, although somewhat less strongly than caffeine. Chocolate can cause insomnia when large amounts are consumed late in the day.

9: Avoid Nicotine: Banish tobacco. Not only is it a highly addictive stimulant that can disturb sleep, nicotine can reset the circadian clock and can reset it to the wrong time.

10: Avoid Alcohol: Although alcohol is often used to self-medicate to help initiate sleep, it is not an effective agent for treating insomnia. Alcohol use decreases deep restorative sleep stages and causes fragmentation of rapid eye movement (REM) sleep. Alcohol consumption desynchronizes circadian rhythms, thus making regular sleep more difficult[109]. Alcohol also prevents light from resetting the circadian clock[110].

When the alcohol begins to wear off, glutamine levels in the brain rebound and acts as a stimulant, causing shallow, non-restorative sleep or wakefulness. Alcohol also blocks vasopressin production in the pituitary, leading to increases urine output, promoting nocturia, increasing sweating, dehydration, and dry mouth. Alcohol depletes glycogen stores in the liver, briefly raising blood sugar, followed by a fall in blood sugar and causes fatigue. Once habituated to alcohol, stopping its consumption can temporarily induce insomnia and nightmares, deterring efforts to avoid it. Alcohol should be avoided for at least 3 hours before expected sleep time. A small drink before a siesta causes a rebound that keeps the nap short.

11. Create a Restful Sleep Environment: The purchase of a well-made, new car, with proper maintenance, care and luck should provide about 4000 hours of service; 4000 hours at an average of 50 MPH gives 200,000 miles and costs about $25 per hour, accounting for typical expenses. A good mattress gives about 30,000 hours of comfortable service at a cost of about six cents an hour.

Make sure your bed is comfortable, and service it frequently (Turn mattress according to the manufacturer's instructions, e.g., twice a year). A comfortable bed with quality sheets and comfortable pillow can be justified as an investment in career productivity if not just for the pleasure.

To help promote sleep, the temperature of the bedroom should pleasant and cooler than the daytime room temperature. The room should be dark, and quiet, without distractions. There should not be a TV or computer in the bedroom; reserve those distractions for a different location.

12. Don't fret: Wanting to fall asleep not only makes it harder to fall asleep, but also increases the chances of wakening during sleep and increases sleep fragmentation[111]. If unable to sleep, just relaxing in a dark, comfortable environment provides benefit.

12: Napping: Napping is a healthy activity for adults, and can be used to increase performance and learning. It can also be used to supplement and catch up on sleep.

Table 43-14: Nap Guide

6 to 30 minutes Stage 2 Sleep	Quick refresher. Avoids SWS and waking groggy. Use an alarm to prevent oversleeping. A cup of coffee taken just before the nap can enhance wakening with energy as it takes about 30 to 40 minutes for the caffeine to be absorbed.
30 to 60 minutes SWS Sleep	Generally avoid naps of this duration; they result in waking during SWS sleep and grogginess which can last for 30 minutes.
60 to 90 minutes Full sleep cycle	Allows a full sleep cycle and waking refreshed during stage1/REM sleep. Use an alarm set for 90 minutes, or use a smartphone app or another device that monitors motion and wakes the sleeper during stage 1 sleep. Phone apps such as "Sleepbot," "Sleep Cycle," or "Sleep" as Android can also be used to monitor sleep at night and even to screen for sleep disorders such as sleep apnea.

A good laugh and a long sleep are the best cures in the doctor's book.

[1] Sleep deprivation: Impact on cognitive performance. Alhola P, Polo-Kantola P. Neuropsychiatr Dis Treat. 2007;3(5):553-67.PMID: 19300585

[2] Fatigue, alcohol and performance impairment. Dawson D, Reid K. Nature. 1997 Jul 17;388(6639):235. PMID: 9230429

[3] Does Abnormal Sleep Impair Memory Consolidation in Schizophrenia? Dara S. Manoach and Robert Stickgold Front Hum Neurosci. 2009; 3: 21. PMCID: PMC2741296

[4] Why we sleep: the temporal organization of recovery. Mignot E. PLoS Biol. 2008 Apr 29;6(4):e106. PMID: 18447584

[5] Paradoxical sleep deprivation impairs spatial learning and affects membrane excitability and mitochondrial protein in the hippocampus. Yang RH, Hu SJ, Wang Y, Zhang WB, Luo WJ, Chen JY. Brain Res. 2008 Sep 16;1230:224-32. Epub 2008 Jul 17.PMID: 18674519

[6] CLOCK and BMAL1 regulate MyoD and are necessary for maintenance of skeletal muscle phenotype and function. Andrews JL, Zhang X, McCarthy JJ, et al. Proc Natl Acad Sci U S A. 2010 Nov 2;107(44):19090-5. Epub 2010 Oct 18.PMID: 20956306

[7] Melatonin signaling and cell protection function. Luchetti F, Canonico B, Betti M, Arcangeletti M, Pilolli F, Piroddi M, Canesi L, Papa S, Galli F. FASEB J. 2010 Oct;24(10):3603-24. Epub 2010 Jun 9. Review.PMID: 20534884

[8] The cumulative cost of additional wakefulness: dose-response effects on neurobehavioral functions and sleep physiology from chronic sleep restriction and total sleep deprivation. Van Dongen HP, Maislin G, Mullington JM, Dinges DF. Sleep. 2003 Mar 15;26(2):117-26. Erratum in: Sleep. 2004 Jun 15;27(4):600. PMID: 12683469

[9] The cumulative cost of additional wakefulness: dose-response effects on neurobehavioral functions and sleep physiology from chronic sleep restriction and total sleep deprivation. Van Dongen HP, Maislin G, Mullington JM, Dinges DF. Sleep. 2003 Mar 15;26(2):117-26. Erratum in: Sleep. 2004 Jun 15;27(4):600. PMID: 12683469

[10] Sleep duration associated with mortality in elderly, but not middle-aged, adults in a large US sample. Gangwisch JE, Heymsfield SB, Boden-Albala B, et al. Sleep. 2008 Aug 1;31(8):1087-96.PMID: 18714780

[11] Mortality associated with sleep duration and insomnia. Kripke DF, Garfinkel L, Wingard DL, Klauber MR, Marler MR. Arch Gen Psychiatry. 2002 Feb;59(2):131-6.PMID: 11825133

[12] Habitual sleep duration and insomnia and the risk of cardiovascular events and all-cause death: report from a community-based cohort. Chien KL, Chen PC, Hsu HC, Su TC, Sung FC, Chen MF, Lee YT. Sleep. 2010 Feb 1;33(2):177-84.PMID: 20175401

[13] Association of sleep duration with mortality from cardiovascular disease and other causes for Japanese men and women: the JACC study. Ikehara S, Iso H, Date C, Kikuchi S, Watanabe Y, Wada Y, Inaba Y, Tamakoshi A; JACC Study Group. Sleep. 2009 Mar 1;32(3):295-301.PMID: 19294949

[14] Sleep duration and all-cause mortality: a systematic review and meta-analysis of prospective studies. Cappuccio FP, D'Elia L, Strazzullo P, Miller MA. Sleep. 2010 May 1;33(5):585-92. Review.PMID: 20469800

[15] Systematic interindividual differences in neurobehavioral impairment from sleep loss: evidence of trait-like differential vulnerability. Van Dongen HP, Baynard MD, Maislin G, Dinges DF. Sleep. 2004 May 1;27(3):423-33.PMID: 15164894

[16] Daytime napping after a night of sleep loss decreases sleepiness, improves performance, and causes beneficial changes in cortisol and interleukin-6 secretion. Vgontzas AN, Pejovic S, Zoumakis E, et al. Am J Physiol Endocrinol Metab. 2007 Jan;292(1):E253-61.PMID: 16940468

[17] The impact of sleep duration and subject intelligence on declarative and motor memory performance: how much is enough? Tucker MA, Fishbein W. J Sleep Res. 2009 Sep;18(3):304-12. PMID:19702788

[18] Enhancement of declarative memory performance following a daytime nap is contingent on strength of initial task acquisition. Tucker MA, Fishbein W. Sleep. 2008 Feb;31(2):197-203. PMID:18274266

[19] Post-sleep inertia performance benefits of longer naps in simulated nightwork and extended operations. Mulrine HM, Signal TL, van den Berg MJ, Gander PH. Chronobiol Int. 2012 Nov;29(9):1249-57. PMID:23002951

[20] Effects of physical positions on sleep architectures and post-nap functions among habitual nappers. Zhao D, Zhang Q, Fu M, Tang Y, Zhao Y. Biol Psychol. 2010 Mar;83(3):207-13. PMID:20064578

[21] Coordinated regulation of circadian rhythms and homeostasis by the suprachiasmatic nucleus. Nakagawa H, Okumura N. Proc Jpn Acad Ser B Phys Biol Sci. 2010;86(4):391-409. PMID:20431263

[22] Leptin and ghrelin levels in patients with obstructive sleep apnoea: effect of CPAP treatment. Harsch IA, Konturek PC, Koebnick C, et al. Eur Respir J. 2003 Aug;22(2):251-7.PMID: 12952256

[23] Advances in the study of histaminergic systems and sleep-wake regulation. Liu TY, Hong ZY, Qu WM, Huang ZL. Yao Xue Xue Bao. 2011 Mar;46(3):247-52. PMID:21626776

[24] Leptin and the regulation of the hypothalamic-pituitary-adrenal axis. Malendowicz LK, Rucinski M, Belloni AS, Ziolkowska A, Nussdorfer GG. Int Rev Cytol. 2007;263:63-102. PMID: 17725965

[25] Resolution of hypersomnia following identification and treatment of vitamin D deficiency. McCarty DE. J Clin Sleep Med. 2010 Dec 15;6(6):605-8.PMID:21206551

[26] Prostaglandin D2 mediates neuronal protection via the DP1 receptor. Liang X, Wu L, Hand T, Andreasson K. J Neurochem. 2005 Feb;92(3):477-86. PMID:15659218

[27] Prostaglandins and adenosine in the regulation of sleep and wakefulness. Huang ZL, Urade Y, Hayaishi O. Curr Opin Pharmacol. 2007 Feb;7(1):33-8. Epub 2006 Nov 28. PMID:17129762

[28] Leptin levels are dependent on sleep duration: relationships with sympathovagal balance, carbohydrate regulation, cortisol, and thyrotropin. Spiegel K, Leproult R, L'hermite-Balériaux M,

Copinschi G, Penev PD, Van Cauter E. J Clin Endocrinol Metab. 2004 Nov;89(11):5762-71.PMID: 15531540

[29] Sleep restriction increases the risk of developing cardiovascular diseases by augmenting proinflammatory responses through IL-17 and CRP. van Leeuwen WM, Lehto M, Karisola P, Lindholm H, et al. PLoS One. 2009;4(2):e4589. Epub 2009 Feb 25.PMID: 19240794

[30] Short sleep duration is associated with reduced leptin, elevated ghrelin, and increased body mass index. Taheri S, Lin L, Austin D, Young T, Mignot E. PLoS Med. 2004 Dec;1(3):e62. Epub 2004 Dec 7.PMID: 15602591

[31] Polysomnographic sleep, growth hormone insulin-like growth factor-I axis, leptin, and weight loss. Rasmussen MH, Wildschiødtz G, Juul A, Hilsted J. Obesity (Silver Spring). 2008 Jul;16(7):1516-21. Epub 2008 May 8.PMID: 18464752

[32] Improved prediction of all-cause mortality by a combination of serum total testosterone and insulin-like growth factor I in adult men. Friedrich N, Schneider HJ, Haring R, et al. Steroids. 2012 Jan;77(1-2):52-8. PMID:22037276

[33] Adverse effects of modest sleep restriction on sleepiness, performance, and inflammatory cytokines. Vgontzas AN, Zoumakis E, Bixler EO, Lin HM, Follett H, Kales A, Chrousos GP. J Clin Endocrinol Metab. 2004 May;89(5):2119-26.PMID: 15126529

[34] Effect of zinc and melatonin supplementation on cellular immunity in rats with toxoplasmosis. Baltaci AK, Bediz CS, Mogulkoc R, Kurtoglu E, Pekel A. Biol Trace Elem Res. 2003 Winter;96(1-3):237-45. PMID:14716103

[35] Influence of melatonin on rat thyroid, adrenals and testis secretion during the day. Zwirska-Korczała K, Kniazewski B, Ostrowska Z, Buntner B. Folia Histochem Cytobiol. 1991;29(1):19-24. PMID:1783094

[36] The hormonal Zeitgeber melatonin: role as a circadian modulator in memory processing. Rawashdeh O, Maronde E. Front Mol Neurosci. 2012 Mar 6;5:27. PMID:22408602

[37] Physiologic calcification of the pineal gland in children on computed tomography: prevalence, observer reliability and association with choroid plexus calcification. Doyle AJ, Anderson GD. Acad Radiol. 2006 Jul;13(7):822-6. PMID:16777555

[38] Pineal concretions in turkey (Meleagris gallopavo) as a result of collagen-mediated calcification. Przybylska-Gornowicz B, Lewczuk B, Prusik M, Bulc M. Histol Histopathol. 2009 Apr;24(4):407-15. PMID:19224443

[39] Correlation of serum trace elements and melatonin levels to radiological, biochemical, and histological assessment of degeneration in patients with intervertebral disc herniation. Turgut M, Yenisey C, Akyüz O, Ozsunar Y, Erkus M, Biçakçi T. Biol Trace Elem Res. 2006 Feb;109(2):123-34. PMID:16444002

[40] Pineal gland calcification, lumbar intervertebral disc degeneration and abdominal aorta calcifying atherosclerosis correlate in low back pain subjects: A cross-sectional observational CT study. Turgut AT, Sönmez I, Cakıt BD, Koşar P, Koşar U. Pathophysiology. 2008 Jun;15(1):31-9. PMID:18215511

[41] Aortic stenosis, atherosclerosis, and skeletal bone: is there a common link with calcification and inflammation? Dweck MR, Khaw HJ, Sng GK, et al. Eur Heart J. 2013 Jun;34(21):1567-74. PMID:23391586

[42] Association of mast cells with calcification in the human pineal gland. Maślińska D, Laure-Kamionowska M, Deręgowski K, Maśliński S. Folia Neuropathol. 2010;48(4):276-82. PMID:21225510

[43] Mast cell distribution, activation, and phenotype in atherosclerotic lesions of human carotid arteries. Jeziorska M, McCollum C, Woolley DE. J Pathol. 1997 May;182(1):115-22. Erratum in: J Pathol 1997 Oct;183(2):248. PMID: 9227350

[44] Gas6/Axl-PI3K/Akt pathway plays a central role in the effect of statins on inorganic phosphate-induced calcification of vascular smooth muscle cells. Son BK, Kozaki K, Iijima K, Eto M, Nakano T, Akishita M, Ouchi Y. Eur J Pharmacol. 2007 Feb 5;556(1-3):1-8. PMID:17196959

[45] α-Lipoic acid attenuates vascular calcification via reversal of mitochondrial function and restoration of Gas6/Axl/Akt survival pathway. Kim H, Kim HJ, Lee K, et al. J Cell Mol Med. 2012 Feb;16(2):273-86. PMID: 21362131

[46] Taurine restores Axl/Gas6 expression in vascular smooth muscle cell calcification model. Liao XB, Peng YQ, Zhou XM, Yang B, Zheng Z, Liu LM, Song FL, Li JM, Zhou K, Meng JC, Yuan LQ, Xie H. Amino Acids. 2010 Jul;39(2):375-83. PMID:20033237

[47] Statins protect human aortic smooth muscle cells from inorganic phosphate-induced calcification by restoring Gas6-Axl survival pathway. Son BK, Kozaki K, Iijima K, Eto M, Kojima T, Ota H, Senda Y, Maemura K, Nakano T, Akishita M, Ouchi Y. Circ Res. 2006 Apr 28;98(8):1024-31. PMID:16556867

[48] Gas6-axl receptor signaling is regulated by glucose in vascular smooth muscle cells. Cavet ME, Smolock EM, Ozturk et al. Arterioscler Thromb Vasc Biol. 2008 May;28(5):886-91. PMID:18292389

[49] Healthy Lifestyle Change and Subclinical Atherosclerosis in Young Adults: Coronary Artery Risk Development in Young Adults (CARDIA) Study. Spring B, Moller AC, Colangelo LA, et al. Circulation. 2014 Jul 1;130(1):10-7. PMID:24982115

[50] Arterial stiffening with ageing is associated with transforming growth factor-β1-related changes in adventitial collagen: reversal by aerobic exercise. Fleenor BS, Marshall KD, Durrant JR, Lesniewski LA, Seals DR. J Physiol. 2010 Oct 15;588(Pt 20):3971-82. PMID:20807791

[51] Morphology and function: MR pineal volume and melatonin level in human saliva are correlated. Liebrich LS, Schredl M, Findeisen P, Groden C, Bumb JM, Nölte IS. J Magn Reson Imaging. 2013 Nov 8. PMID:24214660

[52] Degree of pineal calcification (DOC) is associated with polysomnographic sleep measures in primary insomnia patients. Mahlberg R, Kienast T, Hädel S, Heidenreich JO, Schmitz S, Kunz D. Sleep Med. 2009 Apr;10(4):439-45. PMID:18755628

[53] Effects of melatonin and epiphyseal proteins on fluoride-induced adverse changes in antioxidant status of heart, liver, and kidney of rats. Bharti VK, Srivastava RS, Kumar et al. Adv Pharmacol Sci. 2014;2014:532969. PMID:24790596

[54] Melatonin as antioxidant, geroprotector and anticarcinogen. Anisimov VN, Popovich IG, Zabezhinski MA, et al. Biochim Biophys Acta. 2006 May-Jun;1757(5-6):573-89. PMID:16678784

[55] Light-at-night-induced circadian disruption, cancer and aging. Anisimov VN, Vinogradova IA, Panchenko AV, Popovich IG, Zabezhinski MA. Curr Aging Sci. 2012 Dec;5(3):170-7. PMID:23237593

[56] Gastrointestinal melatonin: localization, function, and clinical relevance. Bubenik GA. Dig Dis Sci. 2002 Oct;47(10):2336-48. PMID:12395907

[57] Role of circadian rhythm and endogenous melatonin in pathogenesis of acute gastric bleeding erosions induced by stress. Brzozowski T, Zwirska-Korczala K, Konturek PC, et al. J Physiol Pharmacol. 2007 Dec;58 Suppl 6:53-64. PMID:18212400

[58] Melatonin, a promising supplement in inflammatory bowel disease: a comprehensive review of evidences. Mozaffari S, Abdollahi M. Curr Pharm Des. 2011 Dec;17(38):4372-8. PMID:22204435

[59] Detection of melatonin and homocysteine simultaneously in ulcerative colitis. Chen M, Mei Q, Xu J, Lu C, Fang H, Liu X. Clin Chim Acta. 2012 Jan 18;413(1-2):30-3. PMID:21763296

[60] Localization and biological activities of melatonin in intact and diseased gastrointestinal tract (GIT). Konturek SJ, Konturek PC, Brzozowska I, et al. J Physiol Pharmacol. 2007 Sep;58(3):381-405. PMID:17928638

[61] Melatonin metabolism in the central nervous system. Hardeland R. Curr Neuropharmacol. 2010 Sep;8(3):168-81. PMID:21358968

[62] Melatonin improves metabolic syndrome induced by high fructose intake in rats. Kitagawa A, Ohta Y, Ohashi K. J Pineal Res. 2011 Dec 7. PMID:22220562

[63] Clinical uses of melatonin: evaluation of human trials. Sánchez-Barceló EJ, Mediavilla MD, Tan DX, Reiter RJ. Curr Med Chem. 2010;17(19):2070-95. PMID:20423309

[64] The potential therapeutic effect of melatonin in Gastro-Esophageal Reflux Disease. Kandil TS, Mousa AA, El-Gendy AA, Abbas AM. BMC Gastroenterol. 2010 Jan 18;10:7. PMID:20082715

[65] The therapeutic potential of melatonin in migraines and other headache types. Gagnier JJ. Altern Med Rev. 2001 Aug;6(4):383-9. PMID:11578254

[66] Potential therapeutic use of melatonin in migraine and other headache disorders. Peres MF, Masruha MR, Zukerman E, Moreira-Filho CA, Cavalheiro EA. Expert Opin Investig Drugs. 2006 Apr;15(4):367-75. PMID:16548786

[67] The association of nocturnal serum melatonin levels with major depression in patients with acute multiple sclerosis. Akpinar Z, Tokgöz S, Gökbel H, Okudan N, Uğuz F, Yilmaz G. Psychiatry Res. 2008 Nov 30;161(2):253-7. PMID:18848732

[68] Sleep depth and fatigue: Role of cellular inflammatory activation. Thomas KS, Motivala S, Olmstead R, Irwin MR. Brain Behav Immun. 2011 Jan;25(1):53-8. PMID: 20656013

[69] Retinoid-related orphan receptors (RORs): critical roles in development, immunity, circadian rhythm, and cellular metabolism. Jetten AM. Nucl Recept Signal. 2009;7:e003. PMID:19381306

[70] Meta-analysis of short sleep duration and obesity in children and adults. Cappuccio FP, Taggart FM, Kandala NB, Currie A, Peile E, Stranges S, Miller MA. Sleep. 2008 May 1;31(5):619-26. PMID: 18517032

[71] Finn L "Chronic insomnia and all cause mortality in the Wisconsin Sleep Cohort Study" Association of Professional Sleep Societies 2010; Poster 607.

[72] Adverse effects of modest sleep restriction on sleepiness, performance, and inflammatory cytokines. Vgontzas AN, Zoumakis E, Bixler EO, Lin HM, Follett H, Kales A, Chrousos GP. J Clin Endocrinol Metab. 2004 May;89(5):2119-26. PMID: 15126529

[73] Prolonged sleep restriction affects glucose metabolism in healthy young men. van Leeuwen WM, Hublin C, Sallinen M, et al. Int J Endocrinol. 2010;2010:108641. PMID: 20414467

[74] Impaired nighttime sleep in healthy old versus young adults is associated with elevated plasma interleukin-6 and cortisol levels: physiologic and therapeutic implications. Vgontzas AN, Zoumakis M, Bixler EO, et al. J Clin Endocrinol Metab. 2003 May;88(5):2087-95. PMID: 12727959

[75] Sleep disturbances and correlates of children with autism spectrum disorders. Liu X, Hubbard JA, Fabes RA, Adam JB. Child Psychiatry Hum Dev. 2006 Winter;37(2):179-91. PMID: 17001527

[76] Prospective associations of insomnia markers and symptoms with depression. Szklo-Coxe M, Young T, Peppard PE, Finn LA, Benca RM. Am J Epidemiol. 2010 Mar 15;171(6):709-20. Epub 2010 Feb 18. PMID: 20167581

[77] "Measuring the cosmic dust swept up by Earth." Royal Astronomical Society (RAS). *ScienceDaily*, 29 Mar. 2012. Web. 13 Feb. 2013.

[78] Self-evaluations of factors promoting and disturbing sleep: an epidemiological survey in Finland. Urponen H, Vuori I, Hasan J, Partinen M. Soc Sci Med. 1988;26(4):443-50. PMID: 3363395

[79] Bathing before sleep in the young and in the elderly. Kanda K, Tochihara Y, Ohnaka T. Eur J Appl Physiol Occup Physiol. 1999 Jul;80(2):71-5. PMID: 10408315

[80] Photoreception for circadian, neuroendocrine, and neurobehavioral regulation. Hanifin JP, Brainard GC. J Physiol Anthropol. 2007 Mar;26(2):87-94. PMID: 17435349

[81] Physiological significance of cyclic changes in room temperature around dusk and dawn for circadian rhythms of core and skin temperature, urinary 6-hydroxymelatonin sulfate, and waking sensation just after rising. Kondo M, Tokura H, Wakamura T, Hyun KJ, Tamotsu S, Morita T, Oishi T. J Physiol Anthropol. 2007 Jun;26(4):429-36. PMID: 17704620

[82] Sleep disordered breathing and metabolic syndrome. Nieto FJ, Peppard PE, Young TB. WMJ. 2009 Aug;108(5):263-5. PMID: 19743760

[83] The significance, assessment, and management of nonrestorative sleep in fibromyalgia syndrome. Moldofsky H. CNS Spectr. 2008 Mar;13(3 Suppl 5):22-6. Review. PMID: 18323770

[84] Evidence for genetic association of RORB with bipolar disorder. McGrath CL, Glatt SJ, Sklar P, et al. BMC Psychiatry. 2009 Nov 12;9:70.PMID: 19909500

[85] Differential association of circadian genes with mood disorders: CRY1 and NPAS2 are associated with unipolar major depression and CLOCK and VIP with bipolar disorder. Soria V, Martínez-Amorós E, Escaramís G, et al. Neuropsychopharmacology. 2010 May;35(6):1279-89. Epub 2010 Jan 13.PMID: 20072116

[86] Sleep disturbances and serum ferritin levels in children with attention-deficit/hyperactivity disorder. Cortese S, Konofal E, Bernardina BD, et al. Eur Child Adolesc Psychiatry. 2009 Jul;18(7):393-9. PMID: 19205783

[87] Effects of Statins on Energy and Fatigue With Exertion: Results From a Randomized Controlled Trial.Golomb BA, Evans MA, Dimsdale JE, White HL. Arch Intern Med. 2012 Aug 13:1-2. PMID:22688574

[88] Phase-dependent treatment of delayed sleep phase syndrome with melatonin. Mundey K, Benloucif S, Harsanyi K, Dubocovich ML, Zee PC. Sleep. 2005 Oct 1;28(10):1271-8.PMID: 16295212

[89] Circadian rhythms and sleep in bipolar disorder. Murray G, Harvey A. Bipolar Disord. 2010 Aug;12(5):459-72.PMID: 20712747

[90] Disruption of the circadian timing systems: molecular mechanisms in mood disorders. Mendlewicz J. CNS Drugs. 2009;23 Suppl 2:15-26. PMID: 19708722

[91] Circadian rhythms and sleep in children with autism. Glickman G. Neurosci Biobehav Rev. 2010 Apr;34(5):755-68. Dec 4. PMID: 19963005

[92] Increased sensitivity to light-induced melatonin suppression in premenstrual dysphoric disorder. Parry BL, Meliska CJ, Sorenson DL, et al. Chronobiol Int. 2010 Aug;27(7):1438-53.PMID: 20795885

[93] Rheumatic manifestations of sleep disorders. Moldofsky H. Curr Opin Rheumatol. 2010 Jan;22(1):59-63. PMID: 19935069

[94] Prevalence and characteristics of restless legs syndrome in patients with pulmonary hypertension. Minai OA, Malik N, Foldvary N, Bair N, Golish JA.J Heart Lung Transplant. 2008 Mar;27(3):335-40.PMID: 18342758

[95] The relationship between sensory hypersensitivity and sleep quality of children with atopic dermatitis. Shani-Adir A, Rozenman D, Kessel A, Engel-Yeger B. Pediatr Dermatol. 2009 Mar-Apr;26(2):143-9.PMID: 19419459

[96] Sleep-associated movement disorders and heart failure. Schaffernocker T, Ho J, Hayes D Jr. Heart Fail Rev. 2009 Sep;14(3):165-70. PMID: 19051011

[97] Intravenous iron dextran for severe refractory restless legs syndrome. Ondo WG. Sleep Med. 2010 May;11(5):494-6. 20371212

[98] The natural history of post-traumatic neurohypophysial dysfunction. Agha A, Sherlock M, Phillips J, et al. Eur J Endocrinol. 2005 Mar;152(3):371-7. PMID:15757853

[99] Sleep alterations and iron deficiency anemia in infancy. Peirano PD, Algarín CR, Chamorro RA, Reyes SC, Durán SA, Garrido MI, Lozoff B. Sleep Med. 2010 Aug;11(7):637-42.PMID: 20620103

[100] Delayed CNS maturation in iron-deficient anaemic infants. Ayala R, Otero GA, Porcayo Mercado R, Pliego-Rivero FB. Nutr Neurosci. 2008 Apr;11(2):61-8.PMID: 18510805

[101] A history of iron deficiency anemia during infancy alters brain monoamine activity later in juvenile monkeys. Coe CL, Lubach GR, Bianco L, Beard JL. Dev Psychobiol. 2009 Apr;51(3):301-9.PMID: 19194962

[102] Children with autism: effect of iron supplementation on sleep and ferritin. Dosman CF, Brian JA, Drmic IE, Senthilselvan A, Harford MM, Smith RW, Sharieff W, Zlotkin SH, Moldofsky H, Roberts SW. Pediatr Neurol. 2007 Mar;36(3):152-8.PMID: 17352947

[103] Improvement of anemia with erythropoietin and intravenous iron reduces sleep-related breathing disorders and improves daytime sleepiness in anemic patients with congestive heart failure. Zilberman M, Silverberg DS, Bits I, et al. Am Heart J. 2007 Nov;154(5):870-6. PMID: 17967592

[104] Iron deficiency and infant motor development. Shafir T, Angulo-Barroso R, Jing Y, et al. Early Hum Dev. 2008 Jul;84(7):479-85. Epub 2008 Feb 12.PMID: 18272298

[105] Circadian rhythm of hormones is extinguished during prolonged physical stress, sleep and energy deficiency in young men. Opstad K. Eur J Endocrinol. 1994 Jul;131(1):56-66.PMID: 8038905

[106] Melatonin decreases delirium in elderly patients: A randomized, placebo-controlled trial. Al-Aama T, Brymer C, Gutmanis I, Woolmore-Goodwin SM, Esbaugh J, Dasgupta M. Int J Geriatr Psychiatry. 2010 Sep 15. PMID: 20845391

[107] Vitamin B12 enhances the phase-response of circadian melatonin rhythm to a single bright light exposure in humans. Hashimoto S, Kohsaka M, Morita N, Fukuda N, Honma S, Honma K. Neurosci Lett. 1996 Dec 13;220(2):129-32.PMID: 8981490

[108] A multicenter study of sleep-wake rhythm disorders: therapeutic effects of vitamin B12, bright light therapy, chronotherapy and hypnotics. Yamadera H, Takahashi K, Okawa M. Psychiatry Clin Neurosci. 1996 Aug;50(4):203-9. PMID: 9201777

[109] Acute ethanol modulates glutamatergic and serotonergic phase shifts of the mouse circadian clock in vitro. Prosser RA, Mangrum CA, Glass JD. Neuroscience. 2008 Mar 27;152(3):837-48. Epub 2008 Jan 29.PMID: 1831322

[110] Habitual moderate alcohol consumption desynchronizes circadian physiologic rhythms and affects reaction-time performance. Reinberg A, Touitou Y, Lewy H, Mechkouri M. Chronobiol Int. 2010 Oct.;27(9-10):1930-1942.PMID: 20969532

[111] High intention to fall asleep causes sleep fragmentation. Rasskazova E, Zavalko I, Tkhostov A, Dorohov V. J Sleep Res. 2014 Jun;23(3):295-301. PMID:24387832

44. Hearing and Balance

Hearing

The inner ear is composed of two sections, the cochlea that is the hearing sensor, and the vestibular organ, a multidirectional accelerometer, helps us with a sense of position, balance, and motion.

The human ear is sensitive to sound frequencies from about 16 to 20,000 pressure wave cycles per second (hertz or Hz), although there is a loss of *range*, especially at from the upper frequencies with age. In addition to the loss of range, there is a loss of hearing *sensitivity* with age and injury. The ear does not hear all sound frequencies at the same dynamic level. Within the range of hearing, the ear is most sensitive to sound pressure waves between 2,000 Hz and 6,000 Hz. Several elements explain the difference in sensitivity at various frequencies:

- The shape of the outer ear (the pinnae)
- The shape of the ear canal
- The transfer of energy pressure energy by the ossicle bones of the inner ear,
- The transmission the traveling wave of energy through the endolymph fluid, and
- The number of hair cells stimulated by different frequencies of sounds.

Pressure measurements recorded at the tympanic membrane and other areas in and near the ear show the pinnae amplifies higher pitched sound between about 1,200 and 6,000 Hz to the front of a listener; this makes speech more intelligible and aids in locating the direction from which sounds emanate. The ear canal mostly acts to dampen sounds at certain frequencies, with slight dampening by about 3 dB at around 1000 Hz, by about 10 to 12 dB of dampening between 7,000 and 10,000 Hz and at about 16,000 Hz. This dampening causes the formation of two distinct ranges of heightened hearing; a broad peak from 1000 to 7000 Hs with an apex at about 3,000 Hz, a second narrower peak with an apex at about 13,000 Hz. Hearing sensitivity falls off above 14,000 Hz; thus, isolation of the third peak in sound wave pressure at about 17,000 Hz likely has little impact on hearing. This amplification and dampening of sound wave pressure at different frequencies creates two sound clusters whose energy is distinct from each other. Different frequencies are reflected differently by objects in the environment, and the higher pitched frequencies are transmitted to hair cells in the cochlea more rapidly. These clusters of sound energy are used to amplify differences in directional information and to give us more information about our environment; the proximity of walls, direction of the sound, whether it is approaching or not. Thus, we can discern if we are in an open space, or the size of a closed space using sound and the delays in processing between the ears as well as within the ear. We rely on frequencies above 1000 Hz for locating the directional source of sounds.

Although we are convinced that we can pinpoint the directional source of a sound, at best, we isolate sound direction to about 10-degree sections in our environment. Try dropping a coin on a table; we hear the sound emanate exactly from the spot where we see the coin. Then, close your eyes, drop the coin and put your finger on the point where you expect the coin to be. When you open your eyes, you may be surprised at the lack of precision in locating the sound source.

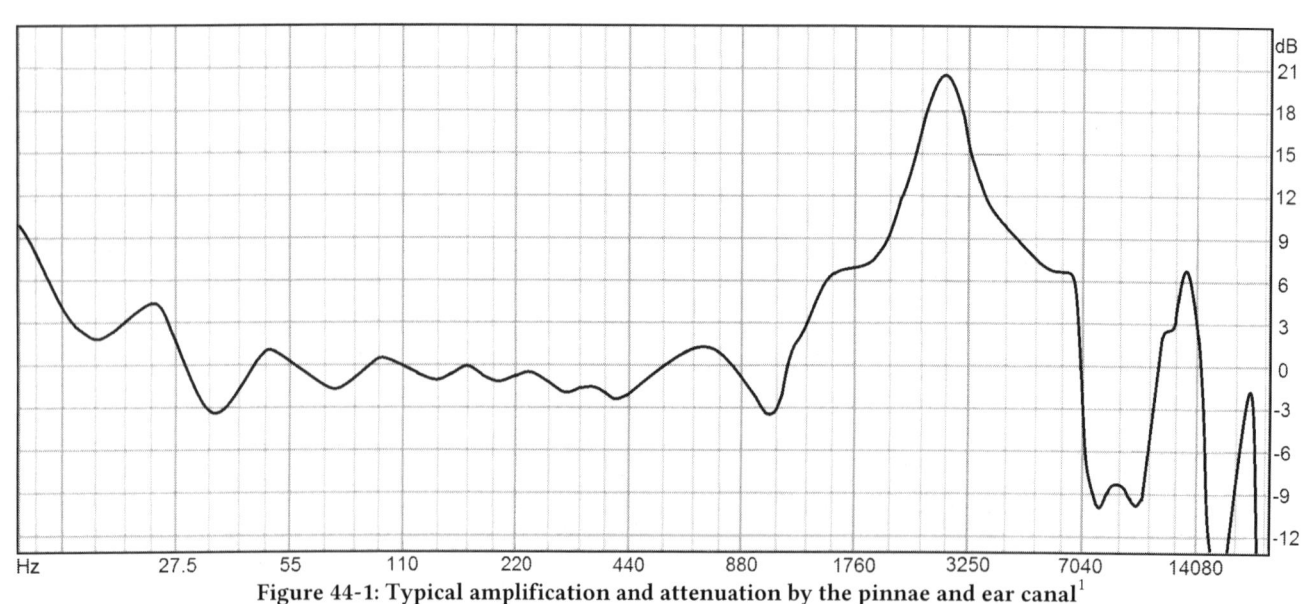

Figure 44-1: Typical amplification and attenuation by the pinnae and ear canal[1]

The cochlea has a spiraled chamber resembling the shape of a snail. If it were to be unwound, it would be about 3.5 cm long. Sound waves from the tympanic membrane are mechanically transduced by the ossicles into shorter and more powerful pressure waves on the oval window of the middle ear; these communicates the pressure waves into the perilymph of the scala vestibuli. Here the pressure waves travel up the spiral through the perilymph, to the top to the spiral and back down through the scala tympani, on either side of another closed fluid space, the scala media. The scala media is filled with endolymphatic fluid.

Depending on the frequencies of the sound, different areas of the basilar membrane, between the perilymph and endolymph resonate. The lower frequencies vibrate the membrane nearer to the apex of the spiral, and higher frequencies resonate the basilar membrane and organ of Corti closer to the base of the cochlea. The pressure wave is allowed to equalize by movement of the membrane at the round window at the end of the spiral.

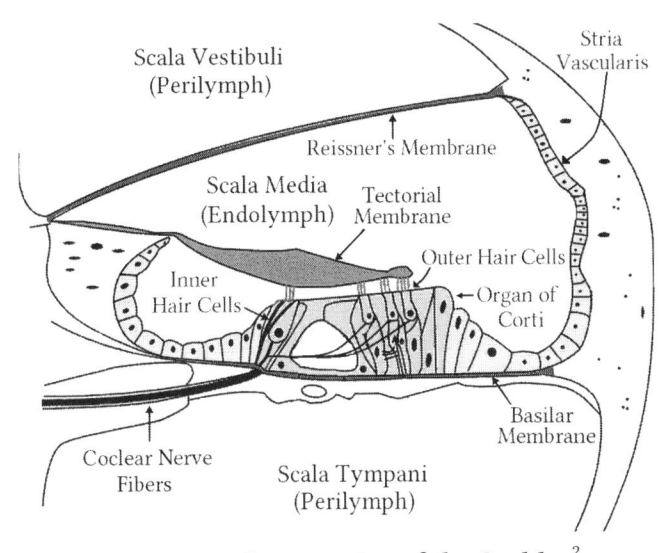

Figure 44-2: Cross section of the Cochlea[2]

The distribution of hair cells in the inner ear also affects the sound dynamics. When low-frequency traveling waves pass through the cochlea, they increase in amplitude and then decay quickly. The apex of the cochlea has a higher mass and is less stiff. When a sound is presented to the human ear, the time taken for the wave to travel through the cochlea is only five milliseconds. Additionally, higher pitched frequencies excite more hair cells. Even a pure sine wave tone excites many hair cells in the ear. We judge pitch by the ranges and level of stimulation of multiple hair cells.

Each individual has uniquely shaped pinnae and canals, and thus each of us person hears a different blend of sounds. These differences make recorded sounds played back through headphones sound different to different individuals, and makes the accurate re-creation of presence and directionality difficult.

The designation dB(A), is a loudness weighting system used to measure loudness. It is based on hearing threshold sensitivity for pure tone sine waves and measures the ability to hear low levels of sound energy. While this useful for testing hearing sensitivity, it is not the best weighting system for determining levels of sound pressure that induce injury to the ears. Nevertheless, dB(A) are the mandated international standard (IEC 61672). Another weighting system, defined in the international standard ISO 226:2003 gives more accurate loudness comparisons. This curve adjusts sound pressure measurements to reflect the greater sensitivity of hearing to frequencies between 1000 and 7000 Hz. This standard recognizes the peak in hearing sensitivity at about 3000 Hz. Loudness perception is important as noise induced hearing losses correlate with the transfer of energy to the cochlea and the perception of loudness. It is this area of hearing, 1000 to 7000 Hz that is most affected by NIHL

The perilymph fluid is similar to cerebral spinal fluid, but endolymph is more similar to intracellular fluid. Hair cells in the ear are unusual in that they use K^+ influx for polarization, rather than Na^+ as do most neurons and muscle cells. The cells of the stria vascularis pump potassium from the perilymph into the endolymph, creating and maintaining an 80 millivolt differential in charge between the perilymph and endolymph. Thus, the endolymph bathes the stereocilia that project into the endolymph in a high K^+ fluid. This gradient maintains a very low threshold for activation of the hair cells, and since all the hair cells share the potassium gradient, continued sound in the same frequency range does not to exhaust the hair cell's electrical potential.

Each human cochlea comes equipped with about 3,500 inner hair cells and 12,000 outer hair cells[3]. This is far smaller number than the number than the million photoreceptors in each eye. The ear needs to be small to concentrate the small amount of mechanical energy available from sound. These cells are polarized, and when depolarized, by the movement of waves in the endolymph in the cochlea, sending nerve impulses to the brain via the eighth cranial nerve.

Each hair bears 30 to 300 stereocilia. The stereocilia are the hair on the hair cells; however, rather than being independent, as are cilia, they are bound together, more like a cluster of bristles than a lock of hair. The multiple stereocilia are fused at their apices and work in concert with each other, providing stability. Pressure waves transmitted through the organ of Corti cause the stereocilia to move in relationship to the tectorial membrane, and this causes depolarization of the hair cells, and the activate neuronal transmission through their depolarization.

The vestibular system has very similar hair cells to those of the auditory system. These are located in the otolithic organs and the semicircular canals. The vestibular hair cells have one tallest cilium, the kinocilium, which is surrounded by a cluster of shorter stereocilia. When the stereocilia move toward the kinocilium, it causes depolarized; when the stereocilia move away from the kinocilium, it causes hyperpolarization that prevents nerve discharge. Changes in the velocity of the fluid in the semicircular canal, with changes in body movement, are perceived as a result of differences in the firing rates of these hair cells.

There are two hair cell types in the organ of Corti. When type I Hair cells (inner hair cells; IHC) are stimulated, they release neurotransmitters and actuate the 8th cranial nerve, sending signals to the brain. These are the hair cells that are doing the hearing.

The Type II (outer hair cells; OHC's) have a different function; they amplify sound. The stereocilia of the OHC extend through a rigid cuticle plate. These unusual cells are actually pressurized so that the stereocilia elongate when the cells are hyperpolarized and relax and contract when they are depolarized. Thus, they push and pull the tectorial membrane as they pressurize and relax. The OHC can contract and relax 70,000 times per second, and by doing so, they amplify the vibrations of the organ of Corti.

This turgor within OHC's relies on the creation of intracellular pressure within the outer hair cells by contraction a transmembrane protein, prestin that encircles the walls of these cylindrical cells. Prestin has two voltage-dependent steps, and thus three different levels of contraction depending on hyperpolarization or depolarization and binding of chloride ions to prestin. Salicylate, the active metabolite of aspirin, can cause reversible hearing loss; it binds to the chloride binding area of prestin, immobilizing it in its elongated state[4].

The nerve fibers that innervate OHC's release the neurotransmitter acetylcholine, which increases the motility of these cells, thereby making them more active[5]. This allows us to tune our hearing and listen to certain sounds.

The movement created by OHC's creates sound that can be recorded as otoacoustic emissions. It is these OHC cells that are most susceptible to noise induced and other types of hearing loss. Measuring otoacoustic emissions can be used to determine if OHC's are functioning normally.

Noise-Induced Hearing Loss

Obviously, noise-induced hearing loss is caused by exposure to loud noise. Less obvious is that noise-induced hearing loss (NIHL) is a disease of mitochondrial dysfunction, caused by oxidative stress.

Unfortunately, mammalian hair cells, unlike those in our fine feathered friends and reptiles, are postmitotic, terminally differentiated cells; they are not known to regenerate in mammals even though some stem cells are retained[6]. Furthermore, the stereocilia of the hair cells are exquisitely sensitive and easily damaged[7]. The stereocilia, although superficially similar in structure to microvilli behave quite differently. Their internal actin skeleton has a very long half-life of at least several months; only the tips of the structures have a more rapid turnover of actin. With age and acoustic injury there is shortening of the stereocilia; this may account for progressive hearing loss[8]. Noise induce hearing loss (NIHL) is accentuated at the same frequencies that we hear best, as these are the areas that sound is best transmitted to the ear.

The frequencies best heard, and most lost in NIHL are those most important for speech intelligibility. Speech contains not only words, but also prosody, or emotional content, which an essential component of language. In some languages, pitch can change the meaning of words. For example in Thai, the word; "Ma" can mean horse, mother or doctor, depending on pitch inflection. A frequency of 3000 Hz can encode ten-times as much information as a frequency of 300 Hz. We also use subtle differences in "presence" to determine when speech is directed to us, or just background noise to ignore. If we lose the sensory cues that the brain uses to detect "presence," it is more difficult to attend focus on those sounds. This is why it is hard to pay attention when sitting in the back of a classroom, church or lecture hall, where reflected sounds with more than a few millisecond delays from the primary sound, not only decrease intelligibility, but also signal the brain to interpret that the speech as background noise, rather than speech directed to us. In a crowded room, we can attend to a single conversation in spite of other dialog; however, with damage to hearing, this becomes more difficult.

Noise-induced hearing loss is commonly seen persons exposed to loud sound levels, such as industrial workers exposed to loud machinery and soldiers that practice shooting rifles without hearing protection. About forty percent of individuals over the age of 65 have hearing loss, and about 16% of hearing impairments are due to exposure to noise.

While the initial mechanisms for NIHL, presbycusis (age-related hearing loss; ARHL), and hearing loss due to ototoxicity vary, all cause apoptosis of hair cells[9]. ARHL and NIHL likely occur through similar mechanisms and show similar susceptibilities. In all these conditions, oxidative stress damages the hair cells, causing mitochondrial damage, leading to apoptosis.

Loud noise, 123 dB for 15 minutes, or 114 dB for two hours in chinchilla, causes disruption of connections of the tips of the stereocilia with the tectorial membrane and of the links between the tips or the hair cells, causing them to be in disarray and causing hearing loss. The fine protein webbing between the tips of the stereocilia, and presumably with the tectorial membrane are sheared immediately. This limited damage can be repaired in about 48 hours, with the recovery of hearing[10]. If acoustic injury is more severe, the stereocilia fall into more severe disarray, and injury progresses over the course several days[11]. The stereocilia can recover from this disarray over several weeks, with recovery of hearing, although some damage and accumulation of toxins appear permanent[12]. Repeated noise-induced injury, especially if it occurs before recovery is completed, is likely to cause more damage than continuous cumulative exposure to lower level loud noise[13].

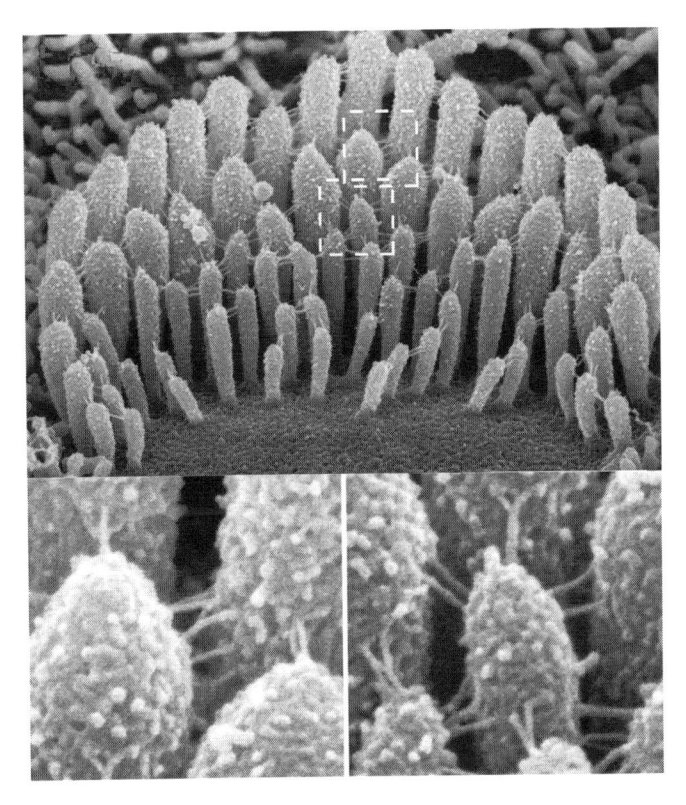

Figure 44-3: Image showing the protein webbing between the tips of hair cells. Images show partial recovery of links after 24 hours after exposure to noise[10].

Orchestra musicians are commonly exposed to high levels of sound pressures, although they would likely take offense if it were referred to as noise. Especially in percussion and horn sections, continuous sound pressure levels of 85 to 90 dB are common, and peak levels commonly reach 125 to 135 dB. Although many of the orchestra musicians studied did have NIHL, most of the hearing loss within the cohort was attributable to ARHL[14]. Noise is just one factor causing NIHL.

Oxidative stress is the principal cause of hearing loss, including noise-induced hearing loss. Cigarettes, alcohol abuse, and malnutrition increase susceptibility to hearing loss[15]. Cigarette smoking increases the risk of severe noise-induced hearing loss by more than seven-fold[16,17]. Exposure to the organic solvents xylene, toluene, and methyl ethyl ketone increases the risk of hearing loss[18] and the risk of noise-induced hearing loss[19].

In ARHL, there is progressive dysfunction of the antioxidant mechanisms. The antioxidant glutathione binds to oxidatively damaged proteins. 4- hydroxynonenal (4-HNE) is the major aldehydic product of lipid peroxidation. 4-HNE is a peroxidative degradation product of arachidonic acid and other n-6 fatty acids, and it is recognized a biomarker of oxidative damage in tissue. The enzyme glutathione S-transferase A4, (GSTA4) is a critical protein that efficiently catalyzed the conjugation of reduced glutathione to 4-hydroxynonenal (4-HNE), in order to detoxify it. 3-nitrotyrosine (3-NT); a marker of peroxynitrite[20]. 4-HNE and 3-NT also increase in the in the cochlea with age. Glutathionylated proteins are a marker of H_2O_2 production; 4-HNE of lipid peroxidation; and 3-NT of peroxynitrite reactions. The level of glutathionylated proteins, 4-HNE, and 3-NT in the cochlea increase with age. Exposure to loud noise causes the formation of 4-hydroxynonenal.

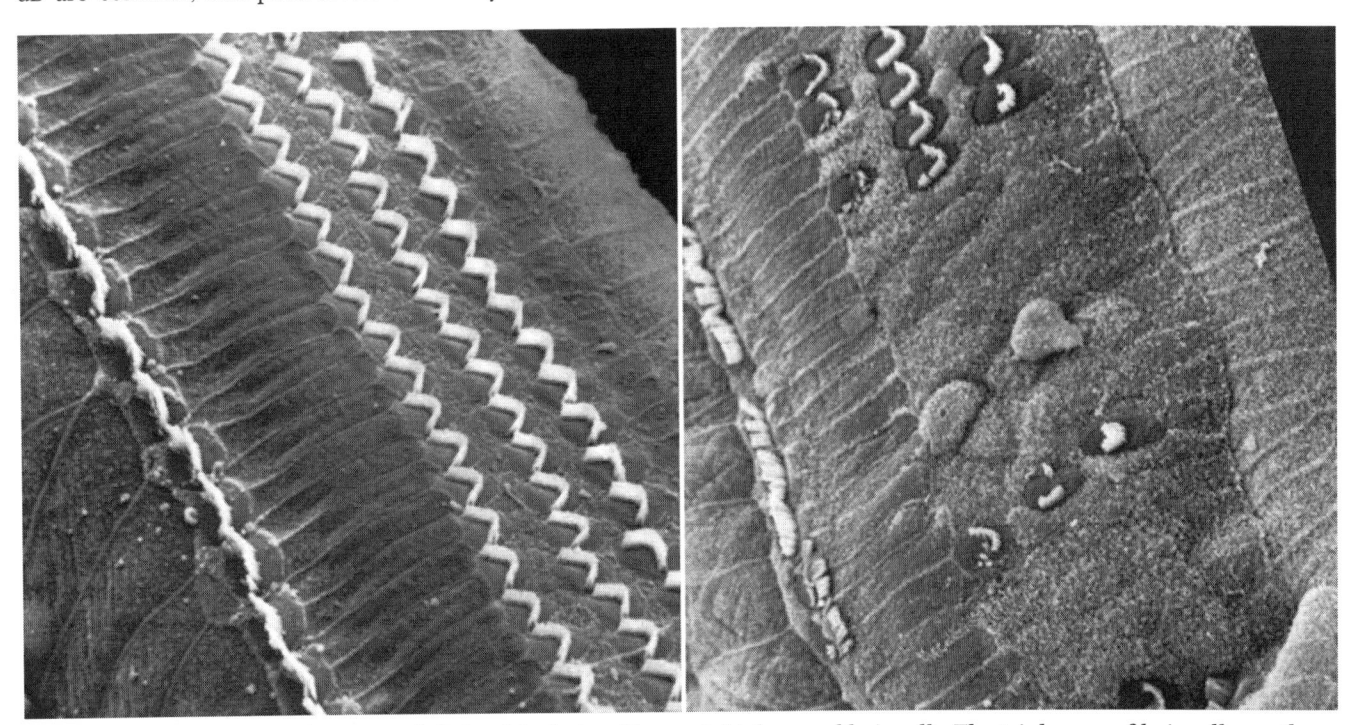

Figure 44-4: The organ of Corti, on left; healthy hair cells, on right damaged hair cells. The triple-row of hair cells are the outer hair cells that mechanically which amplify the sound pressure waves. The single-row of hair cells are the inner hair cells that transform sound vibrations into nerve impulses that are relayed by the cochlear nerve[21].

With aging, the mitochondria become less efficient, due to the accumulation of mtDNA errors and insufficient culling of effete mitochondria. The cochlea is exquisitely sensitive to disturbances in energy metabolism and thus susceptible to oxidative injury from mitochondrial inefficiency. NIHL occurs as a result of free radical damage that triggers apoptosis of hair cells in the cochlea[22]. The OHC's are active cells that require a constant source supply of potassium ions potential. They don't get to take breaks when they get fatigued during a workout. The diuretic furosemide can be ototoxic as it impedes the stria vascularis from adequately creating the potassium gradient the hair cells depend on for polarization.

Gap junction proteins form channels between cells that communication between adjacent cells. Gap junctions are common in many neurons and allow electrical coupling, the passage of calcium or other ions, and even the passage of tumor suppressor genes. Gap junction β2 protein (GJB2, also known as connexin 26; Cx26) is found between stria vascularis cells in the cochlea. Here it allows the diffusion of ions between cells that facilitate the transport of potassium into the endolymph. Genetic defects in this protein are one of the most frequent causes of congenital deafness. Exposure to animals to 110 dB of sound pressure causes an immediate and prolonged decrease in the expression the Cx26 protein, along with a decrease in sodium-potassium ATPase activity and reduce gap junction coupling between these cells[23]. Oxidative stress will also cause this decline in Cx26. Use of free radical scavengers, such as alpha lipoic acid, will prevent both free radical and noise-induced declines in Cx26 expression and activity[22].

In ARHL mtDNA mutations in the cochlear cells accumulate, leading to mitochondrial dysfunction. The resulting inefficiencies impair energy metabolism of the hair cells, promoting the induction of mitophagy, and the death of hair cells and neurons through apoptosis[24]. An estimated twenty percent of genetic diseases that cause post-lingual hearing loss, occurring after the acquisition of language, are genetic disorders of either the mitochondrial-DNA or of host-DNA incorporated into the mitochondria.

For example, autosomal dominant optic atrophy and deafness (ADOAD) is caused by a defect in OPA1, dynamin-related GTPase, required for mitochondrial fusion. Progressive external ophthalmoplegia, (PAO), which causes hearing loss, is caused by a defect in the gene DNA polymerase-γ, which results in mitochondrial DNA instability. MELAS, (myoclonic epilepsy, lactic acidosis, and stroke-like episodes), MERRF, (myoclonic epilepsy with ragged red fiber) and MIDD, (maternally inherited diabetes and deafness), are diseases caused by point mutations in the mitochondrial DNA that result in age-related hearing loss. In MELAS and MERRF, the hearing loss can begin by the age of three[25].

In lab rats, a 30% lifetime caloric restriction prevents mitochondrial DNA damage and reduces age-related hearing loss. Supplementation with vitamin E or vitamin C also prevented these changes, however, less efficiently than does caloric restriction[26]. In another study, alpha-lipoic acid reduced age-related deterioration of hearing; acetyl-carnitine improved auditory thresholds, and both compounds reduced mtDNA age-related deletions[27]. In a separate study, a 50 mg/kg of L-carnitine daily was found to be effective in reducing presbycusis in rats[28]; this would be equivalent to 500 of L-carnitine for a 60 kg adult man.

NIHL appears to be the result of noise-induced oxidative stress. Oxidative stress from homocysteine may increase the risk of hearing loss; otherwise healthy women that had lower levels of vitamin B_{12} and folate had higher more hearing loss[29], and tinnitus[30] and folate supplements appear to slow that rate of hearing loss[31]. Vitamin B_{12} replacement after the injury, however, was not effective in the treatment of tinnitus[32]. The antioxidant alpha-lipoic acid has been found to be more effective than vitamin E in preventing acoustic trauma-induced hearing loss[33].

One source of this oxidative stress is glutamate excitotoxicity. In animals, noise-induced hearing loss can be blocked by the use of compounds that antagonize glutamate activity. When guinea pigs were exposed to noise sufficient to cause hearing loss and a loss of outer hair cells, there was an increase 4-HNE measure indicating increased levels of ROS.

Magnesium level in the cochlea is inversely correlated to ROS formation and to hearing loss[34,35]. Mg mitigates glutamate excitotoxicity, and inversely, low Mg levels exacerbate catecholamine release, increase thromboxane A2 levels, and decrease endothelial NO release; these factors reduce blood flow to the cochlea[3,36].

Magnesium has been demonstrated to protect the ear from NIHL, even when the administration begins an hour after the noise exposure[37]. Similar to traumatic brain injury, hearing loss is an inflammatory process that results in apoptosis, principally of OHC. The damage to the hair cells progresses over several days; thus, there is an opportunity even after the noise insult to prevent the inflammatory damage.

NIHL can also be prevented by L-carnitine, which protects the mitochondria from oxidative damage and by other nutrients that replenish glutathione[38]. Under excitotoxic stress, GSH becomes oxidized to GS:SG, and thus depleted. Glutathione availability in the cochlea increases it ability to "toughen," the ability to become more resistant to loud noise after exposure[39]. N-acetyl cysteine, which helps form glutathione has been found helpful in preventing blast injury to the ear[40].

Phenolic compounds[41,42] and melatonin prevent NIHL, ototoxicity and loss of OHC's, by reducing TNF-α expression[43] and by preventing the activation of NF-κB[44]. Melatonin and phenolic compounds may also prevent cochlear damage as antioxidants[45]. N-acetyl cysteine and vitamins A, C, and E, and magnesium prevent NIHL[46].

Both ARHL and NIHL are diseases of mitochondrial dysfunction, and they can be prevented by maintaining mitochondrial health, and avoiding loud noise and toxins that cause oxidative stress.

Circadian Influence

Hearing does not turn off at night, but during sleep listening should. The decrease in cholinergic efferent stimulus on the outer hair cells should decrease the discharge rate and metabolic demand on the hair cells during sleep, giving the cells an opportunity for recovery from the day's activities and metabolic demands.

The ear may be more sensitive to NIHL from noise at night. BDNF levels are higher in response to daytime noise than nighttime noise[47]. BDNF protects the IHC's and the nerve cells and innervation to both populations of hair cells[48]. Like the HPA axis, the cochlea both makes and responds to ACTH and CRH and other hormones that are under circadian influence[49]. Melatonin levels within the cochlea are higher during dark periods[50],

Vestibular function also is also responsive to circadian cycles[51]. Not only does sleep deprivation decrease vestibular function, but even without sleep deprivations, postural sway varies during the circadian cycle[52].

Tinnitus

Tinnitus is the perception of sound from within the ear. Ten to fifteen percent of adults report it and about for one to two percent of the population, its symptoms seriously reduce their quality of life[53]. Tinnitus is most commonly a high-pitched whine, but can also be ringing, hissing, buzzing, clicking, a low roar, the sound of crickets or other noises. Tinnitus can be caused by cerumen or a hair up against the tympanic membrane, or middle ear problems such as infection, otosclerosis, or spasms of the tiny muscles in the ear. Pulsatile tinnitus may be caused by a vascular tumor in the area of the ear.

The most common form of tinnitus is a high-pitched whine, and the most cause is hearing loss, commonly NIHL. In this case, the tinnitus appears to be a compensatory response to the loss of hearing, and the pitch of the tinnitus is in the frequency area of hearing loss. The decrease in activity of the auditory nerve for that frequency area appears to be counteracted by a gain in neuronal response[54]. With damage or loss of activity or the inner hair cells, the neuronal networks that amplify spontaneous activity become hyperexcitable[55].

In hearing loss due to dysfunction, damage or loss of OHC's, prestin levels rise to help accommodate. Treatment with salicylate, which blocks prestin activity, also increases prestin transcription and protein levels within a several days[56]. Prolonged treatment with salicylate can also inhibit GABAergic activity and results in excitotoxic, oxidative damage to the spiral ganglion neurons of the cochlea.

Salicylate is thought to causes tinnitus, by impairment of OHC activity and a shift in neuronal sensitivity towards 16,000 Hz[57]. The rapid onset of tinnitus and recovery after removal in acute salicylate overdose, suggests that OHC dysfunction is an important cause of tinnitus.

Since hearing loss is the principal cause of tinnitus, preventing hearing loss is essential to the prevention of it. Like hearing loss, risk factors for tinnitus include obesity, smoking, hypertension, and hyperlipidemia[58].

Magnesium helps prevent excitotoxicity. Mg also protects the ear from NIHL[59] and helps in the recovery after acoustic trauma[60] and idiopathic hearing loss[61]. Patients and with tinnitus. In an open-label study, Mg gave significant relief of tinnitus[62].

Melatonin has been shown to be helpful in the treatment of tinnitus[63]. Additionally, it helps prevent ototoxicity from gentamycin and the chemotherapeutic agent, cisplatin, in lab animals, protecting both IHC's and OHC's from oxidative damage and apoptosis. Three milligrams of melatonin daily taken for 30 days reduces tinnitus[64].

Antioxidants[65] and L-carnitine[66] may be helpful for tinnitus, especially in combination with melatonin and magnesium. Tinnitus may be prevented by protecting the ears from injury especially injury to OHC's by preventing oxidative damage, mitochondrial dysfunction and avoiding stressors such as loud noise.

Listening for tinnitus may train the ear to hear it better. This may explain why anxious patients have more problems with tinnitus. Alternatively, anxiety may be associated with hyperexcitability.

Vestibular Dysfunction

Hearing loss, from ARHL, NIHL, or from ototoxic agents is commonly, perhaps nearly universally, accompanied by damage to vestibular function. Ironworkers that have NIHL have been found to have impaired vestibular function[67], as do soldiers with NIHL associated with the use of firearms[68]. The vestibular damage usually goes unrecognized, as these individuals accommodate; they increase reliance on visual cues, muscular proprioception and have increased body sway, which amplifies the remaining vestibular function. The loss of vestibular function, however, is not without consequence. In a study of audiology patients over 60 years of age, 50% reported that they had fallen during the previous 12 months[69].

To find subjects for a genetic linkage study of Usher Syndrome I, a disease that causes deafness, vestibular problems, and night-blindness, I visited a school for the deaf. The principal gathered the student body into a large room and the screening process for the entire student population the student took a total of about 20 seconds. I instructed the children to stand on one leg and close their eyes. The six children with Usher I, immediately stood out from the other deaf children, as they were, much to their own surprise, incapable of performing this task. Even though these children had severe vestibular dysfunction, they accommodated well enough not to recognize this deficit. When I was looking the homes of adult Usher I patients, their neighbors were often as aware of their neighbor's stumbling in low light situations as they were of their neighbor's deafness.

Individuals may accommodate vestibular function well enough that it is not readily apparent and may not be aware of it, especially if it has progressed slowly; nevertheless, this disability greatly increases the risk of falls and injury. Vestibular dysfunction often impacts visual function during motion[70] and thus, may affect driving safety.

Summary

We only have 3,500 inner hair cells and 12,000 outer hair cells in each ear, and they are irreplaceable. It is essential that we treat them well. Hearing loss is associated with loss of vestibular function; damage to our hearing is usually accompanied by impaired balance and risk of falls and accidents.

Like traumatic brain injury, noise-induced hearing damage can be mitigated by immediate treatment to reduce inflammation and prevent apoptosis even after exposure to loud noise; however, prevention is a far better long-term strategy. It is not only preventing exposure to acoustic stress that is important: maintaining health, avoiding oxidative stress, and healthy mitochondria are essential to auditory health and preventing are related hearing loss. Noise levels that are tolerated without damaging hearing in healthy, well-nourished individuals can easily cause hearing loss in those whose health is compromised by high oxidative stress and sluggish mitochondria.

1. Magnesium: Mg is the most common nutrient deficiency in the Western diet, and the one most clearly related to hearing loss. Mg is the central ion in chlorophyll; much like iron is in heme. Green vegetables are a great source of Mg. Mg is also found in fruits, nuts, legumes and whole grains. For treatment, magnesium supplements may be required. Magnesium supplementation is discussed in Chapters 30 and 40.

2. Maintain Mitochondrial Health: See Chapter 21. Avoid oxidative stress, and get sufficient exercise. L-carnitine supports mitochondrial energy transport.

3. Avoid Oxidative Stress: Folate and vitamin B12 deficiencies are associated with ARHL, likely as a result of homocysteine-induced oxidative damage. Alpha lipoic acid supplements may reduce this risk. Dietary Phenols, melatonin, other antioxidants and vitamin D help prevent the inflammatory cascade the results in apoptosis.

4. Peace and Quiet: A good night's rest, in the quiet, should help the ears recover from the day. Melatonin, taken at night helps with tinnitus, and endogenous or exogenous melatonin likely helps protect the ear from damage.

---

[1] Adapted from research by David Griesinger

[2] Adapted from image by Oarih Ropshkow

[3] Magnesium therapy in acoustic trauma. Sendowski I. Magnes Res. 2006 Dec;19(4):244-54. PMID:17402292

[4] Evidence that prestin has at least two voltage-dependent steps. Homma K, Dallos P. J Biol Chem. 2011 Jan 21;286(3):2297-307. PMID:21071769

[5] Regulation of electromotility in the cochlear outer hair cell. Frolenkov GI. J Physiol. 2006 Oct 1;576(Pt 1):43-8. PMID:16887876

[6] Recent advances in hair cell regeneration research. Collado MS, Burns JC, Hu Z, Corwin JT. Curr Opin Otolaryngol Head Neck Surg. 2008 Oct;16(5):465-71. PMID:18797290

[7] An actin molecular treadmill and myosins maintain stereocilia functional architecture and self-renewal. Rzadzinska AK, Schneider ME, Davies C, Riordan GP, Kachar B. J Cell Biol. 2004 Mar 15;164(6):887-97. PMID:15024034

[8] β-Actin and fascin-2 cooperate to maintain stereocilia length. Perrin BJ, Strandjord DM, Narayanan P, Henderson DM, Johnson KR, Ervasti JM. J Neurosci. 2013 May 8;33(19):8114-21. PMID:23658152

[9] Apoptosis in acquired and genetic hearing impairment: the programmed death of the hair cell. Op de Beeck K, Schacht J, Van Camp G. Hear Res. 2011 Nov;281(1-2):18-27. PMID:21782914

[10] Molecular remodeling of tip links underlies mechanosensory regeneration in auditory hair cells. Indzhykulian AA, Stepanyan R, Nelina A, Spinelli KJ, Ahmed ZM, Belyantseva IA, Friedman TB, Barr-Gillespie PG, Frolenkov GI.PLoS Biol. 2013;11(6):e1001583. PMID:23776407

[11] Changes of hair cell stereocilia and threshold shift after acoustic trauma in guinea pigs: comparison between inner and outer hair cells. Chen YS, Liu TC, Cheng CH, Yeh TH, Lee SY, Hsu CJ. ORL J Otorhinolaryngol Relat Spec. 2003 Sep-Oct;65(5):266-74. PMID:14730182

[12] Structure of the stereocilia side links and morphology of auditory hair bundle in relation to noise exposure in the chinchilla. Tsuprun V, Schachern PA, Cureoglu S, Paparella M. J Neurocytol. 2003 Nov;32(9):1117-28. PMID:15044843

[13] Adjustment of dose-response relationship of industrial impulse noise induced high frequency hearing loss with different exchange rate. Zhao YM, Chen SS, Cheng XR, Li YQ. Zhonghua Yi Xue Za Zhi. 2006 Jan 3;86(1):48-51. PMID:16606538

[14] Evaluation of sound exposure and risk of hearing impairment in orchestral musicians. Pawlaczyk-Łuszczyńska M, Dudarewicz A, Zamojska M, Sliwinska-Kowalska M. Int J Occup Saf Ergon. 2011;17(3):255-69. PMID:21939598

[15] Contribution of the N-acetyltransferase 2 polymorphism NAT2*6A to age-related hearing impairment.

Van Eyken E, Van Camp G, Fransen E, et al. J Med Genet. 2007 Sep;44(9):570-8. PMID:17513527

[16] Interaction of smoking and occupational noise exposure on hearing loss: a cross-sectional study. Pouryaghoub G, Mehrdad R, Mohammadi S. BMC Public Health. 2007 Jul 3;7:137. PMID:17605828

[17] Cigarette smoking and occupational noise-induced hearing loss. Mohammadi S, Mazhari MM, Mehrparvar AH, Attarchi MS. Eur J Public Health. 2010 Aug;20(4):452-5. PMID:19887518

[18] Organic solvent exposure and hearing loss in a cohort of aluminium workers. Rabinowitz PM, Galusha D, Slade MD, Dixon-Ernst C, O'Neill A, Fiellin M, Cullen MR. Occup Environ Med. 2008 Apr;65(4):230-5. PMID:17567727

[19] Combined effects of ototoxic solvents and noise on hearing in automobile plant workers in Iran. Mohammadi S, Labbafinejad Y, Attarchi M. Arh Hig Rada Toksikol. 2010 Sep;61(3):267-74. PMID:20860967

[20] Oxidative imbalance in the aging inner ear. Jiang H, Talaska AE, Schacht J, Sha SH. Neurobiol Aging. 2007 Oct;28(10):1605-12. PMID:16920227

[21] Electron micrograph courtesy of the House Ear Institute, Los Angeles, California

[22] Disruption of ion-trafficking system in the cochlear spiral ligament prior to permanent hearing loss induced by exposure to intense noise: possible involvement of 4-hydroxy-2-nonenal as a mediator of oxidative stress. Yamaguchi T, Nagashima R, Yoneyama M, Shiba T, Ogita K. PLoS One. 2014 Jul 11;9(7):e102133. PMID:25013956

[23] Radix astragali inhibits the down-regulation of connexin 26 in the stria vascularis of the guinea pig cochlea after acoustic trauma. Xiong M, Zhu Y, Lai H, et al. Eur Arch Otorhinolaryngol. 2014 May 25. PMID:24858698

[24] Age-related hearing loss in C57BL/6J mice is mediated by Bak-dependent mitochondrial apoptosis. Someya S, Xu J, Kondo K, Ding D, et al. Proc Natl Acad Sci U S A. 2009 Nov 17;106(46):19432-7. PMID:19901338

[25] Mitochondrial oxidative damage and apoptosis in age-related hearing loss. Someya S, Prolla TA. Mech Ageing Dev. 2010 Jul-Aug;131(7-8):480-6. Apr 29. PMID:20434479

[26] Effects of dietary restriction and antioxidants on presbyacusis. Seidman MD. Laryngoscope. 2000 May;110(5 Pt 1):727-38. PMID: 10807352

[27] Biologic activity of mitochondrial metabolites on aging and age-related hearing loss. Seidman MD, Khan MJ, Bai U, Shirwany N, Quirk WS. Am J Otol. 2000 Mar;21(2):161-7. PMID: 10733178

[28] The effects of L-carnitine on presbyacusis in the rat model. Derin A, Agirdir B, Derin N, et al. Clin Otolaryngol Allied Sci. 2004 Jun;29(3):238-41. PMID: 15142068

[29] Age-related hearing loss, vitamin B-12, and folate in elderly women. Houston DK, Johnson MA, Nozza RJ, Gunter EW, Shea KJ, Cutler GM, Edmonds JT. Am J Clin Nutr. 1999 Mar;69(3):564-71. PMID:10075346

[30] The role of plasma melatonin and vitamins C and B12 in the development of idiopathic tinnitus in the elderly. Lasisi AO, Fehintola FA, Lasisi TJ. Ghana Med J. 2012 Sep;46(3):152-7. PMID:23661829

[31] Effects of folic acid supplementation on hearing in older adults: a randomized, controlled trial. Durga J, Verhoef P, Anteunis LJ, Schouten E, Kok FJ. Ann Intern Med. 2007 Jan 2;146(1):1-9. PMID:17200216

[32] Vitamin B12 levels in patients with tinnitus and effectiveness of vitamin B12 treatment on hearing threshold and tinnitus. Berkiten G, Yildirim G, Topaloglu I, Ugras H. B-ENT. 2013;9(2):111-6. PMID:23909117

[33] Comparison of the Protective Effects of Radix Astragali, α-Lipoic Acid, and Vitamin E on Acute Acoustic Trauma. Xiong M, Lai H, Yang C, Huang W, Wang J, Fu X, He Q. Clin Med Insights Ear Nose Throat. 2012 Nov 29;5:25-31. PMID:24179406

[34] The cochlea magnesium content is negatively correlated with hearing loss induced by impulse noise.Xiong M, Wang J, Yang C, Lai H. Am J Otolaryngol. 2013 May-Jun;34(3):209-15. PMID:23332299

[35] Dependence of noise-induced hearing loss upon perilymph magnesium concentration. Joachims Z, Babisch W, Ising H, et al. J Acoust Soc Am. 1983 Jul;74(1):104-8. PMID:6886192

[36] Biochemical mechanisms affecting susceptibility to noise-induced hearing loss. Günther T, Ising H, Joachims Z. Am J Otol. 1989 Jan;10(1):36-41. PMID:2655464

[37] Long-term administration of magnesium after acoustic trauma caused by gunshot noise in guinea pigs. Abaamrane L, Raffin F, Gal M, Avan P, Sendowski I. Hear Res. 2009 Jan;247(2):137-45. PMID:19084059

[38] Candidate's thesis: enhancing intrinsic cochlear stress defenses to reduce noise-induced hearing loss. Kopke RD, Coleman JK, Liu J, Campbell KC, Riffenburgh RH. Laryngoscope. 2002 Sep;112(9):1515-32. PMID: 12352659

[39] The role of antioxidants in protection from impulse noise. Henderson D, McFadden SL, Liu CC, Hight N, Zheng XY. Ann N Y Acad Sci. 1999 Nov 28;884:368-80. PMID:10842607

[40] Mechanisms and treatment of blast induced hearing loss. Choi CH. Korean J Audiol. 2012 Dec;16(3):103-7. PMID:24653882

[41] Therapeutic window for ferulic acid protection against noise-induced hearing loss in the guinea pig. Fetoni AR, Eramo S, Troiani D, Paludetti G. Acta Otolaryngol. 2011 Apr;131(4):419-27. PMID:21198344

[42] Resveratrol protects auditory hair cells from gentamicin toxicity. Bonabi S, Caelers A, Monge A, Huber A, Bodmer D. Ear Nose Throat J. 2008 Oct;87(10):570-3. PMID:18833534

[43] An experimental comparative study of dexamethasone, melatonin and tacrolimus in noise-induced hearing loss. Bas E, Martinez-Soriano F, Láinez JM, Marco J. Acta Otolaryngol. 2009 Apr;129(4):385-9. PMID:19051071

[44] (-)-Epigallocatechin-3-gallate protects against NO-induced ototoxicity through the regulation of caspase- 1, caspase-3, and NF-κB activation. Kim SJ, Lee JH, Kim BS, So HS, Park R, Myung NY, Um JY, Hong SH. PLoS One. 2012;7(9):e43967. PMID:23028481

[45] Efficacy of three drugs for protecting against gentamicin-induced hair cell and hearing losses. Bas E, Van De Water TR, Gupta C, Dinh J, Vu L, Martínez-Soriano F, Láinez JM, Marco J. Br J Pharmacol. 2012 Jul;166(6):1888-904. PMID:22320124

[46] Uniform comparison of several drugs which provide protection from noise induced hearing loss. Tamir S, Adelman C, Weinberger JM, Sohmer H. J Occup Med Toxicol. 2010 Sep 1;5:26. PMID:20809938

[47] TrkB-mediated protection against circadian sensitivity to noise trauma in the murine cochlea. Meltser I, Cederroth CR, Basinou V, Savelyev S, Lundkvist GS, Canlon B. Curr Biol. 2014 Mar 17;24(6):658-63. PMID:24583017

[48] Lack of brain-derived neurotrophic factor hampers inner hair cell synapse physiology, but protects against noise-induced hearing loss. Zuccotti A, Kuhn S, Johnson SL, et al. J Neurosci. 2012 Jun 20;32(25):8545-53. PMID:22723694

[49] The cochlea as an independent neuroendocrine organ: expression and possible roles of a local hypothalamic-pituitary-adrenal axis-equivalent signaling system. Basappa J, Graham CE, Turcan S, Vetter DE. Hear Res. 2012 Jun;288(1-2):3-18. PMID:22484018

[50] Levels of the pineal hormone melatonin and its circadian variations in the cochlea of Wistar rats. López González MA, Guerrero JM, Ceballo Pedraja JM, Mata Maderuelo F, Delgado Moreno F. Acta Otorrinolaringol Esp. 1998 Oct;49(7):509-12. PMID:9866214

[51] Genetic evidence for a neurovestibular influence on the mammalian circadian pacemaker. Fuller PM, Fuller CA. J Biol Rhythms. 2006 Jun;21(3):177-84. PMID:16731657

[52] Circadian amplitude and homeostatic buildup rate in postural control. Forsman P, Hæggström E. Gait Posture. 2013 Jun;38(2):192-7. PMID:23245641

[53] General review of tinnitus: prevalence, mechanisms, effects, and management. Henry JA, Dennis KC, Schechter MA. J Speech Lang Hear Res. 2005 Oct;48(5):1204-35. PMID:16411806

[54] Predicting tinnitus pitch from patients' audiograms with a computational model for the development of neuronal hyperactivity. Schaette R, Kempter R. J Neurophysiol. 2009 Jun;101(6):3042-52. PMID:19357344

[55] Tinnitus with a normal audiogram: physiological evidence for hidden hearing loss and computational model. Schaette R, McAlpine D. J Neurosci. 2011 Sep 21;31(38):13452-7. PMID:21940438

[56] Long-term administration of salicylate enhances prestin expression in rat cochlea. Yang K, Huang ZW, Liu ZQ, Xiao BK, Peng JH. Int J Audiol. 2009 Jan;48(1):18-23. PMID:19173110

[57] Review of salicylate-induced hearing loss, neurotoxicity, tinnitus and neuropathophysiology. Sheppard A, Hayes SH, Chen GD, Ralli M, Salvi R. Acta Otorhinolaryngol Ital. 2014 Apr;34(2):79-93. PMID:24843217

[58] Clinical observations and risk factors for tinnitus in a Sicilian cohort. Martines F, Sireci F, Cannizzaro E, et al. Eur Arch Otorhinolaryngol. 2014 Sep 5. PMID:25190254

[59] Preventive effect of magnesium supplement on noise-induced hearing loss in the guinea pig. Scheibe F, Haupt H, Ising H. Eur Arch Otorhinolaryngol. 2000;257(1):10-6. PMID:10664038

[60] Therapeutic efficacy of magnesium after acoustic trauma caused by gunshot noise in guinea pigs. Sendowski I, Raffin F, Braillon-Cros A. Acta Otolaryngol. 2006 Feb;126(2):122-9. PMID:16428187

[61] Magnesium: a new therapy for idiopathic sudden sensorineural hearing loss. Gordin A, Goldenberg D, Golz A, Netzer A, Joachims HZ. Otol Neurotol. 2002 Jul;23(4):447-51. PMID:12170143

[62] Phase 2 study examining magnesium-dependent tinnitus. Cevette MJ, Barrs DM, Patel A, et alJ. Int Tinnitus J. 2011;16(2):168-73. PMID:22249877

[63] The effects of melatonin on tinnitus and sleep. Megwalu UC, Finnell JE, Piccirillo JF. Otolaryngol Head Neck Surg. 2006 Feb;134(2):210-3. PMID:16455366

[64] Drug-mediated ototoxicity and tinnitus: alleviation with melatonin. Reiter RJ, Tan DX, Korkmaz A, Fuentes-Broto L. J Physiol Pharmacol. 2011 Apr;62(2):151-7. PMID:21673362

[65] Antioxidant therapy in idiopathic tinnitus: preliminary outcomes. Savastano M, Brescia G, Marioni G. Arch Med Res. 2007 May;38(4):456-9. PMID:17416295

[66] An in vitro model for testing drugs to treat tinnitus. Wu C, Gopal K, Gross GW, Lukas TJ, Moore EJ. Eur J Pharmacol. 2011 Sep 30;667(1-3):188-94. PMID:21718695

[67] Are hearing loss and balance dysfunction linked in construction iron workers? Kilburn KH, Warshaw RH, Hanscom B. Br J Ind Med. 1992 Feb;49(2):138-41. PMID:1536822

[68] Postural body sway and exposure to high-energy impulse noise. Juntunen J, Matikainen E, Ylikoski J, Ylikoski M, Ojala M, Vaheri E. Lancet. 1987 Aug 1;2(8553):261-4. PMID:2886727

[69] Falls in the audiology clinic: a pilot study. Criter RE, Honaker JA. J Am Acad Audiol. 2013 Nov-Dec;24(10):1001-5. PMID:24384085

[70] Clinical evaluation of dynamic visual acuity in subjects with unilateral vestibular hypofunction. Dannenbaum E, Paquet N, Chilingaryan G, Fung J. Otol Neurotol. 2009 Apr;30(3):368-72. PMID:19318888

45. Enteroimmune Disease and Public Health

The things that proceed from the mouth may defile the soul, but those that enter it defile the body. Most of the disease burden and years of life lost in industrialized countries results from foods, beverages, alcohol and tobacco products; causing cancer, heart disease, diabetes, and stroke. Most of the major causes of death in developed countries are implicitly nutritional diseases. Furthermore, the common morbidities affecting younger people; asthma acne, depression, migraines, irritable bowel syndrome, bladder pain syndrome, autism, fibromyalgia, and autoimmune diseases are enteroimmune diseases; with diet and immune reaction to proteins in the diet at the core of their causation.

In the last hundred years, the world's population has grown from 1.75 billion to 7 billion people and is expected to grow to eight billion by the year 2025. Our modern lifestyle, the good and the not so good, are dependent on the ability of the agricultural sector to provide food for the human population. Nevertheless, over the last century, the world's population has largely migrated away from farms, and into urban environments. During this time, women have become more empowered. Most children now survive the first two years of life and have access to education. Up into the 1930's in the United States orphan children in the cities were shipped off to farms as cheap labor and as a cost savings mechanism for the cities. Large families were needed just for farm labor. These changes and advances in technology rely on a critical mass of educated individuals, which could not have occurred without cities and highly productive farms to feed them.

Mechanized monoculture, intensive use of fertilizers, pesticides, and irrigation have allowed for very efficient high-yield agriculture that can feed seven billion people. Corn, largely through corn subsidies in the United States, is a key element of this great feat. Without corn, food prices would be considerably higher, and even now, competition for corn for use in making fuel alcohol has raised the price of many foods. Meat, inexpensively and quickly raised in feedlots and industrial sized chick coups, are dependent on cheap corn. Inexpensive mass-produced chicken feed based on corn and industrialized soy farming also keep egg prices low.

But there are associated costs with this. If there ever was, there is now little natural about farming. We are depleting the phosphate supply, polluting rivers with fertilizer, pesticides, and antibiotics, consuming fossil fuels, depleting the aquifers, limiting diversity, destroying wildlife, and causing dead zones in the sea with our farms.

Another cost is human health.

Our corn and soy-based diet provides an unhealthy and undesirably high levels of proinflammatory linoleic acid. Although, as individuals, we can buy grass fed beef and free range chicken eggs, as a population, it cannot be done; there is not enough land, and the costs are too high. Seven billion people cannot eat salmon three times a week to supply sufficient EPA and DHA for their health requirements; the oceans are already overfished.

In this book, I have advocated the consumption of a healthier diet; high in vegetables and fruits, whole grains and fish. While agricultural production is sufficient to supply the world's population with calories and protein, it cannot supply the quality of food recommended herein for even a large fraction of that population. The Western diet is a high-protein, high-fat diet based on food from highly productive industrialized farming, but this is not a healthy diet. This is everyone's concern, not only as a humanitarian issue, but as an economic issue. Society can ill-afford the rising healthcare costs associated with chronic diseases caused by our faulty diet. The U.S. Congressional Budget Office estimates that healthcare costs consume 17 percent of the gross domestic product, and these costs are projected to increase to 30 percent by the year 2035[1]. This tax on health is unsustainable, and as the population ages, the cost becomes untenable.

The major risk factors for obesity, diabetes, cancer, heart disease, stroke, and COPD are inappropriate diet, alcohol and tobacco use. These diseases create the vast majority of medical care costs. Yet, almost all the resources expended in caring for the afflicted goes to treatments that maintain these diseases, rather than avoiding or reversing them.

As in the tale of the men who spent their day rescuing people who were being washed down the river, it is uneconomic, imprudent, and even harmful to focus on treating one patient at a time. While the rescue may feel noble and exhilarating, it is irresponsible not to repair the bridge, and continue to allow our family members, and those of our neighbors to fall through; many are not saved.

Our food supply needs to deliver healthful food. This goal needs to look to technologies that can provide healthy and economical food. This may involve developing new foods perhaps from algae and duckweed, or by genetically modifying corn to make it produce α-linolenic acid. Genetically engineered, stearidonic acid enriched soy has been developed which produces soy oil with high levels of this n-3 fatty acid. This crop may present a sustainable terrestrial of source n-3 fats for human and animal nutrition[2]. We need a new wheat which does not have the toxicity of gliadin, but which allows for our favored foods, including bread, pizza, croissants, and cupcakes.

New farming practices are needed to economically produce a wider variety of vegetables than currently available on most grocery shelves. Perhaps we can find a way to treat cattle in a healthier manner; simply allowing feedlot cattle to graze on grass one day per fortnight, would greatly reduce their need for antibiotics and decrease the risk of antibiotic resistance in human disease. Like us, cattle need real food with fiber to have a healthy enteric biome.

Feeding cattle corn, which are in turn are used as food, is an inefficient method of producing food. Grass-fed cattle require less intensive farming practices, but use more agricultural land, and take several times longer to raise. This would require consumption of smaller quantities of meat than typically consumed in the American Western diet. This would be a healthier choice, but it may be hard to get than to give up their burgers.

Some changes towards health are easy to make. In the late 1990's food fortification with the B vitamin, folic acid was mandated for some processed foods in the U.S. As a result, the average person's folate level in the U.S. doubled, and now, is adequate for most of the population; the incidence of neural tube defects, neuroblastoma, and some other cancers, and the incidence of heart disease have fallen. Vitamin B_{12} levels remain low in half of the U.S. population, and vitamin B_6 levels are lower than optimal to prevent inflammation and disease in a large percentage of the population. Fortification of grain-based products (breakfast cereal, bread, pasta) with vitamins B_{12} and B_6 should be considered.

The current normal reference range, lower-limit for vitamin B_{12} levels in adults is 200 pg/ml (148 pmol/L); a level associated with risk of elevated homocysteine, increased risk of cancer, and decreased regeneration of SAMe and CoQ_{10}. This standard also prevents the reimbursement for treatment of the elderly with suboptimal vitamin B_{12} status, but in whom levels are above the current inappropriate lower reference level. The lower level for the cyanocobalamin should be set at a level which prevents adverse metabolic changes; about 500 pg/ml[3].

The current reference range lower-limit for vitamin B_6, is 20 nmol/L. However, levels need to be above 70 nmol/L to prevent an elevated risk of colon cancer. Even without fortification of the food supply, changing the reference values to reflect levels associated with lower risk of common diseases would help prevent these diseases; as it would acknowledge levels required for health. Currently, the norms are based on levels required to prevent acute deficiencies and upon the normal distribution of levels found in a population plagued with chronic disease.

Vitamin D_3 levels are also low in much of the population. Seventy percent of Americans have vitamin D levels lower than 80 nm/L of 25OHD3[4]. The level of fortification of vitamin D_3 in milk was set to prevent, not to replicate the amount produced in a natural lifestyle when most of the day was spent in the sunshine. Most adults consume little milk. If vitamin D supplementation is a public policy, it should be provided in foods other than just milk, a food poorly digested by most adults. The cost of medical care for the elderly would likely be substantially lower if vitamin D_3 supplements were supplied at no cost to all Medicare recipients as it would lower the risk of fractures, diabetes, cancer and other diseases.

Most cancer is caused by carcinogens in food, with tobacco-use being the second largest source of carcinogens. We have somehow accepted that this is a lifestyle choice. The largest sources of food carcinogens for Americans are heterocyclic amines (HCA). The largest source of these of HCA are from cooking meat, using poor cooking technique. Meat can be prepared with minimal HCA levels. Several methods can be used to decrease HCA production, (see Chapter 40), most improve the quality of the food and improve flavor. This is not a lifestyle choice; this is a matter of education.

Factories and vehicles which pollute the air or water are examples of economic policies that externalize the costs. It is not that the pollution does create an economic burden; for example, air pollution causes asthma, medical care cost, lost days of education and productivity. However, this burden is externalized. The polluters do not pay the cost, so they have little economic incentive to prevent their pollution. The cost instead is borne by those in society who live downwind or downstream of the polluter. It is easy to see the economic advantages of free, unregulated markets when you turn a blind eye to the cost borne by others.

Economic incentives can be used as a method to internalize the cost of things that damage health. Most disease factors externalize the costs. Cigarette smoking has a high economic burden on society from the damage it does to children in terms of ill health and behavioral problems associated with its exposure in utero or in infants, the decreased academic performance in children of smokers. Additionally, smokers are sick more frequently, less productive and consume place a higher economic burden on the health care system. Alcohol increases the risk of social failure, behavioral problems and incarceration, and disease burden. Most of these costs are externalized. Society pays the extra costs incurred by tobacco and alcohol use through higher taxes, higher medical insurance premiums, supporting prisons and having less efficient classrooms.

Taxing cigarettes and alcohol at levels equivalent to the costs they incur onto the general public would mitigate these costs, shifting them back from society, to those who use or produce these products. Anything short of this should be understood as a subsidy to the industry that promotes the use of these products and damages us.

At present, government corn subsidies finance cheap food, (beef, chicken, eggs) and corn syrup. As discussed in

Chapter 9, corn syrup is an important contributor to metabolic syndrome. Although it may unpopular, taxation on corn syrup would promote lower utilization of this product.

IgG to foods, specifically IgG$_4$, is an important contributor to enteroimmunopathic disease. These anterigies can be easily tested for; however, at present, almost no insurance companies pay for these tests. At $10 per food item tested, a 150-food panel, which covers a large enough spectrum of foods to be helpful, costs $1500. This is a large out-of-pocket cost for a patient. The negotiated insurance price is about a quarter of this.

Since food elimination cost nothing to the medical insurance companies, failure to pay for this test is financially short-sighted, as the treatment cost (alternate foods) is borne by the individual, and thus is obviously much less expensive than other treatments and disability from ongoing disease and palliative treatments. It is in the interest of the patients, other policyholders, and the insurance companies to effectively diagnose anterigies as the treatment is very cost effective and efficacious.

We have long treated obesity as personality deficit; a combination of gluttony and sloth. In the enteroimmune paradigm, obesity can be understood as an inflammatory disease which affects appetite, hormones, and fat deposition. Providing patients with a dietary prescription that controls the inflammatory response, thus decreasing the appetite gives a much better chance of successful disease mitigation than telling a patient to curtailment of caloric intake and, go hungry; impart stress and a sense of failure upon the patient. The caloric deprivation strategy inevitably fails, yet it is accepted practice in medicine.

Similarly, the medical community has a maladaptive approach to the prevention of domestic violence, in that it has ignored the most significant factors in this scourge, the perpetrators of violence. If we are to decrease the incidence of domestic violence and child abuse, we need to screen for perpetrators of domestic violence, and offer them medical treatment to help with this problem and offer non-accusatory therapy for non-medical behavioral issues. CNS inflammation and injury often causes rage, PTSD, impulsiveness, and aggression; often resulting from traumatic brain injury. Since these are often young men that may have limited contact with physicians, screening should be included in new patient exams and done annually for even if for incidental visits. Screening may, alternatively, be done outside of medical situations.

Although there is no excuse for abuse, there are causes. These causes can and should be treated. Perpetrators of domestic violence frequently have a history of having been abused as children. Traumatic brain injury, drug abuse, alcohol abuse, PTSD, rage disorder, depression, bipolar disorder, chronic pain, and irritability caused by inflammation can increase the likelihood of domestic violence. These conditions need to be diagnosed and adequately treated to decrease the risk of domestic violence. If the transgressor is offered non-judgmental, non-punitive assistance to overcome their problems, they are much more likely to seek the treatment they require. Self-loathing, self-recrimination, and shame are ineffective preventive treatments for domestic violence.

Elimination or control of the underlying problems promotes a milieu favorable to personal growth and self-control A screening tool for perpetrators of domestic violence is provided in Appendix D.

Our jails are filled with patients with histories of TBI and the diagnosis of schizophrenia. These are inflammatory diseases. If we would like to live in a safer, less violent society, perhaps it should be routine to screen arrested persons, at least those involved in violence, for treatable neurologic dysfunction. Surely, at a cost of $40,000 to $60,000 per year to imprison a criminal, treatment for those who might respond, would be less costly. Incarceration is rarely curative.

Nutrition Deserts

There are many food deserts (not to be confused with dessert foods). These are locations where there is limited local access to grocery stores that carry fresh fruits or vegetables. In the United States, a food desert is defined as a rural county in which all residents have to travel more than 10 mile to the nearest grocery store that carries fresh fruits and vegetables, or as an urban area where residents have to travel more than one mile to a grocery store that carries these items. In urban areas, it is more common for residents not to own a vehicle, thus buying and transporting groceries is difficult. The U.S. Department of Agriculture has documents 5,629 food desert areas in the continental U.S., affecting 23.5 million residents[5], with over 80% or these people living in urban environments[6]. The residents of these areas then rely on convenience stores for food. Especially for the poor, it becomes difficult to get quality nutrition.

In these areas, poor nutrition is common; it is not just a lack of fresh fruits and vegetables; about 30% of residents consume an inadequate amount of protein, as access to fresh meat and dairy are also limited[7]. For the poor, it thus becomes easier to fulfill caloric demands with low-cost calories in the form of processed foods, high caloric, fatty snack foods and soda pop. Although the focus herein is on the U.S., nutritional deserts are documented to contribute to obesity, metabolic syndrome and poverty in Canada, Great Britain, and other European nations[8],[9].

In the United Sates, the Supplemental Nutrition Assistance Program (SNAP) program, formerly known as the Food Stamp Program, provides funding for the purchase of groceries for families and individuals in poverty. In 2013, 47.6 million Americans, fifteen percent of the total population, received SNAP benefits[10]. Those receiving SNAP are among those with the least access to transportation, and most affected by transportation costs.

For example, 70% of SNAP eligible Mississippians travel more than 30 miles to reach a supermarket. In the U.S., low-income areas have 30% more convenience stores than middle-income areas. Food shopping in food deserts is items done in convenience stores and gas stations. These stores are motivated to put in a shelf of canned foods, to supplement the snack foods and colas so that they can qualify to accept SNAP payments. These low-income, low-grocery-store areas have higher rates of obesity and diabetes[5]. Low-cost, high caloric density foods, increase the rate of obesity, diabetes and metabolic syndrome among the less affluent[11].

The USDA cost estimate for cooking food at home for one month for a family of four with two young children is $821.00 using a "low-cost plan," and they estimate it costs a minimum of $168 to feed a teenage boy[12]. The average SNAP assistance is $133 per month. Thus, food budgets are tight, and low-cost, convenience foods are often selected.

The SNAP program was originally developed, equally, to aid farmers that produced perishable crops, and broaden the market for these foods and low-income consumers. The US Department of Agriculture, (USDA) still administers this program. Their rules state that SNAP benefits are for the purchase of fruits and vegetables, bread and cereals, dairy products, meat, poultry, and fish.

Nevertheless, $4 billion; six percent of the $63 billion dollars in SNAP food aid is spent on soda pop alone[13]. The processed food maker, Kraft Foods, earns one-sixth its revenues from the SNAP program. These are sources of cheap, easy to consume calories. There is, however, only very limited place for these calories in a healthy diet.

Legislation that was introduced, in 2012, to prevent SNAP benefits from being spent on sodas, candy, chips and other junk food was contentiously lobbied against by Coca-Cola, other "snack food" companies, and the convenience store industry[14]. Ironically, the junk-food industry lobbies the legislature heavily, often preaching that they are defending the "personal freedom" of the poor to make their own choices. The choice they provide is between dozen flavors of carbonated, artificially colored sodas and several styles of chips.

If SNAP food assistance were be restricted to the purchase of real foods, with minimums set for the percent of SNAP dollars of fresh produce sold in a given store, it would provide an incentive for grocers to locate in foods deserts, or for existing stores to provide nutritious food and fresh produce. This would benefit not only those receiving SNAP assistance, but also other members of these communities.

My Public Health Wish List:

1. Supplemental Nutrition Assistance Program purchases should be limited to exclude processed snack foods such as potato chips and soda pop. Stores taking SNAP payments should have to demonstrate significant provision and sales of fresh produce. Nowadays, when most fruits and vegetables have bar code labels, and SNAP credit is computerized, it is not a technological challenge to monitor the sales of goods paid for with SNAP funds to assure that stores are making these healthy foods available. This indirect funding of grocers would support better access to nutrition to millions of Americans.

3. Vitamin D_3 should be supplied at daily doses of at least 2000 IU to individuals on Medicare without charge. To simplify administration, the vitamin could be given as a once-weekly dose format. The improved health of the elderly receiving these supplements would likely lower medical care costs, and thus, this should provide savings to Medicare.

Foods, in addition to milk, should be fortified with vitamin D_3. Supplementing all processed foods with one or two units of vitamin D per calorie, would be too little to create risk of toxicity, even for those on a purely processed food diet, but would help reduce disease.

3. New food sources of n-3 fatty acids need to be developed. We cannot depend on harvesting fish from the sea to fulfill the n-3 needs of seven to ten billion people. Farmed salmon, raised in enclosed netted areas at sea, are fed wild-caught fish; thus, they deplete the sea just as much as wild caught salmon do. Genetically engineered foods or fats harvested from large-scale, commercial algae production are likely needed to support sufficient n-3 fats a population of over seven billion healthy persons. The need for n-3 fats can also be mitigated through diets with less consumption of n-6 fats.

4. The lower accepted healthy range for serum vitamin B_{12} level should be changed to reflect levels that prevent elevations in plasma homocysteine; about 500 pg/ml, however, the reference range is 210-911 pg/ml. This allows nearly half of the population to have inadequate levels to provide for optimal health and prevents payment for treating for those with inadequate levels due to malabsorption. Reference levels for nutrients should be set to levels associated with health, rather than setting them to a minimal level required to prevent overt disease. A separate set of levels should be used for diagnosing nutrient-related diseases.

5. Many people have marginal vitamin B_6 intake. The levels associated with decreased risk of colon cancer, heart disease, or to prevent elevations in CRP are greater than those currently recommended for health. The current RDA for vitamin B6 is 1.3 to 1.7 mg/day; an intake greater than 2 mg daily is needed to prevent elevated CRP levels, a marker of inflammation[15]. A significant portion of the population has pyridoxal-5-phosphate levels too low to prevent elevations in the toxic kynurenine metabolite, 3-HK[16]. Supplementation designed to add one or two extra milligrams of vitamin B_6 to the diet would likely decrease the incidence of inflammatory disorders.

6. The costs created by pollution should be borne by the polluter, not those who live downstream. Allowing these indirect costs to be externalized and ducked by those who create them, creates a false economy were the product's true costs are hidden, and those downstream pay the costs, too often with their health or their lives. Similarly, alcoholic beverages and tobacco products should have taxes assessed upon them based on their costs to society. The intent is not to penalize their users, but rather to remove the inherent subsidy society pays for their production and use.

Beverages sweetened with high fructose corn syrup should also be taxed at a rate which recovers, at a minimum, the cost of the agricultural subsidy used to produce it. Alcoholic beverages and soda-pop should not be classified as food for sales tax or SNAP purposes.

8. IgG testing of food reactivates should be reimbursed by medical insurance.

9. Nutritional supplements shown to be effective in the treatment of disease and prescribed by licensed physicians should be covered by medical insurance.

10. Much of the violence in our society, especially domestic violence, results from disease, such as TBI, and lead toxicity and neuroinflammatory diseases. All perpetrators of a buse and violence should be screened for neurologic and inflammatory disorders, and treated when possible to lower the risk society and to themselves. Patients should be screened not just for being victims of domestic violence; it is as more important to identify those who peretrators, and who need of treatment so that the violence can be stopped.

Much of the disease burden in developed countries comes from what we eat and how our enteric immune system interfaces with our enteric environment. Addressing enteroimmune disease is a public health issue, and less troublesome than the results of ignoring it.

---

[1] The Long-Term Outlook for Health Care Spending. Congress of the United States Congressional Budget Office, Nov. 2007.

[2] Conclusions and recommendations from the symposium, Heart Healthy Omega-3s for Food: Stearidonic Acid (SDA) as a Sustainable Choice. Deckelbaum RJ, Calder PC, Harris WS, Akoh CC, Maki KC, Whelan J, Banz WJ, Kennedy E. J Nutr. 2012 Mar;142(3):641S-643S. PMID:22323767

[3] Tutorial in biostatistics: Analyzing associations between total plasma homocysteine and B vitamins using optimal categorization and segmented regression. Bang H, Mazumdar M, Spence D. Neuroepidemiology. 2006;27(4):188-200. PMID:17035715

[4] Assessing the vitamin D status of the US population. Yetley EA. Am J Clin Nutr. 2008 Aug;88(2):558S-564S. PMID:18689402

[5] The Grocery Gap. Treuhaft S, Karpyn A. The Food Trust http://thefoodtrust.org/uploads/media_items/grocerygap.original.pdf

[6] http://www.ers.usda.gov/dataFiles/Food_Access_Research_Atlas/Download_the_Data/Archived_Version/archived_documentation.pdf USDA. Accessed July 2014

[7] Starved for Access: Life in Rural America's Food Deserts. Morton LW, Blanchard, TC. Rural Realites. Vol 1:4. Missisipp State Univ. 2007

[8] Good Neighbores? Community impacts of supermarkets. Friends of the Earth. http://www.foe.co.uk/sites/default/files/downloads/good_neighbours_community.pdf

[9] Food environments and obesity--neighbourhood or nation? Cummins S, Macintyre S. Int J Epidemiol. 2006 Feb;35(1):100-4. Epub 2005 Dec 7. PMID:16338945

[10] http://www.fns.usda.gov/pd/supplemental-nutrition-assistance-program-snap

[11] Poverty and obesity: the role of energy density and energy costs. Drewnowski A, Specter SE. Am J Clin Nutr. 2004 Jan;79(1):6-16. PMID:14684391

[12] Official USDA Food Plans: Cost of Food at Home at Four Levels, U.S. Average, January 2012 http://www.cnpp.usda.gov

[13] http://www.cnbc.com/id/40452370 Accessed July 2014.

[14] http://www.northescambia.com/2012/02/house-puts-candy-chips-soda-back-in-public-assistance-bill Accessed July 2014

[15] Vitamin B-6 intake is inversely related to, and the requirement is affected by, inflammation status. Morris MS, Sakakeeny L, Jacques PF, Picciano MF, Selhub J. J Nutr. 2010 Jan;140(1):103-10. PMID:19906811

[16] Low plasma vitamin B-6 status affects metabolism through the kynurenine pathway in cardiovascular patients with systemic inflammation. Midttun O, Ulvik A, Ringdal Pedersen E, et al. J Nutr. 2011 Apr 1;141(4):611-7. PMID:21310866

Appendix A: Cross Immunogens

Individuals that are allergic to environmental allergens often have cross-reacting food allergies. Risk is generally lower for foods that have been cooked, and thus, are more likely to have had their proteins denatured. If a food allergy provoked in an individual by a "common element" in one food in that group, they are also likely to react to other foods containing the related antigen.

A single food may contain several antigens; an individual may react to one or more of these, but is unlikely to react to all of the antigens present in that food. Thus, they would be expected to react to other foods that share the same antigen that they react to, but not to the others. Bananas, for example, have several antigenic proteins, and an individual with an immune response to banana may also react to foods with cross-reacting antigens. They would not be expected to react to other cross-reacting antigens present in banana or to plants which share these other antigens.

Environmental Antigen	Related Allergies	Common Elements or Antigen	Foods with Cross Reacting Antigens
Dust Mites Cockroaches Moths	Mite contaminated flour	Tropomyosin	Shrimp, squid, snails, mollusks. lobster
Alternaria alternata; mold	Other molds		Raw mushrooms
Latex from the rubber tree; Hevea brasiliensis. Hev b's common in: Children: 1 and 3 Healthcare Workers: 2, 5, 6, 7, and 13	Potato, tomato, sweet pepper, and avocado, banana, kiwi[1] Olive tree pollenosis (Ole e9 and 10)	Hevein ((Hev b 1-13; several different proteins)[2]	Hev b 5: Kiwi Hev b 6: Avocado, banana, kiwi Hev b 7: Potato, tomato Hev b 8 and 9: Molds Hev b 11 and 12: fruit allergens - papaya, chestnut, peach, grapefruit carrot, chestnut, custard apple, passion fruit, fig, melon, mango, paprika, celery, strawberry, pineapple, peach, and tomato[3]
Latex Hev b 8 Birch pollen Bet v 2 Ragweed	Ragweed	Profilin	Bell peppers, banana, pineapple
Poison Oak or Poison Ivy	Cashews Mango (skin) Pistachio	Anacardiaceae family, Urushiol	Contact with mango skin during consumption may cause circumoral vesicular rash
Tree Pollen (Birch Alder, Hazelnut)	Hazelnuts, Walnut	Betulaceae family	Kiwi fruit, pomaceous fruits: e.g.; cherry, peach, plums, almond, also apple, pear, certain spices
Alder pollen			Almonds, apples, celery, cherries, hazelnuts, peaches, pears, parsley, strawberry, raspberry
Birch pollen			Almonds, apples, apricots, avocados, bananas, carrots, celery, cherries, chicory, coriander, fennel, fig, hazelnuts, kiwifruit, nectarines, parsley, parsnips, peaches, pears, peppers, plums, potatoes, prunes, soy, strawberries, wheat
Feathers	Eggs, chickens	Bird Proteins	
Grass, grass pollen	Wheat, rye, oats	Grasses	Tomato, kiwi, celery, fig, melon, tomatoes
Mugwort pollen	Composites (Aster, Sunflower family) chamomile	Art v 1, a 28 kDa protein, a defensin	Honey, sunflower seeds, chamomile, pistachio, hazelnut, lettuce, beer, almond, peanut, tree nuts, carrot, pine nuts[4], and apple
Molds	Bread and brewer's yeast		

Environmental Antigen	Related Allergies	Common Elements or Antigen	Foods with Cross Reacting Antigens
Ragweed Pollen	Sunflower seeds Sunchoke (Jerusalem Artichoke)	Helianthus Tribe	Melons, zucchini cucumbers, squash, dandelions, hibiscus, chamomile, banana
Woodworm	Tarragon, Celery, Carrot, Cumin, Dill, Coriander, Fennel, Caraway, Parsnip, Anise, Parsley	Aster Family	Apple, melons
Mugwort Art v 1 Ragweed	Banana Pineapple	Profilin	Apple, Celery, Carrot
Birch (Bet v 1)			Cherry, apple, hazelnut, peach, carrot, celery, soya bean
	Sesame Seed		Peanut, papaya, kiwi, brazil nut, poppy seed, buckwheat, hazelnut, almond, pecan, walnut
Ficus benjamina (A house plant)	Fig	Proteinase?	Kiwi fruit, papaya, and avocado, pineapple, banana
Buckwheat	Polygonaceae		Garden sorrel, rhubarb, sea grape
Lupin	Peanut		
Che a 3, lambs quarters Phl p 7, timothy grass Bet v 4, white birch Amb a 9, ragweed Aln g 4, alder Ara t 1/2, mouse-ear cress Art v 5, mugwort Bra n 1/2, rape Bra r 1/2, turnip Cyn d 7, Bermuda grass Nic t 1/2, tobacco Ole e 3, common olive Ory s 7, rice Syr v 3, common lilac Vit v CBP, grape	Olive Rice, Grape, turnip, rape (Canola)	Polcalcin[5]	
Percent IgE Inhibition to rPyr c 5[6] Birch pollen: 89% Pyr c 5: 82% Bet v 6: 80% Mugwort pollen: 51% Grass pollen: 18%	**Percent IgE Inhibition to rPyr c 5**[7] Pear: 82% Nectarine: 76% Lychee: 64% Orange: 63% Apple: 59% Zucchini: 58% Carrot: 55% Peach: 52% Strawberry: 50% Soya: 49% Hazelnut: 49% Potato: 40% Persimmon: 35% Mango: 36% Melon: 30% Banana: 22% Cherry: 15% Kiwi: 13% Pea: 9% Milk: 5%	Phenylcoumaran Benzylic ether reductase	

[1] Latex type I sensitization and allergy in children with atopic dermatitis. Evaluation of cross-reactivity to some foods. Tücke J, Posch A, Baur X, Rieger C, Raulf-Heimsoth M. Pediatr Allergy Immunol. 1999 Aug;10(3):160-7.PMID: 10565556

[2] Thermo Scientific http://www.phadia.com/Products/Allergy-testing-products/ImmunoCAP-Allergen-Information/Occupational-Allergens/Allergen-Components/rHev-b-1-Latex/

[3] "Latex-fruit syndrome": frequency of cross-reacting IgE antibodies.Brehler R, Theissen U, Mohr C, Luger T. Allergy. 1997 Apr;52(4):404-10. PMID: 9188921

[4] Anaphylaxis to pine nut: cross-reactivity to Artemisia vulgaris? Rodrigues-Alves R, Pregal A, Pereira-Santos MC, Branco-Ferreira M, Lundberg M, Oman H, Pereira-Barbosa M. Allergol Immunopathol (Madr). 2008 Mar-Apr;36(2):113-6. PMID: 18479664

[5] Three-dimensional structure of the cross-reactive pollen allergen Che a 3: visualizing cross-reactivity on the molecular surfaces of weed, grass, and tree pollen allergens. Verdino P, Barderas R, Villalba M, Westritschnig K, Valenta R, Rodriguez R, Keller W. J Immunol. 2008 Feb 15;180(4):2313-21.PMID: 18250440

[6] Phenylcoumaran benzylic ether and isoflavonoid reductases are a new class of cross-reactive allergens in birch pollen, fruits and vegetables. Karamloo F, Wangorsch A, Kasahara H, Davin LB, Haustein D, Lewis NG, Vieths S. Eur J Biochem. 2001 Oct;268(20):5310-20.PMID: 11606193

[7] Phenylcoumaran benzylic ether and isoflavonoid reductases are a new class of cross-reactive allergens in birch pollen, fruits and vegetables. Karamloo F, Wangorsch A, Kasahara H, Davin LB, Haustein D, Lewis NG, Vieths S. Eur J Biochem. 2001 Oct;268(20):5310-20.PMID: 11606193

APPENDIX B: RESOURCE LINKS

Irritable Bowel Syndrome:

Rome III Diagnostic Questionnaire for Irritable Bowel Syndrome: www.romecriteria.org/pdfs/IBSMode.pdf

Additional Rome III Diagnostic Questionnaires: www.romecriteria.org/questionnaires/

Sleep Deprivation Evaluation:

The Epworth Sleepiness Scale: http://epworthsleepinessscale.com/epworth-sleepiness-scale.pdf

Cleveland Adolescent Sleepiness Questionnaire (CASQ):
http://www.sleepeducation.com/resources/lessons/teensdrowsydriving/teensleepquestionnaire.pdf

Osteoporosis Risk:

Osteoporosis Risk Calculator (United States): http://riskcalculator.fore.org/

Osteoporosis Risk Calculator (International: see "Calculation Tool"): http://www.shef.ac.uk/FRAX/

Breast Cancer Risk Evaluation for BRCA1 and BRCA2 carriers: http://brcatool.stanford.edu

Mood Disorder Evaluation:

A Brief, Self-Rated Screen for Depressive, Bipolar, Anxiety, and Post-Traumatic Stress Disorders in Primary Care[1]

http://www.mymoodmonitor.com/User/DiagnosisQues.aspx

Paper form: http://www.annfammed.org/content/suppl/2010/03/04/8.2.160.DC1/Gaynes_Supp_App.pdf

Vitamin Intake Recommendations by the Institute of Medicine:

Dietary Reference Intakes: Vitamins,
http://www.iom.edu/Global/News%20Announcements/~/media/474B28C39EA34C43A60A6D42CCE07427.ashx

PUBMED:

Find references in the U.S. National Library of Medicine website, by entering the articles PMID:
http://www.ncbi.nlm.nih.gov/pubmed/.

Reporting Errors:

If the reader comes across any errors in content or presentation, including typos, it will be greatly appreciated if they are sent by email to Enteroimmunology★gmail.com so that they can be corrected in updated printings. Please include the book's edition number (3.03), page number, the error observed, and the recommended revision.

---

[1] Feasibility and diagnostic validity of the M-3 checklist: a brief, self-rated screen for depressive, bipolar, anxiety, and post-traumatic stress disorders in primary care. Gaynes BN, DeVeaugh-Geiss J, Weir S, Gu H, MacPherson C, Schulberg HC, Culpepper L, Rubinow DR. Ann Fam Med. 2010 Mar-Apr;8(2):160-9. PMID: 20212303

APPENDIX C: LAB TESTS

Test	Notes	CPT Code	Labcorp	Quest
Tissue Transglutaminase (tTG), IgA and IgG	Gluten enteropathy, celiac disease	83516 (x2)	164640 164988	8821 IgA 11070 IgG
Omega-3 and -6 Fatty Acids, Plasma		82541	N/A	91001
Vitamin D, 25-OH, 25-Hydroxycalciferol	40 – 80 ng/mL or 100 - 200 nmol/L	82306	081950	17306
Saccharomyces cerevisiae Antibodies (ASCA) (IgA, IgG)		86671 (x2)	164657	17609
Inflammatory Bowel Disease Differentiation Panel: ASCA IgG and IgA ANCA Screen with Reflex to ANCA Titer, Myeloperoxidase Ab (MPO) Proteinase-3 Antibody	Differentiation panel is different between labs; both include ASCA and give p-ANCA results, as well as a "probable or indeterminate" UC or CrD assessment.	86671 (x2) (ASCA) plus other tests	164830 or 162045	16503
Food Allergies (IgE) Usually small panels or specific test for suspect allergy	Small test panels of the most common allergens, also for many individual foods	86003	Many	Many
IgG comprehensive foods panel	Immunolabs.com – 154 food panel	86001	N/A	Many
Plasma Citrulline – see page 14.	Uric acid cycle amino acids	82136	700182	N/A
	Gives full amino acid profile	82139	700068	767
Trypsin	Pancreatic Exocrine Insufficiency	83519	010355	30329
Stool Tests:				
Reducing Substances, Stool	(Malabsorption of sugars)	84376-7	016766	5022
Fecal Fat, Total	(Malabsorption of fats)	82710	001354	455
Eosinophil Protein X Stool	Available from Genova Diagnostics		N/A*	N/A*
Calprotectin, Stool		83993	123255	16796
Lactoferrin, Quantitative, Stool	Useful to differentiate IBS from IBD	83631	123016	17321
Pancreatic Elastase-1, Stool	Low in severe PEI (Chapter 8)	82656	123234	14693
Chymotrypsin, Stool	More sensitive to intestinally caused PEI?	84311	N/A	11235
Stool culture of Salmonella, Shigella, and Campylobacter. Detection of enterohemorrhagic E coli (EHEC) and Shiga toxin by EIA.	Mostly used in acute and febrile diarrhea rather than chronic disease. May be helpful when the onset of IBS or IBD is recent.	87045; 87046; 87427	008144	10108
Occult Blood, Fecal, Immunoassay (For Medicare Screening)		82274 (G0328)	182949	11293
Ova and Parasites Examination with Giardia antigen		87177; 87209	008623	1748
Giardia lamblia, Direct Detection EIA		87329	182204	8625
Helicobacter pylori Antigen, EIA, Stool		87338	180764	34838
Mast Cell Activation Tests:				
Plasma Histamine		83088	144600	36586
Mast Cell Tryptase (plasma or serum)		83520	004280	34484
Heparin (Heparin Anti-Xa)		85520	117101	30292
Serum chromogranin A*		86316	140848	16379
Urinary tests for N-methylhistamine, prostaglandin D_2, leukotriene E_4	Tests not widely available		N/A*	N/A*
Other Tests:				
Serum FGF19, fecal bile acids, and 7 α-hydroxy-4-cholesten-3-one (C4)	Tests not widely available		N/A*	N/A*
Bile acids (serum)	May show shift to secondary bile acids	82542	503640	4668
Low growth of commensal bacteria: Lactobacillus, Bifidobacterium	Available at Genova Diagnostics		N/A*	N/A*
Fecal Calgranulin C, tryptase, serine protease, Eosinophil Cationic Protein	Stool tests for these markers are not widely available		N/A*	N/A*
Eosinophil Cationic Protein (ECP)	Serum test		004180	37914

* Tests considered to be investigational by Medicare and other carriers are often not offered at the major labs; thus these tests are usually not an insurance covered benefit for patients.
Refer to the laboratory's websites for details on interpretation, limitations, collection, storage and shipment of specimens.

Appendix D: Domestic Violence Screening

The HITS questionnaire (Hurts – Insults – Threatens and Screams) for victims of domestic violence[1] is a validated, brief questionnaire for determining domestic violence. Also provided below are two adaptations of the HITS tool intended to help identify domestic violence.

Although the first concern in situations of domestic violence is to remove the victims from imminent harm, prevention of domestic violence includes self-identification of the transgressor. If physicians can identify patients who are perpetrators of domestic violence, they can offer them treatment. Many perpetrators of domestic violence were themselves victims of abuse, and physicians can offer treatment which may avert intergenerational propagation of violence. Perpetrators of domestic violence may suffer from PTSD, traumatic brain injury, rage disorder, depression, bipolar disorder, excessive irritability associated with inflammatory conditions such as fibromyalgia, chronic pain, alcohol or drug abuse, or another medical condition that has gone undiagnosed or inadequately treated.

I encourage screening of patients for domestic violence transgressions as well as for victims a routine part of new patient interviews and annual physical exams. If nothing else, it helps to send the messages that corporal punishment, verbal abuse, and violence are neither normal nor acceptable behaviors. When assistance is offered in a non-judgmental manner, it teaches patients that help and alternatives are available.

On the original HITS test, each item was ranked from one to five; if the total score from the four items was ten or greater, it indicated that intimate partner violence was occurring. The Home Life Survey on the following page has modified so that it uses a range from zero to four. This was done to emphasize that zero is the appropriate amount of domestic violence.

Thus, a score of six or greater is evidence of domestic violence for this HITS tool. The HITSP and HITSC have not yet been validated. Nevertheless, a similar score of six or greater should be regarded as problematic, and be used as a tool to open discussion with the patient about violent behaviors, thier possible underlying causes, and as a opening to offer treatment.

---

[1] HITS: a short domestic violence screening tool for use in a family practice setting. Sherin KM, Sinacore JM, Li XQ, Zitter RE, Shakil A. Fam Med. 1998 Jul-Aug;30(7):508-12. PMID:9669164 Used with author's permission.

HOME LIFE SURVEY

If you are in an intimate relationship, please fill in the circle that best indicates the frequency with which you and your partner engage in the following behaviors.

How often does your partner?

	Never 0	Rarely 1	Sometimes 2	Fairly Often 3	Frequently 4
Physically hurt you	○	○	○	○	○
Insult or talk down to you	○	○	○	○	○
Threaten you with harm	○	○	○	○	○
Scream or curse at you	○	○	○	○	○

HITS Score[2] _____

How often do you?

	Never 0	Rarely 1	Sometimes 2	Fairly Often 3	Frequently 4
Physically hurt your partner	○	○	○	○	○
Insult or talk down to your partner	○	○	○	○	○
Threaten your partner with harm	○	○	○	○	○
Scream or curse at your partner	○	○	○	○	○

HITSP Score _____

If you have a child or children staying in your home:
How often do you?

	Never 0	Rarely 1	Sometimes 2	Fairly Often 3	Frequently 4
Physically hurt the child, including spanking or other corporal punishment	○	○	○	○	○
Insult or talk down to or berate the child	○	○	○	○	○
Threaten the child with physical or emotional harm	○	○	○	○	○
Scream or curse at the child	○	○	○	○	○

HITSC Score _____

---

[2] The HITS Tool, © Kevin Sherin, 2003, ksherin@yahoo.com

Appendix E: Exercise Assessment

Please complete the following table. It refers only to exercise that you have done in the last week and that that has lasted more than 10 minutes during those occasions.

Please note both, the number of occasions over the last 7 days that you walked or done more than 10 minutes of vigorous or moderate exercise at a time. Then note the cumulative time of those occasions.

Vigorous activities are those which make a healthy person breathe much harder than at rest, and may include work or leisure activities such as jogging, heavy lifting, digging, aerobics or fast bicycling, and which under normal conditions cause heavy sweating.

Moderate physical activities are those that make ah healthy person breathe more quickly than at rest, but that could be sustained for longer periods. Some examples include carrying light loads, vacuuming, bicycling at a regular pace, hiking up and down hills with a backpack, fast walking, or doubles tennis. Do not include exercise that is including in the walking section.

Walking, for this assessment, refers walking at a comfortable on level or fairly level ground at a speed of about three miles per hour (about 5 kilometers per hour); This is a walking speed that a healthy person can sustain for hours[1].

Exercise lasting more than 10 minutes during the last 7 days:

Your Exercise During the Last 7 Days	Number of Occasions	Total time for those occasions
Walking		
Vigorous Exercise		
Moderate Exercise		

---

[1] Adapted from: Reliability and validity of a brief physical activity assessment for use by family doctors. Marshall AL, Smith BJ, Bauman AE, Kaur S. Br J Sports Med. 2005 May;39(5):294-7; PMID:15849294

Appendix F: Pelvic Pain and Urgency/Frequency Patient Symptom Scale

Please circle the answer that best describes how you feel for each question. The last 2 columns are for your doctor to assess your score. Please do not mark anything in these columns. Be sure to bring this questionnaire with you into the examination room so that you can review your answers with your doctor.

		0	1	2	3	4	SYMPTOM SCORE	BOTHER SCORE
1	How many times do you go to the bathroom during the day?	3-6	7-10	11-14	15-19	20+		
2	a. How many times do you go to the bathroom at night?	0	1	2	3	4+		
	b. If you get up at night to go to the bathroom, does it bother you?	Never Bothers	Occasionally	Usually	Always			
3	a. Do you now or have you ever had pain or symptoms during or after sexual intercourse?	Never	Occasionally	Usually	Always			
	b. Has pain or urgency ever made you avoid sexual intercourse?	Never	Occasionally	Usually	Always			
4	Do you have pain associated with your bladder or in your pelvis (vagina, labia, lower abdomen, urethra, perineum, testes, or scrotum)?	Never	Occasionally	Usually	Always			
5	a. If you have pain, is it usually		Mild	Moderate	Severe			
	b. Does your pain bother you?	Never	Occasionally	Usually	Always			
6	Do you still have urgency after going to the bathroom?	Never	Occasionally	Usually	Always			
7	a. If you have urgency, is it usually		Mild	Moderate	Severe			
	b. Does your urgency bother you?	Never	Occasionally	Usually	Always			
8	Are you sexually active? Yes___ No___							

	SYMPTOM SCORE = (1, 2a, 3a, 4, 5a, 6, 7a)
	BOTHER SCORE = (2b, 3b, 5b, 7b)
TOTAL SCORE (Symptom Score + Bother Score) =	

©2000 C. Lowell Parsons, M.D.

Total score ranges from 1 to 35.
A total score of 10-14 = 74% likelihood of positive PST; 15-19 = 76%; 20 or above = 91% likelihood of positive PST.

Revised 11/17/2003

Permission for use granted by Lowell Parsons, MD

Appendix G: Trauma Screening Questionnaire (TSQ)

These questions relate to reactions you may be having now to a past event.

This questionnaire is concerned with *your personal reactions* to the traumatic event that happened to you. Please consider the following reactions which sometimes occur after a traumatic event.

Please indicate (Yes/No) whether or not you have experienced any of the following, at least twice, in the past week.

	No	Yes
1. Upsetting thoughts or memories about the event that have come into your mind against your will		
2. Upsetting dreams about the event		
3. Acting or feeling as though the event were happening again		
4. Feeling upset by reminders of the event		
5. Bodily reactions (such as fast heartbeat, stomach churning, sweatiness, dizziness) when reminded of the event		
Score for items 1 through 5		
6. Difficulty falling or staying asleep		
7. Irritability or outbursts of anger		
8. Difficulty concentrating		
9. Heightened awareness of potential dangers to yourself and others		
10. Being jumpy or being startled at something unexpected		
Score for items 6 through 10		
Total Score		

Positive response to three or more of re-experiencing questions 1 – 5, or to arousal questions 5-10, or a combination of any 6 items gives a strong positive predictive value for PTSD when applied at least 3 weeks after the traumatic event.[1]

---

[1] Brief screening instrument for post-traumatic stress disorder. Brewin CR, Rose S, Andrews B, Green J, Tata P, McEvedy C, Turner S, Foa EB. Br J Psychiatry. 2002 Aug;181:158-62. PMID:12151288 Used with permission.

Appendix H: Methionine Restriction for Mitochondrial Health

In animals, life span can be increased with a 40% restriction in calories, proteins or methionine. Methionine appears to be the key element. Diets in which methionine intake is restricted by 40 percent decrease mitochondrial ROS production and free radical leak measured in the brain and kidneys of laboratory animals[1], while increasing intake of dietary methionine increases oxidative damage to the liver and heart[2]. In animals, every-other-day (EOD) dietary restriction also decreases mitochondrial oxidative stress by decreasing free radical leak in the complex I mitochondrial respiratory chain proteins and increases longevity[3].

Thus, I speculated in Chapter 21 that EOD methionine restricted diets may decrease oxidative damage, and improve mitochondrial health. Diets with a 40 percent methionine restriction can achieve mitochondrial ROS reduction. Such a diet may allow the benefit of caloric restriction without fasting or caloric deprivation through adherence to an every-other-day, modified, vegan diet. The typical mitochondrial life cycle is only seven days, thus, a methionine restriction two to three times a week may be sufficient to force the retirement of weak ones. Alternatively, a 41-hour methionine restricted diet once or twice a week may also be sufficient to provide such benefits. The 41-hour diet restricts methionine-rich foods for only four meals: from 7 P.M. after supper on one evening, during the next day and the following morning, returning to a regular lunch time meal at noon.

The World Health Organization promulgates a daily intake of 0.45 grams of protein per kilogram (0.204 grams per pound) ideal body weight as the minimum daily protein intake required for maintaining nitrogen balance[4].

Ideal Body Weight

Men: 106 lbs. + (6 lbs per inches over 60" in height)
48 kg + (1 kg per cm over 150 cm in height)

Women: 100 lbs. + (5 lbs per inches over 60" in height)
45 kg + (0.85 kg per cm over 150 cm in height)

A 5'8" tall man would have an ideal body weight of 154 pounds (70 kg) and would have a 31.5 gram daily protein requirement. One extra gram of dietary protein is required for individuals doing endurance training.

A 40 percent methionine restricted diet would supply 60 percent of the dietary methionine requirement; equivalent to 8.37 mg of methionine per kg ideal body weight, (3.8 mg per pound). Thus, a 70-kg (154 lb.) ideal body weight individual could consume up to 586 mg of methionine a day on the 40% restricted methionine diet. The methionine requirement is about three percent of the protein requirement. Methionine makes up 3.1% of the protein in chicken eggs, which is considered to be a balanced protein. On average, meals with proteins containing less than 1.86 percent methionine (60% of 3.1%) would work for this diet.

Assuming a daily dietary intake of 2200 calories for a 70-kg man; a 586 mg methionine restriction would limit meals to an average of less than 0.106 percent of the calories coming from methionine. Table H, below, shows that there are only a limited number of foods that have methionine at 0.11% or lower. Thus, low-methionine foods, such as fruits, tubers, vegetables, and fats are needed in this diet. Adding butter or olive oil to mashed potatoes and squash can be used to add required calories.

This diet is not recommended for growing children, adolescents, nor for pregnant and lactating women.

Table H gives methionine content of a sample of foods, ranked from low to high methionine content. Unless otherwise noted, the portion size is 100 grams of prepared food. Nutrition data for specific foods can be found online at http://nutritiondata.self.com/tools/nutrient-search.

A diet high in fruits and vegetables helps to fill out caloric intake in a methionine restricted (MR) diet. Added fats (olive oil as in salad dressing, for example, can help add non-protein calories Use of almond milk or coconut milk are useful in MR diets, and can be used with breakfast cereal or to make smoothies. Foods in which methionine makes up less than 0.1% of calories (most fruits and vegetables) can be thought of as "low-MR foods" as they lower the methionine ratio in the diet.

Some example of methionine restricted meals are:

Breakfast: Almond milk or coconut milk with rice or corn based dry cereal, Porridge with a bit of butter and honey to add calories. Serve fruit with the meal.

Lunch: An almond butter and banana sandwich made with whole-wheat bread (25 mg of methionine per slice) or potato bread. Fresh fruit. Almond veggie burger sandwich.

Supper: A baked sweet potato with butter, along with lentils and rice, served with a salad with tomatoes and avocado. Winter squash, cream of cauliflower and potato soup.

Table H: Methionine Content of Some High Protein Foods[5][6]

Food Item: 100 grams	Calories per 100g [kcal]	Grams Protein: Grams/100g	Methionine mg per 100g	Methionine: percent of protein	Protein as percent of Calories	Methionine as percent of Calories
Apple	52	0.03	1	3.33	0.23	0.01
Macadamia nuts	718	7.91	23	0.29	4.41	0.01
Plantains	116	1	10	1.00	3.45	0.03
Sweet Potato	144	0.9	21	2.33	2.50	0.06
Coconut	354	3.33	62	1.86	3.76	0.07
French Fried Potatoes	319	3.8	58	1.53	4.76	0.07
Orange (naval)	49	0.9	9	1.00	7.35	0.07
Carrots	36	0.8	7	0.88	8.89	0.08
Avocado	167	2	37	1.85	4.79	0.09
Winter Squash (Acorn)	40	0.8	10	1.25	8.00	0.10
Almonds	575	21.22	151	0.71	14.76	0.11
Pecans	691	9.17	183	2.00	5.31	0.11
Pumpkin	36	1	11	1.10	11.11	0.12
Potatoes	100	2.1	33	1.57	8.40	0.13
Filberts (hazelnuts)	628	14.95	221	1.48	9.52	0.14
Cantaloupe	34	0.8	12	1.50	9.41	0.14
Lettuce, iceberg	14	0.9	5	0.56	25.71	0.14
Walnut, English	654	15.23	236	1.55	9.31	0.14
Butternut Squash	39	1.2	15	1.25	12.31	0.15
Pine nuts	673	13.69	259	1.89	8.14	0.15
Spaghetti (wheat)	158	5.8	64	1.10	14.68	0.16
Beans, baked	94	5.15	40	0.78	21.91	0.17
White Rice	130	2.4	56	2.33	7.38	0.17
Corn Pasta	126	2.6	55	2.12	8.25	0.17
Shitake mushrooms	56	1.56	25	1.60	11.14	0.18
Rye, Whole	338	10.34	153	1.48	12.24	0.18
Cheerios (oats)	367	11.63	167	1.44	12.68	0.18
Rice, brown	362	7.5	169	2.25	8.29	0.19
Corn	362	8.12	170	2.09	8.97	0.19
Peanut butter	549	24.1	262	1.09	17.56	0.19
Soy Milk	54	3.27	27	0.83	24.22	0.20
Buckwheat	343	13.25	172	1.30	15.45	0.20
Corn Grits	59	1.4	30	2.14	9.49	0.20
Oats	379	13.15	207	1.57	13.88	0.22
Cream of wheat cereal	62	1.8	34	1.89	11.61	0.22
Peanuts, Virginia	578	25.87	317	1.23	17.90	0.22
Lima Beans, immature	123	6.81	68	1.00	22.15	0.22
Bulgur, dry	342	12.29	190	1.55	14.37	0.22
Millet	378	11.02	221	2.01	11.66	0.23
Pistachio	562	20.27	335	1.65	14.43	0.24
Tomatoes	10	0.9	6	0.67	36.00	0.24
Rye, dark flour	325	15.91	199	1.25	19.58	0.24
Wheat, winter red	327	12.61	201	1.59	15.43	0.25
Peas, Pigeon (red gram)	121	6.76	76	1.12	22.35	0.25
Popcorn	387	12.94	252	1.95	13.37	0.26
Cashew	553	18.22	362	1.99	13.18	0.26
Lentils	116	9.02	77	0.85	31.10	0.27

Food Item: 100 grams	Calories per 100g [kcal]	Grams Protein: Grams/100g	Methionine mg per 100g	Methionine: percent of protein	Protein as percent of Calories	Methionine as percent of Calories
Barley	354	12.48	240	1.92	14.10	0.27
Wheat, spring red	329	15.4	230	1.49	18.72	0.28
Garbanzo (chick pea)	164	8.86	116	1.31	21.61	0.28
Peas, Green, Split	341	24.55	251	1.02	28.80	0.29
Beans, navy	140	8.23	111	1.35	23.51	0.32
Oats	389	16.89	312	1.85	17.37	0.32
Beans, pinto	143	9.01	117	1.30	25.20	0.33
Quinoa	368	14.12	309	2.19	15.35	0.34
Sunflower seeds	584	20.78	494	2.38	14.23	0.34
Lima Beans, large	115	7.8	99	1.27	27.13	0.34
Beans, Black	132	8.86	133	1.50	26.85	0.40
Peas, Green	81	5.4	82	1.52	26.67	0.40
Sesame	573	17.73	586	3.31	12.38	0.41
Beans, kidney	127	8.67	130	1.50	27.31	0.41
Soy Flour	436	34.54	466	1.35	31.69	0.43
Pumpkin seeds	559	30.23	603	1.99	21.63	0.43
Broccoli florets	28	3	34	1.13	42.86	0.49
Milk (Whole) 8 oz.	146	7.9	183	2.32	21.64	0.50
Soybeans	173	16.64	224	1.35	38.47	0.52
Portabella mushrooms	22	2.11	29	1.37	38.36	0.53
Brazil Nuts	656	14.32	1008	7.04	8.73	0.61
Cheddar Cheese	403	24.9	652	2.62	24.71	0.65
Spinach (3 cups)	23	2.9	53	1.83	50.43	0.92
Soy Protein	331	58.13	814	1.40	70.25	0.98
Sardines	185	20.86	476	2.28	45.10	1.03
Eggs (2, large, chicken)	142	12.52	379	3.03	35.27	1.07
Pork, chop	247	27.94	724	2.59	45.25	1.17
Cottage Cheese	86	11.83	286	2.42	55.02	1.33
Chicken, thigh	195	25	692	2.77	51.28	1.42
Liver, Pork	165	26.02	645	2.48	63.08	1.56
Liver, beef or calf	191	29.08	759	2.61	60.90	1.59
Beef, sirloin	178	29.42	766	2.60	66.11	1.72
Turkey, dark	188	28.57	828	2.90	60.79	1.76
Salmon	154	25.82	764	2.96	67.06	1.98
Chicken, light meat	159	28.88	799	2.77	72.65	2.01
Turkey, white	157	29.9	866	2.90	76.18	2.21
Shrimp	99	20.91	589	2.82	84.48	2.38
Tuna	116	25.51	755	2.96	87.97	2.60

[1] Forty percent methionine restriction decreases mitochondrial oxygen radical production and leak at complex I during forward electron flow and lowers oxidative damage to proteins and mitochondrial DNA in rat kidney and brain mitochondria. Caro P, Gomez J, Sanchez I, Naudi A, Ayala V, López-Torres M, Pamplona R, Barja G. Rejuvenation Res. 2009 Dec;12(6):421-34. PMID:20041736

[2] Effect of methionine dietary supplementation on mitochondrial oxygen radical generation and oxidative DNA damage in rat liver and heart. Gomez J, Caro P, Sanchez I, Naudi A, Jove M, Portero-Otin M, Lopez-Torres M, Pamplona R, Barja G. J Bioenerg Biomembr. 2009 Jun;41(3):309-21. PMID:1963393

[3] Effect of every other day feeding on mitochondrial free radical production and oxidative stress in mouse liver. Caro P, Gómez J, López-Torres M, Sánchez I, Naudi A, Portero-Otín M, Pamplona R, Barja G. Rejuvenation Res. 2008 Jun;11(3):621-9. PMID:18593280

[4] Protein and Amino Acid Requirements in Human Nutrition: Report of a Joint WHO/FAO/UNU Expert Consultation. World Health Organization ISBN-13: 9789241209359 December 2007

[5] USDA Nutrion Database

[6] http://nutritiondata.self.com/tools/nutrient-search accessed June 2012.

Appendix I: How Vegetable Oil is Made

In Chapter 6, it was suggested that vegetable oils were not a natural product and that their use should be limited in the diet. The method used to produce extra virgin olive oil involves squeezing the juice from olives, and then allowing the oil to float to the top, and separating it from the aqueous portion of the juice. It is usually filtered to remove fine particles.

Corn oil, soy oil, and other commercially made oils are prepared in an ever-so-slightly differently manner, which might be of interested to consumers. The following describes the process used for commercial soy oil, which is similar to that used for most other vegetable oils.

The dry soybeans are cracked, and a vacuum machine is used to separate the hulls (the seed coat) from the endosperm and cotyledon. The hulls are shaken over a fine screen to recover fine pieces of the soy seed generated during cracking, and the cracked soybean endosperm and cotyledon are processed into flakes to rupture oil cells in the seed, in a process similar to rolling oats to make oatmeal; however, the high pressure creates heating of the soy flakes.

These thin flakes have a large surface area, which allows for efficient solvent extraction of oils. The soybean flakes undergo solvent extraction, typically using isohexane/hexane to yield crude soybean oil. The soybean meal which remains is used as livestock feed or for human consumption.

The crude soy oil is then further refined through several steps. The first step is known as "degumming." During this process, phospholipids are removed through a process in which the oil is mixed with water or acid solution, to form "gums." This mixture is centrifuged to separate layers and remove the water and gum from the rest. Fatty acids that remain in the degummed oil are neutralized by adding caustic lye (sodium hydroxide) which forms soap with the free fatty acids. The resulting liquid is again passed through a centrifuge to remove the soap. Washing and centrifugation, or treatment with an adsorbent, followed by filtration, removes soaps to levels compatible with bleaching.

The oil is then bleached by mixing it with a citric acid solution. Next, the oil is treated with adsorbent clay that removes peroxides, phosphatides, color bodies and traces of soap. The pigments are adsorbed and removed by filtration under vacuum, to inhibit oxidation of the oil.

The oil is then deodorization to remove "flavor components" and "odoriferous components" by steam distillation. This process also further removes some remaining free fatty acids from the oil. Steam distillation is done at high temperatures, typically at 225°C to 255°C (437F° to 491°F), again, under vacuum.

As a final step antioxidants, such as Tenox-20, are utilized to inhibit oxidation of the oil. Tenox-20 is a combination of propylene glycol, citric acid, and tertiary butylhydroquinone[1].

The resulting oil is ready for use in food preparation.

---

[1] GRAS Notice for Stearidonic (SDA) Omega-3 Soybean Oil. Food and Drug Administration. February 2009
http://www.accessdata.fda.gov/scripts/fcn/gras_notices/grn000283.pdf

Appendix J: Trigger Point and Periarticular Injections

Trigger point injections are very useful in the treatment of somatic pain. Somatic pain is generally dull, aching, and often poorly localized, in contrast to the sharp, well-defined, stabbing of radicular pain. Somatic pain can often be elicited by palpation and extension while radicular pain is reproduced by flexion, such as straight leg raising.

Note: Loss of strength, sensation or severe radicular pain may indicate nerve root compression or spinal stenosis that may require prompt surgical intervention. With spinal stenosis, the patient may complain of rubbery feeling legs that may feel cold, numb, or weak, and may cause pain at night relieved with walking and pain with walking that improves with rest.

Often patients receive gratifying, long relief of pain, even chronic pain with this simple procedure. Trigger point myalgia often results from injuries to the neck and back and are typified by tender areas. These are often found in the trapezius, rhomboid in the upper back, and lumbar and gluteal muscles and in the low back. Trigger points often cause referred pain; for example, treating those in the trapezius will often provide headache relief. Trigger point compressive treatment of the biceps often provides lasting relief for carpal tunnel syndrome[1], apparently by reducing irritation to the nerve.

Trigger points are taut bands of muscle, that can be found by palpation, and which contain proinflammatory mediators[2] and byproducts of muscular ischemia. The pain may result from involuntary muscular guarding after an injury. Muscular spasm causes pain and that pain and spasm. Breaking the cycle of spasm and pain, can allow increased blood flow to the area and allow the patient increased range of motion.

Trigger points are found in myofascial pain syndrome, in contrast to the "tender points" found in fibromyalgia. Nevertheless, TPI to tender points is also helpful in the treatment of fibromyalgia, although here, there may be a delay in benefit and post injections soreness[3].

There are many variations of trigger point injections (TPI), with multiple different medications or without the use of any medications. Dry needling alone gives relief of pain. The needle needs to be introduced into the affected, spastic muscle, and if treatment is effective, the muscle will discharge after about 30 seconds.

Even a needle is not required. Trigger point release can be done through the application of a constant "thumb" pressure over the spastic muscle[4,5]. It generally takes about 60 seconds of constant pressure, before the practitioner feels the muscle give way, and felt to relax; at this time the patient also feels relief of pain and typically has improved range of motion of the affected area.

Bupivacaine, which is longer lasting than lidocaine can be used; however, there may be no therapeutic advantage to it; it is more toxic than lidocaine, and may present more risk of injury to the patient, if the patient ignores painful stimuli that were not a true trigger point lesion. Steroids offer no therapeutic benefit in TPI. Saline solution can also be used but has no benefit over dry needling. Lidocaine is more effective than dry needling and more effective and less expensive than botulinum toxin[6].

Lidocaine has additional advantages. Most patients have had it in the past for dental procedures, know if they tolerate it and recognize that it helps with pain. They are thus, more willing to allow treatment. Therapeutically, lidocaine gives the advantage that even if the needling does not discharge the muscle, the introduction of the medication can. Even failing this, the local anesthetic effect allows a decrease in local pain that facilitates manual trigger point release of the area. When compared to dry needling, there is less pain to that area in the hours following the procedure[7].

I recommend a triple technique that has been validated for its efficacy[8]. After carefully localizing the tender muscle through palpation and cleansing of the area, the needle on a syringe is advanced into the muscle to elicit a local twitch response. For most areas, 1 cc of one percent lidocaine is gently infused into the muscle. After withdrawing the needle, I usually wait about one minute, and then place about 5 pounds (2.5 kg) of pressure with a thumb onto the muscle for about 60 to 90 seconds, until I feel it relax. The amount of pressure depends on the amount the patient tolerates. The pressure is used to fatigue the muscle, rather than to overpower it. Use more time, and sometimes less pressure, when needed, rather than more pressure to get the muscle to relax. Other areas that feel taut in the immediate area are then also treated with compression until they relax.

I generally limit treatment to 3 areas during a visit. On the next visit, usually a week later, I reassess and may treat the same area or other affected areas if the patient benefited from the treatment.

Periarticular Injections

Similar to TPI, periarticular injections may provide long-term pain relief and increase mobility to certain injured joints. Please note, these are periarticular injections; care is taken to avoid injecting into the joint capsule.

Periarticular injections the sacroiliac joint area[9], the facet joints of the spine[10],[11], and the acromial clavicular joint[12] provide relief just as well, if not better than that do intra-articular injections. Note that these joints are similar in their limited range of motion.

Similar to TPI, the addition of corticosteroids to these periarticular injections is no more effective than using local anesthetic alone[13]. It is very possible that injections of the facet joints of the spine only provide relief when the volume of medicine injected is sufficient to leak and bathe the surrounding tissues. These joint capsules easily rupture using small volumes of medication[14].

Although TPI are generally done into the belly of the muscle, treatment to the area of the insertion of the muscles is also helpful. The nerve endings are the probable target of effective treatment. This is likely the case here as well. The injection needs to target the tender area, not the interior of the joint capsule.

Facet joint pain is responsible for about 15% of all low back pain. Periarticular facet joint injections provide lasting relief to about a third of patients. While not a panacea, it is a simple, low risk, inexpensive treatment that often can provide relief and help the patient avoid the chronic use of opiates or toxic medications. It can also help the patient avoid surgical treatment that would be unhelpful, if indeed, the facet area was the source of the pain.

About 20% of low back pain is caused by injury to the SI joint[15]. SI sprains often cause referred pain down the back of the thigh.

The SI distraction test can be used to localize SI pain: with patient supine, the practitioner, using crossed arms, puts pressure on the iliac crests with the heel of the hands, stretching the SI ligaments. Direct pressure or palpation of the SI joint also usually elicits the pain.

Periarticular injections into the posterior SI can be performed by injecting into the tender area, and are superficial, and do not require fluoroscopy to guide injection placement as do intra-articular injections. Since this area is large, it may take four 1 cc injections to cover a bilateral sprain.

---

[1] A randomized controlled (intervention) trial of ischemic compression therapy for chronic carpal tunnel syndrome. Hains G, Descarreaux M, Lamy AM, Hains F. J Can Chiropr Assoc. 2010 Sep;54(3):155-63. PMID:20808615

[2] Mechanisms of muscle pain : significance of trigger points and tender points. Brezinschek HP. Z Rheumatol. 2008 Dec;67(8):653-4, 656-7. PMID:19015861

[3] Difference in pain relief after trigger point injections in myofascial pain patients with and without fibromyalgia. Hong CZ, Hsueh TC. Arch Phys Med Rehabil. 1996 Nov;77(11):1161-6. PMID:8931529

[4] Effect of acupressure and trigger points in treating headache: a randomized controlled trial. Hsieh LL, Liou HH, Lee LH, Chen TH, Yen AM. Am J Chin Med. 2010;38(1):1-14. PMID:201280

[5] Changes in a patient with neck pain after application of ischemic compression as a trigger point therapy. Montañez-Aguilera FJ, Valtueña-Gimeno N, Pecos-Martín D, et al. J Back Musculoskelet Rehabil. 2010;23(2):101-4. PMID:20555123

[6] Comparison of lidocaine injection, botulinum toxin injection, and dry needling to trigger points in myofascial pain syndrome. Kamanli A, Kaya A, Ardicoglu O, Ozgocmen S, Zengin FO, Bayik Y. Rheumatol Int. 2005 Oct;25(8):604-11. PMID:15372199

[7] Lidocaine injection versus dry needling to myofascial trigger point. The importance of the local twitch response. Hong CZ. Am J Phys Med Rehabil. 1994 Jul-Aug;73(4):256-63. PMID:8043247

[8] Ischemic compression after trigger point injection affect the treatment of myofascial trigger points. Kim SA, Oh KY, Choi WH, Kim IK. Ann Rehabil Med. 2013 Aug;37(4):541-6. doi: 10.5535/arm.2013.37.4.541. Epub 2013 Aug 26. PMID:24020035

[9] Sources of sacroiliac region pain: insights gained from a study comparing standard intra-articular injection with a technique combining intra- and peri-articular injection. Borowsky CD, Fagen G. Arch Phys Med Rehabil. 2008 Nov;89(11):2048-56. PMID:18996232

[10] Lumbar facet joint syndrome. A randomised clinical trial. Lilius G, Laasonen EM, Myllynen P, Harilainen A, Grönlund G. J Bone Joint Surg Br. 1989 Aug;71(4):681-4. PMID:2527856

[11] Imaging findings predicting the outcome of cervical facet joint blocks. Hechelhammer L, Pfirrmann CW, Zanetti M, Hodler J, Boos N, Schmid MR. Eur Radiol. 2007 Apr;17(4):959-64. Epub 2006 Oct 3. PMID:17180331

[12] Intra-articular versus periarticular acromioclavicular joint injection: a multicenter, prospective, randomized, controlled trial.Sabeti-Aschraf M, Stotter C, Thaler C, et al. Arthroscopy. 2013 Dec;29(12):1903-10. PMID:24140142

[13] Corticosteroids in peri-radicular infiltration for radicular pain: a randomised double blind controlled trial. One year results and subgroup analysis. Tafazal S, Ng L, Chaudhary N, Sell P. Eur Spine J. 2009 Aug;18(8):1220-5. MID:19387704

[14] Fluoroscopic percutaneous lumbar zygapophyseal joint cyst rupture: a clinical outcome study. Allen TL, Tatli Y, Lutz GE. Spine J. 2009 May;9(5):387-95. PMID:18809358

[15] Evaluation of sacroiliac joint interventions: a systematic appraisal of the literature. Rupert MP, Lee M, Manchikanti L, et al. Pain Physician. 2009 Mar-Apr;12(2):399-418. PMID:19305487

Appendix K: Postconcussion Evaluation

Section I: History of Concussion	Have you ever had a head injury or been in an accident, sporting event or other situation where there was an impact that caused a loss of consciousness or that caused you to be dazed or confused even for ten seconds? Has this occurred on more than one occasion? (Details) At the time of the injury was there: A loss of consciousness ☐ A feeling of being Disoriented, ☐ Dazed ☐ or Confused ☐ even for a few seconds? Did it take some time to gather your wits? Or to figure out what happened? ☐ Did you feel an adrenaline rush or very excited? ☐
Section II	Postconcussive Symptoms and Signs
Headaches (Migrainous)	Increased frequency of headaches ☐ Severity? Location? What helps? Blurred vision ☐ Double vision ☐ Sensitivity to noise ☐ Sensitivity to light ☐ Accompanied by nausea ☐ or vomiting ☐
Neurological	Tinnitus (ringing in the ears) ☐ Dizziness ☐ Difficulty with balance ☐ Vertigo ☐ Falls or near falls? ☐ Muscular Weakness ☐ Tremor ☐ Seizures ☐ Syncope or near syncope ☐
Sleep	Restless sleep ☐ Insomnia ☐ Daytime Sleepiness ☐ Fatigue ☐ Recurrent dreams ☐
Emotional	Frequent frustration ☐ Easily Irritable ☐ Explosive Temper ☐ Frequent upsets ☐ Easily emotional or cry over little things ☐
Cognitive	Forgetfulness ☐ Poor concentration ☐ Depression ☐ Fidgety ☐ Take longer to think ☐ Frequent worry ☐ Anxiety ☐
Ideation	Thoughts of hurting self or others ☐ Suicidal thoughts ☐ Recurrent troubling thoughts ☐
Drug and Alcohol use	Is there an increase or inappropriate use of alcohol or drugs? ☐
Intellectual Function	Has there been a decline in academic or intellectual performance? ☐
Vestibular Function	Young and healthy people should be able to stand on one leg, eyes closed for 10 seconds. Older individuals and those with orthopedic problems need to be evaluated using less difficult tests. <div align="right">Abnormal</div>One leg stand, eyes closed 10 seconds ☐ Standing, feet together, eyes closed; Is there increased head sway? ☐ Heel to toe walk (Sobriety test) ☐ Recent difficulty hearing ☐ Recent difficulty understanding speech ☐
Cognition	These tests (listed most to least difficult) should be evaluated in light of the person's education, trade, and premorbid abilities. <div align="right">Abnormal</div>Serial seven subtractions ☐ The alphabet backward ☐ Months of the year backward ☐
Nocturia	Average frequency ____ (Normal is 0 – 1)
Language	Difficulty with word finding ☐ Slurring or slowing of the speech ☐

Patients with an injury with followed by a loss of consciousness or any of the symptoms listed in Section I may have had a concussion. Patients with signs or symptoms from 3 or more areas of sections II should be considered as having postconcussion syndrome (PCS). Items in bold type are common in PCS. Increases in drug or alcohol abuse, suicidal ideation, tremor, loss of motor control and language difficulty suggest more severe or more advanced disease.

Injured patients *without* postconcussion syndrome (PCS) or chronic traumatic encephalopathy (CTE) can also have sleep impairment, due to pain or discomfort from their injuries. Injuries of the cervical spine may cause cervicogenic headaches in patients with or without PCS. Injured patients may have anxiety, depression and frustration from the loss of health and fear of new injury. If these symptoms last more than three weeks but lack neurologic manifestations, it is suggestive of PTSD (See Appendix G for the Trauma Screener).

Noise-induced hearing loss, ototoxic drugs or other damage to the ears can cause tinnitus and vestibular dysfunction. (Chapter 44). There are many causes of nocturia; all merit investigation.

The abrupt onset of this cluster of symptoms following an impact, even when there was no direct head injury, suggests post-concussive syndrome. Side impact car accidents often cause post-concussive injury even without the head hitting any object due to acceleration-deceleration injury.

Appendix L: Car Seat Safety

Car seats are an important safety device; nevertheless, they only provide the driver and passengers protection when properly adjusted to the person seated in them. This is a guide for properly adjusting the driver and front passenger seats. Adjust the seat in the following order.

1. Adjust the seat angle: The car seat back should be adjusted to support the back. The optimal angle if for the seat is usually leaning back 10° from vertical, or 100° back from level. At the correct positions, the front of the shoulders is just behind the hips.

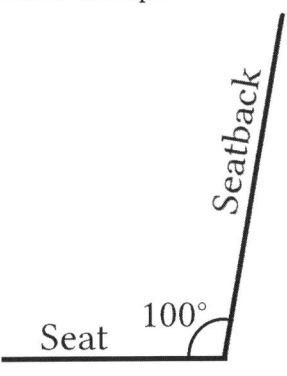

2. Adjust the headrest: The head rest protects the neck from whiplash injury, especially in rear-end collisions. The top of the headrest should be set to be about the same height as the top of the head. The protuberance at the back of the head should be at the same height as the forward curve of the head rest. Most importantly, the distance between the back of the head and the headrest when driving should be ½ to 2 inches (1 to 5 cm). Distances greater than an inch, increase head movement during deceleration and increase the risk of whiplash injury.

3. Adjust the seat distance from the steering wheel: Air bags need time and space to deploy. Leave at least 10, but no more than 18 inches between the center of the steering wheel and the base of the sternum. Leave 20 to 28 inches from the dashboard to the passenger's chest. Being too close can cause injury. If the car fits the driver well, the driver should be able to plant their left foot firmly on the floorboard foot rest on the left side of the driver's foot area. (Race car drivers are trained to press their foot into this area to force their back into their seat if their car is about to roll, to keep them in the seat and prevent serious injury that can occur during a rollover.)

4. Make sure you have lumbar support. The low back area should rest snugly on the seatback. Your hand should not fit between the seatback and your low back. Among the most common injuries seen in accidents are lumbar disk herniations that occur when cars are rear-ended. If the lumbar spine is not supported, the impact can snap the lumbar spine into hyperflexion at the speed at which the car is hit. This can cause herniation or rupture of the disks into the spinal canal. Sacroiliac injuries also commonly result. The low back may not be supported it the seat is set too far back. This is especially common in the passenger seat. Old seats may have lost their support, and individuals with more anterior curvature of the low spine (lordosis) may need more support. Add lumbar support pad if your seat does not provide adequate support. *Avoid sliding down in the seat or sitting with the hips away from the seat back, as this greatly increased risk of lumbar spine injury in rear-end collisions.* This is especially important in stop-and-go traffic where rear-end accidents are most common.

4. Adjust seat height: In cars that allow adjustment of seat height, there should be at least two inches of headroom between the top of the head and the roof. Ideally the eyes of the driver should be about mid-height of the windshield.

5. Adjust the steering wheel. If the steering wheel angle can be adjusted, is should be set so that the driver can easily see the dashboard through the upper half of the steering wheel. The steering wheel should be angled so that it is flat to the driver's chest when the driver leans forward. The steering wheel should be set at a height that when the hands properly grip the wheel just above the horizontal bar, (at about 9:30 and 2:30). The fingers should comfortably wrap around the wheel, and the hands should be just lower than the shoulders.

6. Adjust the mirrors for best visibility. After adjusting the seat, set the rearview mirror so that it is centered on the back window. The driver should be able to glance up and see the entire back window without moving their head from the forward-looking position. Adjust the side mirrors, so the side panels of the vehicle are just visible, as this helps in judging distances. They should be adjusted vertically, so they center on the horizon behind the vehicle.

7. Adjust the shoulder strap height: The shoulder strap height should be adjusted so that the center of the strap lies over the outer tip of the collarbone, over the acromial clavicular joint. If the belt is set too high, it may cross close to the neck and cause injury; if set too low, it may not restrain the driver in some accidents. Having it set low, over the shoulder increases the risk of acromioclavicular injuries in an accident.

NOTE: Some vehicles will not fit large or small people properly. When choosing a car – make sure you find one that fits you correctly.

WARNING: Children under the age of 12 should not ride in the front seat of passenger vehicles. The air bag, which is designed to protect adults, can injure or kill an infant or child.

Appendix M: Functional Inhibitors of Acid Sphingomyelinase

This is a non-comprehensive list of functional inhibitors of acid SMase (FIASMA), medications that prevent the conversion of sphingomyelin from the lipid membrane into ceramide, which can then be converted into sphingosine-1-phosphate (S1P). Ceramide promotes apoptosis and S1P activates inflammatory cell proliferation and prevents their apoptosis. FIASMA decrease both aspects of inflammatory activation. The dynamic balance between ceramide and S1P is an important mediator of cell growth and death.

The enzyme acid SMAse is attached to the inner liposomal membrane. FIASMA act indirectly, dislodging the enzyme from the membrane and promoting its degradation. Activity is listed as the residual of normal activity so that a score of 12 indicates that SMAse is only 12% of normal activity. These medications may promote inflammatory quiescence and prevent apoptosis.

These represent the most active functional inhibitors of SMAse from a list of over 2000 medications[1]. The effects of FIASMA are additive used in combination; thus use of two or more medications, at low doses, may avoid side effects while providing more FIASMA activity. The antihistamine clemastine has high FIAMSA activity while that of fexofenadine is low. In addition to these, etidronic acid and amiodarone are direct inhibitors of acid SMase.

Medication	Residual Activity	Medication	Residual Activity	Medication	Residual Activity	Medication	Residual Activity
Emetine	0.4	Perphenazine	20.1	Pimozide	30.6	Bromocriptine	67.5
Tamoxifen	4.1	Conessine	20.8	Paroxetine	31.7	Idarubicin	68.9
Trifluoperazine	8.3	Mibefradil	20.8	Mebeverine	31.8	Pergolide	69.2
Perhexiline	8.5	Drofenine	20.8	Promethazine	32.2	Benfluorex	69.7
Cepharanthine	9.2	Zolantidine	21.6	Imipramine	32.6	Butorphanol	69.8
Thioridazine	10.4	Camylofin	21.7	Flunarizine	32.7	Vinblastine	70.3
Amitriptyline	11.7	Alverine	21.7	Promazine	33.6	Rimantadine	70.3
Sertindole	12	Terfenadine	21.8	Fluvoxamine	37.4	Barnidipine	70.6
Amlodipine	12	Clomipramine	21.8	Dilazep	41.6	Chloropyramine	71.4
Sertraline	12.3	Desloratadine	21.9	Mebhydrolin	41.9	Azaperone	71.4
Clemastine	12.6	Suloctidil	21.9	Chlorpromazine	42.4	Tripelennamine	71.7
Protriptyline	12.7	Penfluridol	22	Hydroxyzine	43	Naproxen	72
Benztropine	12.7	Solasodine	22.2	Dimebon	44.1	Spiperone	72.6
Fluoxetine	13	Cyproheptadine	22.2	Mepacrine	44.3	Brompheniramine	72.7
Clomiphene	13	Carvedilol	22.4	Doxepin	46.6	Spiramycin	73.3
Nortriptyline	13.3	Chlorprothixene	22.4	Loratadine	48.5	Diphenhydramine	73.4
Maprotiline	13.5	Norfluoxetine	22.5	Cinnarizine	48.9	Trifluperidol	74
Trimipramine	13.8	Clofazimine	23.7	Ritanserin	51.2	Carbamazepine	74.2
Astemizole	14.3	Loperamide	24.4	Amorolfine	57.1	Orphenadrine	74.6
Amiodarone	14.5	Fendiline	25.2	Mesoridazine	59.5	Azithromycin	74.8
Desipramine	15.6	Biperiden	26.2	Dutasteride	61	Indomethacin	75
Tomatidine	15.8	Cyclobenzaprine	26.2	Opipramol	61.3	Oxeladin	75.2
Fluphenazine	16.5	Cloperastine	26.7	Buclizine	62.7	Lercanidipine	75.4
Pimethixene	16.5	Bepridil	27.1	Sibutramine	63.2	Memantine	75.6
Flupenthixol	18.2	Aprindine	27.5	Ibuprofen	63.3	Fexofenadine	76.3
Dicyclomine	18.6	Triflupromazine	29.5	Chloroquine	63.3	Chlorpheniramine	77.6
Lofepramine	19.2	Profenamine	29.7	Oxybutynin	63.4	Sulindac	81.3

---

[1] Identification of novel functional inhibitors of acid sphingomyelinase. Kornhuber J, Muehlbacher M, Trapp S, et al. PMID:21909365

INDEX

Acne and Antioxidants.....Table 37-2
Acne Vulgaris.....406, 434, 334, 481
Active Transport.....16
ADHD.....497, 130, 401, 423
Aflatoxin.....461
Age Related Hearing Loss.....508
Aging.....192
AgRP.....71
Alcohol.....86
Alcohol and Cancer.....453, 465
Alcohol as a Sexual Lubricant.....165
Alcohol during pregnancy.....164
Allergens, Food.....Table 11-2
Allergens, Seasonal.....Table 11-3
Allergic Rhinitis.....97, 107, 113, 143, 153, 159
Allergy Prevention.....110
Allergy Testing.....112
Allometric Conversions.....Table 40-2
Alpha lipoic acid.....440, 88, 144, 357, 361, 510
Alpha-linolenic acid.....45, 46, 154, 340, 364
Alveolar Bone.....480
Alzheimer's disease.....356, 294, 299, 363
Amine Oxidase Copper Containing: See AOC1
Amino acids.....57, Table 7-1
Ammonia.....25, 389
Amygdala.....399
Anaerobes.....18
Anger Attacks.....397
Angiotensin-Receptor Blockers.....302
Anisakis.....108
Antergies.....174, 264, 420, 424
Antergies and Depression.....339
Antergies and IBS.....258
Antergies and Migraine.....271
Antergies in Autoimmune Disease.....371
Antergies in Bladder Pain.....264
Antergies and Crohn's Disease.....378
Antigen Presentation.....210
Antioxidant Levels in Food.....524
Antioxidants and Cofactors.....Table 21-4
Anxiety.....362, 238, 338, 406
Anxiety: Mediators for Learning.....Table 32-5
AOC1.....130, Table 13-16
Appetite.....71
Apoptosis.....197, Figure 41-2
Apoptotic Signaling.....Figure 21-4
Arachidonic Acid.....47
Archae.....18
ASCA.....376

Aspirin Hypersensitivity.....Chapter 15
Aspirin Related Compounds.....Table 15-3
Aspirin Sensitive Asthma.....148
Asthma.....107, 143, 148
Attention.....128, 294, 306, 324, 353, 366
Attention Deficit Hyperactivity.....See ADHD
Autophagy Inducing Flavonoids.....Table 21-3
Autism.....387, 119, 245
Autism Causality.....Figure 35-1
Autoimmune Disease.....370
Autophagy.....198
B Cells.....95
Bacteria Density in the Intestine.....Table 24-1
Bacteria of the GI tract.....20
Bacterial Translocation.....245
Balance and Vestibular Function.....511
Basophils.....94
BDNF.....297-308, 327, 357, 363, 511
Beer.....85, 458
Belching.....28
Beta Carotene.....411
Beta glucuronidase.....23
Betaine.....300, 439
Betaine in Food.....Table 40-9
Bile.....5
Bile Acids.....5, 463, 467, Table 2-4
Bile acid malabsorption.....255
Bioamine Enzymes and Inhibitors.....Table 13-13
Bioamine Food Reactions.....Table 13-14
Bioamine Toxicosis.....126, 132
Bioamines Reactions from Food.....Table 13-8
Biofilm.....218, 408, 478, 173, 376, 388
Biogenic Amine Catabolic Enzymes.....Table 13-7
Biogenic Amines.....Table 13-2
Biogenic Amines from Fermentation.....Table 13-3
Biome of the Colon.....73
Biotin.....434, 69, 429
Bipolar Disorder.....323, 330, 334, 500
Bipolar Prodrome.....Table 31-7
Bladder Pain Scale.....528
Bladder Pain Syndrome.....263
Blood-brain barrier.....298
Bone Loss form Medication.....Table 42-1
Boron.....29, 337, 412, 420, 467, 477
Botox for Migraine.....275
Brain-Derived Neurotrophic Factor: See BDNF
Breast Cancer.....448, 464
Breast Milk.....27, 49, 52, 126, 280, 499
Breastfeeding.....110, 213, 250
Cadaverine.....135
Caffeine.....134, 161, 202, 256, 334,
Caffeine Levels in Foods and Drinks.....Table 43-13

Calcium.....186, 292, 295, 304, 334, 427
Campylobacter jejuni.....255
Cancer Genes.....449
Cancer Induction.....448
Cancer Prevention.....448
Cancer Promotion.....450
Candida albicans.....376
Cannabinoids.....301, 77, 145, 353
Car Seats.....536
Carbohydrates.....15
Carcinogens and Mutagens.....Table 41-1
Carotenoids.....431
CCK: See Cholecystokinin
Cecal Transit Time.....232
Celiac Disease (CD).....208
Celiac-Related Immune Diseases.....Table 22-4
Cell Proliferation.....Figures 41-1, 41-2
Central Sensitization of pain.....352
Ceramide.....102, 329, 356
CGRP (Calcitonin Gene-Related Peptide).....268
Cheese Reaction.....133
Chitin.....24
Chlamydia.....98, 272, 335, 482
Chocolate.....161, 410, 134, 256, 359, 410
Chocolate Dosing.....Table 17-1
Cholecalciferol.....183
Cholecystokinin (CCK).....70, 13, 33, 63, 68, 74, 353
Cholecystokinin; pain.....353
Cholelithiasis 74
Choline.....439, 307
Choline in Food.....Table 40-9
Choline/Betaine and Methionine.....Figure 40-2
Cholelithiasis....
Chronic Fatigue Syndrome.....356
Chronic Prostatitis.....263
Chronic Traumatic Encephalopathy.....293
Crohn's Disease.....376
Chymotrypsin.....391, 6, 69, 224, 381, 384
Circadian Influences.....227, 234, 237, 285, 334, 394
Circadian Rhythm Disorders.....497, Table 43-11
Citrulline.....12, 58, 213, 377
Clostridia.....20, 27, 66, 101, 173, 220, 226
Clostridia and Autism.....389
Cochlea.....507
Cochlea Cross-Section.....Figure 44-2
Coenzyme Q10.....194, 204, 357, 421, 438,
Colic.....239
Colon Cancer.....429, 29, 379, 450, 453,
Colonic Bacteria Genera.....Table 4-1
Colonic Transit Time.....28
Colorectal Cancer.....See Colon Cancer
Commensal Microbia.....223

Constipation.....232, 254, 304, 389, 392
Cooking oils.....53
Cooking, Effect on Allergenicity.....159
Coronary Artery Disease: 87, 332, 438, 478, 491,
Coronary Heart Disease: .....See Coronary Artery Disease
Corticotropin Releasing Hormone.....284
Corticotropin Releasing Hormone (CRH).....402
Corticotropin-Releasing Hormone (CRH).....247
Creatine Formation.....Table 35-1
Cross-reacting Immunogens.....520
Cruciferous Vegetables.....26, 122, 282, 458, 461
Cutaneous Mastocytosis.....117
Cystic Fibrosis.....60, 76,103,
Cytokines.....451, Table 10-6
Cytokines in Fibromyalgia and Pain.....355
Cytokines in Rage Disorder.....402
Cytotoxic T Cells.....96
Delayed Sleep-Phase Syndrome.....497
Delayed Sleep-Phase Therapy.....Table 43-10
Delta Cells.....4, 14, 69, 77
Demodex.....411
Dendritic Cells.....96
Dental Hygiene.....483
Dental Root Resorption.....Figure 42-2
Depression.....322
Depression and Neurohormones.....Table 31-3
Depression Causal Web.....Figure 31-1
Depression in Fibromyalgia.....357
Dermatitis herpetiformis.....212
Diabetes, Type 1.....12, 17, 110, 173, 210, 246
Diabetes, Type 2.....53, 71, 81, 84, 86, 220, 491
Digestion of Carbohydrates.....15
Disaccharides.....Table 3-2
Docosahexanoic Acid in Fish.....Table 6-6
Docosahexaenoic Acid (DHA).....44, 47, 302
Domestic abuse.....191, 399, 517, 525
Domestic Abuse Screening Tool.....525
Dosing: Animals to Human.....Table 40-2
Drug and Alcohol Abuse in CTE.....308
Dysmenorrhea....420
Dysbiosis.....219
ECL Cells.....4, 13
Eicosanoid Biosynthesis.....Figure 15-1
Eicosanoid Pathway.....Figure 6-5
Eicosanoids.....45, Table 6-2
Eicosapentaenoic Acid (EPA).....48
Eicosapentanoic Acid in Fish.....Table 6-6
Electron Transport Chain Cofactors.....Table 21-5
Electron Transport.....194, Figure 21-2, 21-3
EMDR (Eye Movement Desensitization and Reprocessing).....362
Emotional Distress.....286

Enterochromaffin Cells in IBS.....257
Enterochromaffin Serotonin Releasers.....Table 26-1
Enterocyte Functions.....Table 2-6
Enterocytes.....8, 67, 127, 243, 245
Enteroendocrine Cells.....7, 260
Enteroimmune symptoms.....Table 1-2
Environmental Antigens.....520
Enzymes Pancreatic.....74
Enzymes, Intestinal.....11
Eosinophils.....94, 100, 108, 149, 155, 169
Epigenetic Reset.....282, Table 29-2
Epigenetic Reset Factors.....Table 29-2
Epigenetics.....118, 154, 246, 281, 338,
Epigenetics of Stress.....281
Errors.....523
Escholar.....109
Esophageal Cancer.....27, 428, 453, 459
Exercise.....202, 306, 477
Exercise Assessment.....527
Exercise Evaluation Tool.....Appendix E
Explosive Disorder.....397
Eye Movement Desensitization and Reprocessing (EMDR).....362
Facet Joints.....535
Farty Foods.....Table 4-7
Fat Smoke Temperatures.....Table 6-9
Fatigue.....497
Fatigue; Common Causes.....Table 43-9
Fats and depression.....330
Fatty acids.....43, Table 6-1
Fatty Acids and Disease.....Tables 6-3, 6-4
Fecal Transplant.....21, 225, 226
Fertility.....419
Fiber.....21, 461, Table 4-2
Fibromyalgia.....351, 237, 419, 497
Fibromyalgia Associated Conditions.....Table 32-1
Fibromyalgia Diagnostic Criteria.....Figure 32-1
Flatulence.....26
Flavonoid Rich Foods.....Table 21-3
Flow (Psychological).....288, Figure 29-3
Folate.....34, 305
Folate and Colon Cancer.....429
Food Additives.....423
Food Allergens.....520
Food Allergies.....107
Food Colorants effect on Nerve growth.....Table 39-2
Food Coloring.....423
Food Colorings.....Tables 39-1, 39-3, 39-4, 39-5, 39-6
Food Oils n3:n6 ratios.....Table 6-5
Food Preservatives.....425
Food Sensitivity Testing.....177
Foods Alleged to Release Histamine.....Table 14-6

Fructans.....22, Table 4-4
Fructo-Oligosaccharides.....22
Fructose.....16, 34, 41, 88
Fructose in Foods.....Table 5-8
Fructose Malabsorption.....37
Fructose Utilization.....Table 9-2, 9-3
G cells.....4, 13
GABA.....355, 403
GABA Metabolism.....Table 28-4
Gallbladder.....5, 74, 77, 225, 234, 463
Gastroesophageal Reflux (GERD).....117, 226, 235, 430, 492,
Gastrointestinal Allergies.....112
Gastrointestinal Hormones.....Table 2-7
Gastrointestinal Motility.....233
Gastrointestinal Motility Hormones.....Table 24-3
Gempylotoxin.....109
GERD: See Gastroesophageal Reflux Disease
Ghrelin.....71, 357, 490
Giardiasis.....36, 41, 131, 138, 224, 259
Glial cell-derived neurotrophic factor, (GDNF).....293
Gliadin.....209
Glucoraphanin.....458
Glutamate.....353, 403
Glutamate Metabolism.....Table 28-4
Glutathione.....144, 203, 331, 409, 440, 509
Glutathione Recycling.....Figure 14-2
Glutathione S-Transferase (GST).....454, 458
Gluten Disease.....208
Gluten Disease, Non-Celiac.....215
Gluten Enteropathy Malabsorption.....Table 22-3
Gluten Enteropathy Symptoms.....Table 22-1
Gluten Hidden in Food.....Table 22-5
Gluten-Related Immune Diseases.....Table 22-4
Glycoproteins.....11, 58 63, Table 7-3
Goblet Cells.....4, 8
Granulocytes.....94
Hair Cells.....Figures 44-3, 44-4
Hair Cells of the Ear.....508
Halitosis.....28
Hay Fever: See Allergic Rhinitis
HCA Production in Cooking.....Table 41-2
Headache.....267
Headache, Posttraumatic.....293
Headache: (also see Migraine)
Hearing.....184, 239, 506
Hearing Loss.....508
Hematopoiesis.....93, Table 10-1
Hemicellulose.....24
Hemochromatosis.....428, 442
Hepatic Encephalopathy.....389
Heterocyclic Amine from Cooking.....Table 41-2
Heterocyclic Amines (HCA).....454

Hexose Transfer Proteins.....Table 3-3
High-Mobility Group Box1 (HMGB1).....307
Histamine Catabolism Cofactors.....Table 13-6
Histamine.....107
Histamine Catabolic Pathway.....Figure 13-1
Histamine Effect by Blood Level.....Table 13-1
Histamine effects on CNS.....Table 36-4
Histamine Intolerance.....131
Histamine Receptors.....Table 13-5
Histamine, GI Absorption.....126
Histamine: Systemic Effects.....Table 13-4
Histocompatibility Proteins.....208
HITS questionnaire.....525
HLA DQ Associated Immune Diseases.....Table 22-2
HMGB1 (High-Mobility Group Box1).....307
HNMT Inhibitors.....Table 13-16
Hormones, GI Motility.....234
Hormones and Sleep.....Table 43-4
Hormones for Hunger and Satiety.....Tables 8-1, 8-2
Hormones in Sleep.....490
Hormones Promoting Direct Mast Cell Activation.....142
Hormones, Gastrointestinal.....13 (Table 2-6)
Hormones, Hunger.....69 (Table 8-2)
Hormones, Pancreatic.....14 (Table 2-7)
Hormones, Satiation.....69 (table 8-1)
Human Metabolic Evolution.....90, (Table 9-4)
Hunger Hormones.....69, (Tables 8-1, 8-2)
Hydrogen Breath Tests.....232
Hydroxybenzoic Acids in Foods.....Table 15-5
Hypersensitivity to Foods.....170
Hypothalamic Pituitary Axis (HPA).....278
Hypothalamic Pituitary Hormones.....Table 29-1
Hypoxic Injury.....196
IBS Constipation or Diarrhea.....Table 26-2
IDO Induction.....Table 31-2
IED (Intermittent Explosive Disorder).....397
IgE and IgG Response to Antigens.....Table 19-1
IgG Food Reactivity Test.....Figure 19-1
IgG Functions.....Table 19-2
IgG Receptors.....Table 19-5
IgG Subtypes.....Table 19-4
Immune Cells.....93
Immune Hypersensitivity.....Table 18-1
Immune Hypersensitivity Reactions.....168
Immune Hypersensitivity to Food.....172
Immunocytotoxicity.....295
Immunoexcitotoxic CNS Injury.....292
Immunoglobulin A (IgA).....172
Immunoglobulin Classes.....Table 10-2
Immunoglobulin G (IgG).....175
Immunoglobulins to Foods and Disease.....Table 19-3
Induction of Cancer.....448

Infantile Colic.....239
Infertility.....47, 52, 165, 213, 265, 283
Inflammation and Cancer.....450
Inflammation and Osteopenia.....477
Inflammation and Sleep.....492
Inflammatory Bowel Disease.....77, 376
Insomnia.....493
Insomnia Causes.....Table 43-7
Insomnia: 136, 161, 171, 300, 493, 499
Insulin Resistance.....81, 89,186
Interferon.....335
Interferon-γ Affecters.....Table 31-5
Interluekin-1 beta.....269
Intermittent Explosive Disorder (IED).....397
Interstitial Cystitis.....263
Intestinal Alkaline SMase.....379
Intestinal gases.....Table 4-6
Intestinal Permeability Factors.....Table 25-1
Intestinal Permeability-Related Diseases.....Table 25-2
Intestinal Structure.....6
Intimacy.....419, 165
Intracellular Pathogens.....Table 10-4
Inulin.....22, 222, 232
Irritable Bowel Syndrome (IBS).....33, 77, 254
Ischemia/Reperfusion Injury.....296
Ischemic Heart Disease: .....See Coronary Artery Disease
Keiorrhea.....109
Kynurenine.....237, 324, 388
Kynurenine and IDO Induction.....Table 31-2
Kynurenine Pathway.....Figure 31-2
Lactose in Dairy Foods.....Table 5-3
Lactose Intolerance.....34, 213
Lactulose.....40, 223, 323. 249, 392
Lariciresinol rich Foods.....Table 41-4
Lead.....403
Leaking Gut Syndrome.....243
Leaky Gut Factors.....Table 25-1
Leaky Gut-Related Diseases.....Table 25-2
Learning.....487
Lectins.....62, Table 7-4
Lectins in Foods.....Table 7-5
Lectins that Bind to Bacteria.....Table 23-2
Lectins, Non-Toxic Dietary.....223
Leptin.....69, 71, 85, 283, 490
Leukotriene Associated Hypersensitivity (LAH).....148
Leukotriene Hypersensitivity.....Table 15-1
Leukotriene Hypersensitivity Prevalence.....Table 15-2
Leukotriene Pathway.....Figure 6-6
Light and Light Therapy.....500
Link list of resources.....523
Lipid Rafts.....101, 309
Lipofuscin.....199

Lipopolysaccharide.....219
Lung Cancer.....448
Lymphocytes.....95
Lymphoma.....187, 197, 208, 210, 376, 458
M Cells.....7, 8
Macrophages.....95
Magnesium.....303
Major Histocompatibility Antigens.....208
Malabsorption.....429
Malabsorption and Osteopenia.....477
Malabsorption in Gluten Disease.....211, Table 22-3
Malnutrition.....429
Management of Antergies.....177
Marijuana.....See Cannabinoids
Marinade.....468, 458
Mast Cell Activation Disorder.....116-123
Mast Cell Activation Disorders.....116, Tables 12-4, 12-6
Mast Cell Activation in Autism.....388
Mast Cell Activation in Fibromyalgia.....358
Mast Cell Activators.....Table 12-3
Mast Cell Degranulating Medications.....Table 14-5
Mast Cell Degranulation.....142
Mast Cell Disorder Manifestations.....Table 12-1
Mast Cell Growth Factors.....Table 12-5
Mast Cell Leukemia.....116
Mast Cell Mediators.....Table 11-1
Mast Cell Sarcoma.....116
Mast Cell Waves.....149
Mast Cells.....95, 107
Mastocytoma.....116
Mastocytosis Triggers: Foods and Drugs.....Table 12-2
Meat and Cancer.....454
Medications Affecting Appetite.....77
Melatonin.....306, 491
Melatonin Synthesis Cofactors.....Table 28-3
Memory.....487
Memory Cells.....93
Menopausal Symptoms.....412, 420
Mercury.....50
Mercury in Fish.....Table 6-7
Metabolic Syndrome.....81
Methionine Homocysteine Pathway.....Figure 31-4
Methionine in Food.....530
Microglia.....95, 296
Microglial Activation.....296
Microtubule-Associated Protein Tau.....294
Microvilli.....8
Migraine Comorbidity.....Table 28-1
Migraine.....267
Migraine and Antergies.....271
Migraine and Glutamate.....271
Migraine and Melatonin.....270

Migraine Effectors.....Table 28-2
Migraine Mitigation Supplements.....Table 28-6
Migraine Prophylaxis.....Table 28-5
Migraine: (see also Headache)
Microglial Activators.....Table 30-4
Minocycline.....299
Minocycline Antiinflammatory Actions.....Table 30-5
Mitochondria.....192, Figure 21-1
Mitochondrial Dysfunction Diseases.....Table 21-3
Mitochondrial Fusion and Fission.....Table 21-2
Mitochondrial Rehabilitation.....361, 530
Molybdenum.....144
Molybdenum Dependent Enzymes.....Table 14-1
Monoamine Oxidase.....130, 401
Monoamine Oxidase Inhibitors.....Table 13-15
Monoclonal Mast Cell Activation Syndrome (MMAS).....116
Monocytes.....94
Mood Disorder Prevalence.....Table 31-1
Mood disorders.....322
Mucosal Enzymes.....Table 2-5
Multiple Sclerosis (MS).....97, 185, 210, 246, 301, 370
Mutagens and Carcinogens.....Table 41-1
Mycotoxins.....461
Myenteric Motility Disorders.....235
Myotonic Dystrophy.....352
Myotonic Dystrophy Type 2.....352
N3 and N6 Fatty Acids.....403, 411
N-Acetyl Cysteine.....299, 440
N-acetyltransferase (NAT).....454, 458
Nap Guide.....Table 43-14
Napping.....489, 501
Narcolepsy.....75, 128, 267, 497
Natural Killer Cells.....96
Neurohormones in Depression.....Table 31-3
Neuroinflammatory Diseases.....Table 1-1
Neuropathic Pain; Nutrients for.....Table 32-4
Neuropeptide Y (NPY).....71, 278
Neurotrophic Factors.....Table 31-4
Neurotrophic factors.....327
Neutrophils.....94
Niacin.....434
Nitric Oxide Synthase Cofactors.....Table 25-3
Nitric Oxide Synthase (NOS).....403
N-Nitrosyl Compounds.....459
NO Signaling.....199
Nocturia.....499
Nocturia; Causes.....Table 43-12
Noise-Induced Hearing Loss.....508
Non-digestible carbohydrates.....22
Non-digestible Polysaccharides.....Table 4-5
Non-Restorative Sleep.....496
Non-Restorative Sleep Conditions.....Table 43-8

Norepinephrine.....354
NSAIDS.....302
Nutrition Deserts.....517
Nutritional Deficiency Causes.....Table 40-1
Nutritional Supplements.....427
Obesity.....68, 80
Obesity and Cancer.....453
Obesity and Sleep.....493
Octopamine.....134
Oligosaccharides.....24, 238, 391
Opiates.....306, 355, 390
Oral Cecal Transit Time (OCTT).....232
Orexin.....72, 490
Orthodontics.....479
Osteoblasts.....476
Osteoclasts.....476, 482
Osteoimmunity.....476
Osteomalacia.....183, 185, 209, 211, 235, 477
Osteoporosis.....33, 117, 162, 184, 211, 353, 437
Osteoporotic Bone.....Figure 42-1
Osteoclast down-regulators.....Table 42-4
Oxidants; Avoiding.....Table 41-5
Oxidative Stress.....357
Oxidative Stress and Cognition.....331
Pain Facilitation Pathway.....Figure 32-2
Pain Sensitization.....351
Pain; Nutrients for Neuropathic Pain.....Table 32-4
Pancreatic Cancer..... 78, 448, 453
Pancreatic Enzymes.....5, 74, Table 8-3
Pancreatic Hormones.....14, Table 2-7
Pancreatic polypeptide (PP)..... 14, 71
Pancreatitis.... 76
Paneth Cells.....8, 11, 13
Paracellular hyperpermeability.....243
Parasomnias; Conditions.....Table 43-12
Parasomnias.....498
Parietal Cells.....4, 434
Parkinson's disease.....293, 308, 328, 334, 337, 353
Paternal alcohol consumption.....165
Pediatric Dosing.....394
Periodontal Ligaments.....Figure 42-3
Pelvic Pain Evaluation Tool.....Appendix F
Pelvic Pain Scale.....528
Periaqueductal Grey Area.....399
Periarticular Injections.....535
Periodontal Ligaments.....479
Periodontitis.....478
Peristalsis.....233
Phenolic Compounds.....364
Phenolic Eicosanoid Inhibitors.....Table 15-4
Phenolic Leukotriene Inhibitors.....Table 15-6
Phenylethylamine Intoxication.....134

Phytates.....430, 481
Phytates in Food.....Table 42-2
Phytohemagglutinin.....8, 63, 179, 244, 247
Pilosebaceous Unit.....Figure 37-1
Pineal Gland.....491
Pituitary Hormones.....Table 29-1
Plant Enzyme Reactions.....159
Plasma Cells.....95
Pollen Food Allergy.....113
Pollinosis.....113
Polyamines in Food.....Table 13-10
Polycyclic Aromatic Hydrocarbons (PAH).....460
Polycystic Ovary Syndrome.....184, 407, 412, 420
Polypharmacy.....307
Polyphenolic Compounds.....24, 88
Polyphenols.....466
Postconcussion Symptoms.....Table 30-1
Postconcussion Syndrome.....292
Posttraumatic Headaches.....293
Post-traumatic stress disorder.....362
Potatoes.....380, 143, 67, 74
PPAR-γ.....300
PPAR-γ Activators.....Table 30-6
PPAR-γ Induced Transcription.....Figure 30-3
PQQ.....129, 203, 204, 270, 274, 300, 356, 413
Prebiotic.....221
Prebiotics.....20, 73, 222
Prefrontal Area.....401
Presbycusis.....508
Prion Disease.....336
Probiotics.....22, 221
Promotion of Cancer.....450
Propionibacterium acnes.....408
Prostaglandin Pathway.....Figure 6-6
Prostate Cancer.....184, 364, 427, 436, 448, 159
Prostatitis.....263
Protein.....57
Protein Function.....60
Protein Half-life.....Table 7-2
Protein Malabsorption.....66, 223
Protein Malfunction.....60
Protein Structure.....Figure 7-3
Proteolytic Enzymes in Fruits.....Table 16-1
Pseudo Allergy.....125
Pseudo-Allergy to Medications.....136
Pseudomembranous Colitis.....21, 27, 64, 224, 226, 295,
PTSD.....362
PTSD Screening Questionnaire.....529
PTSD Screening Tool.....Appendix G
Public Health.....515
Putrescine.....135
Pyridoxine.....274, 327, 360, 433, 464

Pyrroloquinoline quinone (See PQQ)
Quercetin Antiinflammatory Actions.....Table 30-5
Quorum Sensing.....221
RAGE (receptor for advanced glycation end-products)...307
Rage (Explosive Disorder).....397
Rage Behavior Model.....Figure 36-1
Rage in Humans and Animals.....Table 36-2
Rage Neurohormones.....Table 36-3
Rage Questionnaire.....Table 36-1
RANKL (Receptor Activator of NF-κβ Ligand).....476
Reactive Oxygen Species.....195, Table 21-1
Regressive Autism.....388
Retinal Activity Equivalents.....Table 40-3, 40-4
Retinoic Acid.....333
Reynaud's Syndrome.....175, 267
Ribosome Protein Synthesis.....Figure 7-2
RNA.....58
Sacroiliac Joints.....535
Saccharide Classes.....Table 3-1
S-Adenosylmethionine.....129, 144, 270, 300, 332, 433
Saliva.....4, Table 2-1
Salt.....87
SAMe: See S-Adenosylmethionine
Sarcoidosis.....212, 220, 235
Satiation.....68
Satiation Hormones.....69, Table 8-1
Satiety.....68
Schizophrenia.....335
Schizophrenia Major Symptoms.....Table 31-6
Schizophrenia-Bipolar Prodrome.....Table 31-7
Scombroid.....125, 131, 135, 402
Scombroid Poisoning.....125
Sebum.....407
Seizures.....38, 48, 161, 267, 271, 303, 400
Serotonin.....403
Serotonin in Food.....Table 13-11
Serotonin Syndrome (Storm).....Table 13-12
Serotonin Synthesis Cofactors.....Table 28-3
Serotonin Toxidrome.....136
Serotonin, Dietary.....135
Sexual Dysfunction.....419
Sphingomyelin.....Figure 6-8
Short Chain Fatty Acids.....Table 4-3
Sugars...34
Sugar Malabsorption....32
SIBO.....231
SIBO and Sleep.....237
SIBO related Diseases.....Table 24-5
SIBO Risk Factors.....Table 24-4
Skin Surface Lipids.....Table 37-1
Sleep.....487
Sleep Apnea.....496

Sleep Deprivation.....489
Sleep Drivers.....Table 43-3
Sleep Disorders.....494, Table 43-6
Sleep Hormones.....Table 43-4
Sleep Requirements by Age.....Table 43-2
Sleep Restriction: Metabolic Effects.....Table 43-5
Sleep stages.....487, Table 43-1, Figure 43-1
Small Intestinal Bacterial Overgrowth Sx.....Table 24-2
Small Intestinal Bacterial Overgrowth (SIBO).....231
Solar Index Map.....Figure 20-2
Sorbitol.....39
Spermidine.....135
Spermine.....135
Sphingolipid Digestion.....Figure 34-1
Sphingolipids.....86
Sphingolipids and Autoimmune Disease.....371
Sphingolipids and depression.....329, 356
Sphingolipids and the Intestinal Mucosa.....104, 379
Sphingolipids in Immune functions.....102
Sphingosine-1-phosphate (S1P).....102
Sphingosine-1-Phosphate Activity.....Table 10-7
Sphingolipid Pathway.....Figure 10-5, Table 31-6
Sphingolipids, dietary.....53
Sorbitol Content in Foods.....Tables 5-5, 5-6, 5-7
Statin Medications.....302
Stomach Cells.....4
Stress.....278, 330
Stress Hormone Pathway.....Figure 29-2
Stroke.....302, 304, 306, 510
Sucrose Intolerance.....38
Sugar Alcohols.....39, Table 5-4
Sugar Malabsorption.....34, Table 5-2
Sugars.....15, 34, Table 5-1
Sulfite Degranulation Prevention.....Table 14-2
Sulfite Sensitivity Testing.....Table 1-7
Sulfites.....143
Sulfites: Food Additives.....Table 14-3
Sulforaphane.....458
Sulfites in Foods.....Table 14-4
Supplement Recommendations.....Table 40-10
Sympathetic Facilitation of Pain.....354
Sympathetic Immune System.....278
Syndrome X.....80
Synephrine.....135
Systemic Mastocytosis.....117
T Cells.....96
T Helper 17 Related Autoimmune Dz......Table 33-1
T Helper Cell Functions.....Table 10-3, 10-5
T Helper Cells.....97
Taurine Enzymes and Cofactors.....Table 35-2
TBI.....See Traumatic Brain Injury
Telomeres.....192

Temperature for Cooking Meat.....Table 41-3
THC.....See Cannabinoids
Theobromine.....161
Thiazolidinediones.....303
Tight Junctions.....244, Figure 25-2
Tinnitus.....117, 200, 293, 510
TNF-α Inducers.....Table 23-1
TNF-α Inhibiting Flavonoids.....Table 32-3
TNF-α Inhibitors.....Table 32-2
Tocopherols and Tocotrienols.....Tables 40-7, 40-11
Toll-Like Receptor Activation.....Figure 10-4
Toll-Like Receptor Activators.....Table 42-3
Toll-like Receptors.....100, 356, Table 10-7
Tooth Root Resorption.....480
Toxoplasmosis.....214, 272, 336, 376
Trace amine associated receptors (TAAR).....134
Trans Fats.....52, Table 6-8
Trauma Screening Questionnaire.....529
Trauma Screening Questionnaire.....Appendix G
Traumatic Brain Injury (TBI).....165, 246, 292, 353, 362, 517
Traumatic Brain Injury Progression.....Table 30-3
Trehalose.....38
Trigger Point Injections.....534
Trimethylglycine (TMG).....See Betaine
Trypsin Inhibitors in Food.....Table 23-3
Tryptamine.....134, 272
Tryptophan.....323
Tumor Necrosis Factor-α.....220
Tuna.....50, 108, 109, 125, 127, 256, 532
Type I Hypersensitivity.....107, 169
Type II Hypersensitivity.....169
Type III Hypersensitivity.....170
Type IV Hypersensitivity.....170
Type V Hypersensitivity.....170
Tyramine in Food.....Table 13-9
Tyramine Intoxication.....132
Ubiquitination.....101, 196, 300, 308, 413, 439
Ulcerative Colitis.....378
Uric Acid.....80-89
Uric Acid Effects.....Table 9-1
Uric Acid Pathway.....Figure 9-5
Urinary Frequency Evaluation Tool.....Appendix F
Urinary Frequency Scale.....528
Vegetable Oil Manufacture.....533
Vestibular Dysfunction.....511
Villi.....7
Vitamin A.....333, 411, 431
Vitamin B Deficiency and Toxicity.....Table 40-5
Vitamin B Recommended Intake.....Table 40-6
Vitamin B12.....305, 306, 434
Vitamin B6.....433, 464
Vitamin C.....434

Vitamin D.....183
Vitamin D and Bipolar Disorder.....332
Vitamin D and Crohn's Disease.....378
Vitamin D Deficiency Diseases.....Table 20-1
Vitamin D3 Molecule.....Figure 20-1
Vitamin E.....436
Vitamin E in Food.....Table 40-11
Vitamin K.....305, 437, 476
Vitamin K Compounds.....Table 40-8
Vitamin Supplements and Cancer.....462
Vitaminers E.....Table 40-7, 40-11
Vitamins B.....432
Vitamin B and Mood Disorders.....332
Wheat.....208
White Blood Cell Differentiation.....Figure 10-1
Wine.....87, 163
Winemaking.....163
Worry in Depression.....495
Xylitol.....34, 38, 481
Yeast (See also Candida).....376
Zinc.....334, 412

Printed in Great Britain
by Amazon.co.uk, Ltd.,
Marston Gate.